'*Foundations of Naturopathic Nutrition* provides a really comprehensive introduction to the building blocks of naturopathic nutrition. In addition to technical explanations, additional information such as case study work helps to bring the theory to life. I thoroughly recommend this book as a learning aid for students, and as an excellent reference guide for experienced practitioners.'

Jackie Day, President Naturopathic Nutrition Association (UK)

'The foundation nutrition text we've all been waiting for. Fay Paxton has drawn from her many years of clinical nutrition experience, combining it with relevant research-based evidence, to produce an exhaustive body of work that is unique in its specific relevance to naturopathic and complementary medicine students and practitioners.'

David Stelfox, Associate Program Leader Naturopathy, Endeavour College of Natural Health

'This is an informative, comprehensive and well-researched practical guide to basic nutrition. A fabulous resource, not only for practitioners but also all those with an interest in nutrition.'

Professor Alan Bensoussan, Director National Institute of Complementary Medicine, University of Western Sydney

Foundations of Naturopathic Nutrition

A comprehensive guide to essential nutrients and nutritional bioactives

Fay Paxton

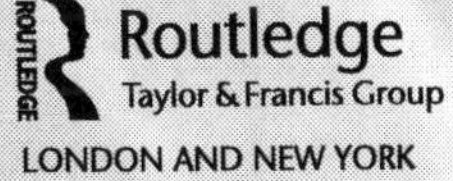
LONDON AND NEW YORK

First published 2015 by Allen & Unwin

Published 2020 by Routledge
2 Park Square, Milton Park, Abingdon, Oxon OX14 4RN
605 Third Avenue, New York, NY 10017

Routledge is an imprint of the Taylor & Francis Group, an informa business

Copyright © Fay Paxton 2015

All rights reserved. No part of this book may be reprinted or reproduced or utilised in any form or by any electronic, mechanical, or other means, now known or hereafter invented, including photocopying and recording, or in any information storage or retrieval system, without permission in writing from the publishers.

Notice:
Product or corporate names may be trademarks or registered trademarks, and are used only for identification and explanation without intent to infringe.

Cataloguing–in–Publication details are available
from the National Library of Australia
www.trove.nla.gov.au

Diagrams by Rod McClean, Midland Typesetters, Australia
Set in 10/11.5 pt Bembo by Midland Typesetters, Australia

ISBN–13: 9781742370408 (pbk)

Contents

List of figures and tables

FIGURES

TABLES

Acronyms and abbreviations

$1,25(OH)_2D$ 1,25-dihydroxycholecalciferol (calcitriol, active vitamin D)
10H2DA 10-hydroxy-2-decenoic acid
25(OH)D 25-hydroxycholecalciferol
AA arachidonic acid
AAA Ca Active Absorbable Algal Calcium
AAS amino acid score
ABG ascorbigen
ACC acetyl-CoA carboxylase
ACE angiotensin converting enzyme
ACh acetylcholine
ACP acyl carrier protein
ACTH adrenocorticotropic hormone
AD Alzheimer's disease
ADH antidiuretic hormone
ADHD attention deficit hyperactivity disorder
ADP adenosine diphosphate
AE acrodermatitis enteropathica
AFA *Aphanizomenon flos-aquae*
AGE aged garlic extract
AGEs advanced glycation end-products
AHCC active hexose-correlated compound
AI adequate intake
AIDS acquired immune deficiency syndrome
AITD autoimmune thyroid disease
Ala alanine
Alcar acetyl-L-carnitine
alpha-LA alpha-lipoic acid
alpha-LNA alpha-linolenic acid
alpha-TE alpha-tocopherol equivalents
alpha-TPP alpha-tocopherol transfer protein
ALS amyotrophic lateral sclerosis (motor neurone disease)
ALU acid lactase unit
AMA American Medical Association
AMP adenosine monophosphate
AN anorexia nervosa
ANP atrial natriuretic peptide
AO aldehyde oxidase
AQIS Australian Quarantine and Inspection Service
AREDS Age-Related Eye Disease Study
Arg arginine
ARMD age-related macular degeneration
ARs adenosine receptors
AsA ascorbic acid
A-SAAs acute-phase serum amyloid A proteins
ASD autistic spectrum disorder
Asn asparagine
Asp aspartic acid
AThDP adenosine thiamin diphosphate
AThTP adenosine thiamin triphosphate
ATN-224 choline tetrathiomolybdate
ATP adenosine triphosphate

ATSDR Agency for Toxic Substances and Disease Registry (USA)
AV anisidine value
AVED ataxia with vitamin E deficiency
Axl receptor tyrosine kinases of the TAM family
BCAAs branched-chain amino acids
BCDO2 beta,beta-carotene 9',10'-dioxygenase
BCMO1 beta,beta-carotene 15,15'-monooxygenase 1
BCRP breast cancer resistance protein
BDMC bisdemethoxycurcumin
beta-CTx beta-C-terminal telopeptide
BGP bone-Gla protein
BH4 tetrahydrobiopterin
BHA breath-holding attacks
BHMT betaine-homocysteine S-methyltransferase
BMD bone mineral density
BMI body mass index
BMR basal metabolic rate
BNCT boron neutron capture therapy
BNP brain natriuretic peptide
BP blood pressure
BPA bisphenol A
BPH benign prostatic hyperplasia
BPs brominated phenols
BSE bovine spongiform encephalopathy (mad cow disease)
BV biological value
CABG coronary artery bypass grafting
cAMP cyclic adenosine monophosphate
CAMs cellular adhesion molecules
CAPE caffeic acid phenethyl ester
Car carnitine
CaR calcium-sensing receptor
CAT chronic autoimmune thyroiditis
CDM copper deficiency myelopathy
CF calcium fructoborate
CFD cerebral folate deficiency syndrome
CFTR cystic fibrosis transmembrane conductance regulator
CFU colony-forming unit
CGF chlorella growth factor
cGMP cyclic guanosine monophosphate
CHD coronary heart disease
Ch-OSA choline-stabilised orthosilicic acid
CI confidence interval
Cit citrulline
CJD Creutzfeldt-Jakob disease
CKD chronic kidney disease
CNS central nervous system
CoA coenzyme A
COMT catechol-O-methyltransferase
CoQ10 coenzyme Q10
COX cyclooxygenase
CP ceruloplasmin
C-PC C-phycocyanin
CPM central pontine myelinolysis
cPMP cyclic pyranopterin monophosphate
CRF chronic renal failure
CRP C-reactive protein
CS chondroitin sulfate
CSD cortical spreading depression
CSF cerebrospinal fluid
CSIRO Commonwealth Scientific and Industrial Research Organisation (Australia)
CU cellulase unit
CVD cardiovascular disease
CV-N cyanovirin-N
CYP cytochrome P450
Cys cysteine
D1 type 1 iodothyronine deiodinase
D2 type 2 iodothyronine deiodinase
D3 type 3 iodothyronine deiodinase
DADS diallyldisulfide
DAS diallylsulfide
DASH Dietary Approaches to Stop Hypertension
DATS diallyltrisulfide
DBP vitamin D binding protein
DCI D-chiro inositol
DFE dietary folate equivalents
DGLA dihomo-gamma-linolenic acid
DHA docosahexaenoic acid
DHAsA dehydroascorbic acid
DHEA dehydroepiandrosterone
DHF dihydrofolate
DHLA dihydrolipoic acid
DHT dihydrotestosterone
DIM diindolylmethane
DMC demethoxycurcumin
DMG dimethylglycine
DMSO dimethyl sulfoxide
DMT1 divalent metal transporter 1
DNA deoxyribonucleic acid
DOPA dihydroxyphenylalanine
DPA docosapentaenoic acid
DTH delayed-type hypersensitivity

dTTP thymidine 5'-triphosphate
dU deoxyuridine
DU dextrinising unit
DUOX2 dual oxidase 2
DVT deep vein thrombosis
DXA dual-energy x-ray absorptiometry
EAR estimated average requirement
ECF extracellular fluid
ECG electrocardiograph
EDLF endogenous digitalis-like factor
EE energy expenditure
EEG electroencephalogram
EER estimated energy requirement
EFA essential fatty acid
EGCG epigallocatechin-3-0-gallate
EGOT erythrocyte glutamic oxalacetic transaminase
EGRAC erythrocyte glutathione reductase activity coefficient
EMO 5-ethoxy-4-methyl-oxazole
ENaC epithelial sodium channel
eNOS endothelial nitric oxide synthase
EO endogenous ouabain
EPA eicosapentaenoic acid
EPO evening primrose oil
ER endoplasmic reticulum
Erk extracellular signal-regulated kinase
ETKA erythrocyte transketolase activity
ETKAC erythrocyte transketolase activity coefficient
FA fatty acid
FAD flavin adenine dinucleotide
FAO Food and Agriculture Organization of the United Nations
FBD fibrocystic breast disease
FCC Food Chemical Codex
FHPP familial hypokalaemic periodic paralysis
FLVCR feline leukaemia virus subgroup C receptor
FMN flavin mononucleotide
FPN1 ferroportin 1
FSANZ Food Standards Australia New Zealand
GABA gamma-aminobutyric acid
GAGs glycosaminoglycans
GAIT Glucosamine/Chondroitin Arthritis Intervention Trial
Gas-6 growth arrest specific gene 6 protein
GD Graves' disease
GHK glycyl-L-histidyl-L-lysine
GI glycaemic index
GIT gastrointestinal tract
GK glucokinase
GL glycaemic load
GLA gamma-linolenic acid
GLM green-lipped mussel
Gln glutamine
Glu glutamic acid
GLUT glucose transporter
Gly glycine
GORD gastro-oesophageal reflux disease
GPx glutathione peroxidase
GRP Gla-rich protein
GSAC gamma-glutamyl-S-allylcysteine
GSH glutathione
GSMC gamma-glutamyl-S-methylcysteine
GSPC gamma-glutamyl-S-propylcysteine
GST glutathione S-transferase
GTF glucose tolerance factor
GTT glucose tolerance test
Hb haemoglobin
HbA_{1C} glycated haemoglobin
HCP hydrolysed casein protein
Hcy homocysteine
HD Huntington's disease
HDL high-density lipoprotein
HF hydrogen fluoride
HH hereditary haemochromatosis
HHC hexahydrocurcumin
His histidine
HIV human immunodeficiency virus
HMG-CoA 3-hydroxy-3-methylglutaryl coenzyme A
HRT hormone replacement therapy
HSH hypomagnesaemia with secondary hypocalcaemia
HSHs hydrogenated starch hydrolysates
HSV *Herpes simplex* virus
HUT haemoglobin unit on a tyrosine basis
HYPP hyperkalaemic periodic paralysis
I3C indole-3-carbinol
IBD inflammatory bowel disease
ICC Indian childhood cirrhosis
ICF intracellular fluid
ICT idiopathic chronic toxicosis
IDA iron deficiency anaemia
IDD iodine deficiency disorders
IDL intermediate-density lipoprotein
IF intrinsic factor
IFN-gamma interferon-gamma

Ig immunoglobulin
IGF-1 insulin-like growth factor-1
IL interleukin
Ile isoleucine
IM integrin-mobilferrin
im intramuscular
iNOS inducible nitric oxide synthase
INR international normalised ratio
IOM Institute of Medicine (USA)
IPs inositol phosphates
IREs iron-responsive elements
IRPs iron regulatory proteins
IU international unit
iv intravenous
KBD Kashin-Beck disease
KF Kayser-Fleischer (rings)
kJ kilojoule
KLF Krüppel-like factor
KSS Kearns-Sayre syndrome
LA linoleic acid
LCAT lecithin:cholesterol acyltransferase
LDL low-density lipoprotein
L-dopa levodopa
Leu leucine
LipU lipase unit
LMWCr low-molecular weight chromium-binding substance
LOX lipoxygenase
LOXL lysyl oxidase-like
LP lipoprotein
LT leukotriene
LTr-1 2-(indol-3-ylmethyl)-3,3'-diindolylmethane
LVH left ventricular hypertrophy
LX lipoxin
Lys lysine
MAOI monoamine oxidase inhibitor
MAPK mitogen-activated protein kinase
mARC mitochondrial amidoxime reducing component
MAS milk-alkali syndrome
Mb myoglobin
MC micellar casein
MCH microcrystalline hydroxyapatite
MCP monocyte chemoattractant protein
MCT monocarboxylate transporter
MCV mean corpuscular volume
MD Menkes disease
MDMA methylenedioxymethamphetamine (ecstasy)
mDNA mitochondrial DNA
MDR1 multi-drug resistance protein 1
MeHg methylmercury
MELAS stroke-like syndrome
Mer receptor tyrosine kinases of the TAM family
MERRF myoclonus epilepsy with ragged red fibres
Met methionine
MGP matrix-Gla protein
MI myocardial infarction (heart attack)
mJ megajoule
MK menaquinone
MMA methylmalonic acid
mmHg millimetres of mercury
MMP matrix metalloproteinase
MMST monomethylsilanetriol
MMT methylcyclopentadienyl manganese tricarbonyl
MoCD molybdenum cofactor deficiency
Moco molybdenum cofactor
MOT2 molybdate transporter type 2
MPACs metal-protein attenuation compounds
MPC milk protein concentrate
MPI milk protein isolate
MRDD maximum recommended daily dose
MRE metal response element
MRI magnetic resonance imaging
MRJPs major royal jelly proteins
mRNA messenger RNA
MS multiple sclerosis
MSG monosodium glutamate
MSM methylsulfonylmethane
MT metallothionein
MTHFR methylene tetrahydrofolate reductase
MTPPT mitochondrial thiamin pyrophosphate transporter
MUFA monounsaturated fatty acid
MUIC mean urinary iodine concentration
MX methylxanthine
Na/K-ATPase sodium/potassium-ATPase
NAAD nicotinic acid adenine dinucleotide
NaBC1 sodium-coupled borate transporter
NAC N-acetylcysteine
NAD nicotinamide adenine dinucleotide
NADP nicotinamide adenine dinucleotide phosphate
NADPH reduced nicotinamide adenine dinucleotide phosphate

NAFLD non-alcoholic fatty liver disease
NAMN nicotinic acid mononucleotide
NaS-1 sodium-dependent sulfate cotransporter
NASH non-alcoholic steatohepatitis
NCC sodium/chloride cotransporter
NEAP net endogenous acid production
NF-kappaB nuclear factor kappaB
NFTs neurofibrillary tangles
NH_2 amino group
NH_3 ammonia
NHF National Heart Foundation (Australia)
NHMRC National Health and Medical Research Council (Australia)
NIS sodium/iodide symporter
NK cell natural killer cell
NKT cell natural killer T cell
NMDA N-methyl-D-aspartate
NMN N'-methylnicotinamide
NO nitric oxide
NOAEL no observed adverse effect level
NOC N-nitroso compounds
NPC1L1 Niemann-Pick C1-like 1 protein
NPU net protein utilisation
Nrf2 nuclear factor erythroid 2-related factor 2
NRVs Nutrient Reference Values
NSAIDs non-steroidal anti-inflammatory drugs
NSPs non-starch polysaccharides
NTBI non-transferrin bound iron
NTDs neural tube defects
NUTTAB Food Standards Australia New Zealand Nutrient Database
OA osteoarthritis
OATP1C1 organic anion-transporting polypeptide 1C1
OCD obsessive-compulsive disorder
OCs organosulfur compounds
OHC octahydrocurcumin
OHS occipital horn syndrome
OPCs oligomeric proanthocyanidins
Orn ornithine
OSPS oral sodium phosphate solution
PA pernicious anaemia
PABA para-aminobenzoic acid
PAF platelet-activating factor
PAHs polyaromatic hydrocarbons
PAM peptidylglycine alpha-amidating monooxygenase
PanK pantothenate kinase
PAPS 3'-phosphoadenosine 5'-phosphosulfate
PARP poly(ADP-ribose)polymerases
PBDEs polybrominated diphenyl ethers
PC phosphatidylcholine
PCBL phenethyl caffeate benzoxanthene lignan
PCBs polychlorinated biphenyls
PCC propionyl-CoA carboxylase
PCFT proton-coupled folate transporter
PCOS polycystic ovarian syndrome
PCOs procyanidolic oligomers
PD Parkinson's disease
PDCAAS protein digestibility-corrected amino acid score
PDE pyridoxine-dependent epilepsy
PDEs phosphodiesterases
PDGF platelet-derived growth factor
PE phosphatidylethanolamine
PEA phenylethylamine
PEM protein-energy malnutrition
PEMT phosphatidylethanolamine methyltransferase
PEPCK phosphoenolpyruvate carboxykinase
PepT1 peptide transporter 1
PER protein efficiency ratio
PG prostaglandin
PGI prostacyclin
pH potential hydrogen
Phe phenylalanine
PI phosphatidylinositol
PIH pregnancy-induced hypertension
PIVKA-II proteins induced in vitamin K absence
PK phylloquinone, vitamin K1
PKAN pantothenate kinase-associated neurodegeneration
PKU phenylketonuria
PL phospholipid
PLF periostin-like factor
PLP pyridoxal 5'-phosphate
PMN polymorphonuclear leukocyte
PMP pyridoxamine 5'-phosphate
PN phosphate nephropathy
PNP pyridoxine 5'-phosphate
PP pellagra preventative factor
PPAR-gamma peroxisome proliferator-activated receptor gamma
PPIs proton pump inhibitors
ppm parts per million
PRGP proline-rich Gla proteins
Pro proline
PrPC prion protein, normal

PrPSc prion protein, abnormal
Prx peroxiredoxin
PS phosphatidylserine
PSA prostate-specific antigen
PSK polysaccharide-K
PSP polysaccharide-peptide
PT prothrombin time
PTH parathyroid hormone
PTPN1 tyrosine-protein phosphatase non-receptor type 1
PU papain unit
PUFA polyunsaturated fatty acid
PV peroxide value
PVP-I povidone-iodine
QCT quantitative computed tomography
QUS quantitative ultrasound
RA retinoic acid
RANK receptor activator of NF-kappaB
RAR retinoic acid receptor
RBP retinol-binding protein
RCPA Royal College of Pathologists of Australasia
RDI recommended dietary intake (per day)
RDS respiratory distress syndrome
RE retinol equivalents
RFVT riboflavin transporter
RH reactive hypoglycaemia
RhA rheumatoid arthritis
RL Ringer's lactate
RLS restless legs syndrome
RNA ribonucleic acid
RNOS reactive nitrogen oxide species
RNS reactive nitrogen species
ROS reactive oxygen species
rRNA ribosomal RNA
RS resistant starch
RXR retinoid X receptor
SAAs sulfur-containing amino acids
SAC S-allylcysteine
SAD seasonal affective disorder
SAH S-adenosylhomocysteine
SAM or SAMe S-adenosylmethionine
SAMC S-allylmercaptocysteine
Sat-1 sulfate/oxalate/bicarbonate anion exchanger
SCC sodium copper chlorophyllin
SCFA short-chain fatty acid
SeBP selenium-binding protein
Sec selenocysteine
SEC S-ethylcysteine
SELECT Selenium and Vitamin E Cancer Prevention Trial
Sep selenoprotein
Ser serine
SFAs saturated fatty acids
SFN sulforaphane
SGLT sodium-glucose transporter
SH sulfhydryl
SIADH syndrome of inappropriate antidiuretic hormone secretion
SIDS sudden infant death syndrome
SIRT sirtuin
SLC solute carrier
SLE systemic lupus erythematosus
SMCT1 sodium-coupled monocarboxylate transporter 1
SMVT sodium-dependent multivitamin transport system
SOD superoxide dismutase
SOX sulfite oxidase
SOZC seaweed oligosaccharide-zinc complex
SPC S-propylcysteine
SPI soy protein isolate
SPs sulfated polysaccharides
SR sarcoplasmic reticulum
SR-B1 scavenger receptor class B type 1
SREBP-2 sterol regulatory element binding protein 2
SSKI supersaturated potassium iodide
SSRIs selective serotonin reuptake inhibitors
STRA6 stimulated by retinoic acid 6
SUDS sudden unexplained death syndrome
SULTs sulfotransferase enzymes
SWL shockwave lithotripsy
Syk spleen tyrosine kinase
T cell thymus-derived lymphocyte
T-2 toxin trichothecene
T3 triiodothyronine
T4 thyroxine
TAN tropical ataxic neuropathy
Tau taurine
TB tuberculosis
TCM Traditional Chinese Medicine
TD tardive dyskinesia
TDP thiamin diphosphate
TDPase thiamin diphosphokinase
TEE total energy expenditure
TF transferrin
TfR transferrin receptor

Tg thyroglobulin
TG triacylglycerol, triglyceride
TGA Therapeutic Goods Administration, Australia
Tg-DIT Tg-3,5-diiodotyrosine
Tg-MIT Tg-3-monoiodotyrosine
TGN trans-Golgi network
Tg-rT3 reverse T3
Tg-T3 Tg-3,5,3'-triiodothyronine
Tg-T4 Tg-3,5,3',5'-tetraiodothyronine
THC tetrahydrocurcumin
THF tetrahydrofolate
ThPP thyrotoxic periodic paralysis
Thr threonine
THTR thiamin transporter
TIBC total iron-binding capacity
TM tetrathiomolybdate
TMAO trimethylamine N-oxide
TMG transmembrane Gla proteins
TMP thiamin monophosphate
TNF-alpha tumour necrosis factor-alpha
TPN total parenteral nutrition
TPO thyroperoxidase
TPP thiamin pyrophosphate
TR thyroid receptor
TRAb thyroid stimulating hormone receptor antibody
TRD treatment-resistant depression
TRH thyrotropin-releasing hormone
TRMA thiamin-responsive megaloblastic anaemia
tRNA transfer RNA
Trp tryptophan
TRPM transient receptor potential cation channel melastatin
Trx thioredoxin
TrxGR thioredoxin reductase-glutathione reductase
TrxR thioredoxin reductase
TSEs transmissable spongiform encephalopathies
TSH thyroid-stimulating hormone
TTFD thiamin tetrahydrofurfuryl disulfide
TTP thiamin triphosphate
TX thromboxane
Tyr tyrosine
Tyro3 receptor tyrosine kinases of the TAM family
UC ulcerative colitis
UDP uridine diphosphate
UFA unsaturated fatty acid
UL upper level of intake
UTI urinary tract infection
UTP uridine triphosphate
UV ultraviolet
Val valine
VDR vitamin D receptor
VKDB vitamin K deficiency bleeding
VLDL very low-density lipoprotein
WHO World Health Organization
WMP whole milk protein
WPC whey protein concentrate
WPH whey protein hydrolysate
WPI whey protein isolate
XDH xanthine dehydrogenase
XLH X-linked hypophosphataemic rickets
XO xanthine oxidase
XOR xanthine oxidoreductase
ZAG zinc alpha 2-glycoprotein

Preface

This text has been designed as a reference for students who are beginning the study of nutritional therapy and complementary medicine. It provides a detailed and comprehensive coverage of important food components and their effects on health, information that is an essential foundation for the use of foods, diets and dietary supplements for health maintenance and disease prevention and treatment. Although it has been written from an Australian perspective, it is based on international research and is applicable to students worldwide.

The text begins by introducing the concepts of a naturopathic approach to health and nutrition, and providing an overview of basic physiological principles and the body's protective systems, including the antioxidant, detoxification and immune systems. Food components covered include essential nutrients (vitamins, minerals and trace elements) and nutritional bioactives (naturally occurring components of food or diet-related substances that affect body function). Information on each food component covers (where applicable) digestion, absorption, transport, metabolism, storage, excretion, regulation of body balance, synthesis, functions, dietary sources, factors influencing body status, daily requirement, deficiency effects, deficiency case reports, assessment of body status, evidence-based therapeutic uses, therapeutic doses, effects of excess, toxicity case reports, supplements and cautions.

Foundations of Naturopathic Nutrition includes discussions of important or controversial nutritional topics, such as water as therapy, obesity, anorexia nervosa, high-protein diets, hypoglycaemia, diabetes, phytosterols, gamma-tocopherol, vitamin E and mortality, vitamin C and cancer, infantile scurvy, acid-forming and alkaline-forming diets, hair analysis, sodium and blood pressure, and coenzyme Q10 and cancer. Summary boxes and quizzes are included to enhance understanding, and recommended nutrient intake tables for Australia, the UK and the US are given in the appendix.

Having worked in the field of naturopathic nutrition for over thirty years, I am more convinced than ever of the central role that food and nutritional supplements play in optimal health. I trust this book will help you, as a student or practitioner, gain new insights into the powerful effects that improved nutrition can have on you and your patients.

Fay Paxton
PhD (Hum Nutr), B App Sci (Health Prom), Grad Dip Hum Nutr, Grad Dip Ed, Dip Nat Ther, Cert IV (A&WT)

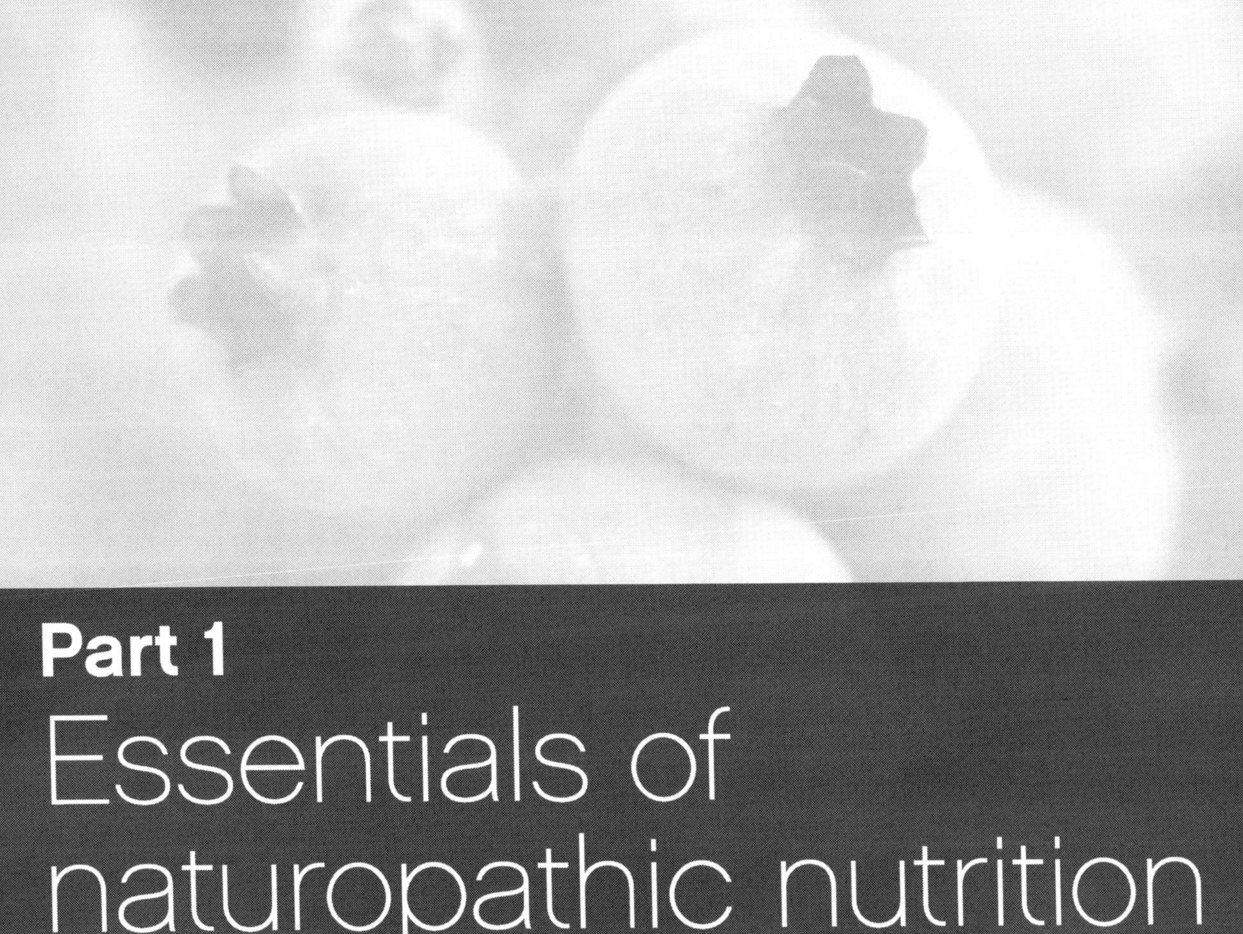

Part 1
Essentials of naturopathic nutrition

1

Introduction to naturopathy, nutrition, naturopathic nutrition, basic physiology, digestion and the body's protective systems

NATUROPATHY

Naturopathy is the use of natural therapies, and diet and lifestyle modifications, that aim to restore health, physiological balance and well-being, and enhance resistance to disease.

History of naturopathy

Natural methods of treating disease—especially physical therapies and medicines based on plant and animal extracts—have been used throughout history. The development and written recording of systematic approaches to treatment is believed to have originated in the ancient Greek, Roman, Indian and Chinese cultures. The modern naturopathic movement began in Germany about 200 years ago, where natural therapists began using therapies such as hydrotherapy, hygiene, fasting, exercise, colonic irrigation, diet and sunlight exposure to restore health. Most early naturopaths practised at sanatoria, where people would stay to take the 'cure'. The nineteenth-century German homeopath John Scheel is credited with first using the term 'naturopathy' to represent treatments based on natural approaches.

Father Sebastian Kneipp (1821–97), a priest turned healer, developed a five-point approach to treatment, based on hydrotherapy, exercise, herbs, nutrition and lifestyle change, and gained fame for his revolutionary and effective health practices. Henry Lindlahr (1862–1924) was cured of diabetes and obesity by Father Kneipp's treatments, and established a sanatorium in the United States dedicated to 'nature cure'; he also wrote several books that popularised this approach to health. Benedict Lust was healed of tuberculosis by Father Kneipp's treatments, and in 1892 settled in the United States, where he opened several health resorts and founded the first naturopathic medical school in the world, the American School of Naturopathy in New York City, in 1902. He wrote extensively about natural treatments, and also introduced America to Ayurveda (traditional Indian medicine) and Yoga. He became known as the 'father of naturopathy' in America.

From these early beginnings, naturopathy became a worldwide movement that was first seen as an alternative to orthodox health care. Some early practitioners actively disparaged orthodox medicine and discouraged its use, but modern naturopaths view naturopathy as complementary to orthodox approaches, and believe it is possible for both approaches to work together for the good of the patient. Modern naturopathy makes use of evidence-based and traditional treatments, and emphasises prevention and patient education as well as cure.

Principles of naturopathy

The principles of naturopathy are based on the twin concepts of boosting the body's natural vital force and removing any blockages or inhibiting factors.

- *The body has an innate healing power.* The body has an innate ability to balance and heal itself (vital force), and naturopaths work to boost the body's natural vitality and remove any impediments to healing.
- *Treatment should work with the body's natural vital force.* Naturopaths use treatments that help to balance and optimise body functions and support and enhance the vital force.
- *Treatment should focus on the underlying cause of the health issue.* Naturopaths compile comprehensive case histories and undertake physical examinations in an effort to identify the true cause of health disorders, rather than treating the symptoms.
- *Treatment should encompass the whole person.* In naturopathy, it is the person with a health disorder who is treated, rather than the disorder. There is no one treatment for every patient with the same disorder because treatment must be tailored to suit the individual. Before deciding on a treatment program, naturopaths investigate a patient's health history, family history, diet, psychological issues, and environmental and lifestyle factors that may contribute to ill-health or increase health risk.
- *Blockages to vitality should be addressed.* Naturopaths believe environmental, lifestyle and dietary factors can lead to a build-up of toxins in the body that contribute to inflammation, and these must be cleared for optimal health and vitality. For detoxification, the liver, kidneys, digestive tract, skin and lymph system are regarded as important targets of treatment.
- *Prevention is as important as cure.* Naturopaths educate patients about the principles of good health, identify an individual's health risks and instigate preventive behaviours to maintain health at its optimal level. They aim to prevent minor, acute complaints from progressing to more serious or chronic conditions.

The three stages of disease

Traditional naturopaths view disease as occurring in three stages: the acute, sub-acute and chronic stages. The acute stage occurs when the body has enough vitality to attempt to resist an illness by developing a fever or acute inflammation, such as a cold, influenza or skin inflammation like eczema. Traditional naturopaths believe that suppressing the acute stage by using treatments that merely give symptom relief can lead to the development of the sub-acute stage. In the case of a respiratory disorder, this may appear as a continual or intermittent mucus discharge. The prolonged disturbance caused by the sub-acute stage may further lower the body's vitality, and suppression of symptoms may lead to the chronic stage of disease, which is marked by destruction of tissue or gross malfunctions of body systems. Chronic inflammatory or autoimmune diseases may then result.

Retracing and the healing crisis

When treating the underlying cause of the disorder with natural therapies, these stages of disease can retrace from the chronic stage back to the acute stage during the healing process. A healing crisis, in which the patient has an acute exacerbation of the original disorder, may occur during this time, indicating that the patient's vitality is now much stronger. Although symptoms flare up, the patient may still feel quite well, and the crisis usually resolves rapidly. Not all patients will show retracing or a healing crisis during their treatment.

Naturopathic practice

Naturopaths work towards improving health on all levels and use a wide range of approaches, including:

- dietary and lifestyle change
- exercise programs
- nutritional supplements
- herbal, homeopathic and flower essence remedies
- detoxification programs
- weight management
- physical therapies, such as massage, breathing exercises, and relaxation and meditation techniques
- stress management
- counselling.

NUTRITION

Genes, environment, lifestyle and diet are important factors that impact on health. The diet provides essential nutrients, which are food components that are vital for normal body function but either cannot be made in the body or cannot be made in sufficient amounts to maintain good health, and therefore must be obtained from a dietary source. A lack or imbalance of essential nutrients can lead to poor health and even death if the deficiency is prolonged and severe enough. In Western countries, it is rare that a nutritional deficiency becomes life-threatening, but subtle, mild deficiencies that impair general health often go unrecognised. Even mild nutritional deficiencies can cause fatigue, reduced resistance to stress, susceptibility to illness and difficulty coping with life's demands, and long-term poor nutrition may lead to cellular and organ dysfunction, resulting in disease.

Poor nutrition can cause a range of adverse effects in the body, including:

- biochemical imbalances, such as excesses of potentially harmful substances and inadequate levels of essential substances
- impaired enzyme function and inefficient energy production
- impaired function of cells, organs and tissues
- impaired or abnormal immune responses
- impaired detoxification
- chronic inflammation and infections
- psychological, physical or oxidative stress caused by reduced resistance to stressors
- cumulative damage to tissues.

Essential nutrients

Essential nutrients are classified according to the amount required to keep the body functioning normally, and are measured in terms of grams (g), milligrams (mg) or micrograms (mcg or μg—'μ' is the Greek letter 'mu' and represents 'micro'). One gram is a thousandth of a kilogram, one milligram is a thousandth of a gram, and one microgram a thousandth of a milligram. Macronutrients are essential nutrients present in foods in gram amounts, and micronutrients are essential nutrients usually present in milligram or microgram amounts.

Macronutrients

Macronutrients are the energy-containing (kilojoule-containing) components of food, such as protein, carbohydrates and lipids. Alcohol also provides energy, but is not regarded as a nutrient.

- *Protein* is the building block of body structures, such as cells, tissues, enzymes, and immune and communication substances.
- *Available carbohydrates* are sugars and starch; these are the major energy providers in the body.
- *Unavailable carbohydrates,* such as dietary fibre, provide little or no energy, but are important for health—especially bowel health.
- *Lipids* are fats and oils, and are required for the structure of cell membranes and the production of cholesterol, fatty acids and eicosanoids, which are local hormone-like substances that regulate many different body processes, including immunity and inflammation. Lipids are also used as a storage form of energy.
- *Water* is used for transporting and excreting substances, for digestion and other chemical reactions in the body, and for cooling the body as sweat.

Micronutrients

Micronutrients include vitamins, macrominerals, trace elements and ultratrace elements that may have structural and/or metabolic roles in the body:

- *vitamins:* vitamins A, B, C, D, E and K
- *macrominerals:* calcium, phosphorus, magnesium, sodium, potassium, chloride and sulfate
- *trace elements:* iron, zinc, copper, manganese, iodine, selenium, chromium, molybdenum and fluoride
- *ultratrace elements:* boron and silicon, which may be essential nutrients, as well as aluminium, arsenic, cobalt, germanium, lithium, nickel, rubidium, tin and vanadium, which have physiological activity in the body but are not regarded as essential.

Recommended amounts of essential nutrients

The Australian and New Zealand governments jointly publish tables of Nutrient Reference Values (NRVs) as a guide to the amounts of macro- and micronutrients that are needed in the diet each day. The *Nutrient Reference Values for Australia and New Zealand Including Recommended Dietary Intakes* can be accessed at <www.nrv.gov.au>. These tables provide figures for the estimated average requirement (EAR) or recommended dietary intake (RDI) per day of each essential nutrient. The EAR is the daily amount of a nutrient that would meet the needs of 50 per cent of healthy individuals in a particular life stage and gender group. The RDI is the average daily amount of a nutrient that would meet the needs of 97–98 per cent of healthy individuals in a particular life stage and gender group. When no RDI has been established, an adequate intake (AI) is given, which is the average daily requirement for a nutrient based on estimates from studies of apparently healthy people. The estimated energy requirement (EER), in terms of the kilojoules needed per day, is also given. This is the average estimated daily energy intake required to maintain energy balance and good health in a healthy adult of a defined age, gender, weight, height and level of physical activity. The upper level of intake (UL) is the highest average daily intake of a nutrient that poses no health risks to almost all individuals in the general population. As intake increases above the UL, the potential risk of adverse effects increases. Note that NRVs are based on the needs of an average healthy population and may not be relevant to individual needs.

Factors that may affect individual nutritional status

These factors include:

- a diet based on highly processed food, which provides excess kilojoules but insufficient micronutrients
- excess alcohol and caffeinated drinks, which can deplete water-soluble nutrients by increasing urinary losses
- special diets for weight loss, body-building, sport, food allergies or intolerances, or cultural or religious practices, which may mean that food intake is unbalanced or restricted
- different life stages, which affect food intake and requirements. Children can be fussy eaters and teenagers often have a high intake of junk foods. Elderly people may have poor teeth and digestion, low energy and/or reduced mobility, which may lead to a restricted 'tea and toast' diet. For women, menstruation, pregnancy, breastfeeding and menopause alter nutritional needs
- poor digestion and digestive disorders, which can limit the ability to obtain nutrients from food
- inborn genetic factors, which may increase the need for specific nutrients
- illness, which can increase the demand for nutrients and decrease appetite
- prescription medications, which may affect the digestion, uptake or metabolism of nutrients
- poor-quality soil, which depletes the mineral content of plant food
- a fast-paced, stressful lifestyle, which increases the need for supportive nutrients
- smoking and exposure to passive smoke or other pollutants, which can increase the need for detoxifying and protective nutrients
- strenuous exercise or heavy physical work, which increases nutrient demand
- lack of sun exposure, which increases the need for vitamin D.

Naturopaths use dietary modification and nutritional supplementation to improve nutritional status and treat cellular and organ dysfunctions that are being expressed as disease. Nutritional therapy is also used to increase energy and improve brain function, mood and attitude; to maintain good health throughout life; to help reduce the risk of diet-related diseases; and to help compensate for genetic predisposition to disease.

Nutritional supplements

Nutritional supplementation provides a quick means of compensating for dietary deficiencies and initiating rapid improvement in impaired body functions. However, nutritional supplements cannot deliver the entire amount of health-promoting factors found in food; nor can they take the place of a well-balanced diet. Dietary improvement must go hand in hand with supplementation.

Nutritional supplements can be derived from plant or animal material, or produced in a laboratory by chemical synthesis or microbial fermentation. The development of methods of synthesising nutrients led to the availability of relatively cheap forms of nutrients that could be put into powder, liquid, tablet or capsule form; this created an industry based on the manufacture and sale of nutritional supplements.

In many cases, the synthetic version of a nutrient is 'nature identical', meaning that it has exactly the same molecular structure as the nutrient that is found in food—for example, ascorbic acid (vitamin C) has the same structure if made synthetically (usually from sorbitol derived from glucose) or if eaten in an orange. Because it is identical, it is believed to have exactly the same role in the body as if it were derived from food. Most commercial products contain synthetic nutrients because they are cheaper and easier to produce than extracting them from food. Methods of producing synthetic vitamins differ between manufacturers. In contrast to manufacturers in other parts of the world, Australian manufacturers are subject to regulation by the Therapeutic Goods Administration (TGA), a government body that regulates manufacturing processes, product ingredients, labelling, advertising and the health claims on product labels.

Production methods

Raw materials are obtained from distributors, and checked for identity, potency and purity. The required weights of ingredients are measured out, placed in a mixer and tested periodically to ensure that mixing is complete. A common method used for making tablet formulations is to mix the nutrient ingredients with excipients and blend them together before compressing the powder into tablets (direct compression). If the material cannot be blended easily, the particles are combined using a binding agent (wet granulation) or by using mechanical force to compact them together to form dry granules (dry granulation). After blending, the mixture is put into a tableting machine that compresses the material into a tablet shape, which is then coated, dried and packaged, or into an encapsulating machine that dispenses it into capsules, which are then polished and packaged. Quality-control testing is carried out throughout the process.

Capsules are made from gelatine derived from animal skin, tendons, ligaments or bones, or from non-gelatine material suitable for vegans, such as carrageenan (from seaweed), hydroxypropyl starch, disodium phosphate or glycerol. Excipients used in tablets are non-active ingredients included for manufacturing or marketing purposes, and may include fillers/diluents, binders, disintegrants, lubricants, anti-adherents, glidants (flow enhancers), wetting/surface active agents, colours, flavours, sweeteners and taste-maskers. Some excipients commonly used in the process of manufacturing tablets include:

- *microcrystalline cellulose*, a purified, modified cellulose prepared by treating cellulose derived from fibrous plant material with mineral acids
- *lactose*, a sugar derived from cow's milk
- *sugars and starches*, such as modified forms of sucrose, modified starch derived from corn, wheat, potato or rice, native starches from corn, wheat, rice and potatoes, starch paste and partially pre-gelatinised starch
- *inorganic salts*, such as dicalcium phosphate, tricalcium phosphate and calcium sulfate
- *polyols* (sugar alcohols), such as sorbitol, mannitol and xylitol, derived from starch or glucose
- *povidone* (polyvinylpyrrolidone), a synthetic polymer, and crospovidone, a cross-linked form of povidone
- *gelatine*, derived from animal skin, tendons, ligaments and bones
- *plant gums*, such as acacia, tragacanth, guar and pectin
- *croscarmellose sodium*, a form of sodium carboxymethylcellulose derived from cellulose, used as a disintegrant
- *sodium starch glycolate*, a sodium salt of a carboxymethyl ether of starch
- *magnesium stearate*, the most commonly used lubricant; other lubricants include calcium stearate, stearic acid, hydrogenated vegetable oils and mineral oil
- *talc* (magnesium silicate), used as an anti-adherent
- *alkali stearates* and *colloidal silicon dioxide*, used as glidants to improve processing.

Coatings may be used to make the tablet easier to swallow, mask an unpleasant taste or colour the tablet for cosmetic purposes. Colours may be synthetic dyes approved for use in food or natural pigments. Tablets are often coated with carnauba wax, derived from the leaves of a tropical palm. Enteric-coated tablets have a pH-sensitive chemical coating that keeps the tablet intact in the stomach, allowing it to release its contents in the intestine where absorption takes place. This is often used for strong-tasting ingredients that may cause reflux or an unpleasant after-taste.

NATUROPATHIC NUTRITION

Naturopathic nutrition is the use of diet and nutritional supplements to prevent and treat health disorders, and improve physical and mental health and general wellbeing.

History of naturopathic nutrition

Nutritional therapy has its origins in ancient systems of medicine, such as Traditional Chinese Medicine (TCM), Ayurvedic (traditional Indian) medicine and ancient Greek medicine as used by Hippocrates. In these traditions, food was recognised as an important part of health, and specific foods and diets were used for illness-prevention and healing purposes.

In the late nineteenth century, it was believed that the only essential nutrients were proteins, carbohydrates, fats, inorganic salts and water, and diseases that we now know result from nutritional deficiencies were generally attributed to toxins or infections. In 1905, the Dutch researcher Cornelis Pekelharing found that animals fed purified diets that comprised only the known essential nutrients failed to grow, lost weight and died unless they were also given small amounts of milk, and concluded that milk contained some unrecognised factor that was necessary for growth and survival. The Polish scientist Casimir Funk is credited with discovering the existence of vitamins in 1912; he called these 'vitamines', coined from the term 'vital amines'. He believed they were all amines, but this was found to be incorrect and the name was altered to 'vitamins'. Following this major breakthrough, many other micronutrients were discovered in food, and their role in healthy body function is still subject to intensive research today.

Modern nutritional therapy began with the discovery of previously unknown micronutrients and their role in health. Pioneers of nutritional therapy in the United States in the period from the 1950s to the 1970s began to use dietary changes and supplementary doses of vitamins, minerals and trace elements to improve health. However, their discoveries were largely ignored and often actively opposed by orthodox medicine. One of the most famous of these early nutritional therapists was Adelle Davis (1904–74), an American biochemist, dietitian and author of four best-selling books, including the ground-breaking *Let's Eat Right to Keep Fit*, published in 1954. Her books have been criticised by health experts for containing many errors and misinterpretations of the facts, and for providing dangerous advice regarding the use of excessive doses of vitamin A and the use of potassium chloride for infantile colic, which even led to the death of one infant. However, she was largely responsible for raising public awareness around the world about the connection between diet and disease, and the possible role of diet and nutritional supplements in disease-prevention and treatment. Other important pioneers were:

- *Dr Evan Shute (1907–82) and Dr Wilfred Shute (1905–78).* The Shute brothers were Canadian doctors who pioneered the use of large doses of vitamin E for heart and burns patients. They reported dramatic improvements in heart patients who were given oral vitamin E supplements and in patients with severe burns who were given oral and topical vitamin E. In burns, they reported that pain was markedly reduced, infection risk was reduced and affected areas healed without the need for skin grafts and with much-reduced scarring.
- *Irwin Stone (1907–84) and Linus Pauling (1901–94).* Irwin Stone was an American biochemist who first proposed the theory that the inability of humans to make vitamin C in their bodies, as most other animal species do, is caused by a genetic disorder. He introduced this concept to the American biochemist Linus Pauling, who followed up with research into vitamin C and became a promoter of its health properties around the world. Linus Pauling won two Nobel prizes, the Chemistry Prize in 1954 for his research into chemical bonding, and the Peace Prize in 1962 for his work advocating a nuclear test ban treaty.
- *Dr Fred Klenner (1907–84).* Dr Klenner was an American general practitioner who became aware of the importance of vitamin C for health, and experimented on himself, his family and his patients using large doses. He used vitamin C extensively for bacterial and viral infections, and was one of the first to realise that the dose needed to be high enough to saturate the tissues or it would not be effective. He used massive doses orally and intravenously for a wide range of diseases—including polio, which was epidemic at that time—and became firmly convinced of its healing powers.
- *Dr Humphry Osmond (1917–2004) and Dr Abram Hoffer (1917–2009).* Dr Osmond and Dr Hoffer were American psychiatrists who developed the theory that schizophrenic symptoms were caused by the body's production of an adrenalin-based hallucinogen (the Hoffer-Osmond adreno-chrome hypothesis). They pioneered the use of very large doses of vitamin C and the B vitamin niacin for schizophrenics, and also discovered that niacin was effective in large doses for lowering serum cholesterol levels.
- *Dr William Kaufman (1910–2000).* Dr Kaufman was an American physician who pioneered the use of large doses of vitamin B3 (as niacin or niacinamide) for arthritis, together with vitamins C, B1 and B2, and documented dramatic improvements in symptoms in his patients.
- *Dr Carl Pfeiffer (1908–88).* Dr Pfeiffer studied the biochemistry of schizophrenia, and identified biochemical abnormalities that could be rectified by vitamin and mineral supplements. He classified schizophrenias into three biochemical groups and designed nutritional supplement programs that helped to balance each group's faulty biochemistry. He founded the Brain Bio Center in Princeton, New Jersey in 1973 to research the effects of nutrients on the brain. He believed that the right combination of nutrients could be as effective as drugs, without the side-effects.

- *Lady Phyllis Cilento (1894–1987).* Lady Cilento was a journalist and medical practitioner working in Queensland, Australia, who became interested in the work of Adelle Davis and others. She was a pioneer of the use of nutritional therapy in Australia, and advocated women's rights, family planning and improved antenatal and childcare practices. She published several popular books about dietary supplements and health.
- *Dr Archie Kalokerinos (1927–2012).* The Australian medical practitioner Dr Kalokerinos pioneered the use of vitamin C to prevent infant deaths in the Aboriginal communities of the Australian outback. His book *Every Second Child*, published in 1981, recorded his quest for a preventive treatment. He became convinced that the vitamin C deficiency disease scurvy was responsible for illness and deaths in children. Together with his colleague, pathologist Glen Dettman, he became a lifelong advocate for the use of supplementary vitamin C to improve health.

Principles of naturopathic nutrition

Naturopathic nutritional therapy is based on the belief that an inadequate or unbalanced nutritional intake is common, and contributes to reduced resistance to stress, reduced cell function and energy production, impaired immunity, tissue damage, accelerated ageing and biochemical imbalances that impact on physical and mental health. Optimum nutrition helps the body to protect and repair itself, resist disease and regain optimum function, as well as improving health, energy, mood and attitude.

Naturopathic nutritional therapists believe that each individual has a unique physiology, and that a diet and supplement program must be tailored to suit individual needs, taking into account dietary, genetic, environmental and lifestyle factors that affect nutritional status. Nutritional supplements are often given in doses many times larger than can be obtained from the diet ('megadoses'). 'Orthomolecular medicine', a term used for this type of nutritional therapy, was coined by Linus Pauling from the Greek word *ortho*, meaning 'correct' or 'right', and the word 'molecule', referring to the simple chemical structures that exist in the body. This approach to health believes in providing the body with the right molecules (nutrients) in the right amounts to allow it to function at an optimum level. Naturopathic nutritional therapists also take into account digestive problems, food sensitivities, allergies and intolerances, and the need to remove or reduce exposure to the 'wrong' molecules, such as toxins, that may interfere with body function.

Naturopathic nutrition in practice

Naturopathic nutritional therapists compile a comprehensive case history of a patient that includes details of dietary, environmental, psychological and lifestyle factors that impact on health. Nutritional deficiencies and imbalances are identified, and dietary and lifestyle recommendations are made that are suited to the unique needs of the patient. Treatment includes the use of specific foods, beverages and diets, and a range of supplements that may include digestive enzymes, essential nutrients and nutritional bioactives (food-related supplements that are not essential nutrients but have an impact on health).

UNDERSTANDING NUTRITION RESEARCH

Research studies can be carried out in a number of ways, and the study design affects the quality of the results. High-quality study designs attempt to avoid any possible bias (distorting factor) that may affect the results. Clinical trials (experimental studies), in which a group of subjects is given treatment over a specified amount of time, are commonly used in nutrition research. Various statistical tests are used to analyse the results of a research study and the results are expressed as significant or non-significant.

A significant result means that it is a reliable finding and there is a high probability that the treatment has a real effect. However, it does not mean that the result is necessarily of clinical importance because the effect may be too small to make a real difference to health. A non-significant effect may mean that the treatment has no effect or that the number of subjects (sample size) was too small to detect an effect.

The confidence interval (CI) is commonly used to measure the range of the likely size of a treatment effect. The 95 per cent CI is commonly used, and means that the CI range will contain the true value of the treatment effect 95 per cent of the time (95 in 100 such experiments will find the true value of the treatment effect). If a CI range does not include '1', the effect is significant (e.g. a CI of 0.75–0.86). If a CI range includes '1', the effect is not statistically significant (e.g. a CI of 0.70–1.23). Another measure is the 'p' value, which is a measure of the probability that the observed difference could have occurred purely by chance. A p value of less than 0.5 indicates that the outcome is statistically significant; $p<0.05$ means that there is a less than 5 per cent likelihood that the effect occurred by chance and $p<0.01$ means that there is a less than 1 per cent likelihood that the effect occurred by chance.

Types of research studies include the following:

Experimental studies (clinical trials)

- *Controlled clinical trial.* A group (or groups) of subjects is given active treatment and a control group (or groups) is given a sham or inert (placebo) treatment that is as similar as possible to the active treatment.
- *Randomised controlled clinical trial.* A group of subjects is given active treatment and a control group is given a placebo treatment. Subjects are allocated to active or control groups by random assignment (by chance)—for example, by a coin toss or other random method.
- *Randomised controlled single-blind clinical trial.* A group of subjects is given active treatment and a control group is given a placebo treatment. Subjects are allocated to active or control groups by random assignment and do not know (are blind) to which group they belong.
- *Randomised controlled double-blind clinical trial.* A group of subjects is given active treatment and a control group is given a placebo treatment. Subjects are allocated to active or control groups by random assignment and both the investigators and the subjects do not know to which group they belong.
- *Randomised controlled triple-blind clinical trial.* A group of subjects is given active treatment and a control group is given a placebo treatment. Subjects are allocated to active or control groups by random assignment and the investigators, the subjects and the statisticians who analyse the data do not know to which group they belong. This is regarded as a very high-quality study design, which attempts to avoid any possible bias that may affect study results.
- *Pseudo-randomised controlled clinical trial.* Subjects are allocated to treatment or control groups by a systematic method rather than purely by chance (e.g. by alternate allocation).
- *Clustered randomised clinical trial.* Groups of subjects, rather than individuals, are randomised (e.g. randomising of community groups).
- *Crossover clinical trial.* Subjects are randomly allocated to study arms, in which two or more treatments are given consecutively and the responses to the different treatments are compared in the same subject.

Comparative (non-randomised) studies

Subjects are chosen without random selection, and there may or may not be a control group.

- *Single arm study.* All subjects are given active treatment with no control group.
- *Case series study:* A single group of subjects is given active treatment with no control group.
- *Post-test study.* The outcome is measured after the active treatment has been given.
- *Pre-test/post-test study.* The outcome is measured before and after active treatment.
- *Interrupted time series study.* The outcome to active treatment is measured over multiple time points before and after the treatment.
- *Case-control study.* Subjects with a specific outcome/health disorder (cases) are compared with control subjects who do not have the outcome/health disorder in order to identify differing characteristics.
- *Cohort study.* Subjects with a common characteristic (a cohort) (e.g. smokers) are observed over time and the incidence of a specific outcome/health disorder is determined and compared with the incidence in a control group without the characteristic (e.g. non-smokers).

Research reviews

- *Literature review.* The scientific material related to a specific topic is read and described, summarised, evaluated and clarified.
- *Systematic review.* The research on a specific topic is reviewed and the results from a number of the highest quality studies are combined in order to obtain an overall conclusion about the effect of the treatment. A defined method is used to determine the studies to be included and the analysis of the results.

- *Meta-analysis.* This is a type of systematic review that uses specialised statistical techniques to analyse the data.

Scientific evidence ranking

Scientific evidence can be ranked according to the way in which the study was designed and carried out, see Table 1.1. The highest quality of evidence is given a ranking of I and the lowest quality has a ranking of IV.

Some nutrients have been the subject of a great deal of research, but others have not. When evidence is lacking, naturopathic nutritional therapists are guided by knowledge about how nutrients work in the body and the results from cell (in vitro) and animal studies, patient case reports and clinical experience.

Table 1.1 Evidence quality rankings

Level of evidence	Study design
I	Evidence obtained from a systematic review or meta-analysis of all relevant randomised controlled trials
II	Evidence obtained from at least one properly-designed randomised controlled trial
III-1	Evidence obtained from well-designed pseudo-randomised controlled trials (trials using alternate allocation or some other method)
III-2	Evidence obtained from comparative studies (including systematic reviews of such studies) with concurrent controls and allocation not randomised, cohort studies, case-control studies, or interrupted time series with a control group
III-3	Evidence obtained from comparative studies with historical control, two or more single-arm studies, or interrupted time series without a parallel control group
IV	Evidence obtained from case series, either post-test or pre-test/post-test

Source: National Health & Medical Research Council (2000), *How to use the evidence: Assessment and application of scientific evidence* (Canberra: Commonwealth of Australia), <www.nhmrc.gov.au/guidelines/publications/cp69>.

BASIC PHYSIOLOGY

At the smallest level, the body is made up of elements, 24 of which are essential for the body to function normally. Elements present in the largest quantities in body structures are oxygen, carbon, hydrogen and nitrogen. Other important elements are macrominerals, trace elements and some ultratrace elements. Most of the elements needed are obtained from food and water, and oxygen comes from the air breathed in.

Elements are made up of atoms that have electrons that are negatively charged, orbiting a nucleus made up of positively charged protons and uncharged neutrons. The number of protons in the nucleus determines which element it is. Electrons have different levels of orbits (shells) that have a maximum number of electrons they can hold. Hydrogen is the simplest element, having one proton, one neutron and one electron.

Elements prefer to exist in a stable, neutral state that requires the maximum number of electrons in the outer shell. Atoms that do not have the required number of electrons in the outer shell will be either positively or negatively charged, and will then give or receive electrons to another element or share electrons with another element to regain stability. The charged form of an element is called an ion. Elements bond together by electron sharing (covalent bonding) or giving and receiving electrons (ionic bonding). An example of covalent bonding is hydrogen gas (H_2), in which two hydrogen atoms share their electrons. An example of ionic bonding is sodium chloride. Sodium (Na) has one electron in its outer shell and needs seven more to be complete, and chlorine (Cl) has seventeen electrons in its outer shell and needs one more to be complete. Sodium becomes the positively charged sodium ion (Na^+) by giving up an electron, and chlorine becomes the negatively charged chloride ion (Cl^-) by receiving one electron from sodium. Negative and positive charges attract each other, so sodium and chlorine become stable partners as sodium chloride (table salt).

The importance of carbon

A carbon atom has four electrons in its outer shell and needs eight to be stable. Therefore, a carbon atom readily forms four covalent bonds with other elements, and also bonds easily with other carbon atoms, forming straight chains, branched chains or rings. This results in the formation of an enormous variety of organic compounds that are vital to health and life. Chemically speaking, 'organic' compounds are those based on carbon atoms bonded together. They typically contain other elements as well, such as hydrogen, oxygen and nitrogen. 'Organic food' has quite a different meaning: it refers to food that is grown in a natural way without the use of artificial chemicals.

Water

About two-thirds of the body is made up of water, which consists of two hydrogen atoms bonded to an oxygen atom (H_2O). It is particularly useful because it is a polar molecule, which means that it has both positive and negative regions. This property means that water molecules can bond with each other, and it allows water to carry heat and act as a dissolving agent (solvent) for many other substances. When substances dissolve in another substance, it is called a solution. Homoeopaths believe that water has the unique capacity to be imprinted with the energy of dissolved substances, and that this energy can be retained even when the solution is extremely dilute.

Acids and bases

Acids and bases need to be balanced for healthy body function. Water solutions that give off hydrogen ions (H^+) are acidic and water solutions that give off hydroxide ions (OH^-) are basic (alkaline). Acidity or alkalinity is measured on a scale called the potential hydrogen (pH) scale. In this scale, measurements run from 0 to 14. A pH of 7 is neutral and one of less than 7 is acidic; the lower the number, the stronger the acid. Measures over 7 are alkaline; the higher the number, the stronger the base. Water has a pH of 7, which makes it neutral. Combining equal concentrations of acids and bases will neutralise a solution. Acids and bases combine to form salts—for example, when hydrochloric acid combines with sodium hydroxide (a base), it forms water and sodium chloride (a salt).

The body requires a neutral environment for its enzymes to function effectively, with the exception of the digestive tract, where hydrochloric acid lowers the pH to about 1 in the stomach and sodium bicarbonate produced by the pancreas increases the pH to about 8 in the upper part of the small intestine. Buffers in the body can maintain a neutral pH even when exposed to acids or bases, and the body has three main buffering systems: bicarbonates in the bloodstream, phosphates in the kidneys and proteins in blood and tissues. Homeostasis is the mechanism by which the body keeps all internal processes in a steady and balanced state compatible with optimum health.

Oxidation-reduction

Oxidation-reduction (redox) reactions are common reactions in the body, and involve the transfer of electrons. Oxidation reactions involve removing hydrogen atoms from a molecule to form a new substance and reduction reactions involve adding hydrogen atoms to a molecule to form a new substance. The reactions are paired so that when a substance is oxidised, another is reduced at the same time.

Enzymes

Enzymes are proteins that enable chemical reactions that build, transform or break down substances in the body to proceed at a faster rate. Their names usually have the suffix 'ase'—for example, sucrase, the enzyme that digests the sugar sucrose. Each enzyme has an active site that has a specific shape into which a similarly-shaped substrate (a substance that needs to be chemically changed) can attach (see Figure 1.1). Only a similarly shaped molecule can attach to the active site, so an enzyme can only work on one particular type of substrate. When the substrate attaches, the enzyme changes the substrate into new substances. For example, protein-splitting enzymes called proteases in the digestive tract split large protein substrates from food into smaller peptides and amino acids so that they can be absorbed.

Cofactors are non-protein substances that are needed for enzymes to function. There are two types of cofactors: those that are part of the enzyme, called prosthetic groups; and coenzymes, which are loosely bound to the enzyme and attach to the active site alongside the substrate only when required. Prosthetic groups can be vitamins, lipids, carbohydrates or minerals, whereas most coenzymes are vitamins. After a reaction that involves a coenzyme, both the substrate and the coenzyme leave the enzyme's active site changed in some way.

Enzyme and substrate

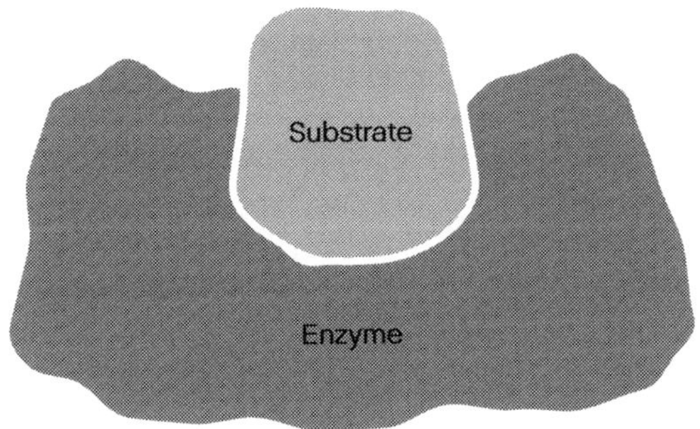

The enzyme binds with a specific substrate and facilitates a chemical reaction

Enzyme with coenzyme and substrate

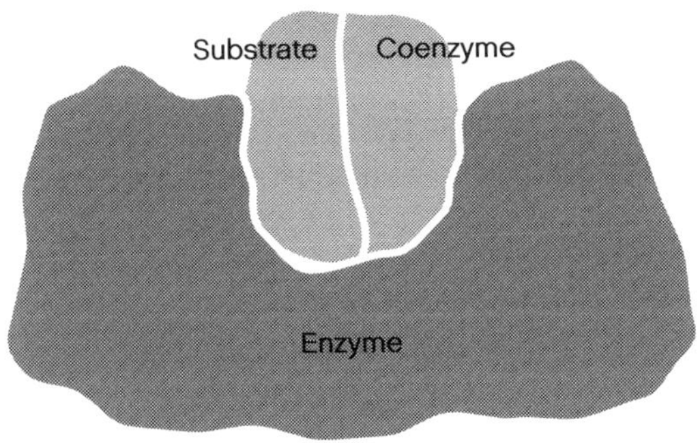

The coenzyme joins with the substrate and the enzyme binds with both, facilitating a chemical reaction

Figure 1.1 Enzymes and coenzymes

Cell structure and function

The cell is the basic unit of all the tissues, organs and structures in the body, and the body is a product of their integrated, specialised functions. Cells are bathed in extracellular fluid (ECF) outside and intracellular fluid (ICF) inside. Each cell is divided into a central nucleus and surrounding cytoplasm. The cell membrane, cell nucleus and organelles embedded in the cytoplasm inside the cell are the functioning units of the cell. Cell structures vary according to their specialised functions.

Cell nucleus

The nucleus contains strands of chromosomes containing deoxyribonucleic acid (DNA), the substance that carries the genes inherited from our parents. DNA allows the cell to replicate and provides the blueprint, or recipe, for making proteins. It is made of two strands, which wind about a common axis to form a double helix. Each strand of DNA consists of a number of nucleic acids joined together. Nucleic acids are large molecules made up of nucleotide units, which comprise nitrogen bases, phosphate and a sugar molecule. A gene is an ordered sequence of nucleotides that is responsible for making a specific type of protein. The entire collection of genes determines all the characteristics of an individual. Genes can be switched on (expressed) or switched off (silenced) as required. To make proteins, a DNA sequence is transcribed (copied) to messenger ribonucleic acid (mRNA), which then relocates to ribosomes in the cell cytoplasm, where the mRNA is translated and a specific protein is assembled.

Cytoplasmic organelles

- *Mitochondria* are the energy-making centres in the cell where protein, lipids and carbohydrates are broken down to make energy for cell activities.
- *Ribosomes* are made in the nucleolus of the nucleus and consist of granules of ribosomal RNA (rRNA). They make proteins and carbohydrate-protein molecules (glycoproteins).
- *Rough (granular) endoplasmic reticulum (ER)* is studded with ribosomes that make proteins and glycoproteins. It also acts as a temporary storage depot for newly made proteins.
- *Smooth (agranular) ER* is where fatty acids, phospholipids and steroids are made.
- *The Golgi complex* receives newly made proteins and lipids from the ER, and sorts, packages and delivers them to the plasma membrane or to vesicles for transport to the membrane and out of the cell.
- *Lysosomes* are membrane-enclosed sacs formed from the Golgi complex, and are the garbage disposal and recycling units of the cell. They contain powerful digestive enzymes that can break down worn-out cell structures and recycle them for further use. They can also deliberately release enzymes into the interior of the cell to destroy the cell when it is severely stressed, infected or behaving abnormally, a process known as apoptosis (cell suicide, or programmed cell death).
- *Centrioles* are paired structures of microtubules that become active during cell division.
- *Cell projections* are specialised parts of the cell membrane of some cells that project out from the cell. Cilia are many short projections, resembling

hairs, that are found in the lining (epithelium) of the respiratory tract. Cilia move in a waving motion to move mucus and inhaled substances out of the body. Microvilli are tiny, finger-like projections found on the villi cells lining the small intestine, which increase the surface area available for absorption of dietary nutrients.

Cell membrane

A plasma membrane surrounds each cell, forming a barrier that controls transport into and out of the cell (see Figure 1.2). It is made of a double layer of specialised fats called phospholipids that have an affinity with water (hydrophilic, water-loving) at the 'head' end and an affinity with lipids (hydrophobic, water-hating) at the 'tail' end. The membrane also contains cholesterol, proteins, glycoproteins and protective antioxidants such as vitamin E. Cholesterol provides rigidity and phospholipids provide fluidity. Proteins act as transport channels across the membrane and glycoproteins are markers that identify the cell to immune cells as being part of the body, rather than foreign. Movement of substances across the membrane can occur by diffusion, in which substances move from an area of higher concentration to one of lower concentration; active transport, in which energy and a transporter are used to pump the substance across; and endocytosis, in which a receptor on the membrane surface binds to the substance and pinches off to form a vesicle that moves into the cell and releases its contents.

Cell metabolism

Metabolism is the term used to describe all the chemical reactions in the body. Catabolism is the breaking down of substances and anabolism is the process of building new ones. Enzymes are essential for enabling chemical reactions to take place at the correct rate, and energy is used up in this process.

Energy production

Cells convert food into energy by oxidation. Glucose from carbohydrates is the preferred fuel, but fats, protein and alcohol are used as well. There are three main stages of energy production (see Figure 1.3):

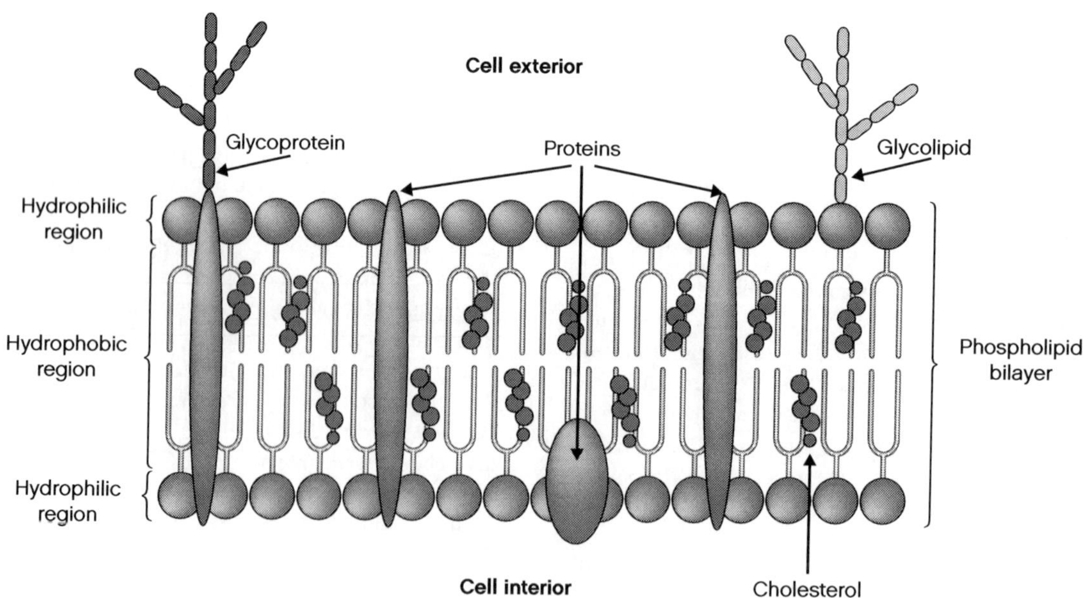

Figure 1.2 Cell membrane structure

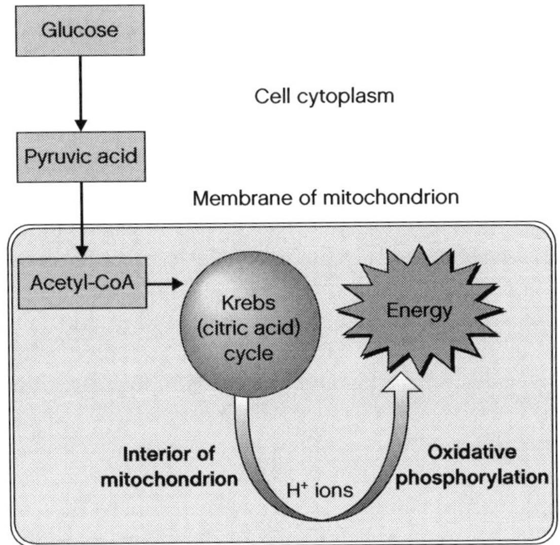

Figure 1.3 Overview of energy production

- *Glycolysis.* This first stage occurs in the cell cytoplasm in the absence of oxygen—that is, in an anaerobic environment. Glycolysis converts the 6-carbon molecule glucose into two 3-carbon molecules of pyruvate, with a net gain of two molecules of energy in the form of adenosine triphosphate (ATP). Pyruvate can then proceed to the next stage of the energy pathway if oxygen is present (aerobic environment) or is converted to lactic acid in an anaerobic environment. Although almost all cells in the body gain most of their energy from aerobic pathways, red blood cells gain all their energy from glycolysis because they do not have mitochondria and some skeletal muscles have few mitochondria and also depend largely on glycolysis. During intense muscle activity, large amounts of lactic acid accumulate in these muscles, causing fatigue and pain.
- *Citric acid (Krebs) cycle.* In this second stage, pyruvate enters the mitochondria and is converted to acetyl coenzyme A (acetyl-CoA), which then enters the citric acid cycle. The acetyl group from acetyl-CoA is transferred to oxaloacetate to form citrate and, through a complex series of biological oxidations, hydrogen atoms are transferred to two coenzymes and carbon dioxide (CO_2) and a small amount of energy (ATP) is produced.
- *Oxidative phosphorylation.* This last stage is the most important energy-producing pathway in most cells, and occurs in the mitochondrial membranes. The hydrogen-containing coenzymes transfer electrons to cytochromes in the inner mitochondrial membranes, generating hydrogen ions (protons). Protons are moved across to the outer side of the mitochondrial membranes, creating a gradient, and the electrons are further transferred along the inner membrane, a process called the electron transport chain. Finally, the electrons are transferred to molecular oxygen, which combines with hydrogen ions to form water; the protons then flow back across the membrane through protein channels, generating ATP.

Cell replication

Cells contain 23 pairs of chromosomes and replicate by dividing into two identical daughter cells, each with 23 pairs of chromosomes, in a series of phases called mitosis. During mitosis, DNA is copied and the cell divides to form two new identical cells.

Body tissues and organs

A tissue is a group of similar cells that work together to perform specialised functions.

- *Epithelial tissue* forms the skin, glands and lining of hollow organs, such as the respiratory, digestive, urinary and reproductive tracts. The blood and lymph vessel linings are similar tissues but are called endothelium. Epithelial cells can be in a single layer or stacked on top of each other in several layers. Their functions include protection against invading micro-organisms, absorption of dietary nutrients, and secretion of substances such as sweat, oil or hormones.

  Exocrine glands make secretions that are sent through ducts to a tissue surface and include the sweat and sebaceous glands in the skin, the mammary glands and the glands that secrete digestive enzymes. Endocrine glands are ductless glands that secrete hormones directly into the blood. Hormones travel to specific target cells and affect the way they function.
- *Muscle tissue* is made up of proteins that are able to contract and relax, which enables body parts to move. Muscles attached to bones are under the control of the conscious mind and other internal muscles work subconsciously. *Smooth muscle* functions involuntarily and is found in internal body structures such as the blood vessels and digestive system. *Skeletal muscle* has a striped appearance and enables voluntary body movements. *Cardiac muscle* is in the heart, and is made

of interconnected muscle cells that contract in a coordinated way to keep the heart beating in rhythm.
- *Connective tissue* is made of cells that produce a matrix of water-holding glycoproteins and fibrous proteins such as collagen. It provides support and strength, and connects different types of tissues and systems together. It includes fat tissue, cartilage, tendons and ligaments, and forms a layer beneath the skin that attaches it to the rest of the body. Connective tissue makes up the framework to which minerals attach in bone. Blood is a specialised type of connective tissue, consisting of liquid plasma in which blood cells and other substances travel through the body.
- *Nervous tissue* is made of nerve cells (neurons) that generate electrical impulses and transmit them around the body, and neuroglia that are supporting cells for neurons. Neuroglia provide nutrients, protect nerves against damage and produce the myelin sheath that insulates nerve fibres to help nerve transmission.

Organs, such as the liver, pancreas and spleen, are made up of combinations of tissues arranged together to perform a specialised function. Body systems are made up of a number of different types of organs arranged together so that they can carry out complex and specific functions. For example, the digestive system is a specialised tube that runs from the mouth to the anus. It has associated organs, and is designed to break down and absorb dietary nutrients and eliminate wastes.

DIGESTION

The digestive tract, also called the gastrointestinal tract (GIT), is responsible for the mechanical and physical breakdown of food and for getting rid of some bodily and dietary substances that are not needed. In order to absorb nutrients from the diet, the large molecules present in food need to be broken down into smaller ones that can be absorbed across the gut wall and into the blood for use by body cells (see Table 1.2).

Saliva functions

In the mouth, food is chewed to mechanically break it down into smaller portions that are more accessible to the digestive enzymes produced further down the GIT. Saliva secreted by salivary glands moistens the food for easier chewing. Amylase, a digestive enzyme in saliva, begins the breakdown of starch. Swallowed food then passes through the throat (oesophagus) to the stomach. Lingual lipase, which is secreted by serous glands in the tongue, travels to the stomach in saliva, where it begins the breakdown of medium- and long-chain fats.

Stomach functions

The stomach acts as a blender to thoroughly combine and liquefy food in preparation for digestion by intestinal enzymes. Gastric glands in the stomach wall secrete gastric juice, containing hydrochloric acid and pepsinogen, the precursor to the protein-digesting enzyme pepsin. Gastric juice has a high concentration of hydrogen ions and a very acid pH of about 1. Hydrochloric acid helps to break down proteins, and also acts as a protective barrier by destroying potentially harmful micro-organisms. Pepsinogen is converted to pepsin by hydrochloric acid, and digests protein by splitting long protein chains into shorter lengths (peptides). The stomach also produces renin, which breaks down milk proteins to peptides; gelatinase, which breaks down connective tissue in meat; gastric amylase, which acts on starch; and intrinsic factor, a glycoprotein that is required for absorption of vitamin B12 in the small intestine. A healthily functioning stomach is vital for initiating the digestive 'cascade', and for absorption of many vitamins and minerals.

Digestive functions of the pancreas

Digestive secretions from both the liver and the pancreas enter the duodenum from the common bile duct. The acidic liquefied food in the stomach is ejected into the duodenum and the pancreas secretes sodium bicarbonate to neutralise the acid and raise the pH to about 8. This provides an alkaline environment that allows pancreatic digestive enzymes to break down carbohydrates, proteins and fats. Pancreatic amylase splits starch into smaller units of glucose. Pancreatic lipase and colipase split dietary fats into fatty acids and into single fatty acids attached to a glycerol molecule (monoacylglycerols, or monoglycerides). Phospholipases break down phospholipids (fatty acid, phosphate and glycerol-containing fats) to fatty acids and monoglycerides. The protein-splitting enzymes trypsin, carboxypeptidase and chymotrypsin break down protein into peptides and amino acids. Trypsin is produced from its precursor trypsinogen and chymotrypsin is produced from its precursor chymotrypsinogen by the enzyme enterokinase, which is present in intestinal juice.

Other functions of the pancreas

Islets of Langerhans in the pancreas consist of four cell types that produce hormones. Alpha cells produce glucagon and beta cells produce insulin, both of which help to regulate blood glucose levels. Delta cells produce somatostatin, which is an inhibitor of hormone activity, and gamma cells produce pancreatic polypeptide, a regulator of somatostatin.

Digestive functions of the liver and gall bladder

The liver produces bile that is stored and concentrated in the gall bladder and secreted in response to fatty food. Bile contains bile acids that emulsify dietary fat into small droplets that are easier for lipase to break down. Bile also contains brown pigments derived from broken-down haemoglobin removed by the liver from old red blood cells.

Other functions of the liver

Dietary nutrients are delivered to the liver after meals, and these are stored, metabolised or transferred into the bloodstream for delivery to other body tissues. The liver stores some of the glucose from carbohydrate foods as glycogen and releases glucose into the bloodstream when blood levels drop. It stores fats and converts some fats to cholesterol; both are then packaged into lipoproteins for transport in the blood. The liver's other functions are to detoxify potentially harmful or unwanted substances,

Table 1.2 Actions of digestive enzymes

Digestive enzyme	Acts on	End-products
Saliva		
Salivary amylase	Starch	Maltose, oligosaccharides
Lingual lipase	Fat (in the stomach)	Fatty acids, monoglycerides
Gastric juice		
Pepsin	Protein	Peptides
Gastric lipase	Fat	Fatty acids, monoglycerides
Renin	Milk protein	Peptides
Gelatinase	Connective tissue protein	Peptides
Pancreatic juice		
Pancreatic amylase	Starch	Maltose, oligosaccharides
Trypsin	Protein	Peptides
Chymotrypsin	Protein	Peptides
Carboxypeptidase	Protein	Peptides, amino acids
Pancreatic lipase, colipase	Fat	Fatty acids, monoglycerides
Phospholipase	Phospholipids	Fatty acids, monoglycerides
Small intestine		
Dextrinase	Oligosaccharides	Glucose
Maltase	Maltose	Glucose
Sucrase	Sucrose	Glucose, fructose
Lactase	Lactose	Glucose, galactose
Peptidases	Peptides	Peptides, amino acids

store fat-soluble vitamins, break down old red blood cells and make plasma proteins for maintaining fluid balance, nutrient transport and blood clotting.

Small intestine functions

Food is passed through the intestines by muscle movements called peristalsis. The walls of the small intestine produce a variety of digestive enzymes that continue the breakdown of carbohydrates, fats and protein. Carbohydrates are broken down to small sugar molecules such as glucose, fructose and galactose. Fats and oils are broken down to fatty acids or monoglycerides. Proteins are broken down to peptides, and finally to amino acids, the smallest units of proteins. The end-products of digestion are simple food units that are absorbed into the villi cells lining the intestine and transported to the liver, from which they are sent to body cells via the bloodstream.

Large intestine (colon) functions

Some mineral salts and water from digestive enzyme secretions are absorbed back into the body in the colon. Dietary fibre is passed undigested from the small intestine into the colon. Soluble fibre, found in most whole grains, legumes, fruits and vegetables, is fermented by naturally occurring bacteria in the colon to form fatty acids. These fatty acids provide energy for the cells lining the colon and help regulate their replication. Insoluble fibre, found mainly in wheat bran, is not fermented but helps bulk up the waste material (faeces), allowing for easier excretion. Faeces are made up of residues of digestion, fibre, bile salts and bacteria, and are excreted via the rectum and anus.

Hormone regulators of digestion

Gastrin, gastric inhibitory peptide, secretin and cholecystokinin are hormones produced by the digestive tract that regulate the secretion of digestive enzymes and coordinate digestive functions.

THE BODY'S PROTECTIVE SYSTEMS

The antioxidant system

Oxygen and nitrogen are essential for body function, but they can also cause damage to body tissues by changing to become highly reactive forms, referred to as reactive species. Free radicals are a common type of reactive species generated during normal metabolism, and especially during energy production, inflammation, immune defence, detoxification, tissue injury and ageing. They can also be created by exercise, cigarette smoking, drinking alcohol, taking drugs, exposure to radiation from sunlight, cosmic rays and medical x-rays, and exposure to ozone, high-oxygen environments and environmental pollution.

Generation of free radicals

A stable molecule in the body is one that has atoms with the full complement of electrons. Sometimes an electron is stripped off and the molecule becomes unstable or 'radical', and must take an electron from another molecule to become stable again. This deprives another molecule of an electron and it, in turn, becomes a radical until it can gain another electron; thus a rapid chain reaction occurs that generates many more radicals. The term 'free radicals' refers to these highly reactive molecules that are trying to replace a missing electron.

Types of reactive species in the body

These include reactive oxygen species (ROS) and reactive nitrogen species (RNS).

ROS

ROS include hydroxyl, peroxyl, hydroperoxyl and superoxide radicals, and their by-products: hydrogen peroxide, singlet oxygen and hypochlorous acid. ROS can cause oxidative damage to DNA, proteins and lipids, especially cell membrane lipids.

- *Hydroxyl radicals* are produced from hydrogen peroxide and also from water during exposure to radiation. They are among the most reactive and destructive species in the body, and can attack all types of molecules and are a major cause of damage to lipids.
- *Peroxyl and hydroperoxyl radicals* are highly reactive and damage polyunsaturated fatty acids (PUFAs) in cell membranes, forming lipid peroxides.
- *Superoxide radicals* are formed in the electron transport pathway during energy production in mitochondria, and during detoxification, immune defence and the metabolism of adrenaline, dopamine and folic acid. They can also react with nitric oxide to generate RNS.

- *Hydrogen peroxide* is not a radical, but is a damaging by-product of free radical activity that is generated during oxidation of compounds and also when oxygen supply to tissue is impaired (ischaemia), which occurs in atherosclerosis. When oxygen flow is restored in ischaemia, the extra oxygen generates more hydrogen peroxide and has damaging effects (reperfusion injury). Hydrogen peroxide can react with the superoxide radical to generate highly reactive hydroxyl radicals and hypochlorous acid.
- *Singlet oxygen* is oxygen in which the electrons spin in opposite directions, creating an 'excited' state. It is generated during lipid peroxidation of cell membranes, immune defence and photochemical reactions.
- *Hypochlorous acid* is produced by phagocytes, and plays a vital role in the killing of a wide range of pathogens (disease-causing microbes), but also contributes to the tissue injury associated with inflammation.

RNS

RNS include nitric oxide and its by-products, nitrate, nitrite, peroxynitrite and 3-nitrotyrosine.

- *Nitric oxide* is important for healthy blood flow and blood pressure by preventing platelet stickiness and relaxing blood vessels. It is relatively unreactive, but its by-products can cause nitrosative damage to proteins and enzymes, and impair the body's regulatory functions.

Effects of ROS and RNS

Reactive species attack lipids, proteins, lipoproteins, DNA, RNA and PUFAs in cell membranes. They can stop the cell functioning properly, cause the cell to become abnormal or even kill the cell. If a cell is badly damaged or develops abnormally, it may destroy itself, a process called apoptosis.

Mitochondria, the energy-producing units in cells, are exposed to higher levels of ROS because they are generated from the oxygen used during energy production. Mitochondrial DNA (mDNA) is simpler than the DNA in the cell nucleus and is more easily damaged because it does not have the same level of protective and repair mechanisms. ROS damage mitochondrial proteins, lipids and mDNA and this can cause disruption to the energy supply, permanent age-related mitochondrial dysfunction and accelerated ageing. Damage accumulation can trigger release of cytochrome c, a protein that transfers electrons in the energy pathway in mitochondria that is also a key trigger of apoptosis. The damaging effects of ROS and RNS are referred to as oxidative stress.

Health disorders that may be related to oxidative stress include:

- inflammatory diseases, such as cardiovascular disease and osteoarthritis
- autoimmune diseases, such as rheumatoid arthritis
- diseases of ageing, such as impaired immunity, stroke, Parkinson's disease, Alzheimer's disease, and the vision disorders cataracts and macular degeneration
- chronic degenerative disease, such as Friedreich's ataxia and amyotrophic lateral sclerosis (ALS, or motor neurone disease)
- fatigue syndromes
- liver damage and alcohol-induced diseases
- lung damage
- male infertility
- cancer.

The protective role of antioxidants

An antioxidant is any substance that has a role in delaying, preventing or removing oxidative damage to a target molecule. Antioxidants can be food components or substances made in the body that protect tissues from free radicals and reactive species. They sacrifice themselves by donating an electron to a free radical in order to save body components from damage, a process referred to as free radical scavenging. The antioxidant then becomes a radical, but not a destructive one, because it can gain an electron from another antioxidant. Many different types of antioxidants are needed for this protective cycle to continue normally, and damage accumulates when there is an imbalance between ROS, RNS and antioxidants.

Types of antioxidants

Antioxidants can be made in the body (endogenous) and obtained from the diet (exogenous). Many of the essential nutrients in food and the colouring pigments in plants, such as fruit, vegetables and many herbs used in cooking and as medicines, have antioxidant activity.

Endogenous antioxidants include:

- *albumin*, which is a plasma protein that binds copper and iron to prevent them catalysing oxidation reactions and contains sulfhydryl groups that trap multiple ROS and RNS, such as hydrogen peroxide, peroxynitrite, superoxide and hypochlorous acid.

- *glutathione*, which is a sulfur-containing protein composed of glycine, cysteine and glutamic acid that is part of the body's primary water-soluble antioxidant system. The glutathione system consists of glutathione and the enzymes glutathione reductase and glutathione peroxidase (GPx), which contains the trace element selenium. This system scavenges ROS and removes hydrogen peroxide, other peroxides and hydroxyl radicals by converting them to water. GPx catalyses the reaction of glutathione with ROS, during which glutathione is oxidised. Glutathione can be regenerated from its oxidised state by glutathione reductase, niacin (vitamin B3) and dihydrolipoic acid (DHLA), formed from alpha-LA. Glutathione can also conjugate (join with) toxic compounds, and is then excreted, requiring additional glutathione to be synthesised.
- *superoxide dismutases* (SODs), which are important antioxidant enzymes that require copper, zinc or manganese for their activity. Copper and zinc are part of SOD in the cytoplasm of body cells (Cu/Zn-SOD, SOD1) and Cu/Zn-SOD (SOD3) is found in the extracellular compartment. SOD in mitochondria contains manganese (Mn-SOD, SOD2). SOD removes superoxide radicals by converting them to hydrogen peroxide.
- *catalases*, which are iron-containing enzymes that remove hydrogen peroxide by converting it to water. They are less active than the glutathione system.
- *the thioredoxin system*, which includes the protein thioredoxin, reduced nicotinamide adenine dinucleotide phosphate (NADPH), and thioredoxin reductase, a selenium-containing antioxidant enzyme. This system provides electrons to thiol-dependent peroxidases in order to remove ROS and RNS.
- *peroxiredoxins*, which act like other antioxidant enzymes such as catalase and GPx, but have lower activity.
- *alpha-LA* and its reduced form, DHLA, which is regarded as a 'super' or universal antioxidant because it has potent water-soluble and fat-soluble activity. DHLA scavenges ROS and RNS, removes hydroxyl radicals and enhances repair of oxidatively damaged proteins.
- *CoQ10* (ubiquinone-10), which can be converted to ubiquinol-10, a fat-soluble antioxidant that scavenges peroxyl radicals that damage mitochondrial membranes and lipoproteins in the bloodstream. It is a superior antioxidant because it protects lipids by preventing initiation of free radicals, as well as preventing their propagation, unlike vitamin E which can only inhibit propagation. It also helps protect proteins and DNA from free radical damage and regenerates vitamin E from its radical form. Ubiquinol-10 is regenerated by DHLA, the thioredoxin system and enzymes in the mitochondrial electron transport chain.

Exogenous antioxidants include:

- *fat-soluble antioxidants*, such as vitamin E, coenzyme Q10 (CoQ10), alpha-lipoic acid (alpha-LA), and carotenoids; they protect PUFAs in cell membranes, fat-soluble vitamins, and steroid hormones, such as the sex and anti-stress hormones
- *water-soluble antioxidants*, such as vitamin C, alpha-LA and many fruit, vegetable and herbal antioxidants; they protect substances in the watery parts of the body, such as the circulation and the fluid inside and outside cells.

Some important dietary antioxidants are:

- *vitamin C*, which is a key water-soluble antioxidant that removes superoxide radicals by converting them to hydrogen peroxide and then to water. It also eliminates hydroxyl radicals and aqueous peroxyl radicals by converting them to water, and converts peroxyl radicals to lipid peroxides, which are then removed by the glutathione system. Vitamin C is regenerated by the glutathione system, DHLA, thioredoxin and the interaction of radical forms of vitamin C.
- *vitamin E*, which is a key fat-soluble antioxidant located in cell membranes. It is a chain-breaking antioxidant that neutralises singlet oxygen and scavenges peroxyl radicals formed from PUFAs to terminate lipid peroxidation in cell membranes. It can be regenerated by vitamin C, ubiquinol-10 and glutathione.
- *zinc, copper, manganese, and selenium*, which are trace elements that are part of the body's antioxidant enzyme systems. Manganese is also able to directly scavenge peroxyl radicals.
- *carotenoids*, which are fat-soluble orange, yellow and red plant pigments that include beta-carotene, lycopene, lutein, beta-cryptoxanthin, zeaxanthin, astaxanthin and others. They work like vitamin E to remove peroxyl radicals and protect PUFAs, and may be more active in the cell interior than in the cell membrane. Carotenoids inactivate singlet oxygen by

absorbing its energy and returning it to its natural state without being chemically changed themselves.

- *resveratrol*, found in grapes, red wine, peanuts, berries and the herb giant knotweed, which is a particularly powerful antioxidant that has direct and indirect antioxidant activity and can scavenge ROS and RNS. It has been shown to extend lifespan in animals, and has anti-ageing, anticancer, anti-inflammatory, anti-diabetic and anti-atherogenic activity.
- *proanthocyanidins*, purple plant pigments found in purple fruits and vegetables, grape skins and grape seed, which are powerful antioxidants that have anti-inflammatory, anticancer and neuroprotective activity. They protect against peroxynitrite species.
- *catechins*, found in green tea, red wine, grape skins and grape seeds, which scavenge ROS and peroxyl radicals and support normal cell replication, liver detoxification and the circulatory system.
- *curcumin*, found in the spice turmeric used in curry powder, which can scavenge superoxide and hydroxyl radicals and hydrogen peroxide. It has anti-inflammatory, antiviral, antibacterial, antifungal and anticancer activity.

The detoxification system

Detoxification is the chemical modification of potential toxins to assist their removal from the body, and is also called biotransformation. Potential toxins can include anything foreign to the body (xenobiotics), as well as naturally occurring metabolites that could cause harm if they accumulate. They include prescription and non-prescription drugs; pollutants, such as air and water pollutants, industrial chemicals, pesticides, herbicides and the toxic metals mercury, lead and cadmium; alcohol; microbial toxins; phytochemicals (bioactive plant compounds); fat-soluble vitamins; steroid hormones; and inflammatory compounds produced by immune activity. Water-soluble toxins can be excreted in urine or perspiration, or breathed out by the lungs. However, fat-soluble toxins need to be chemically changed into more water-soluble forms before they can be excreted. Some fat-soluble toxins can be stored relatively harmlessly in fat tissue, and may be mobilised during weight loss, putting an extra load on detoxification systems.

Detoxification pathways

The iron-containing cytochrome P450 enzymes catalyse several types of oxidation reactions and are the most important of the detoxification enzymes. The liver is the key site for detoxification and acts by converting fat-soluble substances into water-soluble substances for excretion by the kidneys in urine or excretion in faeces via bile secretions into the gut. In the intestine, the antiporter system pumps toxins out of the intestinal lining cells and back into the gut and cytochrome P450 enzymes in the intestinal epithelium help to detoxify substances before they reach the bloodstream. Detoxifying enzymes are also present in the skin, lungs, nasal mucosa, eyes, kidneys, adrenal glands, pancreas, spleen, heart, brain, testes, ovaries, placenta, plasma, blood cells and aorta. Detoxification occurs in two phases (see Figure 1.4):

- *Phase I detoxification (oxidative phase).* Phase I reactions involve hydrolysis, reduction and oxidation. Fat-soluble compounds are oxidised by cytochrome P450 enzymes to form an activated oxygen-toxin-cytochrome complex. This complex is then broken down to generate an oxidised toxin plus oxidised cytochrome P450 and water. A by-product of phase I detoxification is the generation of free radicals that are highly reactive, with the potential to damage liver cells; a range of antioxidants are needed to convert them to stable compounds.
- *Phase II detoxification (conjugative phase).* Phase II reactions use enzymes such as glutathione S-transferases and UDP-glucuronosyltransferase, and involve glucuronidation (adding glucuronic acid), sulfation (adding sulfate), acetylation (adding an acetyl group), methylation (adding a methyl group), conjugation (combining) with glutathione and conjugation with amino acids such as glycine, taurine and glutamic acid. In this pathway, the oxidised toxin arising from the phase I pathway is combined with a water-soluble compound such as an amino acid to form an excretable water-soluble compound. Some toxins bypass phase I and are directly detoxified by the phase II pathway.

Removal of toxin end-products

Small water-soluble compounds are transported to the kidneys and then excreted in urine. Large water-soluble compounds are excreted from the liver in bile, which is secreted into the digestive tract and removed in faeces. However, some bacteria in the colon can have an adverse effect by producing toxins themselves or reconverting conjugated toxins to their original forms, which can then be reabsorbed.

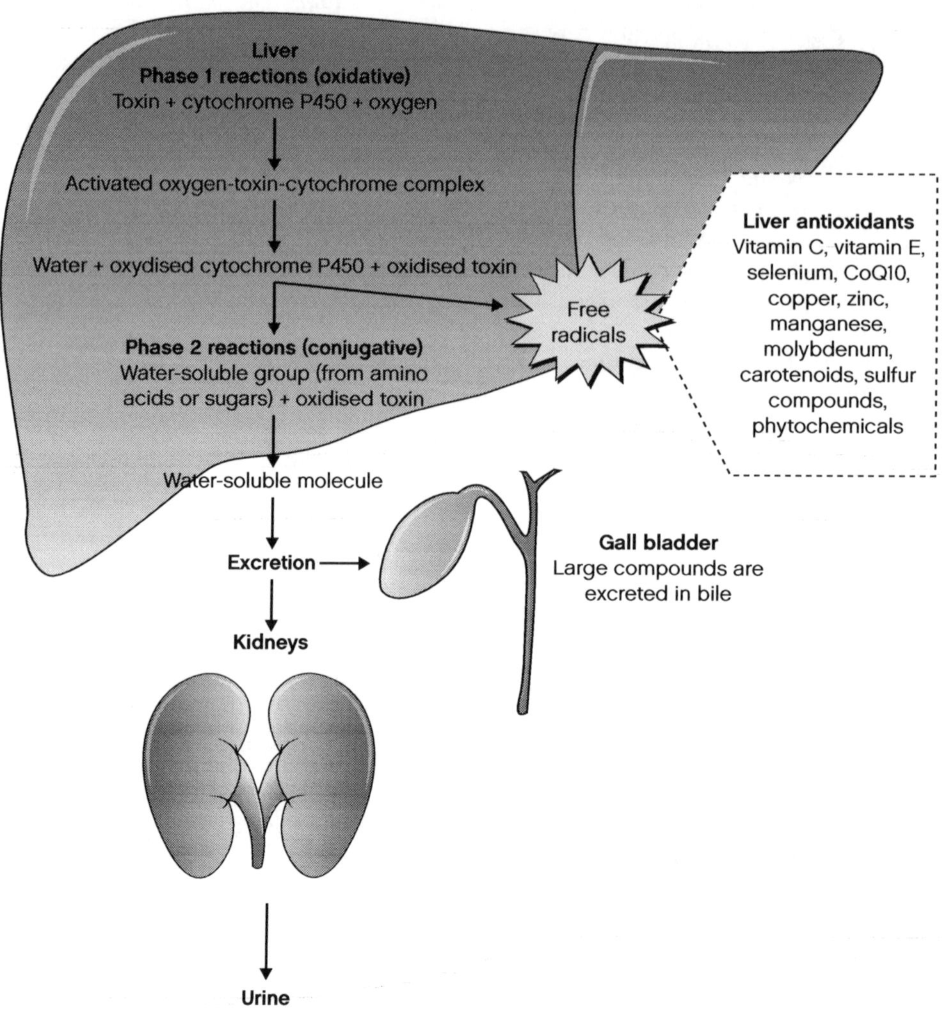

Figure 1.4 Liver detoxification

Induction of detoxifying enzymes

Detoxification requires healthy activity of the phase I and phase II pathways. When the body is exposed to a substance that is potentially toxic, phase I enzymes are induced (activated). Induction of phase I enzymes can occur without phase II induction, leading to a build-up of partially detoxified compounds and damaging free radicals that are generated by phase I reactions. Substances in cigarette smoke and char-grilled meat have been found to induce phase I only. Adverse drug reactions may occur because of reduced phase I detoxification activity. Induction of phase I with a lower phase II activity is a feature of cancer, systemic lupus erythematosus and Parkinson's disease.

Phase II inducers that allow detoxification to be completed include many phytochemicals in fruit, vegetables and herbs. Enhancing phase II activity is believed to protect against many cancers.

Antioxidants are vital to protect body tissues, cell membranes and DNA in liver and intestinal cells from free radical damage due to phase I induction. Important antioxidants include the body's antioxidant enzyme systems and dietary antioxidants, such as vitamin C, vitamin E, selenium, CoQ10, copper, zinc, manganese, molybdenum and a variety of phytochemicals, including carotenoids and flavonoids. The activity of many detoxification enzymes requires nutritional co-factors, including B vitamins, magnesium and iron.

Inhibitors of detoxification

Fasting, some phytochemicals and a number of prescription drugs, such as the contraceptive pill, benzodiazepines (tranquillisers), selective serotonin reuptake inhibitors (SSRIs, or antidepressants), antihistamines, cimetidine and other drugs that block production of stomach acid, ketoconazole (antifungal) and sulfaphenazole (antibacterial) can impair detoxification. Fasting, together with the drug acetaminophen (paracetamol) found in many cold, flu and pain-relief medications, has been shown to decrease blood levels of the sulfate needed for phase II detoxification. The drug cimetidine, used for stomach ulcers and gastro-oesophageal reflux disease, blocks all phase I activity by binding to the active site on cytochrome P450. Intestinal detoxification of many drugs is inhibited by naringenin, formed in the gut from the flavonoid naringin in grapefruit juice. A larger amount of the drug then reaches the bloodstream, elevating body levels.

The immune system

The immune system includes the physical barriers of the skin, mucous membranes and lining tissues that resist entry by invading micro-organisms, as well as the internal immune defence of white blood cells, antibodies (immunoglobulins) and other immune proteins, such as complement, interferons and cytokines (cell-signalling proteins), that defend against them. Innate immunity involves non-specific immune responses that are the first line of defence, and adaptive immunity involves humoral immunity, mediated by antibodies produced by B lymphocytes, and cell-mediated immunity, mediated by T lymphocytes.

The immune system displays a coordinated response to any threat to tissues by producing, marshalling and directing immune cells to destroy any invading micro-organisms and any infected cells. This internal defence system is able to distinguish between body cells and foreign cells, and can remember previous exposures to micro-organisms and react accordingly when the next exposure occurs. When triggered, the immune response causes local or systemic inflammation, according to the severity of the attack. Symptoms may include pain, fever, chills, muscle aches, headaches and fatigue.

Immune cells include the following:

- *Granulocytes*, which include monocytes, dendritic cells, neutrophils, eosinophils, basophils and mast cells. Monocytes are white blood cells that move into tissues at the site of injury and become macrophages. They engulf pathogens, digest them and display bits of their distinctive proteins (antigens) on the outside of their cell membranes, triggering immune activity. Dendritic cells are found in the bloodstream, thymus, lymph nodes and spleen, and help transport antigens to immune organs. Neutrophils, eosinophils and basophils are white blood cells that contain granules of digestive enzymes. They engulf pathogens and release their enzymes to destroy them. Mast cells stay in connective tissue and become active in inflammatory and allergic responses.
- *Lymphocytes*, which include thymus-derived cells (T cells), B cells, memory cells and natural killer (NK) cells. T cells are white blood cells that develop in the thymus gland. Helper T cells activate other immune cells and cytotoxic T cells directly destroy body cells infected with a pathogen by a free radical burst. B cells are white blood cells that, when activated, form plasma cells that produce specific antibodies to antigens displayed by other immune cells. These antibodies lock on to the pathogen and to infected body cells, and trigger an immune attack. Memory cells develop after recovery from a disease and quickly generate an attack on the pathogen if it invades again, providing future immunity. NK cells are lymphocytes that can bind to target cells and release a lethal burst of chemicals that damage the cell's membrane and destroy the cell. They are particularly effective against tumour cells and pathogens.

Immune organs include the following:

- *Bone marrow*, which produces all the immune cells from stem cells, which differentiate into specialised cells with specific functions as they develop.
- *The thymus gland*, which produces mature T cells from immature cells made in bone marrow and releases them into the bloodstream.
- *The spleen*, which receives antigen-carrying macrophages and dendritic cells from the bloodstream. Antigens are presented to T cells and B cells, which triggers an immune response. The spleen also acts as a filter to remove antigens.

- *The lymph system*, which drains fluid from the tissues and the lymph nodes (glands), which in turn filter out antigens. As in the spleen, antigen-carrying macrophages and dendritic cells in the lymph nodes present their antigens to T and B cells, triggering an immune response. Tonsils at the back of the throat and adenoids at the back of the nose are part of the lymph system. Peyer's patches are clumps of lymphoid tissue on the walls of the small intestine.

Infections

Pathogens are present in the environment and, in most cases, have little impact on health because the immune system keeps them under control. They include viruses, bacteria, fungi, parasites and prions.

- *Viral infections.* Viruses are molecules of genetic material (DNA or RNA) that cannot replicate independently. They invade cells and use the cell's machinery to produce copies of themselves, forming multiple duplicates that invade and take over other cells. Some viruses can incorporate their DNA into the host cell's DNA and change the cell, possibly causing cancer to develop. Viruses can change their form (mutate) and sometimes jump from one species to another, such as the bird and swine flu viruses. Viruses are responsible for influenza, colds, warts, cold sores, genital herpes, polio, hepatitis, chicken pox, shingles and AIDS.
- *Bacterial infections.* Bacteria are single-celled microbes that can be useful or pathogenic. They can enter the body through air, water or food, or via contact with an infected person. Poor toilet hygiene can contaminate hands and spread bacteria to food. Most bacteria require water to stay alive and breed, and many common food-preserving methods tie up or remove water by adding salt or sugar, or drying the food. In general, cold conditions, such as refrigeration, slow bacterial growth; however, some bacteria—such as *Listeria monocytogenes* and *Yersinia enterocolitica*, common bacteria that cause food poisoning—like cold conditions. Many bacteria like to live in the conditions present in the human body. Some of these are helpful, such as the lactobacilli and bifido species that live in the bowel. Others can cause disease if their numbers increase too much, such as *Escherichia coli* (*E. coli*), a common bowel bacteria that can cause food poisoning symptoms if it is present in large numbers. Pathogenic bacteria cause illness by directly attacking a specific part of the body or by producing toxins.
- *Fungal infections.* Fungal diseases are called mycoses, and often affect the skin. Fungi are micro-organisms that exist in one of two forms: as unicellular yeasts or as branching moulds. Fungi can grow on the surface of the skin, and particularly in areas kept warm and moist by clothing and shoes. Fungal infections are usually mild, but will trigger immune responses and sometimes cause hypersensitivity reactions. People with lowered immunity are more likely to get chronic fungal infections that can be fatal. Some mould forms of fungi can form highly potent toxins (mycotoxins), such as aflatoxin and ochratoxin, which are the most significant natural food contaminants in the world. Exposure to mycotoxins can cause kidney, nerve and circulatory damage, as well as cancer.
- *Parasitic infections.* Parasites more commonly affect people in contact with animals or travellers to areas where parasites are prevalent. They include single-celled protozoa, flukes and worms.
- *Prion infections.* Prions are newly discovered infectious proteins that contain no genetic material. The gene for making prion protein is in all mammals, and is mainly active in nerve cells. This gene normally produces a harmless protein but, very rarely, a genetic or environmental factor causes the protein to flip into a different shape, converting it to a prion. A prion is infectious in a way that is not well understood, but it seems to be able to cause a normal protein to convert to the abnormal shape and become another prion in a chain-reaction effect. Prions are extraordinarily resistant to all forms of sterilisation, including radiation.

  Prion diseases are called transmissable spongiform encephalopathies (TSEs) and, although very rare, cause a fatal, progressive degeneration of the central nervous system (CNS) in which clumps of prion protein accumulate in the brain and kill off brain cells, leaving 'holes' in the brain. TSEs include kuru, a disease affecting natives of New Guinea that is related to cannibalism; Creutzfeldt-Jakob disease (CJD), a human fatal degenerative disease affecting the CNS; bovine spongiform encephalopathy (BSE, or mad cow disease) in cattle; and scrapie, a similar disease to BSE that affects sheep. Prion diseases in animals have not been detected in Australia and New Zealand.

Inflammation

Inflammation is a local response to tissue damage, characterised by swelling, heat, redness and pain, which is caused by the release of inflammatory chemicals. Inflammatory chemicals are molecules that act at the damage site and coordinate the inflammatory response. They stimulate immune activity and increase blood flow, which facilitates delivery of immune cells and nutrients to the affected area to protect against infection and heal damaged tissue.

Cytokines are inflammatory chemicals, and include lymphokines (made by lymphocytes), monokines (made by monocytes), chemokines (chemoattractants made by various immune cells) and interleukins (ILs, made by leukocytes). Important inflammatory proteins include complement, a system of plasma proteins that form the membrane-attack complex when activated, interferon-gamma (INF-gamma), produced by T cells and NK cells, and acute-phase blood proteins, such as C-reactive protein and acute-phase serum amyloid A proteins (A-SAAs), which are produced by the liver. The release of inflammatory chemicals is a sequential, ordered process that involves multiple pathways, which act like cascades, with the activation of one part triggering the activation of the next.

Nuclear factor-kappaB (NF-kappaB) is a protein in cellular cytoplasm that translocates to the nucleus upon activation, where it induces transcription of multiple genes for inflammatory substances. It acts like an early warning damage detector, and can turn inflammation on and off in the body. Among the first genes switched on are those for IL-1, IL-6 and tumour necrosis factor-alpha (TNF-alpha). These chemicals then activate multiple biochemical pathways that promote inflammation.

Acute inflammation

There are three stages of acute inflammation:

- *Stage 1.* When injury occurs, the complement system is activated and triggers mast cells and basophils to release histamine. This attracts immune cells (chemotaxis), dilates blood vessels and increases their permeability. Bradykinin is formed to enhance dilation and permeability of blood vessels, and is a major cause of the pain of inflammation. Dilated and leaky blood vessels increase blood flow and delivery of immune cells and chemicals to the damaged area. Water, salts and small proteins, such as fibrinogen, migrate into injured tissue. Fibrinogen forms fibrin networks to trap micro-organisms and form a clot, which seals the wound and prevents blood loss. All this activity results in pain, heat, redness and swelling.
- *Stage 2.* This stage involves white blood cells moving into damaged tissue and engulfing or destroying microbes. Cellular adhesion molecules (CAMs), including vascular cellular adhesion molecule 1 (VCAM1) and intercellular adhesion molecule 1 (ICAM1), are expressed to assist immune cells to stick to the blood vessel wall and move through it to enter tissue. Complement activation attracts neutrophils that accumulate and squeeze through blood vessel walls. Neutrophil activation has three phases: phase 1 (margination), in which neutrophils are recruited and form bridges made of selectins with endothelial cells; phase 2 (rolling), in which neutrophils roll along the endothelium because the bridges are initially loose; and phase 3 (diapedesis), in which the bridges become firm and allow neutrophils to migrate into tissue. Neutrophils release TNF-alpha, INF-gamma and IL-1 and IL-6, and also engulf invading microbes before dying off. Monocytes follow neutrophils and transform into macrophages that engulf microbes, dead neutrophils and damaged tissue. Pus may accumulate, and is largely made up of white blood cells that have died while fighting infection.

  Cytotoxic immune cells release an 'oxidative burst' of ROS, such as superoxide radicals, hypochlorite and hydroxyl radicals, to destroy microbes. The complement-derived membrane-attack complex attaches to a microbial membrane and creates holes that allow water and salts to enter and kill the microbe. If a cell is infected by a virus, it releases interferon into the surrounding ECF, which binds to receptors on nearby cell membranes and stimulates production of antiviral enzymes.
- *Stage 3.* This is the healing stage, during which the capillary network is restored, new tissue forms and growth factors stimulate fibroblasts to produce large amounts of collagen to strengthen the damaged area. If the damage is severe, a scar may form.

Chronic inflammation

In the process of defending the body, the immune attack creates an inflammatory 'firestorm', which destroys infected cells but also damages surrounding tissues. Usually, this is short lived and tissues are rapidly repaired. In some circumstances, inflammation does not switch off and becomes persistent, which damages tissue in the affected area and may cause chronic pain, swelling and loss of function. The cause is not clear, but it may be triggered or enhanced by the presence of microbes, ROS, RNS, toxins or allergens.

Chronic inflammatory disorders are common in Western countries, and include osteoarthritis, eczema, asthma, cardiovascular disease, Alzheimer's disease, inflammatory bowel diseases such as colitis and Crohn's disease, autoimmune disorders such as multiple sclerosis, systemic lupus erythematosus (SLE) and rheumatoid arthritis, diseases of ageing and obesity, which is now thought to have a chronic inflammatory component. Factors contributing to chronic inflammation include NF-kappaB, TNF-alpha, CAMs, ILs, interferons, nitric oxide (NO), platelet-activating factor (PAF) and eicosanoids. Eicosanoids are produced from the polyunsaturated omega-3 and omega-6 fatty acids in cell membrane phospholipids. They include prostaglandins (PGs), thromboxanes (TXs) and leukotrienes (LTs), some of which promote inflammation and some of which suppress it. Overall, omega-6 fats have inflammatory effects and omega-3 fats have anti-inflammatory effects and the correct balance of omega-3 and omega-6 fats in cell membranes is vital for keeping inflammation under control.

Part 2
Macronutrients

2

Water, energy and protein

WATER

WATER STATUS CHECK

1. Do you drink mainly tea or coffee and don't often drink plain water?
2. Do you fail to increase your water intake in hot weather and when you exercise?
3. Do you usually pass urine only two or three times a day?
4. Is your urine usually dark in colour?

'Yes' answers may indicate inadequate water status. Note that a number of nutritional deficiencies or health disorders can cause similar effects and further investigation is recommended.

FAST FACTS . . . WATER

- Water is found in all liquids and most foods.
- It is needed for metabolic activities, transport, body form and structure, regulation of body temperature, lubrication, elimination and excretion.
- Water losses are increased by activity, warm temperatures, air travel, diuretics, vomiting, diarrhoea, hormone imbalances and diabetes.
- Early signs of dehydration include thirst, headache, sleepiness, fatigue, impaired thinking ability, dizziness, infrequent urination and darker-coloured urine.
- Excessive water intake within a short space of time can lead to water intoxication, which overloads the brain, the heart and circulation.

Oxygen, water, food . . . if the key elements that are essential for life were prioritised, this is the order in which they would be placed. Life stops in a few minutes without oxygen, in a few days without water and in a few weeks without food. Water consists of the elements hydrogen and oxygen (H_2O), and makes up about 55–65 per cent of an adult's body weight. Body cells are bathed in it and body functions rely on it. Most of the body's water is in the blood and lymph vessels, the extracellular fluid (ECF), the intracellular fluid (ICF) and lean tissues. Water makes up about 90 per cent of blood plasma, about 70 per cent of muscle, brain tissue and skin, 20–30 per cent of fat tissue, about 20 per cent of bones and fifteen per cent of teeth. Generally, a man's body has about ten per cent more water than a woman's because of a higher percentage of lean tissue. Body water content declines with age. An infant's body contains about 72 per cent water, and a child's body about 60 per cent, but an elderly person's body may only contain 45–50 per cent.

Regulation of water balance

When water losses are greater than intake, the osmotic pressure of ECF increases. This activates osmoreceptors in the hypothalamus which trigger release of anti-diuretic hormone (ADH). ADH acts on the kidneys to conserve water and urinary frequency decreases. Less water in urine means that it is more concentrated in solutes and the colour intensifies. ADH and increased osmotic pressure of ECF cause the sensation of thirst. By reducing urinary losses and increasing thirst, water balance is re-established.

When water intake is greater than losses, there is a decrease in plasma osmolality (a measure of the moles of solute per kg of solvent) and a suppression of ADH secretion. This causes the kidneys to produce a large volume of dilute urine. Urinary frequency increases and urine colour becomes very pale. Loss of excess water re-establishes water balance.

Functions

The functions of water include:

- *Cell function.* Water is a solvent for water-soluble compounds, and a constant amount of water inside and outside cells is necessary for cell function. Together with minerals, water maintains the osmotic gradient necessary for movement of substances across cell membranes.
- *Hydrolytic (water-splitting) reactions.* Hydrolysis is the process of adding a water molecule to a bond between two molecules to separate them. One hydrogen from water becomes attached to one of the molecules and the hydroxyl (OH) group is attached to the other. Hydrolytic reactions are important for breaking down nucleic acids and for digestion. During digestion, water from the body is passed into the gut along with digestive enzymes, and is used to split food components into smaller absorbable units.
- *Transport.* In the bloodstream, water is the transporter that carries blood cells, oxygen, hormones, immune chemicals, waste products, secretions and nutrients to and from body tissues. Water is also part of lymph, which transports dietary fats and fat-soluble nutrients from the digestive tract to the bloodstream, drains ECF and transports immune cells.
- *Regulation of body temperature.* Water has a large capacity for absorbing heat, which helps limit changes in body temperature in a warm environment. Water evaporates out of the skin as sweat in hot conditions, providing a cooling effect.
- *Lubrication and shock absorption.* Water in saliva helps chewing, the process of physically breaking down food to prepare it for digestion. Water is an important component of joint cartilage that provides a smooth surface over the ends of bones to stop them rubbing together during movement. Water is part of the mucus that protects the epithelial linings of the respiratory passages and digestive, urinary and reproductive tracts, and water in tears helps lubricate the eyeballs and protect them from damage. Water fills up body spaces, plumps up the skin, maintains cellular shape and acts as a shock absorber during movement. It protects the joints, brain and spinal cord, and is particularly important for protection of the foetus.
- *Elimination of wastes.* Water is important for the proper consistency of faeces, which enables normal movement and expulsion of waste material from the bowel. Water helps flush water-soluble waste materials out of the body in urine.

Dietary sources

Water is found in all liquids and most foods. Fruit and vegetables are about 80–95 per cent water, cooked rice about 70 per cent, cooked meat about 60 per cent, bread about 40 per cent, butter about 16 per cent, dry cereals less than 5 per cent and vegetable oils have no water content.

Factors influencing body status

These factors include:

- *Skin loss.* More water is lost through increased sweating in hot weather and during a fever or physical activity. Daily sweat loss increases by about 500 mL per 1°C rise in environmental temperature, and sweat loss during moderate exercise can range from 1000 to 3000 mL per hour. Electric blankets, central heating and excessive bed coverings can cause over-heating during sleep, increasing sweating and leading to disturbed sleep and aggravation of skin disorders. Considerable amounts of water are lost through damaged skin in severe burns.

- *Lung loss.* Dry climates, air-conditioned or heated environments, and air travel causes dry air to reach the lungs and body water is used up moistening the air for effective oxygen and carbon dioxide transfer. About 500 mL of water is lost every hour during air travel.
- *Urinary loss.* The kidneys have a major role to play in maintaining the body's fluid balance. They filter blood to remove wastes and excrete them in urine, and also reabsorb water to prevent dehydration. Diuretic drugs, alcohol, theophylline in tea and caffeine in coffee, tea and caffeinated drinks stimulate the kidneys to increase urine output. A high sodium intake causes increased urination because of the need to excrete the excess and a high protein diet causes formation of increased amounts of urea, the waste product of protein metabolism, that need to be excreted in urine. In diabetes mellitus, glucose cannot be used for energy, and ketones, formed from protein and fat, are used instead. Ketones are acidic and more urine is produced in order to excrete the excess and keep body pH stable.
- *Gastrointestinal loss.* Vomiting and diarrhoea can lead to large water losses. This is particularly dangerous in infants because of their higher body water content, and can cause life-threatening dehydration.
- *Hormone activity.* Female sex hormones, ADH, produced in the posterior pituitary gland, aldosterone, produced in the adrenal glands, and thyroxine, produced in the thyroid gland, act to conserve water in the body. Pregnancy and breastfeeding increases the need for water. In diabetes insipidus, ADH activity is impaired and the body loses large amounts of water as urine.

Daily requirement

For adequate hydration, water input needs to be balanced with output. On average, intake of water is about 1000 mL a day from food and 1200 mL from drinks, and about 350 mL is produced by metabolic activities, totalling about 2550 mL. About the same amount is lost daily: about 1300 mL of water is lost in urine, 100 mL in faeces, 750 mL from the skin and 400 mL from the lungs.

Government recommendations by age and gender (see Table 2.1) can be found in the National Health and Medical Research Council's (NHMRC) *Nutrient Reference Values for Australia and New Zealand Including Recommended Dietary Intakes*, available at <www.nhmrc.gov.au>.

Table 2.1 Adequate intake (AI) of water (as fluid) (L/day)

Age (years)	Female AI	Male AI
1–3	1.0	1.0
4–8	1.2	1.2
9–13	1.4	1.6
14–18	1.6	1.9
19–70	2.1	2.6
>70	2.1	2.6
Pregnant women		
14–18	1.8	
19–50	2.3	
Lactating women		
14–18	2.3	
19–50	2.6	

Source: Nutrient Reference Values for Australia and New Zealand Including Recommended Dietary Intakes, Canberra: National Health and Medical Research Council, Australian Government Department of Health and Ageing, Canberra and Ministry of Health, New Zealand, Wellington, 2006.

Deficiency effects

If the body's fluid output exceeds intake, dehydration develops. Dehydration may be isotonic, in which both salt and water levels are equally low; hypertonic, in which body water is lower than salt and there is an increased concentration of salt in body fluids; or hypotonic, in which salt concentration is lower than water and there is a decreased concentration of salt in body fluids. Inadequate water intake mainly leads to hypertonic dehydration. Thirst is an after-effect of dehydration; in chronic mild dehydration, thirst signals may not always be recognised. A loss of 1 per cent of body water triggers thirst, a loss of 5–10 per cent of body water causes fatigue, mental confusion, apathy and collapse, and a loss of more than 20 per cent of body water can result in death.

Early effects of dehydration include thirst, headache, sleepiness, fatigue, impaired thinking ability, dizziness, dry lips, mouth and eyes, dry nasal membranes, longitudinal cracks on the tongue, heat intolerance, loss of appetite, nausea, a burning sensation in the stomach, constipation, infrequent urination, darker-coloured urine and increased susceptibility to urinary tract infections and kidney stones. More advanced dehydration can cause rapid weight loss, a fever, dry tongue, difficulty swallowing, vomiting, diminished flow of dark, strong-smelling urine, thirst, dry, shrivelled skin, diminished skin turgor (reduced skin elasticity), areas of numbness on the skin, sunken eyes, cold extremities, lethargy, aggressive behaviour, mental confusion, dizziness, loss of balance and falls, weakness, reduced capacity for physical exertion, and muscle cramps and spasms. Heart rate, pulse rate and blood pressure can increase, but blood pressure may drop when changing posture, especially on standing. Severe dehydration causes a rise in body core temperature, loss of coordination, hallucinations, rapid pulse, raised blood pressure, collapse of peripheral veins, kidney failure, shock and coma, and may lead to death. Exertional rhabdomyolysis (acute muscle damage, also known as 'muscle meltdown') has occurred in people exercising without adequate hydration, especially if they are unused to exercise or if the exercise is very intense. Deep vein thrombosis (DVT) occurring during air travel may be linked to dehydration and immobility.

Infants and older people are more at risk of dehydration, which is often associated with vomiting and diarrhoea. In infants, dehydration is indicated by sunken fontanelles (the soft spots on the top of an infant's head), extreme fussiness or sleepiness, and infrequent dark-coloured urine. Older people have the same thirst signals as younger people, but the signals switch off too early, before they have taken in enough fluid, causing them to remain permanently dehydrated.

Assessment of body status

Water balance can be assessed by measuring serum albumin, plasma or urine osmolality, or body weight changes, or by bioelectrical impedance, which measures the resistance of body tissue and water to an electrical current. Serum albumin is elevated and plasma and urine osmolality increase in dehydration, and weight drops by 1 kg for every litre of fluid lost. Other indicators include:

- *Urine colour.* Urine should be a pale straw colour if hydration is adequate, and dark, orange-coloured urine indicates dehydration. However, urine colour will change to a strong golden-yellow if B vitamin supplements are taken; this colour is the natural colour of B vitamins, particularly vitamin B2, and indicates that residual amounts of vitamins are being eliminated.
- *Skin turgor.* Gently pinch the skin on the back of the hand or over the breastbone, release it and observe how fast it flattens down again. If fully hydrated, the skin should instantly flatten. In dehydration, the skin remains in the pinched position for two or more seconds before flattening. In elderly people, pinch the skin on the forehead or breastbone rather than the hand because age-related loss of skin elasticity can make the hand test unreliable.
- *Blood pressure.* Measure blood pressure while lying down and again when standing. A drop in systolic blood pressure of more than 20 mmHg when standing indicates possible dehydration.
- *Pulse rate.* A pulse rate greater than 100 beats per minute may indicate dehydration. Take the pulse while lying down and then when standing. An increase of 10–20 beats per minute when standing indicates possible dehydration.

Case reports—water deficiency

- *A boy, 16 years of age,* participated in a three-day pre-season wrestling camp consisting of intense fitness training.[1] On the second evening, he developed dark brown urine and, subsequently, severe pain in his quadriceps muscles. He was found to have greatly elevated creatine kinase levels, an indicator of muscle damage, and was diagnosed with exertional rhabdomyolysis. He was hospitalised for six days and given intravenous saline for rehydration, which led to his recovery.
- *A man, 36 years of age,* developed heat cramps, profuse sweating and dehydration after working outdoors for more than six hours in summer.[2] He was found to have elevated serum albumin and calcium. The raised serum calcium level was found to be a consequence of dehydration, rather than a reflection of disturbed calcium balance. After he was treated with intravenous saline rehydration, his calcium level returned to normal in 24 hours and his symptoms resolved.

REFERENCES

1 Cleary, M.A., et al., Exertional rhabdomyolysis in an adolescent athlete during preseason conditioning: A perfect storm, *J Strength Cond Res* (2011), 25(12): 3506–13.

2 Ma, T.K., et al., Pseudohypercalcaemia in patients with heat cramps: Implications on clinical practice, *QJM* (2012), 105(10): 997–9.

Effects of excess

Taking a lot more fluids than are needed will increase urine output, and can also increase losses of water-soluble nutrients, such as vitamins and minerals. Drinking a large amount in a short period of time can cause water intoxication, in which water intake exceeds the capacity of the kidneys to excrete it, overloading the brain, heart and circulation. Binge drinking, the party drug methylenedioxymethamphetamine (MDMA, also known as ecstasy) and excess aldosterone production can all cause a potentially fatal water overload. Effects of water intoxication include mental confusion, dizziness, impaired coordination, headache, nausea, vomiting, weakness, tremors, congestive heart failure, kidney failure, seizures, coma and death. Rarely, rhabdomyolysis can occur in association with water intoxication.

Case reports—water intoxication

- *A man, 39 years of age*, with bipolar disorder developed recurring headaches, confusion and agitation, and had a seizure followed by semi-consciousness.[1] He was found to have very low sodium levels and cerebral oedema caused by excessive fluid intake. For several months, he had been in the habit of drinking 8–10 litres of Diet Coke and 15–20 cups of coffee a day, as well as several cups of water every few minutes. He developed rhabdomyolysis, greatly elevated creatine kinase levels, and acute kidney failure. He was treated with diuretic therapy to reduce his water overload, which led to resolution of his rhabdomyolysis and normalisation of his kidney function.
- *A man, 34 years of age*, became sleepy and developed seizures requiring intubation and mechanical ventilation.[2] It was discovered that he had drunk 40 glasses of water (about 8 L) during a period of a few hours, the penalty of losing a bet with his friends. He was found to have low sodium levels and cerebral oedema, and was treated with a slow infusion of a concentrated saline solution. Fast salt replacement is dangerous because it can lead to osmotic demyelination syndrome of the central nervous system, a form of brain damage. He no longer required mechanical ventilation after three days and he made a full recovery after five days.

REFERENCES

1 Katsarou, A. & Singh, S., Hyponatraemia associated rhabdomyolysis following water intoxication, *BMJ Case Rep* (2010), 9 September 2010.

2 Santos-Soares, P.C. et al., Excessive water ingestion and repeated seizures, *Arq Neuropsiquiatr* (2008), 66(3-A): 552–3.

WATER AS THERAPY—NOVEL THEORIES ON DEHYDRATION AND HEALTH DISORDERS

Dr Batmanghelidj was an Iranian doctor who claimed to have discovered the healing power of water during imprisonment in Iran in the 1980s. He reported being able to relieve severe peptic ulcer pain in another prisoner in eight minutes by giving him two glasses of water.[1] After many further experiments using water as a treatment for his fellow prisoners, he became convinced that dehydration was a vastly underestimated factor in disease. After his release and move to the United States, he worked as a naturopath, promoting the concept that chronic dehydration causes heartburn, gastrointestinal ulcers, abdominal colic, hiatus hernia, chronic inflammation, arthritis, back and neck pain, osteoporosis, headaches, heart disease, elevated serum cholesterol, high blood pressure, overweight, asthma and allergies.[2]

Naturopath Christopher Vasey claims that some of the common symptoms of chronic, mild and unrecognised dehydration are:[3]

- fatigue due to reduced cellular enzyme function
- constipation because the colon reabsorbs water to conserve it for vital body functions
- digestive disorders, gastritis and stomach ulcers due to reduced secretion of digestive juices and a reduced amount of protective mucus in the stomach lining

- high or low blood pressure due to reduced blood volume and the consequent constriction of blood vessels
- respiratory disorders due to lack of protective mucus
- overweight or obesity because of a craving for food as a source of water and because thirst signals are misinterpreted as hunger
- eczema because sweat output is insufficient to clear toxins and irritants from the skin
- elevated serum cholesterol because cholesterol is the waterproofing material in cell membranes and more is produced to try to prevent water loss
- cystitis and urinary tract infections due to the toxins in concentrated urine remaining in contact with the urinary tract and bladder for prolonged periods
- joint inflammation due to lack of water in cartilage and increased concentration of toxins that may irritate the joints
- premature ageing because a decline in body water content causes cell dysfunction and accelerates the ageing process.

These claims are controversial because supporting evidence is limited. However, hydration is often a neglected factor in health disorders, and hydration status should be assessed in all patients. In older patients, water intake should be increased slowly over several days to avoid putting extra strain on the circulation and kidneys. Intake of large amounts of water within a short space of time may overload the kidneys, and is not recommended. Patients with serious illness or kidney disease require medical supervision during rehydration.

REFERENCES

1 Batmanghelidj, F., A new and natural method of treatment of peptic ulcer disease. *J Clin Gastroenterol* (1983) 5: 203–5.
2 Batmanghelidj, F., *Your body's many cries for water* (2nd ed.), Global Health Solutions, Falls Church, VA, 1995.
3 Vasey, C., *The water prescription,* Inner Traditions, Rochester, VT, 2006.

ENERGY

ENERGY STATUS CHECK

1 Do you often feel tired and sluggish?
2 Do you find it hard to get started in the morning?
3 Do you find that your fitness does not improve much when you exercise regularly?
4 Do you rely on stimulants like caffeine to keep you going through the day?

'Yes' answers may indicate inadequate energy status. Note that a number of nutritional deficiencies or health disorders can cause similar effects and further investigation is recommended.

FAST FACTS . . . ENERGY

- All macronutrients provide energy.
- Energy is needed for all metabolic activities.
- The body's total energy expenditure (TEE) equals the basal metabolic rate (BMR) plus the energy expenditure (EE) of metabolic activities related to eating and the EE of physical activity.
- A prolonged low energy intake leads to ketosis.
- Excess energy intake, especially when combined with inactivity, leads to weight gain.

Energy, in a nutritional sense, refers to the fuel that can be burnt in the body to release energy for the body's functions, rather than the feeling of being energetic. However, there is a close relationship between the two because impaired energy production in the body will be reflected in impaired body functioning, leading to fatigue, and poor stamina and endurance. Ultimately, all energy comes from the sun. Solar energy is captured by plants and used for making protein, carbohydrates and fats, and animals obtain their energy from eating these macronutrients in plants or the tissues of other animals. Cellular energy mainly comes from the oxidation (burning) of carbohydrates, but protein, fats and alcohol can also be used for energy.

Units of energy

Energy is measured as joules, with 1 joule equalling the energy used when 1 kg is moved 1 m by a force of 1 Newton. In Australia, the potential energy in food is measured in kilojoules (kJ) and sometimes megajoules (mJ): 1 kJ = 1000 joules and 1 mJ = 1000 kJ. In some countries, the kilocalorie (kcal), usually referred to as a calorie (cal), is the unit used for measuring potential food energy: 1 kJ = 0.239 cal and 1 cal = 4.184 kJ.

Kilojoules in food represent the potential ability of that food to provide the body with energy after it is eaten, digested and absorbed. The amount of potential energy, or fuel, in a food can be measured by a bomb calorimeter, a chamber filled with oxygen and surrounded by water, designed to mimic the body's oxidation process. A portion of food is burnt in the central chamber and the energy released heats the water. The temperature rise of the surrounding water is measured and indicates the amount of energy contained in the food. One cal (4.184 kJ) represents the amount of heat needed to raise the temperature of one kilogram of water by 1°C.

Functions

In the body, chemical energy is used for active transport across cell membranes and for metabolism, which involves both breaking down and building molecules. Mechanical energy is used for muscle function and physical activity, and electrical energy is used for brain and nerve function. As energy is produced, heat is generated as a by-product.

The rate at which energy is produced to support involuntary activities that keep the body ticking over, such as breathing, heartbeat, circulation and kidney function, is called the basal metabolic rate (BMR).

Dietary sources

Fat is the most energy-dense macronutrient, followed by alcohol, protein and carbohydrate (see Table 2.2). Water, vitamins, minerals and trace elements are not oxidised for energy, so do not provide kilojoules. In general, dietary fibre cannot be digested and absorbed and therefore does not have a kilojoule value. However, some types of fibre, such as soluble fibre, can be fermented by bacteria in the large intestine and the end-products absorbed into the body or used for energy by the intestinal lining cells.

Some of the energy in food is not fully available because it needs to be digested, absorbed and oxidised in cells, and these processes are not totally efficient. Also, about 60 per cent of the energy from food is lost as heat during oxidation. However, this heat generation is vital because it keeps the body temperature normal and allows metabolic activities to proceed.

Table 2.2 Energy value of dietary components (kJ) per gram (g)

Water	0 kJ (0 cal)
Dietary fibre (insoluble)	0 kJ (0 cal)
Dietary fibre (soluble)	13 kJ (3 cal)
Carbohydrate	16 kJ (4 cal)
Protein	17 kJ (4 cal)
Alcohol	29 kJ (7 cal)
Fat	37 kJ (9 cal)

Access the Food Standards Australia New Zealand nutrient database (NUTTAB) at <www.foodstandards.gov.au> for the amounts found in specific foods.

Recommended proportion of dietary kilojoules from protein, carbohydrate and fat

The required amounts of kilojoules derived from protein, carbohydrate and fat in the diet vary according to individual needs, and are usually expressed as a percentage of the total kilojoules in the diet. Note that dietary fibre is not usually included in these calculations, because the amount of fibre in grams eaten per day is regarded as more relevant to health. The acceptable macronutrient distribution ranges to reduce chronic disease risk recommended by the National Health and Medical Research Council (NHMRC), Australia, are:

- protein—15–25 per cent of total kJ
- carbohydrate—45–60 per cent of total kJ
- total fat—20–35 per cent of total kJ, made up of no more than 10 per cent as saturated fat and trans fatty acids (commercially modified fats) and up to 10 per cent as essential fatty acids (linoleic acid and alpha-linolenic acid).

The higher level of carbohydrate is more suitable for individuals who are very physically active. An increased proportion of protein and a reduced proportion of carbohydrate and fat may be helpful for weight loss.

Energy production

The primary, immediate energy source for cells is carbohydrate in the form of glucose, which is converted to energy by anaerobic and aerobic pathways in body cells. Alcohol, if available, is an alternative energy source that is used preferentially. Energy is made in cells by breaking down glucose in a series of processes that occur in the cell's cytoplasm and mitochondria (see Chapter 1: Basic physiology). Energy is stored as adenosine triphosphate (ATP), a high-energy compound that is broken down to release energy as needed for cell activities. Micronutrients needed for efficient energy production include B vitamins, coenzyme Q10 (CoQ10), magnesium, iron, zinc and manganese.

Energy storage

Carbohydrate can be stored as glycogen in the liver and muscles, and converted back to glucose for energy. However, glycogen is a bulky molecule, limiting the amount that can be stored, and there is only enough to provide about one day of energy when fasting. Fat can be formed from excess carbohydrate, protein and fat, and stored in adipose tissue, a more compact and efficient way of storing energy for longer-term use.

Factors influencing energy status

The body's total energy expenditure (TEE) equals the BMR, plus the energy expenditure (EE) of metabolic activities related to eating and the EE of physical activity. The BMR is measured when a person has fasted, and is lying down and completely still. It is related to the rate of oxygen consumption and is largely driven by the body's lean mass, which is more metabolically active than fat tissue. The brain, liver, heart and kidneys are highly metabolically active, and account for about 50 per cent of the BMR; muscles account for about 25 per cent; bones, endocrine glands, the intestine and the skin for about 20 per cent; and fat tissue for about 5 per cent. BMR varies according to gender and age. In adults, the average BMR is about 101 kJ per kg body weight per day.

Factors that increase BMR

The process of digesting, absorbing, transporting, metabolising and storing food uses energy, and can raise EE by about 5–30 per cent. This process lasts for about four hours after eating, with the maximum effect after about one hour. Protein has the greatest effect, increasing EE by up to 30 per cent, carbohydrates by up to 10 per cent and fat by up to 5 per cent. In general, physical activity accounts for about 20–40 per cent of TEE, but varies widely according to the intensity, duration and frequency. Exercise also boosts energy expenditure for some hours afterwards. During light activity, the body uses about 5–6 kJ per kg body weight per hour and about 33–35 kJ per kg body weight per hour during intense exertion. Other factors that boost BMR include:

- younger age—the metabolic rate is naturally higher in children and teenagers
- male gender—men in general have more lean tissue than women
- stress, anxiety—stress hormones such as adrenaline boost metabolism as part of the 'fight or flight' reaction
- use of stimulants—catechins in green tea; capsaicinoids in cayenne, chillies, paprika, capsicum and mustard; stimulants in herbs, such as oxedrine in bitter orange and hydroxycitric acid in brindle berry; xanthines such as caffeine, theophylline and theobromine in tea, coffee, cocoa products and guaraná; nicotine; or amphetamines. Unless use is excessive, these have a relatively mild and short-term stimulating effect on metabolic rate
- hyperthyroidism—thyroid hormones boost the metabolic rate of every cell; if the thyroid gland is over-active and producing excess hormones, it can cause tremors, nervousness, restlessness and weight loss
- illness and trauma, such as severe infection, fever, injury, surgery, tumours or burns—immune activity and repair processes boost metabolic rate
- pregnancy and lactation—metabolic activities increase due to additional demands.

Factors that reduce BMR

These factors include:

- a higher level of fat tissue and lower level of lean tissue
- a lower level of physical activity

- older age—in ageing, metabolic activities are not as efficient and muscle tissue is replaced by fat
- female gender
- fasting and starvation, in which metabolism slows to conserve energy
- hypothyroidism—if the thyroid gland is underactive and producing too few hormones, metabolism slows down, resulting in weight gain, fluid retention, a dull expression, constipation, hair loss and mental and physical sluggishness.

Daily requirement

Government recommendations by age and gender (see Table 2.3) can be found in *Nutrient Reference Values for Australia and New Zealand Including Recommended Dietary Intakes*, available at <www.nhmrc.gov.au>.

Table 2.3 Estimated energy requirements (EER) per day (kJ/day)*

Age (years)	Female EER	Male EER
1–3	3200–5300	3500–5600
4–8	5500–6900	5900–7300
9–13	7300–8900	7800–10 000
14–18	9200–9700	10 600–12 500
19–30	8200–11 100	10 300–13 500
31–50	8400–10 000	10 200–12 600
51–70	7900–9600	9300–11 700
>70	7400–9200	8300–10 800
Pregnant women		
All ages: 2nd trimester	additional 1400	
All ages: 3rd trimester	additional 1900	
Lactating women		
14–18 19–50	additional 2000–2100	

* Variable according to body mass index (BMI) and activity level, values given are for a light activity level

Source: Nutrient Reference Values for Australia and New Zealand Including Recommended Dietary Intakes, National Health and Medical Research Council, Australian Government Department of Health and Ageing, Canberra and Ministry of Health New Zealand, Wellington, 2006.

Assessment of energy balance

Maintaining energy balance, as indicated by a stable body weight, requires that the dietary intake equals TEE. If the dietary intake is greater than TEE, weight gain will result, and if it is less, weight will be lost. A common measure used to assess whether body weight is in the healthy range is body mass index (BMI). BMI is calculated by dividing body weight in kg by height in metres squared.

$$\text{BMI} = \frac{\text{Weight (kg)}}{\text{Height (m)}^2}$$

For example, a person weighs 80 kg and is 160 cm tall.

160 cm = 1.6 metres.

1.6 m squared is 1.6 multiplied by itself (1.6) = 2.56. 80 kg divided by 2.56 = a BMI of 31.25 (Obese Class 1, see Table 2.4).

BMI can be used to assess whether an individual is underweight, in the healthy weight range, overweight or obese. Although BMI is a good indicator of weight status for many people, it is not accurate for the very young or very old, or for those with a large amount of muscle. Athletes or body builders will have a heavier weight due to well-developed muscles, and this may cause an increased BMI.

Abdominal fat is more risky for health, and waist circumference is a convenient measure of abdominal obesity. In men, a waist measurement of 94 cm or greater confers an increased health risk and 102 cm or

Table 2.4 Body mass index (BMI) classifications

BMI	Classification	Risk of comorbidities (related illnesses)
Underweight	<18.50	Low
Normal range	18.50–24.99	Average
Overweight	>25.00	See classifications below
Pre-obese	25.00–29.99	Increased
Obese class 1	30.00–34.99	Moderate
Obese class 2	35.00–39.99	Severe
Obese class 3	>40.00	Very severe

Source: Reproduced from WHO, *Obesity: Preventing and Managing the Global Epidemic*, WHO, Geneva, 2000.

more confers a substantially increased risk. In women, a waist measurement of 80 cm or greater confers an increased health risk and 88 cm or more confers a substantially increased risk.

Deficiency effects

A low kJ intake triggers adaptive changes that allow the body to continue to function by using stored energy and converting body tissues into energy substrates.

Short-term adaptation to reduced energy intake

When energy intake is reduced, as in fasting, starvation or dieting for weight loss, the first adaptive change is the breakdown of stored glycogen in the liver and its release as glucose into the bloodstream for use by cells as fuel. The liver also steps up the conversion of lactate into glucose. Muscle glycogen stores can be broken down as well, but this glucose can only be used within the muscle itself, and cannot be released into the bloodstream for use by other cells.

Long-term adaptation to reduced energy intake

Glucose is rapidly used up, especially by the brain and central nervous system, and, if fasting continues, the glycogen supply is exhausted after about one day and blood glucose levels decline. When the brain and nerves are deprived of fuel, fatigue, sleepiness, irritability, temper outbursts, mental confusion, loss of concentration, headaches, dizziness, faintness and blackouts can result.

When blood glucose drops, the pancreas releases the hormone glucagon, made in the alpha cells, that stimulates gluconeogenesis (glucose formation) in the liver from lactate, pyruvate, glucogenic amino acids and glycerol from fats. If fasting persists, the kidneys also begin gluconeogenesis. Eventually the body switches to starvation mode, in which it tries to continue providing fuel for energy while conserving vital proteins, preventing a life-threatening breakdown of the body's organs.

When eating normally, the hormone insulin, made by the beta cells of the pancreas, is released in response to elevated blood glucose. During fasting, blood glucose levels drop and the absence of insulin allows triglyceride stores in fat tissue to be broken down and free fatty acids and glycerol to be released into the bloodstream. Protein is also mobilised from muscle cells, and fatty acids and amino acids serve as the main fuel for the heart, liver and skeletal muscles. Fat is converted to acetyl-CoA and then to ketones (acetoacetate, beta-hydroxybutyrate and acetone), which can be oxidised in the citric acid cycle. Muscle amino acids have the nitrogen component removed (deamination), and the remaining carbon skeletons are used to make glucose or ketones. Nitrogen released by deamination is excreted in urine as urea. This process can continue as long as there are sufficient fat and protein stores, allowing a person of normal body weight to survive about twelve weeks in starvation conditions.

Ketones are an emergency source of energy that have some undesirable effects. They are acidic and can disturb the body's pH balance, moving it towards acidity. Ketones are removed in urine and acetone also is breathed out through the lungs, giving a distinctive smell to the breath. A shift towards acidity can cause nausea, constipation, irritability, headaches, weakness and fatigue. Water is lost because extra urine is produced to help excrete ketones, also causing losses of electrolytes such as sodium, and possibly leading to dehydration.

Effects of excess

Taking in more energy than can be used, especially if combined with inactivity, will lead to weight gain, particularly in people with a lower BMR. This will be reflected in a higher BMI but, in terms of health, the distribution of fat around the body is an important factor. If fat is mainly confined to the buttocks, hips and thighs, referred to as gynoid obesity or 'pear' body shape and more common in women, there are no known health risks associated. Large amounts of fat deposited around the abdomen, termed android obesity or 'apple' body shape and more common in men ('beer belly'), are associated with significant health risks. Abdominal fat, also called visceral fat, is associated with various metabolic abnormalities, especially those that increase risk of coronary heart disease (CHD) and type 2 diabetes. Abdominal obesity is associated with an increased risk of:

- mortality, especially for the younger age group, in which being overweight or obese increases the risk of premature death
- metabolic syndrome (syndrome X), which features elevated blood lipids and blood pressure, elevated

serum cholesterol and low-density lipoprotein (LDL) cholesterol, and reduced high-density lipoprotein (HDL) cholesterol
- cardiovascular disorders, such as atherosclerosis, CHD, stroke and varicose veins
- type 2 diabetes, also associated with metabolic syndrome, featuring increased blood insulin levels, reduced insulin sensitivity (insulin resistance), glucose intolerance and elevated blood glucose
- cancer, especially cancer of the colon, gall bladder, prostate, breast, endometrium, ovaries and cervix
- fatty liver and gall bladder disorders
- osteoarthritis, gout and back pain
- oedema and cellulitis
- breathlessness, asthma, snoring and sleep apnoea, which is linked to an increased risk of high blood pressure, stroke, heart attack and heart failure
- hormonal dysfunction and reduced fertility, low testosterone levels and impotence in men, and abnormal menstrual cycles and polycystic ovarian syndrome (PCOS) in women.

A WEIGHTY ISSUE

Australia is in the grip of an obesity epidemic, with the number of adults who are overweight and obese doubling over the past two decades.[1] In 2004–05, about 40 per cent of men and one-quarter of women were overweight (BMI 25–30), and a further 18 per cent of men and 17 per cent of females were obese (BMI greater than 30). Overweight and obesity are also increasing in prevalence in younger age groups, affecting about a quarter of children.[1]

Fat gain in early life can affect weight in later life. A quarter of obese preschool children and half of obese six-year-olds are obese in adulthood.[2] If an obese sixteen-year-old has one obese parent, there is an 80 per cent chance that they will be an obese adult.[3] Fat cells enlarge in the first year of life (hypertrophy) and then decrease in size in lean children, but remain enlarged in obese children, enabling more fat to be stored. During periods of rapid growth from one to two years and twelve to fourteen years of age, more fat cells develop (hyperplasia), and this also permits more fat storage. As fat tissue builds up and lean tissue reduces, BMR slows down.

There are many factors blamed for the overweight crisis, including genetic factors, eating too much fat and too many kJ, and a sedentary lifestyle providing insufficient exercise. Genetic factors may account for individual variations in BMR and the distribution of fat stores.

The simplistic view of weight gain is that it occurs because more kilojoules are taken in than can be used up and the excess is stored as fat. This view arises from the standard scientific view that a kilojoule is converted to a defined amount of energy in the body, regardless of the food source. However, low-carbohydrate diets can be as effective or work better for weight loss than low-fat diets because they effectively 'waste' kilojoules by increasing thermogenesis, the heat generated in processing the extra protein or fat that substitutes for carbohydrate in the diet. Basically, this means that the body is 'wasting' extra kilojoules by converting them to heat, rather than body fat.

As a consequence of the 'dietary fat phobia' resulting from research into the role of saturated fat in heart disease, high carbohydrate intakes are now common and regarded as healthy. Unfortunately, processed carbohydrates are used to excess in such diets, and these can cause a sharp rise in blood glucose levels. In response, insulin is released to promote glucose uptake by cells for use as fuel and, as a consequence, fat synthesis and storage are enhanced and fat breakdown inhibited. In this way, insulin acts like a jailer by pushing fat into fat cells and turning the key. The hormone glucagon has the opposite effect, mobilising fuel stores to boost blood glucose when levels drop. Overall, high-protein, low-carbohydrate foods will moderate insulin release and have less effect on fat synthesis.

The neuroendocrine system also affects body weight. The hypothalamus has a key role in defending the existing body weight, called the set-point, and it does this by changing eating behaviour in response to a variety of neurotransmitters and the hormone leptin. In animals, damage to the ventromedial hypothalamic nucleus increases appetite and weight, and damage to the lateral hypothalamic nucleus reduces appetite and weight.[4]

The thyroid gland, controlled by the hypothalamus and the pituitary gland, plays a major part in weight control by boosting the metabolic rate of all body cells. The amino acid tyrosine, together with the trace element iodine, as iodide, are the basic building blocks of thyroid hormones. Iodide combines with tyrosine and is then further converted to the active thyroid hormones T3 and T4, also known as thyroxine. A lack of dietary iodine may inhibit production of thyroid hormones, causing a slowing down of metabolism, weight gain, low energy, low mood and a reduced body temperature.

For weight loss, a high-protein, low-fat diet may be equally or more effective than a high-carbohydrate, low-fat diet, and have more beneficial effects on risk factors for cardiovascular disease.[5,6] In an Australian study, 100 middle-aged, obese women were divided into two groups and given a kilojoule-controlled diet, one being high in protein and low in fat and the other being high in carbohydrate and low in fat.[6] Both groups lost an average of about 7 kg over twelve weeks. Subjects with higher serum fat levels at the start of the trial lost more fat on the high-protein diet than on the high-carbohydrate diet. In both groups, serum fasting LDL cholesterol, HDL cholesterol, glucose, insulin and free fatty acids decreased with weight loss but serum fats decreased more in those on the high-protein diet. Vitamin B12 levels increased on the high-protein diet but decreased on the high-carbohydrate diet, and folate and vitamin B6 increased with both diets. These results show that many heart disease risk factors improve with weight loss and that a high-protein, low-fat diet may be preferable for people with elevated blood fats.

REFERENCES

1. Commonwealth of Australia, Department of Health, *Promoting healthy weight*, available at <www.health.gov.au>.
2. Garn, S.M. & LaVelle, M., Two-decade follow-up of fatness in early childhood, *Am J Dis Child* (1985), 139: 181–5.
3. Whitaker, R.C., Wright, J.A., Pepe, M.S. et al., Predicting obesity in young adulthood from childhood and parental obesity, *N Engl J Med* (1997), 337: 869–73.
4. Kalra, S.P., Dube, M.G., Pu, S. et al., Interacting appetite-regulating pathways in the hypothalamic regulation of body weight, *Endocr Rev* (1999), 20(1): 68–100.
5. Claessens, M., van Baak, M.A., Monsheimer, S. & Saris, W.H., The effect of a low-fat, high-protein or high-carbohydrate ad libitum diet on weight loss maintenance and metabolic risk factors, *Int J Obes (Lond)* (2009 January): 20.
6. Noakes, M., Keogh, J.B., Foster, P.R. & Clifton, P.M., Effect of an energy-restricted, high-protein, low-fat diet relative to a conventional high-carbohydrate, low-fat diet on weight loss, body composition, nutritional status, and markers of cardiovascular health in obese women, *Am J Clin Nutr* (2005), 81(6): 1298–306.

ANOREXIA NERVOSA

Anorexia nervosa (AN) is an eating disorder in which sufferers undergo self-inflicted starvation to achieve an extremely low BMI. It is a complex illness that especially affects children and young people with low self-esteem, a perfectionist attitude and a perceived lack of control over their life, and may be triggered by an episode of unintentional weight loss or other people's attitudes and comments about body weight. AN affects about 0.5 per cent of girls and young women in developed societies, and has a high mortality rate, with about 20 per cent of people with the disorder dying within twenty years.[1] It is eight times more common in people whose relatives have the disorder.[2]

As AN progresses, sufferers develop a distorted body image and perceive themselves to be fat even though they may be extremely emaciated. People with AN become phobic about weight gain, obsessive about their food intake and counting kilojoules, and may exercise to excess. They may voluntarily exist on a very low food intake or binge eat and then induce vomiting or use laxatives and/or diuretics in an attempt to rid themselves of the food (bulimia nervosa). In contrast to AN, bulimia nervosa may also be present in people who are of normal weight or overweight.

Features of anorexia nervosa[3]

- Change of eating pattern, avoidance of certain food types and a narrowed range of food choices
- Avoidance of socialising that involves food
- Compulsive or ritualistic behaviours related to eating
- Control of appetite by drinking water or diet drinks or smoking cigarettes

- Binge-eating, followed by self-induced vomiting or purging.

Effects of AN[2]

AN is a condition of starvation and has similar effects to protein-energy malnutrition (PEM). Growth slows down, and fat and muscle mass are lost. Digestion is impaired, resulting in bloating and constipation, and fluid may build up in peripheral tissues. Body temperature drops, the heart is weakened and hair on the head becomes thinner. A downy covering of fine hair (lanugo) covers the skin. If vomiting is habitual, the oesophagus is damaged by stomach acid and tooth enamel is eroded. In females, the menstrual cycle stops (amenorrhoea) and the absence of three consecutive menstrual periods is indicative of the disorder. Over time, calcium is lost from bones and teeth, leading to premature osteoporosis, stress fractures and tooth loss.

About 40 per cent of all people with AN recover, about 40 per cent continue to have AN but function reasonably well and about 20 per cent remain severely symptomatic and are chronically disabled.[3] Death can result from suicide, malnutrition or medical complications. It is a serious illness that requires specialist help and may need long-term institutional care. Because micronutrient deficiencies may be severe and can aggravate dysperceptions that contribute to a distorted body image, it is important to use dietary supplements, especially B vitamins, magnesium, iron and zinc to help normalise cognitive and perceptual functions. As micronutrients do not contain kilojoules, this approach may be more acceptable to the AN patient than increasing macronutrient intake. However, because the risk of suicide and life-threatening malnutrition is very high, AN patients with a severe form of the disorder should always be referred for urgent medical treatment.

REFERENCES

1 Australian Government, Department of Health & Ageing, *Anorexia nervosa: Australian treatment guide for consumers and carers*, 2005, available at <www.health.gov.au>.

2 MedlinePlus Medical Encyclopedia, *Anorexia nervosa*, 2008, available at <www.nlm.nih.gov/medlineplus/ency/article/000362.htm>.

3 Gilchrist, P.N., Ben-Tovim, D.I., Hay, P.J. et al., Eating disorders revisited. I: Anorexia nervosa. *Med J Aust* (1998), 169(8): 438–41.

PROTEIN

PROTEIN STATUS CHECK

1 Do you often feel run down and do you catch infections easily?
2 Do you feel bloated and uncomfortable after eating?
3 Are your hair and nails weak and brittle?
4 Are your muscles weak, and do you have poor posture?

'Yes' answers may indicate inadequate protein status. Note that a number of nutritional deficiencies or health disorders can cause similar effects and further investigation is recommended.

FAST FACTS . . . PROTEIN

- Sources of high-quality protein include animal foods, soybeans and soy products (tofu, tempeh, soy milk, soy cheese, soy yoghurt), amaranth, quinoa and spirulina.
- Protein is important for tissue growth, repair and maintenance, metabolism, immunity, transport and fluid and pH balance.
- It supports brain function, energy production, detoxification and antioxidant protection.
- A deficiency can cause poor growth, underweight, muscle wasting, a round, puffy (moon) face and miserable expression, oedema, fatty deposits in the liver, and skin and hair disorders.

Protein is a core element of the diet that, together with water, makes up a major part of the body. Named after the Greek word *proteios*, meaning 'primary' or 'taking first place', it is crucial for a vast range of vital body functions and essential for growth, repair and maintenance of body structures. Nearly half of the protein in the body is in skeletal muscles, about 15 per cent is in the skin, another 15 per cent is in blood and the remainder is mainly in organ tissue.

Protein structure

Proteins are made up of a large number of amino acids that contain carbon, hydrogen and oxygen, as well as nitrogen, the characteristic element not present in fats and carbohydrates. Some proteins also incorporate the elements sulfur, phosphorus, iron, copper and iodine into their structure. Nitrogen makes up about 16 per cent of proteins. Eating protein from plants or animals is a way of obtaining nitrogen in a usable form because, unlike plants, animals cannot use nitrogen from the soil or air.

Proteins are amino acids linked in chains by peptide bonds. Simple molecules containing up to 100 amino acids are referred to as peptides. Dipeptides consist of two amino acids, tripeptides have three amino acids and polypeptides have 50–100 amino acids. Proteins can contain hundreds to many thousands of amino acids in varying combinations. The type and sequence of amino acids control the final shape of the protein and its function in the body, and are determined by DNA in the nucleus of cells. There are more than 100 000 different proteins (different amino acid sequences) in the body, which have four basic structures:

- *primary protein structure*—this is the basic structure of proteins, and consists of a chain of amino acids bonded together in a specific sequence
- *secondary protein structure*—the amino acid chain is folded and held in shape by disulfide bonds and forms a coiled shape by hydrogen bonding
- *tertiary protein structure*—additional bonds twist the protein into a complex folded structure
- *quaternary protein structure*—two or more peptide or protein sub-units are held together by various types of bonds to form a specific shape required for the function of the protein.

Types of body proteins

- *Fibrous proteins.* These have a secondary structure, and are linear and rope-like in shape, made up of intertwined polypeptides held together by hydrogen bonds that provide strength and disulfide cross-links that provide elasticity. They are relatively insoluble, and resist acids, bases and moderate heat. Examples include collagen in tendons, cartilage and bone, elastin in ligaments and joint capsules, keratin in hair and nails, myosin in muscle and fibrin in blood clots.
- *Globular proteins.* These have a tertiary structure and are spherical in shape, made up of folded strands of polypeptides held together by various bonds that leave the hydrophilic (water-loving) side chains exposed on the outside. This property makes them soluble in water and able to be transported around the body in the bloodstream. However, they are easily denatured by acids, bases and heat. Examples include albumins and globulins in blood plasma, enzymes, hormones, glutelins and prolamines in plants, and protamines and histones in the nuclei of cells.
- *Conjugated proteins.* These contain non-protein components, such as glycoproteins that contain carbohydrates; lipoproteins that contain lipids; and metalloproteins that contain metals.

Amino acid structure

Amino acids contain one or more basic amino groups (NH_2), an acidic carboxyl group (COOH), hydrogen (H) and a radical (R) group that is unique to each amino acid and is responsible for its characteristics. Amino acids in food and supplements are commonly in the 'L' (laevorotatory) form (the form that rotates plane-polarised light anti-clockwise), indicated by 'L' before the name (e.g. L-histidine). This form is well absorbed and utilised. 'D' (dextrorotatory) amino acids are in the form that rotates plane-polarised light clockwise and, in general, are poorly absorbed and utilised.

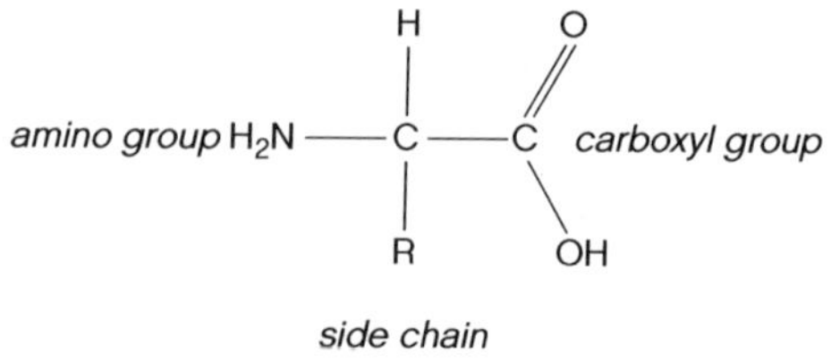

Figure 2.1 Amino acid structure

Types of amino acids

Twenty-one amino acids are the building blocks of all proteins in the body (structural amino acids), and all are required to be present in the correct ratio in order to make the proteins needed for forming body structures and for growth, repair and maintenance of tissues. Six other amino acids are not required for protein synthesis, but are required for other functions in the body, such as synthesis of the neurotransmitters essential for brain function.

Essential (indispensable) amino acids

There are nine amino acids that are essential in the diet because they cannot be made in the body at a rate that is sufficient for the body's requirements. These are:

- Histidine (His)
- Isoleucine (Ile)
- Leucine (Leu)
- Lysine (Lys)
- Methionine (Met)
- Phenylalanine (Phe)
- Threonine (Thr)
- Tryptophan (Trp)
- Valine (Val).

Semi-essential (conditionally dispensable) amino acids

These amino acids may become essential in the diet during times when they cannot be made in sufficient quantities because of increased needs, such as during growth in childhood, adolescence and pregnancy, or in major illness. These are:

- Arginine (Arg) (essential for infants)
- Carnitine* (Car)
- Citrulline* (Cit)
- Cysteine (Cys)
- Taurine* (Tau)
- Tyrosine (Tyr)

* Non-structural amino acids

Non-essential (dispensable) amino acids

Twelve amino acids can be synthesised in the body, provided that sufficient nitrogen is available from other amino acids, and they are therefore not essential in the diet. However, they are essential for normal body function. These are:

- Alanine (Ala)
- Aspartic acid (Asp)
- Asparagine (Asn)
- Gamma-aminobutyric acid* (GABA)
- Glutamic acid (Glu)
- Glutamine (Gln)
- Glutathione* (GSH)
- Glycine (Gly)
- Ornithine* (Orn)
- Proline (Pro)
- Serine (Ser)
- Selenocysteine (Sec)

* Non-protein-forming amino acids

Arg, Cys, Pro, Tau, Tyr and Gly are essential in the diet of preterm infants.

Protein digestion, absorption and transport

Digestion of proteins in food is dependent on hydrochloric acid in the stomach, which activates the protein-digesting enzyme pepsin and denatures proteins by breaking apart the bonds in the secondary, tertiary and quaternary structures. Pepsin breaks down protein chains to form polypeptides, oligopeptides (smaller peptides) and free amino acids. In the small intestine, polypeptides and oligopeptides are broken down further by protease enzymes, which include trypsin, chymotrypsin, carboxypeptidases A and B, proteolase, collagenase, aminopeptidases, dipeptidyl aminopeptidases and tripeptidases. The end-products of protein digestion are dipeptides, tripeptides and free amino acids.

Small peptides are the form in which most dietary proteins are absorbed, and they are absorbed more rapidly than amino acids. They have a number of specific transport systems, such as peptide transporter 1 (PepT1), that work in association with movement of hydrogen ions across the intestinal epithelial cell (enterocyte) membrane. Amino acids are absorbed into the intestinal wall by a range of carrier systems involving sodium-dependent and sodium-independent mechanisms. Amino acids compete with each other for absorption, and essential amino acids are absorbed faster than non-essential amino acids. In enterocytes, peptides are broken down to amino acids that can be used within enterocytes or can be transferred into the bloodstream by diffusion and sodium-independent transport systems and are then taken up by the liver.

Metabolism, storage and excretion

Amino acids in the liver are used for production of proteins and nitrogen-containing compounds for use in the liver and release into the bloodstream. Non-essential amino acids are made from other amino acids as required. Protein is taken up into tissue cells by sodium-dependent, sodium-independent and glutathione-dependent carrier systems. The body maintains a constant pool of free amino acids in plasma and tissues that consists of dietary amino acids and amino acids derived from tissue breakdown. There is no mechanism for the excretion of protein.

Production of non-essential amino acids

Amino acids are made in the body by making a carbon skeleton (keto acid) and attaching a nitrogen-containing amino group to it, using vitamin B6 as a co-factor for the enzymes involved. There are two methods via which this can be accomplished:

- *Transamination.* This involves the transfer of an amino group (NH_2) from one amino acid to a keto acid to make a different amino acid—for example, pyruvic acid can act as a carbon skeleton and accept an amino group from glutamic acid; it then becomes the amino acid alanine and, as glutamic acid no longer has an amino group, it becomes a keto acid.
- *Deamination.* An amino group is removed from an amino acid, commonly glutamine, and converted to ammonia (NH_3). Ammonia is then converted to back to NH_2 and attaches to a carbon skeleton to form a new amino acid—for example, glutamine loses one amino group and becomes glutamic acid; the lost amino group is converted to NH_3 and then back to NH_2, which joins a keto acid to form a new amino acid.

There is no specific storage depot for protein in the body, and the amino acid pool must be replenished daily. Muscles comprise an accessible store of amino acids that can be mobilised in a deficiency. Cellular proteins are broken down primarily by enzyme systems in lysosomes and proteasomes. Amino acids can be broken down by deamination to form ammonia, which is then broken down in the liver to urea and excreted in urine.

Protein functions

Protein is the major functional and structural component of body cells. The functions of protein include the following:

- *Tissue growth, repair and maintenance.* Protein is an essential component of body structures, especially muscle, skin and connective tissue.
- *Cell structure.* Protein is an essential component of cell structures and membranes.
- *Regulation of metabolism.* Enzymes are proteins that facilitate biochemical reactions in the body, including energy production and digestion. Many of the hormones that regulate cell activities are proteins, including insulin, oxytocin and growth hormone. Insulin regulates glucose metabolism, oxytocin stimulates uterine contractions during childbirth, and growth hormone stimulates protein production in muscle cells.
- *Muscle contraction.* Actin and myosin are contractile proteins found in muscles that allow muscle movements.
- *Immunity.* Protein is required for the formation of white blood cells and immune proteins, such as antibodies, complement and interferons, that protect against pathogens.
- *Transport.* Proteins in cell membranes transport substances into and out of the cell. Protein carriers in the bloodstream transport insoluble substances such as lipids, fat-soluble nutrients and trace elements, and haemoglobin is a globular protein that transports oxygen and carbon dioxide in red blood cells.
- *Fluid balance.* Plasma proteins exert an osmotic pressure that draws fluid from the tissues back into the bloodstream to maintain normal blood pressure.
- *pH balance.* Some amino acids have extra acidic groups (COOH) or extra basic groups (NH_2) in their side chains that are used to buffer acids and bases.
- *Brain function.* Some amino acids can convert to neurotransmitters that regulate brain function, cognition and mood—for example, Trp can convert to serotonin, a neurotransmitter that can have effects on appetite, sleep, memory, learning, mood and behaviour.
- *Energy production.* Every gram of protein supplies 17 kJ of energy, which is derived from the

carbon skeleton of amino acids that remains after deamination. Some amino acids are converted to glucose (glucogenic amino acids), while others are converted to ketones (ketogenic amino acids) and used in the energy cycle. Surplus amino acids are deaminated, and the carbon skeleton is converted to fat and stored in adipose tissue.

- *Detoxification and antioxidant protection.* Glutathione is a sulfur-containing tripeptide important for cellular defence against heavy metals, reactive oxygen species, hydrogen peroxide and other peroxides, and hydroxyl radicals. The enzymes cytochrome P450, glutathione S-transferases and UDP-glucuronosyltransferase take part in the breakdown of potentially toxic chemicals and metabolites.

Dietary sources

If a protein is to be useful in the body, it needs to contain all the essential amino acids in the ratio the body needs. If even one is missing or present in an amount that is too low, protein synthesis stops. Like threading beads on a wire in a particular pattern, when one type of bead runs out, the chain cannot be completed.

Foods that contain all the essential amino acids in approximately the right ratio are classed as first-class (complete) proteins, and foods that are missing or low in one or more essential amino acids are regarded as second-class (incomplete) proteins. To assess the adequacy of protein intake, it is important to know both the quality, in terms of the essential amino acid content, and the quantity of protein the diet supplies.

Sources of first-class (complete) proteins include:

- *animal sources:* eggs, dairy products, organ meats, meat, fish, poultry
- *plant sources:* soybeans and soy products (tofu, tempeh, soy milk, soy cheese, soy yoghurt), the grains quinoa and amaranth, and the microalgae spirulina.

Sources of second-class (incomplete) proteins include:

- *animal source:* gelatine
- *plant sources:* legumes (except soy), most grains, seeds, nuts, fruit, vegetables.

Access the Food Standards Australia New Zealand nutrient database (NUTTAB) at <www.foodstandards.gov.au> for the amounts of protein found in specific foods.

Limiting amino acids

The protein value of a food is reduced according to the level of the essential amino acid present in the smallest amount. This essential amino acid is called the limiting amino acid because it limits the usefulness of the protein in the body. Common limiting amino acids in plant foods are Lys, Thr, Trp and Met. In grains, Lys is the common limiting amino acid and Lys, Trp and Thr are limiting in corn and rice. Met and Trp are limiting amino acids in legumes and Met and Lys in peanuts.

Protein complementing to compensate for limiting amino acids

By combining two or more second-class proteins or first-class and second-class proteins in a meal, it is possible to increase the protein value of the meal by compensating for the limiting essential amino acid(s). A protein food low in an essential amino acid can be combined with a food high in that same essential amino acid or, alternatively, combined with a food that is a first-class protein (contains all the essential amino acids).

Vegetarians and vegans (who do not eat animal foods) are more likely to have diets higher in second-class protein and protein complementing can increase the quality of the protein in such diets. However, it is not necessary to protein complement at every meal. A range of different types of protein foods eaten within a twelve-hour period should provide a source of first-class protein.

Protein combinations that increase protein quality are:

- *grains with dairy foods*—for example, porridge with milk, cheese sandwich, rice custard
- *grains with legumes*—for example, chick pea and cracked wheat salad, rice and bean dishes
- *seeds with legumes*—for example, sunflower seeds or pumpkin seeds added to dishes containing beans, lentils, chick peas or peas.

Measuring protein in food

Measuring protein quantity

The quantity of protein in a food is measured in grams (g), often expressed as a percentage, which is equivalent to protein g per 100 g of food. The amount of protein in selected foods is given in Table 2.5.

Table 2.5 Amount of protein (g) per 100 g of food (approximate values)

Food	Amount of protein (per 100 g)
Spirulina powder	60–70
Egg, dried	47
Soy flour, low fat	46
Skim milk, dried	36
Cheese, cheddar	24
Meats, nuts, seeds	20–30
Legumes, dried	20–25
Quinoa	14
Egg, hard-boiled	12
Milk, fresh, skim	4
Grains	2–3

Measuring protein quality

The quality of a protein is assessed by measuring the amount and proportion of essential amino acids it contains. Measurement methods include amino acid score, protein efficiency ratio, biological value, net protein utilisation, and protein digestibility-corrected amino acid score.

- *Amino acid score.* The amino acid score (AAS), also called the chemical score, measures the essential amino acid content of a protein food by chemically analysing the food and then comparing it to a high quality reference protein, usually a hen's egg. It is calculated by dividing the milligrams of the limiting amino acid in 1 g of the test protein by the milligrams of the same amino acid in 1 g of reference protein. AAS is expressed as a percentage; the hen's egg has the highest value (100 per cent). However, this method fails to assess the digestibility of a food; if a food is poorly digested, the essential amino acids will not be able to be absorbed and used.
- *Protein efficiency ratio.* The protein efficiency ratio (PER) measures the effect of a protein food on growth rate in terms of weight gain of a test animal—usually a rat. The animal's weight gain is divided by the amount of protein consumed. PER is expressed as a range between 0 and 4. A good-quality protein food is more than 2, an intermediate-quality food is 1.5–2, and a poor-quality food is less than 1.5. The PER value is 3.92 for the hen's egg (the highest value) and 0 for gelatine. However, assessments using animals may not be applicable to humans.
- *Biological value.* Rather than just chemically analysing a food, the biological value (BV) measures its usefulness in the body, which is the per cent of absorbed protein that the body uses. In essence, BV measures the amount of essential amino acids that are absorbed from the protein food and then used to form proteins for body tissues. Because no food is fully utilised without wastage, the hen's egg scores 97 per cent, the highest score possible. Although a better measure than AAS, BV fails to assess digestibility.
- *Net protein utilisation.* Net protein utilisation (NPU) measures the digestibility, as well as the usefulness of a protein food. To obtain the NPU score, BV is multiplied by digestibility and expressed as a percentage, with the hen's egg scoring 94 per cent.
- *Protein digestibility-corrected amino acid score.* The protein digestibility-corrected amino acid score (PDCAAS) uses a variation of the AAS multiplied by a digestibility factor, and is regarded as the best available method of predicting the protein quality of foods for humans. Amino acids in the test food are determined by chemical analysis, and true digestibility is determined by nitrogen balance studies using animals. The AAS is calculated by dividing the amount of each essential amino acid in the food by the amount specified for children aged two to five years (obtained from the Food and Agriculture Organization of the United Nations (FAO) standard values). The essential amino acid present in the lowest amount in the food (the limiting amino acid) determines the AAS. The PDCAAS is calculated by multiplying the AAS by true protein digestibility—for example, wheat has an AAS of 47 per cent (0.47) and true digestibility of 91 per cent (0.91). Therefore, 0.47×0.91 = a PDCAAS of 0.42. PDCAAS can range from 0, which is very poor, to 1, which is the best possible protein quality score. The PDCAAS for egg white is 1—see Table 2.6.

Factors influencing body status

Nitrogen is lost in urine as urea, a by-product of protein deamination. Undigested protein from food and sloughed off epithelial cells may be removed in

Table 2.6 PDCAAS for some common foods

Food protein	PDCAAS
Egg white	1.00
Milk powder	1.00
Soy protein concentrate	0.99
Beef	0.92
Soybean	0.91
Chick pea	0.80
Pea flour	0.69
Kidney bean	0.68
Rolled oats	0.57
Lentils	0.52
Whole wheat	0.42

faeces, and protein is lost during menstruation, blood loss, seminal emissions and when skin cells, hair and nails are lost.

- *Digestion and absorption are reduced* by inadequate production of stomach acid, impaired protease production and chronic gastrointestinal disorders such as coeliac disease, Crohn's disease and other inflammatory bowel disorders. Tannins in tea and red wine can form complexes with various digestive enzymes and reduce digestive activity, and also complex with protein in food and reduce digestibility.
- *Metabolism is impaired* by a diet deficient in first class protein, a carbohydrate-deficient diet, a kilojoule-deficient diet or liver damage. Second class proteins are deaminated, and the carbon skeleton is used for energy or stored as fat. If carbohydrate or kilojoule intake is inadequate, protein is diverted to energy pathways rather than used for structural functions. Protein synthesis in the liver may be impaired by alcohol, drugs, toxins or infections such as hepatitis.
- *Losses are increased* by kidney disease, in which proteins may be lost in urine.
- *Needs are increased* by body and muscle growth occurring in pregnancy, infants, children and adolescents, and by weight training, trauma, surgery and prolonged physical or emotional stress that causes the breakdown of body proteins for energy.

Daily requirement

Government recommendations by age and gender (see Table 2.7) can be found in *Nutrient Reference Values for Australia and New Zealand Including Recommended Dietary Intakes*, available at <www.nhmrc.gov.au>. The minimum amount of dietary protein to support basic tissue maintenance is about 22 g a day. About 0.8–1 g per kg/body weight per day is needed to supply sufficient protein for optimal body function.

Table 2.7 Recommended daily intake (RDI) of protein (g/day)

Age (years)	Female RDI	Male RDI
1–3	14	14
4–8	20	20
9–13	35	40
14–18	45	65
19–70	46	64
>70	57	81
Pregnant women		
14–18	58	
19–50	60	
Lactating women		
14–18	63	
19–50	67	

Source: Nutrient Reference Values for Australia and New Zealand Including Recommended Dietary Intakes, National Health and Medical Research Council, Australian Government Department of Health and Ageing, Canberra and Ministry of Health, New Zealand, Wellington, 2006.

Deficiency effects

When kilojoules are adequate but protein is severely inadequate, kwashiorkor can result. Kwashiorkor particularly affects children, and can occur in poor areas of Asia and Africa, where a single grain such as rice is the main food and other foods—especially animal foods—are in limited supply. There is a sufficient kilojoule intake to provide energy, but there is not enough protein to support growth, immunity, pH balance and maintenance of tissues such as skin and hair. The features of kwashiorkor are poor growth, underweight, muscle wasting (which may not be obvious due to fatty deposits), a round, puffy (moon) face and miserable expression, oedema, fatty deposits in the liver, and skin and hair disorders.

When both protein and kilojoules are inadequate, starvation—also called protein energy malnutrition (PEM), or marasmus—results. This is very common in developing countries when the food supply is interrupted, often because of conflict or drought. Young children are most affected because of their increased demand for protein to support growth. The features of PEM are weight loss, severe underweight, very thin limbs, loss of fat under the skin, muscle wasting and a wizened face. However, in contrast to kwashiorkor, hair may have normal texture and oedema may be absent.

Indicators of a severe protein deficiency may include:

- failure to grow in children, wasting of muscles, pot belly, sunken chest, flat feet
- skin, hair and nail abnormalities, such as depigmentation of skin, dry and peeling skin (flaky paint appearance), skin ulceration and thinning hair with loss of pigment (the outer layer of hair is absent and the inner red-coloured core is revealed)
- poor brain development, apathy, irritability
- reduced production of stomach acid and digestive enzymes, loss of appetite, vomiting, diarrhoea
- enlargement of the liver
- anaemia
- reduced immunity, susceptibility to infections.

Effects of a mild or moderate protein deficiency may include:

- susceptibility to infections
- poor digestion, bloating after eating, heartburn
- oedema
- poor posture and muscle tone
- low blood pressure
- anaemia
- reduced kidney function
- brittle or thinning hair
- brittle or peeling nails.

Assessment of body status

Body protein status is measured by nitrogen balance studies, in which nitrogen intake from the diet is measured and compared with nitrogen losses in faeces and urine:

- *Nitrogen balance*, in which nitrogen intake equals excretion, is normal for adults.
- *Positive nitrogen balance*, in which intake is greater than excretion, is normal for growth periods.
- *Negative nitrogen balance*, in which excretion is greater than intake, is abnormal and indicates a breakdown of protein for energy production. This can occur when kilojoule intake is insufficient, such as during fasting, dieting for weight loss or starvation.

High-protein, low-carbohydrate diets

High-protein, low-carbohydrate diets may be useful in the following conditions:

- *Metabolic syndrome (syndrome X).* This is a genetic disorder with a high risk of CHD that features abdominal obesity, elevated blood lipids and blood pressure, elevated serum cholesterol and low-density lipoprotein (LDL) cholesterol, reduced high-density lipoprotein (HDL) cholesterol, and type 2 diabetes, associated with increased blood insulin levels, reduced insulin sensitivity and elevated blood glucose. It is triggered or worsened by a diet high in sugar, processed carbohydrates and salt, and an increased protein and reduced carbohydrate intake may help to reduce weight and normalise blood lipids and glucose metabolism.
- *Obesity.* A reduced carbohydrate intake mobilises body fat for conversion to ketones that are used for energy. Protein is also used for energy production in the absence of adequate carbohydrate, and a higher protein intake helps conserve muscle protein that would otherwise be used for energy. Protein also reduces hunger sensations by stabilising blood glucose.
- *Hypoglycaemia (low blood glucose).* This can be triggered by carbohydrate foods—especially those that are high glycaemic index and high glycaemic load—by causing a rapid rise in blood glucose that leads to a rebound lowering of blood glucose in susceptible people. Reducing carbohydrate and increasing protein intake helps to prevent blood glucose swings that contribute to hypoglycaemia symptoms, binge eating, and food, alcohol, drug, caffeine and nicotine cravings.

Effects of excess

Proteins in foods are responsible for food allergies and intolerances, but these do not occur as a consequence of the amount of protein eaten. They are caused by a genetic predisposition to idiosyncratic immune reactions to specific proteins in foods or food groups. Although the liver and kidneys are important for protein metabolism, there is no evidence that this is damaging—on the contrary, organs like the heart and lungs develop increased efficiency when regularly forced to work hard by intense physical activity. High-protein diets do not have adverse effects on people with healthy kidneys, but protein must be restricted in patients with kidney disease. Eating large amounts of protein, especially if these are not balanced by adequate plant foods, has the potential to cause adverse effects, including:

- *Reduced bone density.* Meat, fish, chicken, eggs and grains are generally high in the acid-forming minerals phosphorus and sulfur (from the sulfur-containing amino acids Met, Cys and Tau) that temporarily and slightly decrease body pH. An increase in acidity leads to calcium loss from bones because calcium is drawn into the bloodstream as a buffer to restore normal pH.
- *Increased need for nutrients.* Protein increases the need for nutrients such as water for excretion of excess urea; zinc and manganese for urea metabolism; and vitamin B6 for amino acid metabolism. High-phosphate (acidic) protein foods may cause an imbalance in body levels of calcium and magnesium.
- *Unbalanced diet.* Excess energy-dense protein may crowd out other types of foods in the diet and lead to nutritional deficiencies, especially deficiencies of dietary fibre, potassium, vitamin C and folic acid.
- *Obesity.* Excess amounts of any kilojoule-containing food can cause obesity because the excess is converted to fat and stored.

Supplements

Most mixed diets are likely to provide sufficient protein. However, extra protein in the form of a supplement may be of temporary use for increasing muscle strength and bulk, healing soft tissue injuries, assisting weight loss, stabilising blood glucose levels, and improving the texture of skin, hair and nails. Pre-digested supplements, such as free-form or hydrolysed amino acids, are available for people who have difficulty digesting high protein foods.

Types of protein supplements include the following:

- *Free-form amino acids* are individual amino acids that are easily absorbed because they do not need to be broken down by digestive enzymes.
- *Hydrolysed amino acids* have been partially pre-digested but still contain peptides that need to be broken down further in the gut.
- *Branched-chain amino acids (BCAAs).* Leu, Ile and Val are BCAAs used by skeletal muscles to provide energy and reduce muscle protein breakdown. They may help muscle recovery and reduce fatigue and soreness after exercise.
- *Whole milk protein (WMP)* is a filtered form of whole milk that concentrates the protein component by removing most of the carbohydrates and fat.
- *Milk protein concentrate (MPC)* is a more concentrated filtered milk protein containing whey proteins and casein, the main milk protein.
- *Milk protein isolate (MPI)* contains whey proteins and casein derived from skim milk.
- *Whey protein concentrate (WPC)* is derived from milk, and is a good source of BCAAs and sulfur-containing amino acids. Whey protein contains lactoferrin and immunoglobulins that support immunity.
- *Whey protein isolate (WPI)* is a more refined whey protein, but the processing method may denature some of the beneficial compounds found in WPC.
- *Whey protein hydrolysate (WPH)* is WPI that is partially pre-digested for improved absorption.
- *Caseinate* is a soluble form of the milk protein casein that can mix easily in drinks.
- *Micellar casein (MC)* is casein that has been removed from milk by micro-filtration. It is slower to digest than caseinate, and is taken before bedtime to help prevent muscle breakdown during sleep.
- *Hydrolysed casein protein (HCP)* is a partially pre-digested form of casein.
- *Soy protein isolate (SPI)* is a concentrated protein derived from soybeans that has no lactose and is very low in carbohydrates and fats. It is useful for people with a dairy allergy or lactose intolerance.

AMINO ACID SUPPLEMENTS

Amino acids are available as individual or combination supplements. In most products, the 'L' form is used because it is the most bio-available form. 'D' forms are usually poorly metabolised or have blocking effects in the body. In general, amino acid supplements are manufactured by microbial fermentation or enzymatic conversion of an appropriate substrate. Amino acids are dependent on vitamin B6 for their metabolism, and should be used with a source of vitamin B6. In most cases, the optimal supplementary dose is unknown and the doses given below are a guide only.

Arginine (Arg)

Arg is important for production of the vasodilator nitric oxide and for endocrine function, particularly for the function of the adrenal and pituitary glands. It stimulates the release of adrenal hormones involved in the stress response; the blood glucose regulators insulin and glucagon; growth hormone; and the hormone prolactin that stimulates breast milk production, immune responses and the cell cycle. Arg is used for lowered immunity, erectile dysfunction, reducing the occurrence of post-surgical infections, maintaining healthy blood pressure and heart function, and relieving symptoms of angina and congestive heart failure.[1] Arg has improved endothelial function and reduced LDL oxidation in heart patients.[2] However, not all studies have found benefits for cardiovascular disease and one recent study found that Arg use was associated with higher mortality.[2] The supplementary dose may be 3–10 g daily.

Branched-chain amino acids (BCAAs)

Ile, Leu and Val are BCAAs that can be used by skeletal muscles for fuel. BCAA supplementation before exercise reduces muscle damage, helps muscle recovery and repair, and reduces muscle soreness and fatigue after exercise.[3] In older people, BCAAs can help maintain muscle mass.[4] They may help support liver function in people at risk of liver failure, and may be of use in surgical and cancer patients to reduce breakdown of muscle protein.[5,6]

In the genetic disorder phenylketonuria (PKU), Phe cannot be converted to tyrosine and builds up to toxic levels. Newborn babies are routinely screened for PKU, and children affected must have a low Phe diet throughout life to prevent brain damage. BCAAs have been used in PKU to elevate plasma concentrations of BCAAs, which inhibit the uptake of Phe by the brain and help protect brain function.[7] The supplementary dose of BCAAs used in athlete studies is 14–21 g daily.

Carnitine (Car) and acetyl-L-carnitine (Alcar)

Car is a conditionally essential amino acid that is part of four enzyme systems that transport medium- and long-chain fatty acids across mitochondrial membranes for energy production. Car also helps transport intermediate toxic compounds out of the mitochondria, supports heart and muscle function and improves sperm motility.[8] Alcar is synthesised from Car and is a precursor to acetyl coenzyme A, which is an integral part of the energy cycle in cells and a precursor to the neurotransmitter acetylcholine, essential for the function of cholinergic nerves. Alcar has been used to restore mitochondrial function in aged animals, returning mitochondrial function to the level of young animals, as well as reducing oxidation of RNA and improving performance on memory tasks.[9,10] Alcar has analgesic properties, and has been shown to promote peripheral nerve regeneration and to improve vibration perception; it is potentially useful for improving nerve function in diabetics and human immunodeficiency virus (HIV) patients.[11] It has been shown to improve blood flow to the brain in stroke patients and improve symptoms of mild cognitive impairment and early Alzheimer's disease.[12] The supplementary dose of Car may be 2–3 g daily and the dose of Alcar may be 1.5–4 g daily.

Cysteine (Cys) and N-acetylcysteine (NAC)

Cys is a sulfur-containing amino acid that can be made from Met and can be converted to Tau and NAC, which is the supplemental form of Cys. NAC has antioxidant activity, is a constituent of the antioxidant glutathione and is a source of sulfhydryl (SH) groups required for detoxification. It is used intravenously as an antidote to paracetamol poisoning, and has mucolytic (mucus-loosening) activity.[13] It may be beneficial for HIV, drug or gambling addiction, obsessive-compulsive disorder, schizophrenia, bipolar disorder, Alzheimer's disease, chronic obstructive pulmonary disease and contrast-induced kidney damage.[13,14] The supplementary dose of NAC may be 1.2–2 g daily.

Glutamine (Gln)

Gln transfers nitrogen between molecules, and helps synthesise amino acids and protect the body from high levels of ammonia. It is essential for immunity, maintaining blood glucose levels and the integrity of the digestive tract and is a constituent of the antioxidant glutathione. Gln is useful for treating inflammation of the mucous membranes resulting from chemotherapy or radiation therapy for cancer, and has enhanced the action of chemotherapy drugs in cancer patients.[15] Gln may be beneficial for intensive care patients, and patients with HIV, muscle-wasting disorders or inflammatory bowel disease.[15,16] Gln supplementation improves the structure and function of the digestive tract lining and inhibits leaky gut (increased permeability of the gut) and movement of pathogens across the gut wall, which can occur in Crohn's disease, sepsis and the development of multi-organ failure in critically ill patients.[17,18] There are reports that Gln may be useful for hypoglycaemia and for reducing alcohol cravings in alcoholics, but supporting evidence is lacking. The supplementary dose may be 3–6 g daily or more.

Glycine (Gly)

Gly is a constituent of glutathione, and is an inhibitory neurotransmitter acting in noradrenaline-responsive nerve cells in the brain that regulate anxiety, arousal, fear and vigilance. By reducing noradrenaline release, Gly may relieve anxiety, insomnia related to anxiety, panic and addictive behaviour.[1] It has anti-spasmodic activity in muscles, and may relieve muscle tension, spasms, cramps and twitches.[1] The supplementary dose may be 4 g or more daily.

Histidine (His) and carnosine

His binds minerals and can help mineral absorption and detoxification of heavy metals. It converts to histamine, which is involved in inflammation, allergic responses, neurotransmission, regulation of gastric acid secretion, sexual function and memory. Carnosine (beta-alanyl-L-histidine) is made from His and found only in animal tissue. It helps to maintain body pH, binds metals, acts as an antioxidant and anti-inflammatory, and protects against the formation of advanced glycation and lipoxidation end-products that are damaging to tissues. Carnosine protects proteins from damage, enhances breakdown of damaged proteins and binds zinc ions, which may help protect against zinc-induced amyloid-beta buildup in the brain, a feature of Alzheimer's disease.[19] Carnosine has extended the lifespan of test animals.[20] It may be useful for improving exercise performance and for eye disease, ageing, neurological disorders, and diabetes and its complications.[19,21] The supplementary dose of His may be 4–5 g daily and the dose of carnosine may be 1 g daily.

Lysine (Lys)

Lys is required for the synthesis of connective tissues such as collagen and elastin, for production of Car that is used for converting fatty acids to energy, and for making antiviral antibodies and maintaining immunity. Proteins synthesised by herpesviruses have been found to contain more Arg and less Lys than normal body cells, and Arg is required for herpesviruses replication. Lys is believed to antagonise Arg by competitive inhibition of Arg absorption in the gut, reducing Arg reabsorption in kidney tubules and reducing its transport into cells. It also induces the enzyme arginase that breaks down Arg. Lys supplementation has been found to reduce the recurrence of herpesviruses outbreaks in some human studies, but not all studies have shown benefits.[22] The supplementary dose may be 1–3 g daily.

Methionine (Met) and S-adenosylmethionine (SAM)

Met is a sulfur-containing amino acid that converts to Cys and Tau, and supports folic acid metabolism, liver function and the detoxification of alcohol, heavy metals, pollutants and drugs. It is required for the formation of body tissues and the metabolism of carbohydrates, lipids and amino acids. Adequate Met is needed to make SAM, the sole methyl donor in a variety of reactions in the body. SAM-dependent methylation reactions are required for the synthesis and inactivation of the neurotransmitters adrenaline, histamine, noradrenaline, serotonin and dopamine, and for the metabolism of DNA, RNA, creatine, proteins within the central nervous system and phosphatidylcholine, which is an important constituent of cell membranes. Glutathione is produced in the liver by Met and SAM metabolism, and is important for antioxidant activity during liver detoxification. SAM has potential for the treatment of cholestasis (blockage of bile flow), hepatitis and cirrhosis.[23] Although SAM is an intermediate in the conversion of Met to homocysteine, a potentially toxic metabolite, oral SAM does not appear to elevate homocysteine levels.[24]

Impairment of methylation reactions affects the metabolism of important neurotransmitters that affect mood and behaviour. SAM has been found to increase the activity of serotonin-dependent pathways and act as an effective antidepressant, having similar efficacy to antidepressant drug therapy and fewer adverse effects.[25] Treatment with SAM has also relieved symptoms of arthritis in depressed patients, having similar efficacy to non-steroidal anti-inflammatory drugs (NSAIDs) but without the adverse effects.[26] The supplementary dose of Met may be 1.5–2.5 g daily and the supplementary dose of SAM for depression is about 1.6 g daily.

Phenylalanine (Phe)

Phe converts to Tyr and adrenal gland hormones, and is part of brain neuropeptides such as somatostatin, vasopressin, melanotropin, ACTH, substance P, enkephalin, angiotensin II and cholecystokinin. It is important for brain function, memory and alertness, and may have antidepressant activity. Unlike most other amino acids, the D form has been shown to be absorbed and converted to the L form in the body. The DL form of Phe has been used to relieve chronic pain, and both the DL and the L forms have been used to relieve depression.[27] The supplementary dose of DL-Phe may be 1–4 g or more daily, and the dose of L-Phe may be 1–14 g daily. Phe supplements should not be used in PKU and in patients on L-dopa for Parkinson's disease.

Taurine (Tau)

Tau, produced from Cys, helps regulate cell volume and mineral content, stabilises cell membranes and regulates calcium flux, thereby maintaining cell stability. It conjugates with cholesterol to form part of bile and has antioxidant and neurotransmitter activity. Like Gly and GABA, it is an inhibitory neurotransmitter. Tau has been shown to possess antioxidant properties and to regulate the release of inflammatory cytokines. Tau deficiency leads to severe cardiomyopathy, kidney and pancreatic dysfunction, and loss of photoreceptors in the retina in the eyes.[28] Tau has anti-diabetic, anti-epileptic and neuro-protective activity in animals, and is especially important for brain development and protection of nerve cells in the retina.[28] Tau is an essential amino acid for cats, and is low in plant foods; cats fed a vegetarian/vegan diet develop severe nerve damage. Tau may help prevent high blood pressure, stroke, atherosclerosis, non-alcoholic liver disease and metabolic syndrome.[29] The supplementary dose may be 1–6 g daily.

Tryptophan (Trp)

Trp was widely used as an effective insomnia treatment in the 1970s, but was banned for many years because of an episode of serious adverse effects from one form of supplement produced by a single manufacturer in Japan in the 1980s. This manufacturer used genetically engineered bacteria to produce Trp, which was sold in the United States and caused many cases of eosinophilia-myalgia syndrome, a nerve and muscle disorder. In severe cases, it resulted in paralysis and respiratory arrest and was linked to 37 deaths and 1500 cases of permanent disability. The cause was eventually traced to a toxic contaminant in the genetically engineered Trp. Trp in supplements on the market today is free of contamination, but the amount permitted in over-the-counter supplements is still restricted.

Trp is converted in the brain to the neurotransmitter serotonin (5-hydroxytryptamine), which helps to regulate the sleep–wake cycle and the emotions of pleasure, anxiety, panic, pain and arousal. Trp has been used for tension and irritability in premenstrual syndrome, insomnia, mood swings and low serotonin depression, and has been used with light therapy for seasonal affective disorder (SAD, depression caused by lack of unltraviolet light during the winter months).[30] It has been found to improve obstructive sleep apnoea but not central sleep apnoea. Trp depletion lowers mood, but the results of supplementation in depression are conflicting. Trp supplementation increases serotonin, and may lead to more cooperative and less argumentative behaviour.[31] It may also help smokers trying to quit by reducing withdrawal symptoms if used with a high carbohydrate diet.[32] Trp is available as L-Trp and the supplementary dose may be 1–6 g daily, but the dose in over-the-counter supplements in Australia is restricted to 100 mg or less daily. High doses of Trp should not be used with serotonin reuptake inhibiting drugs because of the possible risk of 'serotonin syndrome', in which excess serotonin levels cause agitation, confusion, delirium, rapid heartbeat, sweating and blood pressure fluctuations.

Tyrosine (Tyr)

Tyr is produced from Phe, and is required for the synthesis of thyroxine and melanin. It is converted to 3,4-dihydroxyphenylalanine (DOPA) and then to the neurotransmitters dopamine, noradrenaline and adrenaline. Tyr supplementation enhances dopamine release in the brain, and may be useful for depression, stress symptoms, cognitive function, Parkinson's disease and PKU.[33] Tyr is an essential amino acid for PKU patients because of their inability to tolerate its precursor, Phe. Tyr has been found to prevent the detrimental effects of stress, such as raised blood pressure, headache, tension, fatigue and impaired working memory and alertness.[33] The supplementary dose used in clinical trials is 100 mg/kg body weight daily.

Cautions

People taking drugs such as monoamine oxidase inhibitors, serotonin reuptake inhibitors, antidepressants and other drugs for psychiatric and neurological conditions should seek medical advice before taking amino acid supplements because some amino acids can interact with these medications. Amino acid supplements are not recommended for children or pregnant women because the effects are unknown.

REFERENCES

1 Meletis, C.D. & Barker, J.E., Therapeutic uses of amino acids, *Altern Compl Ther* (2005), 11(1): 24–8.

2 Böger, R.H., L-Arginine therapy in cardiovascular pathologies: Beneficial or dangerous? *Curr Opin Clin Nutr Metab Care* (2008), 11(1): 55–61.

3 Shimomura, Y. et al., Nutraceutical effects of branched-chain amino acids on skeletal muscle, *J Nutr* (2006), 136(2): 529S–32S.

4 Fujita, S. & Volpi, E., Amino acids and muscle loss with aging, *J Nutr* (2006), 136(1 Suppl): 277S–80S.

5 Charlton, M., Branched-chain amino acid enriched supplements as therapy for liver disease, *J Nutr* (2006), 136(1 Suppl): 295S–8S.

6 Choudry, H.A. et al., Branched-chain amino acid-enriched nutritional support in surgical and cancer patients, *J Nutr* (2006), 136(1 Suppl): 314S–18S.

7 Fernstrom, J.D., Branched-chain amino acids and brain function, *J Nutr* (2005), 135 (6 Suppl): 1539S–46S.

8 Kelly, G.S., L-Carnitine: Therapeutic applications of a conditionally-essential amino acid, *Altern Med Rev* (1998), 3(5): 345–60.

9 Hagen, T.M., Ingersoll, R.T. et al., Acetyl-L-carnitine fed to old rats partially restores mitochondrial function and ambulatory activity, *Proc Natl Acad Sci USA* (1998), 95(16): 9562–6.

10 Liu, J., Head, E. et al., Memory loss in old rats is associated with brain mitochondrial decay and RNA/DNA oxidation: Partial reversal by feeding acetyl-L-carnitine and/or R-alpha-lipoic acid, *Proc Natl Acad Sci USA* (2002), 99(4): 2356–61.

11 Chiechio, S., Copani, A., Nicoletti, F. & Gereau, R.W. IV, L-acetylcarnitine: A proposed therapeutic agent for painful peripheral neuropathies, *Curr Neuropharmacol* (2006), 4(3): 233–7.

12 Montgomery, S.A., Thal, L.J. & Amrein, R., Meta-analysis of double blind randomized controlled clinical trials of acetyl-L-carnitine versus placebo in the treatment of mild cognitive impairment and mild Alzheimer's disease, *Int Clin Psychopharmacol* (2003), 18(2): 61–71.

13 Kelly, G.S., Clinical applications of N-acetylcysteine, *Altern Med Rev* (1998), 3(2): 114–27.

14 Dean, O., Giorlando, F. & Berk, M., N-acetylcysteine in psychiatry: Current therapeutic evidence and potential mechanisms of action, *J Psychiatry Neurosci* (2011), 36(2): 78–86.

15 Miller, A.L., Therapeutic considerations of L-glutamine: A review of the literature, *Altern Med Rev* (1999), 4(4): 239–48.

16 Shabert, J.K., Winslow, C., Lacey, J.M., Wilmore, D.W., Glutamine-anti-oxidant supplementation increases body cell mass in AIDS patients with weight loss: A randomized, double-blind controlled trial, *Nutrition* (1999), 15: 860–4.

17 Hardy, G., Does glutamine enable severely ill intensive care patients to cope better with infection and increase their chance of survival? *Nutrition* (2002), 18: 712–13.

18 Den Hond, E., Hiele, M., Peeters M. et al., Effect of long-term oral glutamine supplements on small intestinal permeability in patients with Crohn's disease, *J Parenter Enteral Nutr* (1999), 23: 7–11.

19 Hipkiss, A.R., Carnosine and its possible roles in nutrition and health, *Adv Food Nutr Res* (2009), 57: 87–154.

20 Gallant, S., Semyonova, M. & Yuneva M., Carnosine as a potential anti-senescence drug, *Biochemistry (Mosc)* (2000), 65(7): 866–8.

21 Sale, C., Artioli, G.G., Gualano, B. et al., Carnosine: From exercise performance to health, *Amino Acids* (2013), 44(6): 1477–91.

22 [No authors listed]. Lysine monograph, *Altern Med Rev* (2007), 12(2): 169–72.

23 Lieber, C.S., S-adenosyl-L-methionine: Its role in the treatment of liver disorders, *Am J Clin Nutr* (2002), 76(5): 1183S–7S.

24 Goren, J.L., Stoll, A.L., Damico, K.E. et al., Bioavailability and lack of toxicity of S-adenosyl-L-methionine (SAMe) in humans, *Pharmacotherapy* (2004), 24(11): 1501–7.

25 Mischoulon, D. & Fava, M., Role of S-adenosyl-L-methionine in the treatment of depression: A review of the evidence, *Am J Clin Nutr* (2002), 76(5): 1158S–61S.

26 Bottiglieri, T., S-Adenosyl-L-methionine (SAMe): From the bench to the bedside: Molecular basis of a pleiotrophic molecule, *Am J Clin Nutr* (2002), 76(5): 1151S–7S.

27 [No authors listed]. Phenylalanine monograph, *Altern Med Rev* (2002): 305–9.

28 Ripps, H. & Shen, W., Review: Taurine—a 'very essential' amino acid, *Mol Vis* (2012), 18: 2673–86.

29 Imae, M., Asano, T. & Murakami, S., Potential role of taurine in the prevention of diabetes and metabolic syndrome, *Amino Acids* (2014), 46(1): 81–8.

30 [No authors listed] L-Tryptophan monograph, *Altern Med Rev* (2006), 11(1): 52–6.

31 Young, S.N., The effect of raising and lowering tryptophan levels on human mood and social behaviour, *Philos Trans R Soc Lond B Biol Sci* (2013), 25: 368(1615): 2011–375.

32 Bowen, D.J. et al., Tryptophan and high-carbohydrate diets as adjuncts to smoking cessation therapy, *J Behav Med* (1991), 14: 97–110.

33 [No authors listed]. Tyrosine monograph, *Altern Med Rev* (2007), 12(4): 364–8.

THE PREHISTORIC PALATE . . . A PREFERENCE FOR PROTEIN?

Evidence from fossils of early man indicates a larger cranium and brain, and smaller mandibles than other primates. Jaw and tooth development shows that early humans were suited to an omnivorous diet. Stone tools used for butchering animals and animal fossils showing butchering marks have been discovered, appearing at about the time of the appearance of early humans (*Homo habilis*). Analysis of the bone proteins in Neanderthals and Palaeolithic humans indicates that they were high-level carnivores, subsisting mainly on animal flesh and some fish. It has been proposed that the development of a larger brain was 'expensive' in terms of nutritional input, and should have required a large digestive system, yet humans have a relatively small digestive system. It is suggested that meat provided the required energy- and protein-dense food to drive the brain's growth, and the ensuing increased intelligence led to the development of more sophisticated tools for hunting, with the additional access to meat further increasing brain growth.[1]

Human genes are prehistoric, showing little evolutionary change over time, whereas there has been a major shift in diets away from high-protein, meat-based diets to high-carbohydrate, grain-based diets, coinciding with the introduction of agriculture. It is estimated that the first 100 000 generations of humans were hunter-gatherers, the next 500 generations were farmers, the next ten were industrialised farmers, and only the last two generations have been eaters of highly processed food.[1]

Professor Loren Cordain, of Colorado State University and author of *The Paleo Diet*,[1] has developed a hypothesis that the move away from an omnivorous hunter-gatherer diet of minimally processed wild plant and animal foods is responsible for many of the diseases prevalent in today's Western societies. He claims that humans have successfully existed on hunter-gatherer diets for 99.5 per cent of their ancestry, and their genome is well-adapted to such diets. He identifies key changes in modern diets compared with prehistoric diets which include:

- a shift from a protein-based to a carbohydrate-based diet
- an increase in glucose load (GL) because of increased carbohydrate intake
- a shift in fatty acid intake towards a higher omega-6 and lower omega-3 fat intake
- a decrease in micronutrient intake
- an increase in acidity in the diet, leading to a slight, chronic metabolic acidosis
- an increase in sodium and decrease in potassium intake
- a decrease in fibre intake, due to an emphasis on refined carbohydrates and sugars.

An analysis of the diets of hunter-gatherers worldwide shows that protein makes up 19–35 per cent of their energy intake, compared with about 15 per cent for modern diets.[2] Professor Cordain's paleo diet is based around foods eaten by hunter-gatherers, and emphasises minimally processed lean meat, chicken, seafood, fresh fruit and non-starchy vegetables, nuts and seeds. No grains, legumes, dairy products or processed foods are included. The diet is promoted for weight control and for reducing the risk of many common diseases such as type 2 diabetes, cardiovascular disease, osteoporosis, digestive disorders, acne, asthma and inflammatory diseases.

Professor Cordain has analysed the paleo diet to determine its ability to provide adequate macro and micronutrients.[3] The paleo diet provides 38 per cent protein, 39 per cent fat (10 per cent of this as saturated fat) and 23 per cent carbohydrate, in contrast to the modern Australian diet, which contains about 14–17 per cent protein, 33 per cent fat and 45–50 per cent carbohydrate.[4] The paleo diet was found to be superior in providing nutrients that help reduce the risk of cardiovascular disease, such as omega-3 fats, antioxidants, dietary fibre and vitamins, and is lower in sodium than regular diets. Vitamin D was an exception, being low in all diets because it is found in very few foods and mostly in very small amounts, but would be amply supplied by a hunter-gatherer lifestyle that involved regularly exposing the skin to the sun.

In a study carried out by Australian researchers, ten full-blood Aboriginal Australians were returned to their traditional country in north-western Australia to live as hunter-gatherers for seven weeks.[5] All were diabetic, middle-aged and overweight. The traditional hunter-gatherer diet they followed was low in kilojoules, 64 per cent of which came from animal foods, and low in fat (13 per cent) because the wild animals they ate had a very low fat content. All subjects lost weight steadily on the traditional diet. At seven weeks, there was a marked drop in fasting plasma triglycerides, decreases in blood glucose and insulin levels, and improved insulin release and glucose clearance after meals.

Typical diet of pre-European Aboriginal Australians[6]

- *Vegetables:* roots, tubers (rich in fructans), bulbs (murnong, vanilla lily, chocolate lily, fringe lily), yams, wild potatoes, native onions, aquatic plants (water ribbons, cumbungi, club rush), bracken—crushed and treated with fire ash before eating to reduce toxicity.
- *Seeds, nuts:* acacia seeds, pandanus nut, bunya bunya nut.
- *Fruit:* desert tomato, desert raisin, quandong, native fig, billygoat plum.
- *Animal foods:* bird's eggs, and the flesh, organs, bone marrow, fat, blood and stomach contents of lizards, small marsupials, rodents, kangaroo, wallaby, emu, turtles, mussels, oysters, crabs, magpie geese. The fat of animal food was highly prized.
- *Insects:* Bogong moth, witchetty grub, Cossid grub, green ant, honey ant.
- *Sugar:* honey, bloodwood apple (tree gall).

Studies of communities eating traditional diets provide evidence that the increasing epidemic of diabetes in Westernised countries, including Australia and the Pacific Islands, may be caused by modern diets high in kilojoules, processed foods and carbohydrates. These diets lead to obesity and metabolic abnormalities that may be corrected by a return to a higher protein, lower carbohydrate and lower kilojoule eating pattern, using 'stone age' diets as a model.

REFERENCES

1 Cordain, L. *The Paleo diet*, John Wiley & Sons, New York, 2002.
2 Cordain L., Eaton, S.B., Miller, J.B. et al., The paradoxical nature of hunter-gatherer diets: Meat-based, yet non-atherogenic, *Eur J Clin Nutr* (2002), 56(Suppl 1): S42–52.
3 Cordain, L., The nutritional characteristics of a contemporary diet based upon Paleolithic food groups, *JANA* (2002), 5(3): 15–24.
4 Australian Bureau of Statistics, *National Nutrition Survey: Nutrient intakes and physical measurements, Australia, 1995*. Available at <www.abs.gov.au>.
5 O'Dea, K., Marked improvement in carbohydrate and lipid metabolism in diabetic Australian Aborigines after temporary reversion to traditional lifestyle, *Diabetes* (1984), 33(6): 596–603.
6 O'Dea, K., Traditional diet and food preferences of Australian Aboriginal hunter-gatherers, *Philos Trans R Soc Lond B Biol Sci* (1991), 334(1270): 233–40; discussion 240–1.

HOW MUCH DO I KNOW?

Choose whether the following statements are true or false. Then review this chapter for the correct answers.

	True (T)	False (F)
1 An adult's body is 55–65 per cent water.	T	F
2 Up to 3000 mL of water per hour is lost during moderate exercise.	T	F
3 Weight drops by 1 kilogram for every litre of fluid lost.	T	F
4 A gram of carbohydrate provides 37 kJ of energy.	T	F
5 Glycogen stores can provide energy for several weeks of fasting.	T	F
6 Eating protein boosts BMR by up to 30 per cent.	T	F
7 Protein contains 16 per cent nitrogen.	T	F
8 Arginine is an essential amino acid for all adults.	T	F
9 Protein efficiency ratio is the best method of assessing protein quality.	T	F
10 A lack of protein can decrease immunity.	T	F

FURTHER READING

Gropper, S.S., Smith, J.L. & Groff, J.L., *Advanced nutrition and human metabolism*, 4th ed., Thomson Wadsworth, Belmont, CA, 2005.

3

Carbohydrates: available and unavailable

CARBOHYDRATE STATUS CHECK

1 Are you on a low-carbohydrate diet, and do you avoid eating grains, legumes, fruit and potatoes?
2 Do you fail to have a bowel movement every day?
3 Are your bowel motions often small, dry and difficult to pass?
4 Do you need laxatives to help your bowels function regularly?

'Yes' answers may indicate inadequate carbohydrate status. Note that a number of nutritional deficiencies or health disorders can cause similar effects and further investigation is recommended.

Carbohydrates are primarily plant substances that are made up of carbon, hydrogen and oxygen in ring-shaped units. Available carbohydrates are those that are digested by human digestive enzymes and serve as a primary fuel for body cells. Unavailable carbohydrates are those that either cannot be digested by human digestive enzymes or are very poorly digested, and therefore pass through to the large bowel (colon) relatively intact, where they are either fermented by bacteria or passed in faeces.

AVAILABLE CARBOHYDRATES

FAST FACTS . . . AVAILABLE CARBOHYDRATES

- Available carbohydrates include starch, found in potatoes, root vegetables, bananas, all types of grains and flour products, legumes, seeds and nuts, and sugars, found in fruit, vegetables, juices, molasses, maple syrup and honey, and added domestically or commercially to many foods and drinks.
- Available carbohydrates are used for energy, energy storage, forming part of the structure of non-essential amino acids, glycoproteins, glycolipids and connective tissue, and for sparing proteins from conversion to energy.
- A severe deficiency can cause ketosis.
- A high sugar intake may cause damage to body proteins, metabolic syndrome, abdominal obesity, fatty liver, elevated serum lipids, cardiovascular disease, hypoglycaemia, diabetes and behaviour problems.

Available carbohydrates are made up of sugar units (saccharides), and are classified according to the number of units they contain. They include monosaccharides (single sugars), disaccharides (two sugars) and polysaccharides (multiple sugars, known as starch). Monosaccharides include glucose, fructose, galactose and ribose; disaccharides include sucrose, lactose, maltose and trehalose; and polysaccharides include starch, dextrin and glycogen. About half of the available carbohydrate in the diet is in the form of starch from grains and starchy vegetables, and the rest is in the form of sugars that are naturally occurring in food—especially fruit—or are added as domestic or commercial sweeteners.

Digestion, absorption and metabolism

Dietary starch must be broken down to single sugar units by the digestive enzyme alpha-amylase before absorption. Disaccharides are broken down by specific enzymes such as sucrase, lactase and maltase to single sugars for absorption. Sugars are absorbed into the gut wall by various transporters, delivered to the bloodstream and taken up by the liver. The liver uses glucose from the diet and from the conversion of other monosaccharides in a number of ways. Some is used for energy in liver cells, some is stored as glycogen, some is converted to triglycerides and stored as fat and some is released into the bloodstream for use by other body cells. This circulating blood glucose, often referred to as blood sugar, is taken up by cells for fuel. Some tissues, such as skeletal and cardiac muscle and fat cells, are dependent on activity of the hormone insulin for the transfer of glucose from blood, whereas other tissues are insulin independent.

Monosaccharides

Monosaccharides, also called single sugars or simple sugars, are made up of one sugar unit. They are the smallest carbohydrate units and, as they do not need digestion, are absorbed intact in the intestine.

- *Glucose*, also called dextrose, is found in honey, maple syrup, fruit and some vegetables, such as corn and carrots, and is part of sucrose (table sugar). It is also used as a commercial sweetener. Glucose requires no digestive activity, and is very quickly absorbed by an active process involving the sodium-glucose transporter 1 (SGLT1). It is then transferred to the bloodstream by diffusion or a carrier, and is taken up by tissue cells via six glucose transporters, GLUT1–5 and GLUT7, which are specific to different tissues. GLUT6 appears to have no transporting activity. GLUT4, found in fat cells, the heart and skeletal muscle, is regulated by insulin. Glucose is used for energy production in cells or stored as glycogen in the liver and muscles.
- *Fructose*, also called laevulose or fruit sugar, is a monosaccharide that is part of sucrose, and is found in fruit and some vegetables. It has a slower and incomplete absorption in comparison to glucose, and the exact mechanism is unclear but appears to be dependent on GLUT5. Absorption of fructose is enhanced if it is eaten together with other sugars in food, which suggests that it may be absorbed also via a disaccharidase-related transport system. Fructose cannot enter most tissue cells because they lack GLUT5, and is delivered to the liver where it is mainly metabolised to triglycerides. In contrast to glucose, dietary fructose does not stimulate insulin release and is sometimes promoted—incorrectly—as a 'healthier' sugar.
- *Galactose* is found as part of other sugars, such as lactose and raffinose and polysaccharides such as galactans, agar and gum arabic. It is absorbed in the gut via SGLT1 and is readily taken up by the liver and converted to glucose. Galactose makes up part of the myelin sheath of nerve fibres in the brain.
- *Ribose* is a sugar found in cells as part of the genetic material ribonucleic acid (RNA) and as deoxyribose in deoxyribonucleic acid (DNA) but only small amounts are ingested in the diet.

Disaccharides

Disaccharides are made up of two monosaccharides joined together. They need to be broken down by digestive enzymes into individual sugar units for absorption. Lack of the enzyme required for digestion of a specific disaccharide leads to intolerance, with associated digestive disturbances such as bloating of the abdomen, colic, flatulence and diarrhoea.

- *Sucrose* consists of one glucose and one fructose unit, and is derived from sugar cane or sugar beets. It is used domestically and commercially as a common sweetener. It is naturally present in fruit and vegetables, but is obtained mainly from its use as an additive in many processed foods and drinks. In the gut, it is broken down by sucrase to glucose and fructose. It has a slower absorption than glucose.

- *Lactose* is made up of glucose and galactose, and is found in dairy products and as a commercial sweetener. In the gut, it is broken down to glucose and galactose by the enzyme lactase.
- *Maltose* is made up of two glucose units, and is found in germinating cereals, malt extract, breakfast cereals, bakery products and beer. It is also used as a commercial sweetener. In the gut, it is broken down to glucose units by maltase.
- *Trehalose* consists of two glucoses joined with a different linkage to that of maltose. The major dietary source is mushrooms, but it occurs naturally in insects, plants, fungi and bacteria, where it is a source of energy, a signalling molecule, and a protein and cell membrane protector. It can be used commercially as a sweetener, humectant (moisture-holder) and texturiser in bakery goods, beverages, confectionery, jams and breakfast cereals. It is rapidly broken down to glucose by the enzyme trehalase in the body.

Polysaccharides

Polysaccharides are made up of thousands of glucose units in straight or branched chains.

- *Starch* is a polysaccharide that is the storage form of energy in plants and a major form of carbohydrate in the diet. The main starchy foods are grains and flour products, legumes, potatoes and bananas. Starch exists in two forms: amylose and the major form, amylopectin, which makes up about 80–85 per cent of starch. Amylose is a straight-chain form containing 500 to 20 000 glucose units, and amylopectin is in the form of highly branched chains containing one to two million glucose units. Starch is found in plant tubers and seeds as granules that contain several million amylopectin and amylase molecules. In the gut, starch is first digested by alpha-amylase to maltose, maltotriose (a trisaccharide made of three maltose units), and branched alpha-dextrins, which are then broken down by maltase to glucose for absorption.
- *Dextrin* is formed from starch when long glucose chains are split into smaller units by heating, toasting bread or browning flour. It is broken down by isomaltase to maltose units during digestion.
- *Glycogen* is the storage form of carbohydrate in animals, and is mainly found in the liver and muscles. It has a similar structure to amylopectin, but has a more branched form. Glucose units can be split off from the ends of the chains when required for energy. It is degraded when animals die, and is not a significant carbohydrate in the diet.

Regulation of available carbohydrate levels

It is vital that there is sufficient glucose circulating in the blood at all times to supply tissues such as the central nervous system and red blood cells that use glucose predominantly but cannot store glycogen. The hormones insulin and glucagon help keep the amount of glucose circulating in the bloodstream within tight limits.

When blood glucose rises

After a meal—especially one rich in carbohydrate—hormones called incretins, produced in the lining of the small intestine, serve as an early warning system for the pancreas that glucose is arriving. These hormones work with the hormone insulin, secreted by beta cells of the pancreas in response to an increase in blood glucose, to lower blood glucose by stimulating glucose uptake by liver, muscle and fat cells (see Figure 3.1). Insulin promotes the use of glucose as fuel and inhibits the use of fat. It enhances glycogen synthesis in the liver and muscles, and encourages fat gain because it allows glucose to enter fat cells, boosts fat synthesis and prevents breakdown of stored fat. In the liver, insulin also decreases the production of ketones and glucose, and increases lipid and protein production. Insulin assists amino acid transport into cells and acts on a genetic level to alter cell messages that regulate protein synthesis, which enhances growth, DNA synthesis and cell replication.

When blood glucose drops

When blood glucose falls between meals or in fasting or starvation, the hormone glucagon is released from the alpha cells of the pancreas (see Figure 3.1). Glucagon boosts blood glucose levels by stimulating the breakdown of liver glycogen to glucose and the production of glucose in the liver; the resulting glucose is then released into the bloodstream to keep levels within normal limits. Glucagon also inhibits liver glycogen synthesis, because its role is to mobilise glucose rather than store it.

Other hormones can also increase blood glucose. In response to stress, adrenaline is released from the

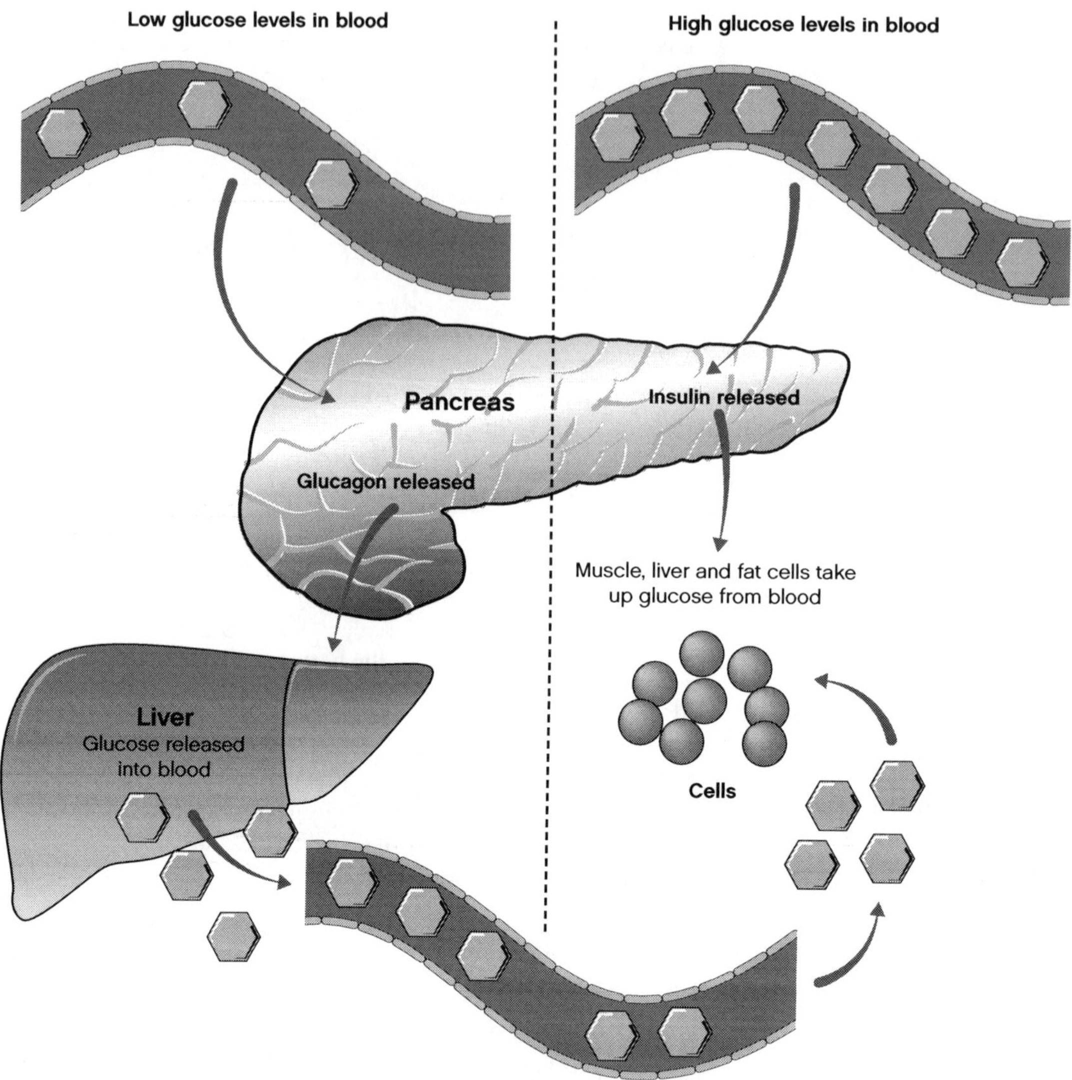

Figure 3.1 Blood glucose regulation

adrenal medulla and sympathetic nerves are activated in the pancreas to inhibit insulin and stimulate glucagon release and glycogen breakdown. In addition, glucocorticoids are released from the adrenal cortex to stimulate glucose synthesis in the liver and muscles. The end-result of the stress response is to make more glucose available for 'fight or flight' activities. Thyroxine produced in the thyroid gland enhances breakdown of glycogen and increases glucose uptake in the gut. Growth hormone, released from the pituitary gland, inhibits the uptake of glucose by tissues other than the liver.

Glycaemic index

The glycaemic index (GI) is a measure of the effect of a specific available carbohydrate food on blood glucose, and reflects the efficiency of digestion of the test food in terms of the amount absorbed and the speed of absorption. To obtain a GI value, a test food containing a set amount of carbohydrate is eaten and the total amount of glucose appearing in the bloodstream in a given time period after eating it (usually two hours) is measured. This value is compared to the GI value obtained over the same time period after eating an identical amount of carbohydrate as glucose (or white bread). As glucose is the standard, it is given a value of 100 and other foods are compared with this. Surprisingly, the GI of maltose is even higher, with a value of 105. Other foods have lower GI values than glucose.

A high GI value indicates that the food causes a fast and steep rise in blood glucose, and will therefore stimulate more insulin release than a lower GI food. For this reason, low GI foods are recommended for health and weight loss and for improving glucose intolerance and elevated insulin levels that are precursors to type 2 diabetes. Carbohydrate foods can be divided into low, intermediate and high GI (see Table 3.1).

Table 3.1 Glycaemic index (GI) categories (glucose = 100)

Low-GI food	=	less than 55
Intermediate-GI food	=	55–70
High-GI food	=	greater than 70

Low GI foods

- *Breakfast cereals:* **whole-grain or bran-based breakfast cereals**
- *Grains:* **buckwheat, bulgur, some white rice varieties, brown rice, pasta, barley**
- *Bread/crackers:* **whole-grain and multi-grain breads, fruit loaf, kibbled barley bread, mixed grain, oat, rye and pumpernickel breads, wholegrain crackers**
- *Cakes:* **most varieties**
- *Vegetables:* **most varieties**
- *Legumes:* **baked beans, most varieties of beans, split peas, chick peas, lentils**
- *Fruit:* **most varieties, raw or canned**
- *Dairy foods:* **whole, skim or flavoured milk, ice cream, yoghurt, custard**
- *Beverages:* **fruit juice, vegetable juice, soy milk**
- *Snack food:* **nuts, potato crisps, muesli bars**
- *Confectionery:* **chocolate**
- *Sugars:* **sucrose, fructose, lactose, honey**

High-GI foods

- *Breakfast cereals:* **most commercial breakfast cereals, instant oatmeal, rice porridge**
- *Grains:* **white rice, tapioca, noodles, gluten-free pasta**
- *Bread/crackers:* **white and wholemeal bread, rice crackers, water crackers, doughnuts, pancakes, pikelets, scones, corn and rice cakes**
- *Sweet snacks*: **some varieties of biscuits and cookies**
- *Vegetables:* **potatoes, sweet potatoes, pumpkin, yams**
- *Legumes:* **broad beans**
- *Fruit:* **melons, canned lychees**
- *Beverages:* **glucose drinks, non-diet soft drinks, sports drinks, rice milk**
- *Snack food:* **corn chips, pretzels, some varieties of fruit bars**
- *Confectionery:* **jelly beans**
- *Sugars:* **rice syrup, corn syrup, glucose, maltose (malt)**

Source: University of Sydney, *Glycemic Index*, <www.glycemicindex.com>.

GI limitations

GI only applies to carbohydrate-containing foods, and only if they are eaten as single foods. Once foods are combined into a meal, the GI value will change according to the presence of other food factors that may affect absorption, such as dietary fibre, protein, acids and fat. Research is incomplete, and the effect of meals rather than single foods has not been well researched.

GI values are obtained from 'normal', apparently healthy, individuals. However, people who are deficient in nutrients required for carbohydrate metabolism, such as magnesium, B vitamins and chromium, or people sensitive to carbohydrates, may react abnormally, making the values unreliable.

Low, intermediate and high GI values are arbitrary cut-off points set by researchers. GI values are merely a comparison of the effect of different carbohydrate foods, and all available carbohydrate foods will cause some increase in blood glucose levels and stimulate insulin responses. Eating a large amount of low-GI foods may be just as unhealthy as eating a small amount of high-GI foods. Also, low-GI foods may not be healthy because GI can be lowered by a high fat or sugar content.

Some foods are low in available carbohydrates, such as non-starchy vegetables, and because foods tested need to have the same carbohydrate quantity as the comparison food, large amounts have to be eaten. For example, if you wanted to compare the effect of 50 g of carbohydrate from broccoli with 50 g of glucose (which is pure carbohydrate), you would need to eat about sixteen cups of cooked broccoli. This is not a common pattern of eating by any means, and makes the GI value somewhat irrelevant. It is equally important to assess the total amount of available carbohydrate ingested, as that will also affect blood glucose levels.

Glycaemic load

Glycaemic load (GL) takes into consideration the GI of the food as well as the amount of carbohydrate consumed per standard serve, and is a more accurate indication of the total effect on blood glucose. To calculate the GL of a food, multiply the GI value of the food by the number of carbohydrate grams it contains and divide by 100—for example, the GI of a raw 120 g Braeburn apple from New Zealand is 32 and the carbohydrate content is 14.6 g, therefore the GL of the apple = (32 × 14.6)/100 = 4.7 (see <www.glycemicindex.com> for an online GI and GL calculator). Foods can be divided into low-, medium- and high-GL categories (see Table 3.2). For a whole day's food intake, a low GL is less than 80 and a high GL is more than 120.

Table 3.2 Glycaemic load (GL) categories

Low-GL food	=	10 or less
Medium-GL food	=	11 to 19
High-GL food	=	20 or more

High-GL foods include sultanas, dates, raisins, potatoes, sweet potatoes, yams, most varieties of pasta and noodles, white and brown rice, refined breakfast cereals, cornmeal, instant oatmeal, pancakes, rice cakes, rice milk, jellybeans and condensed milk. Low-GL foods include most fruit and vegetables, whole-grain/bran cereals, oatmeal, muesli, most varieties of bread, whole-grain crackers, yoghurt, soy milk and whole, low fat or skim milk.

Functions

The main function of available carbohydrates is to provide an immediate source of fuel for cell metabolism. Available carbohydrate functions include the following:

- *Energy production*. Available carbohydrates, as glucose, are a prime source of energy. One gram of available carbohydrate provides 16 kJ of energy. In normal conditions, there is about 3.5–7.8 mmol/L of glucose circulating in the bloodstream, with levels fluctuating throughout the day according to food intake. Body tissues dependent on glucose as a primary fuel include the brain, nervous system, red blood cells, mammary glands and testes.
- *Energy storage*. The liver stores about 100 g of glycogen, which can last for about a day if not replenished by eating. This is converted to glucose and released into the bloodstream when blood glucose levels drop. The body also stores about 400 g of glycogen in muscles for use only by muscle cells, and this storage capacity increases with exercise training. Glucose is the prime fuel for muscles during extended exercise, and is especially important for endurance activities. Excess available carbohydrates—especially fructose—are converted to triglycerides and stored in adipose tissue.

- *Synthesis of non-essential amino acids.* Available carbohydrates can be used to provide the carbon skeleton to which an NH_2 group from an amino acid is added to make a new amino acid.
- *Part of the structure of some tissues.* Ribose is part of nucleic acids in DNA and RNA and other available carbohydrates are part of glycoproteins in cell membranes that help cell identification, glycolipids in cell membranes that are responsible for defining the blood group in red blood cells, immunoglobulins that take part in immune responses and some connective tissue structures, such as the glycosaminoglycans in joint cartilage.
- *Protein-sparing activity.* If sufficient available carbohydrate is present, protein is spared from energy pathways, and can be used for its primary purpose of growth, repair and maintenance.

Dietary sources

Starch is found in potatoes and root vegetables, bananas, all types of grains and flour products, legumes, seeds and nuts. Sugars are naturally found in fruit, vegetables, juices, molasses, maple syrup and honey, and are added domestically or commercially to many foods and drinks. Table sugar (sucrose), glucose, lactose, maltose, fructose and grain syrups such as high-fructose corn syrup are common food additives, especially in bakery products, breakfast cereals, confectionery, soft drinks, fruit juice, cordials and snack foods.

Access the Food Standards Australia New Zealand Nutrient Database (NUTTAB) at <www.foodstandards.gov.au> for the amounts found in specific foods.

Factors influencing body status

Overall, available carbohydrates are well absorbed, and inhibiting factors have minor effects. Some of the monosaccharides and disaccharides in food can be lost through leaching out into processing or cooking water. When carbohydrates are heated, monosaccharides and amino acids—especially lysine—interact in the Maillard reaction, causing browning and flavour changes—for example, toasting bread, browning flour or roasting coffee. In the process, the carbohydrate and protein quality of the food is reduced.

The crystalline structure of starch granules affects digestibility. Granules with a larger A-type crystal structure, found in most grains, are better able to absorb water, swell up and lose their crystal form, which enhances absorption. B-type starch crystals are smaller and are not able to swell up as effectively, and are less digestible. Uncooked starch is less digestible than cooked starch because cooking causes the starch granules to break down, absorb water and become gelatinised, which improves digestibility. The presence of sugar—especially fructose—binds water and inhibits gelatinisation. Freshly cooked starchy food is absorbed better than raw starch, or starch that has been cooked and then cooled. Starch in intact whole grains (except for most varieties of rice) and starch with a high amylose content is less digestible, and the use of extrusion cooking in commercial food processing reduces digestibility.

Dietary fibre, which is indigestible, can surround other food components and partially block the action of digestive enzymes. Fat and protein can interact with starch, and phytate (myo-inositol hexaphosphate) in whole grains reduces starch absorption. Tannins in some cereals and legumes, tea and red wine form complexes with various digestive enzymes and reduce digestive activity. Dietary fibre, acids, protein and fat reduce emptying of the stomach and delay carbohydrate digestion. Deficiencies of B vitamins, magnesium, potassium, iron, zinc, copper, manganese or chromium may affect carbohydrate metabolism.

Daily requirement

There are no Australian government recommendations for daily carbohydrate intake, as insufficient data are available. It is estimated that the minimum amount of dietary carbohydrate to support basic energy production is about 50–100 g a day. The average Australian intake is 255 g a day, of which about 25 per cent is sugar. The National Health and Medical Research Council (NHMRC) of Australia recommends that carbohydrates make up about 45–60 per cent of total kilojoules. The lower level is more appropriate for people who are overweight and the upper level for people with additional needs, such as endurance athletes.

Deficiency effects

When carbohydrate intake is reduced and body stores of glycogen are depleted, the body produces ketones to provide energy (see Chapter 2: Energy). Adverse effects of ketosis induced by a low carbohydrate intake include:

- dehydration, because ketone excretion in urine also causes a loss of sodium and water
- a pH shift towards acidity that can lead to nausea, constipation, loss of appetite, irritability, headaches, weakness and fatigue. Calcium is mobilised from bones into the bloodstream in order to buffer the acidity, increasing the risk of osteoporosis and calcium-based kidney stones.
- constipation caused by dehydration and a low fibre intake.

Beneficial effects of a low carbohydrate intake include:

- weight loss because fat stores are mobilised to make ketones
- more loss of fat than lean tissue, which is a healthier form of weight loss
- reduced blood pressure, increased serum LDL cholesterol particle size, lower serum triglycerides and higher serum HDL cholesterol levels, possibly reducing heart disease risk
- reduced fasting blood glucose and improved insulin sensitivity, possibly reducing the risk of type 2 diabetes.

Effects of excess

Excess intake of sugars

It is estimated that Australians consume 119–136 g of sugar per person per day. Thirty per cent of the total sugar in Australian diets now comes from soft drinks and the rest mainly comes from prepared foods, with sugar intake from sweetened soft drinks, ice cream and cereals increasing markedly in recent years. Fructose intake has also climbed with the introduction of high-fructose corn syrup as a commercial sweetener in soft drinks, fruit juices and bakery products, and the use of apple juice, which contains 65 per cent fructose, as a sweetener. In Stone Age ('Paleo') diets, fructose was obtained from fruit and honey, and daily consumption is estimated to have been 16–20 g, but now intakes greater than 100 g a day are common.

Fructose may be considered suitable for diabetics because it has a relatively low GI and has less impact on blood glucose levels, but it should be avoided because it can contribute to metabolic syndrome, which is associated with abdominal obesity, cardiovascular disease (CVD), elevated blood glucose (hyperglycaemia), insulin resistance and type 2 diabetes. In contrast to glucose, fructose can encourage over-eating by suppressing release of the hormone leptin, which signals the brain to stop eating.

Fructose is readily taken up by the liver, where it bypasses an important regulatory step in glycolysis, leading to increased production of lactate and pyruvate. Elevated lactic acid may lead to anxiety attacks, fatigue and irritability. Excess pyruvate drives fat synthesis because the extra acetyl-CoA produced from pyruvate that is not used in the citric acid cycle is converted to triglycerides, which then build up in the bloodstream and accumulate in liver tissue. Fatty infiltration damages the liver and causes reduced sensitivity of liver cells to insulin (insulin resistance) and elevated levels of blood fats, cholesterol and homocysteine, a toxic metabolite of the amino acid methionine that is implicated in heart disease. A very high fructose intake can induce insulin resistance in as little as six days. A large, long-term population study in America found that one or more soft drinks or fruit punch drinks a day increases the risk of type 2 diabetes by 32 per cent.

Both fructose and glucose can damage body proteins if present in excessive amounts. These sugars bind to proteins, causing protein glycation and the formation of advanced glycation end-products (AGEs) that cause irreversible loss of protein function. AGEs may cause haemoglobin damage, capillary damage and accelerated ageing. They play a role in cataract development and in the disorders of the cardiovascular system, nerves, kidneys and retina that are complications of type 2 diabetes. Fructose also elevates uric acid levels, a risk factor for heart disease, and may trigger gout. Fructose intake has been linked to chronic diarrhoea, irritable bowel syndrome and other bowel disorders. As sucrose contains fructose, it can have similar adverse effects.

Excessive glucose can also cause undesirable effects because it leaves the stomach rapidly and quickly elevates blood glucose levels, stimulating insulin release and fat synthesis, and elevating triglyceride levels. Glucose stimulates inflammatory responses after ingestion, and these responses are heightened in people with metabolic syndrome. Elevated blood glucose levels in diabetics increase AGE formation, in a similar manner to fructose. Maltose has a slightly higher GI than glucose, and quickly elevates blood glucose levels and stimulates insulin release.

Sugar may be addictive. Animal studies show that a high sugar intake causes changes in the reward and pleasure centres of the brain similar to those caused by drugs of addiction, and animals fed sucrose are more likely to self-administer these drugs. Removing sugar from the diet can improve behaviour dramatically. Juvenile offenders in Los Angeles institutions were put on low-sugar diets, with one study showing a reduction in antisocial behaviour of 44 per cent and another study in rehabilitation camps showing a 54 per cent reduction. Another US study of institutionalised juvenile offenders, in which junk foods were replaced with healthy foods, showed a 100 per cent drop in suicide attempts, a 75 per cent drop in the use of restraints to prevent self-harm, a 42 per cent drop in the incidence of disruptive behaviour and a 25 per cent drop in fights and assaults. Studies on sugar and children with behaviour problems have shown conflicting results, but many parents and teachers remain convinced that low-sugar diets lead to calmer, more cooperative children.

Excess high-GL foods

Blood glucose abnormalities are related to a high-GL diet. In some individuals, reactive hypoglycaemia may occur, possibly because of an over-response of the body to insulin and a subsequent fast and steep drop in blood glucose (see 'Sugar lows'). Glucose intolerance and insulin resistance, characterised by elevated fasting blood glucose and insulin levels, and type 2 diabetes are possible outcomes of a long-term high GL diet.

Frequent sugar consumption and sticky forms of sugary foods that adhere to the teeth are associated with a higher risk of dental caries. Sugars and other carbohydrates are fermented by oral bacteria to produce acids that cause tooth erosion. Processed carbohydrates and sugars can deplete the body of micronutrients by a parasitic effect because they use up vitamins and minerals for their metabolism but cannot supply them because they have largely been removed or destroyed during the manufacturing process. Nutrients that may be depleted include B vitamins, magnesium, potassium, iron, zinc, copper, manganese and chromium.

A number of health disorders may be associated with high-GL diets, including CVD, metabolic syndrome, obesity, gout, joint pain, dental caries, behavioural disorders in children and adolescents, such as attention deficit hyperactivity disorder (ADHD), anti-social behaviour, hostility and aggression, and some cancers, such as colorectal, gastric and breast cancer. However, these disorders are multifactorial, and genetic factors play an important part. It may be that these disorders only occur in individuals who have either inherited or acquired a sensitivity to high carbohydrate intakes. Even if the diet is based around high-fibre foods and is low in simple sugars, a high carbohydrate intake can elevate serum triglyceride levels by as much as 60 per cent in individuals predisposed to this condition. High-fibre foods do not drive triglyceride synthesis to the same extent as simple sugars, but may reduce clearance of fats from the bloodstream.

SUGAR LOWS: REACTIVE HYPOGLYCAEMIA

Reactive hypoglycaemia (RH), also called 'postprandial reactive hypoglycaemia', 'functional hypoglycaemia', 'relative hypoglycaemia' or 'essential hypoglycaemia', refers to a condition in which blood glucose temporarily drops to a low level, usually in reaction to a meal, and deprives the brain and nerves of their main energy source, causing impairment of function. Hypoglycaemic episodes can also occur in diabetics who are given too much insulin and as a result of stomach surgery, a pancreatic tumour or pancreatic enlargement, but RH is not related to any pathology. For this reason, RH is considered to be a phantom disease by many medical practitioners because it is particularly hard to identify and symptoms may be dismissed as 'all in the mind'. The mind is certainly affected, but the condition is a real one, and its existence and mechanisms have been identified.

RH occurs more commonly in very lean individuals, in people who have lost a significant amount of weight, in women when fasting, and in women who carry excess weight on the hips and thighs (gynoid obesity).[1] Episodes are often triggered by carbohydrates, especially high-GL meals or snacks. In response to carbohydrate intake, blood glucose levels rise and insulin is released causing a drop in blood glucose to lower than normal levels, usually about two to four hours after eating. The brain and nerves are temporarily deprived of fuel when blood glucose drops. The body perceives this as an emergency, and sends signals to eat sweet food to restore blood glucose to normal. Symptoms occur because the drop in blood glucose affects brain and nerve function (neuroglucopenic symptoms) or because of the hormonal response to this (adrenergic symptoms). Neuroglucopenic symptoms include headaches, hypothermia, visual disturbances, slurred speech, cognitive impairment and seizures. Adrenergic symptoms result from the release of adrenal gland hormones such as adrenaline in response to the stress of low blood glucose, and include hunger, weakness, sweating, flushing, rapid heart rate, palpitations and tremors. Adrenergic symptoms are prominent in RH.

Low-blood glucose episodes often occur mid-morning and mid-afternoon, and can occur in the middle of the night, first thing in the morning or when meals are delayed or missed. Symptoms are usually improved or abolished by eating.

Symptoms reported in RH[2]

- Nervousness, irritability, exhaustion
- Faintness, dizziness, tremors, cold sweats
- Depression, migraine headaches, insomnia, digestive disturbances
- Forgetfulness, mood swings, anxiety, aggression, violence, anti-social behaviour
- Sugar addiction, drug addiction, alcoholism
- Mental confusion, limited attention span, lack of concentration, learning disability
- Low libido
- Itching and crawling sensation on the skin
- Blurred vision
- Phobias, fears, nightmares, neurodermatitis, restless legs syndrome
- Bedwetting and hyperactivity in children.

Key features of RH

- Sudden episodes of fatigue or sleepiness, often mid-morning or mid-afternoon
- Mood swings, mental confusion, depression, episodes of panic, crying, irritability, anger
- Headaches
- Nausea, weakness, blackouts, speech difficulties, incoordination, heart palpitations
- Insomnia, which features disturbed sleep, waking in the early morning, night hunger episodes and needing to eat in order to go back to sleep
- Over-eating, binge eating, cravings for sweet foods, sugar, confectionery, alcohol, drugs or stimulants.

A number of health disorders may be associated with RH, including food allergies, premenstrual syndrome, Ménière's disease, tinnitus, alcoholism, drug addiction, epilepsy, behaviour problems in children, anti-social or criminal behaviour, and obesity.

Causes of RH

The cause of RH has been difficult to determine. People who experience RH symptoms without abnormally low blood glucose levels may have an increased adrenergic sensitivity.[3] Others, whose symptoms occur when blood glucose is abnormally low, may have a dysfunction of glucose regulation—in some cases, an exaggerated insulin response and in others an increased sensitivity to insulin and a reduced glucagon release and sensitivity. It is estimated that increased insulin sensitivity accounts for 50–70 per cent of RH cases,[1] and this is worsened by a high-carbohydrate, low-fat diet and also by a very low-kilojoule diet. Alcohol can be a trigger, especially if taken together with a sugar-containing beverage—for example, a gin and tonic—causing increased insulin response and reduced glucose release from the liver. Alcohol directly inhibits glucose production, and it may also inhibit the release of glucose precursors—particularly alanine—from muscles.

Deficiencies of nutrients required for carbohydrate metabolism, such as low levels of vitamins B1, B2, B3 and B5, chromium, magnesium, manganese, zinc or potassium, may aggravate the condition. Stress, physical or mental exhaustion, drugs, stimulants, allergies and hormonal changes related to the menstrual cycle may also contribute.

Diagnosing RH

RH symptoms often occur when blood glucose levels drop below 3.3 mmol/L. The standard two-hour glucose tolerance test (GTT) is not regarded as a suitable test, although it is the one most commonly used, because it tests blood glucose under the artificial conditions of being given 75 g of oral glucose on an empty stomach. It is designed to detect diabetes, and patients are required to follow a diet containing 150 g of carbohydrate for three days prior to the test, with a fast for eight hours beforehand. Blood glucose levels are assessed before the glucose is ingested and at one hour and two hours afterwards, usually not a long enough time period for detecting an RH episode.

Indicators of RH that may occur during the GTT include a fasting blood glucose level below normal, a sharp fall in blood glucose during the test that occurs simultaneously with symptoms, and a slow return of blood glucose to normal. However, pure glucose appears to trigger a stronger insulin response than that of mixed meals, and may lead to an RH episode in people who do not experience RH in everyday life. Dr George Samra, an Australian medical practitioner specialising in RH, recommends using a four-hour GTT, with no dietary restrictions or fasting beforehand, and readings taken before the test and then every half-hour.[2]

Dr Samra's guidelines for diagnosing hypoglycaemia during a four-hour GTT[4]

- A sudden drop in blood glucose, with a rate of descent greater than 2.6 mm/L in any hour, or greater than 1.6 mm/L in any half-hour
- A fasting reading or any other reading less than 3.4 mm/L
- No reading greater than 1.3 mm/L above fasting, possibly indicating a low metabolic rate and hypothyroidism
- A normal GTT but the presence of hypoglycaemic symptoms, possibly caused by nutritional deficiencies.

The hyperglucidic breakfast test

This test is recommended as a more accurate diagnostic procedure in RH.[1] The breakfast consists of 80 g of bread with 10 g of butter and 20 g of jam, and coffee containing 2.5 g of powdered coffee, 80 g of skim milk and 10 g of sugar. This provides about the same amount of carbohydrate as is given before a GTT. In a study using this breakfast as a diagnostic tool, blood glucose dropped below 3.3 mmol/L in almost half of subjects suspected of having RH but in only 2.2 per cent of control subjects.

Treating RH

The overall approach to RH is to use a low-GL diet based on high protein, moderate fat and low carbohydrate with five to six small meals eaten at three-hour intervals throughout the day. By the time hunger occurs, blood glucose levels may already have dropped, so it is important to eat by the clock rather than waiting until hungry. Fibre helps to slow down the release of glucose into the bloodstream, and also prevents constipation. Because a low-carbohydrate diet can be lower in fibre unless legumes are eaten regularly, a fibre supplement can be used with meals.

The following foods and drinks should be avoided completely during the initial few weeks of treatment; when symptoms have improved, they can be included very occasionally but always as part of a mixed meal:

- caffeine-containing and alcoholic beverages
- sugar, fructose, honey, molasses, treacle, golden syrup, maple syrup, malt extract, rice syrup, fructose and all simple sugars
- processed carbohydrates such as white flour, white rice and foods containing these ingredients, such as crackers, pretzels, crisps, dry biscuits, sweet biscuits, pastries, cakes
- potatoes
- fruit, canned, stewed or fresh—especially bananas, grapes and dried fruit
- fruit and vegetable juices, sweetened beverages, soft drinks
- confectionery, desserts, sweet snack foods.

The diet should consist mainly of low GL foods, including:

- legumes—beans, peas, chickpeas, lentils
- seeds, nuts
- meat, fish, poultry, eggs
- dairy foods or soy substitutes
- non-starchy vegetables
- whole grains and fresh fruit, in small quantities only and as part of a mixed meal
- supplementary fibre added to foods, such as linseeds, guar gum, glucomannan, psyllium husks.

Recommended eating habits for RH

- Have five or six small meals per day.
- Eat every two to three hours.
- Have a protein-containing or savoury snack between meals.
- Have a substantial low-GI breakfast soon after rising.
- Never skip meals or snacks.
- Never fast or go too long without eating.
- Eat according to the clock, not according to hunger pangs—for example, breakfast at 7 a.m., snack at 10 a.m., lunch at 1 p.m., snack at 4 p.m., dinner at 7 p.m. and snack at 10 p.m.

For most people with RH, correcting the diet can relieve or totally abolish symptoms, but the diet must be continued long term. Nutritional supplementation with vitamins B1, B2, B3 and B5, chromium, magnesium, manganese and zinc is recommended, especially if symptoms persist. By ensuring an adequate supply of nutrients to support carbohydrate metabolism, occasional lapses in the diet will have less impact.

REFERENCES

1 Brun, J.F., Fedou, C. & Mercier, J., Postprandial reactive hypoglycemia, *Diabetes Metab* (2000), 26(5): 337–51.
2 Hypoglycemic Health Association of Australia, *What is hypoglycaemia?* Available at <www.hypoglycemia.asn.au>.
3 Berlin, I., Grimaldi, A., Landault, C., et al., Suspected postprandial hypoglycemia is associated with beta-adrenergic hypersensitivity and emotional distress, *J Clin Endocrinol Metab* (1994), 79(5): 1428–33.
4 Samra, G., *The hypoglycemic connection* (1984) MINT, Sydney.

SUGAR HIGHS: THE EMERGING EPIDEMIC OF DIABETES MELLITUS

Like an iceberg, the true number of diabetics is hidden because about 50 per cent of people with diabetes do not know they have it.[1] Worldwide, there are about 150 million people with diabetes, and this is expected to soar to 300 million by 2025.[2] In Australia, the number of people with diabetes has doubled over the last twenty years; more than 7 per cent of Australian adults have diabetes and 16 per cent have a pre-diabetic condition.[1]

What is diabetes?

Diabetes means that blood glucose levels remain above normal, even when fasting, and rise dramatically after eating. When blood glucose levels rise after eating, insulin is needed to transfer glucose into muscle and fat cells. When something goes wrong with this mechanism, a high proportion of glucose remains in the bloodstream, and is unable to be completely reabsorbed in the kidneys, leading to glucose in the urine.

About 10–15 per cent of diabetics have type 1 diabetes, in which the cells in the pancreas that make insulin are destroyed by autoimmune attack and insulin cannot be secreted.[2] It is common in young people under the age of 30 years, and may be triggered by a viral infection or chemical exposure in people with a genetic predisposition. Recent research indicates that a lack of sun exposure, with a consequent vitamin D deficiency, may be an important factor. A worldwide study found that type 1 diabetes was virtually non-existent in regions with high sunlight.[3] Children in Finland given 2000 IU vitamin D daily from one year of age had about 80 per cent lower risk of developing type 1 diabetes over the next 30 years, and children with symptoms of rickets, the classic vitamin D deficiency disease, at one year of age had three times the risk of subsequently developing type 1 diabetes.[4]

In the more common form, type 2 diabetes, body cells become resistant to insulin. In the early stage, the body tries to produce more insulin and insulin levels increase. However, it is less effective and blood glucose is higher than normal, but not high enough to be diagnosed as diabetes. This is called 'pre-diabetes', and includes impaired fasting glucose (high blood glucose not related to food intake) and impaired glucose tolerance (an abnormally large rise in blood glucose after ingestion of glucose). Over time, blood glucose rises into the diabetic range and a formal diagnosis is made, usually by urine testing and a two-hour GTT, in which blood glucose levels are taken before and during the two hours after a drink containing 75 g of pure glucose.

Standard two-hour GTT values[5]

- *Normal:* fasting blood glucose less than 5.5 mmol/L; blood glucose less than 7.8 mmol/L at two hours.
- *Impaired glucose tolerance:* fasting blood glucose less than 5.5 mmol/L; blood glucose 7.8–11.0 mmol/L at two hours.
- *Impaired fasting glycaemia:* fasting blood glucose 5.5–6.9 mmol/L; blood glucose less than 7.8 mmol/L at two hours.
- *Diabetes mellitus:* fasting blood glucose greater than 7.0 mmol/L; blood glucose greater than 11.1 mmol/L at two hours.

Eventually, the beta cells in the pancreas may fail altogether, and insulin injections are required. The end result is the same as for type 1 diabetes, but it is possible to re-sensitise cells to insulin in the early stage while the beta cells are still working.

Who is at risk of diabetes?

Type 2 diabetes is largely a lifestyle and genetic disease. The main lifestyle factors are lack of activity, weight gain—especially around the waist (abdominal obesity)—and a poor diet. It is strongly associated with metabolic syndrome, a cluster of disorders that includes diabetes or pre-diabetes together with high blood pressure, obesity, abnormal blood fat and cholesterol levels and protein in the urine (proteinuria).[6]

During pregnancy, some women develop high blood glucose levels (gestational diabetes) and deliver large babies (over 4 kg). Although blood glucose returns to normal after the baby is born, this condition increases the risk of type 2 diabetes later in life. Women with polycystic ovarian syndrome (PCOS), in which they develop ovarian cysts and are infertile because they fail to ovulate, are at increased risk. About 30–50 per cent of women with PCOS develop pre-diabetes or type 2 diabetes by the age of 30 years.[2] Diabetes risk is also higher in Aboriginal Australians, Pacific Islanders and people of Asian and Indian backgrounds.

How do you know if you have diabetes?

The short answer is that you probably won't know. If you have a family history of diabetes, carry a lot of weight around your waistline or have any of the following symptoms, it is essential to visit a health care practitioner for a blood glucose check.

Some common symptoms of diabetes[2]

- Increased thirst
- Increased hunger
- Tiredness
- Increased urination
- Increased appetite, weight loss (more common in type 1 diabetes), overweight (more common in type 2 diabetes)
- Blurred vision
- Sores that do not heal
- Susceptibility to infections, such as thrush.

How diabetes causes damage

Because diabetics have a shortage of glucose at the cell level and cannot make energy in the normal way, the body's emergency systems for coping with starvation switch on, and fats and protein are converted to ketones that are used for energy instead. This can lead to ketoacidosis, a buildup of acidic ketones that can cause irritability, nausea, headaches, weakness and fatigue, more commonly affecting type 1 diabetics. The body can become too acidic, tissues are damaged and, because glucose and ketones are excreted in urine, urine frequency increases and losses of water, sodium and potassium occur. In severe cases, ketoacidosis, dehydration or hypoglycaemia caused by an overdose of diabetic medication can result in a coma.

High levels of glucose in the blood inhibit protein function by causing protein glycation and the formation of AGEs. Glucose binds to haemoglobin in red blood cells, forming glycated haemoglobin (HbA_{1c}), and this is used as a measure of diabetes control. Diabetes can lead to atherosclerosis, heart disease, stroke, blindness, kidney disease, skin ulcers, gum infections and poor circulation in the extremities, possibly leading to amputation of limbs.

Reducing the risk of type 2 diabetes

- *Weight control.* Obesity is a global epidemic, increasing along with the rise in diabetes. A body mass index (BMI) in the overweight or obese range increases risk significantly (see Chapter 2: Table 2.4). A large Australian study found that 60 per cent of adults were overweight or obese, with more women obese than men.[7]
- *Waist control.* Waist measurement is an even better indicator of risk than BMI. Fat stored around the waist is linked to glucose intolerance and high blood pressure, blood fats and cholesterol. There is an increased risk of diabetes and CVD in people with a waist measurement of more than 80 cm for women and 94 cm for men. A Canadian study found that, in subjects with elevated blood fat levels, more than half of men and nearly 80 per cent of women with abdominal obesity had glucose intolerance or type 2 diabetes, and they developed heart disease symptoms five years earlier than those with normal waistlines.[8] In contrast, large hips and thighs are associated with a lower risk of type 2 diabetes.[9]
- *Replace high-GL carbohydrates with protein and low-GL carbohydrates.* Meals high in quickly absorbed carbohydrate foods drive blood glucose levels higher and cause large demands on insulin. All carbohydrates, even low GL types, have some impact on blood glucose because they break down to glucose during digestion. Diabetic men who increased their intake of protein and reduced

carbohydrates had dramatically improved glucose tolerance and a reduced amount of HbA_{1c}.[10] High-protein diets may improve glucose tolerance by reducing demand for insulin and providing more of the branched chain amino acid leucine that helps regulate insulin function.[11] Dr Manny Noakes, of the Commonwealth Scientific and Industrial Research Organisation (CSIRO) in Australia, compared a high-protein, low-fat diet with a high-carbohydrate, low-fat diet in overweight and obese women, and found that the high-protein diet resulted in greater weight and fat loss and there were fewer drop-outs. This diet became the basis of the best-selling book *The Total Wellbeing Diet*[12] that is recommended for weight loss and reducing diabetes risk.

- *Drink coffee.* Regular heavy coffee drinkers have 35 per cent less risk of developing type 2 diabetes compared with those with the lowest consumption.[13] Consumption of decaffeinated coffee is also associated with a reduced risk, although the effect is not as pronounced.[14] Although coffee intake increases insulin resistance in the short term, long-term intake appears to be protective. Coffee contains important nutrients, including potassium, magnesium, vitamin B3 and antioxidants, such as tocopherols and phytochemicals, including chlorogenic acid. Chlorogenic acid improves glucose tolerance and decreases blood cholesterol and fat levels, and a high magnesium intake has been shown to reduce risk of type 2 diabetes.[13]
- *Exercise.* During exercise, glucose uptake by working muscles rises many times higher than the resting level. Regular exercise improves sensitivity to insulin, stabilises blood glucose, assists weight loss and lowers blood fat levels and can delay or prevent type 2 diabetes and diabetes-related mortality. Exercise and modest weight loss have been shown to lower the risk of type 2 diabetes by up to 58 per cent in high-risk populations.[15]

REFERENCES

1 Dunstan, D., Zimmet, P., Welborn, T., et al., The rising prevalence of diabetes and impaired glucose tolerance: The Australian Diabetes, Obesity and Lifestyle Study, *Diabetes Care* (2002), 25: 829–34.

2 International Diabetes Institute, What is Diabetes Fact Sheet. Available at <www.diabetes.com.au>.

3 Mohr, S.B., Garland, C.F., Gorham, E.D. & Garland, F.C., The association between ultraviolet B irradiance, vitamin D status and incidence rates of type 1 diabetes in 51 regions worldwide, *Diabetologia* (2008), 51(8): 1391–8.

4 Hypponen, E., Läärä, E., Reunanen, A. et al., Intake of vitamin D and risk of type 1 diabetes: A birth-cohort study, *Lancet* (2001), 358(9292): 1500–3.

5 Royal College of Pathologists of Australasia, *RCPA manual*, available at <www.rcpamanual.edu.au>.

6 Zimmet, P., Alberti, K. & Shaw, J., Global and societal implications of the diabetes epidemic, *Nature* (2001), 414: 782–7.

7 Cameron, A.J., Welborn, T.A., Zimmet, P.Z. et al., Overweight and obesity in Australia: The 1999–2000 Australian Diabetes, Obesity and Lifestyle Study (AusDiab), *Med J Aust* (2003), 178(9): 427–32.

8 St-Pierre, J., Lemieux, I., Perron, P. et al., Relation of the 'hypertriglyceridemic waist' phenotype to earlier manifestations of coronary artery disease in patients with glucose intolerance and type 2 diabetes mellitus, *Am J Cardiol* (2007), 99(3): 369–73.

9 Snijder, M.B., Dekker, J.M., Visser, M. et al., Associations of hip and thigh circumferences independent of waist circumference with the incidence of type 2 diabetes: The Hoorn Study, *Am J Clin Nutr* (2003), 77(5): 1192–7.

10 Nuttall, F.Q. & Gannon, M.C., The metabolic response to a high-protein, low-carbohydrate diet in men with type 2 diabetes mellitus, *Metabolism* (2006), 55(2): 243–51.

11 Layman, D.K. & Baum, J.I., Dietary protein impact on glycemic control during weight loss, *J Nutr* (2004), 134(4): 968S–73S.

12 Noakes, M. & Clifton, P. (2005), *The CSIRO Total Wellbeing Diet*, Ringwood: Penguin.
13 van Dam, R.M. & Hu, F.B., Coffee consumption and risk of type 2 diabetes: A systematic review, *JAMA* (2005), 294(1): 97–104.
14 Salazar-Martinez, E., Willett, W.C., Ascherio, A. et al., Coffee consumption and risk for type 2 diabetes mellitus, *Ann Intern Med* (2004), 140(1): 1–8.
15 Colberg, S.R., Albright, A.L., Blissmer, B.J. et al., American College of Sports Medicine, American Diabetes Association, Exercise and type 2 diabetes: American College of Sports Medicine and the American Diabetes Association: Joint position statement. Exercise and type 2 diabetes. *Med Sci Sports Exerc* (2010), 42(12): 2282–303.

UNAVAILABLE CARBOHYDRATES

FAST FACTS . . . UNAVAILABLE CARBOHYDRATES

- Unavailable carbohydrates include sugar alcohols, oligosaccharides, resistant starch, chitin, chitosan and dietary fibre.
- They assist bowel function, protect the bowel lining and enhance the growth of beneficial bowel bacteria.
- They also increase excretion of dietary cholesterol, have anti-inflammatory activity, reduce the risk of obesity and improve glycaemic control.
- They may be beneficial for irritable bowel syndrome and inflammatory bowel disease, and for the prevention of bowel cancer and diverticular disease.

Unavailable carbohydrates are plant substances that are either indigestible or partially digestible because they are resistant to human digestive enzymes. Many unavailable carbohydrates pass through to the colon, where they are fermented by bacteria, and others are neither digested nor fermented; these pass through the digestive tract intact, and are excreted in faeces. Unavailable carbohydrates include sugar alcohols, oligosaccharides, resistant starch and dietary fibre.

Sugar alcohols

Sugar alcohols (polyols) are carbohydrates with a chemical structure similar to that of sugar and alcohol. Chemically, polyols are hydrogenated sugars, having an additional hydroxyl group (-OH), and they have a slower rate of absorption than sugars. Hydrogenated monosaccharides include dulcitol, erythritol, mannitol, sorbitol and xylitol, and hydrogenated disaccharides include isomalt, lactitol and maltitol. Polyols occur naturally in small amounts in fruit and vegetables, and are also commercially produced from available carbohydrates. Although they are called sugar alcohols, they do not contain ethanol and have no alcoholic effect.

Most polyols cannot be fully digested, and only provide about half the kilojoules of other sugars. They have less effect on blood glucose levels than sugars and a low GI. For this reason, they are used commercially in diabetic foods and sugar-free foods as low-kilojoule sweeteners. As well as tasting sweet, they add bulk and texture, retain moisture and provide a cooling sensation when used in food products. Polyols are resistant to metabolism by oral bacteria, and do not increase the acidity of the mouth after ingestion. Therefore, they do not erode tooth enamel and cause caries. Because polyols, with the exception of erythritol, are not digested completely, some of them pass into the colon where they can be fermented by bacteria.

A drawback of most polyols is that large amounts have a laxative effect because their presence draws fluids into the colon and bowel movements are stimulated in order to remove them from the body. This can lead to bloating, flatulence, colic and diarrhoea, and may contribute to irritable bowel syndrome. A warning about this laxative effect is required on food labels if the total content exceeds 2 g per maximum recommended daily dose.

Polyols include the following:

- *Erythritol* occurs naturally in fruit such as pears, melons and grapes, as well as mushrooms and fermented foods such as wine, soy sauce and cheese. It tastes like sucrose but is only 70 per cent as sweet.

In contrast to other polyols, erythritol is well absorbed and is not fermented by bacteria in the colon, so has very little laxative effect. After absorption, it is not metabolised and passes out of the body within 24 hours. It provides only 0.84 kJ per gram, and is used as a sweetener in low-kilojoule or reduced-kilojoule foods designed for weight control.

- *Mannitol* occurs naturally in exudates from trees, and in mushrooms and seaweed. It has about half the kilojoules and sweetness of sucrose, and is used commercially in the powder coating of stick chewing gum and chocolate-flavoured coatings because it does not pick up moisture (non-hygroscopic activity) and helps retain moisture (humectant activity).
- *Sorbitol* is found in fruit, and is formed naturally in the body from glucose by the enzyme aldose reductase. It is about 60 per cent as sweet as sucrose, with about two-thirds of the kilojoules, and is made commercially from corn syrup for use as a low-kilojoule sweetener, humectant and texturising agent. Sorbitol is used in diabetic foods as a sugar substitute, and as an ingredient in sugar-free gums and confectionery. In the body, elevated sorbitol production—which is associated with high blood glucose levels—can cause damage to the nerves and retina of the eyes, and contribute to cataract formation.
- *Xylitol* is also called 'wood sugar', and occurs naturally in corn cobs, fruit, vegetables, mushrooms and some cereals. It has the same relative sweetness as sucrose, with about 40 per cent fewer kilojoules. Produced commercially from trees and vegetable fibre, it is found in chewing gum, gum drops and hard confectionery, and in health products such as throat lozenges, cough syrups, chewable vitamin supplements, toothpastes and mouthwashes. Xylitol appears to be particularly useful for the prevention of tooth decay because it reduces the growth of *Streptococcus mutans* (the main tooth decay-causing bacterium), stimulates saliva flow and reduces plaque formation. Studies show that chewing gum containing xylitol reduces the formation of new dental caries in children.
- *Isomalt* is made up of glucomannitol and glucosorbitol. It has similar properties to sucrose, but is only 45–65 per cent as sweet as sucrose and more stable. It does not tend to lose its sweetness or break down when heated. Isomalt absorbs little water, so it is often used in hard confectionery, toffee, cough drops and lollipops.
- *Lactitol* is a derivative of lactose that is about 40 per cent as sweet as sucrose. It is used as a low-kilojoule sweetener in sugar-free ice cream, chocolate, confectionery, baked goods, sugar-reduced jams and chewing gums. It has a less laxative effect than xylitol and sorbitol.
- *Maltitol* is about 90 per cent as sweet as sucrose. It is used in sugar-free hard confectionery and chewing gum, and, because it has a creamy texture, can be used to replace fat in foods such as chocolate-flavoured desserts, baked goods and ice cream.
- *Hydrogenated starch hydrolysates (HSHs)* contain a mixture of polyols, and are syrups produced by the partial hydrolysis of corn. They are often named after the dominant polyol present, such as sorbitol syrup, maltitol syrup or hydrogenated glucose syrup. HSHs are 40–90 per cent as sweet as sucrose. HSHs do not crystallise, and are used extensively in confectionery, baked goods and mouthwashes.

Oligosaccharides

Oligosaccharides (meaning 'few sugars') are typically made up of between three and ten monosaccharides, and are found mainly in legumes, grains and tubers. Up to 90 per cent of dietary oligosaccharides are undigested, and pass into the colon, where they are fermented by bacteria. They act as food sources for probiotics, the beneficial bacteria that colonise the bowel. Oligosaccharides include fructans (1 glucose + 3–50 fructose units), raffinose (1 sucrose + 1 galactose), stachyose (1 sucrose + 2 galactose), and verbascose (1 sucrose + 3 galactose). Fructans are found in chicory roots, grains, Jerusalem artichokes, onions, garlic and asparagus, and include the sub-types inulins, oligofructose and fructooligosaccharides. They are primarily fermented by bifidobacteria in the colon. Fructans have a sweet taste, and are used commercially as low-kilojoule sweeteners and fat replacers.

Resistant starch

In certain forms, starch can become more resistant to human digestive enzymes and is only partially digested. The undigested portion passes into the colon and is fermented. There are three main types of resistant starch (RS) in the diet, and a fourth type is produced commercially by chemical modification of starch.

- *RS1* is physically inaccessible starch found in granular form in whole, partly milled or coarsely ground grains.

- *RS2* is starch that has a B-type or C-type crystalline structure that is less digestible than the A-type structure found in grains. RS2 is found in raw potato, green bananas and legumes.
- *RS3* is retrograded starch that forms when starch has been cooked and cooled. Retrograded amylose is irreversibly changed, whereas retrograded amylopectin can be reversed by reheating.
- *RS4* is starch that has been chemically modified by cross-linking, esterification or etherification, and is used for commercial applications as a functional fibre.

Chitin and chitosan

Chitin is an aminopolysaccharide (sugar and protein molecule) that contains linked glucose units that are largely indigestible, although chitinase, the enzyme that breaks down chitin, has been detected in human gastric juice. Chitosan is a derivative of chitin. They are both found in fungi and some human parasites, and make up the exoskeleton of insects and shells of crustaceans but are not found in mammalian tissue. Chitin can stimulate immune and anti-inflammatory responses, and bind cholesterol in the colon, and chitin and chitosan are mainly used as supplements for reducing serum cholesterol levels. Chitosan supplements have been shown to decrease blood glucose and serum cholesterol levels, increase HDL cholesterol, lower LDL cholesterol and increase total plasma antioxidant activity.

Dietary fibre

Dietary fibre includes lignins and non-starch polysaccharides (NSPs) that are found in plant cell walls, tissues and exudates. They consist of chains of glucose with bonds that are indigestible by human digestive enzymes. Some types are fully or partially fermented by colonic bacteria.

Types of dietary fibre

Dietary fibre is classed as insoluble or soluble.

- *Insoluble fibre.* Insoluble fibre is insoluble in water. It is mainly found in plant cell walls, especially in mature plants, and is either not fermented or poorly fermented in the colon. It includes cellulose, found in wheat bran, legumes, nuts, peas, root vegetables and the cabbage family of vegetables; hemicelluloses, found in whole grains, nuts and vegetables; and lignins, found in wheat, mature root vegetables, berries and older, woody parts of plants and vegetables. Insoluble fibre provides bulk to the bowel contents to assist elimination.
- *Soluble fibre.* Soluble fibre includes glucomannan, pectins, beta-glucans, gums and mucilages. It is water-soluble, and most types are fermented by colonic bacteria. Soluble fibre absorbs water and swells up in the intestinal tract to form a viscous gel. Glucomannan, a mannose and glucose-containing soluble fibre derived from konjac root, has the most water-absorbing properties, absorbing up to 200 times its own weight in water to form a highly viscous gel. Pectins are part of the intercellular connective tissue between plant cell walls, and are found in fruit, especially apple pulp and citrus rind, vegetables and sugar beet. They are gel-forming and almost completely fermented in the colon. Commercially, pectins are extracted from fruit and used as gelling agents, especially for fruit products such as jam. Beta-glucans are readily fermented and are found in oats and barley. Gums and mucilages are hydrocolloids found as part of cell walls or as exudates secreted by plants at a site of injury. Exudates include gum arabic, gum tragacanth, gum karaya and gum ghatti. Seed gums, such as guar gum and locust bean gum, have high water-absorbing capacity, swelling by many times their own weight when exposed to liquids. Xanthan gum is produced by bacterial fermentation, and is used commercially as a thickener and stabiliser. Mucilages include ispaghula from psyllium seeds and alginates, carrageenans and funorans from seaweed. Seaweed mucilages are used commercially as texture modifiers because of their high viscosity and gelling properties.

Functions

The connection between health and unavailable carbohydrates in food was first uncovered in the 1970s by Dr Denis Burkitt and Dr Hugh Trowell, who were medical practitioners working in Africa. They found that many of the diseases common in Western countries were not common in Africans living a rural lifestyle. These diseases included CVD, varicose veins, obesity, diabetes, constipation, diverticulosis and diverticulitis, gallstones, appendicitis, haemorrhoids, bowel polyps and bowel cancer. Dr Burkitt noted that his African patients who had high fibre intakes had more frequent and bulkier stools and less illness, and he formed the theory that the high dietary fibre intake of rural Africans had protective effects. He believed that the increase in CVD and digestive tract disorders in the United States and United Kingdom in the nineteenth century was linked to the switch to low-fibre, finely milled white flour as a staple food. Since Burkitt and Trowell's discoveries, a large amount of research has established the important role of dietary fibre in health.

The beneficial health effects of unavailable carbohydrates include:

- *Facilitation of faecal elimination.* Dietary fibre absorbs water in the colon, and softens and enlarges faeces. Insoluble fibre is especially effective as a bulking agent because very little is broken down by fermentation, and most is excreted intact. A larger faecal mass facilitates the action of the peristaltic muscles of the colon, decreasing the bowel transit time of faecal material.
- *Protection of the bowel lining.* Faecal material contains toxins from food components and lithocholate and deoxycholate, potentially harmful by-products of bile. Dietary fibre binds harmful substances and reduces their contact with the epithelial lining of the bowel. It also speeds up the movement of faeces through the colon, reducing the time available for the formation of toxins.
- *Prebiotic activity.* Soluble fibre and oligosaccharides are a fermentable food (prebiotic) for probiotic bacteria in the colon. Probiotics are beneficial bacteria that ferment fibre for energy and produce the short-chain fatty acids (SCFAs) acetic, propionic and butyric acids and also lactic acid, methane, hydrogen and carbon dioxide. SCFAs can be absorbed by diffusion into the colonic epithelium and used as fuel for colonocytes (colon lining cells). Butyrate has a role in regulating colonocyte replication, and may have anticancer effects, although recent research in this area has yielded mixed results, with studies showing that it can have anti- and pro-tumour activity. Some probiotics can synthesise some B vitamins and vitamin K. Synthesis by colonic bacteria is believed to be a source of vitamin K for the body, but it is not known whether B vitamins can be absorbed effectively from the colon.
- *Increased cholesterol excretion.* Bile acids are made from cholesterol in the liver, and this is the major pathway for removal of cholesterol from the body. However, about 95 per cent of the bile acids entering the duodenum are absorbed back into the bloodstream and returned to the liver for recycling. Deoxycholate is formed from bile by bacterial activity when the transit of faeces is slow and, when reabsorbed, can contribute to cholesterol saturation in the gall bladder, a risk factor for gallstone formation. Dietary fibre binds bile acids, reduces reuptake and increases bile (cholesterol) excretion in faeces. This may act as a stimulus to convert more cholesterol into bile, further enhancing cholesterol removal. Soluble dietary fibre has been shown to lower serum total cholesterol and LDL cholesterol levels.
- *Anti-inflammatory activity.* Dietary fibre and soluble fibre are associated with lower levels of C-reactive protein, a marker of inflammation and an independent risk factor for CVD. Butyrate also appears to have anti-inflammatory activity and, in animal studies, lactulose, inulin, oligofructose and insoluble fibre from germinated barley have been shown to have anti-inflammatory effects in inflammatory bowel diseases.
- *Anti-obesity activity.* High-fibre diets may assist weight control by providing bulk in the digestive tract and slowing down digestion, increasing post-meal satiety (satisfaction) and delaying subsequent hunger. Dietary fibre absorbs water and increases the viscosity of gut contents, holding nutrients in the central lumen of the digestive tract and reducing contact with digestive enzymes and the wall of the small intestine, thereby inhibiting nutrient digestion and absorption.
- *Improved glycaemic control.* Dietary fibre slows down nutrient digestion and absorption, and can lower the GI of food and inhibit insulin release, stabilise blood glucose and improve insulin sensitivity and glucose tolerance. Intake of soluble or insoluble fibre is associated with reduced risk of type 2 diabetes.

Dietary sources

Good sources of dietary fibre include whole grains such as whole wheat, rolled oats, barley, rye, triticale, sorghum, brown rice, corn, millet, quinoa, wholemeal pasta and bran; legumes, such as beans, peas, chick peas and lentils; nuts; seeds, such as linseeds (flaxseeds), sunflower seeds, pumpkin seeds, pine nuts and sesame seeds; fruit; vegetables; and seaweed. Commercial dietary fibre supplements may contain psyllium seed husks, glucomannan, guar gum or chicory root fibre.

Access the Food Standards Australia New Zealand nutrient database (NUTTAB) at <www.foodstandards.gov.au> for the amounts found in specific foods.

Daily requirement

Government recommendations by age and gender (see Table 3.3) can be found in *Nutrient Reference Values for Australia and New Zealand Including Recommended Dietary Intakes*, available at <www.nrv.gov.au>.

The average Australian intake of dietary fibre is 18–25 g per day. The Australian National Health and Medical Research Council suggests that it would be prudent to have a daily intake of 38 g of dietary fibre for men and 28 g for women to reduce the risk of CVD.

Table 3.3 Adequate intake (AI) of dietary fibre (g/day)

Age (years)	Female AI	Male AI
1–3	14	14
4–8	18	18
9–13	20	24
14–18	22	28
19–70	25	30
>70	25	30
Pregnant women		
14–18	25	
19–50	28	
Lactating women		
14–18	27	
19–50	30	

Source: Nutrient Reference Values for Australia and New Zealand Including Recommended Dietary Intakes, National Health and Medical Research Council, Australian Government Department of Health and Ageing, Canberra and Ministry of Health, New Zealand, Wellington, 2006.

Deficiency effects

Adverse effects of a low dietary fibre intake include:

- *Gastrointestinal disorders.* Inadequate dietary fibre reduces faecal size, increases the toxin content of faeces, slows down faecal transit time and leads to small, dry stools that are harder to pass. Movement of faeces requires stronger muscle action that can lead to a build-up of pressure inside the colon. Inadequate fibre may contribute to constipation, diverticular disease (bowel pockets), colitis, irritable bowel syndrome, appendicitis and bowel cancer. Straining on the toilet increases pressure on the abdominal contents and can aggravate a hiatus (stomach) hernia. Increased fibre intake may be of benefit in gastro-oesophageal reflux disease and duodenal ulcer.
- *Bowel cancer.* High-fibre diets have been found to protect against colon cancer, with a large European study concluding that they lower the risk by 25 per cent. There have been mixed results in studies of colorectal cancer and intake of fibre from grains, whereas fruit and vegetable fibre appears to be protective.
- *Circulatory disorders.* A lack of fibre is associated with elevated serum total cholesterol and LDL cholesterol, lower HDL cholesterol and increased risk of atherosclerosis and coronary heart disease. Straining on the toilet increases pressure on the veins of the anus and legs, which can aggravate varicose veins and haemorrhoids.
- *Type 2 diabetes.* Most high-fibre foods are low GI and improve glycaemic control by improving glucose tolerance and reducing insulin resistance.
- *Gallstones.* Dietary fibre encourages bile flow, reduces reuptake of bile and boosts cholesterol excretion. People with cholesterol gall bladder stones often have a high percentage of deoxycholic acid in gall bladder bile, which is thought to result from its enhanced formation in the colon during prolonged colonic transit time.
- *Dental caries and gum disease.* Chewing fibrous particles stimulates blood flow in the gums, strengthens gum tissue and increases the flow of saliva that neutralises acids that cause tooth decay.
- *Obesity.* Dietary fibre has a lower kilojoule content than available carbohydrates, and causes less insulin release, reducing insulin's effect of enhancing fat synthesis and storage. Fibrous foods also take time to eat, provide satiety by their bulking effect in the gastrointestinal tract and slow digestion and absorption.

Effects of excess

Excess intake of polyols can cause diarrhoea. Excess intake of dietary fibre may have the following effects:

- *Increased water needs.* Fibre absorbs water in the gut and speeds transit time, reducing the amount of water that can be reabsorbed in the colon.
- *Reduced nutrient availability.* High-fibre foods form a viscous gel in the digestive tract that can trap nutrients and reduce their exposure to digestive enzymes. Legumes contain haemagglutinins (lectins) and enzyme inhibitors, such as trypsin inhibitors in soybeans and kidney beans, that impair the activity of protein-digesting enzymes, although most are denatured by cooking. Lectins are found in raw or undercooked grains, peas and beans, especially red kidney beans. Lectins bind to glycoproteins in cell membranes and attach to the cells lining the digestive tract, causing cell damage, increased intestinal permeability, increased mucus production and reduced nutrient absorption. When absorbed, they stimulate immune responses and bind to glycoproteins on red blood cells, causing them to clump together. As few as four to five raw kidney beans may trigger acute digestive symptoms, such as severe nausea, vomiting and diarrhoea, which usually resolves rapidly. Moist cooking can inactivate lectins, but slow cooking at low temperatures, as in a crock-pot, may be inadequate. To reduce lectin content, kidney beans must be soaked for at least five hours, the water discarded and then the beans boiled in fresh water for 30–45 minutes. There is preliminary evidence that galactose in fruit and vegetables can bind lectins and help counteract their adverse effects.

  Tannins in some cereals and legumes, and phytate in whole grains, bran and seeds, can bind protein and reduce its digestibility. Phytate in whole grains binds to digestive enzymes and inhibits their activity, and also binds proteins and minerals, such as calcium, potassium, magnesium, iron and zinc, making them insoluble and inhibiting their absorption. Minerals can be released from phytate by the enzyme phytase that becomes active during fermentation, sprouting and soaking.
- *Intestinal obstruction.* An extremely high fibre intake may result in the formation of phytobezoars (fibre balls) in the gut, which may cause obstruction, but this is very rare.

THERAPEUTIC USES OF DIETARY FIBRE

Irritable bowel syndrome

Irritable bowel syndrome (IBS) is abdominal pain or discomfort, a change in bowel habits (diarrhoea or constipation), bloating and incomplete evacuation of faeces, in the absence of detectable physiological abnormalities. It is associated with hyperactivity of the gut, sugar malabsorption, excessive gas production and increased intestinal permeability. It is aggravated by stress, and may be caused by excessive serotonin levels, the neurotransmitter that regulates muscle contractions in the gut.

Wheat bran may exacerbate symptoms but methylcellulose, partially hydrolysed guar gum and psyllium appear to have beneficial effects. Food intolerances or allergies are linked to IBS, and elimination diets that remove the most common allergens from the diet may relieve symptoms. IBS symptoms may be triggered by gluten, wheat, dairy products, eggs, coffee, yeast, potatoes and citrus fruits. A high intake of fat, fructose, sorbitol and other sugar alcohols may contribute to flatulence, abdominal discomfort and diarrhoea. A higher fibre intake from fruit and vegetables is linked to a reduction in bloating.[1] However, wheat bran has not been shown to be effective.[2] Insoluble fibre, in the form of nuts and whole grains, is not as effective and may worsen symptoms. Psyllium fibre may be of help in some individuals and soluble fibre is useful for relief of most IBS symptoms, especially constipation, but not for relief of abdominal pain.[3] To minimise adverse effects in IBS, less allergenic types of soluble fibre should be used, and it should be introduced in small amounts and gradually increased while monitoring symptoms.

Bowel cancer

Some clinical trials have shown that fibre is protective against colon cancer. In a large European observational study, higher dietary fibre from foods was associated with an estimated 25 per cent reduction in risk for colon cancer.[4] In this study, an increase in fibre intake from 15 g per day to 35 g per day was associated with a 40 per cent decrease in colon cancer, but not rectal cancer. However, not all studies have found a protective effect.

A key protective factor is believed to be the formation of liberal amounts of butyrate from fibre by bacterial fermentation in the colon. Butyrate inhibits the gene-regulating enzymes histone deacetylases, and has been shown to produce cell cycle arrest, differentiation and/or programmed cell death (apoptosis) of cancer cells in cell studies. The type of fibre eaten and variations in colonic bacteria between individuals affect the amount of butyrate produced, which may help explain the conflicting results about the protective effect of fibre against bowel cancers. Also, sub-types of colorectal cancers respond differently to butyrate. It appears that fibre may be more protective against benign tumours (polyps) and in the early stages of colorectal cancer rather than in advanced tumours.[5]

Diverticular disease

Diverticular disease (DD) is the presence of diverticula (pockets) in the bowel that may become inflamed. Diverticula may not cause symptoms but inflammation (diverticulitis) causes abdominal pain, changes in bowel habits and bleeding. Intake of fruit and vegetable fibre reduces the risk of DD, with fibre from fruit reducing the risk by 38 per cent and fibre from vegetables reducing the risk by 45 per cent.[6] Insoluble fibre, particularly cellulose, was strongly associated with decreased risk (a reduction of 45 per cent) but fibre from grains did not decrease risk.[6] People with a high meat and low vegetable intake have been found to have a 50-fold higher risk of DD than those with a high vegetable and low meat intake.[6] A dietary study found that the incidence of DD was 33 per cent among non-vegetarians whose mean dietary fibre intake was 21.4 g per day but only 12 per cent among vegetarians whose mean dietary fibre intake was 41.5 g per day.[6]

Inflammatory bowel disease

Inflammation may affect the small intestine (Crohn's disease) or the colon (colitis), and symptoms—which can occur intermittently—may include abdominal pain, diarrhoea, loose stools, urgency, bloating, incomplete evacuation, mucus and constipation. Inflammatory bowel disease is associated with reduced production of SCFAs, and impaired utilisation of butyrate by colonocytes. Butyrate suppresses the inflammatory immune response by inhibiting activation of nuclear factor kappaB (NF-kappaB), which triggers production of inflammatory chemicals. Patients treated with butyrate enemas have shown a marked decrease in inflammation in the bowel.[7] Germinated barley has been found to reduce inflammation in the bowel and psyllium husks have been shown to reduce risk of relapse in colitis patients.[8,9]

REFERENCES

1 Levy, R.L., Linde, J.A., Feld, K.A. et al., The association of gastrointestinal symptoms with weight, diet, and exercise in weight-loss program participants, *Clin Gastroenterol Hepatol* (2005), 3: 992–6.

2 Ford, A.C., Talley, N.J., Spiegel, B.M.R. et al., Effect of fibre, antispasmodics, and peppermint oil in the treatment of irritable bowel syndrome: systematic review and meta-analysis, *BMJ* (2008), 337: 2313.

3 Bijkerk, C.J., Muris, J.W., Knottnerus, J.A. et al., Systematic review: The role of different types of fibre in the treatment of irritable bowel syndrome, *Aliment Pharmacol Ther* (2004), 19: 245–51.

4 Bingham, S.A., Day, N.E., Luben, R. et al., Dietary fibre in food and protection against colorectal cancer in the European Prospective Investigation into Cancer and Nutrition (EPIC): An observational study, *Lancet* (2003), 361: 1496–501.

5 Peters, U., Sinha, R., Chatterjee, N. et al., Dietary fibre and colorectal adenoma in a colorectal cancer early detection programme, *Lancet* (2003), 361: 1491–5.

6 Aldoori, W. & Ryan-Harshman, M., Preventing diverticular disease: Review of recent evidence on high-fibre diets, *Can Fam Physician* (2002), 48: 1632–7.

7 Scheppach, W., Sommer, H., Kirchner, T. et al., Effect of butyrate enemas on the colonic mucosa in distal ulcerative colitis, *Gastroenterology* (1992), 103: 51–6.

8 Bamba, T.I., Kanauchi, O., Andoh, A. & Fujiyama, Y.J., A new prebiotic from germinated barley for nutraceutical treatment of ulcerative colitis, *Gastroenterol Hepatol* (2002), 17(8): 818–24.

9 Fernández-Bañares, F., Hinojosa, J., Sánchez-Lombraña, J.L. et al., Randomized clinical trial of Plantago ovata seeds (dietary fiber) as compared with mesalamine in maintaining remission in ulcerative colitis. Spanish Group for the Study of Crohn's Disease and Ulcerative Colitis (GETECCU), *Am J Gastroenterol* (1999), 94(2): 427–33.

HOW MUCH DO I KNOW?

Choose whether the following statements are true or false. Then review this chapter for the correct answers.

	True (T)	False (F)
1 Maltose is a monosaccharide.	T	F
2 Fructose drives production of triglycerides in the liver.	T	F
3 The glycaemic index measures how much carbohydrate is in a food.	T	F
4 Low-carbohydrate diets can help improve insulin sensitivity.	T	F
5 Increased hunger, thirst and urination may be symptoms of type 2 diabetes.	T	F
6 Most sugar alcohols provide about half the kilojoules of other sugars.	T	F
7 Insoluble fibre can be fermented by bacteria in the colon.	T	F
8 Ispaghula in psyllium seed is a type of mucilage.	T	F
9 Dietary fibre protects the bowel lining by binding toxins and harmful by-products of bile.	T	F
10 Glucomannan and guar gum are good sources of dietary fibre.	T	F

FURTHER READING

Gropper, S.S., Smith, J.L. & Groff, J.L., *Advanced nutrition and human metabolism*. 5th ed., Thomson Wadsworth, Belmont, CA, 2009.

4

Lipids, cholesterol and lipotropic nutrients: choline and inositol

LIPIDS

ESSENTIAL FATTY ACID STATUS CHECK

1 Are you always thirsty and do you perspire a lot?

2 Do you have atherosclerosis or a heart disorder?

3 Do you have a chronic inflammatory or auto-immune disease?

4 Do you have dry skin and hair, skin rashes or weak fingernails that break easily?

'Yes' answers may indicate inadequate essential fatty acid status. Note that a number of nutritional deficiencies or health disorders can cause similar effects and further investigation is recommended.

FAST FACTS . . . LIPIDS

- Lipids commonly consist of glycerol with attached fatty acids and are found in the diet mainly in the form of triglycerides (a glycerol unit with three attached fatty acids).
- The omega-3 fatty acid alpha-linolenic acid and the omega-6 fatty acid linoleic acid are essential fatty acids that must be included in the diet.
- Essential fatty acids are part of phospholipids in cell membranes that can break down to produce eicosanoids, powerful chemicals that regulate functions within the cell and neighbouring cells.
- A deficiency of essential fatty acids may lead to excessive thirst, perspiration, skin rashes, dry skin and hair, weak fingernails and chronic inflammation.
- Omega-3 fatty acids may be useful for cancer prevention, the prevention and management of cardiovascular disease, and the management of inflammatory disorders as well as cognitive, mood and behavioural disorders.

Lipids are fats and oils made of carbon and hydrogen chains that are insoluble in water but can dissolve in alcohol. Fats usually have a solid consistency at room temperature—for example, butter and meat fat—and oils are usually liquid—for example, most vegetable oils. The most common dietary lipids are made of a glycerol 'backbone', with one, two or three fatty acid molecules attached by ester bonds. Fatty acids are carbon chains of varying lengths with attached hydrogen atoms.

TYPES OF LIPIDS

Lipids include glycerolipids, phospholipids, sphingolipids, sterols and prenols.

- *Glycerolipids* include:
  - *Monoacylglycerols* (more commonly called monoglycerides), which consist of a glycerol with one fatty acid attached.
  - *Diacylglycerols* (more commonly called diglycerides), which consist of a glycerol with two fatty acids attached.
  - *Triacylglycerols* (TGs, more commonly called triglycerides), which consist of a glycerol with three fatty acids attached (see Figure 4.1). TGs are the most common form of lipids in food, and can be solid or liquid at room temperature according to the fatty acids they contain. Fatty acids in TGs may be all one type or a mix of different types.
- *Phospholipids (PLs)* consist of a glycerol with one or two fatty acids and one phosphate group bonded to a choline (phosphatidylcholine, PC), ethanolamine (phosphatidylethanolamine, PE), serine (phosphatidylserine, PS) or inositol (phosphatidylinositol, PI). PLs are important components of cell membranes, where they have a structural role, and the fatty acids they contain can break down to form powerful, cell-regulating chemicals (eicosanoids). Cardiolipins are PLs that are part of inner mitochondrial membranes, where they act to stabilise enzymes involved in energy production.
- *Sphingolipids* have the long-chain amino-alcohol sphingosine as their backbone instead of glycerol and include sphingomyelin, cerebrosides and gangliosides. They are found in high quantities in brain and nervous tissue. Sphingomyelin, found in cell membranes and the myelin sheath of nerves, consists of sphingosine together with one fatty acid and phosphorylcholine or phosphorylethanolamine. Cerebrosides and gangliosides are lipids with a sphingosine backbone and a carbohydrate component. They are found in cell membranes, blood cells, the brain and the medullary sheath of nerves, and take part in intercellular communication and define ABO blood groups.
- *Sterols* are fat-soluble alcohols that consist of four interlocking rings of carbon atoms with an attached hydroxyl group (-OH) that has water-soluble properties. The major sterol in the body is cholesterol, which is an important part of cell membrane structure together with PLs and sphingomyelins. Vitamin D, bile salts and steroid hormones, such as sex and adrenal hormones, are derived from cholesterol.
- *Phytosterols* are plant equivalents of animal sterols, most of which contain 28 or 29 carbons and one or two carbon–carbon double bonds and include beta-sitosterol, campesterol, stigmasterol, brassicasterol and ergosterol. Plants also contain stanols, which are sterols with no double bonds in the ring structure. The most common stanols in the diet are sitostanol and campestanol.
- *Prenols* (isoprenoid alcohols) are precursors of isoprenoids, a class of natural substances that includes carotenoids, vitamin E, vitamin K and co-enzyme Q10 (CoQ10).

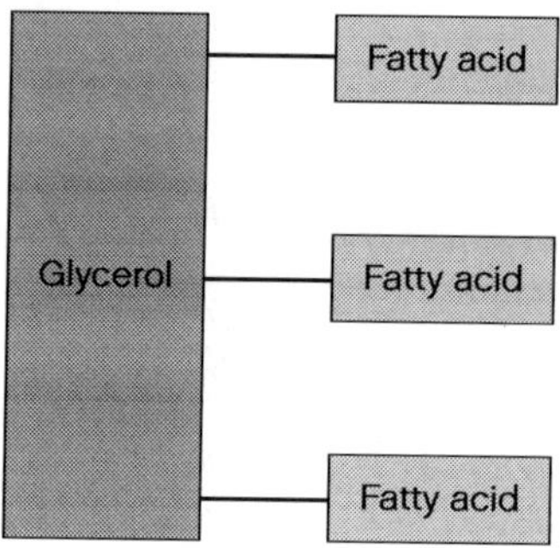

Figure 4.1 Triacylglycerol structure

Fatty acids (FAs)

Fatty acids (FAs) (also called fatty acyls) are carbon chains of varying lengths, with a methyl group (CH_3) at one end and a carboxyl group (COOH) at the other. Each carbon in the chain has the potential to form four bonds. Commonly, each carbon has a bond between itself and the two adjacent carbons, and the other two bonds are attached to hydrogen atoms. Some FAs have double bonds between adjacent carbons in certain positions in the chain; in this case, two hydrogen atoms are missing. FAs can be classified into short-, medium- or long-chain FAs according to the number of carbons in the chain.

- *Short-chain FAs* have four to six carbons, and are found in dairy fats and are also produced by bacterial

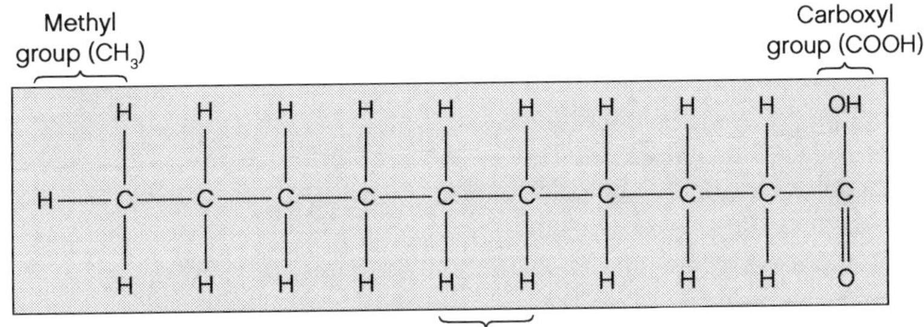

Saturated fatty acid: single bonds between each carbon

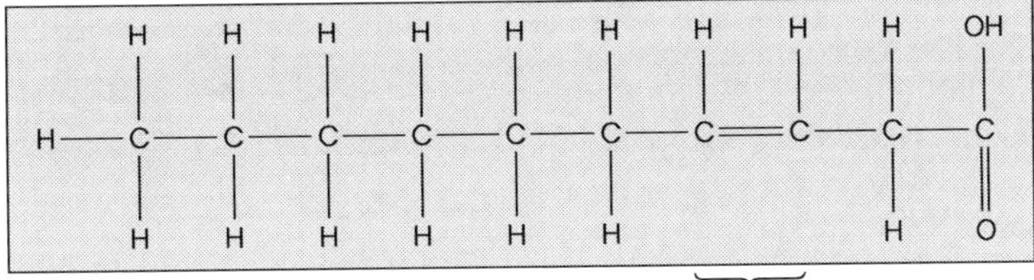

Monounsaturated fatty acid: 1 double bond

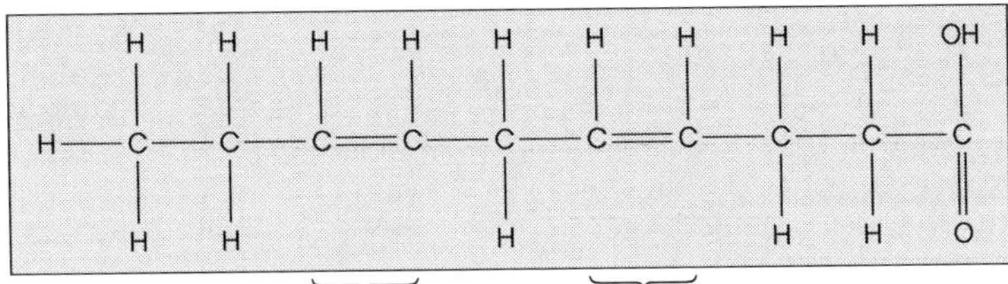

Polyunsaturated fatty acid: more than 1 double bond

Figure 4.2 Fatty acid structures

fermentation in the colon. They are relatively easily digested and absorbed.

- *Medium-chain FAs* have eight to ten carbons, and are found in dairy and tropical fats, such as palm and coconut oil. They are relatively easily digested and absorbed.
- *Long-chain FAs* have twelve to 24 carbons, and are found in most plant and animal fats. They are the most common type of FA found in food, and require more digestive activity before absorption.

The type of bonding between carbons in a fatty acid affects the way they are metabolised in the body and they are divided into groups accordingly (see Figure 4.2).

- *Saturated FAs (SFAs)* have single bonds between carbon atoms, which gives them a straight shape, and they have hydrogen atoms attached to every carbon. They are solid at room temperature if more than ten carbons long and are resistant to oxygen attack (oxidation). They are not essential in the diet because they can be made in the body.
- *Unsaturated FAs (UFAs)* have one or more double bonds between carbon atoms and the two carbons at the site of the double bond are each lacking a hydrogen atom. The double bond gives these FAs a flexible, curved shape that is metabolically useful. However, the double bond site is susceptible to oxidation, and the more double bonds in the chain the more easily they oxidise and form harmful free radicals. Unsaturated FAs consist of:
  - *monounsaturated FAs (MUFAs)*, which have one double bond in the chain. They are liquid at room temperature but semi-solid when refrigerated

and are fairly resistant to oxidation. They are not essential in the diet because they can be made in the body.

– *polyunsaturated FAs (PUFAs),* which have two or more double bonds in the chain and are classified according to the position of the first double bond, counting from the methyl (CH_3), or omega, end. They are liquid at room temperature, and also when refrigerated, and are susceptible to oxidation. Two types of PUFAs are essential in the diet, as they cannot be made in the body. PUFAs are found in the 'cis' shape in most foods, which is a flexible, curved shape. The more double bonds a PUFA has, the more curved its shape. Some types of food processing, such as converting a vegetable oil into margarine, converts some of the 'cis' forms into 'trans' forms, straighter, less flexible structures that cannot be metabolised in the same way as the 'cis' forms. Trans FAs act like SFAs in the body.

Biochemical notation for FAs

In biochemical shorthand, FAs are written as the number of carbons they contain, followed by the number of double bonds (if any) and then the position of the first double bond, which is important because it determines how the FA is metabolised. The position of the first double bond is prefixed by 'omega-' (often written as 'n' or 'ω') and followed by the double bond position. For example, the SFA butyric acid has four carbons and all single bonds and is written as 4:0; the MUFA oleic acid has eighteen carbons and one double bond and is written as 18:1(n-9) because the double bond is after the ninth carbon atom; the PUFA linoleic acid has eighteen carbons and two double bonds and is written as 18:2(n-6) because the first double bond is after the sixth carbon atom; and the PUFA alpha-linolenic acid has eighteen carbons and three double bonds and is written as 18:3(n-3) because the first double bond is after the third carbon atom. Double bonds are always separated by three carbons. The omega-3 (n-3) and omega-6 (n-6) classes of FAs are particularly important for regulating inflammatory processes in the body, and play a role in many chronic health disorders.

Essential FAs (EFA)

Two PUFAs are essential in the diet because they are needed to make vital metabolites, but the body cannot insert the first double bond into the correct position. These are:

- *linoleic acid (LA)*, the essential precursor for the n-6 class of PUFAs
- *alpha-linolenic acid (alpha-LNA)*, the essential precursor for the n-3 class of PUFAs. (A common abbreviation for alpha-linolenic acid is ALA, but alpha-LNA will be used in this text to avoid confusion with alpha-lipoic acid (alpha-LA), which is also commonly abbreviated to ALA.) If sufficient alpha-LNA and LA are present, other PUFAs of the same class can then be made in the body. However, it has been suggested that docosahexaenoic acid (DHA), which is made from alpha-LNA in the body, is more essential than alpha-LNA because DHA production in humans is limited and it is incorporated into cell membrane PLs much more readily than alpha-LNA. DHA appears to be essential in pregnancy and for infants.

Table 4.1 Some types of fatty acids in food

SFAs		Biochemical notation
Short chain	Butyric acid	4:0
	Caproic acid	6:0
Medium chain	Caprylic acid	8:0
	Capric acid	10:0
Long chain	Lauric acid	12:0
	Myristic acid	14:0
	Palmitic acid	16:0
	Stearic acid	18:0
MUFAs		
Long chain	Oleic acid	18:1(n-9)
	Elaidic acid (trans form of oleic acid)	18:1 (n-9)
PUFAs		
Long chain	Linoleic acid (LA)	18:2(n-6)
	alpha-linolenic acid (alpha-LNA)	18:3(n-3)
	Arachidonic acid (AA)	20:4(n-6)
	Eicosapentaenoic acid (EPA)	20:5(n-3)
	Docosahexaenoic acid (DHA)	22:6(n-3)

Lipid digestion, absorption and transport

Dietary fats are mainly in the form of TGs, with smaller amounts of phospholipids and sterols, such as cholesteryl esters. TGs are digested by lingual lipase, produced by glands under the tongue and active in the stomach, and pancreatic lipase, active in the small intestine. Lingual lipase digests short- and medium-chain FAs. Long-chain FAs are first emulsified by bile and digested by pancreatic lipase, with the assistance of pancreatic colipase. The end-products of TG digestion are diglycerides and monoglycerides. PLs are broken down by phospholipase A_2 to produce lysolecithin and FAs, and cholesteryl esters are broken down by cholesterol esterase to cholesterol and FAs. The products of lipid digestion combine with bile salts to form micelles, which release the lipids into the cells lining the small intestine (enterocytes), where they are made into TGs, PC and cholesteryl esters.

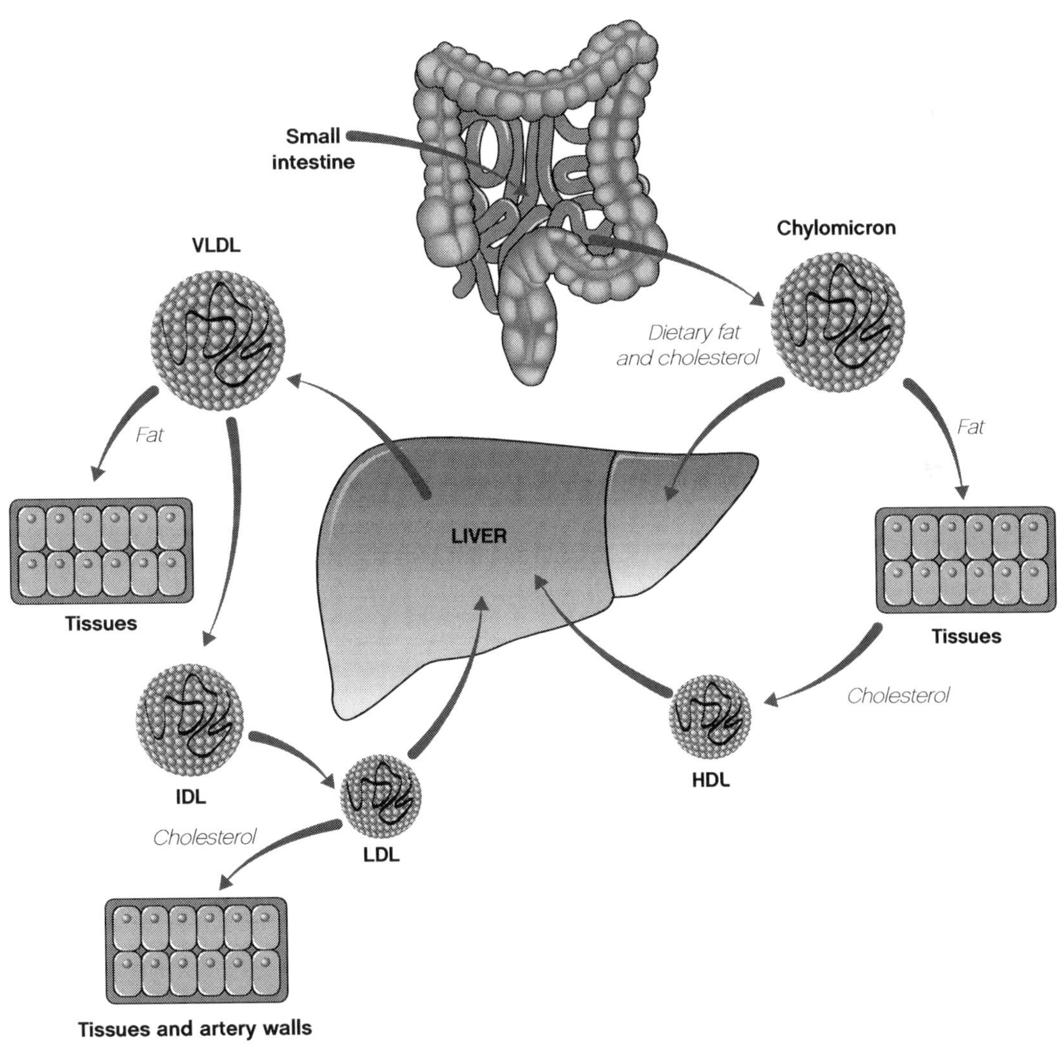

Figure 4.3 Lipid transport

As lipids are not soluble in water, they need water-soluble protein carriers (lipoproteins) for transport around the body in the bloodstream and lymphatic system. The protein components of lipoproteins are apolipoproteins, which act to stabilise the lipoprotein and regulate enzyme and receptor activity. These proteins are classified according to their function and the lipoprotein in which they are found, and have been given alpha-numeric names preceded by 'apo'—for example, apoA-1, apoB-100, apoC-2. The core of lipoproteins contains lipids and the outer shell contains proteins and PLs. The ratio of protein to fat regulates the density of the lipoprotein. If there is more protein and less fat, it has a higher density, and less protein and more fat give it a lower density.

Lipid transport from the intestine to the liver

- *Chylomicrons* transport dietary TGs, together with a smaller amount of dietary cholesterol and PLs, from the intestine to the lymphatic system and then to the bloodstream for delivery to the liver, muscles and fat cells (see Figure 4.3). Density is extremely low, as they contain a lot of fat and only about 2 per cent protein. The enzyme lipoprotein lipase in adipose and muscle tissue releases FAs and diglycerides from chylomicrons for uptake by cells. When FAs have been given off, the chylomicron remnants are taken up by the liver, where the remaining lipids are broken down and resynthesised. The liver can also make lipids from glucose and amino acids.

Lipid transport from the liver to tissues

- *Very low-density lipoproteins (VLDLs)* transport TGs, PLs and cholesterol made in the liver to the rest of the body (see Figure 4.3). They are about 10 per cent protein. As VLDLs circulate around the body, FAs are taken up by cells by the action of lipoprotein lipase and their density increases, rapidly converting them to intermediate-density lipoproteins.
- *Intermediate-density lipoproteins (IDLs)* are very short-lived and, as more fat is lost to body cells, they quickly become low-density lipoproteins.
- *Low-density lipoproteins (LDLs)* mainly transport cholesterol to tissue cells, because the TGs have been already given off from the VLDL and IDL forms. The protein content is now about 20 per cent. ApoB-100 in LDL binds with LDL receptors on cell membranes and LDL is taken into the cell by endocytosis (engulfment by a portion of the cell membrane) and the cholesterol is released for use by the cell.

  LDL cholesterol is sometimes referred to as 'bad' cholesterol because it increases heart disease risk by delivering cholesterol to the artery walls, where it can build up and cause thickening (plaque) and atherosclerosis. However, this is an over-simplification because there are other factors that appear to be more important, such as the size of the LDL particles, the type of protein found in LDL and the degree of LDL oxidation. Oxidised LDL cholesterol, small, dense LDL particles and a type of lipoprotein called lipoprotein (a) (LP(a)) increase the risk of heart disease.

Cholesterol transport from tissues to the liver

- *High-density lipoproteins (HDLs)* are made in the liver and small intestine, and their role is to pick up cholesterol from body tissues and take it back to the liver for recycling or excretion as bile (see Figure 4.3). They are about 45 per cent protein. ApoE in HDLs can bind to LDL receptors on cell membranes, and may compete with LDL for access to the cell. ApoA-1 in HDLs activates the enzyme lecithin-cholesterol acyl-transferase (LCAT), which converts free cholesterol in the cell to cholesteryl esters that are taken up by HDL and delivered to the liver, where they are broken down by cholesteryl esterase to free cholesterol. Free cholesterol is converted to bile and excreted into the duodenum, some of which is reabsorbed. HDL is sometimes called 'good' cholesterol because it takes cholesterol away from plaques in artery walls and reduces the risk of heart disease.

Lipid storage and mobilisation

Lipids are stored in fat cells (adipocytes) in adipose tissue as TGs. TGs in lipoproteins in the bloodstream are first broken down by lipoprotein lipase produced by endothelial cells to form glycerol and free FAs. Adipocytes take up free FAs and glycerol via a transport protein and the FAs are combined with coenzyme A to form thioesters which are then re-esterified to form TGs, using glycerol made from glucose. Most of the glycerol taken up by adipocytes is returned to the bloodstream. TGs stored within adipocytes can be broken down to free FAs and glycerol, and released into the circulation as required. Mobilisation of fat stores occurs in response to hormone-sensitive triglyceride lipase, and is inhibited by insulin and stimulated by a number of hormones, including adrenaline, noradrenaline, adrenocorticotropic hormone, thyroid-stimulating hormone, glucagon, growth hormone and thyroid hormone.

Synthesis of FAs in the body

Many types of FAs can be made in the body by adding extra carbons to increase their length and inserting double bonds to desaturate them. FAs are mainly made in the liver and adipocytes, but also can be made by the kidneys, brain, lungs and mammary glands. First, acetyl coenzyme A (acetyl-CoA), formed from glucose or deaminated amino acids, is converted to SFAs—mainly palmitic acid and a smaller amount of stearic acid—which are then lengthened by the addition of carbons. SFAs can be unsaturated by the addition of a double bond to make MUFAs, and further double bonds are inserted to make some types of PUFAs. In the body, the position of the first double bond cannot be placed at the third or sixth carbon position and n-3 and n-6 PUFAs cannot be synthesised but can be metabolised further if eaten in the diet.

Regulation of FA synthesis

FA synthesis is inhibited by the hormone glucagon, adrenal hormones, high levels of free FAs in plasma, dietary PUFAs—especially n-3 PUFAs—and diets containing more that 10 per cent fat. FA synthesis is increased by the hormone insulin, high-carbohydrate and very low-fat diets, and a high glucose, fructose or sucrose intake. Fructose bypasses an important rate-limiting step in carbohydrate metabolism and loads fat-synthesis pathways and glucose stimulates insulin release, which increases fat synthesis and prevents fat mobilisation from storage.

FA breakdown

Fatty acids are broken down by beta-oxidation, a process that removes carbons to produce acetyl-CoA, which then enters the citric acid cycle with the assistance of the amino acid carnitine to participate in energy production. If more acetyl-CoA is produced than can be used for energy, the excess is converted to ketones, which can be used by tissues in energy pathways.

General functions of lipids

- *Formation of body structures.* Lipids are incorporated into the structure of cell membranes, membranes of intracellular organelles and the myelin sheath of nerve fibres.
- *Energy storage, insulation and protection.* Lipids are stored in fat tissue as TGs containing mainly MUFAs and SFAs, and act as an energy store. Stored lipids can be mobilised as required for use in energy-production pathways. Fat tissue also serves to insulate the body from temperature changes and to protect body organs.
- *Production of energy for cell metabolism.* FAs—particularly SFAs and MUFAs—are used for energy, especially by muscles while resting or lightly exercising; about 40 per cent of the energy used by the body while at rest comes from FAs. Short-chain FAs in the gut can be used for energy by the cells lining the intestine.
- *Cholesterol synthesis.* SFAs can be converted into cholesterol, which is used for cell membrane structure and for making steroid hormones, vitamin D and bile salts.
- *Cell signalling.* Sphingolipids and PLs, such as PI and PC, act as second messengers that relay signals from receptors to target molecules inside the cell. They are involved in regulating many aspects of cell metabolism, including cell growth, proliferation, motility and apoptosis, enzyme activation, calcium mobilisation and immune cell activity.
- *Digestive tract function.* Dietary lipids help absorption of fat-soluble vitamins, increase the palatability of foods, provide a feeling of satiety after eating, and stimulate bile production and secretion. Unabsorbed lipids that reach the colon may help to support the growth of beneficial intestinal bacteria.

Specific functions of EFAs

These include the following:

- *Membrane structure.* AA, its metabolite dihomo-gamma-linolenic acid (DGLA), EPA and DHA are the main PUFAs in PLs in cell membranes, mitochondrial membranes and the membranes of intracellular organelles, where they maintain fluidity and flexibility, and support membrane structure and function. DHA, in particular, increases cell membrane flexibility.

- *Lipid digestion, transport and metabolism.* EFAs in PLs help to emulsify fat and cholesterol to enable digestion and transport. EFAs regulate transcription of genes involved in lipid transport, lipid synthesis and FA oxidation, and have anti-obesity activity by inhibiting lipid synthesis and increasing FA oxidation.
- *Cell division.* EFAs help maintain the stability of chromosomes and regulate gene expression that affects cell division.
- *Brain and nerve function.* EFAs form part of the structure of the brain and the myelin sheath of nerve fibres, and help generate electrical potentials in nerve membranes that enable nerve transmission. They are important for brain development and vision in infants.
- *Formation of lung surfactant.* EFAs form part of PLs that combine with protein to form the surfactant in lungs that prevents air sacs from sticking together when they collapse as the lungs deflate while breathing out.
- *Regulation of skin permeability.* EFAs help reduce skin permeability and reduce water losses from the skin.
- *Calcium and bone metabolism.* EFAs increase calcium absorption, reduce urinary excretion, increase calcium deposition in bone and improve bone strength.
- *Eicosanoid synthesis.* Eicosanoids are 20-carbon metabolites primarily produced from AA and EPA in cell membrane PLs that regulate cell function and body homeostasis. They include prostanoids, which consist of prostaglandins (PGs), prostacyclins (PGIs) and thromboxanes (TXs), as well as leukotrienes (LTs), lipoxins (LXs), resolvins and protectins. They are divided into groups (series) according to the number of double bonds they contain. Specific eicosanoids are produced in different types of cells, and they act as very potent short-acting local chemicals that regulate cell activities. They affect most body functions, including circulation, blood clotting, immunity, reproduction and inflammatory responses.

n-6 PUFA metabolism

In the body, the essential n-6 PUFA, LA, is converted to gamma-linolenic acid (GLA) and then DGLA (see

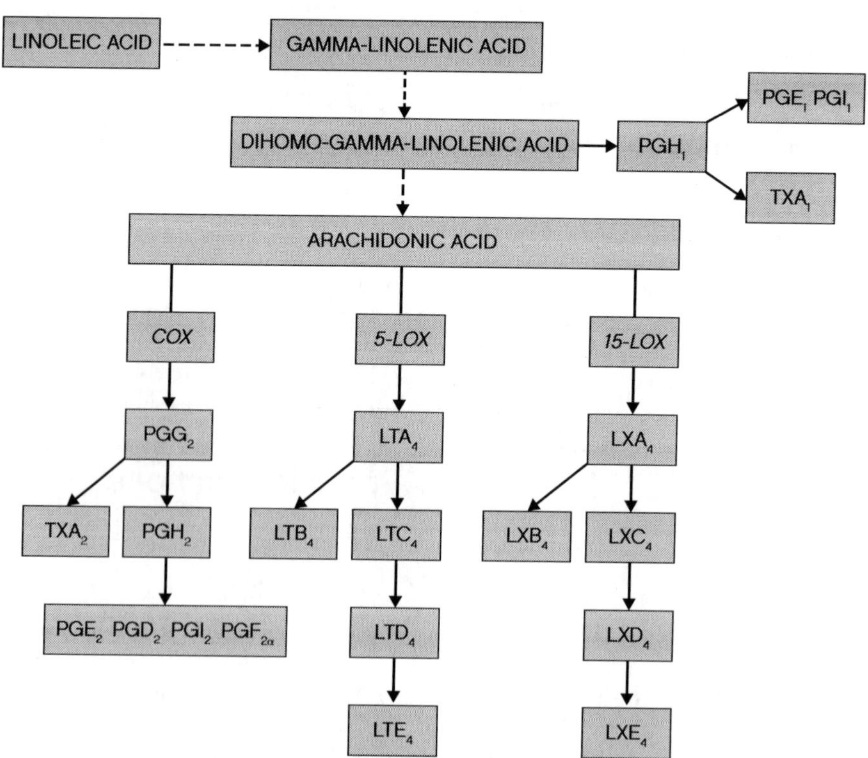

Figure 4.4 Omega-6 fatty acid metabolism

Figure 4.4). DGLA is converted to AA, which can also be obtained from the diet, and there is some evidence for direct conversion of LA to AA. DGLA and AA are incorporated into cell membrane PLs.

AA and DGLA metabolism

In response to stimuli, such as injury or stress, AA is released by the enzyme phospholipase A_2 and then further metabolised to eicosanoids by the enzymes cyclooxygenase (COX) and lipoxygenase (LOX) (see Figure 4.4). AA is converted by COX to PGG_2, which then converts to PGH_2 and finally to the end-products, which are the 2-series prostanoids, PGE_2, PGD_2, PGI_2, $PGF_{2\alpha}$ and TXA_2. The enzyme 5-LOX converts AA to LTA_4, a 4-series LT, and is then converted to LTB_4 and LTC_4. LTC_4 then converts to LTD_4, which produces LTE_4. AA is converted also by 15-LOX to the 4-series LX, LXA_4, which converts to LXB_4 and LXC_4. LXC_4 forms LXD_4 and then LXE_4. DGLA converts to PGH_1, which forms the 1-series prostanoids, such as PGE_1, PGI_1 and TXA_1.

COX enzymes exist in two forms, COX-1 and COX-2. COX-1 is expressed in most cells and is the main source of prostanoids for regulating body homeostasis. COX-2 is expressed by inflammatory stimuli, hormones and growth factors and is an important source of prostanoids in inflammation and cancer, and can contribute to tissue destruction, pain and loss of function. Epimeric 4-series LXs, such as epi-LXA_4 and epi-LXB_4, are produced by COX-2 activity in response to aspirin.

AA-derived 2- and 4-series prostanoids have potent inflammatory and anti-inflammatory effects. In general, anti-inflammatory PGs reduce abnormal clotting and dilate blood vessels, lowering blood pressure and improving circulation. They regulate immunity and calcium metabolism, decrease cholesterol synthesis and protect against heart disease. Inflammatory PGs increase clotting and constrict smooth muscles in blood vessels, respiratory passages, the digestive tract and the uterus. Constriction of blood vessels increases blood pressure. LXs and TXs increase clotting and permeability of blood vessels and constrict smooth muscles.

Functions of n-6 eicosanoids

- *PGE_1* regulates circulation by reducing platelet aggregation (clumping or stickiness) and thinning the blood, dilating blood vessel walls, increasing red blood cell flexibility, decreasing heart valve stiffness by reducing production of excess collagen and lowering atherosclerosis risk by decreasing cholesterol synthesis and decreasing smooth muscle proliferation in artery walls. It has anti-inflammatory, anticancer, diuretic and erectile activity, regulates T lymphocyte function and regulates calcium movement across cell membranes, which affects nerve transmission and muscle function.
- *PGI_1* inhibits production of LTs and has anti-inflammatory effects.
- *PGE_2* is one of the most abundant PGs in the body, and mediates immune responses, blood pressure, gastrointestinal integrity and fertility. It increases platelet aggregation and increases blood pressure by constricting smooth muscles in arteries and increasing sodium and water retention in the kidneys. It is inflammatory and causes pain, heat and fever, and enhances cell growth and proliferation. It constricts airways, enhances loss of calcium from bone, and may cause uterine contractions and menstrual cramping. PGE_2 is broken down by the enzyme 15-hydroxyprostaglandin dehydrogenase (15-PGDH).
- *PGI_2* is an important regulator of cardiovascular function. It is a potent anti-inflammatory, reduces allergic inflammation, reduces platelet aggregation, dilates blood vessels and controls embryo implantation in pregnancy.
- *PGD_2* is the main prostanoid released by mast cells during allergic reactions. It promotes allergic inflammation but inhibits inflammation in other contexts. It reduces platelet aggregation, dilates blood vessels, regulates pain perception and promotes sleep.
- *$PGF_{2\alpha}$* is important for female reproduction by regulating ovulation, breakdown of the corpus luteum, contraction of uterine smooth muscle and initiation of labour in pregnancy. It has a role in kidney and cardiovascular function.
- *4-series LTs* increase leukocyte aggregation, which increases clotting. LTC_4, LTD_4 and LTE_4 constrict smooth muscles, especially in the respiratory system, promote allergic inflammation and anaphylaxis, and increase the permeability of blood vessels.
- *2-series TXs*, especially TXA_2, are inflammatory, increase platelet aggregation and constrict smooth muscles in the respiratory system and blood vessels.
- *TXA_1* inhibits the inflammatory activity of TXA_2.
- *4-series LXs* dilate blood vessels and are anti-inflammatory, with an important role in terminating inflammation. They inhibit movement of leukocytes

to the site of inflammation, block superoxide and peroxynitrite production, stimulate phagocytosis (engulfment) of dead cells by macrophages and inhibit fibrosis (scar formation).

n-3 PUFA metabolism

The essential n-3 PUFA, alpha-LNA, is converted to stearidonic acid, then to eicosatetraenoic acid and then to EPA (see Figure 4.5). EPA can be converted to docosapentaenoic acid (DPA) and then to DHA. EPA and DHA are incorporated into cell membrane PLs. In humans, alpha-LNA has relatively poor conversion to EPA and even poorer conversion to DHA. About 8–20 per cent of alpha-LNA is converted to EPA and between 0.5 and 9 per cent to DHA. Women of reproductive age convert alpha-LNA to EPA at a two and a half times higher rate than healthy men. A diet high in n-6 PUFA reduces conversion by 40–50 per cent. However, there is some evidence from studies of vegans that production of DHA is increased if there is no dietary source.

EPA and DHA metabolism

In response to stimuli, EPA is released from cell membrane PLs by the enzyme phospholipase A_2. EPA uses the same COX and LOX enzymes used in AA metabolism and produces 3- and 5-series prostanoids (see Figure 4.5). EPA is converted by COX to PGH_3, which then produces the 3-series prostanoids, PGE_3, PGD_3, PGI_3, $PGF_{3\alpha}$ and TXA_3. EPA is also converted by 5-LOX to LTA_5, a 5-series LT, and is then converted to LTB_5 and LTC_5. LTC_5 then converts to LTD_5, which produces LTE_5. EPA can be converted also by 15-LOX to the 5-series LXs, LXA_5 and LXB_5, which then produces LXC_5, LXD_5 and LXE_5.

EPA can produce E-series resolvins by 5-LOX activity and DHA can produce resolvin D by 5-LOX activity and protectin D_1 by 15-LOX activity. When COX-2 is expressed, the use of aspirin triggers production of resolvin E_1 by 5-LOX. Resolvin E_1 can be made also by activity of cytochrome P450 enzymes.

Functions of n-3 eicosanoids

- *PGI_3* is anti-inflammatory and reduces platelet aggregation.
- *3-series PGs* have similar actions to their 2-series counterparts, but generally have weaker effects.
- *TXA_3* has similar functions to TXA_2, but weaker effects.

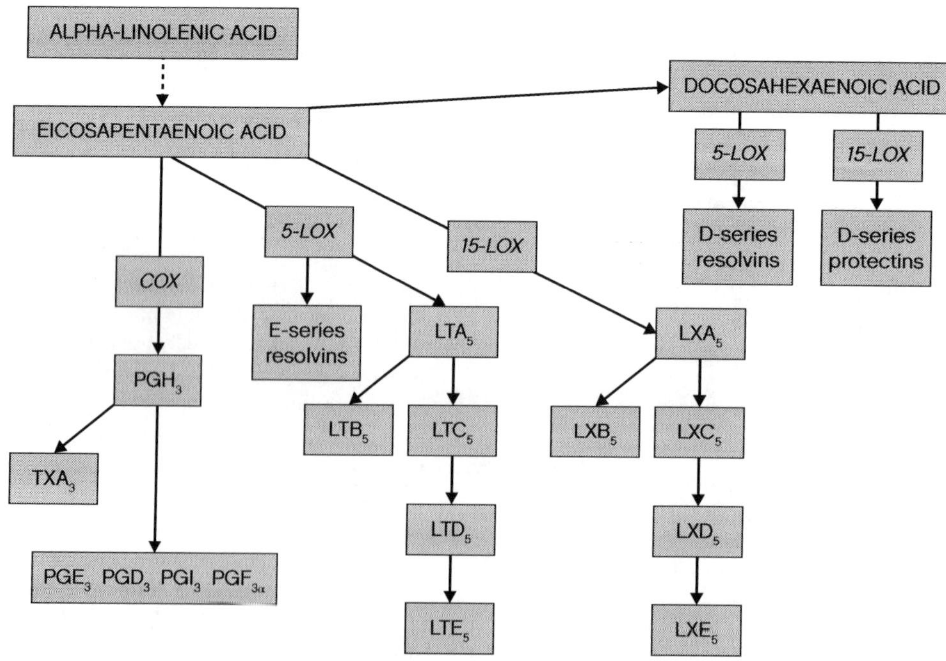

Figure 4.5 Omega-3 fatty acid metabolism

- *5-series LTs* have similar actions to their 2-series counterparts, but generally have weaker effects.
- *5-series LXs* have similar actions to their 4-series counterparts, but have weaker effects.
- *Resolvins*, which include E-series resolvins derived from EPA and D-series resolvins derived from DHA, have inflammation-suppressing and immunomodulating activity in neutrophils, macrophages, dendritic cells and T cells. They assist removal of inflammatory cells and restoration of tissue integrity after an inflammatory response.
- *Protectins*, such as neuroprotectin D_1, derived from DHA, have potent suppressive effects on neutrophils, macrophages, T cells and microglia (nervous system macrophages), protecting nervous tissue from inflammatory immune reactions. Neuroprotectin D_1 has inflammation-suppressing effects in the brain and nervous system, and protects retinal epithelial cells from oxidation damage.

Prostaglandin I_3, resolvins and protectins are strongly anti-inflammatory, and the inflammatory eicosanoids produced from EPA are relatively weak; therefore, the overall effect of n-3 metabolism is to suppress inflammation. AA eicosanoids are synthesised soon after an injury or stress, whereas EPA eicosanoids are formed at a slower rate and generally act to suppress the effects of AA eicosanoids. Both AA and EPA pathways are dependent on the same enzyme systems, but prefer to act on EPA rather than AA and the n-3 pathway will become active if sufficient EPA is available in cell membranes. Eating foods containing n-3 PUFAs results in EPA and DHA replacing some of the AA in cell membranes and producing n-3 eicosanoids.

The correct balance between n-3 and n-6 PUFAs is vital for keeping inflammation under control. Eating a lot more n-6 PUFAs than n-3 PUFAs, which is common in Western diets, is considered to promote chronic inflammation, autoimmune diseases, cardiovascular disease (CVD), cognitive, mood and behavioural disorders, rheumatoid arthritis, cancer and osteoporosis.

Specific functions of n-3 PUFAs

- *Cardiovascular system.* n-3 PUFAs may be useful for moderating inflammation and reducing some of the risk factors for CVD. n-3 PUFAs have blood-thinning activity, dilate blood vessels, stabilise heart rhythm, reduce serum TG levels and have a modest blood pressure-lowering effect. They lower serum TGs by reducing synthesis of TGs and VLDLs in the liver and increasing liver uptake of TGs from VLDLs and chylomicrons, but do not appear to lower serum cholesterol levels. n-3 PUFAs decrease clotting by reducing platelet aggregation and fibrinogen formation, and reduce blood pressure by inhibiting production of TXA_2, increasing production of the vasodilator nitric oxide, improving vascular reactivity and compliance, and moderating autonomic nerve function. n-3 PUFAs increase the content of DHA in the membranes of cardiac mitochondria, which prevents increases in membrane permeability that can lead to cell death.
- *Metabolic syndrome.* Metabolic syndrome is a collection of physiological abnormalities that increases the risk of developing CVD and diabetes. These include abnormal blood lipids and cholesterol, abdominal obesity, high blood pressure and glucose intolerance. n-3 PUFAs may improve insulin sensitivity, enhance weight loss and protect against circulatory disorders in patients with metabolic syndrome.
- *Anticancer activity.* n-3 PUFAs reduce tumour growth by reducing the ability of cancer cells to bind to basement membranes of tissues and reducing collagenase activity by cancer cells that breaks down surrounding connective tissue and assists the spread of cancer. They help to inhibit tumour metastases and development of pre-cancerous bowel polyps, increase the effectiveness of chemotherapy and radiotherapy, and reduce cancer cachexia (wasting).
- *Anti-inflammatory activity.* n-3 PUFAs decrease production of PGE_2, TXA_2 and LTB_4, and increase production of TXA_3, LTB_5, PGI_3, resolvins and protectins while maintaining PGI_2 levels. The overall result is to dampen inflammatory reactions. They also inhibit production of inflammatory substances such as interleukins (ILs), tumour necrosis factor-alpha (TNF-alpha), platelet-activating factor (PAF), monocyte chemoattractant protein-1 (MCP-1), platelet-derived growth factor (PDGF) and cellular adhesion molecules (CAMs). n-3 FAs may inhibit autoimmune inflammation in disorders such as rheumatoid arthritis, asthma, chronic obstructive pulmonary disease, Crohn's disease, ulcerative colitis, systemic lupus erythematosus, IgA nephropathy and psoriasis.
- *Bone health.* n-3 PUFAs have been found to increase bone formation, improve peak bone mass in adolescents and reduce bone loss. They interact with the receptor activator of NF-kappaB (RANK) that stimulates development of the cells that break

down bone (osteoclasts). Resolvins and LXs inhibit inflammation-induced bone resorption.

- *Brain function.* DHA has 22 carbons and six double bonds, a structure that gives it unique structural and functional properties in cell membrane PLs, particularly in the retina and the nerve synapses in the brain. Tissues rich in DHA include the cerebral cortex, retina, testes and sperm. Brain tissue contains a particularly high concentration of DHA, which makes up 40 per cent of total PUFAs in the brain and 50 per cent of nerve cell membranes, where it is incorporated into PS and PE in cell membrane PLs. Brain levels of DHA are conserved at the expense of other tissue if dietary intake is inadequate. However, pregnancy, lactation and alcohol intake cause significant losses from the brain.

  DHA maintains cell membrane function, enhances nerve transmission and nerve development, and protects brain tissue from oxidative stress. It produces eicosanoids that can act in signalling pathways and as transcription factors for genes. It appears to help regulate cognitive function and mood, has anti-depressant properties and can promote a sense of wellbeing.

  DHA is important for brain development, particularly during the third trimester of pregnancy and the first two years of life, when brain growth is rapid. DHA in breast milk is vital for the development of an infant's brain and nervous system, and for visual acuity.

Dietary sources

- *SFAs* are found mainly in animal fats, butter, cream, full-fat dairy products, cheese, lard, suet, dripping, meat, poultry, chocolate, egg yolk and tropical oils such as coconut oil, palm oil and cocoa butter.
- *MUFAs* are found mainly in olive oil, canola oil and flaxseed (linseed) oil.
- *PUFAs* are found mainly in vegetable oils, nuts, seeds, whole grains, legumes, seafood, seaweed and fish oils.
- *LA* is found mainly in corn oil, safflower oil, evening primrose oil, sunflower oil, cottonseed oil, soy oil, sesame oil and most commercial vegetable oils.
- *AA* is found mainly in animal fats (eggs, meats, dairy food) and peanut oil.
- *GLA* is found mainly in evening primrose oil, borage (starflower) oil and blackcurrant seed oil.
- *alpha-LNA* is found mainly in flaxseed, canola, walnut and soy oils, as well as flaxseeds, walnuts, butternuts, pumpkin seeds, redcurrant and blackcurrant seeds, wheat germ, beans, seaweed, microalgae and green vegetables, such as purslane and spinach. Small amounts are found in seafood, fish oil and fish liver oils, but fish liver oils should be used with caution due to their high vitamin A content.
- *EPA and DHA* are mainly found in seaweed, microalgae, fish oil and cold-water seafood, especially oily fish such as Atlantic salmon, bream, sea perch (orange roughy), mullet, pilchards, some varieties of tuna, sardines, anchovies, mackerel, herring and gemfish, as well as crab, prawns, lobster, shellfish, octopus, squid and fish roe (caviar). Smaller amounts are found in poultry, eggs and meat, especially if animals are pasture-grazed or supplied with n-3 fats in their feed. n-3 FAs remain liquid at cold temperatures and act like anti-freeze in fish; therefore, fish from cold ocean waters are better sources. Tropical fish and freshwater fish are generally poor sources.

  Fish that are higher in the food chain are more likely to accumulate toxins such as mercury, other heavy metals, dioxins and polychlorinated biphenyls (PCBs). These fish are predators that live on smaller fish and accumulate the toxins that are in their prey. They also tend to live longer, which means that when they are caught, toxin levels will have built up over a longer period and can reach higher levels. Fish that are lower in the food chain eat mainly algae and plankton, a diet that exposes them to fewer toxins, and they tend to have shorter lifespans over which to accumulate them. To reduce mercury exposure, it is preferable to take fish oil because it is processed to reduce contaminants, or to eat small species of fish, such as sardines. Large species of fish, especially flake, swordfish and marlin, should not be eaten frequently.
- *PLs* are found mainly in egg yolk, organ meats, lean meats, seafood, shellfish, roe, grains, soybeans and seeds. Lecithin is a concentrated source derived from soybeans.

Access the Food Standards Australia New Zealand nutrient database (NUTTAB) at <www.foodstandards.gov.au> for the amounts found in specific foods.

Factors influencing lipid status

Lipid absorption may be reduced in disorders of the pancreas, liver and gall bladder. Other disorders inhibiting lipid absorption include coeliac disease (gluten intolerance), tropical sprue, Crohn's disease, giardia bowel infections, overgrowth of abnormal bacteria in the bowel and cystic fibrosis. People on very low-fat diets will have a low intake of EFAs. A high intake of n-6 PUFAs (from most of the commonly used vegetable oils) may be associated with an inadequate intake of n-3 PUFAs or an imbalance of EFAs. Vegans and people who do not eat seafood must rely on the relatively inefficient production of EPA and DHA from alpha-LNA in the body, which may lead to inadequate production of n-3 PUFA eicosanoids. The obesity drug orlistat (Xenical) selectively inhibits lipase activity and reduces fat absorption by 70 per cent.

Daily requirement

Government recommendations by age and gender (see Tables 4.2, 4.3 and 4.4) can be found in *Nutrient Reference Values for Australia and New Zealand Including Recommended Dietary Intakes*, available at <www.nrv.gov.au>. In general, the NHMRC of Australia recommends that the total dietary fat content should be between 20 and 35 per cent of total kilojoules (approximately 30–60 g daily) and should be made up of no more than 10 per cent SFAs and trans FAs and up to 10 per cent EFAs. The remainder should be made up of MUFAs.

Table 4.2 Adequate daily intake (AI) of linoleic acid (g/day)

Age (years)	Female AI	Male AI
1–3	5	5
4–8	8	8
9–13	8	10
14–18	8	12
19–70	8	13
>70	8	13
Pregnant women		
14–18	10	
19–50	10	
Lactating women		
14–18	12	
19–50	12	

Source: Nutrient Reference Values for Australia and New Zealand Including Recommended Dietary Intakes, National Health and Medical Research Council, Australian Government Department of Health and Ageing, Canberra and Ministry of Health, New Zealand, Wellington, 2006.

Table 4.3 Adequate daily intake (AI) of alpha-linolenic acid (g/day)

Age (years)	Female AI	Male AI
1–3	0.5	0.5
4–8	0.8	0.8
9–13	0.8	1.0
14–18	0.8	1.2
19–70	0.8	1.3
>70	0.8	1.3
Pregnant women		
14–18	1.0	
19–50	1.0	
Lactating women		
14–18	1.2	
19–50	1.2	

Source: Nutrient Reference Values for Australia and New Zealand Including Recommended Dietary Intakes, National Health and Medical Research Council, Australian Government Department of Health and Ageing, Canberra and Ministry of Health, New Zealand, Wellington, 2006.

Table 4.4 Adequate daily intake (AI) of combined EPA, DHA and DPA (mg/day)

Age (years)	Female AI	Male AI
1–3	40	40
4–8	55	55
9–13	70	70
14–18	85	125
19–70	90	160
>70	90	160
Pregnant women		
14–18	110	
19–50	115	
Lactating women		
14–18	140	
19–50	145	

Source: Nutrient Reference Values for Australia and New Zealand Including Recommended Dietary Intakes, National Health and Medical Research Council, Australian Government Department of Health and Ageing, Canberra and Ministry of Health, New Zealand, Wellington, 2006.

Deficiency effects

Fat malabsorption leads to steatorrhoea (fat in the faeces), which manifests as pale, greasy, foul-smelling stools that float in the toilet and are difficult to flush. Although lipid intake is often higher than recommended in Western countries, intake of EFA is often inadequate, especially n-3 PUFAs. General indications of inadequate lipid status may include liver and kidney disorders; increased water permeability of the skin leading to excessive perspiration or thirst; frequent urination; dry, itchy skin; dry hair; dandruff; weak, splitting, flaking or brittle fingernails; gooseflesh appearance of the skin (hyperfollicular keratosis); fluid retention; susceptibility to infections; poor wound healing; gallstones; reproductive disorders; reduced metabolic rate; and deficiencies of fat-soluble vitamins (vitamins A, D, E and K).

Indicators of inadequate levels of n-3 PUFAs may include:

- *cardiovascular disorders*, such as elevated serum TGs, elevated blood pressure, atherosclerosis, thrombosis, heart enlargement, oedema, irregular heart rhythm
- *autoimmune diseases*, such as systemic lupus erythematosus, multiple sclerosis, rheumatoid arthritis, Sjögren's syndrome
- *infections*
- *neurological disorders*, such as mood disorders, depression, schizophrenia, and learning and psychiatric disorders
- *skin disorders*, such as inflammation, dermatitis, psoriasis, increased perspiration, reduced sebum production, overgrowth of epithelial cells, poor wound healing
- *chronic inflammatory disorders*, such as osteoarthritis, asthma, hay fever
- *reproductive disorders*, such as infertility, miscarriage, irregular menstrual cycles, premenstrual syndrome, menstrual cramps
- *osteoporosis*
- *infants*: impaired brain and nerve development, poor vision
- *children*: stunted growth, food sensitivities, excessive thirst, frequent urination, dry skin and hair, eczema, dandruff, brittle nails, rough, gooseflesh appearance of the skin, asthma, poor coordination, hyperactivity, behaviour problems, reduced learning ability, poor school performance.

Assessment of body status

Assessment of FA status is undertaken rarely except in research settings. Serum concentrations of FAs can be used to assess the adequacy of dietary intake or absorption. The plasma ratio of eicosatrienoic acid:arachidonic acid (triene:tetraene ratio) can be used to assess EFA status; a ratio greater than 0.2 indicates EFA deficiency. The reference (normal) serum ranges given by the Mayo Medical Laboratories (USA) are listed in Table 4.5.

The n-3 index has been proposed as a measure of risk of death from coronary heart disease (CHD). It is derived from the total amount of EPA and DHA in red blood cell membranes expressed as a percentage of the total amount of FAs. An index of 8 per cent or more is believed to be cardioprotective. An index of 4 per cent or lower is believed to be associated with the greatest risk of CHD death.

Table 4.5 Serum reference range for fatty acids

	1–17 years	18 years and over
LA	1600–3500 nmol/mL	2270–3850 nmol/mL
Alpha-LNA	20–120 nmol/mL	50–130 nmol/mL
EPA	8–90 nmol/mL	14–100 nmol/mL
DHA	30–160 nmol/mL	30–250 nmol/mL
Total n-3 PUFAs	0.1–0.5 mmol/L	0.2–0.5 mmol/L
Total n-6 PUFAs	1.6–4.7 mmol/L	3.0–5.4 mmol/L
Triene:tetraene ratio	0.013–0.050	0.010–0.038

Source: Mayo Medical Laboratories, available at <www.mayomedicallaboratories.com/test-catalog/Clinical+and+Interpretive/82426>.

Case reports—EFA deficiency

- *A girl, six years of age*, had received an accidental gunshot wound in her abdomen and was placed on a parenteral (intravenous) lipid emulsion providing safflower oil that was almost entirely lacking in n-3 PUFAs but had a very high content of n-6 PUFAs.[1] After five months, she developed episodes of numbness, tingling, weakness and leg pain, an inability to walk, psychological disturbances and blurred vision. She was found to be deficient in n-3 PUFAs and was changed to a soybean preparation that provided n-3 PUFAs, after which her symptoms resolved and her n-3 PUFA status normalised.
- *A boy, seventeen years of age*, developed severe complications after a bone marrow transplant and required parenteral feeding.[2] He had a severe soy allergy and was not able to have the fat emulsions available at the time because they all contained soy oil. He was maintained on a fat-free preparation. After some months, he was still very ill and developed a skin rash. He was found to be deficient in EFAs and was changed to an experimental parenteral fish oil emulsion. His skin rash resolved in ten days, his general health improved and he continued in relatively good health until oral feeding could be resumed.

REFERENCES

1 Holman, R.T., The slow discovery of the importance of omega-3 essential fatty acids in human health, *J Nutr* (1998), 128: 427S–33S.

2 Gura, K.M., Parsons, S.K., Bechard, L.J., et al, Use of a fish oil-based lipid emulsion to treat essential fatty acid deficiency in a soy allergic patient receiving parenteral nutrition, *Clin Nutr* (2005), 24(5): 839–47.

THERAPEUTIC USES OF n-3 PUFAS

Cardiovascular disease (CVD)

Populations of people in northern Canada and Alaska who traditionally eat large amounts of seafood in their diet have much lower CVD mortality than expected for the amount of fat consumed and Japanese populations on traditional diets rich in seafood have a low prevalence of CVD.[1] Medical guidelines for the management of patients after myocardial infarction (MI, heart attack) commonly recommend increased intake of n-3 PUFAs.[2]

n-3 PUFAs have been shown to improve several CVD risk factors, including lowering serum TG levels, stabilising heart rhythm, decreasing platelet aggregation and modestly reducing blood pressure (0.66 mmHg systolic and 0.35 mmHg diastolic blood pressure reduction per 1 g of n-3 PUFAs).[1,3] Supplementary intake of 1–4 g of marine n-3 PUFAs daily is estimated to lower serum TGs by 25–30 per cent and increase HDL cholesterol levels by 1–3 per cent.[2]

Fish oil is used to improve cardiovascular outcomes in patients with CVD. Fish and fish oil intake has been associated with significantly reduced mortality in survivors of an MI, as well as reduced CVD mortality and reduced incidence of MI, sudden death, non-fatal MI and non-fatal stroke.[1] In patients with CHD, 850 mg daily of marine n-3 PUFAs has reduced the risk of CHD mortality and 1800 mg daily has reduced the risk of major coronary events.[1] A review of clinical trials concluded that n-3 PUFAs lowered the risk of overall mortality by 20 per cent and cardiac mortality by 30 per cent in patients with CHD.[4] However, not all trials have found positive effects. A study of men with angina found that n-3 PUFAs, oily fish or fish oils increased the risk of cardiac death by 26 per cent and the risk of sudden cardiac death by 54 per cent.[5] Most of the risk was associated with men taking n-3 PUFAs as fish oil capsules. However the quality of this trial has been criticised.[6]

Increased fish intake is associated with reduced risk of death due to heart failure, and trials of fish oil have found similar protective effects. There are conflicting reports on the benefits of n-3 PUFAs for ventricular arrhythmias, and it is suggested that patients who have had a recent MI and heart failure could benefit, whereas those with ischaemic heart disease but no previous MI could have an increased risk.[7] There are conflicting reports about the effects of n-3 PUFAs in atrial fibrillation.

A study of patients with atherosclerotic plaques in the carotid artery found that n-3 PUFA supplementation was able to stabilise the plaque, which may reduce the risk of rupture.[7] Consumption of fish and n-3 PUFAs appears to have a moderate effect on reducing the risk of cerebrovascular disease (stroke).[8] Although individual studies have found that n-3 PUFAs are associated with benefits in various types of CVD, a review of 20 clinical trials concluded that, overall, n-3 PUFAs have not been shown to improve major cardiovascular outcomes.[9] However, doses of n-3 PUFAs used in most of the studies included in this review were well below the recommendations for patients with CVD.

Diabetes

A review of 23 clinical trials using n-3 PUFA supplementation for diabetic patients found that supplementation lowered serum TG levels by 0.45 mmol/L, lowered VLDL cholesterol by 0.07 mmol/L and raised LDL cholesterol levels by 0.11 mmol/L.[10] There was no significant effect on total or HDL cholesterol, glycated haemoglobin, fasting glucose, fasting insulin or body weight.

Cancer

In general, n-6 PUFAs appear to be cancer-promoting and n-3 PUFAs appear to have anticancer activity. A number of animal studies have shown that animals given supplementary n-3 PUFAs have a 20–50 per cent reduction in tumour incidence and a 30–70 per cent reduction in tumour growth compared with animals given supplementary n-6 PUFAs or a low-fat diet.[11] Exposure of human cancer cells to either EPA or DHA has caused reduced cellular proliferation and increased apoptosis.

In animals, n-6 PUFAs increase the risk of breast cancer, and epidemiological studies have found a similar association in women. Women with a genetic abnormality affecting the LOX enzyme have been found to have an increased breast cancer risk if their diets have a high level of LA.[12] Reducing their LA intake has been shown to abolish the increased breast cancer risk. In two dietary trials investigating CVD, subjects who increased their intake of n-6 PUFAs had an increased cancer rate, and subjects who reduced their intake had a reduced risk.[12]

Studies of n-3 PUFA intake and cancer risk have found that a higher intake may be protective against some cancers, such as breast and colorectal (bowel) cancer, and n-3 PUFAs may improve the effectiveness and tolerability of cancer chemotherapy drugs.[13] EPA is protective against colorectal cancer in animals and has been found to reduce the incidence of bowel polyps in patients with familial bowel polyps.[14] DHA inhibits production of n-6-derived pro-inflammatory eicosanoids and may be particularly protective against cancer because it has anti-proliferative effects on cancer cells and in animals, and can work in conjunction with cancer drugs.[15] Patients with advanced breast cancer treated with chemotherapy together with DHA were assessed for their ability to incorporate DHA into blood cells and plasma.[16] Those who were high incorporators had delayed tumour progression and longer overall survival compared with the low incorporators.

Cognitive and psychiatric disorders

A variety of psychiatric disorders may be associated with PUFA deficiencies, such as ADHD, autism, major depression, post-natal depression, seasonal affective disorder, bipolar disorder, schizophrenia, dementia, aggression, hostility and criminality. Low levels of EFAs have been correlated with suicide attempts, impulsive behaviour and a more severe level of depression. A review of fourteen clinical trials concluded that levels of EPA, DHA and total n-3 PUFAs were significantly lower in depressive patients, but there was no relationship between depression and levels of AA or total n-6 PUFAs.[17] A small study of children with depression found that n-3 PUFAs led to considerable symptom improvement and large doses of n-3 PUFAs together with standard treatment in patients with major depression more than doubled blood levels of DHA and resulted in reduced depression scores.[18]

A small trial of men with substance abuse found that three months of treatment with n-3 PUFAs relieved anger and anxiety.[18] Several studies have found that a combination of n-3 and n-6 PUFAs is effective in improving symptoms of ADHD in children and a review of ten clinical trials concluded that n-3 PUFA supplementation, particularly with higher doses of EPA, had a modest effect on improving symptoms of ADHD.[19] However, a rigorous review of thirteen trials concluded that there was little evidence that PUFA supplementation was of benefit for ADHD.[20]

People with the highest plasma DHA concentration have been found to have a 47 per cent lower risk of dementia.[21] In older patients with memory loss, 900 mg/day of DHA for 24 weeks improved cognitive function[21] and, in healthy older women, 800 mg/day of DHA for four months improved verbal fluency.[22] A review of clinical trials of dementia patients identified a trend in favour of n-3 PUFAs for reducing the incidence of dementia and improving cognitive function, but this did not reach statistical significance.[23] A review of the use of EPA for schizophrenia found that it may help relieve symptoms and reduce the need for standard anti-psychotic drugs.[24] However, the data are limited, and no conclusions can be made about the effectiveness of EPA for this condition.

Rheumatoid arthritis (RhA)

A review of twelve trials using fish oil for the management of RhA concluded that fish oil consistently provided benefits, including relief of pain and morning stiffness, fewer tender and swollen joints, and lower global arthritis activity.[25] In some of the trials, patients on fish oil were able to reduce their use of non-steroidal anti-inflammatory drugs (NSAIDs).

Asthma

Fish oil supplementation has been found to improve lung function in adult asthma patients undergoing exercise, and was associated with reduced use of bronchodilators and reduced markers of inflammation.[26] Other studies of asthma patients have revealed conflicting results and a review of ten clinical trials concluded that it was not possible to determine the effectiveness of n-3 PUFA therapy for asthma.[26]

Osteoporosis

A review of ten clinical trials found four studies reporting that n-3 FA had favourable effects on bone mineral density (BMD) or bone turnover markers.[27] Three of these trials combined n-3 FA supplementation with a high calcium intake. Five studies reported that n-3 PUFAs had no effect and one was inconclusive. It appears that there is a potential benefit of n-3 PUFAs together with calcium on bone health.

Inflammatory bowel disease

Clinical trials in patients with ulcerative colitis have found that fish oil supplements reduce inflammation and LTB_4 production in the bowel, improve bowel histology, decrease the need for anti-inflammatory drugs and promote normal weight gain.[28] However, reported compliance is poor. A review of six clinical trials that used fish oil for ulcerative colitis found that several studies reported benefits, but that study quality was generally too poor to form conclusions about its effectiveness.[28]

A review of six clinical trials that used fish oil for maintaining remission of Crohn's disease found that three studies reported a reduction in the rate of relapse over a twelve-month period.[29] However, the two largest studies did not find that fish oil reduced relapse incidence. A more recent review of nine studies found that fish oil was associated with a small reduction in relapse rate in patients with inflammatory bowel disease.[30]

REFERENCES

1 Lavie, C.J., Milani, R.V., Mehra, M.R. & Ventura, H.O., Omega-3 polyunsaturated fatty acids and cardiovascular diseases, *J Am Coll Cardiol* (2009), 54(7): 585–94.

2 National Heart Foundation of Australia, *Review of evidence: Fish, fish oils, n-3 polyunsaturated fatty acids and cardiovascular health*, National Heart Foundation, Canberra, 2008.

3 Morris, M.C., Sacks, F. & Rosner, B., Does fish oil lower blood pressure? A meta-analysis of controlled trials, *Circulation* (1993), 88(2): 523–33.

4 Bucher, H.C., Hengstler, P., Schindler, C. & Meier, G., n-3 polyunsaturated fatty acids in coronary heart disease: A meta-analysis of randomized controlled trials, *Am J Med* (2002), 112(4): 298–304.

5 Burr, M.L., Ashfield-Watt, P.A., Dunstan F.D. et al., Lack of benefit of dietary advice to men with angina: Results of a controlled trial, *Eur J Clin Nutr* (2003), 57: 193–200.

6 von Schacky, C. & Harris, W.S., Cardiovascular benefits of omega-3 fatty acids, *Cardiovasc Res* (2007), 73: 310–15.

7 Saravanan, P., Davidson, N.C., Schmidt, E.B. & Calder, P.C., Cardiovascular effects of marine omega-3 fatty acids, *Lancet* (2010), 376(9740): 540–50.

8 Chowdhury, R., Stevens, S., Gorman, D. et al., Association between fish consumption, long-chain omega-3 fatty acids, and risk of cerebrovascular disease: Systematic review and meta-analysis, *BMJ* (2012), 345: e6698.

9 Rizos, E.C., Ntzani, E.E., Bika, E. et al., Association between omega-3 fatty acid supplementation and risk of major cardiovascular disease events: A systematic review and meta-analysis, *JAMA* (2012), 308(10): 1024–33.

10 Hartweg, J., Perera, R., Montori, V. et al., Omega-3 polyunsaturated fatty acids (PUFA) for type 2 diabetes mellitus, *Cochrane Database Syst Rev* (2008), 1: CD003205.

11 Cockbain, A.J., Toogood, G.J. & Hull, M.A., Omega-3 polyunsaturated fatty acids for the treatment and prevention of colorectal cancer, *Gut* (2012), 61(1): 135–49.

12 de Lorgeril. M. & Salen, P., New insights into the health effects of dietary saturated and omega-6 and omega-3 polyunsaturated fatty acids, *BMC Med* (2012), 10: 50.

13 Gerber, M., Omega-3 fatty acids and cancers: A systematic update review of epidemiological studies, *Br J Nutr* (2012), 107 (Suppl 2): S228–39.

14 West, N.J., Clark, S.K., Phillips, R.K. et al., Eicosapentaenoic acid reduces rectal polyp number and size in familial adenomatous polyposis, *Gut* (2010), 59(7): 918–25.

15 Gleissman, H., Johnsen, J.I. & Kogner, P., Omega–3 fatty acids in cancer, the protectors of good and the killers of evil? *Exp Cell Res* (2010), 316(8): 1365–73.

16 Bougnoux, P., Hajjaji, N., Ferrasson, M.N. et al., Improving outcome of chemotherapy of metastatic breast cancer by docosahexaenoic acid: a phase II trial, *Br J Cancer* (2009), 101(12): 1978–85.

17 Lin, P.Y., Huang, S.Y. & Su, K.P., A meta-analytic review of polyunsaturated fatty acid compositions in patients with depression, *Biol Psychiatry* (2010), 68(2): 140–7.

18 Sinn, N., Milte, C. & Howe, P.R., Oiling the brain: A review of randomized controlled trials of omega–3 fatty acids in psychopathology across the lifespan, *Nutrients* (2010), 2(2): 128–70.

19 Bloch, M.H. & Qawasmi, A., Omega-3 fatty acid supplementation for the treatment of children with attention-deficit/hyperactivity disorder symptomatology: Systematic review and meta-analysis, *J Am Acad Child Adolesc Psychiatry* (2011), 50(10): 991–1000.

20 Gillies, D., Sinn, J.K.H., Lad, S.S. et al., Polyunsaturated fatty acids (PUFA) for attention deficit hyperactivity disorder (ADHD) in children and adolescents, *Cochrane Database Syst Rev* (2012), 7: CD007986.

21 Cole, G.M. & Frautschy, S.A., DHA may prevent age-related dementia, *J Nutr* (2010), 140(4): 869–74.

22 Johnson, E.J., McDonald, K., Caldarella, S.M. et al., Cognitive findings of an exploratory trial of docosahexaenoic acid and lutein supplementation in older women, *Nutr Neurosci* (2008), 11(2): 75–83.

23 Issa, A.M., Mojica, W.A., Morton, S.C. et al., The efficacy of omega-3 fatty acids on cognitive function in aging and dementia: A systematic review, *Dement Geriatr Cogn Disord* (2006), 21(2): 88–96.

24 Joy, C.B., Mumby-Croft, R. & Joy, L.A., Polyunsaturated fatty acid supplementation for schizophrenia, *Cochrane Database Syst Rev* (2003), 2: CD001257.

25 De Silva, P.V., Efficacy of fish body oil in the treatment of rheumatoid arthritis: A systematic review, *Galle Med J* (2012), 17(1): 18–22.

26 Reisman, J., Schachter, H.M., Dales, R.E. et al., Treating asthma with omega-3 fatty acids: Where is the evidence? A systematic review, *BMC Complement Altern Med* (2006), 6: 26.

27 Orchard, T.S., Pan, X., Cheek, F., Ing, S.W. & Jackson, R.D., A systematic review of omega-3 fatty acids and osteoporosis, *Br J Nutr* (2012), 107 (Suppl 2): S253–60.

28 De Ley, M., de Vos, R., Hommes, D.W. & Stokkers, P., Fish oil for induction of remission in ulcerative colitis, *Cochrane Database Syst Rev* (2007) 4: CD005986.

29 Turner, D., Zlotkin, S.H., Shah, P.S. & Griffiths, A.M., Omega-3 fatty acids (fish oil) for maintenance of remission in Crohn's disease, *Cochrane Database Syst Rev* (2009), 1: CD006320.
30 Turner, D., Shah, P.S., Steinhart, A.H. et al., Maintenance of remission in inflammatory bowel disease using omega-3 fatty acids (fish oil): A systematic review and meta-analysis, *Inflamm Bowel Dis* (2011), 17(1): 336–45.

Therapeutic dose of n-3 FAs

Suggested doses for adults are as follows:

- *General health maintenance:* 3 g daily
- *Mild deficiency:* 6 g daily
- *Severe deficiency:* up to 9 g daily
- *Chronic inflammatory disorders:* up to 9 g daily
- *Cognitive, mood and behaviour disorders:* 3–9 g daily. In clinical trials, doses of up to 6 g daily of EPA and doses of up to 3 g daily of DHA have been used.

Recommendations for CVD

The National Heart Foundation of Australia (NHF) and the Cardiac Society of Australia and New Zealand recommend that all patients with CHD should replace SFAs with MUFAs and PUFAs and consume:[1]

- 1 g daily of combined EPA and DHA through a combination of oily fish (two to three serves per week of 150 g of fish), fish oil capsules or liquid, and food and drinks enriched with n-3 PUFAs, plus
- 2 g daily of alpha-LNA, which can be obtained by eating canola or soybean-based oils and margarine spreads; seeds, especially flaxseeds (linseeds); nuts, especially walnuts; legumes, including soybeans; eggs; and green leafy vegetables.

All patients with elevated serum TGs are recommended to take 1.2 g daily of combined EPA and DHA, which can be increased gradually to 4 g daily if target serum TG levels are not reached.

To prevent heart disease, the NHF recommends that the adult population should consume:[2]

- 500 mg daily of combined DHA and EPA, and
- at least 2 g daily of alpha-LNA.

REFERENCES

1 National Heart Foundation of Australia and the Cardiac Society of Australia and New Zealand, *Reducing risk in heart disease: an expert guide to clinical practice for secondary prevention of coronary heart disease*, National Heart Foundation of Australia, Melbourne, 2012.
2 National Heart Foundation of Australia. *Review of evidence: Fish, fish oils, n-3 polyunsaturated fatty acids and cardiovascular health*, National Heart Foundation of Australia, Melbourne, 2008.

Effects of excess

Excess intake of lipids, especially SFAs, has been associated with overweight, abdominal obesity, type 2 diabetes, elevated serum cholesterol, CVD, inflammatory disorders, gall bladder disease and cancer. Replacing SFAs in the diet with PUFAs has been shown to reduce LDL cholesterol but replacing SFAs with carbohydrates, particularly refined carbohydrates and sugar, increases blood triglycerides, reduces HDL and increases the amount of small LDL particles, which leads to an elevated heart disease risk. However, new research has raised questions about the heart disease/SFA connection and a recent review concluded that there was no significant evidence for linking dietary SFAs with an increased risk of CHD or CVD.

It appears that the type of SFA eaten affects the health risk. Lauric, myristic and palmitic acids increase total serum cholesterol and LDL. Stearic acid has little effect on blood cholesterol or CVD risk, which may be because it is rapidly converted to MUFAs in the body. Short- and medium-chain fatty acids also have little effect. Myristic acid may have beneficial effects because it appears to activate the conversion of alpha-LNA to DHA. Butyric acid appears to regulate cell growth and have anticancer activity. More research is required to clarify the health effects of individual SFAs.

People with liver or gall bladder disorders should use fat or oil supplements with caution because they may cause nausea and vomiting. Adverse effects of large doses of fish oil (more than 6 g daily) include fishy breath, belching, reflux and diarrhoea. PUFAs are susceptible to oxidation, especially those with more double bonds, such as n-3 PUFAs. Excess intake of PUFAs is linked to increased free radical formation and cell membrane and DNA damage, and excess n-6 PUFAs relative to n-3 PUFAs may increase the risk of cancer. Excess n-6 PUFAs may enhance tumour growth, increase inflammation, aggravate insulin resistance and reduce HDL cholesterol as well as LDL cholesterol. A small amount of vitamin E is usually added to oil supplements to protect the fats from oxidation during storage. However, it is advisable to take a vitamin E supplement for extra antioxidant activity when taking increased amounts of PUFAs. Excess n-3 PUFAs can thin the blood and prolong bleeding time, and large amounts are not recommended before surgery or for people on anticoagulant (blood-thinning) therapy.

Supplements

Most lipids are easily obtained from food, especially SFAs, MUFAs and n-6 PUFAs, and supplements are usually not required. However, n–3 PUFAs are harder to obtain from food, and may be inadequate if no seafood is eaten. PUFA sources used as supplements in Australia include evening primrose oil (for LA and GLA), lecithin (for PC and PLs), PS, flaxseed oil (for LA and alpha-LNA), and fish, calamari and krill oils (for EPA and DHA), and are available in capsule or liquid forms.

Cautions

Oil supplements may cause diarrhoea in large doses, and may cause nausea and vomiting in people with liver or gall bladder disorders. Usually, n-6 PUFAs are over-supplied in the diet and excess may deplete n-3 PUFAs; n-6 PUFA supplements should be used with caution. PUFAs should not be exposed to heat, air or light during storage, and are best kept in cool conditions or in the fridge and used within a short space of time. They should not be used as cooking oils; MUFAs should be used instead. Antioxidant intake should be increased if high doses of PUFAs are used.

Fish, calamari and krill oils should not be used in people with seafood allergy. High doses of n-3 PUFAs have a blood-thinning effect, so should be avoided before surgery. People taking blood-thinning medication should seek medical advice before taking supplementary doses of n-3 PUFAs.

Vegetable oil processing

PUFAs are sensitive to heat, light and air, and sensitive FAs may be damaged by standard processing methods. In the standard process of making vegetable oils, seeds are cleaned, de-hulled and softened by steaming at a temperature of about 72°C. The oil is removed from the seed material by a solvent, typically hexane, which removes about 99 per cent of the oil. The solvent is removed by steaming the seed material several times at about 182°C. The end product should contain less than 100 ppm of hexane.

Oils are refined in a number of steps. Oils high in phosphatides, such as soybean, corn and sunflower oils, may be de-gummed at 60–80°C prior to refining. Neutralisation in an alkaline solution at temperatures of about 75°C removes free FAs, proteins, carbohydrates and resins. The oil is then bleached by mixing with a bleaching clay at about 110°C to remove pigments, oxidation products, phosphatides, soaps and trace metals, and to improve the colour. Hydrogenation or fractionation may be used to stabilise the oil's taste and smell during storage, and to extend shelf life, during which temperatures may reach 163°C or higher. Hydrogenation or fractionation can also be used to change the functional characteristics of the naturally occurring fats to suit commercial purposes. The oil is next deodorised by injecting steam at a temperature of about 260°C in order to vaporise free fatty acids and odoriferous compounds. Bulk oils are stored under nitrogen to reduce oxidation.

An alternative to solvent oil extraction is expeller pressing, which uses mechanical pressure without external heat and reduces heat damage to sensitive fatty acids. However, expeller pressing can generate friction temperatures of up to 135°C for brief periods. An alternative method of extraction is the use of supercritical fluid extraction with carbon dioxide.

Cold-pressing is a term that may be used for expeller pressing but true cold-pressing is expeller pressing in a controlled temperature environment that should not exceed 50°C. Cold-pressed oil has been defined as oil that has undergone mechanical extraction without pre-cooking or heating, and without subsequent chemical (solvent) extraction and/or chemical refining. After pressing, the oil is purified by sedimentation, filtration or centrifugation processes that may involve heating to 20–30°C. The cold-pressing process removes phosphates and the oil does not require de-gumming and refining. However, some cold-pressed oils may undergo further non-chemical refining, bleaching, deodorising and hydrogenation or fractionation to enhance shelf life, taste and smell. Cold-pressing is more effective for seeds with a very high oil content, such as olives and sunflower seeds. It removes only about 83–88 per cent of the oil and the resulting oil has a limited shelf life but it has the advantage of preserving flavour and colour, as well as sensitive PUFAs, antioxidants and fat-soluble vitamins.

n-6 PUFA supplements

n-6 PUFA supplements include evening primrose oil, lecithin, PC and PS. See 'Choline' for information on lecithin and PC.

Evening primrose oil (EPO)

EPO is derived from the seeds of the evening primrose plant (*Oenothera biennis*). It is a rich source of n-6 FAs, especially LA and GLA, that also can be made in the body from LA. The GLA content of EPO averages about 9–10 per cent. Supplements usually are standardised to contain 10 per cent GLA. In the body, GLA is metabolised rapidly to DGLA, which is then converted to PGE_1, a potent anti-inflammatory that inhibits the inflammatory activity of other n-6 eicosanoids. DGLA converts to AA, but this conversion appears to proceed slowly, which may reduce the production of AA-derived eicosanoids.

GLA is not commonly present in foods, and is believed to be responsible for the health benefits of EPO. It is theorised that conversion of LA to GLA may not operate efficiently in some people, and a dietary intake may be useful. GLA, via PGE_1 production, thins the blood and relaxes blood vessels to improve blood flow.[1] It also helps regulate female reproductive cycles and maintain the healthy functioning of smooth muscles in the digestive system, blood vessels, the female reproductive tract and respiratory passages.[1]

EPO has been found to improve blood flow[2] and sterols in EPO have been found to inhibit some markers of inflammation in animal studies.[3] As an anti-inflammatory, EPO may help reduce pain, swelling and stiffness due to chronic inflammation in joints.[4] It has been found to improve symptoms of mild diabetic neuropathy.[5] EPO is used for reducing the symptoms of premenstrual syndrome, such as headaches, low mood, irritability, breast pain and bloating, relieving menstrual cramps, and relieving dry, scaly skin and rashes. However, good-quality evidence is lacking. It may be useful for maintaining health of the skin, hair and nails. Oral EPO has been found to reduce water loss from the skin and improve skin moisture, elasticity and firmness, and reduce roughness.[6]

Most trials have involved small numbers of subjects, and have used a wide dose range (80–640 mg GLA/day), and evidence supporting the health effects of EPO is conflicting. A review of 27 clinical trials of EPO and borage oil for eczema found no evidence of effectiveness,[7] but a subsequent trial found that 160 mg and 320 mg of EPO daily improved symptoms of atopic dermatitis, the higher dose being more effective.[8] A standard dose of EPO is 3–6 g daily.

Cautions[9]

EPO is generally well tolerated, but headache, abdominal pain, nausea and loose stools have been reported. One case report suggested that using EPO for more than one year may lead to inflammation, clotting and immunosuppression. EPO has blood-thinning activity and may increase bleeding. EPO increased bleeding in people on anticoagulant medication and a pregnant woman who took a total of 6.5 g of EPO during the week before giving birth delivered an infant with extensive but transient bruises and petechiae (broken blood vessels in the skin). EPO taken during pregnancy may be associated with birth complications, including a more protracted labour, increased incidence of premature rupture of membranes, arrest of descent, oxytocin use and vacuum extraction. Early reports of EPO exacerbating epilepsy appear to be unfounded. In fact, it has been demonstrated to be protective against seizures in animals and PGE_1 has anti-convulsant activity.

REFERENCES

1 Horrobin, D.F., Nutritional and medical importance of gamma-linolenic acid, *Prog Lipid Res* (1992), 31(2): 163–94.
2 Ford, I., Cotter, M.A., Cameron, N.E. & Greaves, M., The effects of treatment with alpha-lipoic acid or evening primrose oil on vascular hemostatic and lipid risk factors, blood flow, and peripheral nerve conduction in the streptozotocin-diabetic rat, *Metabolism* (2001), 50(8): 868–75.
3 Kunkel, S.L., Ogawa, H., Ward, P.A. & Zurier, R.B., Suppression of chronic inflammation by evening primrose oil, *Prog Lipid Res* (1981), 20: 885–8.
4 Belch, J.J. & Hill, A., Evening primrose oil and borage oil in rheumatologic conditions, *Am J Clin Nutr* (2000), 71(1) (Suppl): 352S–6S.
5 Horrobin, D.F., Essential fatty acids in the management of impaired nerve function in diabetes, *Diabetes* (1997), 46 (Suppl 2): S90–3.
6 Muggli, R., Systemic evening primrose oil improves the biophysical skin parameters of healthy adults, *Int J Cosmet Sci* (2005), 27(4): 243–9.
7 Bamford, J.T., Ray, S., Musekiwa, A. et al., Oral evening primrose oil and borage oil for eczema, *Cochrane Database Syst Rev* (2013), 4: CD004416.
8 Chung, B.Y., Kim, J.H., Cho, S.I., Ahn, I.S., Kim, H.O., Park, C.W. & Lee, C.H., Dose-dependent effects of evening primrose oil in children and adolescents with atopic dermatitis, *Ann Dermatol* (2013), 25(3): 285–91.
9 National Toxicology Program, National Institute of Environmental Health Sciences, National Institutes of Health, US Department of Health and Human Services, *Chemical information review document for evening primrose oil (Oenothera biennis L)* [CAS No. 90028-66-3], Research Triangle Park, NC, 2009.

Phosphatidylserin

Phosphatidylserine (PS) is a component of lecithin that is also made in the body and is particularly concentrated in the brain. PS is part of the structure of the myelin sheath of nerves and nerve cell membranes, and plays an important role in communication between cells and transmission of biochemical messages into the cell interior. PS helps regulate nerve cell metabolism and the function of neurotransmitters, such as acetylcholine, noradrenaline, serotonin and dopamine. It can enhance glucose utilisation in brain tissue, and may have protective antioxidant activity.

During ageing, PS may help maintain mood and mental functions, such as memory, learning, vocabulary skills and concentration.[1] In older people, PS (300 mg/day) has been found to improve motivation, initiative, interest in the environment, socialisation, memory and learning.[2,3] In Alzheimer's disease, PS has been shown to improve anxiety, motivation, memory and cognition.[4] In children with ADHD, PS significantly improved symptoms and short-term auditory memory.[5]

Cortisol is produced during exercise and stimulates muscle breakdown, which is counter-productive for athletic training. PS inhibits the release of the hormone cortisol after intense exercise, and may relieve muscle soreness.[6] PS is available as PS-enriched soy lecithin powder or liquid that is made by enzymatically reacting soybean lecithin with the amino acid L-serine. A standard dose is 200–800 mg daily.

REFERENCES

1 [No authors listed], Phosphatidylserine monograph, *Altern Med Rev* (2008), 13(3): 245–7.
2 Cenacchi. T., Bertoldin, T., Farina C. et al., Cognitive decline in the elderly: A double-blind, placebo-controlled multicenter study on efficacy of phosphatidylserine administration, *Aging (Milano)* (1993), 5: 123–33.

3 Crook, T.H., Tinklenberg, J., Yesavage, J. et al., Effects of phosphatidylserine in age-associated memory impairment, *Neurology* (1991), 41(5): 644–9.
4 Crook, T., Petrie, W., Wells, C. & Massari, D.C., Effects of phosphatidylserine in Alzheimer's disease, *Psychopharmacol Bull* (1992), 28: 61–6.
5 Hirayama, S., Terasawa, K., Rabeler, R. et al., The effect of phosphatidylserine administration on memory and symptoms of attention-deficit hyperactivity disorder: A randomised, double-blind, placebo-controlled clinical trial, *J Hum Nutr Diet* (2013), 27 (Suppl. 2), 284–91.
6 Starks, M.A., Starks, S.L., Kingsley, M. et al., The effects of phosphatidylserine on endocrine response to moderate intensity exercise, *J Int Soc Sports Nutr* (2008), 5: 11.

n-3 PUFA supplements

Flaxseed oil

Flaxseed oil is derived from the seeds of the flax plant (*Linum usitatissimum*). It contains unsaturated fatty acids, including oleic acid (12–30 per cent of total unsaturated fats), LA (8–29 per cent), and alpha-LNA (35–67 per cent). It is used as a source of n-3 FAs for vegans and people who do not eat seafood. Unlike fish oil, flaxseed oil lacks ready-made EPA and DHA. Flaxseed oil has been shown to increase EPA, total n-3 PUFAs and the ratio of n-3 to n-6 PUFAs when given to vegetarian men, but does not appear to increase DHA levels.[1] Fish and fish oil are preferred sources of n-3 fatty acids in non-vegetarians.

Flaxseed oil has been reported to have anti-inflammatory, anti-arthritic, antiulcer, antidiabetic, anti-allergic, anti-atherosclerotic, anti-arrhythmic and blood-thinning activity.[2] It is popular for maintaining healthy skin, hair and nails, but supporting evidence is lacking. However, topical flaxseed oil has been found to accelerate wound repair in animals.[3] Alpha-LNA has beneficial effects on central nervous system function and behaviour, and inhibits inflammation induced by AA, PGE_2, LTB_4, histamine and bradykinin.[4] In Sjögren's syndrome, flaxseed oil has reduced eye inflammation and dryness of the eyes.[5]

Flaxseed oil improves artery function, lowers blood pressure and has protective effects against MI.[6] A review of 28 clinical trials found that flaxseed reduces total cholesterol and LDL cholesterol levels, but the effect is small.[7] The review found that flaxseed is more potent than the oil, which appears to be because of the lignan content in the seeds. Unlike fish oil, flaxseed oil does not lower serum TG. Flaxseed oil is available as a liquid or capsules. The standard dose is 3–6 g daily.

REFERENCES

1 Brenna, J.T., Salem, N. Jr, Sinclair, A.J., Cunnane, S.C., International Society for the Study of Fatty Acids and Lipids, ISSFAL, alpha-Linolenic acid supplementation and conversion to n-3 long-chain polyunsaturated fatty acids in humans, *Prostaglandins Leukot Essent Fatty Acids* (2009), 80(2–3): 85–91.
2 Stark, A.H., Crawford, M.A. & Reifen, R., Update on alpha-linolenic acid, *Nutr Rev* (2008), 66(6): 326–32.
3 de Souza Franco, E., de Aquino, C.M., de Medeiros, P.L. et al., Effect of a Semisolid Formulation of *Linum usitatissimum* L. (Linseed) oil on the repair of skin wounds, *Evid Based Complement Alternat Med* (2012), 270752.
4 Kaithwas, G., Mukherjee, A., Chaurasia, A.K. & Majumdar, D.K., Anti-inflammatory, analgesic and antipyretic activities of *Linum usitatissimum* L. (flaxseed/linseed) fixed oil, *Indian J Exp Biol* (2011), 49(12): 932–8.
5 Pinheiro, M.N. Jr, dos Santos, P.M., dos Santos, R.C. et al., Oral flaxseed oil (*Linum usitatissimum*) in the treatment of dry-eye Sjögren's syndrome patients, *Arq Bras Oftalmol* (2007), 70(4): 649–55 [Article in Portuguese].
6 Prasad, K., Flaxseed and cardiovascular health, *J Cardiovasc Pharmacol* (2009), 54(5): 369–77.
7 Pan, A., Yu, D., Demark-Wahnefried, W. et al., Meta-analysis of the effects of flaxseed interventions on blood lipids, *Am J Clin Nutr* (2009), 90(2): 288–97.

Fish oil

Fish oil comes from the flesh of cold-water oily fish, such as salmon, mackerel, herrings, sardines and anchovies, and is a very good source of the pre-formed n-3 fatty acids EPA and DHA that are difficult for humans to make. Most of the fish oil found in supplements is produced from small fish, such as sardines and anchovies, that are currently abundant and are fished well below mandated limits. They have short reproductive cycles that ensure sustainability. Fish oil supplements can be used to supply n-3 fatty acids for people who are unable to eat seafood regularly or for people who wish to ensure a regular, standard intake of n-3 PUFAs. Fish oil is available in capsule or liquid forms. Encapsulation helps to protect the n-3 fats from oxidation. Liquid fish oil should be kept refrigerated and the cap should be replaced immediately after use to minimise oxidation. The functions and uses of fish oil are described in 'Specific functions of n-3 PUFAs' and 'Therapeutic uses of n-3 PUFAs', covered previously in this chapter.

To produce fish oil, crude oil is extracted from the flesh of fish by steam rendering, separating and cold filtering. Fish oil then undergoes purification in vacuum conditions to minimise oxidation. Purification involves de-gumming to remove phosphatides and mucilaginous materials, neutralisation to remove acids, winterisation (cooling and filtering) and stripping to remove some SFAs, distillation to remove contaminants, bleaching and deodorising. The oil is then blended with antioxidants, such as natural mixed tocopherols (about 1 mg/g), and filtered. It is transported and stored under nitrogen in sealed drums to prevent oxidation damage.

During the refining process, most fish oil is molecularly distilled to remove pollutants such as arsenic, cadmium, lead, mercury, PCBs, pesticides, dioxins, furans, polyaromatic hydrocarbons (PAHs) and polybrominated diphenyl ethers (PBDEs). This process removes contaminants without damaging sensitive fats. Third-party testing in accredited labs should be used to ensure that the final product meets relevant standards for contaminant levels, which are:

- PCBs—not more than 0.1 ppm
- dioxins—not more than 2 pg/g
- arsenic—less than 0.1 ppm
- cadmium—less than 0.1 ppm
- lead—less than 0.1 ppm
- mercury—less than or equal to 0.01 ppm.

Purification of fish oil can require repeated heating at high temperatures (90–95°C and even up to 180°C) and n-3 PUFAs are susceptible to oxidation. Initially, fatty acids react with oxygen to form odourless compounds such as peroxides, which can then decompose to form secondary substances, such as aldehydes, that give an 'off' smell and rancid taste. The quality of a batch of fish oil is checked by measuring the hydroperoxide content using the peroxide test (which gives the peroxide value, or PV), and the level of secondary oxidation products is checked by the anisidine test (giving the anisidine value, or AV). The PV indicates the current oxidation state of an oil, whereas the AV indicates the oxidation history of the oil. This is important because, if oil is bought and sold using the PV as the sole measurement of the oxidation status of the batch, older oils that are quite badly damaged can be sold as high quality to unsuspecting buyers because the PVs are low. The lower the values of PV and AV, the higher the quality of the oil. These values are sometimes combined to form the Totox number where: Totox = AV + (2 × PV). The Joint FAO/WHO food standards program has proposed draft standards for fish oil (2013) as follows:

- peroxide value (PV)—max. permitted: 5 meq/kg
- anisidine value (AV)—max. permitted: 20 meq/kg
- totox number—max. permitted: 26.

The amount and type of n-3 PUFAs in fish vary according to their diet, and each batch of fish oil will have a different ratio. This is standardised by mixing oil from different batches of fish oil to achieve the desired EPA:DHA ratio.

- *Regular fish oil* has a 1.5:1 ratio of EPA to DHA, and a 1 g capsule will generally contain 180 mg of EPA and 120 mg of DHA, a total of 300 mg. The ideal ratio of EPA to DHA is not fully understood. Higher EPA may be useful for inflammation and higher DHA may be useful for brain and nerve function. Most research studies have used supplements with the ratio of EPA to DHA that is found in regular fish oil. The standard dose is 3–6 g daily.
- *Concentrated fish oil* contains more EPA and DHA, and is a more convenient form of supplement if a high dose is required. The ratio of EPA to DHA may vary between products.
- *Reflux-free fish oil* is regular or concentrated fish oil that has been emulsified with natural orange oil to form micro-droplets that disperse in the stomach,

reducing reflux and disguising the fishy after-taste. The small droplet size improves absorption, which is helpful for people who have trouble digesting fats. It is available as a liquid or capsules; capsules can be pierced and squeezed into juice or water if desired.

Krill oil

Krill is a small, shrimp-like marine organism that feeds on phytoplankton. Antarctic krill (*Euphausia superba*) is found in the waters of the Southern Ocean and Pacific krill (*Euphausia pacifica*) is found in the northern Pacific Ocean. Krill oil is made up of n-3 PUFAs incorporated into PLs and TGs and smaller amounts of LA, SFAs, MUFAs and antioxidants. In krill oil, 30–65 per cent of the n-3 PUFAs, which are mainly EPA and DHA, are in PLs, whereas most of the FAs in fish oil are in TGs. The most abundant PL in krill oil is PC. Krill oil generally contains 7–24 per cent EPA and DHA; the DHA content of krill oil is similar to that of fish oil but the EPA content is usually higher.

Krill oil contains about 0.2 per cent astaxanthin, a red carotenoid pigment that is a powerful antioxidant, and is more stable during storage than fish oil. However, krill undergoes decomposition within two to three hours after being caught because of its natural content of enzymes, and decomposes much more rapidly than fish. To reduce decomposition and oxidation, krill need to be kept alive in water tanks or frozen until processed to remove the oil. The processing and refining procedure for krill oil is similar to fish oil.

The bioavailability of n-3 PUFAs from krill oil PLs is equal to or possibly greater than that of n-3 PUFAs from fish oil TGs. Smaller amounts of EPA and DHA given as krill oil have been shown to be just as effective in elevating plasma levels as greater amounts of EPA and DHA given as fish oil.[1] In animals, EPA and DHA from krill oil also have been found to be taken up efficiently by plasma PLs and target tissues. Blood levels of AA appear to increase during krill oil intake, but decrease with fish oil intake, and it is possible that AA is mobilised from cell membranes into the blood by EPA and DHA in krill oil PLs.[1] The relevance of this to health is unclear.

Krill oil has been found to reduce serum cholesterol in a clinical trial: low-dose krill oil (1.0–1.5 g/day) decreased total cholesterol by 13–14 per cent and high-dose krill oil (2–3 g/day) decreased it by 18 per cent.[1] Low-dose krill oil reduced LDL cholesterol by 32–36 per cent and high-dose krill oil decreased it by 37–39 per cent; and low-dose krill oil increased HDL cholesterol by 43–44 per cent and high-dose krill oil increased it by 55–60 per cent. Krill oil appears to be more effective at a lower dose than fish oil for abnormal blood lipids and a 500 mg maintenance dose of krill oil appears effective for long-term management.[2]

Krill oil has been found to relieve symptoms of chronic inflammation. Supplementation with 300 mg per day has lowered levels of C-reactive protein (CRP), a key marker of inflammation, by 30 per cent, and the same dose has been associated with relief of rheumatoid arthritic pain, stiffness and functional impairment.[3] Krill oil is reported to relieve breast tenderness, joint pain, swelling and bloating in premenstrual syndrome (PMS), and provide pain relief for menstrual cramps.[4] It has enhanced learning in animals and appears to have anti-depressant effects.[5] Krill oil is associated with improved markers of brain function in elderly people.[6] It has prevented TG and cholesterol buildup in the liver in animals on high-fat diets, and may be beneficial for the prevention of fatty liver.[7] As krill oil provides a dietary source of PLs, it would be expected to provide the same health benefits as PLs in lecithin. The standard dose of krill oil is 1–3 g daily.

REFERENCES

1 Ulven, S.M., Kirkhus, B., Lamglait, A. et al., Metabolic effects of krill oil are essentially similar to those of fish oil but at lower dose of EPA and DHA, in healthy volunteers, *Lipids* (2011), 46(1): 37–46.

2 Bunea, R., El Farrah, K. & Deutsch, L., Evaluation of the effects of Neptune Krill Oil on the clinical course of hyperlipidemia, *Altern Med Rev* (2004), 9(4): 420–8.

3 Deutsch, L., Evaluation of the effect of Neptune Krill Oil on chronic inflammation and arthritic symptoms, *J Am Coll Nutr* (2007), 26(1): 39–48.

4 Sampalis, F., Bunea, R., Pelland, M.F. et al., Evaluation of the effects of Neptune Krill Oil on the management of premenstrual syndrome and dysmenorrhea, *Altern Med Rev* (2003), 8(2): 171–9.

5 Wibrand, K., Berge, K., Messaoudi M. et al., Enhanced cognitive function and antidepressant-like effects after krill oil supplementation in rats, *Lipids Health Dis* (2013), 12: 6.
6 Konagai, C., Yanagimoto, K., Hayamizu, K. et al., Effects of krill oil containing n-3 polyunsaturated fatty acids in phospholipid form on human brain function: A randomized controlled trial in healthy elderly volunteers, *Clin Interv Aging* (2013), 8: 1247–57.
7 Ferramosca, A., Conte, A., Burri, L. et al., A krill oil supplemented diet suppresses hepatic steatosis in high-fat fed rats, *PLoS One* (2012), 7(6): e38797.

POTENTIALLY HARMFUL LIPIDS

Trans FAs and hydrogenated oils

Trans FAs are produced industrially during the hydrogenation process that converts vegetable oils to the solid texture required for margarine. In this process, oils are partially hydrogenated, a process in which hydrogen (H^+) is artificially added to some of the unsaturated carbons. This has the side-effect of altering the configuration of the molecule from the natural 'cis' form to the 'trans' form, which has a straighter shape and is metabolised like SFAs in the body (see Figure 4.6). It increases the SFA content and reduces the EFA content. Trans FAs are also produced in limited amounts in the digestive tracts of cows and sheep by bacterial activity, and are present in the fat of milk, butter, cheese and beef at levels of 2–9 per cent.[1] Trans FAs in foods include vaccenic acid (C18:1 trans-11) and small amounts of conjugated linoleic acid (cis-9, trans-11 18:2) (CLA). CLA is also formed in the body from ingested vaccenic acid.

A meta-analysis of research concluded that manufactured trans FAs increase the risk of atherosclerosis by increasing serum levels of LDL cholesterol, reducing levels of HDL cholesterol and increasing the total cholesterol:HDL cholesterol

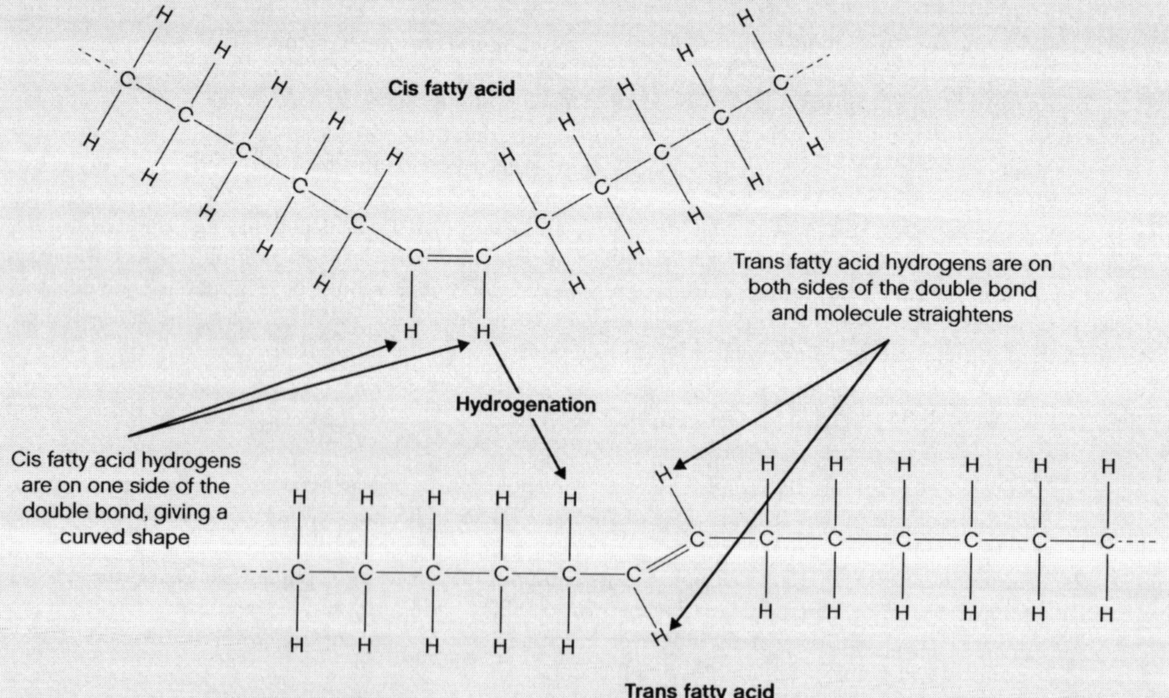

Figure 4.6 Formation of a trans fatty acid

ratio.[2] All trans FAs were found to raise the serum LDL:HDL cholesterol ratio and cause greater adverse cardiovascular effects than SFAs. Trans FAs were also found to have pro-inflammatory effects by increasing activity of TNF-alpha, interleukin-6 (IL-6) and CRP, and causing endothelial dysfunction in arteries. Trans FAs may also increase insulin resistance and possibly contribute to diabetes and weight gain. This meta-analysis found that, when trans FAs were substituted for cis PUFAs in the diet, there was a 32 per cent higher risk of heart attack or death from coronary heart disease for every 2 per cent of energy derived from trans FAs. Naturally occurring trans FAs have not been linked to adverse effects.

CLA modulates immunity and blood clotting, lipid metabolism, eicosanoid production and gene expression in the liver, muscle and adipose tissues. It is promoted as a supplement for weight loss, after initial animal studies found that it had beneficial effects in obesity, and for inflammatory disorders, atherosclerosis, metabolic syndrome, diabetes, cancer and rheumatoid arthritis. However, results from human studies have been conflicting, with some studies showing no effect on body fat and adverse effects on HDL cholesterol levels, glucose metabolism, lipid oxidation, inflammation and endothelial function.[3] In a study of women consuming oleic acid, manufactured trans FAs, or CLA, the total cholesterol:HDL cholesterol ratio was 11.6 per cent higher after trans FAs and 10 per cent higher after CLA compared to the oleic acid diet.[4] A review concluded that intake of CLA from supplements can easily reach 3 g a day, which has the potential to increase the LDL: HDL cholesterol ratio by 0.05, giving a 3–12 per cent increase in the risk of CVD.[1]

Many Australian table margarines are now made by a fractionation process that blends different types of FAs to achieve the right consistency, making them much lower in trans FAs. Hard margarines used in commercial bakery products have higher levels of trans FAs. Trans FA food sources include fried foods, takeaway foods, processed meats and commercial pastry products, with smaller amounts in meat and dairy products.

In Australia and New Zealand, intakes of trans FAs from commercial food products are estimated to have declined by 25–45 per cent since 2007.[5] The 2009 mean intake of industrial trans FAs is estimated at 0.4 g per day or less for Australians and 0.6 g per day or less for New Zealanders. Higher trans FAs in Australian diets are linked to a higher intake of pastry products, sausages, luncheon meats and creamy pasta dishes, and in New Zealanders, a higher intake of pastry products, creamy pasta dishes, cheese, popcorn, doughnuts and takeaway fish products. A 2009 analysis by *Choice* magazine found that Australian foods particularly high in trans FAs were doughnuts, bagel crisps, packaged pastry, meat pies, sausage rolls and quiches, with some brands containing more than 4 per cent as a percentage of total fat.[6]

Oxidised and rancid oils

PUFAs are susceptible to oxidation, especially when unsaturated FAs are exposed to heat, light, air or metals that enhance oxygen attack at the site of double bonds. Oxidation causes the formation of damaging lipid peroxides that further break down into secondary oxidation products such as aldehydes, ketones and alkenals, and finally to short-chain free FAs. Oxidation products are implicated in inflammation, cancer and atherosclerosis.

Oils can also be damaged by hydrolytic rancidity that occurs when micro-organisms in food break down TGs and release free FAs. These oils are referred to as ‘rancid’. They have an unpleasant odour and taste, and contain harmful peroxides and other breakdown products.

Heated oils

Heating increases oxidation damage, especially in highly unsaturated n-3 PUFA oils. Oils containing SFAs and MUFAs are more heat stable, and MUFA-containing oils, such as olive oil, are preferred for cooking. Heating oils to the smoke-point can convert glycerol to acrolein. Acrolein—also emitted in smoke, including cigarette smoke, and present in car exhaust and industrial pollution—is a highly toxic compound that is a respiratory irritant and cancer-causing agent. Severe toxicity has occurred in people exposed to acrolein from over-heated cooking oil.[7] Emission of acrolein from wok cooking is linked to the high incidence of lung cancer in Chinese women.[8]

In a study of the effects of cooking temperature on vegetable oils, the content of lipid oxidation products increased considerably, as measured by alkenal content, which is a measure of the amount of secondary oxidation products present.[9] Olive oils had the lowest alkenal content after heating, which is to be expected as they contain mainly MUFAs. Oils with the highest alkenal content after heating were sunflower oil, soybean oil and one variety of corn oil, all of which contained more than 60 per cent PUFAs.

Oils that are used for deep-frying are particularly subject to oxidation, and can damage antioxidants, essential amino acids and FAs in foods.[10] Oxidation is enhanced by a high frying temperature, reusing oils, a higher unsaturated fatty acid content and the presence of metals. Antioxidants are protective, but their effectiveness decreases as the temperature increases; however, lignan compounds in sesame oil have been found to be effective antioxidants during deep-frying.

To protect the nutritional content, oils should be purchased in opaque or dark glass containers, stored in a cool, dark environment, used within a short space of time and sealed from air immediately after use. Oils high in MUFAs, such as olive oil, should be used for cooking and any excess should be discarded after use. PUFA-rich foods such as nuts and seeds, if shelled, also should be stored in a cool, dark environment and used within a short space of time.

REFERENCES

1 Brouwer, I.A., Wanders, A.J. & Katan, M.B., Effect of animal and industrial trans fatty acids on HDL and LDL cholesterol levels in humans: A quantitative review, *PLoS ONE* (2010), 5(3): e9434.

2 Mozaffarian, D., Aro, A. & Willett, W.C., Health effects of trans-fatty acids: Experimental and observational evidence, *Eur J Clin Nutr* (2009), 63 (Suppl 2): S5–21.

3 Salas-Salvadó, J., Márquez-Sandoval, F. & Bulló, M., Conjugated linoleic acid intake in humans: A systematic review focusing on its effect on body composition, glucose, and lipid metabolism, *Crit Rev Food Sci Nutr* (2006), 46(6): 479–88.

4 Wanders, A.J., Brouwer, I.A., Siebelink, E. & Katan, M.B., Effect of a high intake of conjugated linoleic acid on lipoprotein levels in healthy human subjects, *PLoS ONE* (2010), 5(2): e9000.

5 FSANZ, *Intakes of trans fatty acids in New Zealand and Australia*, review report—2009 assessment, FSANZ, Canberra, 2009.

6 Hidden danger—trans fats in foods, *Choice*, 2009, June, available at <www.choice.com.au/reviews-and-tests/food-and-health/food-and-drink/nutrition/trans-fats-in-foods.aspx>.

7 Beauchamp, R.O. Jr, Andjelkovich, D.A., Kligerman, A.D. et al., A critical review of the literature on acrolein toxicity, *Crit Rev Toxicol* (1985), 14: 309–80.

8 Gao, Y.T., Blot, W.J., Zheng, W. et al., Lung cancer among Chinese women, *Int J Cancer* (1987), 40(5): 604–9.

9 Halvorsen, B. & Blomhoff, R., Determination of lipid oxidation products in vegetable oils and marine omega-3 supplements, *Food Nutr Res* (2011), 55: 10.3402/fnr.v55i0.5792.

10 Choe, E. & Min, D.B., Chemistry of deep-fat frying oils, *J Food Sci* (2007), 72(5): R77–86.

CHOLESTEROL

FAST FACTS . . . CHOLESTEROL

- More cholesterol is made in the body than is eaten in the diet.
- LDL cholesterol delivers cholesterol to tissues and HDL cholesterol recycles it to the liver.
- Cholesterol is essential for formation of steroid hormones, vitamin D, cell membrane structure, brain and nerve function and skin hydration.
- Elevated serum LDL cholesterol and low HDL cholesterol are risk factors for heart disease.
- Plant sterols help reduce cholesterol absorption.

Cholesterol is a waxy, fat-like substance that is an essential component of cell membrane structure, together with PLs and sphingomyelins, and is essential for body function. It is a fat-soluble alcohol (sterol) and consists of four interlocking rings of carbon atoms with an attached hydroxyl group (-OH) that has water-soluble properties. Steroid hormones are derived from cholesterol; female hormones (oestrogens) are 18-carbon steroids, male hormones (androgens) are 19-carbon steroids, and progestogens, glucocorticoids and mineralocorticoids are 21-carbon steroids. Vitamin D and its metabolites are secosteroids that have a cleavage of the B ring of the core structure. Phytosterols are the plant equivalents of animal sterols. Most plants, except for marine macroalgae (seaweed), are not able to make cholesterol, and animal food is the main dietary source.

Cholesterol synthesis

Cholesterol is not essential in the diet because about 1 g of cholesterol is made daily in the body—much more than is usually eaten in the diet. It is made in the liver, and the amount made varies according to dietary intake; if more is eaten, less will be made. Cholesterol is also made in the brain by glial cells because cholesterol in the bloodstream does not cross the blood–brain barrier. In the same way that FAs are made, cholesterol is made from acetyl-CoA produced by glycolysis, the first part of the energy-producing pathway in cells. A series of steps converts acetyl-CoA to 3-hydroxy-3-methylglutaryl-coenzyme A (HMG-CoA) and the enzyme HMG-CoA reductase converts HMG-CoA to mevalonate, which is then converted to farnesyl pyrophosphate in a further series of steps (see Figure 4.7). Farnesyl pyrophosphate is converted to squalene and then to cholesterol. This pathway also makes part of the coenzyme Q10 (CoQ10) molecule.

Digestion, absorption and transport

Dietary cholesterol is in the form of cholesteryl esters that are digested by the pancreatic enzyme cholesterol esterase to free cholesterol and fatty acids. These then combine with other lipid digestion products and bile salts to form micelles that release their contents into enterocytes. Cholesterol absorption by enterocytes appears to be dependent on the presence of Niemann-Pick C1-like 1 (NPC1L1) protein. Cholesterol is converted into cholesteryl esters within enterocytes and incorporated into chylomicrons for transport in the circulation.

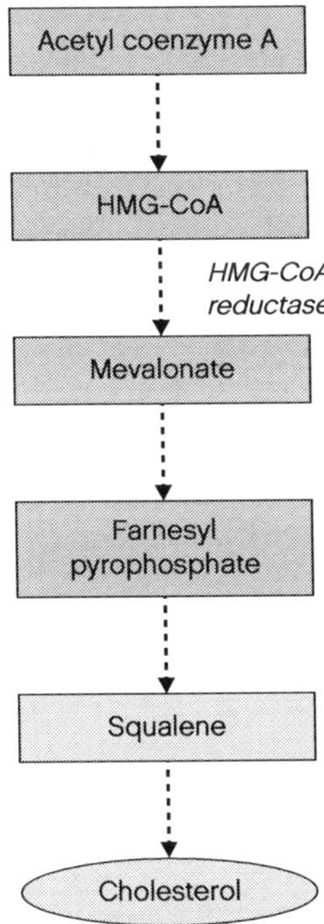

Figure 4.7 Cholesterol synthesis

Transport of cholesterol is discussed more fully in 'Lipid digestion, absorption and transport' in the 'Lipids' section of this chapter. LDL is the main lipoprotein that carries cholesterol in the bloodstream to body tissues. LDL receptors in cell membranes bind with apoB-100 in LDL and transport LDL to the interior of the cell, where the cholesterol is released by lysosomal enzymes. The receptor then travels back to the cell membrane to pick up more cholesterol. Genetic abnormalities in the LDL receptor may impair binding of LDL and lead to elevated plasma cholesterol levels. Small, dense LDL particles are associated with high plasma TGs, reduced HDL cholesterol levels, abdominal obesity, insulin resistance, impaired endothelial function in arteries, and abnormal blood clotting and a three-fold increased risk of coronary heart disease (CHD).

HDL removes cholesterol from tissues and takes it back to the liver for conversion to bile and excretion in faeces. ApoE in HDL cholesterol binds to the LDL receptor on cell membranes and apoA-1 activates the enzyme LCAT which forms cholesteryl esters that are taken up by HDL. High levels of HDLs are associated with reduced risk of CHD.

Regulation of body levels

There is a feedback mechanism that reduces cholesterol synthesis in the liver when cells have adequate amounts, and also reduces the manufacture of LDL receptors in cells so that uptake from the bloodstream is inhibited. A higher dietary intake of SFAs can increase blood levels of LDL cholesterol by reducing synthesis of LDL receptors in the liver, inhibiting clearance from blood.

Cholesterol synthesis is reduced by a higher dietary intake of cholesterol and activity of the hormones glucagon, made by the pancreas, and glucocorticoids, made by the adrenal glands. Cholesterol synthesis is increased by activity of the pancreatic hormone insulin and thyroid gland hormones.

Functions

Cholesterol is not used for energy in the body, but has a number of important functions, including:

- *Formation of steroid hormones.* Cholesterol is converted into steroid hormones, such as male and female sex hormones, as well as glucocorticoids and mineralocorticoids that are made in the adrenal cortex as part of the stress response.
- *Formation of vitamin D.* In the skin, a derivative of cholesterol (7-dehydrocholesterol) is converted to vitamin D on exposure to sunlight.
- *Formation of bile acids.* The liver converts cholesterol into the bile acids chenodeoxycholic acid and cholic acid, which emulsify fats in the gut to assist lipase activity. Part of the cholesterol in bile is excreted in faeces and part is reabsorbed into the bloodstream and returned to the liver for recycling as bile.
- *Structure of cell membranes.* Cholesterol provides solidity and a 'waterproofing' effect in cell membranes, preventing fluids from leaking out of the cell, and is essential for membrane integrity and normal function.
- *Brain and nerve function.* Cholesterol is made in the brain, and is part of brain structure and the myelin sheath of nerve fibres. It supports the activity of neurotransmitters in the brain, such as serotonin that elevates mood.
- *Skin hydration, protection and repair.* Cholesterol helps retain water in the skin, prevents excessive water loss and helps repair wounds.

Dietary sources

Food sources include dairy fats, such as cheese, cream, butter, ice cream and whole milk; egg yolk; organ meats, such as brains, kidneys and liver; meat; poultry; seafood; fish roe and caviar. There are small amounts in red and brown varieties of marine macroalgae (seaweed). A vegan diet is low in cholesterol, but a dietary intake is not important because adequate amounts can be made in the body. Cholesterol is in animal cells and is not stored in the fat of meat; eating lean meat does not reduce cholesterol intake.

Access the Food Standards Australia New Zealand nutrient database (NUTTAB) at <www.foodstandards.gov.au> for the amounts found in specific foods.

Daily requirement

There is no dietary requirement for cholesterol because it is not an essential dietary nutrient. Dietary intake averages 300 mg a day in non-vegetarians.

Deficiency effects

The effect of a low serum cholesterol level is not well understood. It may be associated with anaemia, low antioxidant levels, low blood serotonin levels and underlying infections. Low levels have been associated with violent behaviour, increased anger and dangerous driving in young men, depression, deaths from suicide and increased mortality from causes other than CVD, such as cancer and chronic obstructive pulmonary disease.

Lowering cholesterol by the use of statin drugs can cause side-effects, such as cognitive and memory problems—possibly related to blocking the brain's synthesis of cholesterol—and also muscle pain—possibly related to blocking CoQ10 synthesis—but is not related to increased mortality.

Effects of excess

High serum levels of LDL cholesterol are a risk factor for heart disease caused by atherosclerosis, the process of plaque building up and thickening artery walls. The coronary arteries that supply the heart muscle with blood are very narrow and more easily blocked than other arteries in the body. It is believed that atherosclerosis is triggered by damage to the artery lining (endothelium). LDL cholesterol from the bloodstream moves through the damaged endothelium to the underlying muscle layer (intima), where it builds up and oxidises. Raised serum LDL levels allow more LDL to enter the intima and can prevent it leaving. Small, dense LDL cholesterol particles are especially likely to build up in artery walls and oxidise. Diets high in SFAs and those with a high glycaemic load can raise blood levels of LDL cholesterol, VLDL cholesterol and small, dense LDL.

Oxidised LDL causes an inflammatory and immune response in the intima. Macrophages and smooth muscle cells in the intima ingest oxidised cholesterol and enlarge to become foam cells. The area of the intima becomes a fat-laden streak in the artery wall, but is not a health risk at this stage. Chronic inflammation can cause a fatty streak to grow and develop into a complex lesion called an atheroma, made up of a fatty core of foam cells, dead tissue, macrophages and activated T cells, covered by a fibrous cap of smooth muscle cells, connective tissue and endothelial cells in which calcium is deposited. If the fibrous cap remains intact, there may be some blockage to circulation but no immediate health risk. Chronic inflammation weakens the cap, which may then break down, causing a clot to form. A clot could block the artery and cause an MI if it occurs in a coronary artery, a stroke if it occurs in an artery in the brain or blockage of circulation to other vital organs.

Target serum cholesterol levels

In the United States, serum cholesterol is measured in milligrams per decilitre (mg/dL). In Australia, it is measured in millimoles per litre (mmol/L). Multiply mg/dL by 0.0259 to convert to mmol/L. Total serum cholesterol is no longer regarded as the most important indicator of heart disease risk. Elevated levels of LDL and TGs and low levels of HDL are seen as more important. Recommended targets for serum lipids are given in Tables 4.6 and 4.7. Note that any lowering of total serum cholesterol and LDL cholesterol and any increase in HDL cholesterol is likely to be beneficial even if the recommended target is not achieved.

Table 4.6 Target serum cholesterol and TG levels for prevention of cardiovascular disease

LDL cholesterol	less than 2.0 mmol/L
HDL cholesterol	at least 1.0 mmol/L
TGs	less than 2.0 mmol/L
Total cholesterol	less than 4.0 mmol/L
Non-HDL cholesterol	less than 2.5 mmol/L

Source: National Vascular Disease Prevention Alliance, *Guidelines for the assessment of absolute cardiovascular disease risk*, NVDPA, Sydney, 2009.

Table 4.7 Target serum cholesterol and TG levels for heart patients

LDL cholesterol	less than 1.8 mmol/L
HDL cholesterol	more than 1.0 mmol/L
TGs	less than 2.0 mmol/L
Non-HDL cholesterol	less than 2.5 mmol/L

Source: The National Heart Foundation of Australia and the Cardiac Society of Australia and New Zealand, *Reducing risk in heart disease: An expert guide to clinical practice for secondary prevention of coronary heart disease*, NHFA and CSANZ, Sydney and Wellington, 2012.

Factors influencing serum levels

Cholesterol levels in the body are maintained by balancing the amount produced with the amount absorbed from the diet. When dietary intake is low, production is increased and vice versa. Obese people have been found to have increased cholesterol synthesis and decreased absorption from the diet, and losing weight decreases cholesterol synthesis but has little or no effect on absorption.

Cholesterol absorption from food is reduced by cholesterol-lowering medication, such as ezetimibe, cholestyramine and probucol. Ezetimibe blocks activity of NPC1L1 protein, which is required for cholesterol absorption in the gut; cholestyramine binds with bile acids to prevent their reabsorption in the gut; and probucol enhances the breakdown of LDL, and has a small inhibiting effect on cholesterol absorption and synthesis. Phytosterols compete with cholesterol for absorption in the digestive tract, and are added to margarine and dairy products to help reduce cholesterol absorption. However, therapies that block cholesterol absorption may lead to a compensatory rise in cholesterol production in the body.

Health professionals no longer place as much emphasis on the need to reduce dietary intake of cholesterol for cardiovascular health because elevated serum cholesterol is usually caused by excess production in the body. Reducing SFAs and trans FA intake is more important, as this drives cholesterol production. Many animal foods are high in SFAs and cholesterol and reducing SFA intake will usually automatically reduce cholesterol intake.

The most common medical approach to lowering serum cholesterol levels is to reduce cholesterol synthesis by the use of statin drugs. These act by blocking HMG-CoA reductase activity, which reduces cholesterol synthesis in the liver. Statin drugs also interfere with CoQ10 synthesis, and can cross the blood–brain barrier and may also reduce cholesterol synthesis in the brain. High-dose slow-release niacin, a form of vitamin B3 available only on prescription, has been used to reduce release of FAs from fat tissue and reduce liver production of VLDL, the lipoprotein precursor to LDL. However, the very high doses of niacin required can cause liver damage, and this treatment has been superseded by statin therapy.

Dietary recommendations for serum cholesterol reduction

Intake of foods high in SFAs, such as cheese, cream, butter, ice cream, whole milk, organ meats, fatty meat and poultry skin, and intake of commercial bakery products containing trans fat margarines, should be minimised. Seafood is recommended for anti-inflammatory n-3 PUFAs, and fruit and vegetables for protective antioxidants.

The National Heart Foundation of Australia advises that moderate intake of eggs is now acceptable in heart disease, and states that the most effective dietary strategies for improving serum cholesterol profile are:

- replacing saturated and trans FAs with MUFAs and PUFAs
- increasing intake of plant sterols
- increasing soluble fibre intake
- increasing soy protein intake
- losing weight.

A summary of the effectiveness of dietary approaches for lowering serum LDL cholesterol can be found in Table 4.8.

Table 4.8 Effectiveness of dietary approaches to cholesterol lowering

Method of lowering blood cholesterol	Can lower LDL cholesterol by …
Replace SFAs with unsaturated fats	10%
Increase plant sterol intake to more than 1.5 g/day	10%
Lose weight (if overweight)	6%
Increase soluble fibre intake	about 3%
Increase soy protein intake	about 3%

Source: Clifton, P. et al., Dietary intervention to lower serum cholesterol, *Aust Fam Physician* (2009), 38(6): 424–9.

PHYTOSTEROLS: NATURAL CHOLESTEROL FIGHTERS

Many people have taken on board the health messages that a low-fat diet is good for heart health. However, as with a lot of dietary messages, this advice has changed in light of more recent research. While it is sensible to reduce intake of foods that are rich in SFAs because they drive cholesterol production in the body, oils from many plants are useful for heart protection and not only because they contain n-3 and n-6 PUFAs essential for health. They are also good sources of natural phytosterols that help cholesterol control.

Phytosterols are natural cholesterol-like compounds found in plants, and include sterols and stanols. The main plant sterols are beta-sitosterol, campesterol and stigmasterol. Stanols, such as campestanol and beta-sitostanol, are formed from sterols by the addition of hydrogen and are present only in trace amounts in foods.

Sterols and stanols have attracted interest because they can compete with dietary cholesterol in the gut and reduce the amount absorbed from food, as well as the amount absorbed back into the body from bile. Researchers have speculated that having a higher intake of phytosterols may help reduce serum cholesterol, and so lower the risk of heart disease.

Phytosterols in the diet

Vegetable oil, margarine and nut butters naturally contain about 100–500 mg of sterols per 100 g.[1] Legumes contain about 220 mg per 100 g and seeds contain about 500–700 mg per 100 g. Stanols are found in trace amounts in rice bran oil and shea butter. Tall oil, derived from wood pulp, is used commercially as a source of phytosterols for food manufacturing. Western diets normally provide 200–400 mg of plant sterols a day, traditional Asian diets provide 350–400 mg a day and vegetarian diets provide 600–800 mg a day.[2]

Serum cholesterol and phytosterols

Researchers first became interested in phytosterols because of their similar structure to cholesterol but much lower absorption, ranging from 5–15 per cent for sterols and less than 1 per cent for stanols. Phytosterols compete with cholesterol for uptake into micelles, the fat 'packages' that assist absorption of fats in the small intestine. Less cholesterol is therefore absorbed from food, and also less is absorbed back into the body from bile, causing the liver to take up more cholesterol from the bloodstream, which lowers serum levels. However, a lowering of dietary intake of cholesterol is accompanied by increased cholesterol synthesis in the body, and the overall effect on heart disease is unclear.

Studies in the 1950s showed that supplementing people with plant sterols lowered serum cholesterol levels.[3] However, early studies used plant sterols in solid crystalline form, and these were difficult to incorporate into food fats and not as effective as fat-soluble forms (sterol esters). The high amounts of sterols used experimentally (up to 50 g a day) also increased blood levels of sterols. Interest then switched to plant stanols because of their very poor absorption and their similar effectiveness in lowering blood cholesterol even at low levels of intake.

Studies have shown that taking 1.6–2.4 g of sterols a day leads to a 10 per cent reduction in serum levels of LDL cholesterol in 90 per cent of people, without affecting HDL cholesterol levels.[4] Taking more than 3 g a day of sterols does not provide additional benefits. Plant stanols are also effective at doses of 1–3 g a day, decreasing serum LDL cholesterol by 6–15 per cent.[5]

A review of studies on the use of sterols and stanols concluded that 2 g of added stanols or sterols per day could reduce serum LDL cholesterol by 10 per cent, and reduce the incidence of heart disease by 12–20 per cent over five years.[6]

Cancer and plant sterols

Animal studies show that plant sterols have anticancer activity.[7] They reduce overgrowth of colonocytes and protect against colon cancer. In cell studies, sitosterol induces apoptosis, reduces the growth rate of human colon cancer and prostate cancer cells, and reduces prostate-specific antigen (PSA) production, a marker for prostate cancer. Sitosterol is incorporated into cell membranes in a similar way to cholesterol, and appears to affect membrane fluidity and enzyme activity, decreasing the activity of the enzyme 5-alpha reductase that drives the conversion of the male hormone testosterone to dihydrotestosterone, an enhancer of prostate cell growth. A study of people with benign prostatic hyperplasia (BPH) who were given 60 mg of sitosterol a day for six months found that symptoms improved,[8] and it is used as a natural treatment for this condition in Europe. Sitosterol was found to inhibit the growth of human breast cancer cells by 66–80 per cent in a cell study.[9] Sitosterol also stimulates the immune response, and may inhibit the conversion of cholesterol and bile into cancer-causing compounds in the gut.

Phytosterol-boosted foods

Since the 1990s, stanols and sterols in ester forms have been incorporated into margarines and other foods for cholesterol-lowering purposes. In Australia, plant sterol esters are permitted as additives in table spreads (margarines), low-fat milk, yoghurt and breakfast cereals. Manufacturers are required to label foods with added sterols using the terms 'plant sterols', 'plant sterol esters' or 'phytosterol esters', and must include the amount in grams per serving.[10] Labels must carry a statement advising that these products should be consumed as part of a healthy diet, they may not be suitable for children under the age of five years and pregnant or lactating women, and plant sterols do not provide additional benefits when consumed in excess of 3 g per day.

How safe are sterols?

In the 1970s, a rare inherited disorder called sitosterolaemia was discovered, which is associated with blood levels of plant sterols up to 60 times greater than normal and accelerated atherosclerosis and heart disease.[11] Large quantities of oxidised phytosterols have been found in the blood of people with sitosterolaemia, with none detected in people without the condition. As with oxidised cholesterol, oxidised phytosterols may be a key contributor to plaque buildup in artery walls. Sterol-fortified foods are not recommended for anyone with this condition.

Because sterols inhibit cholesterol uptake, there were concerns that they could reduce absorption of fat-soluble nutrients, like vitamins A, D, E and K and carotenoids, the fat-soluble pigments in plants that are important antioxidants. Beta-carotene is particularly important as an antioxidant and plant source of vitamin A. An eight-week study was carried out, in which 3, 6 and 9 g of plant sterol esters were given to healthy people.[12] There was no evidence of side-effects, although blood concentrations of sterols increased. Fat-soluble vitamins and carotenoids remained within the normal range, but beta-carotene reduced in the group on the highest intake of sterols. An Australian study has shown that the reduction in carotenoid levels can be counteracted by eating one extra serve a day of high-carotenoid fruit or vegetables, such as carrots, sweet potatoes, pumpkin, tomatoes, apricots, spinach or broccoli.[13]

Information on the long-term safety of sterol- and stanol-fortified foods is not yet available. Blood levels of plant sterols increase when sterol-fortified foods are included in the diet, whereas they decrease on stanol-fortified foods. As the health implications of this increase in blood sterols are not known to date, stanols may be a safer choice.

Phytosterols and cholesterol-lowering drugs

Statin cholesterol-lowering drugs act to reduce cholesterol production in the body, something that sterols and stanols cannot do. However, statins are associated with an increase in blood levels of plant sterols. Stanol esters help prevent this increase but plant sterol esters do not. A warning statement is included on sterol-fortified foods that people on cholesterol-lowering medication should seek medical advice before using them. However, advice from Food Standards Australia New Zealand (FSANZ) is that it is safe to eat foods fortified with sterols while taking cholesterol-lowering drugs.[10]

Are phytosterols needed if you are already eating a diet low in cholesterol?

The issue is whether sterols will still work if you do not eat cholesterol-containing foods, considering that the way they act is to reduce dietary cholesterol absorption. This was tested in an Australian study, and adding sterols to a diet low in saturated fat and cholesterol was still able to lower serum LDL cholesterol by 7.7–9.6 per cent.[13] This decrease may have been due to the inhibiting effect of sterols on reabsorption of cholesterol from bile.

Should everyone eat sterol-fortified foods?

Sterol-fortified foods can be expensive, and natural sterol-containing foods are relatively cheap and widely available. To increase intake of sterols, eat more nuts, seeds and legumes, such as beans, peas, chick peas and lentils. Natural sterols are also found in medicinal herbs such as saw palmetto, fenugreek, wild yam, sarsaparilla, withania and guggul. However, it is hard to get the effective amount of about 2 g a day from plant foods. People on a heart healthy diet and lifestyle program who are still struggling to control their cholesterol levels may find sterol-fortified foods useful but the emphasis should be on improving intake of natural sterols, antioxidants, seafood and fish oil, dietary fibre and other protective foods.

REFERENCES

1 Institute of Food Science & Technology (IFST), Updated Information Statement on Phytosterol Esters (Plant Sterol and Stanol Esters), January 2005, available at <www.ifst.org>.

2 National Heart Foundation of Australia, Plant sterols and stanols, position statement, August 2003, available at <www.heartfoundation.com.au>.

3 Law, M., Plant sterol and stanol margarines and health, *BMJ* (2000), 320: 861–4.

4 Nestel, P.J., The role of fats in the lifecycle stages. Adulthood—treatment: Cholesterol-lowering with plant sterols, *Med J Aust* (2002), 176 Suppl: S122.

5 Thompson, G.R. & Grundy, S.M., History and development of plant sterol and stanol esters for cholesterol-lowering purposes, *Am J Cardiol* (2005), 96(1A): 3D–9D.

6 Katan, M. et al., Efficacy and safety of plant stanols and sterols in the management of blood cholesterol levels, *Mayo Clin Proc* (2002), 78: 965–78.

7 Awad, A.B. & Fink, C.S., Phytosterols as anticancer dietary components: Evidence and mechanism of action, *J Nutr* (2000), 130(9): 2127–30.

8 Berges, R.R. et al., Randomized, placebo-controlled, double-blind clinical trial of β-sitosterol in patients with benign prostatic hyperplasia, *Lancet* (1995), 345: 1529–32.

9 Downie, A., Fink, S.C. & Awad A.B., Effect of phytosterols on MDA-MB-231 human breast cancer cell growth, *FASEB J* (1999), 13: A333.

10 FSANZ. Plant sterol fact sheet, available at <www.foodstandards.gov.au>.

11 Patel, M.D. & Thompson, P.D., Phytosterols and vascular disease, *Atherosclerosis* (2006), 186(1): 12–19.

12 Davidson, M.H. et al., Safety and tolerability of esterified phytosterols administered in reduced-fat spread and salad dressing to healthy adult men and women, *J Am Coll Nutr* (2001), 20(4): 307–19.

13 Noakes, M. et al., An increase in dietary carotenoids when consuming plant sterols or stanols is effective in maintaining plasma carotenoid concentrations, *Am J Clin Nutr* (2002), 75(1): 79–86.

LIPOTROPIC NUTRIENTS

Choline

CHOLINE STATUS CHECK

1 Do you have fatty liver disease?
2 Do you have elevated homocysteine levels?
3 Do you have a high alcohol intake?
4 Are you on a low-fat diet?

'Yes' answers may indicate inadequate choline status. Note that a number of nutritional deficiencies or health disorders can cause similar effects and further investigation is recommended.

FAST FACTS . . . CHOLINE

- Choline is found in lecithin, brains, egg yolk, liver, kidneys, fish, meat, full-fat milk, wheat germ, soy beans, brewer's yeast, peanuts and green leafy vegetables.
- It is required for the structure of cell membranes, fat digestion and transport, and liver, nerve, brain, kidney and muscle function.
- It provides methyl groups that have an important role in DNA metabolism and gene expression.
- A deficiency can lead to a buildup of fat in the liver.
- Supplementation may be useful for foetal development during pregnancy, cognitive disorders and tardive dyskinesia.

Choline is a lipotropic (fat-metabolising) nutrient. It is a nitrogen-containing water-soluble amine that can be made in the body, in which it is more commonly found as phosphorylcholine, phosphatidylcholine (PC), and acetylcholine (ACh). Although it is often included in vitamin B complex supplements, it is not a B vitamin. Lecithin is a concentrated form of PC that was identified in egg yolk in 1844 by French pharmacist Nicolas Gobley. Choline was discovered by German chemist Adolf Strecker in 1849. Choline was not thought to be essential in the diet for many years until some healthy people on choline-deficient diets were found to develop depleted body levels, and liver and muscle disorders. It was officially recognised as an essential dietary nutrient by the US Institute of Medicine (IOM) in 1998, and appears to be particularly essential in the diet when levels of methionine and folic acid are inadequate. Tissues that accumulate choline include the liver, kidneys, mammary glands, placenta and brain.

Choline synthesis

Choline synthesis is associated with the function of the methionine cycle that regenerates the amino acid methionine from its metabolite homocysteine, and is dependent on vitamin B12 and folic acid. The precursor to choline synthesis is the amino acid serine, which is first converted to phosphatidylserine (PS), then to phosphatidylethanolamine (PE) and subsequently to PC by the enzyme phosphatidylethanolamine methyltransferase (PEMT) that adds methyl groups donated by S-adenosylmethionine (SAM) (see Figure 4.8). SAM is produced from the amino acid methionine during the methionine cycle. PC can be broken down to free choline and phosphatidic acid by phospholipase D.

Digestion, absorption and transport

Choline is found in foods as free choline and as phosphocholine, glycerophosphocholine, sphingomyelin and PC. Dietary choline appears to be absorbed in the small intestine by facilitated diffusion, sodium-dependent transport and specific choline transporters belonging to the choline-like transporter family (SLC44 family). These transporters are also believed to transport choline across cell membranes. Some dietary choline is broken down by gut bacteria to methylamines and betaine (trimethylglycine), which can be absorbed. Free choline is transferred to the bloodstream after absorption and PC is transported in chylomicrons and enters the bloodstream via the lymph system.

Metabolism, storage and excretion

Choline is formed during the conversion of PE to PC, which is an alternative pathway for PC synthesis; the main pathway is the addition of phosphate groups to choline and conversion to cytidine diphosphocholine, which then combines with diglyceride to form PC and cytidine monophosphate. PC and the lipid ceramide combine to form sphingomyelin. PC can be broken down by phospholipase A_2 to lysophosphatidylcholine, which can be converted to platelet-activating factor (PAF) during inflammation, or to glycerophosphocholine (also known as choline alphoscerate), which can be further metabolised to glycerol-3-phosphate and choline. In the nervous system, choline and acetyl-CoA are converted to the neurotransmitter ACh by the action of the enzyme choline acetyltransferase.

Choline can be oxidised irreversibly in the liver and kidneys to betaine, which acts as a donor of methyl groups (CH_3). Betaine has choline-sparing effects by participating in the methionine cycle, and can also be metabolised to dimethylglycine. Choline is found in PLs in all cell membranes, which may act as a reserve supply. It can be removed from PLs as required, and recycled to the liver and brain when choline supply is low. Choline is broken down in the kidneys and liver to trimethylamine N-oxide (TMAO), which is excreted in urine.

Functions

Choline, as PC, is an integral part of cell membrane PLs. The functions of choline include:

- *Cell membrane function.* PC and sphingomyelin are important PLs in cell membranes that maintain membrane fluidity and transport functions and produce lipid-derived second messenger signalling molecules that influence cell functions.
- *Fat and cholesterol digestion and transport, liver protection.* PC is part of bile, which acts as an emulsifier of fats in the digestive tract. It keeps cholesterol in solution in bile and assists the digestion and absorption of dietary fats. PC is an important component of lipoproteins that transport lipids in the bloodstream, and is important for removing fats from the liver after synthesis, protecting the liver from fat accumulation and damage.
- *Nerve and brain function.* Choline is part of the neurotransmitter ACh, produced by mitochondria at the ends of nerve fibres in order to transmit nerve impulses between neurons. Choline is also present in nerve cell membranes as PC, and PC is a component of sphingomyelin in the myelin sheath that surrounds nerve fibres and ensures normal transmission of nerve impulses.
- *Muscle and heart function.* Choline helps retain the amino acid carnitine in the body by reducing urinary excretion. Carnitine is important for transporting fatty acids into muscle cells, where they are used for energy. Choline appears to have anti-inflammatory activity and, by its role in the methionine cycle, helps lower levels of homocysteine, a toxic product of methionine metabolism that is implicated in heart disease.
- *Mitochondrial function.* Choline as PC is part of the structure of mitochondrial membranes, and helps to maintain mitochondrial function and energy production.
- *Methyl donor.* Choline can be oxidised irreversibly to betaine, which donates methyl groups to other substances such as DNA and histones (proteins associated with DNA). Methylation of DNA and histones is a key step in the regulation of gene expression, and is required for brain development of the foetus during pregnancy and in infancy, and for the expression of genes involved in synaptic plasticity, a process important for learning and memory throughout life.

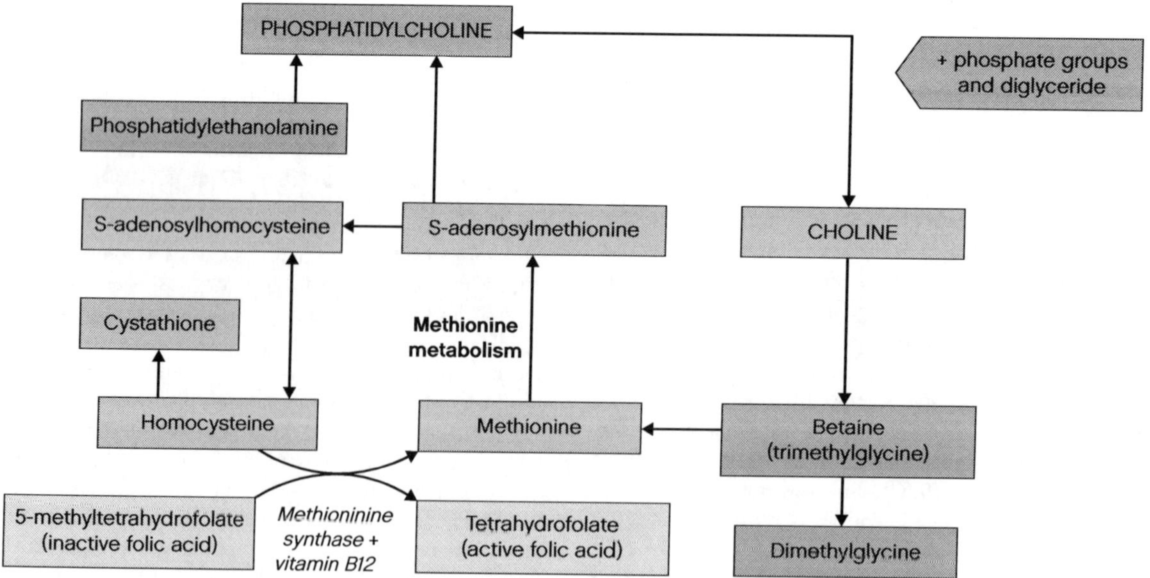

Figure 4.8 Choline synthesis

- *Kidney function.* Choline is used by the kidneys to synthesise betaine and glycerophosphocholine, which act as organic osmolytes to facilitate the reabsorption of water.

Dietary sources

Choline is found in lecithin, brains, egg yolk, liver, kidneys, fish, meat, full-fat milk, wheat germ, soy beans, brewer's yeast, peanuts and leafy green vegetables. Lecithin contains about 10–20 per cent PC, and is found in soybeans, unrefined oils, seeds, nuts, whole grains, egg yolk, liver and brains, and as an emulsifier in mayonnaise, salad dressings, chocolate, frozen desserts and baked goods. Betaine spares choline, and can contribute indirectly to maintaining body levels of choline. Sources of betaine include wheat germ, spinach, sunflower seeds and chicken liver.

Factors influencing body status

A low-fat diet may have inadequate levels of choline. Although choline is water-soluble, PC is a phospholipid that requires the presence of bile in the intestine for digestion. People with inadequate bile production may have impaired absorption of choline from PC. Vitamin B2, B3, B6, B12 and folic acid are required for the function of the methionine cycle that synthesises choline. Vitamin B3 is required for the oxidation of choline to betaine, and zinc is required for betaine metabolism. Maternal choline levels are depleted during pregnancy and lactation. Alcohol impairs the methionine cycle and lowers brain concentrations of choline. Genetic differences in genes related to choline metabolism that increase the dietary requirement for choline have been identified, and have been found to vary between ethnic groups. Low-choline diets have caused organ damage in some individuals with certain genetic variants and muscle damage in others with different variants.

Daily requirement

Government recommendations by age and gender (see Table 4.9) can be found in *Nutrient Reference Values for Australia and New Zealand Including Recommended Dietary Intakes*, available at <www.nrv.gov.au>. The daily requirement of choline appears to vary widely between individuals, with some requiring more than the recommended adequate intake and others requiring less than 50 mg/day.

Table 4.9 Adequate intake (AI) of choline (mg/day)

Age (years)	Female AI	Male AI
1–3	200	200
4–8	250	250
9–13	375	375
14–18	400	550
19–70	425	550
>70	425	550
Pregnant women		
14–18	415	
19–50	440	
Lactating women		
14–18	525	
19–50	550	

Source: Nutrient Reference Values for Australia and New Zealand Including Recommended Dietary Intakes, National Health and Medical Research Council, Australian Government Department of Health and Ageing, Canberra and Ministry of Health, New Zealand, Wellington, 2006.

Deficiency effects

If choline is deficient, TG transport from the liver is impaired, levels of serum TGs reduce, serum fatty acid levels increase and fats build up in the liver, causing liver damage that may lead to liver cancer. Choline deficiency may impair synthesis of apolipoproteins or impair incorporation of TGs into apolipoproteins. In animals, a deficiency causes decreased serum choline, mitochondrial and liver dysfunction and an increase in hydrogen peroxide and oxidised lipids, DNA and proteins. It is also associated with behavioural changes, bone abnormalities and growth retardation, as well as kidney dysfunction and haemorrhage. Men fed a choline-deficient diet containing adequate methionine, folate and vitamin B12 for three weeks developed decreased plasma choline and PC levels and liver damage. Individuals on total parenteral nutrition (TPN, non-oral feeding) devoid of choline but adequate in methionine and folate also have developed fatty liver and liver damage. Replacement of choline leads to a marked increase in plasma choline and reduction of fat in the liver.

Choline deficiency may lead to a deficiency of sphingomyelin and PC in nerve cell membranes and inhibit ACh production, leading to impaired brain and nerve function. Inadequate choline may contribute to a build up of homocysteine, which is toxic to nerves and the cardiovascular system and is believed to contribute to atherosclerosis. However, lowering homocysteine levels does not appear to impact on atherosclerosis and choline supplementation has not been shown to be of benefit. Impaired production of methyl groups for DNA and RNA methylation may lead to abnormal cell replication, birth defects and cancer. Choline deficiency in pregnant animals is associated with offspring that have growth retardation, altered brain function, skeletal abnormalities, liver and muscle damage, orofacial defects and neural tube defects (NTDs), such as spina bifida, in which the spinal cord fails to develop properly. Choline deficiency leads to apoptosis in animal cell cultures, and cells that survive choline deficiency transform into cancer cells. Other effects of choline deficiency include kidney and muscle damage.

Indicators of inadequate levels may include:

- fatty liver, liver damage, cirrhosis, liver cancer
- nerve disorders, memory loss
- elevated homocysteine levels
- kidney damage
- muscle weakness
- abnormal foetal development in pregnancy and birth defects
- cancer.

Assessment of body status

Choline status can be assessed by measuring fasting plasma choline, but the level rarely drops below half the reference value because choline is liberated from PLs when levels are inadequate. The reference range given by the US National Research Council is 7–20 μmol/L.

THERAPEUTIC USES OF CHOLINE

Choline may be useful for the treatment of fatty liver and kidney damage, but evidence from human studies is lacking. Betaine supplementation has been shown to improve non-alcoholic fatty liver disease. There are conflicting reports about the effect of choline on cancer. Therapeutic uses of choline include the following.

Foetal and infant development

Increased maternal intake of choline is associated with a reduced risk of birth defects such as NTDs.[1] Choline appears to be important for brain development and memory processing in animal offspring, and a deficiency during pregnancy has been shown to irreversibly impair cognitive function and memory later in life.[2]

Cognitive function

In animals, adequate prenatal choline has been shown to improve cognitive function in adult offspring and maintain memory during ageing, and supplementation of old animals has improved cognitive function.[3] In humans, a higher choline intake is associated with better cognitive performance.[4] In Alzheimer's disease (AD), there is a loss of cholinergic (choline-dependent) nerve cells, and this was thought to contribute to impaired learning and memory. However, this theory has not been confirmed by research and the relationship between choline and AD is not well understood. In people with mild to moderate AD, various choline treatments have improved cognitive function, but only temporarily. The exception may be glycerophosphocholine (choline alphoscerate), a precursor to ACh, which increases the release of ACh in animal brains and facilitates learning and memory. Glycerophosphocholine has improved memory and attention in dementia disorders.[5] There is some evidence that high-dose choline and lecithin retard the onset and relieve the symptoms of the degenerative nervous system disorders Huntington's disease and Friedrich's ataxia, but not all studies have shown benefits.[6]

Cancer

A low choline intake is associated with an increased incidence of spontaneous liver cancer and increased sensitivity to carcinogenic chemicals in animals.[1] A high choline intake in women has been linked to a 24 per cent lower risk of breast cancer, but a doubling of plasma choline levels in men has been associated with a 46 per cent greater risk of prostate cancer.[1] It appears that choline levels are increased in cancer cells, and it may have a role in promoting cell proliferation once a cancer has been established.

Tardive dyskinesia (TD)

TD is a Parkinson's disease-like condition that may occur in patients as a side-effect of long-term use of anti-psychotic medication. In the 1970s, a small study of mentally ill patients given 13–15 g of choline daily found that almost half had improvements in TD symptoms.[6] Similar improvements were reported in patients given 8–11 g of choline chloride or 12–15 g of lecithin.[6]

Asthma

A study of asthma patients found that 1000 mg of choline three times daily improved markers of respiratory function.[7]

REFERENCES

1 Ueland, P.M., Choline and betaine in health and disease, *J Inherit Metab Dis* (2011), 34(1): 3–15.
2 Zeisel, S.H., The fetal origins of memory: The role of dietary choline in optimal brain development, *J Pediatr* (2006), 149(5) (Suppl): S131–6.
3 Blusztajn, J.K. & Mellott, T.J., Choline nutrition programs brain development via DNA and histone methylation, *Cent Nerv Syst Agents Med Chem* (2012), 12(2): 82–94.
4 Poly, C., Massaro, J.M., Seshadri, S. et al., The relation of dietary choline to cognitive performance and white-matter hyperintensity in the Framingham Offspring Cohort, *Am J Clin Nutr* (2011), 94(6): 1584–91.
5 Scapicchio, P.L., Revisiting choline alphoscerate profile: A new, perspective, role in dementia? *Int J Neurosci* (2013), 123(7): 444–9.
6 Rosenberg, G.S. & Davis, K.L., The use of cholinergic precursors in neuropsychiatric diseases, *Am J Clin Nutr* (1982), 36(4): 709–20.
7 Gupta, S.K. & Gaur, S.N., A placebo controlled trial of two dosages of LPC antagonist: Choline in the management of bronchial asthma, *Indian J Chest Dis Allied Sci* (1997), 39(3): 149–56.

Therapeutic dose

Suggested doses for adults are as follows:

- *health maintenance:* 250–500 mg daily
- *mild deficiency:* 500–1000 mg daily
- *severe deficiency, disease treatment:* 3000 mg or more daily.

Effects of excess

Choline intake in excess of needs is excreted in urine. Very high doses of choline (10 g or more) may cause a 'fishy' or ammonia odour of the body or breath because of its conversion to trimethylamine by intestinal bacteria. Trimethylamine made in the gut is absorbed and converted to TMAO. Increased plasma TMAO levels have been strongly associated with atherosclerosis in human and animal studies, and it appears that TMAO alters cholesterol metabolism, increasing the deposition of cholesterol in artery walls and reducing its removal.

A dose of 7.5 g of choline per day was reported to have a slight blood pressure-lowering effect. Other reported effects of high doses include vomiting and increased sweating and salivation. Inappropriate sexual behaviour has been reported in an elderly man on choline treatment for mild cognitive impairment. The behaviour disappeared after choline was withdrawn.

Supplements

The permitted form of choline in Australian supplements is choline bitartrate, and it is also available as PC in lecithin supplements. Choline bitartrate is produced by reacting trimethylamine with ethylene oxide followed by treatment with tartaric acid.

Lecithin

Lecithin is available as granules or capsules, and is usually extracted from soybeans. It contains 65–75 per cent PLs, including PC (10–20 per cent), PE, PS and inositol-containing phosphatides. Other constituents include TGs, carbohydrates, pigments, sterols and sterol glycosides. Pure lecithin supplements may contain more than 90 per cent PLs. Lecithin is produced commercially as a product of soy oil processing, and is separated out as a lecithin and water emulsion during the de-gumming process. The emulsion may be bleached with hydrogen peroxide to lighten the colour and fluidising additives such as soy oil, fatty acids or calcium chloride can be added to improve viscosity. The dried product is called 'natural lecithin' or 'unrefined lecithin'. Refined lecithin (lecithin granules) is natural lecithin that has had oil removed by extraction with a solvent—usually acetone.

Lecithin is used for similar health purposes to choline. PC supports liver and kidney health and nerve, muscle and brain function. High-dose lecithin has been used for symptoms of AD, TD, Huntington's disease and Friedrich's ataxia. A meta-analysis found that, although there was no strong supporting evidence for the use of lecithin for AD, a moderate effect could not be discounted.[1] In animals with experimental ulcerative colitis, PC reduces inflammatory cytokines and enzymes and supports repair of bowel tissue.[2] It reduces fat levels in the liver in animals fed a high-fat diet,[3] and may help reverse alcoholic liver damage.[4] PC has been shown to enhance exercise performance when exercise has lowered circulating choline concentrations.[5] PC lowers levels of homocysteine[6] and dietary PLs reduce serum cholesterol and TGs and increase HDL cholesterol and levels of apoA-1, the major protein component of HDLs.[7]

The standard dose of lecithin is half to one tablespoon (3–6 g) daily and the standard dose of PC is 800–2400 mg daily. Unlike choline, high-dose lecithin supplementation does not cause a fishy or ammonia body or breath odour.

REFERENCES

1 Higgins, J.P. & Flicker, L., Lecithin for dementia and cognitive impairment, *Cochrane Database Syst Rev* (2003), 3: CD001015.

2 Kovács, T., Varga, G., Erces, D. et al., Dietary phosphatidylcholine supplementation attenuates inflammatory mucosal damage in a rat model of experimental colitis, *Shock* (2012), 38(2): 177–85.

3 Tandy, S., Chung, R.W., Kamili, A. et al., Hydrogenated phosphatidylcholine supplementation reduces hepatic lipid levels in mice fed a high-fat diet, *Atherosclerosis* (2010), 213(1): 142–7.

4 Kidd, P.M., Phosphatidylcholine, a superior protectant against liver damage, *Altern Med Rev* (1996) 1(4): 258–74.

5 Jäger, R., Purpura, M. & Kingsley, M., Phospholipids and sports performance, *J Int Soc Sports Nutr* (2007), 4: 5.

6 Olthof, M.R., Brink, E.J., Katan, M.B. & Verhoef, P., Choline supplemented as phosphatidylcholine decreases fasting and postmethionine-loading plasma homocysteine concentrations in healthy men, *Am J Clin Nutr* (2005), 2(1): 111–17.

7 Sahebkar, A., Fat lowers fat: Purified phospholipids as emerging therapies for dyslipidemia, *Biochim Biophys Acta* (2013), 1831(4): 887–93.

Inositol

INOSITOL STATUS CHECK

1 Do you have fatty liver disease?

2 Do you have diabetes, chronic kidney failure, galactosaemia (elevated levels of galactose), multiple sclerosis or polycystic ovarian syndrome?

3 Are you on a low-fat diet?

4 Is your diet low in fibre?

'Yes' answers may indicate inadequate inositol status. Note that a number of nutritional deficiencies or health disorders can cause similar effects and further investigation is recommended.

FAST FACTS . . . INOSITOL

- Inositol is found in fibre-containing plant foods, such as whole grains, legumes, seeds and nuts, and also in oranges, grapefruit, cantaloupe, raisins, liver, brewer's yeast and lecithin-containing foods.
- It is required for the structure of cell membranes, fat digestion and transport, and cell signalling.
- It is important for DNA repair, regulation of gene transcription, RNA metabolism and brain and nerve function.
- A deficiency can lead to a buildup of fat in the liver.
- Supplementation may be useful for psychiatric disorders, polycystic ovarian syndrome, respiratory distress syndrome in preterm infants, birth defects in infants, gestational diabetes, kidney stones and cancer.

Like choline, inositol (also referred to as *myo*-inositol) is a water-soluble lipotropic nutrient. It was identified by the German chemist Johann Scherer in 1849 and synthesised in 1915. Like choline, it is often included in B-complex supplements but it is not a B vitamin. It is not believed to be essential in the diet because it can be made in the body. In plants, inositol is found as *myo*-inositol hexaphosphate (IP6) and other inositol phosphates, collectively known as phytates, which are a storage form of energy abundant in fibre-containing plant foods. IP6, also called phytic acid, has six reactive phosphate groups that exert a strong negative charge that binds cations, especially calcium, potassium, magnesium, iron and zinc, and inhibits their absorption. In the body, inositol is found as phosphatidylinositol (PI) and a variety of inositol phosphates (IPs) containing different numbers and combinations of phosphate groups. PI shares many functions with phosphatidylcholine (PC).

Inositol synthesis

Inositol is made from glucose-6-phosphate by conversion to inositol-1-phosphate by the enzyme inositol-3-phosphate synthase and subsequent removal of phosphate groups to form free inositol. Several grams daily are synthesised in the body, mainly in the testes, brain, liver and kidneys. PI is present in all tissues, and particularly high levels are found in the brain. In men, inositol is concentrated in semen but its function there is not well understood.

Digestion, absorption and transport

Inositol is present in food as PI and phytate, which need to be broken down to release free inositol for absorption. Free inositol is absorbed by active transport across the intestinal wall by a sodium-dependent co-transporter. Inositol circulates as free inositol in the bloodstream, and is taken up by tissues via a similar sodium-dependent co-transporter process.

Metabolism, storage and excretion

Inositol and cytidine diphosphate diacylglycerol are combined by the activity of the enzyme phosphatidylinositol synthase to form PI, and PI can be broken down by phospholipase C to form IP and diglycerides. Inositol is excreted in urine.

Functions

Like choline, inositol is an integral part of cell membrane PLs. The functions of inositol include:

- *Formation of PI and cell membrane function.* PI is a key component of PLs in cell membranes, and provides fluidity that allows transport across the membrane. It is the primary source of arachidonic acid that breaks down to form n-6 eicosanoids in inflammation. Glycosylphosphatidylinositol in cell membranes binds proteins to the cell surface.
- *Cell function.* IPs are involved in gene regulation, DNA repair, cell signalling, calcium mobilisation, protein metabolism, oocyte maturation and cell division and differentiation. PI and IPs are part of the PI cycle that produces diglycerides, which act as second messenger signalling molecules in cells. These messengers regulate the activity of protein kinase C, a family of enzymes involved in protein phosphorylation, a process that controls a wide range of cell activities, including metabolism, growth, cell survival, differentiation, proliferation and apoptosis. Inositol triphosphate (IP_3) is a second messenger responsible for the release of calcium ions from intracellular stores in the endoplasmic reticulum.
- *Liver function and fat metabolism.* Together with PC, PI is an important component of PLs in lipoproteins that transport lipids in the bloodstream and remove lipids from the liver after synthesis.
- *DNA and RNA metabolism.* IPs are important components of cell nuclei, and are involved in DNA repair, regulation of gene transcription and RNA metabolism.

- *Nerve and brain function.* PI is also part of nerve cell membranes and the myelin sheath that surrounds nerve fibres. The PI cycle generates second messengers that translate hormone messages arriving at brain cells, and it has a role in the release of calcium in nerve cells that is required for nerve impulse transmission.
- *Blood glucose regulation.* D-chiro inositol (DCI), a metabolite of inositol, is part of inositol phosphoglycans that mediate insulin activity in cells, and may help to maintain normal blood glucose levels.
- *Immunity.* IPs increase natural killer (NK) cell function and activity, and activate neutrophils.

Dietary sources

Phytates are found in fibre-containing plant foods, such as whole grains, legumes, seeds and nuts, and particularly the bran component of cereals. Inositol is found in oranges, grapefruit, cantaloupe, raisins, liver and brewer's yeast, and as PI in lecithin and lecithin-containing foods, such as soybeans, unrefined oils, seeds, nuts, whole grains, egg yolk, liver, brains, mayonnaise, salad dressings, chocolate, frozen desserts and baked goods. Inositol and PI are well-absorbed forms.

Factors influencing body status

Although inositol is water-soluble, PI is a phospholipid that requires the presence of bile in the intestine for digestion. People with inadequate bile production may have impaired absorption of inositol from PI. There is limited bioavailability of dietary phytate, but it appears that the enzyme phytase, present in food, can break down about 55–66 per cent of ingested phytate. If no phytase is present, absorption drops markedly. Phytate also can be broken down by phytase produced by bacteria during fermentation, by yeast during bread-making, and by sprouting or prolonged soaking of the plant food prior to eating. Dietary phytate absorption is inhibited by its incomplete liberation from the food matrix. In contrast, oral sodium phytate supplements are rapidly absorbed in humans, and lead to increased levels of phytate in plasma and enhanced urinary phytate excretion. Animal and cell studies have found some evidence for the absorption of intact phytate, and it is suggested that absorption may occur by pinocytosis (engulfment by the cell membrane to form a vesicle that releases its contents in the cell lysosome). Patients with diabetes, chronic kidney failure, galactosaemia (elevated levels of galactose), multiple sclerosis and polycystic ovarian syndrome have been found to have altered metabolism of inositol. Diabetics have increased excretion of inositol in urine.

Daily requirement

Inositol is made in the body and is not an essential dietary nutrient. Therefore, no recommended daily intake has been established.

Deficiency effects

Inositol deficiency in animals causes a loss of fat in the intestines (intestinal lipodystrophy) and accumulation of fats in the liver, leading to liver damage. This may be caused by impaired release of plasma lipoproteins, increased fatty acid mobilisation from adipose tissue and enhanced fatty acid synthesis in the liver. Rats placed on a diet of yellow corn, soybean oil meal, calcium, manganese, sodium chloride and alfalfa hay developed widespread loss of fur that was reversed by inositol supplementation. Subsequently, inositol gained a reputation as a promoter of hair growth in humans, but there is no evidence that it is effective. Inadequate levels of free inositol and PI have been implicated in the impaired nerve conduction associated with diabetes.

Assessment of status

Testing for inositol status is usually confined to clinical trials. It is suggested that the level of plasma inositol is about 52 μmol/L in healthy adults.

Source

Sauberlich, H.E., Skala, J.H. & Dowdy, R.P., *Laboratory tests for the assessment of nutritional status*, CRC Press, Cleveland, OH, 1999.

THERAPEUTIC USES OF INOSITOL

Psychiatric disorders

Inositol deficiency or abnormal inositol metabolism may be associated with psychiatric disorders such as bipolar disorder, depression, panic disorder, obsessive-compulsive disorder (OCD), eating disorders and schizophrenia. Supplementation is reportedly beneficial for depression (12 g/day), panic attacks and agoraphobia related to panic attacks (12 g/day) and OCD (18 g/day).[1] A review of four trials concluded that there was insufficient evidence to show that inositol is effective for depression.[2] Alzheimer's disease patients given 6 g/day of inositol for 30 days had a small improvement on some parameters of cognitive function, but the low dose and short trial duration may have limited its effectiveness.[1]

Polycystic ovarian syndrome

Polycystic ovarian syndrome (PCOS) features elevated male hormones, irregular menstrual cycles, ovarian cysts, excessive body hair growth, acne, obesity, reduced fertility, insulin resistance and increased risk of diabetes. Inositol has been shown to restore ovarian activity and fertility in women with PCOS.[3] Both inositol and DCI have been found to be effective. DCI appears to increase insulin sensitivity and enhance glucose metabolism. However, increasing the dose of DCI progressively worsens oocyte quality and ovarian response, and inositol appears to be primarily responsible for improving oocyte and embryo quality. A review of six trials concluded that inositol was effective for PCOS by improving insulin sensitivity, reducing elevated insulin levels and restoring hormonal balance and ovulation.[3]

Respiratory distress syndrome in preterm infants

Respiratory distress syndrome (RDS) is impaired lung function in infants born preterm that is caused by absence of the surfactant that stops the air sacs from sticking together. A review of three trials concluded that inositol supplementation reduces adverse outcomes in preterm infants, such as bronchopulmonary dysplasia (abnormal cell growth in the breathing passages), retinopathy of prematurity (eye damage), intraventricular haemorrhage (bleeding in the brain) and death.[4]

Prevention of birth defects

Inositol has been found to prevent cleft lip and palate in animals, and to reduce the risk of NTDs, apparently by activating protein kinase C.[5] Up to 30 per cent of NTDs in human infants are not prevented by folic acid use in pregnancy (folate-resistant NTDs) and inositol has been found to prevent folate-resistant NTDs in animals.[6] DCI has been shown to have a more potent effect than inositol in animals, reducing spina bifida by 73–86 per cent compared with a 53–56 per cent reduction with inositol use.[7] Lower blood levels of inositol have been found in pregnant women carrying foetuses with NTDs and the use of folic acid together with inositol has reduced the incidence of NTDs in women who have had a previous pregnancy affected by an NTD.[6]

Diabetes

In experimental diabetes in animals, impaired nerve function has been corrected by inositol supplementation. Inositol supplementation in pregnant women with a family history of type 2 diabetes has reduced the incidence of gestational diabetes and the delivery of an abnormally high body weight infant.[8]

Cardiovascular disease

Plasmalogens are a class of membrane glycerophospholipids associated with protective effects in atherosclerosis. In patients with elevated blood lipids and metabolic syndrome, inositol supplementation increased serum plasmalogens and decreased levels of small, dense low-density lipoproteins that are associated with increased risk of atherosclerosis.[9] Dietary phytate has lowered blood lipids and cholesterol levels in an animal study.[10]

Kidney stones

Phytate has inhibited the formation of deposits of calcium oxalate crystals in urine, and may be protective against kidney stones.[11]

Cancer

IP6 has been found to inhibit the growth of a wide range of cancers in cell studies, and IP6 given in drinking water has been shown to inhibit growth of cancers of the colon, liver, lung, breast and skin in animals.[12] Inositol alone and in combination with IP6 also has anticancer activity, and inositol appears to potentiate the effects of IP6. IP6 reduces metastases (spread of tumours) by inhibiting activity of matrix metalloproteinases that break down connective tissue and allow tumours to spread.[12] It also inhibits angiogenesis (the formation of new blood supply to tumours), does not affect normal cells and can be used with chemotherapy.[13]

Lithium-related psoriasis

Lithium carbonate is a common treatment for bipolar disorder, but can trigger or exacerbate psoriasis. Inositol supplementation has been reported to improve lithium-related psoriasis in one study but has no effect on psoriasis not related to use of lithium.[14]

REFERENCES

1 Colodny, L. & Hoffman, R.L., Inositol: Clinical applications for exogenous use, *Altern Med Rev* (1998), 3(6): 432–47.
2 Taylor, M.J., Wilder, H., Bhagwagar, Z. & Geddes, J., Inositol for depressive disorders, *Cochrane Database Syst Rev* (2004), 2: CD004049.
3 Unfer, V., Carlomagno, G., Dante, G. & Facchinetti, F., Effects of myo-inositol in women with PCOS: A systematic review of randomized controlled trials, *Gynecol Endocrinol* (2012), 28(7): 509–15.
4 Howlett, A. & Ohlsson, A., Inositol for respiratory distress syndrome in preterm infants, *Cochrane Database Syst Rev* (2003), 4: CD000366.
5 Cogram, P., Hynes, A., Dunlevy, L.P. et al., Specific isoforms of protein kinase C are essential for prevention of folate-resistant neural tube defects by inositol, *Hum Mol Genet* (2004), 13(1): 7–14.
6 Cavalli, P., Tonni, G., Grosso, E. & Poggiani, C., Effects of inositol supplementation in a cohort of mothers at risk of producing an NTD pregnancy, *Birth Defects Res A Clin Mol Teratol* (2011), 91(11): 962–5.
7 Cogram, P., Tesh, S., Tesh, J. et al., D-chiro-inositol is more effective than myo-inositol in preventing folate-resistant mouse neural tube defects, *Hum Reprod* (2002), 17(9): 2451–8.
8 D'Anna, R., Scilipoti, A., Giordano, D. et al., myo-Inositol supplementation and onset of gestational diabetes mellitus in pregnant women with a family history of type 2 diabetes: A prospective, randomized, placebo-controlled study, *Diabetes Care* (2013), 36(4): 854–7.
9 Maeba, R., Hara, H., Ishikawa, H. et al., Myo-inositol treatment increases serum plasmalogens and decreases small dense LDL, particularly in hyperlipidemic subjects with metabolic syndrome, *J Nutr Sci Vitaminol (Tokyo)* (2008), 54(3): 196–202.
10 Lee, S.H., Park, H.J., Chun, H.K. et al., Dietary phytic acid improves serum and hepatic lipid levels in aged ICR mice fed a high-cholesterol diet, *Nutr Res* (2007), 27(8): 505–10.
11 Grases, F. & Costa-Bauzá, A., Phytate (IP6) is a powerful agent for preventing calcifications in biological fluids: usefulness in renal lithiasis treatment, *Anticancer Res* (1999), 19(5A): 3717–22.
12 Vucenik, I. & Shamsuddin, A.M., Cancer inhibition by inositol hexaphosphate (IP6) and inositol: From laboratory to clinic, *J Nutr* (2003), 133(11 Suppl 1): 3778S–84S.
13 Kapral, M., Wawszczyk, J., Jurzak, M. et al., The effect of inositol hexaphosphate on the expression of selected metalloproteinases and their tissue inhibitors in IL-1β-stimulated colon cancer cells, *Int J Colorectal Dis* (2012), 27(11): 1419–28.
14 Allan, S.J., Kavanagh, G.M., Herd, R.M. & Savin, J.A., The effect of inositol supplements on the psoriasis of patients taking lithium: A randomized, placebo-controlled trial, *Br J Dermatol* (2004), 150(5): 966–9.

Therapeutic dose

Suggested therapeutic doses for adults are as follows:

- *Psychiatric disorders:* 2–18 g/day
- *PCOS:* 2–4 g/day; DCI: 1200 mg/day
- *Lithium-related psoriasis:* 6 g/day
- *RDS (preterm infants):* 70–100 mg/kg/day.

Effects of excess

Clinical trials have used doses of 4–30 g/day of inositol for periods of one to twelve months, and doses of 12 g/day or more have been associated with mild gastrointestinal adverse effects such as nausea, flatulence and diarrhoea. These adverse effects do not increase with increasing doses. Doses below 12 g/day have not been reported to cause adverse effects.

Supplements

The permitted form of inositol in Australian supplements is inositol, and it is also present in lecithin supplements. Inositol is produced by inositol-secreting micro-organisms or made from rice bran or corn steep liquor. Phytin, an impure phytic acid salt, is extracted from rice bran or corn by a weak acid and is then hydrolysed to free inositol and calcium and magnesium phosphates.

HOW MUCH DO I KNOW?

Choose whether the following statements are true or false. Then review this chapter for the correct answers.

	True (T)	False (F)
1 Triglycerides are the most common form of lipids in food.	T	F
2 Polyunsaturated fatty acids have one double bond.	T	F
3 PGE_1 is an eicosanoid produced from omega-3 metabolism.	T	F
4 Omega-3 fats have blood thinning and blood vessel dilating activity.	T	F
5 Trans fatty acids increase the risk of atherosclerosis.	T	F
6 Cholesterol is transported to cells by high-density lipoprotein.	T	F
7 Cholesterol is needed to make steroid hormones and vitamin D.	T	F
8 Very low-density lipoproteins take dietary fats from the small intestine to the liver.	T	F
9 A choline deficiency may lead to fatty liver.	T	F
10 Inositol may be useful for polycystic ovarian syndrome.	T	F

FURTHER READING

Gropper, S.S., Smith, J.L. & Groff, J.L., *Advanced nutrition and human metabolism,* 5th ed., Thomson Wadsworth, Belmont, CA, 2009.

Part 3
Vitamins

5

Introduction to vitamins and fat-soluble vitamins: vitamins A, D, E and K

INTRODUCTION TO VITAMINS

FAST FACTS . . . VITAMINS

- **Vitamins are essential, naturally occurring micronutrients found in relatively small amounts in food and beverages.**
- **They must be obtained from the diet because they either cannot be made in the body or cannot be made in sufficient amounts (the exception to this is vitamin D).**
- **They usually act as co-factors that support enzyme activity in the body.**
- **They are divided into two main groups: fat-soluble and water-soluble vitamins.**
- **Most vitamins have specific deficiency signs and symptoms associated with them.**
- **A severe deficiency of a vitamin can cause death.**
- **Most vitamins are harmless in large amounts but some can cause toxicity.**

Vitamins are classed as micronutrients because they are only required in milligram or microgram amounts. In contrast to macronutrients, vitamins do not provide energy (kilojoules). However, they are essential for body function and must be eaten in the diet because they either cannot be made in the body or cannot be made in sufficient amounts (the exception to this is vitamin D). Inadequate intake leads to vitamin deficiency disorders, and severe deficiencies may result in death. Age, pregnancy, breastfeeding, exercise training, stress and illness, as well as lifestyle, environmental and inherited genetic factors, may vary the need for certain vitamins. Many vitamins act as cofactors for enzyme systems in the body.

Discovery of vitamins

In 1890, the Dutch doctor Christiaan Eijkman, working in Indonesia, discovered that the disease known as polyneuritis in animals and beriberi in humans could be induced in chickens by feeding them a diet based solely on white rice, and could be cured by feeding them rice bran or brown rice. He believed that this was due to a toxin or microbe in white rice that was inhibited by a factor in brown rice. His assistant, Gerrit Grijns, continued the work, and eventually concluded that the disease was linked to the polishing process used to convert brown rice to white rice, which removed an important nutritional factor in the outer coating of rice.

In 1911, the Polish researcher Casimir Funk isolated a substance from rice polishings that cured polyneuritis in pigeons. This was actually nicotinic acid, which we know now as the anti-pellagra vitamin B3, contaminated with the anti-beriberi factor, which we now know as vitamin B1. Around this time, US researchers Elmer McCollum and Marguerite Davis discovered a fat-soluble food factor essential for the growth of rats. They named it 'fat-soluble A', and found that it was able to cure xerophthalmia (an eye disorder) and rickets (a bone disorder in children). Cod liver oil was found to be a rich source, and, subsequently it was found that cod liver oil contained two separate vitamins: vitamin A (for healthy vision) and vitamin D (for healthy bones).

In 1753, the British naval surgeon James Lind reported curing scurvy using orange and lemon juice, and in 1907, Norwegian researchers produced a scurvy-like disorder in guinea pigs by feeding them a cereal diet with no fresh animal or vegetable foods. The Hungarian researcher Albert Szent-Gyorgyi isolated the anti-scurvy factor in 1928, and named it ascorbic acid (vitamin C). These early discoveries led to the identification of the entire range of vitamins with which we are now familiar, the identification of vitamin deficiency diseases and the synthesis of vitamins for use as supplements for prevention and treatment of deficiencies.

Vitamin groups

- *Fat-soluble vitamins* include vitamins A, D, E and K. They dissolve in alcohol but not in water, and act in the fatty parts of the body, such as cell membranes. Because they do not dissolve in water, they need to be incorporated into water-soluble protein carriers for delivery to body cells via the bloodstream. Amounts in excess of daily needs can be stored and released for use as required. However, a regular daily intake is recommended to ensure that body needs are met. Fat-soluble vitamins are absorbed best if taken with food containing some fat. People on low-fat diets or those who have difficulty absorbing fats may have lower levels of these vitamins. Vitamin D is an unusual vitamin because it is the only vitamin that can be made in the body.
- *Water-soluble vitamins* include vitamin C and the B vitamin group, consisting of B1 (thiamin), B2 (riboflavin), B3 (niacin), B5 (pantothenic acid), B6 (pyridoxine), B12 (cobalamin), folic acid and biotin. These dissolve in water and act in the watery compartments of the body, such as the blood and the fluid inside and outside cells, and are more easily transported in the bloodstream. Most water-soluble vitamins cannot be stored in significant amounts in the body, and are readily excreted in urine, so they need to be ingested regularly. Losses are increased by factors that increase urine flow, such as diuretic drugs, stimulants, alcohol and natural stimulants, such as caffeine, theobromine and theophylline (xanthines) found in coffee, tea, cocoa, chocolate and the herb guaraná. Water-soluble vitamins are leached from food by methods of processing and cooking that involve water, and some are destroyed by exposure to heat and light, and break down during storage—especially prolonged storage at room temperature.

FAT-SOLUBLE VITAMINS

Vitamin A (retinol)

VITAMIN A STATUS CHECK

1 Do you have rough, dry skin, especially on the backs of your arms, thighs or buttocks?
2 Do you have difficulty seeing in dim light conditions?
3 Are your eyes sensitive to glare, and do you need to wear sunglasses when outdoors?
4 Is your hair dry and are your fingernails weak, with longitudinal ridges?

'Yes' answers may indicate inadequate vitamin A status. Note that a number of nutritional deficiencies or health disorders can cause similar effects and further investigation is recommended.

FAST FACTS . . . VITAMIN A

- Vitamin A (retinol) is found in fatty animal foods, and beta-carotene (a retinol precursor) is found in dark-green, orange and red vegetables and fruit.
- Vitamin A is required for the normal replication and development of epithelial tissues.
- It supports immunity and vision in dim light conditions.
- Supplementation may be helpful for skin and eye health, and during infections.
- Pregnant women should avoid taking large amounts of vitamin A.

Vitamin A (retinol) was identified in 1913 as a fat-soluble accessory food factor found in butter and cod liver oil. This factor was later found to be two different fat-soluble vitamins: vitamins A and D. A method of synthesising vitamin A was discovered in the 1940s.

Retinol is a fat-soluble alcohol only found in animal foods, but plant foods contain the naturally occurring pigments beta-carotene, alpha-carotene and beta-cryptoxanthin, belonging to the carotenoid family, that have provitamin A activity and can be converted to retinol in the body. Beta-carotene has the highest rate of conversion to retinol. People who eat vegan diets (devoid of animal products) must depend on beta-carotene as a source of retinol. Beta-carotene conversion to retinol is relatively inefficient and reduces if retinol status is high. Theoretically, one molecule of beta-carotene can convert to two molecules of retinol in the body but, because the body only absorbs about a third of beta-carotene and converts about half of that to retinol, it was initially estimated that 12 mcg of dietary beta-carotene were required to make 1 mcg of retinol. However, studies from the developing world now suggest that the rate of conversion is even less efficient, and it may require 21 mcg of beta-carotene to make 1 mcg of retinol (see Table 5.1). For beta-carotene as a supplement delivered in an oil form, 2 mcg is equivalent to 1 mcg of retinol, and for dietary alpha-carotene and beta-cryptoxanthin, 24 mcg is equivalent to 1 mcg of retinol. Conversion rates appear to vary between individuals.

Digestion, absorption and transport

Retinol in animal foods is present as retinyl esters of fatty acids—for example, retinyl palmitate—and carotenoids are bound to cellular lipids and proteins embedded in complex cellular structures in plants. Both require the presence of fat in the digestive tract for absorption. During digestion, retinol and carotenoids are split from their associated lipids and incorporated into water-soluble droplets (micelles), together with fatty acids, monoglycerides and phospholipids, by bile activity. Micelles are then absorbed into the epithelium of the small intestine. Carotenoid absorption appears to occur via the transporter scavenger receptor class B type 1 (SR-BI) and retinol absorption occurs at low doses via a transporter, possibly the protein stimulated by retinoic acid 6 (STRA6) and by passive absorption at high doses. Retinol is digested and absorbed more efficiently than beta-carotene, having about 70–90 per cent absorption, whereas beta-carotene absorption from raw foods is less than 5 per cent. Absorption increases if the food source is preserved in oil or eaten with fat, and if the food source is chopped or cooked, which breaks down some of the plant structures in which it is bound.

Most of the conversion of beta-carotene to retinol occurs in epithelial cells in the intestine after absorption. Retinol is reformed into retinyl esters and carotenoids, and retinyl esters are incorporated into

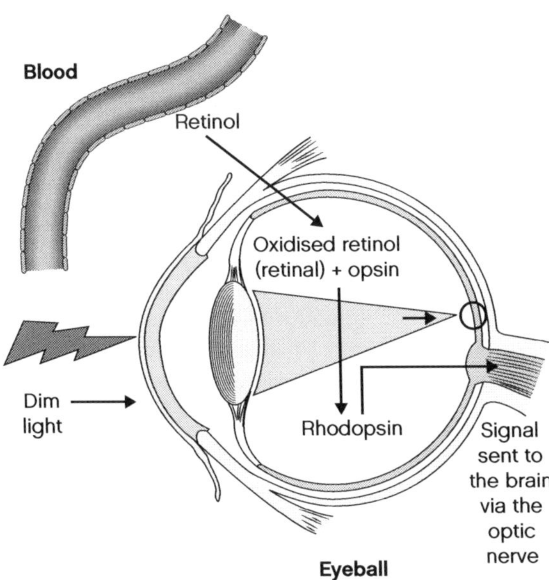

Figure 5.1 Retinal metabolism in the eye during dim light

chylomicrons (transport lipoproteins) together with dietary lipids, and transferred to lymph vessels and then to the bloodstream. As chylomicrons circulate around the body, lipids, retinyl esters and carotenoids are taken up by tissues and the remaining retinyl esters are delivered to the liver in chylomicron remnants.

Metabolism, storage and excretion

In the liver, retinol is removed from retinyl esters and a proportion is transported in the bloodstream to tissues by retinol-binding protein (RBP), synthesis of which depends on zinc. RBP transports retinol in combination with the protein transthyretin and bound to the hormone thyroxine, with the large size of this complex preventing its excretion in urine. Inside cells, a small reserve of retinyl esters is formed to supply the cell's needs. During metabolism, retinol is oxidised to retinal and then converted to retinoids, including retinoic acid (RA), in an irreversible reaction.

Carotenoids reaching the liver can be stored, converted to retinol, or packaged into very low density lipoproteins (VLDLs) for delivery to tissues and for storage in fat cells. Pro-vitamin A carotenoids can be released into the bloodstream from fat stores when required, and converted to retinol in the liver.

Some of the retinol in the liver is converted back into retinyl esters—mainly retinyl palmitate—for storage. The liver is the major storage organ, with a small amount stored as retinyl esters in the body's fatty tissue. Of the proportion of retinol absorbed, 20–60 per cent is metabolised and excreted within one week and 30–60 per cent is stored. The liver regulates the concentration of retinol in the circulation by releasing stores when needed, and serum retinol levels fall only when liver reserves are nearly exhausted. Excess retinol is broken down by the cytochrome P450 pathway in the liver to a number of polar metabolites, such as 4-hydroxyretinol, which are excreted in urine.

Functions

- *Epithelial cell growth and development.* Vitamin A is important for the health of the skin, hair and nails, and the mucous membrane linings (epithelium) of the digestive, respiratory, reproductive and urinary tracts. Retinoids, including RA, are forms of retinol that interact with genes by binding to the nuclear receptors, RA receptor (RAR) and retinoid X receptor (RXR). Retinoids regulate gene expression, and control cell growth and development. RA is particularly important for regulating the growth of epithelial cells, enabling them to develop normally into their mature, functional form. Retinoids maintain gap junctions that enable communication between cells and control cell growth, and retinol and retinoids help produce glycoproteins on cell surfaces that are involved in cell recognition, adhesion and differentiation.
- *Anticancer activity.* Retinoid signalling is impaired early in carcinogenesis. Retinoids can help reduce tumour growth and spread by inhibiting cell proliferation, enhancing cell differentiation, restoring normal differentiation in tumour cells and enhancing apoptosis of abnormal cells. They can prevent development of a tumour by suppressing the invasion and motility of pre-malignant cells and inhibiting angiogenesis (growth of new blood vessels to supply a tumour).
- *Eye health and night vision.* Retinol maintains the health of epithelial tissues that are the outer covering of the eyes, and enables vision in dim light. In the photoreceptor rod cells of the retina of the eye, retinol is converted to retinal, which then binds with the protein opsin to form rhodopsin, also called visual purple—the eye pigment that allows vision in dim light. Rhodopsin is made during dark conditions, and enables the adjustment of vision quickly when moving from well-lit areas to dark. When light hits rhodopsin, it breaks down to retinal and opsin, and a signal is sent to the brain that is registered as an image. The breaking down of rhodopsin is referred to as bleaching because the pigment is lost in the process. Rhodopsin must then be regenerated to enable the visual process to continue, and the speed at which it is regenerated is related to the availability of retinal.
- *Immunity.* Vitamin A is required for a healthy immune response. RA helps activate immune cells such as phagocytes and T lymphocytes, and boosts production of immune cells, immune-activating chemicals (cytokines), natural killer cells (NK cells) and antibodies. It also maintains mucus production in epithelial cells, which acts as a first line of defence against invading pathogens, and helps make the identifying glycoproteins on cell membranes that immune cells use to distinguish between normal body cells and foreign cells. Vitamin A requirements increase rapidly during infections—especially measles. If levels are already low, measles can precipitate a severe acute deficiency.

- *Growth.* RA may stimulate growth by increasing the number of cell receptors for growth factors. It appears to have a regulating role in bone development.
- *Reproduction.* Vitamin A is essential for normal reproduction in animals. In male animals, RA works with follicle-stimulating hormone and testosterone to stimulate sperm production. It is important for production and differentiation of sperm. In females, vitamin A is needed for the health of epithelial tissue in the reproductive tract, initiation of cell division in ovarian germ cells, conception and normal development of the embryo. However, excessive amounts may have adverse effects on embryonic development.

Dietary sources

- *Retinol* is found in fat-containing animal foods, such as fish liver oils, including cod, halibut, salmon and shark liver oils; liver; kidneys; egg yolks; fatty fish such as sardines, mackerel, herring and salmon; and full-fat dairy products, such as butter, cream, full-fat milk and cheese. Low-fat dairy foods are not good sources. Fish oil is low in retinol because it is made from the flesh of fish, not the liver.
- *Beta-carotene* is an orange pigment made by plants. Good sources are yellow, orange and red brightly coloured fruit and vegetables, and also dark-green vegetables, in which the colour is masked by chlorophyll. It is found in vegetables such as parsley, carrots, spinach, broccoli, peas, pumpkin, alfalfa, sweet potato, sweet corn, turnip tops, watercress and seaweed, and also fruit such as apricots, peaches, mango, rockmelon (cantaloupe) and papaya (pawpaw). The only vegetable oil source is red palm oil. Beta-carotene is used as a natural food colouring (additive number 160a).

Access the Food Standards Australia New Zealand nutrient database (NUTTAB) at <www.foodstandards.gov.au> for the amounts found in specific foods.

Factors influencing body status

Dietary fat is needed for absorption of retinol and beta-carotene, and people on low-fat diets and those who do not absorb fats well may have inadequate levels. Digestive disorders associated with impaired fat absorption, such as gall bladder or pancreatic disorders, inflammatory bowel diseases and cystic fibrosis, reduce absorption of vitamin A, and absorption is also decreased by mineral oil taken as a laxative, drugs that inhibit cholesterol uptake, such as cholestyramine and colestipol, and the weight-loss drug orlistat. Plant sterols and stanols added to foods to inhibit cholesterol uptake appear to reduce beta-carotene absorption, but have not been shown to affect retinol, vitamin D or Vitamin E levels in the body.

Retinol in foods can oxidise if exposed to light (particularly UV light), heat, air, acids and metals. A lack of zinc will impair synthesis of RBP and prevent mobilisation of vitamin A from storage. Liver damage can impair storage and kidney damage may lead to urinary losses. Clinical and sub-clinical infections cause the loss of large amounts of the RBP/retinol complex in urine, and can lower serum levels of vitamin A by 25 per cent, independently of vitamin A intake.

Carotenoids from raw foods are poorly absorbed, and cooking helps to break down cell walls and increase bioavailability. Dietary fat (at least 2.4 g fat per meal) is required for carotenoid absorption. Beta-carotene from supplements is absorbed more readily than that from dietary sources. Beta-carotene in microalgae appears to have greater bioavailability than beta-carotene in fruit and vegetables. Conversion of beta-carotene to vitamin A may be impaired in patients with diabetes or hyperthyroidism.

VITAMIN A MEASUREMENT

Vitamin A is measured in micrograms (mcg) or international units (IU) of retinol equivalents (RE). RE are a measure of the total vitamin A potentially obtainable from a substance, including both retinol and pro-vitamin A carotenoids.

Table 5.1 Retinol equivalents guide

1 mcg RE	= 1 mcg retinol
	= 2 mcg beta-carotene derived from oil-containing supplements
	= 12–21 mcg dietary beta-carotene
	= 24 mcg other pro-vitamin A carotenoids
	= 3.33 IU retinol

Source: Institute of Medicine, available at <www.iom.edu>.

Table 5.2 Vitamin A international unit (IU) conversion guide

1 IU retinol	= 0.3 mcg RE
1 IU beta-carotene derived from oil-containing supplements	= 0.15 mcg RE
1 IU dietary beta-carotene	= 0.05 mcg RE
1 IU other pro-vitamin A carotenoids	= 0.025 mcg RE

Source: National Institutes of Health, Office of Dietary Supplements, available at <www.ods.od.nih.gov/factsheets/VitaminA-HealthProfessional>.

Daily requirement

Government recommendations by age and gender (see Table 5.3) can be found in *Nutrient Reference Values for Australia and New Zealand Including Recommended Dietary Intakes*, available at <www.nhmrc.gov.au>.

Table 5.3 Recommended dietary intake (RDI) of retinol equivalents (mcg/day)

Age (years)	Female RDI	Male RDI
1–3	300	300
4–8	400	400
9–13	600	600
14–18	700	900
19–70	700	900
>70	700	900
Pregnant women		
14–18	700	
19–50	800	
Lactating women		
14–18	1100	
19–50	1100	

Source: Nutrient Reference Values for Australia and New Zealand Including Recommended Dietary Intakes, National Health and Medical Research Council, Australian Government Department of Health and Ageing, Canberra and Ministry of Health, New Zealand, Wellington, 2006.

Deficiency effects

Severe vitamin A deficiency is rare in Australia, but it is common in developing countries, affecting up to 250 million children under five years of age around the world and causing a dramatically increased risk of death, blindness and infections, especially measles and diarrhoea. Vitamin A deficiency is a major cause of preventable blindness worldwide. A deficiency leads to xerophthalmia (dry eye), in which the conjunctiva and cornea of the eyes dry out and keratin is deposited. An early symptom is night blindness and, in more advanced xerophthalmia, Bitot's spots may form on the surface of the eyes, which are hard, white, foamy-looking deposits of dead cells. The tissue of the cornea and conjunctiva may ulcerate, leading to scarring and loss of vision. In severe cases, so much eye tissue is destroyed that the eye lens falls out, causing irreversible blindness. Measles precipitates an acute vitamin A deficiency and rapid destruction of the cornea, and blindness can develop within hours in malnourished populations.

A lack of vitamin A causes mucus-secreting cells in epithelial tissue to be replaced by keratin-producing cells. Epithelial cells develop abnormally by failing to differentiate and dying off, and a thick, flattened layer of dead cells and keratin develops on the surface. The number of goblet cells decrease and mucous secretions diminish. The skin becomes dry (xerosis), and plugs of keratin may accumulate and block hair follicles, causing a rough, gooseflesh appearance, known as follicular keratitis or 'toad skin' (phrynoderma). Hair and nails become dry and weak, and nails may develop longitudinal ridges. A loss of protective mucus and lowered immunity contribute to increased risk of infections, especially affecting the skin and mucous membranes.

Animal studies of vitamin A deficiency have shown that epithelial tissues in the male reproductive tract become abnormal and sperm production ceases. In female animals, a deficiency causes abnormal epithelial tissue in the vagina and failure of implantation of the ovum after conception or death of the embryo. Birth defects may occur, especially affecting the eyes and also the genitourinary tract, kidney, diaphragm, lung, aortic arch and heart. However, too much RA at critical stages can result in death of the embryo or malformations.

Indicators of inadequate levels may include:

- poor night vision and reduced ability to see in dim light and darkness, especially after exposure to bright light; poor vision when driving at night, especially noticeable when oncoming headlights cause dazzling that interferes with vision immediately afterwards;

dry, irritated or watery eyes; sensitivity to glare and the need for sunglasses when outdoors; eye fatigue, pain and infections
- hard, cracked skin, especially on the heels; 'toad skin' which has the appearance of permanent gooseflesh and feels rough to the touch, especially affecting the buttocks, thighs and upper arms; dry, rough, flaky skin or scalp; dandruff; acne; poor wound healing; and sun-damaged skin
- skin and mucous membrane infections
- dry, brittle hair
- weak, peeling fingernails with longitudinal ridges (this can also be caused by an iron deficiency)
- abnormal cell growth, especially affecting the skin and mucous membranes.

Assessment of body status

A number of tests can be used to assess vitamin A status:

- *Serum retinol.* The reference range given by the Royal College of Pathologists of Australasia (RCPA) is 0.7–2.8 μmol/L (micromoles per litre) for adults. However, serum retinol level is not a good indicator of adequate retinol stores in most people because it does not start to decline until liver reserves are almost exhausted. Serum retinol can be used to detect very low or very high retinol levels. Serum retinol and RBP concentrations fall during infections, and the RBP:transthyretin ratio may help to determine whether serum retinol concentrations are depressed by infection.
- *Stable isotope dilution.* This is a more accurate measure of total body and liver vitamin A stores, and involves administering an oral dose of vitamin A labelled with a stable isotope and collecting a blood sample after the labelled vitamin A has mixed with the body pool of vitamin A. The plasma ratio of labelled to unlabelled vitamin A is measured and the total amount of vitamin A in the body is estimated using a prediction equation.
- *Conjunctival impression cytology.* This test involves taking an impression of the cells of the conjunctiva of the eye and testing for larger, irregular, keratinised epithelial cells and the absence of goblet cells, which indicates retinol deficiency.
- *Relative dose response (RDR).* A test dose of retinol (about 450 mcg of retinyl acetate) is given and retinol deficiency is indicated if there is a marked rise in serum retinol. The RDR is calculated as the ratio of the difference between serum retinol concentration five hours after the dose and the baseline concentration. A ratio of 20 per cent or more suggests inadequate liver stores.

Case reports—vitamin A deficiency

- *A pregnant woman, 24 years of age,* developed progressive loss of vision, particularly at night.[1] On examination, she had numerous Bitot's spots and keratitis of her eyes, with rod-cone dysfunction. Her serum vitamin A level was less than 0.002 μmol/L. The patient was found to have anorexia nervosa and had limited her diet to white onions, white potatoes and red meat for the past seven years. On vitamin A supplementation, her vision and eyes returned to normal. No information was reported on the pregnancy outcome.
- *A woman, 46 years of age,* developed a red, itchy left eye over the course of one week.[2] She attended an ophthalmologist, who discovered a bacterial infection in the left eye and a large defect in the corneal epithelium of her right eye. She was given a left corneal scrape and commenced antibiotic therapy. Two days later, the left cornea had perforated, requiring further referral for medical treatment. Both conjunctiva appeared thickened with Bitot's spots and her serum vitamin A levels were less than 0.1 μmol/L. The patient reported having experienced severe dry eyes and night blindness for the last three years, during which she had consumed only white fish and beer. Her weight had fallen from 96 kg to 50 kg over the preceding year. Oral and intramuscular (im) vitamin A supplements were given, together with an improved dietary intake. The right corneal epithelial defect had resolved by day six and the left corneal epithelial defect by one month. However, corneal scarring and an early-stage cataract remained.

REFERENCES

1 Braunstein, A., Trief, D., Wang, N.K. et al., Vitamin A deficiency in New York City, *Lancet* (2010), 376(9737): 267.

2 Connell, B.J., Tullo, A.B., Parry, N.R. et al., Vitamin A deficiency presenting with microbial keratitis in two patients in the UK, *Eye (Lond)* (2006), 20(5): 623–5.

THERAPEUTIC USES OF VITAMIN A

Cancer

Epidemiological and animal studies have found that inadequate vitamin A is associated with increased risk of cancer. Although vitamin A in the form of retinol or beta-carotene supplementation has not been found to be effective in cancer treatment or prevention, retinoids have been shown to prevent cancers of the skin, oral cavity, lung, mammary glands, prostate, bladder, liver and pancreas in animals exposed to carcinogens, and to suppress the spread of existing skin, oral, lung, breast, bladder, ovarian and prostate tumours.[1] In human studies, retinoids have reversed premalignant epithelial lesions, induced the differentiation of myeloid cells and prevented lung, liver and breast cancer.[1] Retinoids inhibit or reverse the carcinogenic process in some blood cancers, and premalignant and malignant lesions in the oral cavity, head and neck, breast, skin and liver.[1] Retinoids are now used as prescription medication for cancer prevention and control, but are not always effective because of the rapid metabolism of some retinoids and the development of retinoid resistance in some cells.[2]

Skin disorders

The retinoid drugs tretinoin, isotretinoin and tazarotene are used as medications for acne. In patients with mild to moderate acne, retinoid therapy has been associated with a decrease in non-inflammatory lesions of up to 81 per cent, a decrease in inflammatory lesions of up to 71 per cent and a decrease in total lesion counts of up to 83 per cent.[3] Acitretin, etretinate and tazarotene are retinoid drugs used as medications for psoriasis, often in combination with UV radiation, which allows dose reduction and decreases the incidence of adverse effects. Oral retinoids are effective in pustular and erythrodermic psoriasis, but are less effective in chronic plaque psoriasis.[4] Acitretin or isotretinoin may also be used for some types of ichthyosis (a skin disorder that features dry, scaly skin) and Darier's disease (a rare genetic skin disorder).[4] Topical or oral retinoid drugs should not be used in pregnancy because of the high risk of birth defects (see 'Effects of excess').

Child health

Vitamin A deficiency is common in developing countries and a deficiency among children worldwide is associated with about 20 per cent of measles-related deaths, 24 per cent of deaths from diarrhoea, 20 per cent of malaria incidence and deaths and 3 per cent of deaths associated with other infectious diseases.[5] Vitamin A supplementation reduces child mortality by 24 per cent overall, and is associated with a reduced incidence of diarrhoea and measles and a reduced prevalence of vision problems, including night blindness and xerophthalmia.[5] Measles depletes vitamin A levels dramatically and can be a life-threatening infection, particularly in malnourished children. Vitamin A supplementation reduces mortality in children less than two years of age who are hospitalised with measles, and also can reduce the risk of secondary infections associated with measles.[6,7]

Retinitis pigmentosa

Long-term vitamin A supplementation (15 000 IU per day) has been found to slow progression of vision loss in patients with retinitis pigmentosa, a genetic disorder that causes blindness.[8]

REFERENCES

1 Bushue, N. & Wan, Y.J., Retinoid pathway and cancer therapeutics, *Adv Drug Deliv Rev* (2010), 62(13): 1285–98.

2 Tang, X.H. & Gudas, L.J., Retinoids, retinoic acid receptors, and cancer, *Annu Rev Pathol* (2011), 6: 345–64.

3 Hsu, P., Litman, G.I. & Brodell, R.T., Overview of the treatment of acne vulgaris with topical retinoids, *Postgrad Med* (2011), 123(3): 153–61.

4 Zouboulis, C.C., Retinoids—which dermatological indications will benefit in the near future? *Skin Pharmacol Appl Skin Physiol* (2001), 14(5): 303–15.

5 Ezzati, M., Lopez, A.D., Rodgers, A. & Murray, C.J. (eds), *Comparative quantification of health risks: Global and regional burden of disease attributable to selected major risk factors,* vol. 1, WHO, Geneva, 2004.

6 D'Souza, R.M. & D'Souza, R., Vitamin A for treating measles in children, *Cochrane Database Syst Rev* (2002), 1: CD001479.
7 D'Souza, R.M. & D'Souza, R., Vitamin A for the treatment of children with measles—a systematic review, *J Trop Pediatr* (2002), 48(6): 323–7.
8 Musarella, M.A. & Macdonald, I.M., Current concepts in the treatment of retinitis pigmentosa, *J Ophthalmol* (2011), Article ID 753547.

Therapeutic dose

Suggested therapeutic doses for adults are:

- *Health maintenance:* 2000–5000 IU daily
- *Mild deficiency:* 10 000–15 000 IU daily, reducing on improvement
- *Severe deficiency:* 20 000–50 000 IU daily or higher, short term only
- In countries where vitamin A deficiency is prevalent, the World Health Organization (WHO) recommends giving vitamin A supplements in the following doses, together with the appropriate vaccinations:
  - 200 000 IU once every four to six months for all mothers up to six weeks post-partum if they have not received vitamin A supplementation after delivery
  - 100 000 IU once every four to six months for infants aged nine to eleven months
  - 200 000 IU once every four to six months for children aged twelve months and older, and
  - 200 000 IU once every four to six months for children aged one to four years.

  WHO recommends a minimum interval between doses of one month. However, the interval can be reduced in order to treat clinical vitamin A deficiency and measles.
- *Cystic fibrosis patients:* recommended daily doses are:
  - 1500–2000 IU from birth to one year
  - 1500–2500 IU from one to three years, and
  - 2500–5000 IU from four years to adulthood.

Effects of excess

Retinol is toxic in excessive amounts. In an overdose, body stores are filled to capacity, RBP becomes saturated and free retinol deposits out in tissues. This may cause fluid buildup in the brain, headaches, drowsiness, irritability, blurred or double vision, vomiting, peeling skin, hair loss and bone and joint tenderness. Effects on the brain may mimic symptoms of a brain tumour. In infants, toxicity signs are a bulging fontanelle, vomiting and irritability. Stopping the source of excessive retinol can reverse the toxicity symptoms, leaving no permanent damage. A high intake of vitamin A over a long period has also been linked to osteoporosis and bone fractures, possibly because high levels may interfere with vitamin D absorption or metabolism.

Retinol toxicity is rare, with only 291 cases reported between 1944 and 2000, and usually results from taking very large doses in supplement form over a long period of time rather than through the diet, although toxicity from eating large amounts of liver has been reported. People living in Arctic regions and early explorers in the Arctic and Antarctic have developed acute toxicity after eating the liver of polar bears, bearded seals, walruses or husky dogs, which can provide 250 000–1 million mcg (832 500–3 330 000 IU) retinol per 100 g. The Antarctic explorers Douglas Mawson and Xavier Mertz were both believed to be poisoned by eating the liver of their sled dogs when they ran out of food, and Mertz subsequently died. Their symptoms included vomiting, headaches, drowsiness, depression, psychosis, diarrhoea and severe peeling of the skin, causing thick layers of skin to separate from the soles of their feet, which they had to bind back on in order to walk. However, Lapps from Scandinavia and Finland are reported to consume 15 000 to 18 600 mcg (49 950–228 271 IU) of retinol from reindeer liver daily without ill-effects. Liver from common animal sources such as calves, lambs and pigs contains about 20 000–25 000 mcg (66 600–83 250 IU) retinol per 100 g. Chicken liver contains about 10 500 mcg (34 965 IU) retinol per 100 g. Eating liver from these animals occasionally is not likely to cause toxicity, but daily intake is not recommended.

The toxic dose of retinol is believed to be 2000 mcg (6660 IU) per kg body weight daily or more if taken as liver or an oil-based supplement for many months or years. This is equivalent to 120 000 mcg (399 600 IU) daily for a person weighing 60 kg. Water-soluble or emulsified supplements of retinol are about ten times as toxic as oil-based supplements, possibly because of increased absorption that leads to higher plasma levels, higher liver concentrations and lower losses than other forms of retinol. Water-soluble or emulsified supplements at doses of 200 mcg (666 IU) retinol per kilogram of body weight daily have caused toxicity after only a few weeks. This is equivalent to 12 000 mcg (39 960 IU) daily for a person weighing 60 kg.

Acute toxicity can occur from a one-off dose of more than 217 800 mcg (660 000 IU) in adults and more than 108 900 mcg (330 000 IU) in infants and children. Symptoms may include drowsiness, lethargy, itchiness around the eyes, vomiting, diarrhoea, coma, convulsions and death. For a single dose, the maximum safe amount of retinol in oil or liver seems to be 4000–6000 mcg (13 320–19 980 IU) per kilogram of body weight, equivalent to 240 000–360 000 mcg (799 200–1 198 800 IU) for a person weighing 60 kg. In developing countries where vitamin A deficiency is common, most young children have been found to tolerate single oral doses of 66 000 mcg (200 000 IU) retinol in oil at intervals of four to six months, with occasional short-term diarrhoea or vomiting but no major adverse effects.

Toxicity thresholds do not appear to vary considerably with age. Toxicity is enhanced by alcohol intake, a low-protein diet, exposure to environmental pollutants and drugs, kidney disease, viral hepatitis and other liver diseases; vitamin D appears to be protective.

Beta-carotene has limited conversion to retinol in the body, and does not cause retinol toxicity, even in large amounts. However, large amounts of beta-carotene can deposit in the skin and cause an orange-yellow discolouration, especially on the palms of the hands and around the mouth. This appears to be harmless but, because it indicates that the body cannot use such a large amount, it would be prudent to reduce intake. Beta-carotene, taken as a supplement in doses of 20 mg or more per day, has been linked to increased risk of lung cancer in smokers.

Birth defects

Although vitamin A is an essential nutrient for a healthy pregnancy, taking larger doses than required may be associated with birth defects. There were five reported cases of presumed or suspected birth defects associated with chronic retinol toxicity from 1944 to 2000. The doses ingested were 120–740 mcg (400–2464 IU) retinol per kilogram body weight per day in the first trimester of pregnancy, equivalent to 7200–44 400 mcg (23 976–147 852 IU) per day for a woman weighing 60 kg. Four cases reported kidney defects in the infant and the fifth case reported a defect in one eye. Two cases with the highest intakes of retinol involved infants with more severe defects that included malformations of the central nervous system. There is a higher risk of birth defects in infants born to women who consume more than 4500 mcg (14 985 IU) retinol per day from food and supplements in pregnancy compared with infants whose mothers consume 1500 mcg (4995 IU) or less daily. In pregnant women taking more than 3300 mcg (10 989 IU) daily of supplementary retinol (an average intake of 6500 mcg (21 645 IU), about one infant in 57 had a malformation possibly linked to the supplement, and there was an increased frequency of defects if supplements were taken before the seventh week of gestation. However, this has not been replicated in other studies, and there is debate about the link between retinol intake and some of the types of birth defects that were reported. Beta-carotene taken in pregnancy has not been linked to birth defects.

Retinoid drugs

Retinoid drugs are used by dermatologists for controlling acne and other skin disorders, and have a high risk of causing severe birth defects in pregnant women. Retinoids are believed to interfere with the activity and migration of cranial neural crest cells during development, leading to malformations of the head and face, thymus gland, heart, bones and central nervous system. It is essential that women taking these drugs do not become pregnant. Women of childbearing age must be absolutely certain that they are not pregnant before starting retinoid therapy, and must not become pregnant while on therapy or in the month following completion of treatment for isotretinoin and for two years after completion of etretinate or acitretin therapy.

Case reports—retinol toxicity

- *A woman, 29 years of age*, a part-time employee of a health food store, developed redness and irritation of her gums and tongue, cracks at the corners of her mouth, dry and itchy skin, headache, muscle aches, bone pain, generalised weakness and malaise, nausea and vomiting.[1] She had been taking 50 000 IU of vitamin A daily for about three months, increasing to 100 000 IU daily for one week before seeking medical advice. On ceasing her vitamin A intake, symptoms of nausea, bone pain and headache disappeared in two to three days. Weakness and dry mouth persisted for approximately seven to ten days. No long-term adverse effects were reported.

- *A woman, eighteen years of age*, developed headache, vomiting, back pain and double vision after ingesting a single high dose of vitamin A (about 10 million IU) in a suicide attempt.[2] Symptoms improved on treatment, but the long-term outcome is not reported.
- *A man, 35 years of age*, developed chronic fatigue, malaise, dry and itchy skin, muscle pain, loss of appetite, nausea, vomiting, mild frontal headache and liver enlargement.[3] He reported consuming between 30 and 50 capsules a day of various commercial fish oil preparations, together with an undetermined number of cod liver oil capsules during the previous year. His serum retinol level was 16.8 μmol/L. Supplements were discontinued and most symptoms gradually disappeared by the end of one week. After one month, he no longer had dry skin and liver enlargement, and his serum retinol had dropped to 2.4 μmol/L. No long-term adverse effects were reported.

REFERENCES

1 Baxi, S.C. & Dailey, G.E. III, Hypervitaminosis A: A cause of hypercalcemia, *West J Med* (1982), 137(5): 429–31.

2 Khasru, M.R., Yasmin, R., Salek, A.K. et al., Acute hypervitaminosis A in a young lady, *Mymensingh Med J* (2010), 19(2): 294–8.

3 Grubb, B.P., Hypervitaminosis A following long-term use of high-dose fish oil supplements, *Chest* (1990), 97(5): 1260.

Supplements

In Australia, the permitted forms of vitamin A in supplements are cod liver oil, halibut liver oil, pollack (pollock) liver oil, shark liver oil, skipjack liver oil, retinol, retinyl acetate and retinyl palmitate.

- *Natural retinol* is found in fish liver oils, such as cod liver oil or halibut liver oil, and these oils also contain vitamin D. Fish liver oils are available as bottled oil or capsules. Vitamin A and D can be extracted from fish liver oils by molecular distillation or solvent extraction, and concentrated to produce products with higher amounts of vitamin A and D and less oil. Note that regular fish oil is quite low in vitamin A and D, providing only about 7.5 mcg (25 IU) retinol per 1000 mg capsule.
- *Nature-identical retinol* can be produced chemically from a derivative of pentadiene (a hydrocarbon consisting of a five-carbon chain with two double bonds). It is usually available in supplements as the more stable ester forms retinyl acetate or retinyl palmitate, mixed with vegetable oil. Acetate is derived from acetic acid and palmitate from palm oil.
- *Synthetic retinol* is derived from lemon grass oil (citral) or pseudoionone (a derivative of citral) by chemical processing, and consists of retinyl acetate or palmitate mixed with vegetable oil.
- *Water-soluble retinol* contains natural or synthetic retinol esters with a solubiliser, such as polysorbate 80, an emulsifier commonly used as a food additive (number 433) and in cosmetics and pharmaceuticals. Polysorbate 80 is generally regarded as inert, but has been found to reduce fertility in animals if injected, and can cause severe non-immunological anaphylactic reactions in sensitive individuals.

Cautions

Excessive amounts of retinol can cause toxicity. Although vitamin A is an essential nutrient for a healthy pregnancy, taking larger doses than required may be associated with birth defects, and it is recommended that pregnant women ingest no more than 3000 mcg RE (9990 IU) daily from all sources. The Therapeutic Goods Administration (TGA) in Australia requires this statement on vitamin A supplements:

> *The recommended daily amount of vitamin A from all sources is 700 micrograms retinol equivalents for women and 900 micrograms retinol equivalents for men. WARNING—when taken in excess of 3000 micrograms retinol equivalents, vitamin A can cause birth defects. If you are pregnant, or considering becoming pregnant, do not take vitamin A supplements without consulting your doctor or pharmacist.*

Vitamin D (calciferol)

VITAMIN D STATUS CHECK

1 **Do you have low bone density, osteomalacia or osteoporosis?**
2 **Do you have weak muscles?**
3 **Do you have aches and pains in your muscles?**
4 **Do you avoid exposure to the sun or wear sunscreen at all times when outdoors?**

'Yes' answers may indicate inadequate vitamin D status. Note that a number of nutritional deficiencies or health disorders can cause similar effects and further investigation is recommended.

FAST FACTS . . . VITAMIN D

- Vitamin D is a steroid compound with hormone activity that is made in the body following exposure of the skin to sunlight.
- It maintains calcium and phosphate levels in the blood to support nerve and muscle function and bone growth.
- It regulates immunity, cell replication and growth.
- Supplementation may be helpful for muscle and bone disorders, autoimmune and inflammatory disorders and cancer protection.

Vitamin D, also called calciferol, is a fat-soluble vitamin that, unusually for a vitamin, is not found in adequate amounts in most foods. It is a steroid (cholesterol-derived) pro-hormone that can be converted to a hormone in the body and is made in the skin when it is exposed to solar ultraviolet B (UVB) radiation. The natural form of vitamin D made in the body is vitamin D3 (cholecalciferol), which is made by animals when exposed to sunlight. The synthetic form is vitamin D2 (ergocalciferol), which is made by phytoplankton, yeasts and fungi from the precursor, ergosterol, when exposed to UV light. Vitamin D2 is not made by other plants or animals, including humans.

Rickets, the bone disease caused by vitamin D deficiency, was common in industrialised nations in the nineteenth century, causing bone weakness and deformities in growing children, and cod liver oil was first used in 1824 as a successful treatment. In 1922, an anti-rickets factor was isolated from cod liver oil, subsequently identified as vitamin D. Sunlight was found to be beneficial for rickets, and researchers in the early twentieth century found that the anti-rickets factor could be produced by irradiating vegetable oils that contain sitosterol and also by irradiating cholesterol from animal tissue. This finding led to the discovery that cholesterol in the skin can be converted to vitamin D by sunlight.

Synthesis of vitamin D3

A cholesterol metabolite, 7-dehydrocholesterol, is made in sebaceous glands in the skin and is secreted onto the skin surface in sebum. When exposed to sunlight, 7-dehydrocholesterol absorbs light wavelengths of 290–310 nm (part of the UVB spectrum that causes sunburn) and is absorbed back into the skin, where it is converted to pre-vitamin D3 (pre-D3) (see Figure 5.2). Over the course of several days after the initial sun exposure, pre-D3 is converted to D3 in the skin, and this is transported in the bloodstream by vitamin D binding protein (DBP) to the liver and other body tissues.

About 10–15 per cent of the skin content of 7-dehydrocholesterol can be converted to pre-D3, after which no more is made. During prolonged sun exposure, 7-dehydrocholesterol is converted to lumisterol and pre-D3 is converted to tachysterol and other metabolites, including suprasterols I and II and 5,6 transvitamin D3, that do not appear to have potent vitamin D activity. This may be a protective pathway for preventing vitamin D toxicity from prolonged sunlight exposure. Lumisterol can be converted back to pre-D3 when sun exposure ceases. Short exposure to sunlight leads to prolonged after-sun production of D3 because of the continued conversion of pre-D3 to D3 and the conversion of lumisterol to pre-D3. The functions of pre-D3 and other UVB-induced sterols are not well understood, but they may have a protective role to play by inhibiting keratinocyte proliferation and regulating cell growth in the skin epidermis.

Digestion, absorption and transport

Dietary vitamin D2 and D3 are absorbed together with dietary lipids and incorporated into chylomicrons or bound by DBP for transport from the intestine to the liver. It appears that D2 and D3 have the same affinity for binding to DBP, but D2 may have a shorter retention in the body. Vitamin D3 from the skin is bound to DBP and delivered to the liver and other tissues that

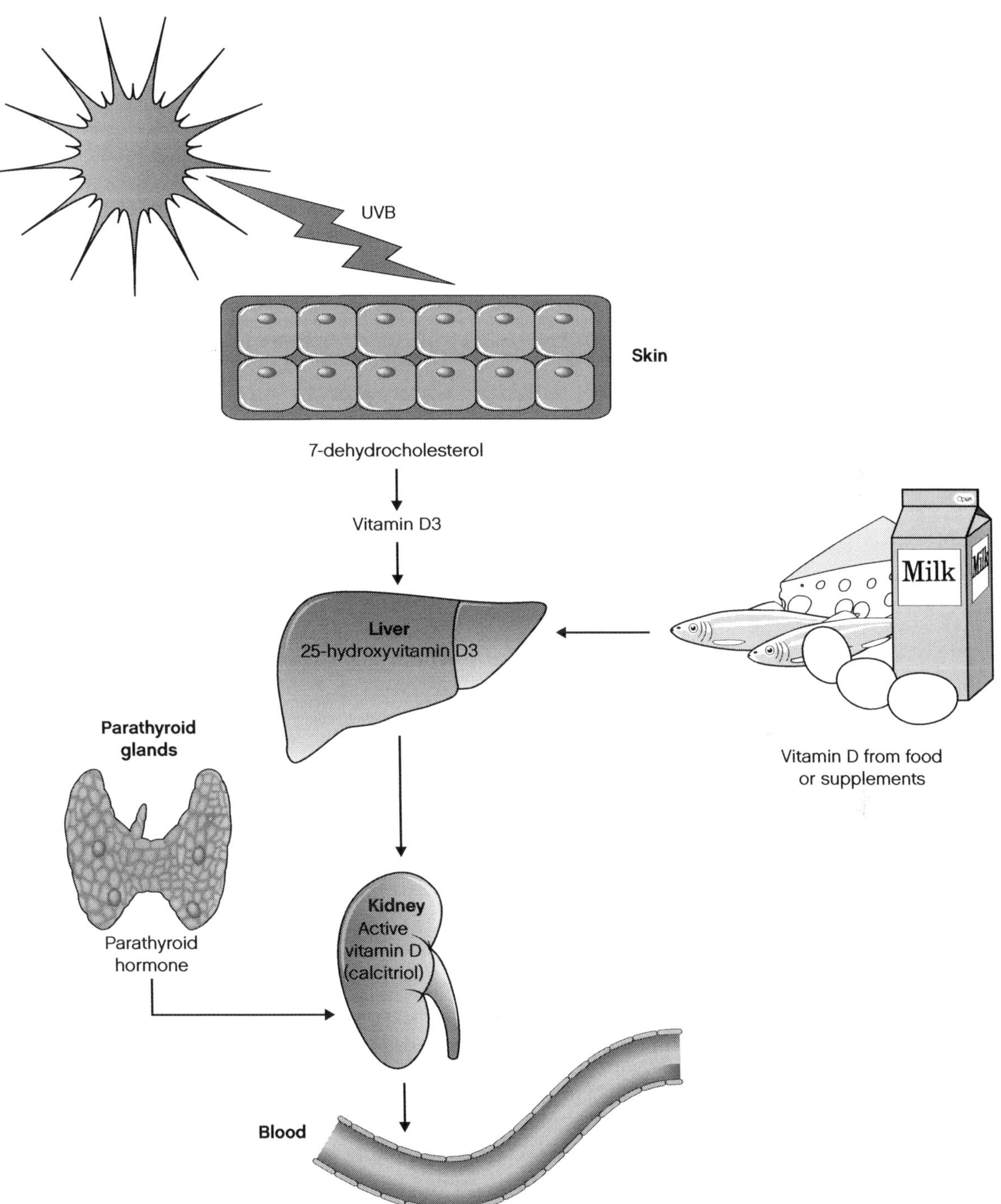

Figure 5.2 Vitamin D synthesis

contain the vitamin D receptor (VDR) in their cell membranes, which include the heart, muscles, pancreas, brain, skin, bones, intestines, parathyroid glands and immune cells.

Metabolism, storage and excretion

Vitamin D2 and D3 require further metabolism in the liver and kidneys to produce the main form of active hormone in the body. In the liver, both forms are converted into 25-hydroxycholecalciferol (25(OH)D) by the enzyme 25-hydroxylase. The liver releases 25(OH)D into the blood stream bound to DBP and it is taken up by the kidneys for conversion by the enzyme 25(OH)D-1alpha-hydroxylase to its major hormonal form, 1,25-dihydroxycholecalciferol (1,25$(OH)_2$D), also called calcitriol or active vitamin D. There is emerging evidence that 25(OH)D has hormone functions as well. Cells can take up 25(OH) D by endocytosis and also via the VDR, and it appears to help regulate cell proliferation and gene expression and works with calcitriol to regulate calcium balance and bone growth.

The blood has the highest concentration of vitamin D, and 25(OH)D originating from the liver has a circulating half life of two to three weeks, with levels regularly replenished from fat stores. Storage sites for vitamin D include the blood, liver, kidneys, muscles and adipose tissue. Vitamin D3 is mainly stored in adipose tissue and vitamin D2 in muscle.

The kidneys and other tissues with VDRs also can produce 24,25$(OH)_2$D from 25(OH)D by the enzyme 24-hydroxylase, but the role of this metabolite is not well understood. It may help to regulate calcitriol levels, support cartilage development, bone growth and fracture repair, and reduce blood pressure by inhibiting renin production in the kidneys.

Calcitriol

Calcitriol produced in the kidneys mainly acts on the digestive tract, kidneys and bones. Its main role is to increase blood calcium and phosphate levels by increasing uptake from food, reducing losses in urine and mobilising minerals from bone. In the small intestine, it stimulates production of the calcium-binding protein calbindin that enhances calcium absorption and in the kidneys, it acts by increasing production of calbindin that enhances calcium reabsorption in kidney tubules. Primarily, calcitriol promotes increased absorption of dietary calcium and reabsorption in the kidneys, but if blood calcium intake remains too low, bone calcium is mobilised.

Synthesis of calcitriol is regulated by the parathyroid glands embedded in the thyroid gland in the neck. These glands primarily monitor blood levels of calcium and release parathyroid hormone (PTH) when levels drop. PTH stimulates the enzyme 25(OH) D-1alpha-hydroxylase in the kidneys, which increases production of calcitriol in order to restore serum calcium levels to normal. PTH also has direct effects on bone by promoting its breakdown to release calcium into the blood.

Circulating calcitriol has a short half-life, and levels vary according to PTH release. Production of calcitriol is regulated by negative feedback; high levels decrease 25(OH)D-1alpha-hydroxylase activity and low levels increase it. High phosphorus levels decrease calcitriol production and bones produce fibroblast growth factor 23 (FGF23) that inhibits calcitriol production when calcium levels normalise. Excess calcitriol is converted to water-soluble calcitroic acid by detoxification enzymes in the liver and excreted in bile.

In other tissues with cell membrane VDRs, 25(OH)D is also converted to calcitriol, which remains in the cell and acts like a local hormone to regulate activities of the cell in which it is produced. Calcitriol acts intracellularly by binding to the VDR in the cell nucleus and works with the receptor RXR, a vitamin A receptor, to regulate the expression of genes. Genes responsive to vitamin D include the gene for calbindin D and those for bone and mineral metabolism, epithelial cell growth and differentiation, hair growth, immunity, detoxification, inflammation control, tumour suppression, apoptosis and DNA repair in the skin.

Functions

- *Bone mineralisation.* Vitamin D is essential for normal bone growth and mineralisation. Although calcitriol mobilises calcium from bones when levels fall, it also enhances bone building by increasing serum levels of calcium for delivery to bones, where it combines with phosphorus to form hydroxyapatite, the major mineral component of bones and teeth that provides rigidity and strength. Calcitriol also stimulates production of bone proteins and enzymes and helps regulate PTH release. 25(OH)D and 24,25$(OH)_2$D also appear to have a role in stimulating bone growth.
- *Muscle and nerve function.* Vitamin D maintains serum levels of calcium for delivery to muscles and

nerves. Calcium regulates the permeability of nerve membranes and the release of acetylcholine, and lowers the resting potential of nerves, which has a calming effect on the nervous system by preventing nerves from firing off too quickly.

- *Brain function*. Calcitriol can cross the blood–brain barrier and is also synthesised in the brain. VDRs are found in the nuclei of a number of cell types in the central nervous system, including microglia, astrocytes and myelin-producing cells. Vitamin D activates receptors on neurons in the brain that regulate behaviour, inhibits age-related changes in brain cells and has protective functions in the brain. It induces nerve growth factor expression, which stimulates release of neurotropins (proteins that assist nerve cell growth and development). It also regulates the expression of genes involved in forming neuron connections and memories, calcium metabolism, neurotransmitter synthesis and control of damaging free radicals. Vitamin D-responsive genes affect learning and memory, motor control, maternal and social behaviour, and ageing processes in animals. Calcitriol has been shown to protect against neurotoxins, increase levels of antioxidants in the brain, block uptake of reactive oxygen species (ROS) by brain cells and enhance apoptosis of abnormal cells, possibly protecting against brain tumours.
- *Cell replication and differentiation, anticancer activity*. Calcitriol has hormone-like activity in cells—especially epithelial cells—and helps regulate cell division and differentiation into the normal, mature form. Keratinocytes in the epidermis synthesise cholecalciferol but can also convert it to calcitriol, which regulates their proliferation and differentiation. Calcitriol inhibits excessive proliferation of fibroblasts, keratinocytes and lymphocytes, and has anticancer activity by blocking proliferation factors in cancer cells, inducing cancer cell maturation and apoptosis, decreasing angiogenesis and promoting repair of sunlight-induced DNA damage in keratinocytes. The VDR appears to have a role in hair follicle cycling by regulating the proliferation and differentiation of cells in the hair root, independent of calcitriol.
- *Immunity*. Calcitriol controls proliferation and activity of dendritic cells, macrophages and lymphocytes, and adaptive and innate immune responses. Calcitriol induces the expression of the antimicrobial peptide cathelicidin which is active in tuberculosis and *Staphylococcus aureus* (golden staph) infections. Adaptive immunity involves T and B lymphocyte activity and immunoglobulin production. Calcitriol suppresses adaptive immune responses, which inhibits autoimmune reactions in which the immune system attacks normal body tissues. It may also help prevent organ transplant rejection.
- *Antioxidant and anti-inflammatory activity*. Vitamin D can increase intracellular levels of the antioxidant precursor glutathione and inhibit production of inflammatory cytokines, such as interleukins, nuclear factor kappaB (NF-kappaB) and tumour necrosis factor-alpha (TNF-alpha), produced during immune responses by monocytes, macrophages and microglia (the counterpart of macrophages in the brain). Calcitriol is anti-inflammatory because it decreases expression of cyclooxygenase-2 (COX-2), the enzyme responsible for production of inflammatory eicosanoids from omega-6 fatty acids, and increases expression of 15-hydroxyprostaglandin dehydrogenase (15-PGDH), the enzyme that breaks down the inflammatory prostaglandin E_2 (PGE_2).
- *Insulin release*. Calcitriol is produced by beta cells in the pancreas that produce insulin in response to elevated blood glucose levels, and appears to have a role in stimulating insulin release.
- *Blood pressure regulation*. Vitamin D inhibits renin production in the kidneys, and thereby reduces activity of the renin-angiotensin system that drives up blood pressure by constricting small arteries and increasing sodium and water retention.

Dietary sources

There is a limited amount of vitamin D in the food supply, and fortification of food is not widespread in Australia. Therefore, it is not possible to maintain healthy blood levels of 25(OH)D solely from dietary intake. UVB exposure and/or supplementation are the most reliable sources.

- *Vitamin D3* is only found in fat-containing animal foods, such as fish liver oils, including cod, halibut, salmon and shark liver oils; liver; kidneys; egg yolks; fatty fish such as sardines, mackerel, herring and salmon; and full-fat dairy products, such as butter, cream, full-fat milk and cheese. Low-fat dairy foods are not good sources. Fish oil is low in vitamin D3, as it is made from the flesh of fish, not the liver. Farmed fish may only contain about 25 per cent of the D3 levels in wild-caught fish because of artificial feeding.

In Australia, it is mandatory that table margarine and low-fat spreads are fortified with vitamin D and must contain no less than 55 mcg/kg. Voluntary fortification is permitted in modified, skim and powdered milk, yoghurt, cheese and some other dairy products. The vitamin D intake of Australian adults from fortified milk and margarine ranges from 3.5–6.4 mcg (140–256 IU) per day.

- *Vitamin D2* may be found in naturally grown field mushrooms and sun-dried mushrooms because they contain ergosterol, which is converted to ergocalciferol if exposed to UV radiation. Most commercially grown mushrooms are grown in dark conditions, and do not contain significant amounts of vitamin D, but commercially grown mushrooms exposed to UVB light are now available, and these contain about 410 mcg of vitamin D per 100 g, which is about 700 per cent higher than the amount in mushrooms grown in the dark.

Access the Food Standards Australia New Zealand nutrient database (NUTTAB) at <www.foodstandards.gov.au> for the amounts found in specific foods.

Factors influencing body status

Most foods are poor sources of vitamin D, and low-fat diets and vegetarian diets are particularly inadequate. About half the vitamin D in food is absorbed. Dietary fat is needed for absorption of vitamin D, and people on low-fat diets and those who do not absorb fats well may have inadequate levels. Digestive disorders associated with impaired fat absorption, such as gall bladder or pancreatic disorders, inflammatory bowel diseases and cystic fibrosis, reduce absorption of vitamin D. Absorption is also decreased by mineral oil taken as a laxative, drugs that inhibit cholesterol uptake, such as cholestyramine and colestipol, and the weight-loss drug orlistat. Disorders affecting the parathyroid gland, the liver or the kidneys may impair vitamin D metabolism.

Serum 25(OH)D levels vary according to the seasons, with the lowest levels at the end of winter and the highest levels at the end of summer. High-altitude regions have greater UVB exposure than lower altitudes. Dietary intake of vitamin D and sun exposure are both inadequate in most Australians, and low vitamin D status is now common—even in young people and Queenslanders at the end of winter. Deficiencies are more common and more severe in dark-skinned, veiled, pregnant women and elderly nursing home and hostel residents. Skin exposure to UVB is restricted by air pollution, indoor lifestyles, nightshift work, excessive clothing and regular sunscreen use.

To make vitamin D effectively, sufficient unprotected bare skin must be exposed and UV radiation must be strong enough. The skin pigment melanin blocks UVB rays from reaching 7-dehydrocholesterol in the skin, and cholecalciferol production is decreased in heavily tanned or pigmented skin. Lower serum 25(OH)D levels are common in people with dark skin pigmentation living in temperate latitudes, and it is estimated that they require ten to 50 times more exposure to UVB in order to make vitamin D compared with people with fair skin types. Sunscreen factor 8 or above, properly applied, reduces the skin's ability to make vitamin D by 95–99 per cent, window glass and covering the skin blocks UVB radiation and skin synthesis declines with age. Bathing or showering straight after sunlight exposure can wash away sebum that produces cholecalciferol before it can be absorbed back into the skin.

During winter in higher latitudes (above 35°), the sun is too weak to make vitamin D effectively, and the body must rely on stores built up over summer. Regular sun exposure during summer can produce the equivalent of 70 mcg (2800 IU) of vitamin D daily. Peak D3 production occurs in the middle of the day when the sun's rays are strongest. One full body exposure to UVB in summer that causes slight reddening of the skin several hours afterwards, called the minimal erythemal dose (MED), can create the same amount of vitamin D as an oral intake of 500 mcg (20 000 IU). It is estimated that ten to fifteen minutes of midday sun exposure on the face, hands, arms, legs or back without sunscreen at least twice a week may be enough to produce adequate vitamin D in summer.

Tanning beds emit mainly UVA radiation with a small amount of UVB (0.5–1.4 per cent). This may be enough to raise serum levels of 25(OH)D somewhat, but use of sun beds has been linked to skin damage and melanoma, and is especially risky in people with fair skin and younger people. People having their first exposure to indoor tanning before the age of 35 years have a 75 per cent increased risk of developing melanoma.

During pregnancy, calcitriol levels increase and reach a peak during the third trimester, with an abrupt decline after the infant's birth. Breast milk has inadequate vitamin D for the infant's needs, and exclusively breastfed infants are at risk of deficiency. Obese people have low serum 25(OH)D, possibly because vitamin D is sequestered in body fat. Severe liver disease impairs vitamin D metabolism and chronic kidney disease can affect production of calcitriol and increase urinary losses. Anti-convulsants, glucocorticoids and HIV and anti-rejection drugs enhance the breakdown of vitamin D to calcitroic acid.

> VITAMIN D MEASUREMENT
>
> Vitamin D is measured in micrograms (mcg) or international units (IU).
> - 1 mcg vitamin D = 40 IU vitamin D
> - 1 IU vitamin D = 0.025 mcg vitamin D

Daily requirement

Government recommendations by age and gender (see Table 5.4) can be found in *Nutrient Reference Values for Australia and New Zealand Including Recommended Dietary Intakes*, available at <www.nhmrc.gov.au>.

Table 5.4 Recommended adequate intake (AI) of vitamin D (mcg/day)*

Age (years)	Female AI	Male AI
1-3	5	5
4–8	5	5
9–13	5	5
14–18	5	5
19–50	5	5
51–70	10	10
>70	15	15
Pregnant women		
14–18	5	
19–50	5	
Lactating women		
14–18	5	
19–50	5	

* Recommendations assume some sun exposure.

Source: Nutrient Reference Values for Australia and New Zealand Including Recommended Dietary Intakes, National Health and Medical Research Council, Australian Government Department of Health and Ageing, Canberra and Ministry of Health, New Zealand, Wellington, 2006.

Many vitamin D researchers consider that government recommendations are too low, and advise sensible sun exposure and supplements providing 400–1000 IU (10–25 mcg) daily for infants, 1000–2000 IU (25–50 mcg) daily for adults and 1500–2000 IU (37.5–50 mcg) daily for pregnant or lactating women and elderly people. Serum 25(OH)D levels should be monitored when using higher doses.

Deficiency effects

Vitamin D deficiency appears to be a worldwide health issue, especially affecting dark-skinned people living at higher latitudes and women wearing traditional Islamic clothing. Vitamin D deficiency has been identified in various population groups, including Middle Eastern women, inner-city young adults in America, elite gymnasts in Australia, young skateboarders in Hawaii and adolescent girls in England. A study in New South Wales, Australia found that 33 per cent of men and 40 per cent of women had low vitamin D levels (less than 50 nm/L). The mean vitamin D levels were 58 nm/L for men and 51 nm/L for women and levels overall decreased with age. However, mean vitamin D levels in people aged 20–29 years were lower than in some older age groups, possibly because of lifestyle factors that reduced their sun exposure. The highest levels occurred in late summer (February) and the lowest in early spring (September/October).

A lack of vitamin D causes serum calcium levels to drop and triggers the release of PTH, which elevates serum calcium by mobilising it out of bones. As the deficiency continues, PTH remains elevated (secondary hyperparathyroidism), serum calcium levels may return to normal or remain low, 25(OH)D and phosphate levels are low and serum levels of the enzyme alkaline phosphatase (a marker of bone metabolism) are elevated. The induced secondary hyperparathyroidism stimulates the kidneys to produce calcitriol, levels of which may be normal or elevated until the vitamin D deficiency is advanced enough to impair calcitriol production. Bones become soft, weak and painful, and fracture more easily. When vitamin D deficiency is combined with calcium deficiency, the bone abnormalities are more rapid and more severe. Elevated PTH is also associated with fatigue, lethargy, depression, constipation, heartburn, peptic ulcers, nausea, vomiting, appetite loss and vague abdominal pains, and may increase the risk of kidney stones, pancreatitis, cancers of the colon and the development of brown tumours (benign growths in bones).

Infants and children

In infants, commonly those between the ages of four and twelve months, a lack of vitamin D causes rickets, in which cartilage in the ends of long bones enlarges but fails to mineralise, inhibiting growth and causing bone deformities. On x-ray, there is widening, cupping and fraying of the metaphyseal regions (growth regions) of long bones, and widened and irregular epiphyseal plates, which are the end regions of bone that remain unfused to the rest of the bone during growth. Bones are soft and deform easily, leading to greenstick fractures, spinal and pelvic deformities, and enlarged joints, and bow legs or knock knees develop when the child is able to stand and walk. Muscle contractions can deform long bones, even before the child has the ability to stand or walk. Growth is retarded and the abdomen enlarges.

Softening of the skull causes bossing, in which the head becomes misshapen, with lumpy overgrowths, flattening of the sides or back of the head, and bulging of the forehead. The fontanelle and skull sutures enlarge and closing of the fontanelle is delayed. The teeth fail to develop normally, eruption is delayed and tooth enamel is defective, leading to the early onset of dental caries. In the ribs, the costochondral junctions (where bones join cartilage) enlarge, causing knobby lumps (beading), known as the rachitic rosary. Muscle contractions deform the ribs and the sternum protrudes (pigeon chest). Ribcage changes and weakness of the thoracic muscles contribute to breathing difficulties and respiratory infections.

Low serum calcium induced by rickets also affects nerve and muscle function, and may cause muscle weakness and pain, as well as delayed motor development—especially delayed walking—and even paralysis. Other effects include sweating of the head, pallor, irritability and lethargy. Convulsions may occur during the infant's first six months, and throat spasms, heart muscle weakness, dysfunction of the left ventricle, congestive heart failure, shock and death may result. Low vitamin D in infancy and childhood has been linked to iron-deficiency anaemia and the development of allergies, multiple sclerosis, type 1 diabetes, schizophrenia and possibly autism.

In Australia, rickets is more common in infants and children with dark skin pigment, especially if they have recently immigrated to Australia, and in those who are not exposed to the sun, who are overdressed, who use excessive amounts of sunscreen or whose mothers are vitamin D deficient. Veiled mothers with dark skin pigment have a higher risk of vitamin D deficiency in their infants.

Some forms of rickets are due to genetic disorders. In vitamin D-dependent rickets type I, the enzyme that produces calcitriol in the kidneys is lacking, and in type II vitamin D-dependent rickets, there are defects in the genes for VDRs. In hypophosphataemic (vitamin D-resistant) rickets, vitamin D supplementation is not effective because of an inherited defect in the reabsorption of phosphate in the kidneys.

Adults

In adults, low vitamin D causes osteomalacia, in which bones are softer, and also osteoporosis, in which bone minerals are lost and bones become porous. Osteomalacia is characterised by an increase in the amount of bone surface covered by osteoid (unmineralised bone) and an increase in osteoid thickness, together with reduced rate of mineralisation and bone formation. Osteomalacia causes generalised bone pain, possibly because of pressure on the periosteum from thickening of osteoid, and is indicated when moderate thumb pressure on the breastbone or shin bone causes pain.

Key symptoms of osteomalacia are pain and muscle weakness, especially in the rib, hip, pelvis, thigh and foot, sometimes causing a waddling gait; diffuse muscular aches and muscle weakness in the limbs and back; and joint or bone pain, most often affecting the shoulders, pelvis, ribs and spine. Subchondral microfractures (small fractures of the bone underlying cartilage in joints), and bone and spinal deformities may develop. In muscles, there is a normal range of type I fibres but a reduced proportion and diameter of type II muscle fibres. Pain symptoms may be misdiagnosed as fibromyalgia or symptoms of depression. Low bone mineral density and fractures may also reflect osteomalacia. In older people, low vitamin D can cause muscle pain and weakness, loss of balance, falls and difficulty walking, standing up from a sitting position and climbing stairs, and may lead to paralysis.

Through its effects on calcium metabolism, vitamin D supports nerve function and a deficiency may cause nervous tension, irritability, anxiety and insomnia. In pregnant women, vitamin D deficiency is associated with pre-eclampsia (high blood pressure and fluid retention), low-birth weight infants, low serum calcium in newborn infants, poor postnatal growth, bone fragility and poorly mineralised bones in children during the first nine years of life, and autoimmune disorders in infants and children.

Vitamin D deficiency activates the renin-angiotensin-aldosterone system, increasing the risk of elevated blood pressure and enlargement of the left ventricle of the heart. By increasing PTH, it contributes to insulin resistance, type 1 and type 2 diabetes and cardiovascular disease. Vitamin D deficiency is also associated with inflammation, autoimmune disorders, infections, allergies, Alzheimer's disease, schizophrenia, depression, psoriasis and cancer.

Indicators of inadequate levels may include:

- bone weakness, pain, fractures, osteoporosis, osteomalacia
- muscle weakness, muscle pain, loss of balance, falls, fibromyalgia, chronic fatigue syndrome, paralysis
- nervous tension, irritability, anxiety, insomnia, mood disorders
- headaches, feeling of pressure in the head
- psoriasis
- lowered immunity, infections, autoimmune disorders such as Crohn's disease, diabetes, multiple sclerosis, asthma and rheumatoid arthritis
- inflammatory and cardiovascular disorders, elevated blood pressure
- dementia, autism, schizophrenia
- cancer
- *pregnant women*: low birth-weight babies, premature labour, preterm birth, infections, pre-eclampsia and toxaemia
- *children*: bow legs, knock knees, beading of ribs, misshapen skull, distended abdomen, sweating of the head during sleep, pallor, irritability, weak muscles, paralysis, convulsions and heart failure.

Assessment of body status

Vitamin D status is assessed by the level of 25(OH)D circulating in serum, which reflects the amount in the liver. Calcitriol is not regarded as an appropriate measure because it is influenced by PTH, and can remain normal or high even when 25(OH)D stores are nearly exhausted. The reference range for serum 25(OH)D given by the RCPA is 40–160 nmol/L (nanomoles per litre) for adults and the reference range for calcitriol for adults is 35–120 pmol/L (picomoles per litre).

Many vitamin D researchers consider that the serum level needed for health and prevention of disorders related to inadequate vitamin D is 75 nmol/L or more, with optimal levels being 90–100 nmol/L. Levels of 50–74 nmol/L are considered to indicate vitamin D insufficiency and levels less than 50 nmol/L indicate a deficiency. A mild deficiency is a level of 26–49 nmol/L, a moderate deficiency is 15–25 nmol/L and a severe deficiency is less than 15 nmol/L. Levels greater than 240 nmol/L may indicate excessive intake.

Most children with rickets and adults with osteomalacia have a high concentration of serum alkaline phosphatase, and low calcium and phosphate levels may be present. Elevation of plasma PTH, indicating secondary hyperparathyroidism, is typical in most patients with osteomalacia, but is not found in mild vitamin D deficiency. Levels of serum alkaline phosphatase and PTH usually start to decline during the first three months of treatment in adults, but may take a year to reach normal values.

Radiographs are used to confirm suspected rickets. Hereditary or renal rickets, indicated by persistent low phosphate, normal alkaline phosphatase or elevated creatinine levels, may not respond to vitamin D supplementation and should be investigated further. People with unusually low vitamin D levels or lack of response to supplementation should be investigated for malabsorption syndromes.

Case reports—vitamin D deficiency

- *A male infant, six months of age* and exclusively breastfed, had a poor growth rate and was diagnosed with failure to thrive.[1] His alkaline phosphatase levels were elevated and 25(OH)D was low. Radiological examinations revealed bone abnormalities indicative of rickets. He was given 2000 IU of vitamin D and 1000 mg of calcium carbonate daily with iron and zinc, which led to improvements in his growth rate and increased serum 25(OH)D levels.
- *An Iranian girl, ten years of age*, living in London, developed a recurring, dull, aching pain in the legs after exercising, which resolved after several hours' rest.[2] She spent very little time outdoors, and when outdoors always wore SPF30 or stronger sun protection on her face and traditional Islamic clothing and head covering. Her serum 25(OH)D level was low (15.8 nmol/L), PTH was raised, and calcium and phosphate levels were low. She was given dietary advice to increase her calcium and vitamin D intake, 6000 IU of supplementary vitamin D daily, and encouraged to expose her arms or legs to sunshine for ten to fifteen minutes several times a week without sunscreen. Her muscle pain disappeared and her exercise tolerance improved.
- *A woman, 54 years of age*, had progressive lethargy, fatigued easily, and had diffuse body pain and weakness of the limbs.[3] She had developed low back and hip pain about two to three years previously,

which had increased in intensity, frequency and duration over time and led to her reducing her physical activity. She was experiencing difficulty climbing stairs, getting up from a sitting position or from bed, and lifting heavy objects. She had also developed headaches with a feeling of pressure in the head ten months previously. She had weakness of muscles in the trunk, generalised muscle tenderness and bone tenderness from very mild pressure on the bones of the shin, forearm and breastbone. A skeletal x-ray showed evidence of osteomalacia. Her alkaline phosphatase levels were elevated and 25(OH)D was low. She was given supplementary vitamin D (1500 IU daily) with calcium (1000 mg daily) and the headache had disappeared completely at four weeks and the diffuse body pain at six weeks. Muscle strength and bone tenderness had improved markedly at four months and vitamin D levels returned to normal.

- *A man, 42 years of age*, had a history of episodic headache for two to three years, described as dull pain over the whole head, mostly mild with occasional exacerbations.[3] He then developed fatigue and pain in the back and both lower limbs, and was having difficulty climbing stairs and getting up from a sitting posture. He had generalised muscle tenderness and bone tenderness affecting the bones of the legs, arms and skull. His alkaline phosphatase levels were elevated and 25(OH)D was low. He was diagnosed with osteomalacia. He was given supplementary vitamin D3 (1500 IU daily) and calcium (1500 mg daily), with an analgesic to be used when required. Within two weeks, his head and body pain started to improve, and in four weeks his headache had gone. His body pain resolved in six weeks and muscle weakness improved to near normal in four months. However, mild bone tenderness was still present at six months. Vitamin D levels normalised after four months.

REFERENCES

1 Stevens, R.L. & Lyon, C., Nutritional vitamin D deficiency: A case report, *Cases J* (2009), 2: 7000.

2 Whyman, J.D., Michie, C., Chan, V.A. et al., Muscle pain and hypovitaminosis D in a 10 year old girl: A case report, *West Lon Med J* (2010), 2(3): 53–7.

3 Prakash, S. & Shah, N.D., Chronic tension-type headache with vitamin D deficiency: Casual or causal association? *Headache* (2009), 49(8): 1214–22.

THERAPEUTIC USES OF VITAMIN D

Bone disorders

Children born to mothers who were sub-clinically deficient in vitamin D during pregnancy have been shown to develop less well-mineralised bones during the first nine years of life.[1] Breast milk is very low in vitamin D, and reflects maternal levels. It is estimated that lactating mothers require at least 2000 IU daily and possibly up to 6000 IU daily to ensure adequate levels in their breast milk.[2] Direct supplementation of breastfed babies with even modest levels of vitamin D in the first year of life (400 IU a day) has been shown to improve bone mineral mass seven to nine years later.[3]

In elderly Australian women, 1000 IU vitamin D with 1200 mg calcium was shown to have long-term beneficial effects on bone density, maintaining bone mineral density in the hip over a five-year period.[4] A meta-analysis of eleven studies found that the risk of hip fracture is reduced by 30 per cent and the risk of any non-vertebral fractures is reduced by 14 per cent at a higher range of vitamin D intake (median intake, 800 IU daily; range, 792 to 2000 IU).[5] Serum 25(OH)D levels of 75 to 110 nmol/L appear to be optimal for protecting against hip fractures in elderly people.[6]

Muscle disorders

In elderly stroke patients with vitamin D deficiency, vitamin D supplementation has been shown to increase the relative content and mean diameter of type II muscle fibres, with the fibre size correlating with serum 25(OH)D levels.[7] Lack of muscle strength in the elderly leads to loss of balance, falls and fractures and is associated with vitamin D deficiency. A meta-analysis of five trials using vitamin D supplementation in elderly people concluded that it can reduce the risk of falls by more than 20 per cent.[8] Elderly nursing home residents given 800 IU daily of vitamin D were found to have a 72 per cent lower rate of falls than those on placebo in a five-month trial.[9] Muscle strength in the legs in elderly people improves with increases in serum 25(OH)D levels, with most of the improvement occurring when 25(OH)D levels rise from 22.5 to 60 nmol/L.[10] Muscle pain, a common adverse effect of statin drugs for lowering serum cholesterol, is reported to improve when serum 25(OH)D levels are normalised.[11]

Multiple sclerosis

Calcitriol interacts with genes relevant to multiple sclerosis (MS). In animal models of MS, vitamin D inhibits inflammation and the development of T helper immune cells that target the myelin coating of nerves, and also induces several regulatory T cells that suppress MS. MS prevalence around the world is highest in regions further away from the equator, believed to be due to differences in sun exposure.[12] In Australia, there is a five-fold increased risk of MS in Tasmania compared with Queensland.[13] Childhood sun exposure may be especially protective, as shown by studies of immigrants. Those who migrate before adolescence acquire the MS risk relating to their new country, while those who migrate after this age retain the risk of their birth country. Tasmanian children with the highest amount of summer sun exposure (averaging two to three hours a day or more on weekends and holidays) have 70 per cent less risk of developing MS later in life compared with those experiencing less than one hour of summer sun exposure daily.[14] MS prevalence is lower at regions of higher altitude (higher than 1000 m) compared with regions of lower altitude, corresponding with UVB intensity.[15]

Low serum levels of 25(OH)D are associated with a higher incidence of MS; it is estimated that there is a 41 per cent decrease in MS incidence for every 50 nmol/L increase in 25(OH)D.[16] Individuals with 25(OH)D serum levels of 99.2 nmol/L or more have a 62 per cent lower risk of MS than those with levels below 63.3 nmol/L.[15] Serum 25(OH)D levels in MS patients are lower during MS relapses than during remissions, and low levels correlate with increased severity of MS.[17]

There are few human studies using vitamin D supplements to treat MS. A small study using 28000–280000 IU oral vitamin D weekly plus 1–2 g calcium daily in MS patients for 28 weeks found no effect on disease severity and activity, but the number of gadolinium-enhancing lesions was reduced, indicating a reduction in inflammatory activity.[18]

Inflammatory disorders

Vitamin D may be protective against rheumatoid arthritis, inflammatory bowel disease, systemic lupus erythematosus (SLE), osteoarthritis and periodontal disease and, in animal models, vitamin D has been shown to prevent and relieve symptoms of SLE, inflammatory bowel disorders and arthritis. Calcitriol has been shown to either prevent or markedly suppress autoimmune encephalomyelitis (inflammation of the brain and spinal cord), rheumatoid arthritis, SLE, type 1 diabetes and inflammatory bowel disease in animal disease models, but only if calcium intake is adequate.[19]

A meta-analysis concluded that people in the highest group of vitamin D intake had a 24.2 per cent lower risk of developing rheumatoid arthritis than those in the lowest group.[20] In animals, vitamin D supplementation is protective during the onset of osteoarthritis but not during the chronic stage.[21] A low intake or low serum levels of vitamin D have been associated with an increased risk for progression of knee osteoarthritis in women,[22] but restoring normal serum vitamin 25(OH)D has not led to improvements in pain and cartilage thickness.[23] Low serum 25(OH)D is associated with a higher risk of periodontal disease and vitamin D reduces risk of tooth loss in elderly people.[24]

Cancer

Animals that are vitamin D-deficient are more likely to develop spontaneous cancers and more susceptible to developing cancer when exposed to cancer-causing (carcinogenic) agents. People living in higher latitude regions (i.e. further from the Equator) have increased risk of breast, colon and prostate cancer, and increased sun exposure reduces the risk of many cancers.[25] In regions of higher UVB, cancer mortality rates are lower for non-Hodgkin's lymphoma, multiple myeloma and cancers of the breast, colon, rectum, ovary, prostate, stomach, bladder, oesophagus, kidney, lung, gall bladder, thyroid, rectum, pancreas and uterus. Overall, low serum 25(OH)D has been found to be predictive of fatal cancer.

Vitamin D supplementation appears to be protective against cancer, and higher serum 25(OH)D levels are associated with reduced incidence of cancer and decreased cancer mortality. Supplementation with calcium (1400–1500 mg/day) plus 1100 IU per day of vitamin D for four years in postmenopausal women was associated with a 60–70 per cent reduction in incidence of all types of cancer.[26] A meta-analysis of seven trials concluded that women within the highest range of serum 25(OH)D have a 45 per cent decrease in breast cancer incidence when compared with those within the lowest range.[27] Another meta-analysis concluded that people within the highest range of serum 25(OH)D have a 50 per cent lower risk of colorectal cancer.[28] It is estimated that maintaining serum 25(OH)D levels of at least 85 nmol/L may prevent about 50 per cent of colon cancers and maintaining levels of at least 105 nmol/L would prevent about 30 per cent of breast cancers.[29] A vitamin D intake of 1100–4000 IU daily and a serum 25(OH)D level of 150–200 nm/L appear to be optimal to reduce cancer risk.[30]

Calcitriol has been found to enhance normal cell growth and suppress cancer by inhibiting cancer cell proliferation, progression and metastasis, reducing angiogenesis and promoting differentiation and apoptosis of cancer cells. Calcitriol also decreases production of aromatase, the enzyme required for oestrogen synthesis in breast cancer. In animal models of cancer, calcitriol or calcitriol analogues have potent anticancer effects on the prostate gland, lung, ovary, breast, bladder, pancreas and neuroblastoma, and also potentiate chemotherapy treatment. Human trials have been hampered because daily high-dose calcitriol leads to excessively elevated calcium levels. However, oral doses given weekly or three days a week are better tolerated.

Excessive sun exposure is linked to photo-ageing and skin cancer. Non-melanoma skin cancers and actinic keratosis (scaly patches on the skin caused by sun damage) are related to UVB exposure, but melanoma may be related to UVA exposure rather than UVB, although the evidence is conflicting. Vitamin D and the skin pigment melanin, which is produced by UVB exposure, may be protective against skin cancer unless exposure is excessive. Older men with serum 25(OH)D levels greater than 75 nmol/L have been shown to have a 47 per cent lower risk of non-melanoma skin cancers.[31]

Cardiovascular disease

Moderate to severe vitamin D deficiency is a risk factor for developing cardiovascular disease (CVD) and low serum 25(OH)D levels are associated with increased risk of high blood pressure, ischaemic heart disease (heart disease caused by narrowing of blood vessels), sudden cardiac death, heart failure and all-cause and cardiovascular mortality.

Vitamin D controls production of the kidney hormone renin, and helps maintain normal blood pressure. Artificial UVB radiation has been shown to increase serum 25(OH)D and reduce blood pressure, but artificial UVA has no effect.[32] Risk of high blood pressure is about threefold higher in people with serum 25(OH)D levels less than 37.5 nmol/L compared with those with levels greater than 75 nmol/L.[33] In people with high blood pressure, those with serum 25(OH)D levels less than 25 nmol/L have been found to have an 80 per cent greater risk of CVD compared with those with levels greater than 37.5 nmol/L.[34] Vitamin D appears to work best with calcium for blood pressure regulation.

Low serum 25(OH)D levels have been found in people with acute myocardial infarction (MI, heart attack), enlargement of the left ventricle of the heart, stroke and congestive heart failure. Low vitamin D levels lead to increased inflammation, which contributes to CVD. Patients with heart failure given 2000 IU/day of vitamin D showed lower concentrations of the inflammatory chemical TNF-alpha and increased concentrations of the anti-inflammatory chemical interleukin-10 (IL-10).[35]

Inflammatory skin diseases

Dysfunction of the vitamin D-dependent antimicrobial peptide cathelicidin is linked to skin diseases, including atopic dermatitis, in which cathelicidin induction is suppressed; rosacea, in which it functions abnormally to induce inflammation and a vascular response; and psoriasis, in which it can trigger autoimmune responses. D3 analogues have been found to relieve psoriasis, possibly by acting to inhibit inflammatory processes in the skin and proliferation of cells in the epidermis, enhancing normal differentiation and keratinisation. Topical calcitriol is used as an effective treatment for reducing the severity and area of psoriatic lesions, with few adverse effects. A review of 51 trials using topical vitamin D analogues for psoriasis reported a satisfactory response rate of 22–96 per cent and a treatment success rate of 4–40 per cent.[36] Exposure to artificial UVB light is also used as an effective treatment.

Diabetes

Vitamin D is required for beta cell function in the pancreas, normal insulin release in response to glucose and maintenance of glucose tolerance. Low vitamin D is associated with insulin resistance, type 2 diabetes and metabolic syndrome, which is a collection of related conditions that include abdominal obesity, elevated levels of blood lipids, cholesterol and glucose, high blood pressure and increased CVD risk. A meta-analysis of 18 trials concluded that people in the highest range of serum 25(OH)D have a 43 per cent lower risk of type 2 diabetes.[37] Two trials of patients with glucose intolerance found that vitamin D supplementation improved insulin resistance. Vitamin D supplementation has been shown to improve beta cell function in people at high risk of type 2 diabetes and reduce fasting blood glucose levels in pregnant women with gestational diabetes, possibly by increasing insulin sensitivity.

Vitamin D supplementation in infants and children has been shown to be protective against the development of type 1 diabetes in later life. A meta-analysis of five studies found that children with symptoms of rickets at one year of age had three times the risk of subsequently developing type 1 diabetes, and it was concluded that vitamin D supplementation in early childhood may protect against the development of type 1 diabetes.[38] Overall, children on any dose of vitamin D supplementation were found to have a 29 per cent reduction in risk of developing type 1 diabetes compared with children not supplemented, but those who were supplemented more regularly or had higher doses had a greater reduction in risk. Children given 2000 IU of vitamin D daily during their first year of life had an almost 80 per cent lower risk of type 1 diabetes developing over the following 30 years, and children of mothers who took cod liver oil during pregnancy also had a lower risk of type 1 diabetes.

Infections and respiratory function

Vitamin D is an important regulator of adaptive and innate immune responses, and is required for the expression of the antibiotic cathelicidin in macrophages. Patients with rickets are more susceptible to infections and low vitamin D levels are associated with impaired lung function, and increased incidence of inflammatory and infectious diseases and cancer. Tuberculosis (TB) has been associated with vitamin D deficiency and cod liver oil was used in the early nineteenth century to enhance recovery. The incidence of many common infections is higher in winter when vitamin D levels are lower and a higher incidence of upper respiratory infections has been found to correlate with lower serum 25(OH)D levels. Vitamin D supplementation has been used to enhance the effectiveness of standard TB treatment[39] and decrease the incidence of colds and influenza.[40]

Low vitamin D is associated with chronic asthma and increased risk of severe episodes, and high vitamin D levels are associated with better lung function, less reactive airways and improved response to glucocorticoid therapy. Maternal vitamin D intake during pregnancy may protect against the infant developing wheezing in childhood.[41] In contrast, one study found that vitamin D levels higher than 75 nmol/L in pregnancy were associated with an increase in the child's susceptibility to eczema at nine months of age and asthma at nine years of age.[42]

Autism

Autism is more common in regions where UVB exposure is limited, such as high latitudes, urban centres and areas of high air pollution or rainfall.[43] Mothers with dark skin pigmentation are more at risk of vitamin D deficiency and their children are at increased risk of autism. In animals, severe vitamin D deficiency during gestation disrupts brain development and causes increased brain size and enlarged ventricles in the offspring, abnormalities similar to those found in some autistic children. Children with vitamin D-deficient rickets may have autistic-type symptoms, such as poor muscle tone, decreased activity, slow motor development, listlessness and failure to thrive, which are relieved by vitamin D treatment. Low consumption of fish during pregnancy is associated with lower IQ and poorer scores for pro-social (helping) behaviour, fine motor skills, communication and social development in infants, which may be because of inadequate omega-3 fats and/or vitamin D.[44] However, there is no good evidence to date that vitamin D supplementation can prevent or treat autism.

Schizophrenia

Low vitamin D in utero and childhood has been proposed as a risk factor for schizophrenia in later life. In animals, low vitamin D in utero leads to persistent changes in brain structure and function, particularly affecting dopamine pathways. The prevalence of schizophrenia is higher in higher latitude and colder climates, particularly in dark-skinned migrant and ethnic groups, and is greater in people with low fish consumption. Prevalence is also greater in infants born in winter and spring. Vitamin D supplementation (2000 IU or more) during the first year of life has been shown to be associated with a reduced risk of schizophrenia in males.[45]

Cognitive decline with ageing

Low 25(OH)D levels among older men and women are associated with a higher risk of cognitive impairment and cognitive decline. Older people with severely deficient 25(OH)D levels have been shown to have a 60 per cent higher risk of cognitive decline compared with people with sufficient levels.[46] Elderly women in the highest 20 per cent of vitamin D intake were found to have 77 per cent less risk of developing Alzheimer's disease over a seven-year period compared with those with lower intakes, and women in the highest 20 per cent of midday sun exposure had half the risk of Alzheimer's disease compared with those with lower sun exposure.[47]

REFERENCES

1 Javaid, M.K., Crozier, S.R., Harvey, N.C. et al., Princess Anne Hospital Study Group, Maternal vitamin D status during pregnancy and childhood bone mass at age 9 years: A longitudinal study, *Lancet* (2006), 367(9504): 36–43.

2 Holick, M.F., Binkley, N.C., Bischoff-Ferrari, H.A. et al., Endocrine Society, Evaluation, treatment, and prevention of vitamin D deficiency: An Endocrine Society clinical practice guideline, *J Clin Endocrinol Metab* (2011), 96(7): 1911–30.

3 Zamora, S.A., Rizzoli, R., Belli, D.C. et al., Vitamin D supplementation during infancy is associated with higher bone mineral mass in prepubertal girls, *J Clin Endocrinol Metab* (1999), 84(12): 4541–4.

4 Zhu, K., Devine, A., Dick, I.M. et al., Effects of calcium and vitamin D supplementation on hip bone mineral density and calcium-related analytes in elderly ambulatory Australian women: A five-year randomized controlled trial, *J Clin Endocrinol Metab* (2008), 93(3): 743–9.

5 Bischoff-Ferrari, H.A., Willett, W.C., Orav, E.J. et al., A pooled analysis of vitamin D dose requirements for fracture prevention, *N Engl J Med* (2012), 367(1): 40–9.

6 Bischoff-Ferrari, H.A., Shao, A., Dawson-Hughes, B. et al., Benefit-risk assessment of vitamin D supplementation, *Osteoporos Int* (2010), 21(7): 1121–32.

7 Sato, Y., Iwamoto, J., Kanoko, R. & Satoh, K., Low-dose vitamin D prevents muscular atrophy and reduces falls and hip fractures in women after stroke: A randomized controlled trial, *Cerebrovasc Dis* (2005), 20: 187–92.

8 Bischoff-Ferrari, H.A., Dawson-Hughes, B., Willett, W.C. et al., Effect of vitamin D on falls: A meta-analysis, *JAMA* (2004), 291(16): 1999–2006.

9 Broe, K.E., Chen, T.C., Weinberg, J. et al., A higher dose of vitamin D reduces the risk of falls in nursing home residents: A randomized, multiple-dose study, *J Am Geriatr Soc* (2007), 55(2): 234–9.

10 Bischoff-Ferrari, H.A., Dietrich, T., Orav, E.J. et al., Higher 25-hydroxyvitamin D concentrations are associated with better lower-extremity function in both active and inactive persons aged > or =60 y, *Am J Clin Nutr* (2004), 80(3): 752–8.

11 Lee, J.H., O'Keefe, J.H., Bell, D. et al., Vitamin D deficiency: An important, common, and easily treatable cardiovascular risk factor? *J Am Coll Cardiol* (2008), 52(24): 1949–56.

12 Ascherio, A., Munger, K.L. & Simon, K.C., Vitamin D and multiple sclerosis, *Lancet Neurol* (2010), 9(6): 599–612.

13 van der Mei, I.A., Ponsonby, A.L., Engelsen, O. et al., The high prevalence of vitamin D insufficiency across Australian populations is only partly explained by season and latitude, *Environ Health Perspect* (2007), 115(8): 1132–9.

14 van der Mei, I.A., Ponsonby, A.L., Dwyer, T. et al., Past exposure to sun, skin phenotype, and risk of multiple sclerosis: Case-control study, *BMJ* (2003), 327(7410): 316.

15 Hayes, C.E., Vitamin D: A natural inhibitor of multiple sclerosis, *Proc Nutr Soc* (2000), 59(4): 531–5.

16 Munger, K.L., Levin, L.I., Hollis, B.W. et al., Serum 25-hydroxyvitamin D levels and risk of multiple sclerosis, *JAMA* (2006), 296(23): 2832–8.

17 Mowry, E.M., Krupp, L.B., Milazzo, M. et al., Vitamin D status is associated with relapse rate in pediatric-onset multiple sclerosis, *Ann Neurol* (2010), 67(5): 618–24.
18 Kimball, S.M., Ursell, M.R., O'Connor, P. & Vieth, R., Safety of vitamin D3 in adults with multiple sclerosis, *Am J Clin Nutr* (2007), 86(3): 645–51.
19 Guillot, X., Semerano, L., Saidenberg-Kermanach, N. et al., Vitamin D and inflammation, *Joint Bone Spine* (2010), 77(6): 552–7.
20 Song, G.G., Bae, S.C. & Lee, Y.H., Association between vitamin D intake and the risk of rheumatoid arthritis: A meta-analysis, *Clin Rheumatol* (2012), 31(12): 1733–9.
21 Castillo, E.C., Hernandez-Cueto, M.A., Vega-Lopez, M.A. et al., Effects of Vitamin D supplementation during the induction and progression of osteoarthritis in a rat model, *Evid Based Complement Alternat Med* (2012), 156563.
22 McAlindon, T.E., Felson, D.T., Zhang, Y. et al., Relation of dietary intake and serum levels of vitamin D to progression of osteoarthritis of the knee among participants in the Framingham Study, *Ann Intern Med* (1996), 125(5): 353–9.
23 McAlindon, T., LaValley, M., Schneider, E. et al., Effect of vitamin D supplementation on progression of knee pain and cartilage volume loss in patients with symptomatic osteoarthritis: A randomized controlled trial, *JAMA* (2013), 309(2): 155–62.
24 Jimenez, M., Giovannucci, E., Krall Kaye, E. et al., Predicted vitamin D status and incidence of tooth loss and periodontitis, *Public Health Nutr* (2014), 17(4): 844–52.
25 Holick, M.F., Vitamin D: Its role in cancer prevention and treatment, *Prog Biophys Mol Biol* (2006), 92(1): 49–59.
26 Lappe, J.M., Travers-Gustafson, D., Davies, K.M. et al., Vitamin D and calcium supplementation reduces cancer risk: results of a randomized trial, *Am J Clin Nutr* (2007), 85(6): 1586–91.
27 Chen, P., Hu, P., Xie, D. et al., Meta-analysis of vitamin D, calcium and the prevention of breast cancer, *Breast Cancer Res Treat* (2010), 121(2): 469–77.
28 Gorham, E.D., Garland, C.F., Garland, F.C. et al., Optimal vitamin D status for colorectal cancer prevention: A quantitative meta analysis, *Am J Prev Med* (2007), 32(3): 210–16.
29 Garland, C.F., Grant, W.B., Mohr, S.B. et al., What is the dose–response relationship between vitamin D and cancer risk? *Nutr Rev* (2007), 65(8 Pt 2): S91–5.
30 Garland, C.F., French, C.B., Baggerly, L.L. & Heaney, R.P., Vitamin D supplement doses and serum 25-hydroxyvitamin D in the range associated with cancer prevention, *Anticancer Res* (2011), 31(2): 607–11.
31 Tang, J.Y., Parimi, N., Wu, A. et al., Osteoporotic Fractures in Men (MrOS) Study Group, Inverse association between serum 25(OH) vitamin D levels and non-melanoma skin cancer in elderly men, *Cancer Causes Control* (2010), 21(3): 387–91.
32 Krause R., Bühring M., Hopfenmüller, W., et al., Ultraviolet B and blood pressure, *Lancet*, (1998), 352(9129): 709-10.
33 Forman, J.P., Giovannucci, E., Holmes, M.D. et al., Plasma 25-hydroxyvitamin D levels and risk of incident hypertension, *Hypertension* (2007), 49: 1063–9.
34 Wang, T., Pencina, M., Booth, S. et al., Vitamin D deficiency and risk of cardiovascular disease, *J Am Heart Assoc* (2008), 117: 503–11.
35 Schleithoff, S.S., Zittermann, A., Tenderich, G. et al., Vitamin D supplementation improves cytokine profiles in patients with congestive heart failure: A double-blind, randomized, placebo-controlled trial, *Am J Clin Nutr* (2006), 83: 754–9.
36 Devaux, S., Castela, A., Archier, E. et al., Topical vitamin D analogues alone or in association with topical steroids for psoriasis: A systematic review, *J Eur Acad Dermatol Venereol* (2012), 26 (Suppl 3): 52–60.
37 Mitri, J., Muraru, M.D. & Pittas, A.G., Vitamin D and type 2 diabetes: A systematic review, *Eur J Clin Nutr* (2011), 65(9): 1005–15.
38 Hyppönen, E., Läärä, E., Reunanen, A. et al., Intake of vitamin D and risk of type 1 diabetes: A birth-cohort study, *Lancet* (2001), 358(9292): 1500–3.

39 Salahuddin, N., Ali, F., Hasan, Z. et al., Vitamin D accelerates clinical recovery from tuberculosis: Results of the SUCCINCT Study [Supplementary Cholecalciferol in recovery from tuberculosis], *BMC Infect Dis* (2013), 13: 22.

40 Yamshchikov, A.V., Desai, N.S., Blumberg, H.M. et al., Vitamin D for treatment and prevention of infectious diseases: A systematic review of randomized controlled trials, *Endocr Pract* (2009), 15(5): 438–49.

41 Camargo, C.A. Jr, Rifas-Shiman, S.L., Litonjua, A.A. et al., Maternal intake of vitamin D during pregnancy and risk of recurrent wheeze in children at 3 y of age, *Am J Clin Nutr* (2007), 85: 788–95.

42 Gale, C.R., Robinson, S.M., Harvey, N.C. et al., Maternal vitamin D status during pregnancy and child outcomes, *Eur J Clin Nutr* (2008), 62: 68–77.

43 Cannell, J.J., Autism and vitamin D, *Med Hypotheses* (2008), 70(4): 750–9.

44 Hibbeln, J.R., Davis, J.M., Steer, C. et al., Maternal seafood consumption in pregnancy and neurodevelopmental outcomes in childhood (ALSPAC study): An observational cohort study, *Lancet* (2007), 369(9561): 578–85.

45 McGrath, J., Saari, K., Hakko, H. et al., Vitamin D supplementation during the first year of life and risk of schizophrenia: A Finnish birth cohort study, *Schizophr Res* (2004), 67(2–3): 237–45.

46 Llewellyn, D.J., Lang, I.A., Langa, K.M. et al., Vitamin D and risk of cognitive decline in elderly persons, *Arch Intern Med* (2010), 170(13): 1135–41.

47 Annweiler, C., Rolland, Y., Schott, A.M. et al., Higher vitamin D dietary intake is associated with lower risk of Alzheimer's disease: A 7-year follow-up, *J Gerontol A Biol Sci Med Sci* (2012), 67(11): 1205–11.

Therapeutic dose

Serum 25(OH)D levels of 75 to 110 nmol/L appear to provide optimal health benefits, with greater benefits occurring at levels of 100 nmol/L or more. In most studies to date, 1800 IU to 4000 IU of supplemental vitamin D daily in adults has achieved levels of 75 to 110 nmol/L, without adverse effects. To maintain optimal serum levels, the suggested doses below should be combined with sensible sun exposure and, in deficiency or disease states, serum 25(OH)D levels should be monitored.

- *Health maintenance:* 400–1000 IU daily for infants, 800–2000 IU for children and adolescents, 1000-2000 IU for adults, 1500–2000 IU for pregnant or lactating women, 2000–4000 IU for obese adults, and 2000 IU for the elderly. It is estimated that about 1700 IU per day is needed to raise blood levels from 50 to 80 nmol/L.
- *Mild deficiency:* 2000–5000 IU daily in the short term for adults until blood levels increase to the optimal range. Alternatively, the dose may be given as 10 000 IU once a week. For children under six months, the daily dose is 800–1000 IU. For children over six months, the daily dose is 2000 IU. Doses should be reduced to maintenance levels when blood levels normalise.
- *Severe deficiency:* 10 000 IU daily in the short term for adults until blood levels increase to the optimal range. A dose of 10 000 IU per day has been used for several months without signs of toxicity. Alternatively, the dose may be given as 50 000 IU once monthly for three months. In adults with severe malabsorption or those unable to take oral medication, an intramuscular injection of 300 000 IU once monthly for three months and then once or twice a year has been used as an alternative. For children under six months, the daily dose is 3000 IU for eight to twelve weeks. For children over six months, the daily dose is 6000 IU daily for eight to twelve weeks. Alternatively, children over twelve months have been given a one-off dose of 300 000 IU. Doses should be reduced to maintenance levels when blood levels normalise.
- *MS patients:* 4000–10 000 IU daily is recommended, in order to maintain serum 25(OH)D levels of 100–150 nmol/L, which should be monitored regularly.
- *Cystic fibrosis patients:* 400–1000 IU is the recommended daily starting dose for all ages.

Effects of excess

Vitamin D toxicity is very rare, and is not known to occur through dietary intake or sun exposure. It can be an outcome of excessively high supplementation, more often because of errors in dispensing or manufacturing vitamin D supplements rather than prescribing errors or deliberate choice. In countries that do not have government regulation of the complementary medicine industry, such as the United States, manufacturing errors may be more common.

According to early studies using massive doses of vitamin D (200 000–500 000 IU daily) for therapeutic purposes, initial symptoms of acute vitamin D toxicity are persistent nausea, increased frequency of urination without increased volume of urine, weakness and increased thirst, which are followed by diarrhoea, abdominal colic and vomiting. Chronic toxicity may lead to vomiting, diarrhoea, loss of weight, headache, thirst, metallic taste, urinary urgency and frequency, irritability, depression, tenderness of bones, joints and muscles, and elevated serum levels of calcium (hypercalcaemia), which can lead to calcium deposits in soft tissues. Hypercalcaemia has been reported in a small number of people with serum 25(OH)D levels greater than 240 nmol/L; however, almost all the reported cases of toxicity had much higher serum levels (525–2070 nmol/L). People with granulomatous disorders (genetic disorders associated with impaired immunity) may show toxicity signs, such as high calcium levels, at levels of 75 nmol/L because of elevated macrophage production of calcitriol.

There are no reports of increases in mean calcium levels in people in clinical trials taking up to 100 000 IU per day of vitamin D. Case reports of people taking vitamin D doses of 50 000–150 000 IU daily, verified by correspondingly high serum 25(OH)D values (up to 1126 nmol/L), have reported that serum calcium levels remained in the normal range. There is no credible evidence linking vitamin D supplementation with kidney stone incidence and oral vitamin D doses of up to 10 000 IU per day have not been associated with calcification of blood vessels in healthy people or dialysis patients. However, the safety of very high doses of calcium used together with vitamin D supplementation has not been established. If vitamin D status is adequate, increased calcium absorption may mean that very high doses of calcium are not required.

Calcitriol is generally not suitable for treatment of vitamin D deficiency because of increased risk of hypercalcaemia or excessive calcium losses in urine (hypercalciuria). Calcitriol may be helpful in patients with renal failure who are unable to produce it from 25(OH)D, but serum calcium levels and renal function must be monitored closely.

Case reports—vitamin D toxicity

- *An American woman, 70 years of age*, with chronic kidney disease, bone weakness, cardiovascular disease and dementia was prescribed 1000 IU of vitamin D daily but had been given a supplement providing a dose of 50 000 IU daily due to a pharmacy dispensing error.[1] After three months of supplementation given by her caregiver, she developed confusion, slurred speech, unstable gait, increased fatigue and acute kidney damage, which were found to be caused by hypercalcaemia. Including other supplements, her total daily dose of vitamin D was 50 400 IU plus 3100 mg of calcium, and her serum 25(OH)D level was 484 nmol/L. Parathyroid function tests were normal. When the vitamin D and calcium supplements were discontinued, her mental status and serum calcium level returned to pre-supplementation values in four days. At five months follow-up, her serum vitamin D level had dropped to 100 nmol/L and renal function had returned to the pre-supplementation level.
- *An American woman, 58 years of age*, with diabetes and rheumatoid arthritis, who had taken a dietary supplement for two months, developed fatigue, constipation, back pain, forgetfulness, nausea and vomiting, and was hospitalised because of slurred speech and an abnormally low blood glucose reading.[2] She had elevated serum calcium and a 25(OH)D level of 1171 nmol/L. Laboratory analysis of the supplement found that she was receiving 186 906 IU of vitamin D3 per recommended dose instead of the intended 400 IU, due to a manufacturing error.
- *An American nutritionist, 65 years of age*, suffered severe acute toxicity from a dietary supplement produced by his own company in 2010.[3] He took two daily servings of the supplement for one month, and reported developing extreme fatigue, pain and cracked, bleeding feet, and became bedridden. Subsequent testing found that the supplement contained one million IU of vitamin D per serving instead of the intended 1000 IU, providing about 60 million IU in total. After discontinuing the supplement, he publicly claimed a return to full health. However, in his $10 million lawsuit filed against the manufacturing company, he claimed to

be still suffering health effects months afterwards, occasionally observed blood in his urine, and claimed that his future health outcome was uncertain.

In addition, a 40-year-old man who took the same defective batch of the supplement for one month developed excessive thirst, frequent urination, muscle aches, nausea, vomiting, mild anaemia and elevated serum calcium, calcitriol and 25(OH)D (1610 nm/L).[4] After discontinuing the product, his serum calcium returned to normal in several days, kidney function normalised in four weeks and vitamin D levels normalised in ten months, but calcitriol levels took a year to normalise. No permanent adverse effects were reported.

REFERENCES

1 Jacobsen, R.B., Hronek, B.W., Schmidt, G.A. & Schilling, M.L., Hypervitaminosis D associated with a vitamin D dispensing error, *Ann Pharmacother* (2011), 45(10): e52.

2 Klontz, K.C. & Acheson, D.W., Dietary supplement-induced vitamin D intoxication, *N Engl J Med* (2007), 357(3): 308–9.

3 Barrett, S., *Gary Null said one of his own products nearly killed him*. Complaint: Supreme Court of the State of New York, County of New York. Gary Null & Gary Null & Associates Inc. plaintiff, against Triarco Industries, Inc. defendant. Case no. 10601070. Complaint filed Apr 26, 2010. Retrieved 10 August 2014 from <www.casewatch.org/civil/null/complaint.shtml>.

4 Araki, T., Holick, M.F., Alfonso, B.D. et al., Vitamin D intoxication with severe hypercalcemia due to manufacturing and labeling errors of two dietary supplements made in the United States, *J Clin Endocrinol Metab* (2011), 96(12): 3603–8.

Supplements

The standard vitamin D dose in most tablets/capsules is 1000 IU, and 8.3 mcg (332 IU) per drop of liquid concentrate. The permitted forms of vitamin D in Australian supplements are cod liver oil, halibut liver oil, pollack (pollock) liver oil, shark liver oil, skipjack liver oil, cholecalciferol and ergocalciferol.

- *Natural vitamin D3 (cholecalciferol)* is available as tablets, capsules or liquid concentrates taken as drops. It is produced commercially by exposing 7-dehydrocholesterol obtained from sheep wool grease (lanolin) to UV light. Vitamin D3 is also found in fish liver oil supplements, such as cod liver oil, halibut liver oil or shark liver oil, and these also contain vitamin A. Fish liver oils are available as capsules, oil or emulsions that have a less fishy taste. Some capsules contain regular fish liver oil and others are fortified to contain higher amounts of vitamin A and D. However, the vitamin A content in fish liver oils is much higher than vitamin D and it is difficult to obtain enough vitamin D without excessive amounts of vitamin A so fish liver oil supplements have limited usefulness.
- *Synthetic vitamin D2 (ergocalciferol)* is available as tablets or capsules, and is usually made by exposing yeast (ergot) that contains the precursor, ergosterol, to UV light. Vitamin D2 is less stable than D3 to temperature changes, humidity and storage and appears to have more potential for toxicity than D3. Vitamin D2 has less affinity for vitamin D enzymes, VDR and DBP, and has a shorter activity life in the body. The liver converts vitamin D3 to 25(OH)D3 five times faster than it converts vitamin D2 to 25(OH)D2, and vitamin D2 is less effective in raising serum 25(OH)D concentrations. Overall, D2 appears to be less than one-third as potent as D3.

Cautions

Very high doses of vitamin D may cause toxicity. People with elevated serum calcium levels, granulomatous disorders, kidney disease or parathyroid hormone disorders should seek advice from a health professional before taking vitamin D.

Vitamin E (alpha-tocopherol)

VITAMIN E STATUS CHECK

1 **Do you have heart disease or a family history of heart disease?**
2 **Do you have a low-fat diet?**
3 **Do you have weak muscles and poor stamina?**
4 **Do you have a chronic inflammatory disorder?**

'Yes' answers may indicate inadequate vitamin E status. Note that a number of nutritional deficiencies or health disorders can cause similar effects and further investigation is recommended.

FAST FACTS . . . VITAMIN E

- **Vitamin E is alpha-tocopherol, which is part of a family of related fat-soluble antioxidants that include tocopherols and tocotrienols.**
- **It is the major fat-soluble chain-breaking antioxidant in the body.**
- **It supports immunity and has anti-inflammatory and anti-atherosclerosis activity.**
- **A deficiency may cause haemolytic anaemia, muscle damage and disorders related to oxidative stress.**
- **Supplementation may be helpful for skin healing, diseases of ageing and cardiovascular disease.**

Vitamin E (alpha-tocopherol) is a fat-soluble alcohol and essential dietary nutrient that was first isolated from wheat germ oil in 1936. A lack of vitamin E in pregnant animals fed on rancid fat was found to be associated with death and resorption of the foetus, and it became known as the fertility vitamin. It was given the name vitamin E because it was the next vitamin discovered after vitamin D, and the name alpha-tocopherol was derived from the Greek *tokos*, meaning 'offspring' and *pheros*, meaning 'to bring forth'. Further research established that alpha-tocopherol was part of a family of related fat-soluble antioxidants called tocochromanols, made by plants from the amino acid tyrosine and the green pigment chlorophyll. These include tocopherols, consisting of alpha-, beta-, gamma- and delta-tocopherol, and tocotrienols, consisting of alpha-, beta-, gamma- and delta-tocotrienol.

Tocotrienols and tocopherols appear to have a similar ability to protect against lipid oxidation but, in the body, alpha-tocopherol is selectively retained and is the predominant tocochromanol antioxidant. The natural form of vitamin E found in food is d-alpha-tocopherol (RRR-alpha-tocopherol) and the synthetic form used in some supplements is dl-alpha tocopherol (all-rac-alpha-tocopherol). Although gamma-tocopherol is the predominant tocopherol in the diet and all forms of tocopherols, and tocotrienols are equally well absorbed, alpha-tocopherol is preferred by body tissues and makes up about 90 per cent of the total tocopherol content. Levels of alpha-tocopherol in the bloodstream and tissues are about ten times higher than levels of gamma-tocopherol. Tocotrienols are potent antioxidants, but they are poorly absorbed and distributed, and are rapidly metabolised and eliminated from the body.

Digestion, absorption and transport

Tocopherols and tocotrienols are released from their ester forms in the digestive tract and are absorbed with dietary fat. They are emulsified by bile and incorporated into micelles together with lipids for absorption into the lining of the small intestine. In the intestinal epithelium, tocopherols and tocotrienols are incorporated into chylomicrons for transport in the lymph vessels to the bloodstream, where they are taken up by tissue cells by the action of the enzyme lipoprotein lipase. The remainder is delivered to the liver in chylomicron remnants.

Metabolism, storage and excretion

In the liver, the alpha-tocopherol transfer protein (alpha-TTP) selectively incorporates the natural form of alpha-tocopherol into very low-density lipoproteins (VLDLs) for circulation in the bloodstream and uptake by tissue cells, with any remaining alpha-tocopherol eventually being transferred to high-density lipoproteins (HDLs). Vitamin E is distributed in plasma lipoproteins and cell membranes, including intracellular membranes, where it plays an essential role in maintaining membrane integrity. It is stored in the liver, and excess or unwanted forms of vitamin E, including gamma-tocopherol, are excreted in bile or undergo metabolism to water-soluble carboxyethyl hydroxychromans (CEHCs) by a cytochrome P450-dependent process in the liver and are excreted in urine. Three to four times more synthetic vitamin E is excreted than the natural form.

Functions

- *Antioxidant activity*. Alpha-tocopherol is the major fat-soluble chain-breaking antioxidant in the body. In lipoproteins, it works with ubiquinol-10, derived from coenzyme Q10 (CoQ10), to protect lipids and cholesterol from oxidative damage. In cells, it is particularly concentrated in the cell membrane and membranes of lysosomes, and its main role is to scavenge peroxyl radicals formed from oxidised polyunsaturated fatty acids (PUFAs) and terminate lipid peroxidation, effectively breaking the chain of free radical generation (see Figure 5.3). Alpha-tocopherol is a very effective protector of cell membranes because it reacts more rapidly with peroxyl radicals than PUFAs do, and a small amount is able to protect a large amount of PUFAs. The ratio of alpha-tocopherol to PUFA molecules in cell membranes is about 1:1000.

  Alpha-tocopherol reacts with nitric oxide, hydroxyl, hydroperoxyl and superoxide radicals to form tocopheryl quinones and other oxidation products. In addition, it can suppress the generation of superoxide and hydrogen peroxide and reduce oxidative damage in mitochondria, and is an effective neutraliser of singlet oxygen. Other forms of tocopherol are less effective against singlet oxygen, with beta-tocopherol having about 50 per cent of the activity of alpha-tocopherol, gamma-tocopherol having about 25 per cent and delta-tocopherol having only about 10 per cent. The trace element selenium, as part of the enzyme glutathione peroxidase, removes hydroperoxides formed by alpha-tocopherol activity.

  Alpha-tocopherol activates the nuclear factor erythroid 2-related factor 2 (Nrf2) signalling pathway that produces protein products involved in enhancing cellular antioxidant capacity and detoxifying and eliminating free radicals. This pathway is a key mediator of the antioxidant response that is important in many physiological and pathological processes. Alpha-tocopherol may also have indirect antioxidant activity by inducing phase II detoxification enzymes in the liver to enhance removal of toxins.

  Alpha-tocopherol has the potential to act as a pro-oxidant because, during its antioxidant activity, the tocopheroxyl radical is formed, which can react with lipids to generate lipid radicals, thereby promoting the free radical chain instead of breaking it. However, this radical can be converted back to alpha-tocopherol by other antioxidants, including vitamin C, ubiquinol-10, and the glutathione system, and can react with other free radicals to form non-radical oxidation products that are conjugated to glucuronic acid and excreted in bile or urine. Alpha-tocopherol has not been found to have a pro-oxidant function in the body because of the presence of other protective antioxidants.
- *Anti-inflammatory activity.* Alpha-tocopherol has been shown to inhibit many key events that promote the inflammation in blood vessel walls that leads to atherosclerosis, including the release of interleukin-1beta (IL-1beta) from monocytes, monocyte adhesion to endothelial cells, production of monocyte reactive oxygen species (ROS), the production of chemotactic proteins, LDL cholesterol-induced

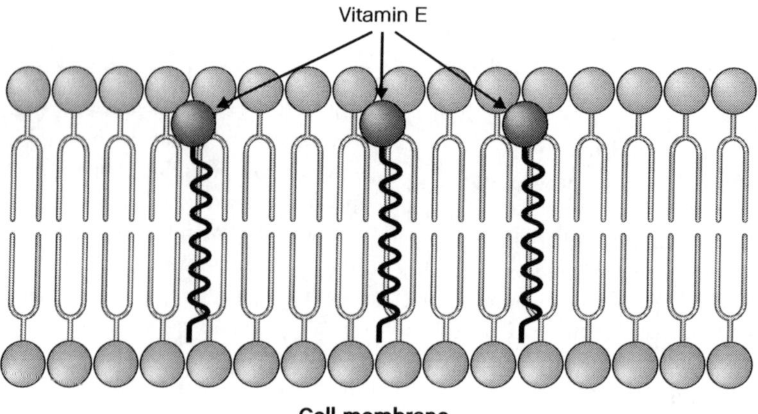

Figure 5.3 Vitamin E in a cell membrane

proliferation of smooth muscle cells, activation of the 5-lipoxygenase (5-LOX) pathway and platelet aggregation. Most of these anti-inflammatory effects are believed to be caused by inhibition of protein kinase C (PKC) activity by alpha-tocopherol.

Vitamin E inhibits activity of COX-2, the enzyme that promotes production of potent inflammatory eicosanoids, such as prostaglandin E_2 (PGE_2), possibly by reducing production of peroxynitrite required for COX activation. Peroxynitrite causes lipid peroxidation, including oxidation of LDL cholesterol, and enhances atheroma formation.

- *Immune and anticancer activity.* Vitamin E helps to protect against free radical damage and inflammation that may contribute to cancer initiation, modulates immune functions and, by inhibiting PKC, reduces abnormal cell proliferation. A deficiency of vitamin E impairs immune function, including both T and B cell-mediated functions. Vitamin E has been shown to restore age-related decreases in immune function and activate detoxification pathways that break down and remove potential carcinogens from the body.
- *Regulation of gene activity.* Alpha-tocopherol appears to regulate expression of genes that control production of connective tissue and muscle proteins, and those that enhance atherosclerosis. These include the liver collagen alpha 1(I) gene that is active in liver cirrhosis, the gene for the connective tissue enzyme collagenase that breaks down collagen, the gene for the muscle protein alpha-tropomyosin and genes for scavenger receptors in cells within artery walls that take up cholesterol, generating lipid-filled foam cells that form an atheroma. Alpha-tocopherol appears to reduce the development of atherosclerosis by its antioxidant activity and by inhibiting smooth muscle cell proliferation and foam cell formation.

GAMMA-TOCOPHEROL: THE MAIN DIETARY TOCOPHEROL

Dietary gamma-tocopherol is well absorbed, and can be delivered to tissues via chylomicrons. It is deposited in skin, muscles, veins and adipose tissue, and levels in these tissues are about 20- to 40-fold higher than those in plasma. However, once it is taken up by the liver in chylomicron remnants, it is largely excreted in favour of alpha-tocopherol. High doses of alpha-tocopherol deplete body levels of gamma-tocopherol.

Gamma-tocopherol acts as an antioxidant, but is less potent than alpha-tocopherol overall; however, it is more effective in scavenging reactive nitrogen oxide species (RNOS), and can work with glutathione in watery compartments of the body. It may protect lipids, DNA and proteins from damage caused by peroxynitrites. It has anticancer activity and promotes nitric oxide (NO) formation, which has vasodilating effects. Gamma-tocopherol and its breakdown product 2,7,8-trimethyl-2-(b-carboxyethyl)-6-hydroxychroman (gamma-CEHC) suppress inflammation by inhibiting COX-2 activity and PGE_2 synthesis, and have more potent anti-inflammatory activity than alpha-tocopherol. Gamma-CEHC appears to promote sodium losses in urine, which may help control blood pressure.

Higher serum levels of gamma-tocopherol are associated with lower CVD morbidity and mortality.[1] Lower plasma levels of gamma-tocopherol have been associated with coronary heart disease[2] and there is preliminary evidence that gamma-tocopherol supplementation may decrease LDL cholesterol and platelet aggregation.[3] Higher plasma levels may be protective against prostate cancer. Men with the highest plasma levels have been found to have a five-fold lower risk of developing prostate cancer than men with the lowest levels.[4]

Gamma-tocopherol may have some adverse effects, although the evidence is controversial. Supplementary gamma-tocopherol has been shown to enhance inflammation in the lungs that was partially or completely reversed by alpha-tocopherol.[5] Gamma-tocopheryl quinone has been shown to induce cell damage and mutagenesis, whereas alpha-tocopheryl quinone does not.[6]

REFERENCES

1 Devaraj S., Jialal I., Failure of vitamin E in clinical trials: is gamma-tocopherol the answer? *Nutr Rev* (2005), 63(8):290–3.

2 Ohrvall, M., Sundlöf, G., Vessby, B., Gamma, but not alpha, tocopherol levels in serum are reduced in coronary heart disease patients, *J Intern Med* (1996), 239(2): 111–17.

3 Singh, I., Turner, A.H., Sinclair, A.J., et al., Effects of gamma-tocopherol supplementation on thrombotic risk factors, *Asia Pac J Clin Nutr* (2007), 16(3): 422–8.

4 Helzlsouer, K.J., Huang, H.Y., Alberg, A.J., et al., Association between alpha-tocopherol, gamma-tocopherol, selenium, and subsequent prostate cancer, *J Natl Cancer Inst* (2000), 92(24): 2018–23.

5 Marchese, M.E., Kumar, R., Colangelo, L.A. et al., The vitamin E isoforms α-tocopherol and γ-tocopherol have opposite associations with spirometric parameters: the CARDIA study, *Respir Res* (2014), 15: 31.

6 Cornwell, D.G., Williams, M.V., Wani, A.A. et al., Mutagenicity of tocopheryl quinones: evolutionary advantage of selective accumulation of dietary alpha-tocopherol, *Nutr Cancer* (2002), 43(1): 111–18.

Dietary sources

Alpha-tocopherol and other tocopherols and tocotrienols are found in nuts, seeds, whole grains, rice bran, wheat germ, wheat germ oil, cold-pressed vegetable oils, vegetables, eggs, butter, margarine, fish oils and cod liver oil. Sunflower seed oil contains mainly alpha-tocopherol, soybean oil contains alpha-, gamma- and delta-tocopherol, and palm oil contains alpha-tocopherol and tocotrienols. Gamma-tocopherol is found in vegetable oils, such as corn, soybean and sesame, and nuts such as walnuts, pecans and peanuts.

Access the Food Standards Australia New Zealand nutrient database (NUTTAB) at <www.foodstandards.gov.au> for the amounts found in specific foods.

Factors influencing body status

Tocopherols can be damaged by oxygen, and this process is accelerated by heat, light, alkaline conditions and metal ions. Vitamin E in food is particularly sensitive to exposure to air, and can also be depleted by light, temperature, food-processing methods, cooking and room-temperature storage.

Dietary fat is needed for absorption of vitamin E, and people on low-fat diets and those who do not absorb fats well may have inadequate levels. Digestive disorders associated with impaired fat absorption, such as gall bladder or pancreatic disorders, inflammatory bowel diseases and cystic fibrosis, reduce absorption of vitamin E. Absorption is also decreased by mineral oil taken as a laxative, drugs that inhibit cholesterol uptake, such as cholestyramine and colestipol, and the weight loss drug orlistat.

Synthetic vitamin E is less bioavailable than the natural form. A deficiency of vitamin C may impair the regeneration of vitamin E from its radical form. Some studies that have shown that vitamin E is ineffective as a treatment for chronic disease have been criticised for using the less bioavailable synthetic form and not using it together with vitamin C and other dietary antioxidants.

VITAMIN E MEASUREMENT

Vitamin E is measured in milligrams (mg), international units (IU) or alpha-tocopherol equivalents (alpha-TE), which are a measure of the total vitamin E potentially obtainable from a substance. The 'd-alpha' form is natural vitamin E and the 'dl-alpha' form is synthetic.

Table 5.5 alpha-tocopherol equivalents (alpha-TE)

Natural vitamin E		
1 mg d-alpha-tocopherol	=	1 mg alpha-TE
1 mg d-alpha-tocopheryl acetate	=	0.91 alpha-TE
1 mg d-alpha-tocopheryl succinate	=	0.81 alpha-TE
Synthetic vitamin E		
1 mg dl-alpha-tocopherol	=	0.74 mg alpha-TE
1 mg dl-alpha-tocopheryl acetate	=	0.67 alpha-TE
1 mg dl-alpha-tocopheryl succinate	=	0.60 alpha-TE

Source: US Pharmacopeia, *Vitamin E*; available at: <www.pharmacopoia.cn/v29240/usp29nf24s0_m88600.html>.

Table 5.6 Relative content of alpha-tocopherol in various forms of vitamin E

Source material (1 mg)	alpha-tocopherol content (IU)
d-alpha-tocopherol	1.49
d-alpha-tocopheryl acetate	1.36
d-alpha-tocopheryl succinate	1.21
dl-alpha-tocopherol	1.10
dl-alpha-tocopheryl acetate	1.00
dl-alpha-tocopheryl succinate	0.89

Source: US Pharmacopeia, *Vitamin E*; available at: <www.pharmacopeia.cn/v29240/usp29nf24s0_m88600.html>.

Daily requirement

Government recommendations by age and gender (see Table 5.7) can be found in *Nutrient Reference Values for Australia and New Zealand Including Recommended Dietary Intakes*, available at <www.nhmrc.gov.au>.

Table 5.7 Daily adequate intake (AI) of alpha-tocopherol equivalents (mg/day)

Age (years)	Female AI	Male AI
1–3	5	5
4–8	6	6
9–13	8	9
14–18	8	10
19–70	7	10
>70	7	10
Pregnant women		
14–18	8	
19–50	7	
Lactating women		
14–18	12	
19–50	11	

Source: Nutrient Reference Values for Australia and New Zealand Including Recommended Dietary Intakes, National Health and Medical Research Council, Australian Government Department of Health and Ageing, Canberra and Ministry of Health, New Zealand, Wellington, 2006.

Deficiency effects

In animals, the most common sign of deficiency is severe muscle damage (necrotising myopathy). However, effects vary between species. In pregnant mice without the gene for alpha-TPP, embryos develop normally until nine and a half days after conception but the labyrinth region of the placenta fails to develop, impairing transport of nutrients to the foetus. Blood vessels fail to form in the embryo, NTDs occur and the embryo dies between eleven and fourteen days.

A severe form of vitamin E deficiency occurs in people who have a genetic inability to make alpha-TTP. This causes low plasma and tissue levels of vitamin E, and leads to the disorder ataxia with vitamin E deficiency (AVED), in which there is a massive accumulation of lipofuscin in dorsal root ganglions in the spine where the cell bodies of sensory neurons are located. Lipofuscin deposits indicate breakdown of the cell membrane and more commonly occur with ageing. Sensory neurons die off, causing peripheral neuropathy, ataxia (incoordination), speech difficulties, impaired nerve reflexes and vibration sense, atrophy of the retina and ultimately death. AVED may be associated with cardiomyopathy and retinitis pigmentosa (damage to the retina, causing vision loss). Symptoms have a striking resemblance to those of Friedreich's ataxia, an inherited neurological disease. Vitamin E supplementation improves symptoms and may prevent disease progression in AVED.

Lower blood levels of vitamin E are associated with more fragile red blood cells that have a shorter lifespan, leading to haemolytic anaemia. In preterm infants, haemolytic anaemia is associated with vitamin E deficiency. Neurological and muscle abnormalities may occur in normal people with impaired absorption of vitamin E.

Indicators of inadequate levels may include:

- haemolytic anaemia
- muscle damage, weak muscles, incoordination, lack of balance, tremors, absence of reflexes, slurred speech, muscle soreness after exercise
- damage to the eyes, nerves, liver, brain and other organs
- increased oxidative stress and diseases related to this, including:
  - inflammatory diseases, such as cardiovascular disease and arthritis
  - diseases of ageing, such as impaired immunity, stroke, Parkinson's disease, Alzheimer's disease, and the vision disorders, cataracts and macular degeneration
  - chronic degenerative disease, such as Friedreich's ataxia and amyotrophic lateral sclerosis (ALS, motor neurone disease)

- fatigue syndromes
- autoimmune diseases, such as rheumatoid arthritis
- liver damage and alcohol-induced diseases
- lung damage
- male infertility
- abnormal cell growth or cancer
- age-related tissue damage and loss of function
- skin damage, wrinkling, slow healing of wounds and burns, and scarring.

Assessment of body status

Vitamin E status is usually assessed by measurement of plasma levels. The reference range given by the RCPA is 7–35 μmol/L for children and 11–46 μmol/L for adults. However, plasma levels of vitamin E are tightly controlled and do not rise more than two- to three-fold with supplementation, even when high doses are used. Red blood cell levels are a better indicator of longer term vitamin E status, and platelet levels are a more sensitive measurement of the dose response to oral vitamin E.

Case reports—vitamin E deficiency

- *A girl, sixteen years of age*, had a history of imbalance while walking, weakness in both lower limbs since five years of age and slurring of speech since three years of age.[1] She had difficulty combing her hair and buttoning clothes, ataxia and nystagmus (involuntary movement of the eyeball). Vibration sense and joint position sense were impaired in the lower limbs, and knee and ankle reflexes were absent. Her serum vitamin E level was 11 μmol/L. She was treated with vitamin E (400 mg three times a day) and showed objective improvement over two weeks. At two months, she had significant objective improvement in gait, upper limb ataxia and sensory signs of the lower limb.
- *A boy, seven years of age*, had developed ataxia with unsteadiness, constant head and hand tremors, and slurred speech at three years of age, with progressive worsening of symptoms.[2] His serum vitamin E level was undetectable. Genetic studies were negative for Friedreich's ataxia, but revealed a mutation of the gene for alpha-TTP. Vitamin E was given by intramuscular injections because oral doses were not effective in raising serum vitamin E levels. Neurological symptoms improved when serum levels rose and worsened when levels dropped. Over time, oral doses were able to be used (3000 mg daily). Symptoms gradually improved, with less gait instability, almost normal walking, less frequent head tremors and fluent speech.

REFERENCES

1 Jayaram, S., Soman, A., Tarvade, S. & Londhe, V., Cerebellar ataxia due to isolated vitamin E deficiency, *Indian J Med Sci* (2005), 59(1): 20–3.

2 Aparicio, J.M., Bélanger-Quintana, A., Suárez, L. et al., Ataxia with isolated vitamin E deficiency: Case report and review of the literature, *J Pediatr Gastroenterol Nutr* (2001), 33(2): 206–10.

THERAPEUTIC USES OF VITAMIN E

Skin disorders, burns and wounds

Canadian doctors Wilfred and Evan Shute pioneered the use of vitamin E supplements in the 1940s, and used oral and topical vitamin E for healing severe burns and minimising scarring, reporting that it relieved pain and speeded up healing of severe and infected burns, and reduced the need for skin grafts.[1] More recent research has shown that cellular oxidative stress appears to be an important factor in burn-mediated injury. Burns patients have been shown to have elevated plasma levels of lipid peroxidation products and reduced levels of vitamin E and other free radical scavengers.[2] Organ failure associated with burn injury may be due to oxidative damage, and supplementation with antioxidants has shown to be protective. Antioxidant treatment for burns has included ascorbic acid, glutathione, N-acetylcysteine (NAC) or vitamins A, E and C alone or in combination, and these treatments have been shown to reduce mortality, protect cell function and microvascular circulation, reduce tissue lipid peroxidation, improve heart performance and reduce the amount of fluid resuscitation required.[3]

Alpha-tocopherol is an important protective antioxidant in human skin. Gamma-tocopherol is also present but in levels ten times lower than alpha-tocopherol.[4] Although vitamin E skin creams are popularly used, it is not known whether topical vitamin E can penetrate through the outer skin layers into the dermis. Alpha-tocopherol may be the more effective form in topical preparations because, although vitamin E esters are more stable, they need to be hydrolysed to the active, free alpha-tocopherol in the skin, which may occur in deeper layers of the skin but not in the outer skin layers.

Even mild doses of UV light deplete alpha-tocopherol levels in the outer stratum corneum of the skin by almost 50 per cent immediately afterwards.[5] Vitamin E applied to the skin prior to sun exposure has been shown to reduce lipid peroxidation, reddening and oedema. Vitamin E acetate, as well as sodium ascorbyl phosphate, can be converted to free vitamin E and C in the epidermis of the skin, and can enhance skin protection when used in sunscreens. Topical formulations have had mixed success in treating scarring, but topical vitamin E with vitamin C has been found to improve pigmented contact dermatitis lesions and the facial pigment chloasma, which often develops in pregnancy.[6] Topical creams containing alpha-tocopherol at concentrations ranging from 0.1–1.0 per cent are likely to be effective in enhancing antioxidant protection of the skin barrier. However, topical vitamin E preparations may cause allergic reactions in the skin in sensitive individuals.

Oral vitamin E (400 mg daily for three weeks) has been found to increase alpha-tocopherol levels of sebum in the skin by 87–92 per cent.[7] Vitamin E supplementation has been recommended for wound healing, yellow nail syndrome (discolouration of the nails and slow growth), vibration disease (numbness, pain, and blanching of the fingers caused by use of vibrating hand tools), skin cancer prevention, cutaneous (skin) ulcers and epidermolysis bullosa (a genetic skin disease that causes blistering). Atopic dermatitis patients taking oral vitamin E (400 IU daily) in the long term have shown an improvement and near remission of symptoms and a 62 per cent decrease in serum immunoglobulin E (IgE) levels, a marker of allergic activity.[8]

Antioxidants, including ascorbic acid, vitamin E and glutathione, have been shown to decrease by 30–40 per cent in skin wounds.[9] In animals with infected wounds, giving vitamin E before infection onset has been found to increase the effectiveness of antibiotic therapy.[10]

Age-related lowered immunity

Ageing is associated with a decline in immune function, especially impaired function of the thymus gland and T cells, which is associated with a higher rate of morbidity and mortality in elderly people. Vitamin E supplementation is associated with enhanced immune response by boosting production of the cytokine interleukin-2 (IL-2), which enhances proliferation of T cells, and decreasing macrophage production of PGE_2, an eicosanoid that suppresses T cell activity at high levels.[11]

Vitamin E supplementation can improve immune functions in old age, including delayed-type hypersensitivity (DTH) skin responses and antibody production in response to vaccination. Supplementation with vitamin E (800 mg daily) in healthy people over 60 years of age has been shown to increase DTH response, T cell proliferation, and IL-2 production, and decrease plasma lipid peroxide concentration and PGE_2 production.[11] Elderly people with a serum vitamin E concentration in the upper third (greater than 48.4 μmol/L) after supplementation have been found to have a higher antibody and DTH response than those with serum levels in the lower third (19.9–34.7 μmol/L).[12] One year of synthetic vitamin E supplementation (200 mg daily) in nursing home residents has been found to reduce the risk of acquiring upper respiratory infections, including the common cold.[13]

Cardiovascular disease

In the 1940s, Drs Wilfred and Evan Shute claimed to have successfully used vitamin E to treat many patients with a variety of cardiovascular diseases (CVD), although its mechanism of action was not understood at that time.[14] A key factor in the development of atherosclerosis is oxidative modification of lipoproteins—especially LDL—which stimulates inflammatory changes in arterial endothelium (the lining of the artery wall). Oxidised LDL promotes production of inflammatory chemicals in artery walls and conversion of smooth muscle cells and macrophages to lipid-filled foam cells, and also inhibits vasodilation induced by nitric oxide. Oxidation of HDL cholesterol impairs its anti-atherosclerotic function.

Alpha-tocopherol has been shown to prevent atherosclerotic plaque formation in animal studies. It is a potent free radical scavenger that increases the resistance of LDL cholesterol to oxidation and decreases the toxic effect of oxidised LDL on the arterial endothelium, although it is not as effective against hypochlorite-mediated oxidation. Alpha-tocopherol also has potent anti-inflammatory activity via inhibition of PKC.

Increased intake of dietary vitamin E has been associated with lower risk of coronary heart disease in middle-aged and older men and women.[15,16] Although animal studies of vitamin E supplementation have shown protective effects in the prevention of CVD, human studies have shown mixed results. Meta-analyses have concluded that vitamin E is not of benefit for the prevention of CVD.[17,18] Another review concluded that alpha-tocopherol has the potential to reduce cardiovascular incidents by 30–60 per cent but the outcome appears to vary with the patient's level of risk, the dose used, the use of natural or synthetic vitamin E, the duration of therapy and the patient's response to vitamin E.[19] It appears that about 20 per cent of subjects do not respond to supplementation with an increased plasma alpha-tocopherol concentration. Studies that failed to show benefits have been criticised for not monitoring the oxidative stress and vitamin E levels of the subjects to identify responders and non-responders, the relatively short treatment times and the use of inappropriate doses or forms of vitamin E, as well as failure to use vitamin C with vitamin E, to ensure supplements were taken with meals and to ensure patient compliance.[20]

The major difference between human and animal studies is that, in animal studies, vitamin E is usually given at the same time as the onset of oxidative stress and the environment and diet are controlled. The main human trials have used patients with existing disease, which may have taken 30 years to develop, and it is unrealistic to expect vitamin E given as a single antioxidant to reverse years of oxidative damage due to multiple causes. It appears that vitamin E supplementation may be more useful in early life or in the early stages of CVD rather than in advanced disease, and it appears to work best when given with vitamin C and possibly other antioxidants. Gamma-tocopherol may also have a protective role because higher serum levels are associated with lower CVD morbidity and mortality.[21]

Cancer

Alpha-tocopherol has antioxidant, immune-boosting and anti-inflammatory activity, and would be expected to be protective against carcinogens. Low vitamin E status is associated with increased risk of some types of cancer.[22] However, studies using vitamin E as the sole supplement for cancer have reported mixed results, and the consensus is that, overall, vitamin E is not beneficial.[23] Supplementation with synthetic vitamin E (50 mg daily) was found to decrease prostate cancer incidence by 32 per cent in one study,[24] but another study using 400 IU daily of synthetic vitamin E found that the risk of prostate cancer increased among healthy men.[25] However, the risk reduced when vitamin E was given with selenium (200 mcg daily). Combined selenium, beta-carotene and vitamin E supplementation has been associated with lower mortality rate and lower cancer mortality.[26]

In contrast to alpha-tocopherol, the vitamin E ester, alpha-tocopheryl succinate, has been shown to be a very potent inducer of apoptosis in tumour cells, and is the most effective form of alpha-tocopherol for inducing cell differentiation, inhibition of proliferation and apoptosis.[27] It appears to work independently of antioxidant activity, and may act by altering gene expression in tumour cells. A major disadvantage of alpha-tocopheryl succinate is that it cannot be used orally, as it breaks down in the digestive tract to alpha-tocopherol and succinic acid, neither of which has strong anticancer properties. Intravenous or skin delivery systems may be necessary.

Cognitive impairment and Alzheimer's disease

Higher intakes of vitamin E and alpha-TE have been associated with a reduced incidence of Alzheimer's disease (AD).[28] A study of dietary intake in older people found that a slower rate of cognitive decline was associated with intakes of vitamin E, alpha-TE and alpha- and gamma-tocopherols.[29] Vitamin E and C supplements in combination are associated with reduced prevalence and incidence of AD.[30]

Studies using alpha-tocopherol as the sole supplement have had mixed results. One study found that synthetic alpha-tocopherol (2000 IU daily) was beneficial in delaying AD progression.[31] However a systematic review of three studies concluded that alpha-tocopherol supplementation in patients with mild cognitive impairment or AD was not effective.[32] Differences in response to vitamin E may explain the mixed results; responders to vitamin E show lower markers of oxidation and maintenance of cognitive scores, whereas non-responders have no change in oxidation markers and a decrease in cognitive function.

Age-related macular degeneration

Age-related macular degeneration (ARMD) is loss of central vision that occurs with ageing because of loss of pigments in the macular of the retina, which may result from oxidative injury to the retinal pigment epithelium. Animals maintained on vitamin E-deficient diets for two years have been found to develop macular degeneration.[33] Higher plasma alpha-tocopherol levels are associated with less risk of ARMD progression, with people with the highest plasma levels having an 82 per cent reduced risk of late (advanced) ARMD compared with those with the lowest levels.[34] However, there is insufficient evidence that vitamin E supplementation is effective in the prevention or treatment of ARMD.

Preterm infants

Preterm infants have increased risk of retinopathy, intracranial haemorrhage, haemolytic anaemia and chronic lung disease, and antioxidant therapy with vitamin E has been used for prevention. A review of 26 trials of vitamin E supplementation in preterm infants concluded that it can reduce the risk of intracranial haemorrhage, severe retinopathy and blindness in very low birth weight infants.[35] However, it may also increase the risk of infections.

Pre-eclampsia of pregnancy

Pre-eclampsia is characterised by high blood pressure and protein in the urine, and is a potentially life-threatening complication of pregnancy, often leading to a preterm delivery. Women with pre-eclampsia have elevated markers of lipid peroxidation and early use of vitamin E (263 mg daily) with vitamin C (1000 mg daily) has been shown to reduce the risk.[36] However, not all studies have been positive, especially if supplementation is begun later in pregnancy. A review of ten trials that used antioxidant supplementation (mainly vitamin E with vitamin C) in pregnant women concluded that there was no effect on pre-eclampsia incidence.[37]

Cystic fibrosis

Supplementation with vitamin E (200–400 IU daily) is a routine treatment for cystic fibrosis patients, who are unable to absorb fat-soluble vitamins, and has been shown to normalise plasma alpha-tocopherol levels.[38]

Arthritis

Vitamin E supplementation may relieve pain and reduce analgesic use in people with osteoarthritis and rheumatoid arthritis.[39]

Male infertility

In men with reduced sperm motility, vitamin E supplementation (100 mg three times daily) for several months led to a significant decrease in lipid peroxidation, an increase in sperm motility and increased pregnancy rates.[40]

REFERENCES

1 Shute, E.V., Notes on the use of alpha-tocopherol in the management of acute and subacute vascular obstructions, as well as in burns, *Ann NY Acad Sci* (1949), 52(3): 358–67.

2 Nguyen, T.T., Cox, C.S., Traber, D.L. et al., Free radical activity and loss of plasma antioxidants, vitamin E, and sulfhydryl groups in patients with burns: The 1993 Moyer Award, *J Burn Care Rehabil* (1993), 14(6): 602–9.

3 Horton, J.W., Free radicals and lipid peroxidation mediated injury in burn trauma: The role of antioxidant therapy, *Toxicology* (2003), 189(1–2): 75–88.

4 Thiele, J.J. & Ekanayake-Mudiyanselage, S., Vitamin E in human skin: Organ-specific physiology and considerations for its use in dermatology, *Mol Aspects Med* (2007), 28(5–6): 646–67.

5 Thiele, J.J., Traber, M.G. & Packer, L., Depletion of human stratum corneum vitamin E: An early and sensitive in vivo marker of UV induced photo-oxidation, *J Invest Dermatol* (1998), 110: 756–61.

6 Hayakawa, R., Ueda, H., Nozaki, T. et al., Effects of combination treatment with vitamins E and C on chloasma and pigmented contact dermatitis: A double blind controlled clinical trial, *Acta Vitaminol Enzymol* (1981), 3: 31–8.

7 Ekanayake-Mudiyanselage, S., Kraemer, K. & Thiele, J.J., Oral supplementation with all-Rac- and RRR-alpha-tocopherol increases vitamin E levels in human sebum after a latency period of 14–21 days, *Ann NY Acad Sci* (2004), 1031: 184–94.

8 Tsoureli-Nikita, E., Hercogova, J., Lotti, T. & Menchini, G., Evaluation of dietary intake of vitamin E in the treatment of atopic dermatitis: A study of the clinical course and evaluation of the immunoglobulin E serum levels, *Int J Dermatol* (2002), 41(3): 146–50.

9 Shukla, A., Rasik, A.M. & Patnaik, G.K., Depletion of reduced glutathione, ascorbic acid, vitamin E and antioxidant defence enzymes in a healing cutaneous wound, *Free Radic Res* (1997), 26(2): 93–101.

10 Provinciali, M., Cirioni, O., Orlando, F. et al., Vitamin E improves the in vivo efficacy of tigecycline and daptomycin in an animal model of wounds infected with methicillin-resistant Staphylococcus aureus, *J Med Microbiol* (2011), 60(Pt 12): 1806–12.

11 Meydani, S.N., Han, S.N. & Wu, D., Vitamin E and immune response in the aged: Molecular mechanisms and clinical implications, *Immunol Rev* (2005), 205: 269–84.

12 Meydani, S.N., Meydani, M., Blumberg, J.B. et al., Vitamin E supplementation and in vivo immune response in healthy elderly subjects: A randomized controlled trial, *JAMA* (1997), 277(17): 1380–6.

13 Meydani, S.N., Leka, L.S., Fine, B.C. et al., Vitamin E and respiratory tract infections in elderly nursing home residents: A randomized controlled trial, *JAMA* (2004), 292(7): 828–36.

14 Shute, E.V., Vogelsang, A.B. et al., The influence of vitamin E on vascular disease, *Surg Gynecol Obstet* (1948), 86(1): 1–8.

15 Rimm, E.B., Stampfer, M.J., Ascherio, A. et al., Vitamin E consumption and the risk of coronary heart disease in men, *N Engl J Med* (1993), 328(20): 1450–6.

16 Stampfer, M.J., Hennekens, C.H., Manson, J.E. et al., Vitamin E consumption and the risk of coronary disease in women, *N Engl J Med* (1993), 328(20): 1444–9.

17 Eidelman, R.S., Hollar, D., Hebert, P.R. et al., Randomized trials of vitamin E in the treatment and prevention of cardiovascular disease, *Arch Intern Med* (2004), 164: 1552–6.

18 Vivekananthan, D.P., Penn, M.S., Sapp, S.K. et al., Use of antioxidant vitamins for the prevention of cardiovascular disease: Meta-analysis of randomised trials, *Lancet* (2003), 361: 2017–23.

19 Kirmizis, D. & Chatzidimitriou, D., Antiatherogenic effects of vitamin E: The search for the Holy Grail, *Vasc Health Risk Manag* (2009), 5: 767–74.

20 Robinson, I., de Serna, D.G., Gutierrez, A. & Schade, D.S., Vitamin E in humans: An explanation of clinical trial failure, *Endocr Pract* (2006), 12(5): 576–82.

21 Devaraj, S. & Jialal, I., Failure of vitamin E in clinical trials: Is gamma-tocopherol the answer? *Nutr Rev* (2005), 63(8): 290–3.

22 Knekt, P., Aromaa, A., Maatela, J. et al., Vitamin E and cancer prevention, *Am J Clin Nutr* (1991), 53(1 Suppl): 283S–6S.

23 Coulter, I.D., Hardy, M.L., Morton, S.C. et al., Antioxidants vitamin C and vitamin E for the prevention and treatment of cancer, *J Gen Intern Med* (2006), 21(7): 735–44.

24 Heinonen, O.P., Albanes, D., Virtamo, J. et al., Prostate cancer and supplementation with alpha-tocopherol and beta-carotene: Incidence and mortality in a controlled trial, *J Natl Cancer Inst* (1998), 90(6): 440–6.

25 Klein, E.A., Thompson, I.M. Jr., Tangen, C.M. et al., Vitamin E and the risk of prostate cancer: The Selenium and Vitamin E Cancer Prevention Trial (SELECT), *JAMA* (2011), 306(14): 1549–56.

26 Blot, W.J., Li, J.Y., Taylor, P.R. et al., Nutrition intervention trials in Linxian, China: Supplementation with specific vitamin/mineral combinations, cancer incidence, and disease-specific mortality in the general population, *J Natl Cancer Inst* (1993), 85(18): 1483–92.

27 Neuzil, J., Vitamin E succinate and cancer treatment: A vitamin E prototype for selective antitumour activity, *Br J Cancer* (2003), 89(10): 1822–6.

28 Morris, M.C., Evans, D.A., Bienias, J.L. et al., Vitamin E and cognitive decline in older persons, *Arch Neurol* (2002), 59(7): 1125–32.

29 Morris, M.C., Evans, D.A., Tangney, C.C. et al., Relation of the tocopherol forms to incident Alzheimer disease and to cognitive change, *Am J Clin Nutr* (2005), 81(2): 508–14.

30 Morris, M.C., Beckett, L.A., Scherr, P.A. et al., Vitamin E and vitamin C supplement use and risk of incident Alzheimer's disease, *Alzheimer Dis Assoc Disord* (1998), 12(3): 121–6.

31 Sano, M., Ernesto. C., Thomas, R.G., et al., A controlled trial of selegiline, alpha-tocopherol, or both as treatment for Alzheimer's disease. The Alzheimer's Disease Cooperative Study, *N Engl J Med* (1997), 336(17): 1216–22.

32 Farina, N., Isaac, M.G., Clark, A.R. et al., Vitamin E for Alzheimer's dementia and mild cognitive impairment, *Cochrane Database Syst Rev* (2012), 11: CD002854.

33 Hayes, K.C., Retinal degeneration in monkeys induced by deficiencies of vitamin E or A, *Invest Ophthalmol* (1974), 13(7): 499–510.

34 Delcourt, C., Cristol, J.P., Tessier, F. et al., Age-related macular degeneration and anti-oxidant status in the POLA study. POLA Study Group. Pathologies Oculaires Liées à l'Age, *Arch Ophthalmol* (1999), 117(10): 1384–90.

35 Brion, L.P., Bell, E.F. & Raghuveer, T.S., Vitamin E supplementation for prevention of morbidity and mortality in preterm infants, *Cochrane Database Syst Rev* (2003), 3: CD003665.

36 Chappell, L.C., Seed, P.T., Briley, A.L. et al., Effect of antioxidants on the occurrence of pre-eclampsia in women at increased risk: A randomised trial, *Lancet* (1999), 354: 810–16.

37 Rumbold, A., Duley, L., Crowther, C.A. & Haslam, R.R., Antioxidants for preventing pre-eclampsia, *Cochrane Database Syst Rev* (2008), 1: CD004227.

38 Brigelius-Flohé, R., Kelly, F.J., Salonen, J.T. et al., The European perspective on vitamin E: Current knowledge and future research, *Am J Clin Nutr* (2002), 76(4): 703–16.

39 Canter, P.H., Wider, B. & Ernst, E., The anti-oxidant vitamins A, C, E and selenium in the treatment of arthritis: A systematic review of randomized clinical trials, *Rheumatology (Oxford)* (2007), 46(8): 1223–33.

40 Suleiman, S.A., Ali, M.E., Zaki, Z.M. at al., Lipid peroxidation and human sperm motility: Protective role of vitamin E, *J Androl* (1996), 17: 530–7.

Therapeutic dose

The health maintenance dose range for vitamin E is 50–100 IU daily. The therapeutic dose range appears to be 200–1000 IU daily. Up to 2000 IU has been used in clinical trials, but the optimum dose is not known. Vitamin E is best used with other supportive antioxidants, such as vitamin C and selenium.

In cystic fibrosis patients, the recommended daily starting doses are 40–80 IU from birth to twelve months, 50–150 IU from one to three years, 150–300 IU from four to seven years, and 150–500 IU from eight years to adulthood.

Effects of excess

There are no recognised toxicity effects of vitamin E. Large doses of alpha-tocopherol (1200 IU daily) have been found to deplete plasma and tissue levels of gamma-tocopherol. However, the impact of this on health is not known. Vitamin E has a mild blood-thinning effect, and was linked to a slight increase in nose bleeds in one study and to increased risk of death from stroke due to haemorrhage in another. However, other studies using higher dosages have not reported this effect on stroke risk and, overall, the risk of stroke appears to be decreased by vitamin E. Patients taking the blood-thinning drug warfarin long term together with vitamin E supplementation have not been shown to have increased risk of bleeding.

Supplements

Vitamin E is available in the following forms in supplements:

Natural vitamin E

The natural d-alpha-tocopherol (RRR-alpha-tocopherol) is commonly derived commercially from methylation of tocopherol mixtures isolated from vegetable oils. It is also available in ester form as d-alpha-tocopheryl acetate (RRR-alpha-tocopheryl acetate) and d-alpha-tocopheryl succinate (RRR-alpha-tocopheryl succinate). Ester forms are less susceptible to oxidation, and are therefore more stable and are more commonly used than the free form. In humans, free and esterified alpha-tocopherols have the same bioavailability.

Synthetic vitamin E

The synthetic dl-alpha-tocopherol (all-rac-alpha-tocopherol) is usually manufactured by the condensation of trimethylhydroquinone with isophytol in the presence of a catalyst and consists of a mixture of eight stereoisomers (molecules that have the same chemical formula but differ in the three-dimensional arrangement of their atoms). It is also available in ester form as dl-alpha-tocopheryl acetate (all-rac-alpha-tocopheryl acetate) and dl-alpha-tocopheryl succinate (all-rac-alpha-tocopheryl succinate). Again, the ester forms are more stable and more commonly used commercially. Synthetic vitamin E has lower bioavailability than natural vitamin E, and is metabolised to alpha-CEHC three to four times faster.

Cautions

Vitamin E supplements are usually well tolerated. No significant adverse effects were reported in healthy older people given up to 800 IU daily for four months or in people taking 3200 IU daily for nine weeks. Vitamin E has mild blood-thinning properties and should be used with caution in people on anticoagulant therapy.

VITAMIN E AND MORTALITY: IS THERE A LINK?

In 2005, a meta-analysis controversially claimed that high-dose vitamin E supplementation increased risk of death.[1] The authors combined the results of nineteen good-quality clinical trials of vitamin E supplementation for various diseases, including heart disease, end-stage renal failure and Alzheimer's disease, and reported that adults who took supplements of 400 IU a day or more were more likely to die of any cause than those who did not take vitamin E supplements. Of these trials, nine used vitamin E alone and ten used vitamin E combined with other vitamins or minerals. The vitamin E dosage ranged from 16.5 to 2000 IU daily (median 400 IU daily). Most trials were small in size, and patients were elderly with various chronic diseases. Causes of death were not given.

The main findings of this meta-analysis were as follows:

- overall, vitamin E supplementation did not affect all-cause mortality
- low-dose vitamin E supplementation (16.5–330 IU daily) slightly reduced all-cause mortality
- all-cause mortality progressively increased as vitamin E dosage rose above 150 IU daily, and the difference remained after controlling for the use of other vitamins or minerals
- high-dose vitamin E (400 IU or more daily for at least one year) increased all-cause mortality.

An independent review of data from this meta-analysis reported that the increased mortality seen in certain trials was not due to the higher dose of vitamin E but rather due to a higher proportion of male patients in these trials.[2] The authors concluded that the causal relationship of vitamin E supplementation and increased mortality is questionable and high-dose vitamin E supplementation has not been proven to increase mortality.

A more recent meta-analysis studied mortality data from 57 randomised controlled trials using vitamin E over a period of at least one year to prevent or treat disease.[3] In total, there were 246 371 subjects and 29 295 all-cause deaths. Duration of supplementation ranged from one to 10.1 years (median 2.6 years). The authors concluded that long-term supplementary vitamin E was not associated with mortality, there was no relationship between dose and risk of mortality and supplementation with vitamin E was not found to effect all-cause mortality at doses up to 5500 IU daily. From the evidence available to date, it appears that there is no credible evidence for a link between increased mortality and vitamin E supplementation.

REFERENCES

1 Miller, E.R. III, Pastor-Barriuso, R., Dalal, D. et al., Meta-analysis: High-dosage vitamin E supplementation may increase all-cause mortality, *Ann Intern Med* (2005), 142(1): 37–46.

2 Gerss, J. & Köpcke, W., The questionable association of vitamin E supplementation and mortality: Inconsistent results of different meta-analytic approaches, *Cell Mol Biol (Noisy-le-grand)* (2009), 55 Suppl: OL1111–20.

3 Abner, E.L., Schmitt, F.A., Mendiondo, M.S. et al.,Vitamin E and all-cause mortality: A meta-analysis, *Curr Aging Sci* (2011), 4(2): 158–70.

Vitamin K

VITAMIN K STATUS CHECK

1 Do you bruise easily?
2 Do you have recurring nose bleeds or prolonged bleeding after injuries?
3 Do you have low bone density?
4 Are you taking anticoagulant, anti-convulsant or anti-tuberculosis medication?

'Yes' answers may indicate inadequate vitamin K status. However, note that 'Yes' answers for points 1 and 2 may indicate inadequate vitamin C status rather than low vitamin K. A number of nutritional deficiencies or health disorders can cause similar effects and further investigation is recommended.

FAST FACTS . . . VITAMIN K

- Vitamin K occurs naturally as phylloquinone and menaquinones.
- It is required for formation of Gla proteins that bind calcium in the body.
- It supports blood clotting, bone and connective tissue metabolism, and brain and nerve function.
- Supplementation may be helpful for preventing haemorrhage in newborn infants, maintaining bone mineral density, preventing calcification of blood vessels and stabilising anticoagulant therapy.

In 1929, Danish biochemist and physiologist Henrik Dam was investigating the role of cholesterol in the diet of chicks, and observed that chicks fed on sterol-free diets developed brain or muscular haemorrhages and slow blood clotting that could not be rectified by giving them any of the vitamins or lipids that had been identified at that time. After further experiments, in 1935 Dam announced the discovery of a new fat-soluble vitamin that he called vitamin K after the German word for clotting, 'koagulation'. Subsequently, other researchers found that they could cure haemorrhagic disease by giving animals either extracts of alfalfa or fish meal and bran preparations that had been subject to bacterial activity. In 1943, Henrik Dam and a US researcher, Edward Doisy, were awarded the Nobel Prize in Physiology or Medicine for their work in discovering vitamin K.

Vitamin K occurs naturally in two forms: phylloquinone (PK) and menaquinones (MKs). PK is referred to as vitamin K1, and is also known as phytomenadione or phytonadione, which is a structurally identical commercially produced form. MKs contain a varying number of 5-carbon (isoprenoid) units in a side chain, and are abbreviated to MK-n, with 'n' referring to the number of isoprenoid units—for example, the most common form in the body, MK-4, has four isoprenoid units and is known as vitamin K2. PK is found in plants and MKs are produced by bacterial activity in food and in the colon. Menadione (referred to as vitamin K3) is a synthetic form that can be converted to vitamin K2 by intestinal bacteria or tissue enzymes.

Digestion, absorption and transport

Dietary vitamin K is in the form of PK and MKs, which are fat-soluble; absorption from food depends on the presence of bile and pancreatic enzymes and is enhanced by dietary fat. After vitamin K is incorporated into micelles together with dietary lipids, it is absorbed across the wall of the small intestine and packaged into chylomicrons for transport in lymph vessels to the bloodstream and then to tissue cells. The remaining vitamin K in chylomicron remnants is taken up by the liver. MKs produced by bacteria in the colon can be absorbed by passive diffusion, but it is not known how much is absorbed in this way.

Metabolism, storage and excretion

In the liver, all forms of vitamin K are packaged into very low-density lipoproteins (LDLs) for transport to tissues, in which PK is converted to MK-4, the dominant form in the body. Menadione conversion to MK-4 occurs in tissues such as the pancreas, salivary glands, brain and sternum, but it is rapidly metabolised and excreted, and only a small amount is converted to MK-4.

Vitamin K metabolism occurs in a cyclic fashion in the rough endoplasmic reticulum membranes inside cells, in which it is activated, inactivated and regenerated many times. Vitamin K is present in the body as the oxidised vitamin K quinone, which must be converted to its reduced hydroquinone form (KH_2) in order to act as an enzyme cofactor in the body. During the vitamin K cycle, the active form, KH_2, is converted to vitamin K2,3-epoxide and then to vitamin K quinone by the enzyme vitamin K epoxide reductase. Vitamin K quinone is then reactivated to KH_2 by the enzyme vitamin K quinone reductase. Vitamin K is stored in the liver, mainly as MK-7, MK-8, MK-10 and MK-11, with about 10 per cent stored as PK. Other storage sites include bones and the heart. Excess vitamin K is mainly excreted via bile in faeces, with a smaller amount excreted in urine.

Functions

Vitamin K is an essential cofactor for the enzyme gamma-glutamyl carboxylase, which adds carboxyl groups to glutamic acid residues in vitamin K-dependent proteins, a process called carboxylation (see Figure 5.4). Carboxylation converts these proteins to active Gla proteins that bind calcium in the body and promote protein–calcium–phospholipid interactions. The liver mainly uses PK for carboxylation, whereas MKs are the main form used in other tissues. The functions of Gla proteins include the following.

- *Regulation of blood clotting.* Blood clotting is dependent on the sequential activation of thirteen blood-clotting proteins, called factors; when activated, these create a web of insoluble fibrin to trap blood cells and pathogens and seal off the site of injury. These clotting factors are made in the liver, and four of them are dependent on vitamin K-dependent carboxylation for activation, namely factor II (prothrombin), factor VII, factor IX and factor X. The major function of Gla residues in clotting factors is to enable the factors to bind to phospholipids on the surface of activated blood platelets. Vitamin K is also required for carboxylation of proteins C, S and Z, which appear to inhibit blood clotting by inactivating specific clotting factors, providing an important regulatory mechanism for keeping blood clotting under control. Protein S also stimulates phagocytosis of dead cells by macrophages.
- *Bone metabolism.* A number of Gla proteins have been identified in bone, including osteocalcin (bone-Gla protein, BGP), matrix-Gla protein (MGP), protein S, Gla-rich protein (GRP), periostin and periostin-like factor (PLF). Gla proteins in bone bind large amounts of calcium and are physically bound to hydroxyapatite, the mineral component of bone. Osteocalcin is a Gla protein secreted by bone-building cells (osteoblasts) that bind calcium and incorporate it into hydroxyapatite crystals in bone, promoting mineralisation. Periostin is a Gla protein in connective tissues that enhances mineralisation in bone and supports connective tissue development, maturation and repair. MK-4 may have a specific role in gene expression in osteoblasts. Vitamin K metabolism in bone is dependent on calcitriol, the active form of vitamin D, which enhances intestinal absorption of calcium and activates the synthesis of osteocalcin.

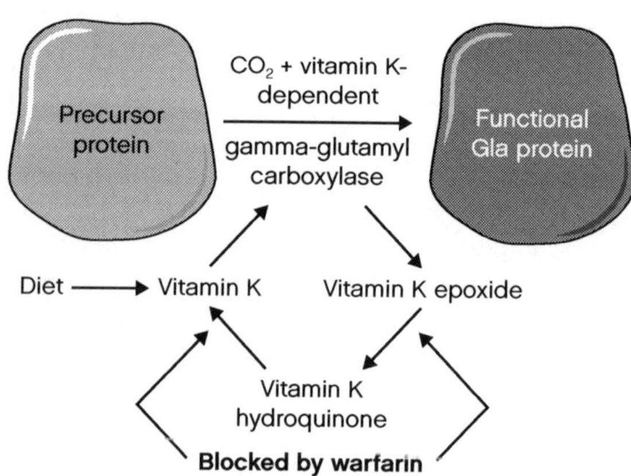

Figure 5.4 Vitamin K metabolism

- *Connective tissue metabolism.* MGP is mainly produced by cartilage-forming cells and smooth muscle cells in blood vessel walls. It is found in the extracellular matrix of soft tissues, such as blood vessel walls, joint cartilage and the heart, lungs and kidneys. It binds to calcium ions and is a powerful inhibitor of calcium buildup in soft tissue, and is particularly important for preventing the calcium accumulation in artery walls that occurs in atherosclerosis. Two other types of Gla proteins have been identified in soft tissue—proline-rich Gla proteins (PRGP) and transmembrane Gla proteins (TMG)—but their functions are unknown.
- *Integrity of blood vessel walls.* Vitamin K is a co-factor for the formation of growth arrest specific gene 6 protein (Gas-6), a Gla protein produced by smooth muscle cells in blood vessel walls. It supports the integrity of the vascular system, regulates growth of cells and inflammation and helps removal of dead cells. Gas-6 prevents smooth muscle cell apoptosis and calcification, and protects against atherosclerotic plaque formation. It has growth factor–like activity by interacting with receptor tyrosine kinases of the TAM family (Tyro3, Axl and Mer), which are cell surface receptors for growth factors, cytokines and hormones. The Gas-6/TAM system regulates many cell functions, including cell survival and proliferation, cell adhesion and migration, blood clot stabilisation and inflammatory cytokine release, and plays a role in the nervous, reproductive and vascular systems, and in autoimmune diseases and cancer.
- *Hormone activity.* About 30 per cent of the osteocalcin produced in bone is secreted into the bloodstream, and acts as a hormone that may influence beta cell function in the pancreas, insulin sensitivity, production of adiponectin (a hormone produced by fat cells that affects glucose and fat metabolism), energy expenditure and body fat levels. It may also enhance synthesis of testosterone.
- *Brain and nerve function.* MK-4 is the predominant form of vitamin K in the brain, and Gas-6 is the predominant Gla protein in the brain. Protein S is present in smaller amounts. Gas-6 is involved in nerve development and MK-4 may prevent oxidative damage to myelin-producing cells (oligodendrocytes) in the brain. Vitamin K is required for production of sphingolipids, lipids in brain cell membranes that help regulate proliferation, differentiation, ageing and interactions between cells. Alterations in sphingolipid metabolism have been linked to age-related cognitive decline and neurodegenerative diseases, such as Alzheimer's disease.

Dietary sources

PK is produced exclusively by plants and some microalgae, in which it functions as an electron carrier during carbon dioxide fixation, assisting chlorophyll metabolism and photosynthesis. Rich sources are cruciferous (cabbage family) vegetables, which include cabbage, broccoli, Brussels sprouts, collards and kale; other dark green vegetables, such as spinach, salad greens and watercress; soybean and canola oil; and microalgae, such as spirulina and chlorella. Smaller amounts are found in cottonseed and olive oils.

Menaquinones—mainly MK-7 through to MK-10—are made in the colon by bacterial activity, but absorption is low. Menaquinone-producing bacteria include lactic acid bacteria, which produce mainly MK-8 and MK-9, and propionic acid bacteria, which produce mainly MK-10. The most common menaquinones in food are MK-4, MK-7, MK-8 and MK-9. Small amounts of menaquinones are found in animal products such as meat, egg yolk, butter and matured cheese, and in legumes such as soybeans. The traditional Japanese food natto, a fermented soybean product, is rich in MK-7, produced by the bacteria *Bacillus subtilis natto*, and matured cheese provides MK-4 through to MK-9.

The Food Standards Australia New Zealand nutrient database (NUTTAB) does not provide any data for the amounts in specific foods.

Factors influencing body status

Vitamin K1 is slowly broken down by exposure to oxygen and more rapidly broken down by exposure to light. It is relatively stable to heat and dilute acids, but breaks down in alkaline conditions. The bioavailability of vitamin K from vegetables is only about 10–20 per cent, and fat is required to optimise uptake. The vitamin K present in oils is substantially more bioavailable.

Dietary fat is needed for absorption of vitamin K, and people on low-fat diets and those who do not absorb fats well may have inadequate levels. Digestive disorders associated with impaired fat absorption, such as gall bladder or pancreatic disorders, inflammatory bowel diseases and cystic fibrosis, reduce absorption of vitamin K. Absorption is also decreased by mineral oil taken as a laxative, drugs that inhibit cholesterol uptake, such as cholestyramine and colestipol, and the weight-loss drug orlistat. Excess vitamin A appears to interfere with vitamin K absorption and a form of vitamin E (tocopherol quinone) may inhibit vitamin K-dependent carboxylase enzymes.

Coumarin-based blood thinners (anticoagulants), such as warfarin, act by blocking the enzyme epoxide reductase that helps regenerate active vitamin K from its inactive form, thereby inhibiting blood clotting. Prolonged use of broad-spectrum antibiotics may destroy intestinal bacteria that synthesise vitamin K. Cephalosporins (antibiotics), salicylates (non-steroidal anti-inflammatory drugs), rifampicin and isoniazid (used for tuberculosis treatment), and anti-convulsants (used for epilepsy) may inhibit vitamin K metabolism. In pregnant women, warfarin, anticonvulsants, rifampicin and isoniazid have been shown to interfere with vitamin K synthesis in the foetus.

Daily requirement

Government recommendations by age and gender (see Table 5.8) can be found in *Nutrient Reference Values for Australia and New Zealand Including Recommended Dietary Intakes*, available at <www.nhmrc.gov.au>.

Table 5.8 Daily adequate intake (AI) of vitamin K (mcg/day)

Age (years)	Female AI	Male AI
0–6 months	2.0	2.0
7–12 months	2.5	2.5
1–3	25	25
4–8	35	35
9–13	45	45
14–18	55	55
19–70	60	70
>70	60	70
Pregnant women		
14–18	60	
19–50	60	
Lactating women		
14–18	60	
19–50	60	

Source: Nutrient Reference Values for Australia and New Zealand Including Recommended Dietary Intakes, National Health and Medical Research Council, Australian Government Department of Health and Ageing, Canberra and Ministry of Health, New Zealand, Wellington, 2006.

Deficiency effects

Vitamin K deficiency may be due to a dietary deficiency or the use of coumarin-based oral anticoagulants that prevent its recycling in the body. A deficiency causes the vitamin K-dependent proteins to be under-carboxylated, with fewer Gla residues and consequent loss of function. The biological half-life of vitamin K is relatively short, and animals deprived of vitamin K develop symptoms of deficiency within a few days. In a deficiency, vitamin K is conserved in the liver to support production of more vital vitamin K-dependent proteins, such as clotting factors, and the early signs of deficiency are under-carboxylation of the Gla proteins made in other tissues. It has been shown that, in apparently healthy subjects, a substantial fraction of osteocalcin and MGP occurs in under-carboxylated forms that have no biological activity, indicating that sub-clinical deficiency of vitamin K may be relatively common. Increased circulating levels of under-carboxylated osteocalcin have been shown to be associated with increased bone loss and osteoporosis in postmenopausal women, and under-carboxylated MGP has been associated with arterial calcification. Inadequate vitamin K is associated with delayed blood clotting, low bone mineral density, increased postmenopausal bone loss, increased risk of fractures, and arterial calcification and cardiovascular disease, particularly in diabetes, end-stage kidney disease and ageing.

Long-term use of coumarin-based anticoagulants, such as warfarin, increases the risk of developing osteoporosis, and arterial and heart valve calcification. The use in pregnancy of coumarin-based oral anti-coagulants or anti-convulsant medication to prevent seizures can result in vitamin K deficiency in the infant. Warfarin use, especially in early pregnancy, is associated with birth defects, including bone deformities, low birth weight, facial and eye abnormalities, and developmental retardation. Use in later pregnancy may result in haemorrhages in the foetus. Heparin does not cross the placental barrier, and is a more suitable anticoagulant in pregnancy.

Vitamin K deficiency bleeding

Newborn infants are usually deficient in vitamin K because of poor transport across the placenta, lack of bacteria in the colon and reduced efficiency of vitamin K recycling. Preterm infants and exclusively breastfed infants are more at risk. Breast milk contains low levels (1–2 mcg/L), but it is mandatory to fortify infant formula milks with at least 30 mcg/L of vitamin K. Vitamin K deficiency bleeding (VKDB) is a potentially life-threatening bleeding disorder in infants that is prevented by routinely injecting infants with vitamin K shortly after birth. In VKDB, bleeding may occur from the umbilicus, gastrointestinal tract, skin punctures, surgical sites and the brain.

- *Early VKDB*, occurring on the first day after birth, is rare and mainly confined to infants born to mothers who have taken medication during pregnancy that interferes with vitamin K metabolism.
- *Classical VKDB* occurs in the first week after birth, and is more common in infants who are unwell at birth or who have delayed onset of feeding.
- *Late VKDB* peaks at three to eight weeks, with most cases occurring at one to three months, although it can manifest up to twelve months of age, with a mortality of about 30 per cent. It usually affects fully breastfed infants, especially infants with underlying liver disease or other malabsorption disorders, indicated by prolonged jaundice, pale stools, and liver and spleen enlargement. The infant may have minor bruising or small bleeds before having a serious haemorrhage.

Indicators of inadequate levels may include:

- easy and pronounced bruising
- bleeding, including nosebleeds, bleeding gums, blood in the urine, blood in the faeces, tarry black faeces or heavy menstrual bleeding
- calcification of artery walls, atherosclerosis
- weak bones, low bone density
- insulin resistance
- age-related cognitive decline
- in infants, bruising, bleeding from the nose or mouth, bleeding within the skull, blood in the faeces, blood in the urine, bleeding from the umbilical cord or excessive bleeding after injections or surgical procedures.

Assessment of body status

Measurement of plasma PK levels is not commonly used because it reflects recent dietary intake and levels fluctuate rapidly; normal levels for adults are reported to be 0.29–2.64 nmol/L. The main assessment method is measurement of the activity of clotting factors. In a vitamin K deficiency, there is decreased activity of the vitamin K-dependent clotting factors II, VII, IX and X, and prolonged clotting time, with normal fibrinogen levels and platelet count. Clotting time is measured by prothrombin time (PT), which measures the time taken for clot formation after thromboplastin and calcium are added to plasma. The reference interval given by the RCPA for PT is eleven to fifteen seconds in adults, two to three seconds longer in newborns, and three to five seconds longer in preterm newborns. A similar test to PT is measurement of under-carboxylated forms of vitamin K-dependent clotting factors. PT is an insensitive and non-specific test for diagnosing vitamin K deficiency. One or more of the Gla clotting proteins has to fall below about 50 per cent of normal before the PT lengthens by 1–2 seconds, at which stage liver stores are severely depleted, and PT only reflects the vitamin K stores in the liver, not the degree of under-carboxylation of Gla proteins in other tissues.

Other tests include measurement of plasma concentrations of under-carboxylated prothrombin (the PIVKA-II test, the term being an abbreviation of 'proteins induced in vitamin K absence'), the percentage of under-carboxylated osteocalcin and urinary levels of gamma-carboxyglutamyl. Antibody tests for under-carboxylated species of osteocalcin and MGP have been developed, and plasma concentration of prothrombin can also be measured, with the reference range being 80–120 mcg/mL.

Case reports—vitamin K deficiency

- *A boy, four and a half years of age*, developed sudden onset left-sided paralysis of unexplained origin.[1] Tests showed that his clotting time was prolonged, and he was given intravenous vitamin K. His symptoms improved within 24 hours and he made a complete recovery within seven days.
- *A male infant, two months of age*, developed crying, progressive pallor, lethargy, poor feeding, abnormal posturing of limbs and asymmetry of eye opening.[2] He had been exclusively breastfed, and it was not known whether he had received vitamin K at birth. Clotting time was prolonged and a computed tomography (CT) scan showed extensive brain haemorrhage, indicating late-onset VKDB. The infant required brain surgery and drug treatment for seizures, and he was given vitamin K, which dramatically improved clotting time. At the time of discharge fourteen days after brain surgery, he was active and feeding well, his pupils were equal and reactive, and he was free of seizures, but he still had mild facial asymmetry and left-sided weakness.

- *A young man, nineteen years of age*, was admitted to hospital because of blood in his urine, low back pain, blood vesicles in the oral cavity and nose bleeds of unexplained origin.[3] He complained of headache and vomiting for three days and a CT scan revealed a brain haemorrhage. Coagulation tests showed prolonged blood clotting, with a PT greater than 120 seconds. He was given 1000 mL blood plasma daily for three days and 80 mg of PK daily. Blood in the urine resolved in one day and, three days after treatment, PT was 17.4 seconds. After administration of 240 mg daily of PK, the brain haemorrhage resolved in two weeks and clotting factors returned to normal in four weeks. After discharge, the patient was injected with 60 mg PK twice per week, but PT time increased and he was then given 240 mg daily of oral MK-4 which improved PT. The cause of his vitamin K deficiency could not be established.

REFERENCES

1 Shah, I.D., Vitamin K deficiency, *Pediatric Oncall* [serial online] (2004), 1: Art #1, retrieved 20 August 2014 from <www.pediatriconcall.com/Journal/Article/FullText.aspx?artid=679&type=J&tid=&imgid=&reportid=85&tbltype=>.

2 Gopakumar, H., Sivji, R. & Rajiv, P.K., Vitamin K deficiency bleeding presenting as impending brain herniation, *J Pediatr Neurosci* [serial online] (2010), 5: 55–8 retrieved 20 August 2014 from <www.pediatricneurosciences.com/text.asp?2010/5/1/55/66681>.

3 Chen, H.F., Wu, T.Q., Jin, L.J. et al., Treatment of vitamin K-dependent coagulation factor deficiency and subarachnoid hemorrhage, *World* (2011), 2(1): 73–6.

THERAPEUTIC USES OF VITAMIN K

VKDB

To prevent VKDB, it is routine practice in Australia to administer a single intramuscular (im) dose providing 1.0 mg of vitamin K to an infant shortly after birth.[1] Newborns with a birth weight of less than 1500 g require a smaller dose of 0.5 mg of im vitamin K. Markers of blood clotting improve at one to seven days after the dose. Intramuscular is the preferred delivery route because it raises plasma concentrations ten times higher than oral dosing. It is recommended that women who are taking medication known to interfere with vitamin K metabolism receive 20 mg of vitamin K daily for at least two weeks before birth and that their newborn infants should be given im vitamin K within four to six hours of birth.

In 1992, a study described an association between im administration of vitamin K and childhood cancer and leukaemia.[2] Although other studies did not confirm this finding, there appeared to be a consistent trend towards a small, increased incidence of acute lymphoblastic leukaemia associated with the product in use at the time, Konakion®, a vitamin K product that also contained cremophor EL, a solubiliser made up of propylene glycol, phenol and polyethylated castor oil. Cremaphor EL-containing preparations have been associated with anaphylaxis following intravenous (iv) use, local irritation when given im and gastrointestinal irritation with oral use.

Because of the controversy, oral doses of vitamin K were introduced in Australia, but this led to the occurrence of some cases of late VKDB. This may have occurred because of failure to adhere to the dosage delivery schedule or because oral doses are not well absorbed, especially if the infant has a digestive disorder, and do not last as long in the body. The Konakion® cremophor formulation has been replaced by a mixed micelles formulation, and im delivery is the preferred method of protection.

Low bone mineral density

Vitamin K deficiency causes under-carboxylation of osteocalcin, low bone mineral density and increased risk of fractures. People with the highest vitamin K intake have been found to have a 65 per cent lower risk of hip fracture than those with the lowest intake.[3] Patients with osteoporotic fractures have been shown to have low serum levels of PK and menaquinone, especially MK-7 and MK-8.[4]

Vitamin K supplementation has been shown to reduce the level of under-carboxylated osteocalcin and improve bone turnover.[5] However, it appears that the amount of vitamin K needed for optimal carboxylation of osteocalcin is significantly higher than can be obtained from the diet alone. Phytonadione (1 mg daily) and menaquinone (45 mg daily) have been shown to rapidly reduce the level of under-carboxylated osteocalcin and, in one study, to reduce fracture risk.[6] A review of thirteen studies concluded that supplementation with PK and MK-4 reduces bone loss and that MK-4 had a strong protective effect against fractures among Japanese patients.[7] Vitamin K appears to work synergistically with vitamin D and female hormone replacement therapy to maintain bone density.

Calcification in blood vessel walls

In atherosclerosis, inflammation in blood vessel walls and accumulation of dead cells leads to calcium deposition, which results in decreased arterial function, enlargement of the left ventricle of the heart and decreased coronary blood flow, as well as instability of atheromas, leading to increased risk of a rupture and clot formation. All these factors increase the risk of fatal complications. Vascular calcification is a strong, independent risk factor for cardiovascular death, and an important predictor of all-cause mortality, vascular complications and heart attack (myocardial infarction, MI).

Arterial calcification is an active, cell-controlled process that has features in common with bone metabolism. In animals, widespread arterial calcification occurs in those that do not express MGP or are unable to carboxylate it.[8] Vitamin K antagonists, such as warfarin, have been shown to cause extensive calcification of the vascular arteries and aortic heart valves.[9] Vitamin K has been shown to increase MGP carboxylation and induce regression of vascular calcification caused by vitamin K antagonists.[10]

Concurrent arterial calcification and osteoporosis occur frequently in postmenopausal women, and has been termed the 'calcification paradox'. In postmenopausal women, daily supplementation with 1 mg of PK, together with 8 mcg of vitamin D3 and minerals (500 mg of calcium, 150 mg of magnesium and 10 mg of zinc) for three years prevented loss of carotid artery elasticity compared with subjects on placebo and those taking vitamin D and minerals without vitamin K.[11] However, it appears that menaquinone supplementation may be more effective than PK for prevention of vascular calcification, possibly because PK is taken up preferentially by the liver and is less available to other tissues. A higher dietary intake of menaquinone has been linked to reduced aortic and coronary calcification, and lower incidence of coronary heart disease.[12,13]

Insulin sensitivity

The level of undercarboxylated osteocalcin in serum has been shown to be associated with fasting plasma glucose, insulin resistance and increased serum osteocalcin, and lowering the amounts of undercarboxylated osteocalcin is associated with an improvement in insulin secretion and sensitivity.[14] A small study of healthy young men found that vitamin K2 supplementation increased insulin sensitivity, which was associated with increased levels of carboxylated osteocalcin.[15]

Stabilising warfarin therapy

Failure of the anticoagulant effect of warfarin can occur with variations in vitamin K intake. Patients on warfarin are often advised to maintain their usual dietary pattern, and to report any planned changes in diet or in the use of supplements. Stability of the diet is more important than avoiding vitamin K-rich foods, and vegetable intake should not be restricted.

Vitamin K supplementation (150 mcg daily) has been found to improve stability in patients with unstable control of anticoagulation, possibly because it leads to a more consistent intake of vitamin K.[16] A limited amount of research has raised the possibility of the potential danger of giving PK in combination with warfarin, because it is preferentially taken up by the liver and the increased warfarin needed to compensate for the higher vitamin K intake may exhaust vitamin K supplies in the vascular system and increase calcification risk. Animals given PK with warfarin have developed widespread arterial calcification within two to four weeks, but the effect in humans is not clear.[17] Menaquinones, which are predominantly used by tissues other than the liver, may be a better choice for use with warfarin therapy.

In warfarin overdose, a prothrombin complex concentrate and fresh frozen plasma are given with vitamin K.[18] Oral or iv vitamin K can be used; the oral dose is usually 1–2 mg or up to 5 mg if required, and the iv dose is usually 0.5–1.0 mg or up to 10 mg if required. Large doses may cause some resistance to re-anticoagulation with warfarin and lower doses are preferred.

REFERENCES

1 National Health and Medical Research Council (NHMRC), *Joint statement and recommendations on Vitamin K administration to newborn infants to prevent vitamin K deficiency bleeding in infancy—October 2010* (the Joint Statement), NHMRC, Canberra, 2010.

2 Golding, J., Greenwood, R., Birmingham, K. & Mott, M., Childhood cancer, intramuscular vitamin K, and pethidine given during labour, *BMJ* (1992), 305(6849): 341–6.

3 Booth, S.L., Tucker, K.L., Chen, H. et al., Dietary vitamin K intakes are associated with hip fracture but not with bone mineral density in elderly men and women, *Am J Clin Nutr* (2000), 71(5): 1201–8.

4 Hodges, S.J., Akesson, K. & Vergnaud, P. et al., Circulating levels of vitamins K1 and K2 decreased in elderly women with hip fracture, *J Bone Miner Res* (1993), 8(10): 1241–5.

5 Bügel, S., Vitamin K and bone health in adult humans, *Vitam Horm* (2008), 78: 393–416.

6 Adams, J. & Pepping, J., Vitamin K in the treatment and prevention of osteoporosis and arterial calcification, *Am J Health Syst Pharm* (2005), 62(15): 1574–81.

7 Cockayne, S., Adamson, J., Lanham-New, S. et al., Vitamin K and the prevention of fractures: Systematic review and meta-analysis of randomized controlled trials, *Arch Intern Med* (2006), 166(12): 1256–61.

8 Luo, G., Ducy, P., McKee, M.D.P. et al., Spontaneous calcification of arteries and cartilage in mice lacking matrix GLA protein, *Nature* (1997), 386(6620): 78–81.

9 Palaniswamy, C., Sekhri, A., Aronow, W.S. et al., Association of warfarin use with valvular and vascular calcification: A review, *Clin Cardiol* (2011), 34(2): 74–81.

10 Schurgers, L.J., Spronk, H.M., Soute, B.A. et al., Regression of warfarin-induced medial elastocalcinosis by high intake of vitamin K in rats, *Blood* (2007), 109(7): 2823–31.

11 Braam, L.A., Hoeks, A.P., Brouns, F. et al., Beneficial effects of vitamins D and K on the elastic properties of the vessel wall in postmenopausal women: A follow-up study, *Thromb Haemost* (2004), 91(2): 373–80.

12 Shea, M.K. & Holden, R.M., Vitamin K status and vascular calcification: Evidence from observational and clinical studies, *Adv Nutr* (2012), 3(2): 158–65.

13 Gast, G.C., de Roos, N.M., Sluijs, I. et al., A high menaquinone intake reduces the incidence of coronary heart disease, *Nutr Metab Cardiovasc Dis* (2009), 19(7): 504–10.

14 Iki, M., Tamaki, J., Fujita, Y. et al., Serum undercarboxylated osteocalcin levels are inversely associated with glycemic status and insulin resistance in an elderly Japanese male population: Fujiwara-kyo Osteoporosis Risk in Men (FORMEN) Study, *Osteoporos Int* (2012), 23(2): 761–70.

15 Choi, H.J., Yu, J., Choi, H. et al., Vitamin K2 supplementation improves insulin sensitivity via osteocalcin metabolism: a placebo-controlled trial, *Diabetes Care* (2011), 34(9): e147.

16 Sconce, E., Avery, P., Wynne, H. & Kamali, F., Vitamin K supplementation can improve stability of anticoagulation for patients with unexplained variability in response to warfarin, *Blood* (2007), 109(6): 2419–23.

17 Price, P.A., Faus, S.A. & Williamson, M.K., Warfarin causes rapid calcification of the elastic lamellae in rat arteries and heart valves, *Arterioscler Thromb Vasc Biol* (1998), 18(9): 1400–7.

18 Baker, R.I., Coughlin, P.B., Salem, H.H. et al., Warfarin reversal: Consensus guidelines, on behalf of the Australasian Society of Thrombosis and Haemostasis, *Med J Aust* (2004), 181(9): 492–7.

Therapeutic dose

The daily intake of PK required for the carboxylation of blood coagulation factors appears to be 90 mcg for adult women and 120 mcg for adult men. A PK dose of 1 mg daily and a menaquinone dose of 45 mg daily have each been used to improve under-carboxylation of osteocalcin without evidence of adverse effects. For prevention of bone loss in postmenopausal women, a dose of 45 mg daily of MK-4 has been found to be effective and a dose of 1.5 mg daily has been found to reduce the amount of under-carboxylated osteocalcin. MK-7 supplementation of 75 mcg daily has been shown to increase the carboxylation of circulating osteocalcin and MGP with no adverse effects on clotting.

- *Infants:* a single im dose providing 1.0 mg of vitamin K soon after birth is recommended. For oral dosing, three doses of 2 mg need to be given, the first on the day of birth, the second three to five days later and the third at four weeks of age.
- *Bleeding disorders caused by vitamin K deficiency:* 2.5–25 mg of phytonadione has been used. To counteract bleeding from a warfarin overdose, 1–5 mg of vitamin K has been used but the precise dose is determined by measuring the international normalised ratio (INR), a blood-clotting test used to assess warfarin dose. The target INR for people maintained on warfarin therapy is 2–3.
- *Cystic fibrosis (CF) patients:* recommended daily doses are 150–500 mcg from birth to three years, and 300–500 mcg from four years to adulthood. However, sub-optimal vitamin K status is common in children and young adults with CF on standard CF supplements. It appears that high-dose vitamin K (at least 1 mg daily) is required to achieve a vitamin K status similar to that of healthy people.

Effects of excess

Natural vitamin K appears to have no adverse effects at doses commonly used. No adverse effects have been reported in mothers or infants after administration of vitamin K during pregnancy. Very high dietary or supplementary intakes of vitamin K may inhibit the anticoagulant effect of vitamin K antagonists. Older formulations of vitamin K used for VKDB have caused adverse effects, apparently caused by the Cremophor EL solubiliser in the preparation, which is no longer used. Synthetic vitamin K (menadione) may damage the liver in high doses and, when given to newborn infants, has been linked to destruction of red blood cells (haemolysis), haemolytic anaemia and jaundice.

Supplements

Vitamin K is available in Australia as phytomenadione (phytonadione), and can be made commercially by condensation of menadione with natural phytol. It has the same biological activity as PK.

Konakion® MM Paediatric

This formulation is used for VKDB. It contains 2 mg per 0.2 mL of phytomenadione, and is a mixed micelles formulation that also contains sodium glycocholate (bile acid) and lecithin, which act to solubilise vitamin K in an aqueous medium.

Cautions

Vitamin K counteracts anticoagulant medication, so people on anticoagulant therapy should seek medical advice before commencing vitamin K supplementation.

HOW MUCH DO I KNOW?

Choose whether the following statements are true or false. Then review this chapter for the correct answers.

	True (T)	False (F)
1 An excess or a deficiency of retinol in pregnancy may cause birth defects.	T	F
2 Retinol helps form the eye pigment rhodopsin.	T	F

		T	F
3	Epithelial cells develop abnormally in vitamin A deficiency.	T	F
4	The active form of vitamin D is 25(OH)D.	T	F
5	Osteomalacia is caused by vitamin D toxicity.	T	F
6	Adequate amounts of vitamin D can be obtained from standard diets.	T	F
7	Gamma-tocopherol is the predominant form of tocopherol in the diet.	T	F
8	Vitamin E has antioxidant and anti-inflammatory activity.	T	F
9	Matrix Gla protein (MGP) is mainly produced by cartilage-forming cells and smooth muscle cells in blood vessel walls.	T	F
10	Vitamin K helps activate some of the clotting factors in the blood.	T	F

FURTHER READING

Braun, L. & Cohen, M., *Herbs & natural supplements: An evidence-based guide,* 3rd ed., Churchill Livingstone Elsevier. 2010.

Gropper, S.S., Smith, J.L. & Groff, J.L., *Advanced nutrition and human metabolism*, 5th ed., Thomson Wadsworth, Belmont, CA, 2009.

Higdon, J., *An evidence-based approach to vitamins and minerals*, Thieme, New York, 2003.

Linus Pauling Institute, *Micronutrient Information Center*, available at <lpi.oregonstate.edu/infocenter>.

6

Water-soluble vitamins: vitamins C, B1, B2 and B3

VITAMIN C (ASCORBIC ACID)

VITAMIN C STATUS CHECK

1. Do your gums bleed when you brush your teeth?
2. Do you have swollen or inflamed gums, gum infections and/or loose teeth?
3. Do you bruise easily and/or have small spots of bleeding underneath your skin?
4. Do you have low resistance to infections?

'Yes' answers may indicate inadequate vitamin C status. Note that a number of nutritional deficiencies or health disorders can cause similar effects and further investigation is recommended.

Vitamin C, also known as ascorbic acid or ascorbate, is a water-soluble six-carbon lactone. A deficiency leads to scurvy, a life-threatening disorder recorded throughout history, especially whenever people were deprived of fresh fruit and vegetables for extended periods of time. Scurvy was particularly prevalent in soldiers during prolonged campaigns and in sailors during the early sea voyages of exploration, killing as many as two million sailors between 1500 and 1800.

FAST FACTS . . . VITAMIN C

- Vitamin C is found in fresh fruit and vegetables.
- It is required for the integrity of connective tissue throughout the body.
- It is a potent antioxidant and supports immunity.
- A deficiency causes scurvy, indicated by spontaneous bleeding and bruising, gum disease, and painful muscles and joints.
- Supplementation may be helpful during infections and for cardiovascular disease, low bone mineral density, brain function and cataract prevention.

In 1747, British naval physician James Lind found that oranges and lemons cured scurvy, but the curative factor in these foods was not identified. In 1928, the Hungarian biochemist Albert Szent-Györgyi isolated a substance from adrenal glands that he called hexuronic acid, and discovered that it was identical to a substance he had isolated from capsicums. It was renamed ascorbic acid (vitamin C), and in 1932 its chemical structure was established and its connection to scurvy was discovered. Szent-Györgyi won the

1937 Nobel Prize in Physiology or Medicine for his work on biological oxidation and vitamin C.

Vitamin C is an unusual vitamin because almost all animals make it in their bodies as required, and they make it in much higher quantities than can be obtained from food. In these animals, glucuronate derived from glucose is converted to gulonate by the enzyme aldehyde reductase, which is then converted to gulonolactone by a lactonase enzyme. Finally, gulonolactone is converted to ascorbic acid by the enzyme gulonolactone oxidase. Some animal species, including humans, apes, guinea pigs, fruit-eating bats, insects, fish and some birds, cannot make the enzyme gulonolactone oxidase, and therefore cannot make vitamin C. Humans have the gene for this enzyme, but research shows that it underwent mutation about 40 million years ago during evolution and no longer functions. Because we lack the enzyme needed to make ascorbic acid, some vitamin C experts claim that humans suffer from a genetic deficiency disorder called 'hypoascorbaemia', meaning 'low levels of vitamin C in the blood', that may contribute to susceptibility to infections and many chronic diseases.

Digestion, absorption and transport

Vitamin C exists in two forms in food and in the body: the reduced form ascorbic acid (AsA) and the oxidised form dehydroascorbic acid (DHAsA). Both forms are absorbed easily. AA is the common abbreviation for ascorbic acid but, to avoid confusion with arachidonic acid which is also abbreviated to AA, the abbreviation AsA will be used for ascorbic acid in this text. AsA absorption in the small intestine and transport into tissue cells is facilitated by two sodium-dependent vitamin C transporters (SVCT1 and SVCT2). SVCT1 has a high capacity but low affinity for AsA, and is found mainly in epithelial cells of the intestine and liver, and also the kidneys, in which it reabsorbs AsA, thereby reducing urinary losses and maintaining body levels. SVCT2 has a lower capacity but higher affinity for AsA, and is found in specialised tissues, such as the brain and eyes, and also the placenta, in which it transports AsA to the foetus during pregnancy. DHAsA is absorbed by passive diffusion or by a sodium-independent process that utilises the glucose transporters GLUT1 and GLUT3. Although DHAsA is absorbed at a higher rate than AsA, it is rapidly converted to AsA in body cells.

In apparently healthy people, absorption of vitamin C decreases with increasing doses, and frequent lower doses appear to be more effective for maintaining body levels. It is estimated that 87 per cent of a one-off 30 mg dose is absorbed, 80 per cent of a 100 mg dose, 72 per cent of a 200 mg dose, 63 per cent of a 500 mg dose and less than 50 per cent of a 1250 mg dose. Assuming a 40 per cent absorption and a dose of 1250 mg, the amount absorbed would be 500 mg, which is still considerably more than is achievable by lower dosing. Absorption of higher doses is reported to increase in disease states, but evidence is lacking.

Plasma concentration is tightly controlled when vitamin C is taken orally. At high doses, production of SVCT1 is reduced in the kidneys, which increases urinary excretion, and less SVCT1 is produced in the intestine, which reduces absorption. The plasma half-life of vitamin C is reported as eight to 40 days during periods of low intake and about 30 minutes at high intake. There is controversy about the point at which plasma becomes saturated with vitamin C, with some researchers suggesting saturation occurs at about 70 μmol/L and others suggesting about 220 μmol/L. It is estimated that a one-off oral dose of 3 g produces a peak plasma concentration of 206 μmol/L and a dose of 1.25 g produces a peak plasma concentration of 187 μmol/L. Intravenous delivery produces plasma concentrations that are 30- to 70-fold higher than are achievable by oral doses.

Absorbed vitamin C diffuses into the capillaries in the intestinal wall and circulates in the bloodstream, mainly in the unbound form. SVCT1 and SVCT2 transport AsA into body cells and GLUT1 and GLUT3 transport DHAsA into body cells, together with GLUT4 in insulin-sensitive tissues. The concentration of AsA inside cells is up to 40-fold higher than the plasma concentration. The pituitary gland and adrenal gland cortex are particularly rich in vitamin C, and high levels are found in white blood cells, the brain, liver, spleen, pancreas, lungs and kidneys.

Metabolism, storage and excretion

Vitamin C acts in body fluids as a potent antioxidant. During metabolism, AsA is oxidised to the ascorbyl radical (semidehydroascorbate), which is relatively unreactive and is rapidly removed by oxidation to form DHAsA or by reaction with another ascorbyl radical to form AsA and DHAsA. DHAsA can be recycled to AsA by dihydrolipoic acid, thioredoxin, or the glutathione enzyme system or it can be irreversibly broken down to 2,3-diketogulonic acid in the liver and kidneys and then to 5-carbon sugars, including xylonate and lyxonate, or to oxalic acid and the 4-carbon sugar threonate. The sugars can be oxidised, releasing carbon dioxide and water, or used as building blocks for cell components. Oxalic acid is excreted in urine. There is no significant storage of vitamin C in the body.

Functions

Vitamin C is an electron donor, which acts as an antioxidant and has a cofactor-like role in a number of enzymes involved in hydroxylation reactions, in which it maintains metal ions in the enzymes in a reduced state necessary for enzyme function. Vitamin C functions include the following.

- *Collagen formation.* Collagen is a fibrous protein that is made by connective tissue cells and is exported to the extracellular matrix to provide structural strength. The amino acids proline and lysine are key components of collagen. Vitamin C is needed to maintain iron in the ferrous state (Fe^{2+}) in the enzymes prolyl 4-hydroxylase, prolyl 3-hydroxylase and lysyl hydroxylase, which hydroxylate proline and lysine. Hydroxylation converts the collagen precursor procollagen to strong, mature collagen. Vitamin C supports wound healing and maintenance of the intercellular matrix (ground substance) in connective tissue. It maintains the integrity of the skin, blood vessels, heart valves, tendons, spinal discs, gums, bones, teeth and the cornea and lens of the eyes. It may also assist production of other connective tissue substances such as elastin and the proteoglycans that are part of joint cartilage, gums, bones and skin.
- *Antioxidant activity.* Vitamin C is a potent water-soluble antioxidant that scavenges almost all reactive oxygen species (ROS) and reactive nitrogen species (RNS). It removes superoxide, hydroxyl, nitroxide, hydroperoxyl and aqueous peroxyl radicals, as well as peroxynitrite, singlet oxygen, ozone, nitrogen dioxide and hypochlorous acid. It converts superoxide radicals to hydrogen peroxide and then to water, converts hydroxyl and aqueous peroxyl radicals to water, and converts peroxyl radicals to lipid peroxides, which are then removed by the glutathione system.

  Vitamin C has been shown to reduce oxidation of protein, nuclear and mitochondrial DNA and lipids, including LDL cholesterol. During detoxification, it activates cytochrome P450 enzymes in the liver and protects microsomal membranes against lipid peroxidation and protein oxidation. It has an important protective role in the bloodstream, because it can prevent damage to plasma lipids and cell membranes by trapping aqueous peroxyl radicals before they can attack lipids and cause peroxidative damage. Once vitamin C has been used up, the remaining water-soluble antioxidants (urate, bilirubin and the protein thiols) can trap only some of the aqueous peroxyl radicals; the remainder diffuse into lipids and initiate lipid peroxidation. Vitamin E is then required as a chain-breaking antioxidant to reduce further free radical damage. Vitamin C maintains vitamin E activity by converting the tocopheroxyl radical back to alpha-tocopherol, and may also regenerate urate, glutathione and beta-carotene from their radical forms.

  Vitamin C has a potential pro-oxidant role by donating electrons to copper (Cu^{2+}) to form Cu^{+} and to ferric iron (Fe^{3+}) to form ferrous iron (Fe^{2+}), which can act as oxidants. However, this function may not have physiological relevance because vitamin C only reacts with free metal ions, and iron and copper are bound to proteins in the body.
- *Immunity and anti-inflammatory activity.* Immune cells accumulate vitamin C at levels up to 100-fold higher than plasma levels, and it is rapidly consumed during infections. Vitamin C increases resistance to infections by increasing the activity of T cells, natural killer (NK) cells and phagocytes, and increasing production of the antiviral protein interferon. It may also increase production of antibodies. Vitamin C has a pro-oxidant and antioxidant role in infections. Phagocytes generate superoxide radicals, which react with hydrogen peroxide generated by vitamin C to form highly reactive hydroxyl radicals that destroy bacteria. Vitamin C also protects phagocytes and other immune cells, as well as body tissues, from free radical damage caused by immune activity. Vitamin C increases production of nitric oxide (NO) in macrophages, which has antibiotic and lymphocyte-regulating functions, and is a cofactor for the production of carnitine, which stimulates immunoglobulin production and immune responses. Vitamin C helps control inflammation by reducing

histamine levels and deceasing production of the inflammatory eicosanoid PGE_2.

- *Anticancer activity.* Vitamin C has antioxidant activity that may protect DNA from damage, and is a cofactor for hydroxylase enzymes that repair DNA damage and reduce the risk of mutations. It supports immune function, stabilises p53 (a protein involved in cell proliferation control), activates apoptosis of abnormal cells and reduces production of insulin-like growth factor, PGE_2 and nuclear factor kappa-B (NF-kappaB), which stimulate tumour growth. Ascorbic acid oxidation products such as DHAsA, hydrogen peroxide, 2,3-diketogulonic acid, 5-methyl 1-3, 4-dehydroxytetrone, gamma-cronolactone and 3-hydroxy-2-pyrone have been shown to have anti-tumour activity. Vitamin C appears to potentiate the actions of cancer chemotherapy.

  The breakdown of ground substance surrounding tumours is identical to the connective tissue breakdown that occurs in severe vitamin C deficiency, and vitamin C may be protective by strengthening ground substance and creating a dense fibrous barrier around tumours, which reduces tumour growth and metastasis. Tumours use anaerobic metabolism (glycolysis) to provide energy and survive in a low-oxygen environment by activating hypoxia-inducible factor 1alpha (HIF-1alpha), and vitamin C promotes oxidative metabolism and reduces expression of HIF-1alpha, which may reduce tumour growth. When present in high levels in extracellular fluid, vitamin C selectively kills cancer cells, which is believed to be due to the generation of hydrogen peroxide by vitamin C and the consequent formation of hydroxyl radicals and aldehydes that damage cell membranes. Hydrogen peroxide has dose-dependent effects on cell function; at low levels, it may stimulate cell growth and at high levels, it may cause growth arrest, apoptosis and eventually cell death (necrosis). Cancer cells may be more susceptible to hydrogen peroxide and its metabolites because of a reduced amount of antioxidant enzymes such as catalases.

  In vegetables belonging to the cabbage (brassica or cruciferae) family, tissue disruption triggers the conversion of glucobrassicin to indole-3-carbinol, which then reacts with vitamin C to form ascorbigen (ABG). ABG induces phase I and II enzymes in detoxification pathways, has immune-stimulating activity that may protect against infections and cancer, and appears to inhibit tumour growth.

  Vitamin C appears to have a protective role in stomach cancer, which is associated with chronic infection with the bacteria *Helicobacter pylori* and the reaction of dietary nitrite with amines and amides in the stomach that produces carcinogenic N-nitroso compounds (NOCs), such as nitrosamines and nitrosamides. *H. pylori* infection increases consumption of vitamin C and reduces its secretion into the gastric lumen. Vitamin C boosts the immune response, has anti-inflammatory activity and acts as a scavenger of ROS formed in the gastric mucosa and inhibits NOC production. NOCs also contribute to cancer of the oesophagus and nasopharynx.

- *Amino acid metabolism and hormone activation.* Production of carnitine from the amino acids lysine and methionine requires vitamin C as a cofactor, together with iron, vitamin B3 and vitamin B6. Carnitine stimulates immune responses and enables transport of fatty acids into mitochondria for use in energy production. Vitamin C is required for histamine breakdown, conversion of phenylalanine to tyrosine and activation of a number of hormones, including aldosterone, cortisol, calcitonin, cholecystokinin, thyrotropin, oxytocin and vasopressin, as well as corticotropin-releasing factor and growth hormone-releasing factor.
- *Neurotransmitter metabolism.* Vitamin C is a cofactor for monooxygenase enzymes that convert dopamine to noradrenaline (norepinephrine) and tryptophan to serotonin. Noradrenaline is a neurotransmitter that increases attention and arousal, and is part of the stress response, and serotonin is a neurotransmitter that regulates sleep, pain perception, body temperature, blood pressure and hormonal activity.

  Vitamin C supports embryonic brain development and differentiation, and is an inhibitor of acetylcholinesterase, the enzyme that breaks down the neurotransmitter acetylcholine. Maintaining acetylcholine levels in the brain promotes cholinergic activity, which affects cognition, memory, learning and behaviour.
- *Circulation.* Vitamin C protects blood lipids and LDL cholesterol from oxidation damage, and reduces serum levels of LDL cholesterol and triglycerides. It lowers serum cholesterol levels by acting as a cofactor for the hydroxylase enzyme that removes cholesterol from the body by converting it to bile acids. Vitamin C increases NO production in blood vessels, which dilates blood vessels, lowers blood

pressure and improves blood flow. It may help to prevent initiation of atherosclerosis by maintaining the integrity of blood vessels and preventing adhesion of monocytes to the endothelium.

- *Iron absorption and folate metabolism*. In the digestive tract, vitamin C donates an electron to ferric iron found in plant foods to convert it to the ferrous form, which is absorbed better. By improving iron uptake, the uptake of the toxic metal lead is reduced. Vitamin C appears to improve folate bioavailability and supports folic acid metabolism by maintaining levels of the active form, tetrahydrofolate.

Dietary sources

Vitamin C is found in rose hips, acerola cherries, blackcurrants, guava, cantaloupe (rockmelon), citrus fruit, kiwi fruit, strawberries, pawpaw (papaya), capsicum, chillies, rosehips, parsley, broccoli, Brussels sprouts, cabbage, cauliflower, chives, mustard greens, horseradish, asparagus, artichokes, radishes, chicory, green leafy vegetables, zucchini and ripe tomatoes. In general, fresh and raw fruit, vegetables and juices are more reliable sources.

The Food Standards Australia New Zealand nutrient database (NUTTAB) at <www.foodstandards.gov.au> provides the amounts found in specific foods.

Factors influencing body status

Vitamin C in food is easily destroyed by exposure to heat, light, air and alkaline solutions, and deteriorates during storage and food preparation—especially when fruit and vegetables are soaked or cut up and left exposed to air. It is leached out of foods by water processing and cooking methods. In general, cooking leads to losses of 50 per cent or more. Acid solutions preserve vitamin C and pickled vegetables, such as pickled cabbage (sauerkraut), retain much of their vitamin C content. Freezing preserves vitamin C, but there are considerable losses during thawing. Contact with copper, bronze, brass, steel or cast iron pots or utensils destroys vitamin C by enhancing its oxidation. To maximise vitamin C intake, use fresh raw foods, cut up vegetables or fruit immediately before eating, avoid dicing vegetables very finely, cook vegetables in the minimum amount of water or stir fry, cook food for the shortest possible time and avoid storing and reheating cooked foods.

Diabetics may have an increased requirement because their plasma levels of vitamin C are about 30 per cent lower than those of non-diabetics, and elevated blood glucose levels may interfere with DHAsA transport into cells by GLUT transporters. Production of the ascorbic acid transporter SVCT1 in the liver has been shown to decline with ageing in animals. Exposure to cigarette smoke and pollutants increases destruction of vitamin C, and it is used up rapidly during stress and infections. Vitamin C enhances iron absorption but high-dose iron supplements can oxidise vitamin C and increase needs.

Bioflavonoids are claimed to increase the absorption of vitamin C. In one study, vitamin C given in a natural citrus extract was found to be more slowly absorbed but 35 per cent more bioavailable than ascorbic acid alone, but another study found no difference in bioavailability between ascorbic acid and ascorbic acid with bioflavonoids.

Daily requirement

Government recommendations by age and gender (see Table 6.1) can be found in *Nutrient Reference Values for Australia and New Zealand Including Recommended Dietary Intakes*, available at <www.nhmrc.gov.au>.

Table 6.1 Recommended dietary intake (RDI) of vitamin C (mg/day)

Age (years)	Female RDI	Male RDI
1–3	35	35
4–8	35	35
9–13	40	40
14–18	40	40
19–70	45	45
>70	45	45
Pregnant women		
14–18	55	
19–50	60	
Lactating women		
14–18	80	
19–50	85	

Source: Nutrient Reference Values for Australia and New Zealand Including Recommended Dietary Intakes, National Health and Medical Research Council, Australian Government Department of Health and Ageing, Canberra and Ministry of Health, New Zealand, Wellington, 2006.

Deficiency effects

A severe lack of vitamin C causes scurvy, in which there is defective connective tissue production and a generalised disintegration of ground substance in the lining tissues of the body. This leads to tissue damage, ulceration, infections, blood vessel breakdown, oedema and haemorrhages, and cells revert to a primitive form because they are unable to differentiate normally. Capillary walls leak blood, leading to red spots or patches of bleeding under the skin (petechiae); extensive bruising; bleeding gums; nose bleeds; bleeding into the skin, muscles and joints; splinter-like haemorrhages under the nails; oedema; back pain; and swollen, painful, tender muscles and joints. Petechiae may affect large areas of the skin and the feet may become red and inflamed. The skin becomes dry and rough, body hair deforms into a coiled shape, scalp hair is lost and red lumps form around hair follicles (perifollicular hyperkeratosis). Wounds fail to heal and old scars may break down. Teeth loosen and fall out, and gums enlarge, forming 'scurvy buds' (gum tissue overgrowth that can extend to cover the teeth), and become spongy, susceptible to infections, and either pale or red and inflamed. A severe deficiency may result in a cerebral or myocardial (heart muscle) haemorrhage, causing sudden death on exertion, which was common among sailors with scurvy centuries ago who were treated as malingerers and forced to work. Anaemia is estimated to occur in 75 per cent of scurvy cases, with iron and folate deficiencies and blood loss as contributing factors.

A vitamin C deficiency may cause mood changes, depression, irritability, lethargy, lowered resistance to stress, gallstones, osteoporosis, joint cartilage and spinal disc disorders, susceptibility to infections and anaemia with pallor, fatigue and shortness of breath. Inadequate vitamin C contributes to atherosclerosis because cholesterol concentrations increase in the liver and bloodstream, LDL cholesterol becomes more susceptible to oxidation, and the lining of arteries is weakened, leading to cholesterol accumulation in artery walls. The development of Sjögren's syndrome, an autoimmune disorder causing dry eyes and mouth, and swelling and tenderness of the glands around the face and neck, has been associated with experimentally induced scurvy.

Scurvy in infants is also called Moeller-Barlow disease. It features irritability, tenderness of the legs, and an unwillingness to move because of pain. Infants cry when picked up and handled, and may adopt a particular posture while lying down, in which the legs are flexed at the knees and splayed out ('frog-leg' position), the head is retracted and the back arched. Infants fail to thrive and may have poor appetite and growth, irritability, hair loss, pale or red gums, swollen gums, bleeding gums during teething, bruises, low resistance to infections, allergies, poor bone development and beading of ribs (called the 'scorbutic rosary' and similar to the beading of the ribs that occurs in the vitamin D deficiency disorder rickets). During growth, bony changes occur at the junction between the end of the bone shaft and the growth cartilage. The collagen-containing bone matrix fails to develop, but the growth plate continues to calcify and thicken. Bones become brittle and develop microscopic fractures, seen on x-ray as a ground glass appearance between the bone shaft and the calcified cartilage. The lateral aspect of the calcified cartilage can project as a spur. The fibrous sheath (periosteum) covering the bone loosens, resulting in subperiosteal haemorrhage at the ends of the long bones.

Early signs of inadequate vitamin C levels in adults are fatigue, lethargy, depression, weakness, irritability, susceptibility to infections, easy bruising, bleeding gums when brushing the teeth, gum infections and vague, dull, aching pains in the legs and feet. In a study of the effects of vitamin C deficiency in the 1940s, subjects given a diet devoid of vitamin C developed undetectable plasma vitamin C levels between weeks four and eleven. Subjects developed hyperkeratoses of hair follicles and haemorrhages between weeks seventeen and twenty. At 30 weeks, gum changes occurred and purplish, swollen, spongy and bleeding gums developed at 36 weeks. At 26 weeks, wounds failed to heal and joints became painful and stiff. One subject developed severe pain and breathing difficulties the day after heavy physical exercise in the 36th week. He was given 1 g of vitamin C and the symptoms disappeared within 24 hours. The other subjects were then given a daily supplement of 10 mg of vitamin C and all showed improvement after two weeks, their skin normalised after eight weeks and their gums recovered after ten to fourteen weeks.

Indicators of inadequate levels may include:

- increased susceptibility to infections, colds and flu
- easy bruising, nose bleeds, bleeding gums when brushing the teeth, swollen spongy gums, red or pale gums, enlargement of gums, gum infections, loosening and loss of teeth
- circulatory disorders, atherosclerosis
- petechiae, poor wound healing, dry, wrinkled skin, dry eyes and mouth
- fluid retention
- low resistance to stress, stress-related disorders
- fatigue, iron-deficiency anaemia, lack of stamina, muscle soreness after exercise
- back, joint or muscle pain and stiffness, disorders of spinal discs

- depression, irritability, lack of appetite
- *infants*: poor appetite and growth, irritability, immobility, frog-leg posture, legs swollen or tender to touch, crying when handled, bruising, infections, bleeding gums during teething.

Assessment of body status

The plasma concentration of ascorbic acid reflects recent dietary intake, and leukocyte concentration is a better measure of the body pool of vitamin C. The reference range for AsA given by the Royal College of Pathologists of Australasia (RCPA) is 30–80 µmol/L for plasma and 1.1–3.0 µmol/10^9 leukocytes for adults. In most cases of scurvy, plasma levels are lower than 11 µmol/L.

Case reports—vitamin C deficiency

- *A man, 45 years of age*, developed anaemia thought to be caused by a bleeding duodenal ulcer.[1] However, the anaemia did not resolve, despite blood transfusions and ulcer treatment. Further investigations revealed lethargy, a painful, swollen right knee causing a limp, swelling and bleeding of the gums, and perifollicular hyperkeratosis. His right leg was swollen and felt as hard as wood, and he had prominent bruising of his thigh with bleeding into the joint of the right knee. He had eaten a very poor diet with no fruit and vegetables for several months. His plasma ascorbic acid level was 5 µmol/L, confirming vitamin C deficiency. He was given vitamin C 250 mg three times daily and his gums, bruising and bleeding improved rapidly and his anaemia resolved.
- *A man, 22 years of age*, reported a four-week history of extensive bruising and a two-year history of petechiae on both legs.[2] He had a large bruise on his left leg that was restricting his mobility, and his gums were swollen and bleeding. Further testing revealed anaemia which was treated by blood transfusions. Eventually, his plasma ascorbic acid was tested and found to be 3 µmol/L, indicating scurvy. His diet consisted entirely of Vegemite, cheese, bread, dry biscuits, chocolate and a cola drink; he was a smoker and he had regular episodes of binge drinking. In spite of his diagnosis, he was reluctant to change his diet. He was prescribed oral vitamin C and iron supplements, and his legs began improving in one week and were almost normal in one month.
- *A girl, nine years of age* with developmental delay, had musculoskeletal pain, pain in both knees, follicular hyperkeratosis, high blood pressure, bone weakness, compression factures of the vertebrae and swollen, purple, spongy and bleeding gums.[3] She was unable to walk unaided. Her diet consisted mainly of water, commercial chocolate puddings and cakes, and small quantities of milk, and she had refused to eat fresh fruit or vegetables for the last five to six years. Scurvy was not immediately recognised, and her plasma vitamin C level—only tested after several weeks of hospital diet—was 27 µmol/L. She was also found to be low in iron and vitamin D. Her family was given dietary education and she was given supplements of 250 mg vitamin C, 800 IU vitamin D, calcium and a multivitamin, together with blood pressure medication. Within one week, her musculoskeletal pain, knee movement, gums and skin had improved, and her blood pressure was normal at six months without medication.
- *An infant, fifteen months of age*, had a history of unexplained bleeding from his gums for several weeks and fever for two days.[4] He had almost no spontaneous movement, he held his legs in a 'frog leg' position and he had swelling and tenderness of the leg bones. His skin was dry and pale and he had bleeding gums and beading of the ribs. He had been fed only cow's milk and oatmeal since four months of age. X-rays revealed bone abnormalities indicative of scurvy. His plasma vitamin D level was normal and his vitamin C level was 28 µmol/L. He was given 100–200 mg vitamin C daily, reducing to 50 mg daily until his symptoms were fully resolved.

REFERENCES

1 Ho, V., Prinsloo, P. & Ombiga, J., Persistent anaemia due to scurvy, *NZ Med J* (2007), 120(1262): U2729.

2 Mapp, S.J. & Coughlin, P.B., Scurvy in an otherwise well young man, *Med J Aust* (2006), 185(6): 331–2.

3 Weinstein, M., Babyn, P. & Zlotkin, S., An orange a day keeps the doctor away: Scurvy in the year 2000, *Pediatrics* (2001), 108(3): E55.

4 Riepe, F.G., Eichmann, D., Oppermann, H.C. et al., Special feature: Picture of the month—infantile scurvy, *Arch Pediatr Adolesc Med* (2001), 155(5): 607–8.

VITAMIN C . . . A CANCER CURE?

Antioxidants in general can improve response to cancer therapy, protect normal tissue from damage and may increase survival. A higher intake of foods rich in vitamin C has been associated with a decreased risk of some cancers, including cancers of the mouth, oesophagus, larynx, stomach, pancreas, rectum, lung, prostate and cervix.[1] Premenopausal women with a family history of breast cancer who had an intake of 205 mg/day of dietary vitamin C were found to have a 63 per cent lower risk of breast cancer than those with an intake of 70 mg/day[2] and overweight women who had an average intake of 110 mg/day of dietary vitamin C were found to have a 39 per cent lower risk of breast cancer compared with overweight women with an average intake of 31 mg/day.[3] Cancer patients have been found to have low plasma vitamin C levels, and low concentrations are associated with increased cancer mortality.[4] However, results are conflicting.

In cell studies, concentrations of vitamin C above 1000 μmol/L are toxic to cancer cells but not to normal cells.[5] Concurrent use of alpha-lipoic acid, which recycles vitamin C, reduces the concentration threshold. In animals, vitamin C injections have been shown to reduce tumour size and growth and prevent the development of metastases; the researchers hypothesised that there is an extracellular 'metalloprotein catalyst', not present in blood, that interacts with vitamin C and causes it to act as a pro-oxidant in extracellular fluid.[6]

The required concentration of vitamin C can be achieved by intravenous (iv) administration, which is more effective than oral supplementation because it bypasses the regulatory absorption mechanisms in the digestive tract and higher circulating levels are achieved for longer periods of time. Oral delivery of 3 g of vitamin C every four hours produces peak plasma concentrations of only 220 μmol/L.[5] Intravenous doses of 50–100 g may result in a peak plasma concentration of about 14 000 μmol/L and concentrations above 2000 μmol/L may persist for several hours.[5]

In the 1970s and 1980s, Scottish surgeon Dr Ewan Cameron, in collaboration with the vitamin C researcher and Nobel prize winner Linus Pauling, studied the use of high doses of vitamin C for terminal cancer patients.[7,8,9] In 50 patients with advanced cancer given iv vitamin C infusions of 5–45 g daily and/or oral doses of 5–20 g daily, 27 patients had no or a minimal tumour response, nineteen patients experienced slowing of tumour growth, cessation of growth or tumour regression, and four patients experienced tumour destruction (necrosis) and haemorrhage, which had a sudden and catastrophic result in one patient with widespread cancer, causing haemorrhaging and death. In Cameron's subsequent studies, he used lower doses of vitamin C in the initial stages of treatment, which prevented this type of reaction. In almost all cases, cancer patients on vitamin C experienced markedly improved quality of life, with pain relief, increased energy and improved mood, and some were able to return home and resume normal life.

In another study, Cameron and Pauling compared survival times between 100 patients with terminal cancer given vitamin C (up to 10 g daily, usually given iv for ten days followed by at least 10 g a day orally) and 1000 matched control patients not given vitamin C.[8] Patients treated with vitamin C survived on average four times longer than the controls, with one patient surviving twenty times longer. A follow-up study reported that patients given vitamin C had a mean survival time that was almost one year longer than matched controls; only 0.4 per cent of controls survived for more than one year compared with 22 per cent of vitamin C patients.[9] Results showed that effects of vitamin C varied between patients, and included no or very minimal change to tumours, slowing of tumour growth, a standstill of tumour growth or regression of tumours and cancer remission.

The Cameron and Pauling studies have been criticised because of poor design; in the first study, classification of patients as terminal appeared to differ between the treatment group and controls, which may have biased the survival data in the vitamin C group. Two studies by the US Mayo Clinic attempted to replicate Cameron and Pauling's research using only oral doses (10 g daily) but survival rates were found to be no different between patients on vitamin C and those on placebo.[10] These studies have been criticised for not using iv treatment as well as oral, as used by Cameron and Pauling.

A more recent study investigated the effect of vitamin C on quality of life in terminal cancer patients.[11] Patients were given 10 g of vitamin C iv every three days and an oral dose of 4 g of vitamin C daily for one week. Although the dose used appears to be inadequate in the light of current research, patients reported significantly less fatigue, nausea, vomiting, pain and appetite loss. A study of 45 cancer patients given 7.5–50 g of iv vitamin C after standard cancer therapy found that it reduced levels of inflammatory chemicals, including interleukins, TNF-alpha, eotaxin (an eosinophil chemoattractant) and C-reactive protein, which correlated with a decrease in tumour markers.[12]

Large-scale, high-quality evidence for the effectiveness of iv vitamin C therapy is lacking, but it appears to be a promising approach for some patients, as shown by the following case reports.

- A man with primary renal cell carcinoma given 30 g of iv vitamin C twice weekly was reported to have disappearance of metastatic lesions in the lung and liver after several weeks.[13]
- A man with a grade I adenocarcinoma of the pancreas with metastasis to one of seven regional lymph nodes had surgery to remove the gall bladder, head of the pancreas, distal stomach and duodenum but not all of the tumour could be removed.[14] He refused chemotherapy and radiotherapy, and chose to have iv vitamin C therapy, which was given as 39 infusions in doses ranging from 57.5 to 115 g over a thirteen-week period. A CT scan of the abdomen six months after surgery showed no progression of the tumour but it recommenced growth when vitamin C treatment was interrupted to allow him to travel to visit family. The patient survived for twelve months after the initial diagnosis and enjoyed a good quality of life until the time of his death.
- An older woman hospitalised and confined to bed with end-stage breast cancer, with metastases throughout her entire skeleton and uncontrollable bone pain, was given iv vitamin C 100 g daily.[15] Her condition improved markedly and she was able to walk about and return home, continuing to receive iv vitamin C three times weekly. Three months after commencement of vitamin C, a bone scan revealed the disappearance of the metastases in her skull. Six months later, she had a fall while shopping that resulted in bone fractures and subsequently died of complications arising from the injury.
- Three patients are reported to have been successfully treated with iv vitamin C: a woman with advanced renal cell carcinoma, a man with bladder carcinoma and a woman with diffuse large B cell lymphoma.[5] All were confirmed by histopathological examination to have a poor prognosis. The study was conducted according to the American National Cancer Institute Best-Case Series guidelines. Two of the patients refused advice to have chemotherapy or radiotherapy, and the patient with lymphoma refused chemotherapy but had one five-week course of local radiotherapy. High-dose iv vitamin C (15–65 g twice weekly) was given, together with a selection of natural remedies, and all patients experienced long-term clinical remission.

REFERENCES

1 Block, G., Vitamin C and cancer prevention: The epidemiologic evidence, *Am J Clin Nutr* (1991), 53(1 Suppl): 270S–82S.

2 Zhang, S., Hunter, D.J., Forman, M.R. et al., Dietary carotenoids and vitamins A, C, and E and risk of breast cancer, *J Natl Cancer Inst* (1999), 91(6): 547–56.

3 Michels, K.B., Holmberg, L., Bergkvist, L., Ljung, H., Bruce, A. & Wolk, A., Dietary antioxidant vitamins, retinol, and breast cancer incidence in a cohort of Swedish women, *Int J Cancer* (2001), 91(4): 563–7.

4 Li, Y. & Schellhorn, H.E., New developments and novel therapeutic perspectives for vitamin C, *J Nutr* (2007), 137(10): 2171–84.

5 Padayatty, S.J., Riordan, H.D., Hewitt, S.M., Katz, A., Hoffer, L.J. & Levine, M., Intravenously administered vitamin C as cancer therapy: three cases, *CMAJ* (2006), 174(7): 937–42.

6 Frei, B. & Lawson, S., Vitamin C and cancer revisited, *Proc Natl Acad Sci USA* (2008), 105(32): 11037–8.

7 Cameron E., Vitamin C and cancer: An overview, *Int J Vitam Nutr Res Suppl* (1982), 23: 115–27.

8 Cameron, E. & Campbell, A., The orthomolecular treatment of cancer. II. Clinical trial of high-dose ascorbic acid supplements in advanced human cancer, *Chem-Biol Interact* (1974), 9: 285–315.

9 Cameron, E. & Pauling, L., Supplemental ascorbate in the supportive treatment of cancer: Reevaluation of prolongation of survival times in terminal human cancer, *Proc Natl Acad Sci USA* (1978), 75: 4538–42.

10 Creagan, E.T., Moertel, C.G., O'Fallon, J.R. et al., Failure of high-dose vitamin C (ascorbic acid) therapy to benefit patients with advanced cancer. A controlled trial, *N Engl J Med* (1979), 301(13): 687–90.

11 Yeom, C.H., Jung, G.C. & Song, K.J., Changes of terminal cancer patients' health-related quality of life after high dose vitamin C administration, *J Korean Med Sci* (2007), 22(1): 7–11.

12 Mikirova, N., Casciari, J., Taylor, P. & Rogers, A., Effect of high-dose intravenous vitamin C on inflammation in cancer patients, *J Transl Med* (2012), 10(1): 189.

13 Riordan, H.D., Jackson, J.A. & Schultz, M., Case study: High-dose intravenous vitamin C in the treatment of a patient with adenocarcinoma of the kidney, *J Ortho Med* (1990), 5: 5–7.

14 Jackson, J.A., Riordan, H.D., Hunninghake, R.E. et al., High dose intravenous vitamin C and long time survival of a patient with cancer of head of the pancreas, *J Ortho Med* (1995), 10(2): 87–8.

15 Riordan, H.D., Riordan, N.H., Jackson, J.A. et al., Intravenous vitamin C as a chemotherapy agent: A report on clinical cases, *P R Health Sci J* (2004), 23(2): 115–18.

THERAPEUTIC USES OF VITAMIN C

Population studies have shown that people with high intakes of vitamin C have a lower risk of chronic diseases, such as heart disease, cancer, eye diseases and neurodegenerative conditions.[1] People within the highest range of plasma vitamin C have been found to have a lower risk of all-cause mortality and mortality from cardiovascular disease (CVD) and coronary heart disease (CHD) compared with people within the lowest range.[2] Men within the lowest range of plasma vitamin C were found to have a higher cancer mortality risk.[2] Vitamin C requirements vary widely according to disease severity and individual needs. In general, vitamin C research has been hampered by the use of inadequate doses and the use of standard doses for every subject. Vitamin C is popularly used for infections, and may have therapeutic activity for the following conditions:

Infections

Vitamin C requirements vary between individuals and increase markedly during infections. Most research studies on vitamin C to date have used a standard low dose for all subjects or a single higher dose, which would be not be expected to be as effective as frequent high doses tailored to individual bowel tolerance or iv therapy (see 'Therapeutic dose'). Severe acute infections, such as Hantavirus, Lassa fever, Marburg virus and Ebola virus, may precipitate acute scurvy. These infections affect mainly humans and apes in Africa, and are classed as haemorrhagic fevers because they feature bleeding, including bleeding under the skin (petechiae and flat or raised red rashes), bleeding in internal organs, such as the lungs and stomach, and bleeding from body orifices, such as the mouth, eyes and ears, conjunctivitis and conjunctival haemorrhages, and muscle and joint pain. Chest pain, shock and death ensue in up to 80 per cent of cases. It is possible that one of the factors causing bleeding is severe acute scurvy, caused by the immune system's dramatically increased requirement for vitamin C in severe infection.[3] In the absence of effective treatments, iv vitamin C may help improve the prognosis, but this has not been attempted to date.

Respiratory tract infections

Vitamin C has been investigated for its role in upper respiratory tract infections, such as the common cold, with variable results. In athletes, pooled data from two trials found that vitamin C supplementation lowered the risk of an upper respiratory tract infection by 51 per cent.[4] In adolescent swimmers, supplementation of 1 g/day of vitamin C reduced the severity of respiratory infections and decreased the duration of infections by 47 per cent, but the effect was seen in male swimmers only.[5] A review of vitamin C trials found that it reduced the incidence of colds by 45 to 91 per cent in five trials of people undergoing intense physical activity and reduced the incidence of pneumonia by 80 to 100 per cent in three other trials.[6] A review of 30 trials that used more than 200 mg of Vitamin C daily to prevent colds found no reduction in the incidence of colds but a slight benefit in reducing symptom severity and duration.[7] One of the trials reviewed, which used a one-off dose of 8 g at the onset of symptoms, found that it shortened the duration of colds. A five-year study using 500 mg of vitamin C daily reported that it reduced the incidence of colds by 66 per cent but did not affect symptom severity or duration.[8]

Tetanus

Vitamin C given to rats either before or after administration of tetanus toxin at twice the minimal lethal dose prevented deaths in all the animals, whereas all the animals not given vitamin C died.[9] In a controlled trial of tetanus patients, subjects were given iv vitamin C 1 g/day together with conventional treatment or conventional treatment only.[10] No child aged one to twelve years died in the vitamin C-treated group but there was a death rate of 74 per cent in the control group. In those aged thirteen to 30 years, there was a death rate of 37 per cent in the vitamin C treated group and 68 per cent in the control group. It could be argued that 1 g daily was an inadequate dose for the older age group.

Vaginal infections

In women with a bacterial infection in the vagina, a tablet of 250 mg ascorbic acid inserted into the vagina once daily for six days was found to be an effective cure, with disappearance of pathogenic bacteria, reappearance of lactobacilli, reduction of vaginal pH and reduced vaginal inflammation.[11]

Gum infections

Several studies have found an association between gum infections (periodontitis) and non-insulin-dependent diabetes, CVD and cerebrovascular disease. The common factor may be underlying vitamin C deficiency, contributing to inflammation and oxidative stress. In a study of periodontitis, people in the highest range of plasma vitamin C were found to have a 47 per cent lower risk of periodontitis compared with those in the lowest range and a 35 per cent reduced risk of severe periodontitis, which increased to 62 per cent reduced risk in those who had never smoked.[12]

Herpes infections

Ascorbic acid has been shown to inactivate a wide range of viruses in cell studies, including *Herpes simplex* virus, and to enhance immune function. A dose of 600 mg of vitamin C given with 600 mg flavonoids was shown to decrease the mean healing time of herpes lesions by 5.5 days to 4.2 days.[13] Vitamin C (iv) has been found to relieve pain and rash in shingles and reduce the risk of post-herpetic neuralgia.[14] It is reported that a combination of oral and iv vitamin C and frequent topical applications of a vitamin C paste made of ascorbic acid or sodium ascorbate mixed with water have helped to heal herpes lesions in AIDS patients.[15]

Cardiovascular disease

Oxidative stress plays a major role in CVD, and antioxidant intake would be expected to help reduce the risk. Vitamin C has been shown to improve endothelial dysfunction, an early indicator of atherosclerosis, and reduce arterial stiffness, platelet aggregation and carotid artery thickness. A high intake of vitamin C (more than 700 mg/day) is associated with a 25 per cent lower risk of CHD.[16] Vitamin C restores activity of the vasodilator NO, and a high dietary intake of vitamin C has been linked to reduced blood pressure.[17] Low plasma levels of vitamin C have been linked to increased risk of myocardial infarction (MI, heart attack).[18] Vitamin C may be particularly beneficial for reducing the risk of CVD in diabetics; it has been shown to lower cellular sorbitol concentrations, strengthen capillaries, improve endothelial function and protect eye tissues, which may reduce the risk of complications.[19]

In older people, mortality from stroke was found to be highest in those with the lowest vitamin C status, as measured by plasma levels and dietary intake.[20] Those in the highest range of vitamin C intake had a 50 per cent reduced risk of mortality from stroke. Vitamin C supplementation (1000 mg daily) has been associated with a 25 per cent reduction in plasma C-reactive protein, an inflammatory marker and risk factor for CVD.[21]

Bone disorders

In animals, vitamin C improves healing of fractures, and a high dietary intake of vitamin C has been linked to higher bone mineral density in human studies. Vitamin C supplementation has improved bone mineral density in postmenopausal women[22,23] and reduced fracture risk.[24] It has also reduced the prevalence of complex regional pain syndrome after wrist fractures in elderly women.[25]

Brain function

Vitamin C is an important antioxidant in the brain, and regulates brain function by producing neurotransmitters and protecting cholinergic function by inhibiting acetylcholinesterase. Alzheimer's disease (AD) is associated with oxidative stress, a buildup of amyloid-beta in the brain and deterioration of the cholinergic system. In an animal model of AD, vitamin C supplementation for six months reduced formation of amyloid-beta and slowed the rate of behavioural decline.[26] Vitamin C injections have been shown to improve learning and memory in aged mice and protect young animals from drug-induced memory loss.[27] AD patients have been found to have low plasma levels of vitamin C[28] and a higher cerebrospinal fluid/plasma ratio.[29] An Australian study of a retirement community found that vitamin C supplementation was associated with a lower prevalence of more severe cognitive impairment.[30] In some studies, a combination of vitamin E and C supplementation was protective against AD.[31,32]

Cataract prevention

Vitamin C is particularly concentrated in the cornea, lens and aqueous humour of the eyes. It acts as an antioxidant in the eye and maintains vitamin E levels by regenerating it from its radical form. Vitamin C intake and elevated blood levels of vitamin C have been associated with a reduced risk of cataracts.[33] In women, use of vitamin C supplements for ten years or more was associated with a 77 per cent lower prevalence of early lens opacities and 83 per cent lower prevalence of moderate lens opacities compared with women who did not use vitamin C supplements.[34]

REFERENCES

1 Jacob, R.A. & Sotoudeh, G., Vitamin C function and status in chronic disease, *Nutr Clin Care* (2002), 5(2): 66–74.

2 Khaw, K.T., Bingham, S., Welch, A. et al., Relation between plasma ascorbic acid and mortality in men and women in EPIC-Norfolk prospective study: a prospective population study, *European Prospective Investigation into Cancer and Nutrition*, *Lancet* (2001), 357(9257): 65763.

3 Hoffer, A. & Saul, A.W., *Vitamin C (ascorbic acid) in orthomolecular medicine for everyone* (Basic Health Books, New York, 2008).

4 Moreira, A., Kekkonen, R.A., Delgado, L. et al., Nutritional modulation of exercise-induced immunodepression in athletes: A systematic review and meta-analysis, *Eur J Clin Nutr* (2007), 61(4): 443–60.

5 Constantini, N.W., Dubnov-Raz, G., Eyal, B.B. et al., The effect of vitamin C on upper respiratory infections in adolescent swimmers: A randomized trial, *Eur J Pediatr* (2011), 170(1): 59–63.

6 Hemila, H., Vitamin C supplementation and respiratory infections: A systematic review, *Mil Med* (2004), 169(11): 920–5.

7 Douglas, R.M., Hemila, H., D'Souza, R. et al., Vitamin C for preventing and treating the common cold, *Cochrane Database Syst Rev* (2004), 4: CD000980.

8 Sasazuki, S., Sasaki, S., Tsubono, Y. et al., Effect of vitamin C on common cold: Randomized controlled trial, *Eur J Clin Nutr* (2006), 60(1): 9–17.

9 Dey, P.K., Efficacy of vitamin C in counteracting tetanus toxin toxicity, *Die Naturwissenschaften* (1966), 53(12): 310.

10 Hemilä, H. & Koivula, T.T., Vitamin C for preventing and treating tetanus, *Cochrane Database Syst Rev* (2008), 2: CD006665.

11 Petersen, E.E. & Magnani, P., Efficacy and safety of vitamin C vaginal tablets in the treatment of non-specific vaginitis. A randomised, double blind, placebo-controlled study, *Eur J Obstet Gynecol Reprod Biol* (2004), 117(1): 70–5.

12 Chapple, I.L., Milward, M.R. & Dietrich, T., The prevalence of inflammatory periodontitis is negatively associated with serum antioxidant concentrations, *J Nutr* (2007), 137(3): 657–64.

13 Terezhalmy, G.T., Bottomley, W.K. & Pelleu, G.B., The use of water-soluble bioflavonoid-ascorbic acid complex in the treatment of recurrent herpes labialis, *Oral Surg Oral Med Oral Pathol* (1978), 45(1): 56–62.

14 Schencking, M., Vollbracht, C., Weiss, G. et al., Intravenous vitamin C in the treatment of shingles: Results of a multicenter prospective cohort study, *Med Sci Monit* (2012), 18(4): CR2.

15 Cathcart, R.F. III, Vitamin C in the treatment of acquired immune deficiency syndrome (AIDS), *Med Hypotheses* (1984), 14: 423–33.

16 Knekt, P., Ritz, J., Pereira, M.A. et al., Antioxidant vitamins and coronary heart disease risk: A pooled analysis of 9 cohorts, *Am J Clin Nutr* (2004), 80(6): 1508–20.

17 Ness, A.R., Chee, D. & Elliott, P., Vitamin C and blood pressure: An overview, *J Hum Hypertens* (1997), 11(6): 343–50.

18 Nyyssönen, K., Parviainen, M.T., Salonen, R.T. et al., Vitamin C deficiency and risk of myocardial infarction: prospective population study of men from eastern Finland, *BMJ* (1997), 314(7081): 634–8.

19 Will, J.C. & Byers, T., Does diabetes mellitus increase the requirement for vitamin C? *Nutr Rev* (1996), 54(7): 193–202.

20 Gale, C.R., Martyn, C.N., Winter, P.D. & Cooper, C., Vitamin C and risk of death from stroke and coronary heart disease in cohort of elderly people, *BMJ* (1995), 310(6994): 1563–6.

21 Block, G., Jensen, C.D., Dalvi, T.B. et al., Vitamin C treatment reduces elevated C-reactive protein, *Free Radic Biol Med* (2009), 46(1): 70–7.

22 Hall, S.L. & Greendale, G.A., The relation of dietary vitamin C intake to bone mineral density: Results from the PEPI study, *Calcif Tissue Int* (1998), 63(3): 183–9.

23 Morton, D.J., Barrett-Connor, E.L. & Schneider, D.L., Vitamin C supplement use and bone mineral density in postmenopausal women, *J Bone Miner Res* (2001), 16(1): 135–40.

24 Sahni, S., Hannan, M.T., Gagnon, D., Blumberg, J., Cupples, L.A., Kiel, D.P. & Tucker, K.L., Protective effect of total and supplemental vitamin C intake on the risk of hip fracture: A 17-year follow-up from the Framingham Osteoporosis Study, *Osteoporos Int* (2009), 20(11): 1853–61.

25 Zollinger, P.E., Tuinebreijer, W.E., Breederveld, R.S. & Kreis, R.W., Can vitamin C prevent complex regional pain syndrome in patients with wrist fractures? A randomized, controlled, multicenter dose-response study, *J Bone Joint Surg Am* (2007), 89(7): 1424–31.

26 Murakami, K., Murata, N., Ozawa, Y. et al., Vitamin C restores behavioral deficits and amyloid-β oligomerization without affecting plaque formation in a mouse model of Alzheimer's disease, *J Alzheimers Dis* (2011), 26(1): 7–18.

27 Parle, M. & Dhingra, D., Ascorbic acid: A promising memory-enhancer in mice, *J Pharmacol Sci* (2003), 93(2): 129–35.

28 Foy, C.J., Passmore, A.P., Vahidassr, M.D. et al., Plasma chain-breaking antioxidants in Alzheimer's disease, vascular dementia and Parkinson's disease, *QJM* (1999), 92(1): 39–45.

29 Bowman, G.L., Dodge, H., Frei, B.C. et al., Ascorbic acid and rates of cognitive decline in Alzheimer's disease, *J Alzheimers Dis* (2009), 16(1): 93–8.

30 Paleologos, M., Cumming, R.G. & Lazarus, R., Cohort study of vitamin C intake and cognitive impairment, *Am J Epidemiol* (1998), 148(1): 45–50.

31 Zandi, P.P., Anthony, J.C., Khachaturian, A.S. et al., Cache County Study Group. Reduced risk of Alzheimer disease in users of antioxidant vitamin supplements: The Cache County Study, *Arch Neurol* (2004), 61(1): 82–8.

32 Morris, M.C., Beckett, L.A., Scherr, P.A. et al., Vitamin E and vitamin C supplement use and risk of incident Alzheimer disease, *Alzheimer Dis Assoc Disord* (1998), 12(3): 121–6.

33 Valero, M.P., Fletcher, A.E., De Stavola, B.L. et al., Vitamin C is associated with reduced risk of cataract in a Mediterranean population, *J Nutr* (2002), 132(6): 1299–306.

34 Jacques, P.F., Taylor, A., Hankinson, S.E. et al., Long-term vitamin C supplement use and prevalence of early age-related lens opacities, *Am J Clin Nutr* (1997), 66(4): 911–16.

INFANTILE SCURVY IN AUSTRALIA

Dr Archie Kalokerinos pioneered the identification of infantile scurvy and the use of vitamin C for infants in Australia.[1] While working as a general practitioner in outback New South Wales in the 1960s and 1970s, he became alarmed at the extraordinarily high incidence of infant deaths, particularly among Aboriginal infants, in which the rate was nearly 50 per cent. Some of the deaths resembled sudden infant death syndrome (SIDS), and others were in apparently well infants or those with a trivial illness. He observed that infants became irritable and apprehensive, and suddenly collapsed with shock or unconsciousness and died. Autopsies failed to reveal a specific cause.

Dr Kalokerinos sent one at-risk infant to a local specialist, who discovered extremely minute haemorrhagic areas around some of the hair roots and diagnosed scurvy, which Dr Kalokerinos initially discounted as the cause of the syndrome. In Australian Aboriginal populations of the time, the staple diet was white bread eaten with golden syrup, jam or honey, and large quantities of sweetened tea. This diet had evolved from the 1920s, when governments established Aboriginal settlements and provided a weekly ration of white flour, sugar and tea. After finally accepting the possibility of scurvy, Dr Kalokerinos investigated the at-risk infants' diets, often consisting mainly of powdered milk, white bread and jam, and found that they were very low in vitamin C, and that vitamin C in large doses given im or iv was able to reverse the syndrome. Over time, he was able to reduce the death rate to zero by vitamin C treatment. His recommendations for supplementation were 100 mg of vitamin C daily for the first month after birth, given in divided doses, increasing by 100 mg daily each month up to ten months and then 1 g daily, increasing by 1 g each year up to ten years of age and then 10 g daily for the rest of life.

Dr Kalokerinos observed that infants with a mild illness could have a sudden collapse involving shock, unconsciousness or sudden death after the routine administration of a vaccine. He theorised that if the vitamin C status of an infant were borderline, the administration of a vaccine could result in endotoxaemia and precipitate acute severe scurvy, which could also be precipitated by a minor illness or series of illnesses. However, this theory was discounted by a 1995 New Zealand study that found that infants were at increased risk of SIDS if they had not been immunised and there was a reduced risk of SIDS in the four days immediately following immunisation.[2] It may be that the discrepancy between findings arises because infants in outback New South Wales in the 1960s and 1970s were much lower in vitamin C than New Zealand infants in 1995; however, in the absence of data on plasma vitamin C levels, it is not possible to establish this.

Dr Kalokerinos believed that the development of acute scurvy may be so rapid that sudden spontaneous bruising and haemorrhage, including brain and retinal haemorrhages, may occur in the absence of other scurvy symptoms. He regarded vitamin C deficiency as an underlying factor in many cases of SIDS and observed that haemorrhage and bone abnormalities due to scurvy may present as 'battered baby syndrome'.

SIDS is more common in infants of mothers who smoke, and it is known that cigarette smoke destroys vitamin C.[3] Up to 80 per cent of SIDS cases have been found to have a mild respiratory viral infection, which would contribute to a lowering of vitamin C levels.[3] Petechiae within the chest area is the most common gross finding in SIDS cases at autopsy, being detected in more than 90 per cent of cases.[4] This has led to the theory that abnormal pressure within the chest—perhaps caused by upper airway obstruction—is a common terminal event. Dr Kalokerinos's experience suggests that the development of petechiae may be a precursor event indicating scurvy. However, his many attempts to promote his theories to the medical profession were met with great scepticism, and there has been no further research to investigate his hypotheses.

REFERENCES

1 Kalokerinos, A., *Every second child*, Keats, New Canaan, CT, 1982.

2 Mitchell, E.A., Stewart, A.W. & Clements, M. Immunisation and the sudden infant death syndrome, New Zealand Cot Death Study Group, *Arch Dis Child* (1995), 73(6): 498–501.

3 Athanasakis, E., Karavasiliadou, S. & Styliadis, I., The factors contributing to the risk of sudden infant death syndrome, *Hippokratia* (2011), 15(2): 127–31.

4 Krous, H.F., Haas, E.A. & Chadwick, A.E., Intrathoracic petechiae in SIDS: A retrospective population-based 15-year study, *Forensic Sci Med Pathol* (2008), 4(4): 234–9.

Therapeutic dose

Suggested doses for adults are as follows:

- *Health maintenance:* 250 mg–3 g daily, preferably in divided doses.
- *Mild deficiency:* 1–3 g daily.
- *Severe deficiency:* 3–10 g daily or higher in the short term.
- *Acute infections:* The bowel tolerance dose is recommended by Dr Robert Cathcart of California (see <www.doctoryourself.com>), who reports using this method in over 20 000 patients over a 23-year period. Bowel tolerance refers to the amount of ascorbic acid that can be tolerated orally without overloading the body's capacity to absorb it. Exceeding this dose will cause diarrhoea because the unabsorbed portion enters the colon and fluid is drawn into the bowel to dilute it, and bowel movements are stimulated in an effort to excrete it. Dr Cathcart reports that a marked clinical improvement or cure can be achieved in many diseases when doses near the threshold of bowel tolerance are given.

According to Dr Cathcart, bowel tolerance increases with the severity of the disease, and may reach 200 g or more over a 24-hour period. A patient who could tolerate 10–15 g of vitamin C orally over a 24-hour period when well may tolerate 30–60 g per 24 hours with a mild cold, 100 g with a severe cold, 150 g with influenza and 200 g or more with glandular fever or viral pneumonia. Doses are usually given four to eight times daily—for example, approximately 4–8 g once an hour for eight hours during a mild cold. One teaspoon of ascorbic acid powder is equivalent to approximately 4 g. It should be noted that bowel tolerance varies widely between individuals and, for people who have not used vitamin C in this manner before, bowel tolerance should be tested by giving a smaller dose initially, which can then be increased cautiously every hour to establish the tolerance level.

Effects of excess

Vitamin C is generally well tolerated. Excess intake is readily excreted in urine.

Oral doses

Taking more vitamin C than can be absorbed leads to the unabsorbed portion passing into the colon, where it can be fermented by bacteria, causing flatulence, bloating and mild diarrhoea. Small frequent oral doses are better absorbed than large, one-off doses. However, the requirement for vitamin C increases in acute infections, and large doses are usually well tolerated.

High doses of vitamin C should be avoided in people with a deficiency of the enzyme glucose-6-phosphate dehydrogenase (G6PD) because it may cause breakdown of red blood cells, and people with iron overload disorders should avoid taking vitamin C with food because it increases absorption of non-haem iron found in plant foods. However, the excess iron in the body destroys vitamin C, so an adequate intake of vitamin C should be maintained.

Contrary to some reports, high doses of vitamin C are unlikely to cause calcium oxalate kidney or bladder stones in healthy people. Although vitamin C can form oxalate during metabolism, there is a ceiling beyond which no further oxalate is formed, even if large amounts of vitamin C are taken. Older reports suggesting a connection between ascorbic acid intake and oxalate levels in urine relied on urinary assays that were contaminated by conversion of ascorbic acid to oxalate during storage and processing of the samples. Large-scale investigations have found that there is either no relationship or a reduced risk of kidney stones with a higher vitamin C intake in people with healthy kidneys. However, it would be prudent to use vitamin C cautiously in people with kidney disease or a history of oxalate kidney or bladder stone formation.

It has been theorised that suddenly stopping high doses of vitamin C could lead to rebound scurvy. However, this has not been shown to occur in humans, and a study of guinea pigs found that mean plasma vitamin C concentrations fell significantly below control values during the second and fifth week following the abrupt withdrawal of vitamin C but remained within the normal range.

Intravenous doses

High-dose iv vitamin C can be used together with conventional cancer treatment, and doses of 150–200 g (up to 1.5 g/kg body weight) over a 24-hour period have been used without adverse effects in patients screened for contraindications. It is generally well tolerated, but is contraindicated in people with a deficiency of G6PD, and in people with poor kidney function, congestive heart failure, oedema or high blood pressure. In people with a deficiency of G6PD, iv vitamin C may cause destruction of red blood cells, and in one case a patient with poor kidney function developed oxalate damage to the kidneys during iv vitamin C treatment. Intravenous vitamin C is given in conjunction with sodium salts and fluid, which may have adverse effects in patients with congestive heart failure, oedema or high blood pressure. To avoid catastrophic necrosis of tumours, the initial dose should be moderate, and then should be increased gradually with careful monitoring—especially in patients at risk, such as those with highly undifferentiated, rapidly growing tumours or multiple tumours.

Supplements

The forms of vitamin C permitted in Australian supplements are ascorbic acid, calcium ascorbate dihydrate, magnesium ascorbate, magnesium ascorbate monohydrate, nicotinamide ascorbate, potassium ascorbate, potassium ascorbate dihydrate, sodium ascorbate and zinc ascorbate. Ascorbic acid is 100 per cent vitamin C, whereas mineral ascorbates have a mineral component and usually contain about 88–90 per cent vitamin C. Vitamin C for oral use is available as flavoured chewable tablets, unflavoured tablets and capsules, and flavoured and unflavoured powders. Most supplements contain ascorbic acid, sodium ascorbate or calcium ascorbate, or a mixture of these. Ascorbic acid has a sour taste, sodium ascorbate has a salty taste, and calcium and other mineral forms have a bitter taste. Vitamin C supplements are available as powder, chewable tablets, non-chewable tablets and slow-release and instant-release forms. All forms are well-absorbed and appear to have equivalent bioavailability.

- *Ascorbic acid.* This is pure vitamin C, which can be derived from food sources or produced chemically from glucose. Manufactured ascorbic acid is nature-identical, having the identical chemical structure to ascorbic acid found in food. Obtaining ascorbic acid from food is a very expensive and wasteful process, and the nature-identical form is used in supplements. During commercial production, glucose is converted to sorbitol by hydrogenation and fermented by micro-organisms, such as the bacteria *Erwinia herbicola*, to produce sorbose, which is then converted to di-acetone sorbose and then to di-acetone keto gulonic acid. Removal of acetone and heating under acid conditions yields pure ascorbic acid.
- *Mineral ascorbates.* These can be made by combining ascorbic acid with a variety of minerals—commonly sodium or calcium—which buffer the acid. Sodium ascorbate contains about 88 per cent vitamin C, and is produced by dissolving ascorbic acid in water, adding an equivalent amount of sodium bicarbonate and then precipitating the sodium ascorbate by the addition of isopropanol alcohol. Calcium ascorbate contains about 90 per cent vitamin C and is made by precipitating ascorbic acid and calcium carbonate in alcohol. Mineral ascorbates are buffered, and therefore less acidic tasting, and may be tolerated better by people with digestive sensitivities. Both the ascorbic acid content and the mineral content appear to be well absorbed.
- *Fat-soluble vitamin C.* Various forms of fat-soluble vitamin C are permitted for topical applications in Australia, but not for oral intake. The main fat-soluble form of vitamin C is ascorbyl palmitate. It can be made by condensing palmitoyl chloride and ascorbic acid in the presence of a dehydrochlorinating agent, such as pyridine, or by a reaction of ascorbic acid and with palmitic acid, catalysed by the enzyme lipase. Ascorbyl palmitate contains about 42 per cent vitamin C and is amphipathic, meaning that one end is water-soluble and the other end is fat-soluble. In theory, this property would allow it to be incorporated into cell membranes, where it may offer protection against oxidative damage. However, in reality, oral ascorbyl palmitate breaks down to palmitate and ascorbic acid in the gut, which are absorbed separately. Ascorbyl palmitate is more commonly used in topical cosmetic preparations because it is well absorbed into the skin and is a more stable form of vitamin C. However, it has been shown to remain on the extracellular surface of skin cells, and does not increase levels of ascorbic acid within the cells. A 15–20 per cent solution of ascorbic acid formulated at a pH of 3.2 has been shown to be the most effective topical preparation, increasing skin vitamin C concentrations by 20 per cent. In studies of human skin cells, ascorbic acid has been shown to stimulate cell growth, whereas equivalent amounts of ascorbyl palmitate are toxic.
- *Vitamin C with metabolites (Ester-C®).* This is a vitamin C supplement that contains mainly calcium ascorbate with smaller amounts of the vitamin C metabolites DHAsA, calcium threonate, xylonate and lyxonate. It contains about 74 per cent vitamin C, 10 per cent calcium, 6 per cent DHAsA and 10 per cent metabolites. This formula is claimed to have improved bioavailability, which was demonstrated in one study; however, another study found no significant differences in plasma vitamin C levels when comparing it with other vitamin C preparations. However, vitamin C with metabolites has been found to increase concentrations of

vitamin C in leukocytes, and another study found that it was associated with reduced urinary oxalate levels compared to ascorbic acid.

- *Intravenous vitamin C.* Health professionals experienced in the use of iv vitamin C state that it should be given by infusion drip as a sodium ascorbate/ascorbic acid mixture containing 0.91 moles of sodium per mole of ascorbate (500 mg AsA/mL, pH range 5.5–7.0). This must be mixed with Ringer's lactate (RL) solution for vitamin C amounts up to 25 g, and mixed in sterile water for larger amounts of vitamin C. Intravenous treatment should commence with a dose of 15 g vitamin C in 250 mL RL given over one hour, and the patient should be observed for any adverse effects. If tolerated, the dose can then gradually be increased over time. The infusion rate should not exceed 1 g of vitamin C per minute. It is reported that 0.5 g/minute is well tolerated by most patients. Intravenous vitamin C should always be administered by an experienced medical practitioner.

Cautions

Some people are sensitive to ascorbic acid, which may cause digestive discomfort, and non-acidic mineral salts of ascorbate may be tolerated better. Large doses of vitamin C taken within a short period of time can cause mild and transient digestive symptoms such as flatulence, bloating and diarrhoea. These symptoms indicate that the dose should be reduced or the time interval between doses increased. Chewable ascorbic acid tablets can damage tooth enamel and should be followed by a drink of water or brushing the teeth. Most chewable tablets combine ascorbic acid with sodium ascorbate to lower the acid content and for palatability. Sodium ascorbate does not appear to increase blood pressure, unlike sodium chloride (table salt).

People with a deficiency of the enzyme G6PD and people with kidney disease or a history of oxalate kidney or bladder stones should use supplements with caution. People taking potassium-sparing diuretics and those with kidney failure should avoid taking extra potassium and should not use large amounts of potassium ascorbate. Precautions relating to administration of iv vitamin C can be found in 'Effects of excess'.

B VITAMINS

The first B vitamin identified was vitamin B1, and further research showed that there are several chemically distinct B vitamins that are often found together in the same foods. B vitamins include B1 (thiamin), B2 (riboflavin), B3 (niacin), B5 (pantothenic acid), B6 (pyridoxine), B12 (cobalamin), folic acid and biotin. A supplement containing all eight B vitamins is referred to as a vitamin B complex. Choline and inositol are water-soluble nutrients that are often included in B complex supplements but are not B vitamins. Many B vitamins are important cofactors for energy production enzymes, and support brain and nervous system function.

Role of B vitamins in energy production

- *Vitamin B1* forms thiamin diphosphate, a cofactor for pyruvic acid, which is the precursor to acetyl coenzyme A (acetyl-CoA), and also for enzymes in the citric acid cycle.
- *Vitamin B2* forms flavin adenine dinucleotide and flavin mononucleotide, cofactors for enzymes in the citric acid cycle and the electron transport chain.
- *Vitamin B3* forms nicotinamide adenine dinucleotide (NAD) and nicotinamide adenine dinucleotide phosphate (NADP), cofactors for enzymes in the citric acid cycle and the electron transport chain.
- *Vitamin B5* is a component of coenzyme A (CoA) and helps form acetyl-CoA.
- *Vitamin B6* forms pyridoxal 5'-phosphate and is a cofactor for enzymes that metabolise amino acids in the citric acid cycle.
- *Vitamin B12* is a cofactor for the enzyme methylmalonyl-CoA mutase, which takes part in the citric acid cycle.
- *Biotin* is a cofactor for carboxylase enzymes that metabolise acetyl-CoA and pyruvate.

B vitamins have no significant storage in the body, and must be included in the diet daily. They are easily excreted in urine and excretion is increased by diuretic drugs, alcohol and stimulants, such as caffeine in coffee, soft drinks, tea and chocolate, theophylline in tea, and theobromine in cocoa and chocolate. They are leached from foods by water processing and cooking methods, and may be destroyed by high-temperature cooking and processing. Cooking with water, boiling foods and adding sodium bicarbonate when cooking vegetables reduces the vitamin B content of foods. B vitamins in food may deteriorate on exposure to light and storage at room temperature. Adequate production of stomach acid is important for absorption of B vitamins.

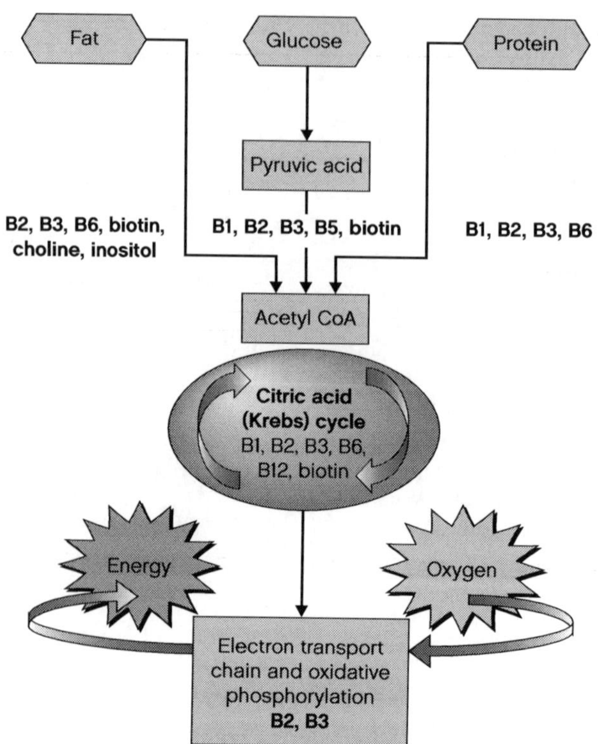

Figure 6.1 Role of B vitamins in energy production

Individual vitamin B supplements are not recommended for long-term therapy. B vitamins work together in many biochemical pathways, and excess amounts of one B vitamin may interfere with the metabolism of others. Single B vitamins should be used in the short term only, and always with a B complex.

All of the B-group vitamins are found in liver. Very few plant foods contain vitamin B12—mainly microalgae, such as spirulina, and fermented plant foods, such as tempeh. Dark-green leafy vegetables, wheat germ, whole grains and brewer's yeast are good sources of most of the B vitamins, except vitamin B12.

Vitamin B1 (thiamin)

VITAMIN B1 STATUS CHECK

1. **Do you have weak muscles and/or numbness, tingling, or pins and needles sensations in your feet or hands?**
2. **Are you moody and irritable, or do you lose your temper easily?**
3. **Is your appetite poor?**
4. **Do you eat a lot of white rice or white flour products, and consume a lot of sweetened food and drinks?**

'Yes' answers may indicate inadequate vitamin B1 status. Note that a number of nutritional deficiencies or health disorders can cause similar effects and further investigation is recommended.

Vitamin B1, also called thiamin or thiamine, consists of a pyrimidine ring and a thiazolium ring joined by a methylene bridge. A deficiency leads to beriberi (meaning 'weakness'), a life-threatening disorder affecting nerves and muscles occurring throughout history and particularly prevalent in Asian countries where white (polished) rice is a staple food. The connection between beriberi and diet was first made by Dr Kanehiro Takaki, a nineteenth-century Japanese

FAST FACTS . . . VITAMIN B1

- **Vitamin B1 is found in brewer's yeast, molasses, whole grains, wheat germ and bran, brown rice, rice bran, nuts, seeds, liver, kidney, pork, legumes, egg yolk and yeast-based spreads.**
- **It is required for energy production in cells.**
- **It supports the production of fatty acids, sterols, nucleic acids and neurotransmitters.**
- **A deficiency causes impaired energy production, elevated lactic acid, and brain and nerve damage.**
- **Supplementation may be helpful for cognitive function, diabetes, congestive heart failure, menstrual cramps and the health of the elderly.**

naval surgeon. In 1883, he observed that more than half of the crew on a naval ship returned to port with beriberi after a long sea voyage. Takaki added dry milk and meat to the provisions of a ship undertaking a similar voyage, and found that the incidence of beriberi was dramatically reduced. He concluded, erroneously, that nitrogenous food was protective against beriberi. He revised the diet in all naval ships and beriberi virtually disappeared from the navy. Unfortunately, Dr Rintaro Mori, the chief medical officer of the Japanese army, continued to believe that beriberi was an infectious disease, and saw no need to change the white rice diet of his troops, causing many more to die from beriberi.

In 1890, the Dutch doctor Christiaan Eijkman, working in Indonesia, made the accidental discovery that chickens fed solely on white rice developed polyneuritis (inflammation of multiple nerves) and died with symptoms that were very similar to beriberi in humans. He found that the polyneuritis could be cured by giving the chickens rice bran or brown rice, and developed the theory that the disorder was caused by a toxin or microbe in white rice that was inhibited by a factor in brown rice. Eijkman's assistant, Gerrit Grijns, eventually concluded in 1901 that the disease was linked to the polishing process used to convert brown rice to white rice, which removed an important nutritional factor in the outer coating of rice. In 1926, the anti-beriberi factor was isolated from rice bran extracts and was named thiamine (vitamin B1). The name thiamine was used because it was thought to be an amine, but this was later found to be incorrect and the final 'e' was deleted from the name. However, the original spelling of the name is still commonly used. Thiamin was chemically synthesised in 1936.

Digestion, absorption and transport

Vitamin B1 is found as free thiamin in plant foods and in phosphorylated form in animal foods, mainly as thiamin diphosphate (TDP), previously known as thiamin pyrophosphate (TPP), which is the active form that functions as a coenzyme in the body. In the digestive tract, phosphates are removed by phosphatase enzymes and free thiamin is absorbed into the enterocytes lining the small intestine. Low concentrations are absorbed by active transport involving two carriers, thiamin transporter-1 (THTR-1) and thiamin transporter-2 (THTR-2). High concentrations are absorbed by passive diffusion, and it appears that doses up to 1500 mg can be absorbed. A third transporter, which transports folate, also appears to be able to transport thiamin monophosphate (TMP) and TDP.

Enterocytes release vitamin B1 into the portal vein for delivery to the liver. Plasma vitamin B1 consists of free thiamin, TMP or TDP bound to a protein such as albumin. Uptake of vitamin B1 by blood cells and other tissues occurs via THTR-1 and THTR-2.

Metabolism, storage and excretion

Vitamin B1 delivered to the liver is converted by the enzyme thiamin diphosphokinase (TDPase) to the major active form, TDP, which makes up about 80 per cent of the body content of vitamin B1. Other forms include thiamin triphosphate (TTP), which makes up about 10 per cent of body content, TMP, free thiamin and the recently discovered adenosine thiamin triphosphate (AThTP) and adenosine thiamin diphosphate (AThDP). Most of the TDP within cells is transported into mitochondria via the mitochondrial thiamin pyrophosphate transporter (MTPPT). Bacteria in the colon have been shown to synthesise vitamin B1 as thiamin and TDP. TDP from this source can be absorbed by colonocytes, and may be used locally or systemically and possibly contribute to body content. There is no significant storage in the body and tissues contain only about two to three weeks' supply. Excess vitamin B1 is excreted in urine as thiamin or its pyrimidine and thiazole metabolites, including 2-methyl-4-amino-5-pyrimidine carboxylic acid, 4-methylthiazole-5-acetic acid and thiamin acetic acid.

Functions

The main active form of vitamin B1 is believed to be TDP, which functions as a cofactor for several key enzymes during cell metabolism. Magnesium is required for TDP activity. TMP appears to be an intermediate in the synthesis of TDP and TTP, and its function and the functions of AThTP and AThDP are not well understood as yet. TTP appears to activate chloride channels in nerves, and to have a role in nerve impulse conduction and brain cell signalling. It may also protect against mitochondrial oxidative stress. AThTP has a similar structure to NAD, important for electron transfer reactions, and has been shown to inhibit the enzyme poly(ADP-ribose) polymerase-1 (PARP-1), over-activity of which is related to various disorders, including diabetes. AThDP may have cell signalling and nervous system functions. Functions of vitamin B1 include:

- *Energy production.* TDP is a cofactor for two important enzymes in the citric acid cycle that produces energy in cells. It is required for activity of the enzyme complex pyruvate dehydrogenase that converts pyruvate to acetyl-CoA, which then condenses with oxaloacetate to form citrate, the first component of the citric acid cycle. It is also required for activity of the enzyme alpha-ketoglutarate dehydrogenase that forms succinyl-CoA in a subsequent step in the cycle. Pyruvate metabolism requires the presence of other B vitamins, including vitamin B2, B3 and B5, as well as alpha-lipoic acid. TDP is a cofactor for the enzyme complex branched-chain alpha-keto acid dehydrogenase, which oxidises alpha-keto acids derived from deaminated branched-chain amino acids used for energy production.
- *Production of nucleic acids, fats and sterols.* Acetyl-CoA formed with the assistance of TDP can also be converted to fatty acids and cholesterol, which then produces steroids such as sex hormones, adrenal cortex hormones and vitamin D. TDP enables activity of the enzyme transketolase in the hexose monophosphate shunt (pentose phosphate) pathway that metabolises some sugars. This pathway is particularly active in adipose tissue, mammary glands and the adrenal cortex, and produces NADPH (the reduced form of NADP), and ribose-5-phosphate. NADPH provides hydrogen atoms required for production of glutathione, coenzymes, sterols, steroid hormones, fatty acids, amino acids and neurotransmitters. Ribose-5-phosphate supports production of complex sugars, coenzymes and nucleic acids for synthesis of RNA and DNA.
- *Nerve and brain function.* Brain tissue cannot use fatty acids for energy, and is dependent on glucose metabolism. Vitamin B1 appears to be particularly important for the function of the thalamus, hypothalamus, mammillary bodies, brainstem and cerebellum in the brain. Vitamin B1 may help regulate sodium channels in nerve membranes, and is required for production of acetyl-CoA that forms the neurotransmitter acetylcholine and supports production of myelin than insulates nerve fibres. Vitamin B1 modulates brain function and mood by promoting production of dopamine, noradrenaline (norepinephrine) and adrenaline (epinephrine), as well as glutamate, glutamine and gamma-aminobutyric acid (GABA). It appears to play a role in the function of serotonin, a neurotransmitter that affects sleep, mood and behaviour.

Dietary sources

Vitamin B1 is found in brewer's yeast, molasses, whole grains, wheat germ and bran, brown rice, rice bran, nuts, seeds, liver, kidney, pork, legumes, egg yolk and yeast-based spreads. In grains, most of the vitamin B1 is found in the germ and the aleurone layer between the starch-containing endosperm and the husk; these nutrient-rich parts are removed during milling of rice and refining of wheat.

In 1991 in Australia, it became mandatory for bread-making flour to be fortified with vitamin B1 at a level of 6.4 mg/kg. Bread fortification was introduced in an attempt to reduce the risk of nerve damage associated with alcohol-induced vitamin B1 deficiency. Organic flour and bread are exempt from mandatory fortification. Vitamin B1 is permitted to be voluntarily added to breakfast cereals and grain and legume products.

The Food Standards Australia New Zealand nutrient database (NUTTAB) at <www.foodstandards.gov.au> provides the amounts found in specific foods.

Factors influencing body status

Vitamin B1 in food is stable at acid pH, and becomes unstable and breaks down at a pH of 7.0 or higher. It can be destroyed if sodium bicarbonate is used in cooking, baking or food processing. It also breaks down when exposed to oxygen and high temperatures during cooking and processing, especially during canning.

Chlorine in tap water and sulfite food preservatives used in dried fruit and wine destroy vitamin B1. It is water soluble and is leached out of foods when they are exposed to water during soaking, cooking and processing. Vitamin B1 is removed when grains are milled to form white rice and white flour. The vitamin B1 content of wheat is reduced by 57 per cent in white flour and by 20 per cent in whole-wheat flour. In bread, the vitamin B1 level is further lowered by 37 per cent in white bread and 31 per cent in whole-wheat bread. Parboiling rice before milling drives some of the vitamin B1 into the inner part of the kernel, and helps to preserve the vitamin B1 content.

Some foods contain anti-thiamin factors that destroy vitamin B1 or reduce its bioavailability. The enzymes thiaminase I and II, mainly found in raw or fermented freshwater fish and shellfish, convert vitamin B1 to an inactive form but are destroyed by cooking. The gut bacteria *Clostridium thiaminolyticus*, an anaerobic bacterium found in the small intestine, and the aerobic bacteria *Bacillus thiaminolyticus* and *Bacillus aneurinolyticus*, found in the colon, also produce thiaminase. In Australia in the 1860s, a group of explorers died of beriberi after eating a fern that has naturally high levels of thiaminase. Aboriginal people who ate the fern used a special preparation method that removed the thiaminase, a method not used by the explorers.

Tropical ataxic neuropathy (TAN) and epidemic spastic paraparesis (konzo) are beriberi-like nerve and muscle disorders prevalent in African countries where cassava is a staple food. Cassava contains cyanide, and has to be intensively processed to be fit for human consumption. When protein intake is low, the body is deprived of sulfur-containing amino acids that inactivate cyanide from improperly processed cassava and the sulfur in thiamin is used instead to inactivate it, leading to thiamin deficiency. Seasonal ataxia (incoordination) in Nigerians is caused by eating the pupae of a silkworm that contains thiaminase.

Polyhydroxyphenols, which include caffeic acid, chlorogenic acid and tannic acid, are heat-stable, anti-thiamin factors found in blueberries, blackcurrants, Brussels sprouts, red cabbage, tea and coffee. Betel nut, which is commonly chewed in some Asian countries, also contains tannins. Polyhydroxyphenols react with thiamin to form the non-absorbable thiamin disulfide, but natural acids in foods, such as citric acid and ascorbic acid, can inhibit this reaction and increase its bioavailability.

Diuretics that stimulate urine flow increase losses of vitamin B1 in urine. Kidney disease, kidney dialysis and loop diuretics, such as frusemide, are known to deplete vitamin B1 levels. Central nervous system stimulants, such as the naturally occurring xanthines, which include caffeine, theophylline and theobromine found in coffee, tea, chocolate products, energy drinks and the herb guaraná, have diuretic effects. Alcohol can also have diuretic effects and, in excessive amounts, inhibits transfer of dietary B1 from the enterocytes to the bloodstream, impairs conversion of thiamin to TDP, promotes the conversion of pyruvic acid to lactic acid and damages the liver, reducing its ability to metabolise vitamin B1. Drugs such as phenytoin used for epilepsy and fluorouracil for cancer also inhibit synthesis of TDP. Absorption of vitamin B1 is impaired in folic acid deficiency.

Low magnesium levels will impair the function of TDP and low levels of vitamin B2, vitamin B3 and vitamin B5 will impair the function of TDP in the citric acid cycle. Carbohydrate foods increase the need for vitamin B1 and, in marginal vitamin B1 status, a high carbohydrate intake—particularly refined carbohydrates that do not provide vitamin B1—can precipitate an acute deficiency. The requirement for vitamin B1 increases during pregnancy, lactation, growth, exercise, diabetes, fever, infections, trauma and surgery. The elderly are particularly at risk of vitamin B1 deficiency.

Daily requirement

Government recommendations by age and gender (see Table 6.2, overleaf) can be found in *Nutrient Reference Values for Australia and New Zealand Including Recommended Dietary Intakes* available at <www.nhmrc.gov.au>.

Deficiency effects

If TDP levels are inadequate, pyruvate conversion to acetyl-CoA is impaired, which impairs the function of the citric acid cycle and reduces energy production. Pyruvic acid builds up and is converted to lactic acid, which damages nerves and impairs brain function. Formation of succinyl-CoA is impaired and an alternative pathway, the GABA shunt, becomes activated, which produces GABA from the amino acid glutamate and converts it to succinate. Activation of this pathway in the hypothalamus leads to loss of appetite.

In thiamin deficiency, branched-chain amino acids and alpha-ketoglutarate are unable to be metabolised effectively, and accumulate in the blood, together

Table 6.2 Recommended dietary intake (RDI) of vitamin B1 (mg/day)

Age (years)	Female RDI	Male RDI
1–3	0.5	0.5
4–8	0.6	0.6
9–13	0.9	0.9
14–18	1.1	1.2
19–70	1.1	1.2
>70	1.1	1.2
Pregnant women		
14–18	1.4	
19–50	1.4	
Lactating women		
14–18	1.4	
19–50	1.4	

Source: Nutrient Reference Values for Australia and New Zealand Including Recommended Dietary Intakes, National Health and Medical Research Council, Australian Government Department of Health and Ageing, Canberra and Ministry of Health, New Zealand, Wellington, 2006.

with pyruvic acid and lactic acid, leading to metabolic acidosis. Alcohol is an exacerbating factor because alcohol metabolism impairs vitamin B1 absorption and metabolism, and promotes the conversion of pyruvic acid to lactic acid, all of which contribute to acidosis. A vitamin B1 deficiency impairs nerve function and brain function, causing a selective loss of neurons in the thalamus, hypothalamus, mammillary bodies, brainstem and cerebellum. It causes a range of brain malfunctions, including decreased glucose utilisation, lowered energy production, increased oxidative stress, lactic acidosis, blood–brain barrier disruption, astrocyte dysfunction, glutamate-induced damage to neurons, deposition of the abnormal protein amyloid-beta and inflammation. In animals, vitamin B1 deficiency causes reduced growth and appetite, marked loss of fur, severe weakness, depression and impaired gait.

Vitamin B1 deficiency in humans (beriberi) is associated with diets that consist mainly of refined carbohydrates, such as white rice, white flour products and sweetened foods and drinks, and can develop within two to three months of a deficient intake. Beriberi is still of concern in Japan, Southeast Asia and western Africa, where white rice is the staple food and food variety is limited. It has re-emerged in some Asian countries with the introduction of sweetened foods and soft drinks to the diet. Exercise may precipitate an acute deficiency in thiamin-depleted individuals.

Vitamin B1 deficiency may occur in Western countries in people who eat mainly refined carbohydrates and/or drink excessive amounts of sweetened soft drinks or alcohol. A deficiency can occur in patients after gastric surgery for weight loss, in patients on long-term parenteral (non-oral) feeding, and in those with severe sepsis, burns, chronic malnutrition, anorexia nervosa, vomiting in pregnancy and neurological disorders with a history of alcohol abuse. Vitamin B1 deficiency should be investigated in unexplained heart failure or lactic acidosis.

A mild (sub-clinical) deficiency of vitamin B1 has been associated with mood swings, uncooperative behaviour, irritability, agitation, anger, aggressive or violent episodes, poor impulse control, fearfulness, sensitivity to criticism, restlessness, poor memory, fatigue, loss of appetite, insomnia, sleep talking or sleepwalking, nightmares, constipation, abdominal or chest pain, and unexplained recurring fevers. Early symptoms of a deficiency may include loss of appetite, weakness, aches and pains, a burning sensation in the hands and feet, indigestion, irritability and depression. Aggressive behaviour appears to be a common early symptom, appearing in animals when a marginal deficiency is induced. Loss of appetite was used in the past as a marker of the severity of the deficiency, and return of appetite after treatment indicated clinical improvement. After a few weeks of a vitamin B1-deficient diet, there may be a slight fall in blood pressure and moderate weight loss. After two to three months, there is marked apathy and weakness, calf muscle tenderness, vomiting, loss of recent memory, confusion and ataxia. Loss of appetite and vomiting may be protective mechanisms that aim to reduce carbohydrate intake because metabolism of carbohydrate is markedly impaired.

Beriberi

Beriberi is the classical deficiency disease, and occurs in chronic and acute forms. Key features of beriberi are peripheral nerve damage (neuropathy) and muscle weakness, with or without cardiac complications. Nerve damage without pronounced cardiac effects is referred to as dry beriberi and the term wet beriberi describes nerve damage with oedema and congestive heart failure.

Infantile beriberi

Beriberi more commonly affects infants at two to three months of age who are breastfed by mothers deficient in vitamin B1. Symptoms may begin with constipation, occasional vomiting, crying and restlessness, and progress rapidly to oedema, breathing difficulties, suspension of breathing (apnoea), decreased urine flow, a loud, piercing cry or hoarseness or loss of voice, poor appetite, persistent vomiting, diminished tendon reflexes, cyanosis, rapid heartbeat (tachycardia), and heart and liver enlargement. In the acute form, cardiac malfunction can result in death within two to 24 hours of onset. In infants aged four to six months, a milder form is more frequent, causing hoarseness and loss of voice due to weakness of the vocal cords. In infants aged seven to nine months, symptoms may mimic bacterial meningitis, such as stiffness and arching of the neck, irritability, restlessness, sweating, vomiting and convulsions. Vitamin B1 deficiency in infancy appears to lead to long-lasting effects on brain function. Almost all of the survivors of children who had been severely vitamin B1 deficient in early infancy were found to have language impairment at five to seven years of age.

Adult beriberi

- *Dry beriberi* causes symmetrical, ascending peripheral neuropathy affecting the limbs, especially the legs, and features glove and stocking numbness, tingling, burning or pins and needles sensations (collectively known as paraesthesia); loss of voice or hoarseness; chest wall pain; muscle weakness and wasting; a feeling of heaviness in muscles; stiff, aching muscles; calf muscle tenderness; difficulty rising from a squatting position; and poor coordination, and may lead to walking difficulties or paralysis. Weak muscles can cause wrist drop and foot drop. Initially, sensory nerve disturbances cause numbness, pain and disturbed temperature sensitivity in the skin, loss of vibratory sense over the big toes and the ankles, paraesthesia in the legs and toes, and increased sensitivity to touch, beginning in the feet and legs and progressing to the fingertips, lower abdomen and mouth region, and gradually expanding. Following this, the motor nerves are affected, beginning with the tips of the toes, then the fingertips and ascending up the limbs. The nerve disturbances are accompanied by loss of appetite, vomiting, abdominal bloating and colic, constipation, fatigue, poor concentration and impaired capacity to work.
- *Wet beriberi* is an acute condition that has the features of dry beriberi together with peripheral vasodilation, oedema of the face, trunk and legs, pulmonary congestion, shortness of breath, heart palpitations, tachycardia, low blood pressure, wide pulse pressure, dizziness and heart enlargement, leading to congestive heart failure and sudden death, especially following exertion. There may be elevated cardiac output combined with low resistance in the peripheral circulation. Another form of wet beriberi features lactic acidosis, low blood pressure, tachycardia and death from pulmonary oedema.
- *Shoshin beriberi* is a very acute, dangerous form of wet beriberi that causes abrupt onset heart failure and sudden death. Its name comes from the Japanese word for 'sudden collapse', and it features a sudden onset of rapid pulse, a drop in diastolic blood pressure, enlarged heart and liver, congested lungs, cyanosis, nausea, vomiting, collapse and death
- *Cerebral beriberi* (Wernicke-Korsakoff syndrome) is mainly induced by chronic alcohol abuse, and is a life-threatening condition characterised by brain damage, ataxia and weakness of the eye muscles causing involuntary repetitive eyeball movements (nystagmus), squint and double vision. Wernicke's encephalopathy features mental confusion, disorientation and vertigo, and Korsakov's psychosis features severe loss of memory for recent events with confabulation (fluent storytelling to cover loss of memory), lack of orientation to place and time, indifference to surroundings, apathy with psychomotor retardation and lack of insight, impaired memory and cognitive function, ataxia, difficulty walking and nystagmus. In cerebral beriberi, eye muscle weakness improves more rapidly on vitamin B1 therapy, but ataxia and mental symptoms are slow to improve and memory may not be completely recovered. About 17 per cent of patients die within three weeks, even with treatment. Binge-drinking of alcohol is particularly dangerous in a vitamin B1 deficiency because it can trigger sudden death from an acute overload of lactic acid (acidosis). Cerebral beriberi may be triggered by administration of glucose to a severely thiamin-deficient patient, and has been observed after gastric surgery for weight loss and in people on strict weight-loss diets, anorexia nervosa patients, kidney dialysis patients and patients on parenteral nutrition.

Thiamin-responsive megaloblastic anaemia

Thiamin-responsive megaloblastic anaemia (TRMA) is a rare genetic disorder affecting thiamin transport or metabolism, and is mainly confined to children of parents who are blood related. It features megaloblastic (large cell) anaemia, insulin-dependent diabetes and nerve deafness. Symptoms include loss of appetite, lack of energy, headaches, pale skin, diarrhoea and paraesthesia in the hands and feet. The disorder is linked to mutations in the SLC19A2 gene that encodes for the vitamin B1 transporter THTR-1. Large doses of vitamin B1 (25–75 mg/day) help to correct the anaemia and reduce the amount of insulin required, but do not appear to reverse deafness or prevent the progression of diabetes.

Indicators of inadequate levels may include:

- fatigue, poor exercise endurance
- low morale, mood swings, headaches, irritability, an uncooperative or argumentative attitude, aggressiveness, anxiety, fearfulness, agitation, disturbed sleep, poor memory and concentration
- heavy, sore, stiff or tender muscles, weak leg muscles, poor coordination, difficulty rising from a squatting position, muscle wasting, difficulty walking, weakness of eye muscles, wrist or foot drop
- nerve pain, 'pins and needles' sensations, numbness, tingling, hypersensitive skin, weak reflexes
- loss of voice, hoarseness
- abdominal or chest pain
- loss of appetite, weight loss, constipation.

Assessment of body status

Vitamin B1 concentration in serum is not regarded as a reliable measure of status because it reflects recent intakes, and levels are low and difficult to measure accurately. About 80 per cent of vitamin B1 is in red blood cells, and the content of whole blood has been shown to be a good indicator of body stores because it reflects the content of major organs. The reference range given by the Biochemistry Department of the Royal Prince Alfred Hospital, Sydney, Australia for vitamin B1 levels in whole blood is 67–200 nmol/L.

The activity of the enzyme transketolase is depressed in vitamin B1 deficiency, and the erythrocyte transketolase activity coefficient (ETKAC) can be used to measure the response of the enzyme when exposed to vitamin B1. An increase in activity of more than 25 per cent after exposure to thiamin indicates a deficiency, a 15–25 per cent increase indicates marginal status and an increase of less than 15 per cent indicates sufficiency. ETKA can be affected by factors other than vitamin B1 deficiency; chronic deficiency and some disease states can lower the amount of transketolase present and cause a lower amount of activation during the test. The response to therapeutic amounts of vitamin B1 may also be used to identify a deficiency.

Case reports—vitamin B1 deficiency

- *A boy, one year of age,* developed eye muscle weakness, involuntary muscle contractions, and became unconscious.[1] He had consumed 1 litre of isotonic (sports) drinks per day for four months after an episode of diarrhoea. He was found to have decreased blood thiamin levels and lesions in the forebrain and thalamus. Levels of lactate in the blood and cerebrospinal fluid were markedly increased and blood sodium levels were low. Thiamin administration led to prompt improvement of symptoms, but the forebrain lesions and involuntary muscle contractions persisted.
- *A boy, eleven months of age,* developed vomiting and sleepiness.[1] Because he suffered from atopic dermatitis, he had been placed on a low-allergenic diet with no eggs, dairy products, meat or fish since early infancy. Thiamin administration rapidly relieved the symptoms.
- *A group of infants, two to twelve months of age,* were identified as vitamin B1 deficient after consuming a soy-based infant formula lacking vitamin B1.[2] Effects included elevated lactate levels, encephalopathy (brain dysfunction), weakness of eye muscles, infections, fever, vomiting, lethargy, irritability, abdominal bloating, diarrhoea, breathlessness, developmental delay and failure to thrive. They were treated with a different formula and im thiamin (50 mg/day for fourteen days). In infants without neurological damage, symptoms disappeared within two to three weeks on vitamin B1 therapy and ETKA tests normalised. Two infants given the formula died of cardiomyopathy during the acute phase and one remained in a persistent vegetative state and died six years later. Ten of the infants have ongoing health issues such as mental retardation, ataxia, hearing loss, swallowing difficulties, movement abnormalities, epilepsy, curvature of the spine and complete atrioventricular block (impairment of nerve conduction between the atria and ventricles of the heart), requiring a pacemaker.[3]

- *A woman, 64 years of age*, developed vomiting and severe diarrhoea, secondary to a bowel infection.[4] In hospital, she developed pneumonia and was unable to eat much food. After fifteen days, she became drowsy and less communicative, and developed generalised weakness in all four limbs with signs of encephalopathy. In spite of no history of alcohol consumption and normal blood TDP levels, radiological tests revealed indicators of Wernicke's encephalopathy. She was given iv vitamin B1 (500 mg three times a day) and made a good recovery over a period of about seven days.
- *A man, 44 years of age*, developed severe flaccid weakness of his arms and legs over a three-week period.[5] On investigation, he revealed that he had a standard diet but had regularly binged on alcohol (up to 20 cans of beer a day with occasional spirits) for more than fifteen years. He had eaten virtually nothing for a week prior to the beginning of limb weakness. He was found to have peripheral neuropathy and acute damage to motor nerve fibres. He was diagnosed with dry beriberi mimicking Guillain-Barré syndrome, a condition that affects peripheral nerves and causes ascending paralysis of the limbs. His symptoms improved with high-dose vitamin B1 replacement and physiotherapy, but he remained dependent on a Zimmer frame for mobility and a splint for wrist drop.
- *A man, 36 years of age* and a chronic alcoholic, was admitted to hospital.[6] Ten days beforehand, he had developed pain in his legs and feet, generalised weakness, and intermittent nausea and vomiting. Two days before admission, he developed sudden severe breathlessness, night sweats, loss of appetite, dark-coloured urine and purple mottling of his hands and feet. For the previous three to four months, his diet had consisted of alcohol (approximately 1.7 litres of vodka a day) and processed snack food. He was found to have severe metabolic acidosis, high output cardiac failure, heart enlargement, markedly low peripheral vascular resistance and reduced ETKA activity. He was diagnosed with Shoshin-type beriberi and treated initially with vitamin B1 (200 mg iv), diuretics, digitalis and oxygen, and had a rapid response. He was then given only vitamin B1 and multivitamins, and all abnormalities had disappeared at ten days.

REFERENCES

1. Saeki, K., Saito, Y., Komaki, H. et al., Thiamine-deficient encephalopathy due to excessive intake of isotonic drink or overstrict diet therapy in Japanese children, *Brain Dev* (2010), 32(7): 556–63.
2. Fattal-Valevski, A., Kesler, A. & Sela, B.A. et al., Outbreak of life-threatening thiamine deficiency in infants in Israel caused by a defective soy-based formula, *Pediatrics* (2005), 115(2): e233–8.
3. Fattal-Valevski, A., Bloch-Mimouni, A., Kivity, S. et al., Epilepsy in children with infantile thiamine deficiency, *Neurology* (2009), 73(11): 828–33.
4. Davies, S.B., Joshua, F.F. & Zagami, A.S., Wernicke's encephalopathy in a non-alcoholic patient with a normal blood thiamine level, *Med J Aust* (2011), 194(9): 483–4.
5. Murphy, C., Bangash. I.H. & Varma, A., Dry beriberi mimicking the Guillain-Barre syndrome, *Pract Neurol* (2009), 9(4): 221–4.
6. Attas, M., Hanley, H.G., Stultz, D. et al., Fulminant beriberi heart disease with lactic acidosis: Presentation of a case with evaluation of left ventricular function and review of pathophysiologic mechanisms, *Circulation* (1978), 58(3 Pt 1): 566–72.

THERAPEUTIC USES OF VITAMIN B1

Cognitive function

The alterations in brain function and structural damage observed in vitamin B1 deficiency have similarities to brain changes in Alzheimer's disease (AD), amyotrophic lateral sclerosis (motor neurone disease), Parkinson's disease, multiple sclerosis, alcoholic brain disease, stroke and traumatic brain injury. Reduced brain glucose metabolism and increased oxidative stress are features of both AD and vitamin B1 deficiency. In AD patients, the activity of thiamin-dependent enzymes is reduced and the reduction correlates with the extent of dementia.[1] Studies have found decreased vitamin B1 levels in plasma or red blood cells and, in a post-mortem investigation, TDP levels were found to be decreased in the brains of AD patients and those with frontal lobe degeneration of the non-Alzheimer's type.[2,3]

In an animal model of AD, vitamin B1 deficiency was found to impair oxidative metabolism, increase oxidative stress, inflammation and amyloid-beta production, and enlarge the area in the brain cortex occupied by plaques by 50 per cent, and in the hippocampus and thalamus by 200 per cent.[4] A study using 8 g/day of vitamin B1 orally found a mild beneficial effect in AD patients but other studies using 3 g/day report conflicting results.[5] A review of three studies using vitamin B1 for AD was not able to come to a conclusion because of poor study quality and limited patient numbers.[6]

Anxiety

A small study of people with anxiety who had low vitamin B1 levels found that intramuscular thiamin therapy improved appetite and wellbeing, reduced fatigue and enabled subjects to discontinue their use of anti-anxiety medication.[1]

Diabetes

Vitamin B1 deficiency is common in people with type 1 and type 2 diabetes. Plasma thiamin concentration has been shown to be decreased by 76 per cent in type 1 diabetics and by 75 per cent in type 2 diabetics, and losses in urine were increased 24-fold in type 1 diabetics and 16-fold in type 2 diabetics.[7] About half of women with gestational diabetes develop a vitamin B1 deficiency during the pregnancy.[8]

Insulin deficiency is associated with impaired thiamin transport across the intestinal wall, and thiamin deficiency leads to a marked impairment of insulin synthesis and secretion. An Australian study reported that vitamin B1 supplementation (4 g/day) normalised red blood cell thiamin levels in people with diabetes, whereas an adequate dietary intake did not.[9] Supplementary vitamin B1 can improve carbohydrate metabolism in diabetes, which reduces glycation and oxidative stress. It can also reduce activation of the protein kinase C isoforms that contribute to damage to blood vessels in retinal, kidney and cardiovascular tissues and reduce activity of the hexosamine pathway, an alternative pathway for metabolising sugars that is implicated in insulin resistance. Vitamin B1 may therefore help to prevent development of diabetes-related damage to the retina, kidneys, blood vessels and nerves.

In diabetic animals, vitamin B1 has been found to reduce fasting glucose and glycated haemoglobin (HbA_{1C}) levels, a marker of damage caused by high blood glucose,[10] and it has improved fasting blood glucose levels in people with type 2 diabetes.[11] Supplementation has reversed excretion of albumin in diabetic animals and in patients with type 2 diabetes, indicating that it may help preserve kidney function.[12] It has also improved blood fat and cholesterol levels and endothelial function in experimental diabetes and may help protect against cardiovascular complications.[13]

Health of the elderly

Vitamin B1 levels decline with ageing. A study of elderly hospitalised patients found that 39 per cent had a moderate vitamin B1 deficiency and 6 per cent had a severe deficiency, and deficiencies were more common in patients admitted from institutions such as nursing homes.[14] Patients with vitamin B1 deficiencies were more likely to be on frusemide diuretic therapy and to have AD, depression or cardiac failure, and to experience falls. In elderly women, vitamin B1 supplementation led to decreased fatigue and increased appetite, energy intake, body weight and general well-being, as well as improved sleep patterns.[15]

Congestive heart failure

Vitamin B1 deficiency can cause oedema and impair heart function, and can mimic the signs and symptoms of congestive heart failure. Loop diuretics are commonly used to relieve oedema and sodium imbalances in these patients, which can increase urinary vitamin B1 losses. In a small study of patients on diuretic treatment for chronic heart failure, vitamin B1 supplementation (300 mg/day) was associated with a small increase in left ventricular ejection fraction (the amount of blood pumped from the left ventricle of the heart).[16] It is recommended that prevention of thiamin deficiency should be a routine component in the overall management of congestive heart failure, especially if loop diuretics are used.

Menstrual cramps

One study of women with moderate to severe menstrual cramps found that vitamin B1 (100 mg/day for three months) abolished pain in 87 per cent, relieved pain in 8 per cent and had no effect in 5 per cent, and the beneficial effects lasted for two months after the supplement was discontinued.[17]

Sudden infant death syndrome (SIDS) and sudden unexplained death syndrome (SUDS)

Sudden unexpected deaths can occur in apparently thriving infants of asymptomatic thiamin-deficient mothers. Like infantile beriberi, SIDS has a peak incidence at two to four months of age, and may be associated with minor episodes of fever. Sleep apnoea has been known to occur in infants with a rare congenital defect of brain TDP. An Australian study found an unexpectedly high incidence of vitamin B1 deficiency in mothers and infants.[18] Deficiency was common in mothers at term, but not in their infants, and apparently healthy older infants were deficient but not their mothers. It appears that vitamin B1 is preferentially delivered to the foetus at the expense of the mother, and levels are restored in mothers after the birth but become depleted in the infant over time. There was a high incidence of thiamin deficiency in infants who had survived a SIDS episode and in their mothers and siblings, and vitamin B1-deficient infants had a high familial incidence of SIDS deaths. One study found that TTP was particularly low in SIDS cases.[19] Other studies have found markedly elevated serum levels of vitamin B1 after death; the importance of this is unknown, but it may indicate impairment of tissue uptake of thiamin and conversion to the active form.[20]

SUDS is a leading cause of death of apparently healthy young men in several Asian populations, and may be related to beriberi.[21,22] The syndrome is known as *bangungut* in the Philippines, *pokkuri* in Japan and *lai tai* in Thailand. Incidence is more common in countries in which white rice is a staple food, and it affects mainly young to middle-aged men. Deaths occur most often during the night, in the hot season and after a period of exertion. Witnesses report groaning, choking or coughing and muscular spasticity or paralysis for a few minutes prior to death. Post-mortem examination has found haemorrhagic congestion or oedema of the lungs, and abnormalities in the cardiac nerve conduction system. Because vitamin B1 deficiency can cause pulmonary congestion and heart malfunction, the possibility of vitamin B1 deficiency deserves to be investigated. However, its role in prevention is unknown.

REFERENCES

1 Lu'o'ng, K. & Nguyen, L.T., Role of thiamine in Alzheimer's disease, *Am J Alzheimers Dis Other Demen* (2011), 26(8): 588–98.

2 Rao, V.L., Richardson, J.S. & Butterworth, R.F., Decreased activities of thiamine diphosphatase in frontal and temporal cortex in Alzheimer's disease, *Brain Res* (1993), 631(2): 334–6.

3 Bettendorff, L., Mastrogiacomo, F., Wins, P. et al., Low thiamine diphosphate levels in brains of patients with frontal lobe degeneration of the non-Alzheimer's type, *J Neurochem* (1997), 69(5): 2005–10.

4 Karuppagounder, S.S., Xu, H. & Shi, Q., Thiamine deficiency induces oxidative stress and exacerbates the plaque pathology in Alzheimer's mouse model, *Neurobiol Aging* (2009), 30(10): 1587–600.

5 Meador, K., Loring, D., Nichols, M. et al., Preliminary findings of high-dose thiamine in dementia of Alzheimer's type, *J Geriatr Psychiatry Neurol* (1993), 6(4): 222–9.

6 Rodríguez-Martín, J.L., Qizilbash, N. & López-Arrieta, J.M., Thiamine for Alzheimer's disease, *Cochrane Database Syst Rev* (2001), 2: CD001498.

7 Thornalley, P.J.J., Babaei-Jadidi, R., Al Ali, H. et al., High prevalence of low plasma thiamine concentration in diabetes linked to a marker of vascular disease, *Diabetologia* (2007 Oct;), 50(10): 2164–70.

8 Bakker, S.J., ter Maaten, J.C. & Gans, R.O., Thiamine supplementation to prevent induction of low birth weight by conventional therapy for gestational diabetes mellitus, *Med Hypotheses* (2000), 55(1): 88–90.

9 Vindedzis, S.A., Stanton, K.G., Sherriff, J.L. & Dhaliwal, S.S., Thiamine deficiency in diabetes: Is diet relevant? *Diab Vasc Dis Res* (2008), 5(3): 215.

10 Thornalley, P.J.B. Jr, Karachalias, N. & Rabbani, N., Prevention of decline in glycaemic control in streptozocin-induced diabetic rats by thiamine but not by benfotiamine, *Diabet Med* (2010), 27(Supplement 1): 74.

11 González-Ortiz, M., Martínez-Abundis, E., Robles-Cervantes, J.A. et al., Effect of thiamine administration on metabolic profile, cytokines and inflammatory markers in drug-naïve patients with type 2 diabetes, *Eur J Nutr* (2011), 50(2): 145–9.

12 Rabbani, N. & Thornalley, P.J., Emerging role of thiamine therapy for prevention and treatment of early-stage diabetic nephropathy, *Diabetes Obes Metab* (2011), 13(7): 577–83.

13 Thornalley, P.J., The potential role of thiamine (vitamin B1) in diabetic complications, *Curr Diabetes Rev* (2005), 1(3): 287–98.

14 Pepersack, T., Garbusinski, J., Robberecht, J. et al., Clinical relevance of thiamine status amongst hospitalized elderly patients, *Gerontology* (1999), 45(2): 96–101.

15 Smidt, L.J., Cremin, F.M., Grivetti, L.E. & Clifford, A.J., Influence of thiamin supplementation on the health and general well-being of an elderly Irish population with marginal thiamin deficiency, *J Gerontol* (1991), 46(1): M16–22.

16 Schoenenberger, A.W., Schoenenberger-Berzins, R., der Maur, C.A. et al., Thiamine supplementation in symptomatic chronic heart failure: A randomized, double-blind, placebo-controlled, cross-over pilot study, *Clin Res Cardiol* (2012), 101(3): 159–64.

17 Gokhale, L.B., Curative treatment of primary (spasmodic) dysmenorrhoea, *Indian J Med Res* (1996), 103: 227–31.

18 Jeffrey, H.E., McCleary, B.V., Hensley, W.J. & Read, D.J., Thiamine deficiency: A neglected problem of infants and mothers—possible relationships to sudden infant death syndrome, *Aust NZ J Obstet Gynaecol* (1985), 25(3): 198–202.

19 Barker, J.N. & Jordan, F., Phrenic thiamin and neuropathy in sudden infant deaths. In H.Z. Sable & C.J. Gubler (eds), *Thiamin: Twenty years of progress, Ann NY Acad Sci* (1982), 378: 449–52.

20 Davis, R.E., Icke, G.C. & Hilton, J.M., High serum thiamine and the sudden infant death syndrome, *Clin Chim Acta* (1982), 123(3): 321–8.

21 Goh, K.T., Chao, T.C., Heng, B.H. et al., Epidemiology of sudden unexpected death syndrome among Thai migrant workers in Singapore, *Int J Epidemiol* (1993), 22(1): 88–95.

22 Munger, R.G. & Booton, E.A., Bangungut in Manila: Sudden and unexplained death in sleep of adult Filipinos, *Int J Epidemiol* (1998), 27(4): 677–84.

Therapeutic dose

Oral vitamin B1 may be absorbed better if taken in divided doses. Vitamin B1 supplements may be more effective if taken with a source of vitamin B2, vitamin B3, vitamin B5 and magnesium, which support vitamin B1 metabolism. Suggested doses for adults are as follows:

Oral doses

- *Health maintenance:* 5–10 mg daily.
- *Mild deficiency:* 10–25 mg daily.
- *Severe deficiency:* up to 300–900 mg daily or higher in the short term. In children with genetic abnormalities of pyruvate dehydrogenase, 100 mg/kg body weight divided into three daily doses may be required. In AD patients, doses of 1000 mg three times daily have been used for periods of two to twelve months. For acute cerebral beriberi (Wernicke-Korsakoff syndrome) in an adult, 50 mg/day of fat-soluble vitamin B1 has been used.

Intramuscular or intravenous doses

For beriberi, 50–100 mg daily is given im or iv for 7–14 days, followed by oral supplementation. For Wernicke-Korsakoff syndrome in an adult, initially vitamin B1 is given as 100 mg by slow iv injection over ten minutes, then 50–100 mg/day im or iv until the patient has improved enough to be transferred to oral thiamin. In research studies, iv thiamin has been used at doses of 500 mg three times daily. Intravenous thiamin should be given before iv glucose solutions because glucose can aggravate an existing vitamin B1 deficiency.

Effects of excess

Vitamin B1 appears to be non-toxic and well tolerated. Intake in excess of needs is excreted in urine. Extremely high doses (up to 8000 mg daily) have been used experimentally over a one-year period to assess tolerance. Two subjects reported nausea and indigestion at doses of 7000–7500 mg daily.

Supplements

Permitted forms of vitamin B1 in Australian supplements are thiamin, thiamin hydrochloride, thiamin nitrate, thiamin phosphate acid ester chloride dihydrate and thiamin phosphoric acid ester chloride.

Water-soluble vitamin B1

Common forms of supplemental vitamin B1 are thiamin nitrate and thiamin hydrochloride. Thiamin can be produced commercially from thiothiamin by oxidisation by hydrogen peroxide to form thiamin sulfate. Thiamin sulfate is then reacted with sodium hydroxide, ammonia and sodium nitrate in an aqueous ethanol solution to produce thiamin nitrate. Thiamin hydrochloride is made from a thiamin sulfate solution acidified by hydrochloric acid.

Fat-soluble vitamin B1

Allithiamin is a fat-soluble disulfide precursor to thiamin that is naturally produced from thiamin in garlic as a result of enzymatic action when a clove is cut or crushed. It can be converted to thiamin in the body, and appears to be more bioavailable than water-soluble thiamin, with higher absorption and retention. Thiamin tetrahydrofurfuryl disulfide (TTFD) is a synthetic counterpart of allithiamin but about half is hydrolysed in the digestive tract and iv delivery may be more effective. Benfotiamine (S-benzoylthiamine O-monophosphate) is another fat-soluble form of thiamin that is well absorbed and has been found to prevent the progression of diabetic complications. Although benfotiamine increases thiamin levels in the blood and liver, it appears to have no significant effect in the brain.

Cautions

Because B vitamins work together in many metabolic pathways in the body, it is possible that individual B vitamins taken alone—especially if taken in high doses—may affect the metabolism of other B vitamins and are not recommended for long-term use, unless supervised by a health-care practitioner.

Vitamin B2 (riboflavin)

VITAMIN B2 STATUS CHECK

1 Do you have cracks or sores at the corners of your mouth?
2 Do you get rashes around your mouth, nose or eyes, or in the genital area?
3 Is your tongue magenta-coloured and sore?
4 Do you have inflamed eyes?

'Yes' answers may indicate inadequate vitamin B2 status. Note that a number of nutritional deficiencies or health disorders can cause similar effects and further investigation is recommended.

FAST FACTS . . . VITAMIN B2

- **Vitamin B2 is found in dairy foods, eggs, liver, kidneys, chicken, meat, fish, brewer's yeast, nuts, broccoli, green leafy vegetables, asparagus, mushrooms, yeast-based spreads and vitamin B2-fortified breakfast cereals and soy milk.**
- **It is required for energy production in cells and antioxidant protection.**
- **It supports the metabolism of vitamin A, vitamin B3, vitamin B6, folic acid, selenium and iron.**
- **A deficiency causes eye inflammation and rashes around the mouth, nose, eyes and genital areas.**
- **Supplementation may be helpful for eye disorders, migraines and elevated serum homocysteine levels.**

A water-soluble growth factor with a distinctive yellow-green fluorescence was identified in milk whey in 1879 and named lactochrome. It was isolated from egg white and yeast in 1934 and identified as a water-soluble vitamin and renamed riboflavin because it contains a derivative of the sugar ribose. It was synthesised in 1935.

Vitamin B2 contains an isoalloxazine ring (flavin) with a 5-carbon sugar alcohol (ribitol) side chain. It is essential for energy production and antioxidant activity in the body, and supports metabolism of other essential nutrients but does not have a clear-cut deficiency syndrome. The most obvious deficiency signs are skin rashes around the mouth and eyes, and in the genital area, termed oculo-orogenital syndrome.

Digestion, absorption and transport

Most of the vitamin B2 in the diet is in the form of the coenzyme flavin adenine dinucleotide (FAD), with a small amount as free riboflavin and the coenzyme flavin mononucleotide (FMN). FAD and FMN in food are protein-bound, and are released by protein-digesting enzymes and then hydrolysed by phosphatases to release riboflavin, which is the absorbed form. Riboflavin is synthesised by bacteria in the colon and absorbed into colonocytes, and may contribute to body levels. Uptake into enterocytes and colonocytes is carrier-mediated at low levels, but passive diffusion may occur at higher levels. Three riboflavin transporters (RFVTs) have been identified: RFVT-1, RFVT-2 and RFVT-3. RFVT-3 acts in the intestine to facilitate absorption of dietary riboflavin, and transport is believed to become saturated at a single dose of about 25 mg.

In enterocytes, riboflavin is phosphorylated by the enzyme riboflavin kinase to form FMN, which is then converted to FAD by FAD synthetase. Vitamin B2 is converted back to riboflavin, transferred into the portal vein by RFVT-2 and bound to a protein—primarily albumin—for transport to the liver, where it is taken up by RFVT-2 and then converted to FMN and FAD.

Metabolism, storage and excretion

Most tissues take up riboflavin from the bloodstream via RFVT-2 and convert it to the coenzyme forms, but the brain is also able to take up FAD. Conversion of riboflavin to the coenzyme forms is stimulated by adrenocorticotropic hormone, aldosterone and thyroid hormones. There is no significant storage of vitamin B2 in the body. Vitamin B2 is excreted in urine mainly as free riboflavin, with a smaller amount of metabolites, such as 7-alpha- and 8-alpha-hydroxymethylriboflavin. When vitamin B2 supplements are taken, the excess that is excreted gives urine a bright yellow colour about two hours afterwards.

Functions

The active forms of vitamin B2 are FMN and FAD, which are incorporated into flavoproteins, enzyme systems that function as hydrogen (electron) carriers for many oxidation-reduction reactions in the body. The main active form is FAD. Functions of vitamin B2 include:

- *Energy production*. FAD is a cofactor for the enzyme complex pyruvate dehydrogenase, which converts pyruvate to acetyl-CoA; for the enzyme succinate dehydrogenase that converts succinate to fumarate in the citric acid cycle; and for activity of the electron transport chain. FAD activates the enzyme fatty acid acyl-CoA dehydrogenase, which oxidises fatty acids, as well as sphinganine oxidase that produces sphingosine, an important component of the sphingolipids that are part of cell membranes.
- *Nutrient metabolism*. FMN is a cofactor for pyridoxine phosphate oxidase, the enzyme that synthesises pyridoxal 5'-phosphate, the active coenzyme form of vitamin B6; FAD activates the enzyme aldehyde oxidase that breaks down vitamin B6 and it enables conversion of vitamin A to retinoic acid, conversion of the B vitamin folic acid to its active form and the synthesis of vitamin B3 from tryptophan. FAD is also required for activity of thioredoxin reductase, a selenium-containing enzyme that takes part in DNA synthesis, cell growth promotion and protection against oxidative stress. Vitamin B2 assists iron absorption, reduces losses in faeces and helps mobilise ferritin, the storage form of iron.
- *Antioxidant protection*. FAD is a cofactor for the enzyme glutathione reductase that regenerates the antioxidant glutathione from its oxidised form. The glutathione system plays an important role in detoxification and protection from ROS. FAD also acts as a coenzyme for the enzyme xanthine oxidase that breaks down purines from DNA and RNA to form uric acid, an important antioxidant in the body.

Dietary sources

Vitamin B2 is found in animal foods—especially dairy foods such as milk, cheese, yoghurt and whey—and also eggs, liver, kidneys, chicken, meat and fish. Plant sources include brewer's yeast, nuts, broccoli, green leafy vegetables, asparagus, mushrooms, yeast-based spreads and vitamin B2-fortified breakfast cereals and soy milk. Cow's milk and dairy products are the richest source but, because it is water-soluble, butter and cream are not good sources. Animal sources are more quickly absorbed, but there is little difference in overall bioavailability between plant and animal sources.

The Food Standards Australia New Zealand nutrient database (NUTTAB) at <www.foodstandards.gov.au> provides the amounts found in specific foods.

Factors influencing body status

Vitamin B2 is unstable at alkaline pH and when exposed to ultraviolet light—which breaks it down to inactive lumiflavin and lumichrome. Packaging of dairy products in clear containers leads to considerable losses. Ten hours of exposure to fluorescent light has been shown to reduce the amount of vitamin B2 in whole milk by 30 per cent and in skim milk by 59 per cent. Adding 0.1 per cent ascorbic acid to milk resulted in 50 per cent less losses in whole milk and 25.5 per cent less losses in skim milk after the same light exposure. A high incidence of vitamin B2 deficiency has been reported in preterm infants receiving breast milk that has been banked, and this is thought to be due to losses from light exposure during storage and delivery. Light therapy for treatment of jaundice in newborn infants depletes vitamin B2 levels because it is destroyed during oxidation of bilirubin.

Sun-drying foods and cooking with alkalising agents such as sodium bicarbonate lead to losses, and it is leached out of foods during water processing and cooking. Alcohol, copper, zinc, iron and manganese inhibit uptake of riboflavin in the digestive tract. Excretion of vitamin B2 is increased by diabetes, trauma and stress, and body levels are reduced by tricyclic antidepressants, phenothiazine anti-psychotic drugs, the anticancer drug doxorubicin, anti-malarial drugs and the anti-gout drug probenecid.

Daily requirement

Government recommendations by age and gender (see Table 6.3) can be found in *Nutrient Reference Values for Australia and New Zealand Including Recommended Dietary Intakes*, available at <www.nhmrc.gov.au>.

Table 6.3 Recommended dietary intake (RDI) of vitamin B2 (mg/day)

Age (years)	Female RDI	Male RDI
1–3	0.5	0.5
4–8	0.6	0.6
9–13	0.9	0.9
14–18	1.1	1.3
19–70	1.1	1.3
>70	1.3	1.6
Pregnant women		
14–18	1.4	
19–50	1.4	
Lactating women		
14–18	1.6	
19–50	1.6	

Source: Nutrient Reference Values for Australia and New Zealand Including Recommended Dietary Intakes, National Health and Medical Research Council, Australian Government Department of Health and Ageing, Canberra and Ministry of Health, New Zealand, Wellington, 2006.

Deficiency effects

A deficiency of vitamin B2 (ariboflavinosis) occurs after three to eight months of an inadequate intake. In animals, a deficiency causes accelerated turnover of enterocytes in the small intestine and a decrease in the number of villi and an increase in villus length, leading to reduced nutrient absorption. This particularly affects iron uptake, causing increased iron losses in faeces and anaemia. In cells, mitochondria enlarge and breaks occur in DNA strands. Animals fail to grow, lose fur and develop scaly red-brown crusty skin rashes, inflamed eyes, vascularisation of the cornea, corneal opacity and cataracts. Nerve damage develops, the liver becomes infiltrated with fat, reproduction is impaired and there is an increased number of birth defects in offspring.

A vitamin B2 deficiency in humans is usually associated with deficiencies of other B vitamins, and may occur in diets low in dairy products and meat. Inadequate vitamin B2 intake impairs metabolism of a number of nutrients, in particular vitamin B3, vitamin B6, folic acid and iron, and also impairs energy production and cell metabolism. Moderate riboflavin deficiency impairs iron absorption, reduces mobilisation of ferritin and reduces red blood cell production and maturation, leading to riboflavin-responsive anaemia, which is associated with increased numbers of immature red blood cells. A deficiency also impairs glutathione metabolism, which causes inflammation by increasing production of the inflammatory prostaglandin PGE_2.

A specific effect of a deficiency of vitamin B2 is oculo-orogenital syndrome, symptoms of which include inflamed, cracked and peeling lips, a sore magenta-coloured tongue, sore throat, mouth inflammation, cracks, sores and rashes at the corners of the mouth, corners of the eyes and around the nostrils, and rashes in the genital area. Inadequate vitamin B2 can cause flaky, scaly rashes (seborrhoeic dermatitis) on oily areas of the skin, such as the scalp, eyebrows, eyelids, creases of the nose, lips, behind the ears, in the outer ear and in the middle of the chest. Night blindness develops and the cornea of the eyes becomes inflamed (keratitis), vascularised and opaque, inhibiting vision. Deficiency symptoms include fatigue, weakness and impaired brain and nerve function.

A genetic defect in the gene for the riboflavin transporter RFVT-2 has been identified recently in patients with Brown-Vialetto-Van Laere syndrome, a progressive neurodegenerative disorder featuring severe weakness of the upper limbs and trunk muscles, hearing loss, optic atrophy, respiratory insufficiency and respiratory failure that usually leads to death during childhood. High doses of vitamin B2 have been found to reverse some of the symptoms, and appear to be especially effective if given early in life.

Indicators of inadequate levels may include:

- rough skin, dry or oily scaly rashes around the nose, eyes or genital areas
- cracks and sores in the corners of the mouth or eyes, flaky cracked lips, sore lips and magenta-coloured tongue, sore throat
- itchiness of the vulva or scrotum
- photophobia (eyes that are sensitive to light), burning and itching of the eyes, eyestrain or rapid visual fatigue, poor distance vision, blurred vision in poor light or twilight, growth of blood vessels in the cornea, sensitive eyes, bloodshot eyes, inflamed eyelids, night blindness
- anaemia, fatigue
- sensations of burning, numbness, and pins and needles.

Assessment of body status

Vitamin B2 concentration in serum is not regarded as a reliable measure of status because it reflects recent intakes, and levels are low and difficult to measure accurately. The measurement of FAD in whole blood is now used to test for a deficiency, as it appears to be a good indicator of tissue levels. The reference range given for FAD levels in whole blood by the Biochemistry Department of the Royal Prince Alfred Hospital, Sydney, Australia is 174–471 nmol/L. The erythrocyte glutathione reductase activity coefficient (EGRAC) has been used as a sensitive measure of vitamin B2 status. It measures the amount of vitamin B2 available to support function of the enzyme glutathione reductase in red blood cells. An increase in activity of 40 per cent or more after exposure to riboflavin indicates a deficiency, a 20 to less than 40 per cent increase indicates marginal status, and a less than 20 per cent increase indicates sufficiency.

Case reports—vitamin B2 deficiency

- *In the 1930s, a group of people* were given an experimental diet deficient in vitamin B2 but supplemented with other vitamins.[1] The first signs to appear were cracking, flaking and inflammation of the lips and corners of the mouth. The skin at the corners of the mouth softened, turned white and became susceptible to infections. Later signs included mild seborrhoeic dermatitis around the nose and occasionally on the ears and eyelids, cracks at the corners of the eyes, ulcers and fissures in the nasal septum and a magenta-coloured tongue with flattened or mushroom-shaped papillae. Subjects were given 0.025–0.075 mg of vitamin B2 per kilogram of body weight and the lesions disappeared within three weeks.
- *A man, 48 years of age,* developed inflammation at the corners of the mouth, a genital skin rash and red, burning eyes over a period of six months.[2] He had been consuming about 150 g of alcohol daily and eating large quantities of beef and pork, but very few cereals or vegetables. He was found to have an enlarged, fatty liver and markedly low serum levels of vitamin B2 and B6. He was treated with 100 mg of riboflavin per day iv and 150 mg of pyridoxine

per day orally. All the skin lesions disappeared within ten days.

- *A woman, 75 years of age*, complained of generally poor health, digestive disturbances, weakness, aches and pains and poor vision.[3] She had early cataracts in both lenses and marked inflammation of the conjunctiva and margins of the eyelids, with constant exudation. Photophobia was especially marked. Her tongue was pale, flabby, clean, moist, burning and sore, with several deep fissures, and enlarged and flattened papillae. She had deep fissures in the corners of her mouth, inflamed lips, and her nose and the neighbouring cheek surfaces showed follicular hyperkeratosis ('toad skin'), giving a swollen, 'doughy' appearance. She had previously been treated with vitamin B1, vitamin C and halibut liver oil but her eye and mouth symptoms persisted. She was then given 2 mg of vitamin B2 by injection three times a week for three weeks, followed by 4 mg a day orally. In four weeks, the cracks around her mouth had healed, her eyes were no longer inflamed, the photophobia had gone and her general health had improved. However, her cataracts and vision impairment showed no response, even when the oral dose of vitamin B2 was temporarily increased to 12 mg daily.
- *A woman, 52 years of age*, developed watering, inflamed eyes and photophobia over a three-month period.[4] She had experienced recurrent episodes of sore eyes for many years. On examination, both eyes looked inflamed and superficial blood vessels could be seen in the cornea, indicative of a vitamin B2 deficiency. No evidence of eye infection was found. Her diet largely consisted of cups of tea with bread and butter. She was given 9 mg of vitamin B2 daily, and reported that her eyes seemed to be entirely normal after about nine days, with improvement occurring within a few days of starting supplementation. The abnormal corneal vascularisation had regressed considerably. Some months later, after improving her diet, she reported no further problems with her eyes.

REFERENCES

1 Sebrell, W.V.H. & Butler, R.E., Riboflavin deficiency in man: A preliminary note, *Pub Health Rep* (1938), 53: 2282; (1939), 54: 2121 as reported in Ellenberg, M. & Pollack, H., Pseudo ariboflavinosis, *JAMA* (1942), 119(10): 790–2.

2 Friedli, A. & Saurat, J.H., Images in clinical medicine. Oculo-orogenital syndrome—a deficiency of vitamins B2 and B6, *N Engl J Med* (2004), 350: 1130.

3 Deeny, J., Riboflavin deficiency: With a case report, *Br Med J* (1942), 212(4272): 607.

4 Jackson, C.R., Riboflavin deficiency with ocular signs: report of a case, *Br J Ophthalmol* (1950), 34(4): 259–60.

THERAPEUTIC USES OF VITAMIN B2

Visual disorders

In animals, a diet low in vitamin B2 leads to corneal vascularisation, corneal opacity and cataracts, and the progression of cataracts can be halted by vitamin B2 supplementation.[1] FAD is a coenzyme for glutathione reductase, a protective antioxidant in the eye lens, and examination of surgically removed human cataracts has found a decrease in activity of glutathione reductase that could be restored by exposure to FAD.[2] A small study found that 80 per cent of patients with cataracts were deficient in riboflavin compared to 12.5 per cent of control subjects.[3] In older people taking a multivitamin supplement, there was a 44 per cent lower risk of nuclear cataract in the group taking riboflavin and niacin.[4] Other studies have not found an association between vitamin B2 and cataracts.[5]

Keratoconus is an eye disorder that begins in early life and is characterised by progressive corneal thinning and stretching that gradually progresses in both eyes, causing the corneas to bulge and form an irregular cone shape, which leads to astigmatism and blurred vision. Vitamin B2 is used as an effective therapy. It involves applying liquid vitamin B2 onto the cornea, which is then exposed to ultraviolet light. The light causes the vitamin B2 to fluoresce, which induces the formation of bonds between collagen molecules (cross-linking). This increases corneal rigidity and has been shown to halt progression of the disorder and may also improve corneal shape and visual function in some patients.[6]

Migraine headaches

Migraines may be associated with reduced cellular energy production, and riboflavin has been proposed as therapy. Several studies have found that a high dose of vitamin B2 (400 mg/day) is helpful for decreasing migraine frequency and duration, and reducing the need for medication, with the effect reaching a peak after three months.[7]

Elevated homocysteine

Homocysteine is formed during metabolism of the amino acid methionine, and is removed by the vitamin B2 and vitamin B12-dependent enzyme methylene tetrahydrofolate reductase (MTHFR) that acts on folic acid. Elevated levels of homocysteine are implicated in cardiovascular disease and stroke, and it is estimated that lowering plasma homocysteine by 25 per cent would reduce the risk of CHD by 11–16 per cent and stroke by 19–24 per cent.[8] Improved vitamin B2 status has been shown to cause a marked lowering of homocysteine in individuals with a gene that produces a variant of the MTHR enzyme (the TT genotype). The TT genotype is associated with lower levels of the vitamin B2 cofactor and reduced MTHFR activity, leading to elevated homocysteine levels. A study of people with the TT genotype has found that vitamin B2 supplementation decreased homocysteine levels by up to 22 per cent overall and, in those with initially lower riboflavin status, decreased homocysteine by 40 per cent.[9] Homocysteine levels in subjects without the TT genotype did not respond, even though their vitamin B2 status was inadequate at the start of the study and improved with supplementation.

Cancer

Vitamin B2 deficiency has been linked to an increased and also a decreased risk of cancer. Vitamin B2-dependent enzymes assist metabolism of some types of carcinogens, and can either increase or weaken their potency. In animals exposed to carcinogens, inadequate vitamin B2 leads to DNA damage but also to induction of repair enzymes, and vitamin B2 supplementation reduces both the DNA damage and repair enzyme activation.[10]

In animals, vitamin B2 deficiency causes abnormal cell development (dysplasia) of the epithelial lining of the oesophagus, and some human studies have found a link between oesophageal cancer and a low intake of vitamin B2 or decreased plasma levels.[11] Inadequate vitamin B2, as well as inadequate vitamin B1, vitamin B12 and folate, has been linked to increased risk of cervical dysplasia.[12]

REFERENCES

1 Day, L., Darby, W.J. & Cosgrove, K.W., The arrest of nutritional cataract by the use of riboflavin, *J Nutr* (1938), 15(1): 83–90.

2 Horwitz, J., Dovrat, A., Straatsma, B.R. et al., Glutathione reductase in human lens epithelium: FAD-induced in vitro activation, *Curr Eye Res* (1987), 6(10): 1249–56.

3 Sperduto, R.D., Hu, T.S., Milton, R.C. et al., The Linxian cataract studies: Two nutrition intervention trials, *Arch Ophthalmol* (1993), 111(9): 1246–53.

4 Bhat, K.S., Nutritional status of thiamine, riboflavin and pyridoxine in cataract patients, *Nutr Rep Inter* (1987), 36: 685–92.

5 Skalka, H.W. & Prchal, J.T., Cataracts and riboflavin deficiency, *Am J Clin Nutr* (1981), 34(5): 861–3.

6 Raiskup-Wolf, F., Hoyer, A., Spoerl, E. & Pillunat, L.E., Collagen crosslinking with riboflavin and ultraviolet-A light in keratoconus: Long-term results, *J Cataract Refract Surg* (2008), 34(5): 796–801.

7 Woolhouse, M., Migraine and tension headache: A complementary and alternative medicine approach, *Aust Fam Physician* (2005), 34(8): 647–51.

8 Homocysteine Studies Collaboration, Homocysteine and risk of ischemic heart disease and stroke: A meta-analysis, *JAMA* (2002), 288(16): 2015–22.

9 McNulty, H., Dowey, R.C., Strain, J.J. et al., Riboflavin lowers homocysteine in individuals homozygous for the MTHFR 677C->T polymorphism, *Circulation* (2006), 113(1): 74–80.

10 Webster, R.P., Gawde, M.D. & Bhattacharya, R.K., Modulation of carcinogen-induced damage and repair enzyme activity by riboflavin, *Cancer Lett* (1996), 98: 129–35.

11 Foy, H. & Kondi, A., The vulnerable oesophagus: Riboflavin deficiency and squamous cell dysplasia of the skin and the oesophagus, *J Natl Cancer Inst* (1984), 72: 941–8.

12 Hernandez, B.Y., McDuffie, K., Wilkens, L.R. et al., Diet and premalignant lesions of the cervix: Evidence of a protective role for folate, riboflavin, thiamin, and vitamin B12, *Cancer Causes Control* (2003), 14(9): 859–70.

Therapeutic dose

Oral vitamin B2 may be absorbed better if taken in divided doses. Suggested doses for adults are as follows:

- *Health maintenance:* 5–10 mg daily.
- *Mild deficiency:* 10–25 mg daily.
- *Severe deficiency:* up to 300–400 mg daily.
- *Migraine prevention:* 400 mg daily.
- *Vitamin B2-responsive anaemia:* 30–50 mg daily.

Effects of excess

Vitamin B2 appears to be non-toxic and well-tolerated. Intake in excess of needs is excreted in urine.

Supplements

Vitamin B2 is available in Australian supplements as riboflavin and riboflavin sodium phosphate. Riboflavin can be produced commercially by fermentation using yeast-like micro-organisms, such as *Eremothecium ashbyii* and *Ashbya gossypii*, or bacteria, such as *Bacillus subtilis* and *Corynebacterium ammoniagenes*, cultured in a medium of D-ribose obtained from glucose. *A. gossypii* is able to make 40 000 times more vitamin B2 than it needs for its own growth. After cultivation, pasteurisation is used to inactivate the micro-organisms, and riboflavin is then separated and extracted. Riboflavin sodium phosphate is produced by phosphorylation of riboflavin with phosphorus oxychloride.

Cautions

Vitamin B2 has specific interrelationships with vitamins B1, B3, B6, B12 and folic acid. Because B vitamins work together in many metabolic pathways in the body, it is possible that individual B vitamins taken alone—especially if taken in high doses—may affect the metabolism of other B vitamins, and such a practice is not recommended for long-term use unless supervised by a health-care practitioner.

Vitamin B3 (niacin)

VITAMIN B3 STATUS CHECK

1. Do you get a scaly, red rash on your skin after being in the sun?
2. Do you have a poor appetite, poor digestion and episodes of diarrhoea?
3. Do you have changeable moods, and are you often irritable, anxious or depressed?
4. Do you get headaches regularly, and have trouble sleeping?

'Yes' answers may indicate inadequate vitamin B3 status. Note that a number of nutritional deficiencies or health disorders can cause similar effects and further investigation is recommended.

FAST FACTS . . . VITAMIN B3

- Vitamin B3 is found in liver, meat, chicken, fish, brewer's yeast, legumes, seeds, nuts, coffee, tea, fortified breakfast cereals and yeast-based spreads.
- It is required for energy production in cells and supports production of fatty acids, sterols and DNA.
- It regulates cell replication and has anti-oxidant and anti-inflammatory activity.
- A deficiency can lead to pellagra, which features dermatitis, diarrhoea, dementia and, eventually, death.
- Supplementation may be helpful for the management of elevated serum cholesterol, arthritis and schizophrenia.

The substance now known as vitamin B3 was discovered by the Austrian chemist Hugo Weidel in 1873 during his studies of nicotine. It was isolated from yeast in 1913 by Casimir Funk and identified as a water-soluble vitamin following research into the disorder pellagra, which was prevalent in the American South during the early twentieth century. Pellagra was characterised by the three 'Ds'—dermatitis, diarrhoea and dementia—leading to the fourth 'D', death, and its name comes from the Italian for 'rough skin'. Pellagra existed for about 200 years in Europe and was first recognised in the United States in 1902. It is estimated that it affected three million people in the American South and caused 100 000 deaths, with many sufferers confined to lunatic asylums.

In 1915, Dr Joseph Goldberger, working for the US government's public health service, observed that pellagra only affected malnourished people, and demonstrated that it was a dietary deficiency disease that could be cured by substituting a corn-based diet with fresh milk, eggs and meat. The epidemic of pellagra appeared to coincide with the increasing use of corn as a staple food by poor people, and the development of new refining methods for corn and other grains that removed far more of the vitamin-containing germ and bran layers.

Goldberger's discovery led to experiments on a similar disease in dogs called 'black tongue' disease. In 1937, the American biochemist Dr Conrad Elvehjem used liver extracts, crystals of vitamin B3 and a synthetic form of vitamin B3, and was able to rapidly cure black tongue disease in dogs. This research was followed up by Dr Tom Spies in the same year, who reported using vitamin B3 to cure four patients with pellagra, which became standard treatment and led to the rapid eradication of the pellagra epidemic. In 1945, American biochemist Dr Willard Krehl discovered that the essential amino acid tryptophan, found in protein foods, can be converted into vitamin B3 in the body. Corn is particularly low in tryptophan, which was a partial explanation of the association between corn-based diets and vitamin B3 deficiency. The complete picture finally emerged in 1951, when it was discovered that vitamin B3 in corn is in a bound form with low bioavailability. Native Americans on corn-based diets did not suffer from pellagra because they used corn that was less intensively milled, and processed it before use by soaking it in water made alkaline by lime (calcium oxide) derived from limestone rock, a centuries-old preparation method called nixtamalisation that liberates the vitamin.

Vitamin B3 was originally called the PP (pellagra preventative) factor, and was found to exist as nicotinic acid (pyridine 3-carboxylic acid) and as the amide form nicotinamide (pyridine 3-carboxamide). Nicotinic acid was renamed niacin, derived from *ni*cotinic *a*c*i*d and vitami*n*, to avoid confusion with nicotine in tobacco. The terms niacin and nicotinic acid are used interchangeably, as are niacinamide and nicotinamide. Niacinamide is the main active form that is the precursor to NAD and NADP, vital cofactors for about 200 enzymes in the body.

Digestion, absorption and transport

Vitamin B3 in food is mainly found as NAD and NADP, which are hydrolysed in the digestive tract to free niacinamide. Low doses are absorbed by the sodium-coupled monocarboxylate transporter 1 (SMCT1) and high doses by passive diffusion. Doses as high as 3–4 g are well absorbed. Vitamin B3 is transported in the bloodstream mainly as niacinamide, but also as niacin bound to plasma proteins. It is taken up by tissue cells via SMCT1.

Metabolism, storage and excretion

In the liver and other tissues, niacinamide and niacin are converted to nicotinic acid mononucleotide (NAMN) and then to NAD. The liver stores vitamin B3 as NAD if excess is available, and converts it to niacinamide for transport to tissues as required. High concentrations of NAD are also found in the heart, kidneys and muscles. Body stores have been shown to become depleted after 50 to 60 days of a low vitamin B3 intake. Vitamin B3 can be excreted in urine as niacin or as metabolites, which include N'-methyl 2-pyridine 5-carboxamide (2PYR) and N'-methylnicotinamide (NMN). In normal conditions, 40 to 60 per cent of urinary vitamin B3 is in the form of 2PYR and 20 to 30 per cent is NMN.

The essential dietary amino acid tryptophan is converted to vitamin B3 in several steps requiring iron, vitamin B2, and vitamin B6 as cofactors. Tryptophan converts to kynurenine and then to quinolinic acid, which converts to NAMN, then to nicotinic acid adenine dinucleotide (NAAD), then to NAD, and finally to niacinamide. It is estimated that 60 mg of tryptophan produces 1 mg of vitamin B3, which increases threefold in late pregnancy. Taking supplementary vitamin B3 does not appear to suppress its synthesis from tryptophan.

Functions

The active forms of vitamin B3 are NAD and NADP, which accept or donate electrons in many of the body's enzyme systems, converting to NADH and NADPH respectively during metabolism. Functions of vitamin B3 include:

- *Energy production.* NAD takes part in many reactions that produce energy, including glycolysis, pyruvate metabolism, acetyl-CoA metabolism and fatty acid and alcohol oxidation. NADH transfers electrons during oxidative phosphorylation, which generates energy in the form of adenosine triphosphate (ATP).
- *Production of fatty acids, sterols and DNA.* NADPH, generated from NADP, acts as a hydrogen donor during synthesis of fatty acids and sterols, such as cholesterol and cholesterol-derived steroid hormones.
- *Cell replication.* NADP is a cofactor for enzymes in the pentose phosphate pathway that oxidises glucose to make NADPH and 5-carbon sugars, such as ribose-5-phosphate used for the production of nucleotides and nucleic acids that are constituents of DNA. NAD works with poly(ADP-ribose)polymerases (PARP), enzymes involved in DNA repair, cell replication and differentiation, cell signalling and apoptosis.
- *Maintenance of the antioxidant network.* Vitamin B3 assists regeneration of the antioxidants glutathione, vitamin C and thioredoxin to maintain antioxidant protection.
- *Vitamin B6 and folic acid metabolism.* NAD is required for the breakdown of vitamin B6 and NADPH takes part in folic acid metabolism.
- *Anti-inflammatory activity.* Niacin has been shown to reduce secretion of a number of cytokines, including TNF-alpha, interleukins, C-reactive protein and monocyte chemoattractant protein–1.

Dietary sources

Vitamin B3 is found in liver, meat, chicken, fish, brewer's yeast, legumes, seeds, nuts, coffee, tea, vitamin B3-fortified breakfast cereals and yeast-based spreads. Niacin is more prevalent in plant food and niacinamide predominates in animal food. In Australia, vitamin B3, as bioavailable free niacin, is permitted to be voluntarily added to some commercial foods, such as breakfast cereals.

The Food Standards Australia New Zealand nutrient database (NUTTAB) at <www.foodstandards.gov.au> provides the amounts found in specific foods.

Factors influencing body status

Vitamin B3 in many plant foods is bound to carbohydrates as niacytin or to peptides as niacinogens, and has limited bioavailability. Only about 10 per cent of the total vitamin B3 content is available in corn and about 30 per cent in other grains and nuts. Corn is a particularly poor source because it has unavailable vitamin B3 and is also low in tryptophan. Soaking corn in an alkaline solution increases bioavailability of vitamin B3. Refining of grains causes considerable losses because of removal of the nutrient-rich bran and germ. Whole-wheat bread is estimated to contain five times more vitamin B3 than white bread.

Vitamin B3 is stable in the presence of oxygen, acids, light and heat, and most is retained during cooking with dry heat, pasteurisation, drying and sterilisation. However, it is water-soluble and can be leached out of food by water processing and cooking methods. Excretion in urine is increased by diuretic drugs, alcohol and stimulants, such as caffeine in coffee, soft drinks, tea and chocolate, theophylline in tea and theobromine in cocoa and chocolate.

About half of the body's requirement is produced from tryptophan, an essential amino acid found in first-class protein foods, such as meat, fish, chicken, dairy and soy products. Therefore, a low-protein intake will reduce intake of both tryptophan and pre-formed vitamin B3. The conversion of tryptophan to niacin may be impaired by a deficiency of vitamin B2, vitamin B6 or iron.

Vitamin B3 deficiency occurs in Hartnup disease, a malabsorption disorder affecting tryptophan, and may occur in carcinoid syndrome, a disorder involving slow-growing cancer-like tumours, in which tryptophan conversion to vitamin B3 is reduced. Vitamin B3 deficiency can occur in chronic alcoholism and malabsorption disorders, and during treatment with anti-tuberculosis (TB) drugs, which are structurally similar to vitamin B3 and can impair its metabolism. TB drugs also impair metabolism of vitamin B6, a cofactor for vitamin B3 synthesis. Other drugs that deplete vitamin B3 include anti-epileptic drugs, the immuno-suppressive drug mercaptopurine, the anti-cancer drug fluorouracil, oestrogen-containing oral contraceptives, the metal chelating drug penicillamine and the antibiotic chloramphenicol.

Daily requirement

Government recommendations by age and gender (see Table 6.4) can be found in *Nutrient Reference Values*

Table 6.4 Recommended dietary intake (RDI) of vitamin B3 (mg/day NE)*

Age (years)	Female RDI	Male RDI
1–3	6	6
4–8	8	8
9–13	12	12
14–18	14	16
19–70	14	16
>70	14	16
Pregnant women		
14–18	18	
19–50	18	
Lactating women		
14–18	17	
19–50	17	

* NE, niacin equivalents: 1 mg niacin equivalent is equal to 1 mg niacin or 60 mg tryptophan.

Source: Nutrient Reference Values for Australia and New Zealand Including Recommended Dietary Intakes, National Health and Medical Research Council, Australian Government Department of Health and Ageing, Canberra and Ministry of Health, New Zealand, Wellington, 2006.

for Australia and New Zealand Including Recommended Dietary Intakes, available at <www.nhmrc.gov.au>.

Deficiency effects

A severe vitamin B3 deficiency causes pellagra, which has commonly been associated with the American South and Southern Europe, where corn was used as a staple food without pre-treatment with an alkalising solution. It was identified among Spanish peasants in 1735 by the physician Don Gaspar Casal, who noted the connection with corn-based diets. It was called 'mal de la rosa' because of the characteristic reddish, shiny rash on the hands and feet.

Pellagra signs and symptoms begin to appear after 50 to 60 days of insufficient vitamin B3. Early symptoms include lassitude, weakness, loss of appetite, weight loss, mild digestive disturbances, anxiety, irritability and depression, followed by the characteristic symptoms of dermatitis, diarrhoea and dementia. Severe untreated pellagra leads to death from multi-organ failure.

Skin effects

A lack of vitamin B3 causes dilation of blood vessels in the skin and proliferation of the endothelial lining, lymphocytic infiltration, excess keratin production and atrophy of the epidermis. Changes occur in areas of skin exposed to sunlight or pressure, and appear symmetrically. Initially, the skin looks as if it is sunburnt, with reddening, blistering and peeling. Over time, the skin becomes a dark reddish-brown, and may be covered with scales and blackish crusts from haemorrhages. Pustules and deep fissures may be present. Lesions often occur on the hands and forearms, feet and lower legs ('glove and boot' distribution), around the base of the neck (casal necklace), and on the forehead, nose and cheeks, which may appear as a butterfly-shaped eruption, similar to that occurring in systemic lupus erythematosus. There is a clear zone of demarcation between the affected and normal skin.

Digestive tract effects

In pellagra, digestive tract changes usually precede skin changes. There is acute inflammation of the lining of the digestive tract, which eventually atrophies, leading to malabsorption. The tongue is inflamed, sore and bright or dark red, and papillae on the tongue atrophy. Gastritis and atrophy of the gastric mucosa are common, and production of hydrochloric acid and digestive enzymes decreases. Symptoms include poor appetite, nausea, excessive salivation, a burning sensation in the stomach and watery diarrhoea.

Nervous system effects

The central and peripheral nervous systems can develop patchy demyelination and degeneration. Early nervous system symptoms of vitamin B3 deficiency may include depression, fatigue, apathy, headache, irritability, poor concentration, insomnia and anxiety. A more severe deficiency causes dizziness after sudden movements, restlessness, nervous tension, argumentativeness, depression, suicidal thoughts and hypersensitivity to stimuli such as noise, smells and bright light, which trigger nausea and vomiting. More severe mental impairment causes tremor, ataxia, muscle spasms, delusions, hallucinations, restlessness, photophobia, stupor, confusion, disorientation, memory loss, delirium, dementia, psychosis and, eventually, coma and death.

Indicators of inadequate levels may include:

- symmetrical patches of dry, scaly, reddened skin or darkened, crusty skin on the neck, face or limbs
- poor appetite, indigestion, red and painful tongue, inflammation of the digestive tract, abdominal or stomach pain, diarrhoea
- depression, fatigue, apathy, headache, irritability, anxiety, poor concentration, mood swings, poor memory, lack of concentration, restlessness, delusions, hypersensitivity to stimuli, confusion, disorientation, dementia, psychosis
- headaches, insomnia, dizziness
- weak muscles, muscle spasms, tremors, poor coordination.

Assessment of body status

The niacin concentration of whole blood has been used to assess vitamin B3 status, with the reference range reported to be 0.9–8.2 µmol/L, and the NAD and NADP concentration in whole blood has also been used; however, both measures are now regarded as unreliable. A more reliable method appears to be measurement of the major urinary metabolites 2PYR and NMN, levels of which decline when vitamin B3 status is inadequate. The reference range given by the Biochemistry Department of the Royal Prince Alfred Hospital, Sydney, Australia is 25–110 µmol/day for 2PYR and 10–75 µmol/day for NMN. The urinary ratio of 2PYR:NMN, obtained from a 24-hour urine collection, is regarded as a reliable indicator of niacin status. The normal ratio is 1.3–4.0 mg/g creatinine and a ratio of less than 1 is indicative of niacin deficiency. Diagnosis of a vitamin B3 deficiency can be confirmed by the response to oral supplementation. Skin symptoms usually improve within two days of treatment.

Case reports—vitamin B3 deficiency

- *A man, 88 years of age*, with chronic obstructive lung disease, developed acute respiratory failure.[1] While hospitalised, he was observed to have a symmetric, scaly, sunburn-like rash extending from his hands to midway up the arms. No previous diarrhoea or dementia were reported. Serum niacin levels were low and a skin biopsy showed evidence of pellagra-like dermatitis. Niacin supplementation was given and there was considerable improvement in the skin lesions over several days. Unfortunately, the patient subsequently died of complications from hospital-acquired pneumonia.
- *A man, 57 years of age*, and a chronic smoker and alcoholic suffering from TB, developed mental confusion and involuntary movements of the hands and legs.[2] He had pallor, a beefy tongue and red, peeling dermatitis with hyperpigmentation. He was already on medication for TB and was taking a multivitamin. He was diagnosed with pellagra encephalopathy, possibly caused by his TB medication and alcohol abuse. Intravenous vitamin B3 was given, which led to a dramatic recovery of his mental faculties and disappearance of his skin rash.
- *A woman, 57 years of age*, had developed a skin rash involving her hands and feet three weeks previously.[3] She was found to have a symmetrical, scaly, reddish-brown eruption on the backs of her hands and tops of her feet, and blisters and marked oedema of the lower legs. The skin lesions were in areas exposed to sunlight and were painful to touch. She also had developed loss of appetite, fatigue, irritability and watery diarrhoea over the last two months, and reported episodic abdominal pain, diarrhoea and considerable weight loss over the last four years. She had been treated with a proton pump inhibitor to reduce gastric acid secretion for several years. She was found to be anaemic, and was diagnosed with Crohn's disease, an inflammatory disease affecting the intestine. She was treated with albumin infusions and an oral multivitamin that contained 200 mg of vitamin B3 daily. Her Crohn's disease was managed with oral prednisolone and metronidazole. Skin lesions resolved within two weeks of beginning the multivitamin.
- *A woman, 32 years of age*, obese and lethargic, had developed an itchy, red, scaly skin eruption over the previous two months, which first appeared on the backs of her hands and tops of her feet, and had spread up her limbs.[4] The rash was strikingly demarcated from healthy skin. She reported a high intake of beer and almost no food for the previous year, during which she had existed on beer and the occasional boiled potato. She also reported cessation of her menstrual cycle, diarrhoea and a sore mouth over the last six months. She was found to have atrophy of the tongue, superficial ulceration of the gums, anaemia and a low thyroxine level. She was given a normal diet, thyroid hormone therapy and a daily supplement of 5 mg of vitamin B2, 100 mg of vitamin B1, 50 mg of vitamin B3 four times daily, and 100 mg of vitamin C three times daily. Before treatment could

take effect, she became acutely psychotic and was admitted to a psychiatric ward. She rapidly improved with treatment, her diarrhoea subsiding in two days and her skin lesions beginning to resolve in two weeks, and she was well enough to be discharged. On investigation, it was found that her high beer intake seemed to supply sufficient amounts of vitamins B1, B2 and B3. It was concluded that malabsorption, the diuretic effect of beer, a slow metabolism caused by an underactive thyroid gland, and lack of tryptophan and vitamin B6 for vitamin B3 synthesis contributed to her severe vitamin B3 deficiency.

REFERENCES

1 Mercieri, M. & Mercieri, A., Images in clinical medicine: A photosensitive dermatitis in the intensive care unit, *N Engl J Med* (2011), 364(4): 361.
2 Das, R., Parajuli, S. & Gupta, S., A rash imposition from a lifestyle omission: A case report of pellagra, *Ulster Med J* (2006), 75(1): 92–3.
3 Rosmaninho, A., Sanches, M., Fernandes, I.C. et al., Letter: Pellagra as the initial presentation of Crohn disease, *Dermatol Online J* (2012), 18(4): 12.
4 DesGroseilliers, J.P. & Shiffman, N.J., Pellagra, *Can Med Assoc J* (1976), 115(8): 768–70.

THERAPEUTIC USES OF VITAMIN B3

Cardiovascular disease

Niacin in high doses (3000 mg/day) has been shown to reduce a number of risk factors for atherosclerosis, including reducing plasma total cholesterol by 21 per cent, triglycerides by 44 per cent, apolipoprotein B by 20 per cent and lipoprotein(a) levels by 26 per cent and increasing HDL cholesterol by 30 per cent.[1] Niacin reduces total and LDL cholesterol levels by reducing the production of VLDL, and consequently LDL, and increasing the clearance of LDL from the bloodstream. It reduces triglyceride synthesis in the liver by inhibiting release of the precursor free fatty acids from adipose tissue and reducing the activity of the liver enzymes that produce triglycerides. Niacin also inhibits the formation of small, dense LDL particles that remain longer in the circulation and are atherogenic (atherosclerosis-promoting). Niacin increases protective factors in the bloodstream, such as HDL cholesterol, apolipoprotein A-I (the main protein in HDL) and the ratio of HDL2:HDL3, and is regarded as the most effective agent for raising HDL cholesterol levels. HDL2, a sub-fraction of HDL, is particularly protective against CVD. All these cardiovascular benefits are specific to niacin, and are not seen with niacinamide supplementation.

Adipose tissue is an active endocrine organ that has a role in inflammation and CVD, and vitamin B3 has been found to suppress inflammatory cytokines and markedly elevate levels of the anti-inflammatory chemical adiponectin in adipose tissue in men with metabolic syndrome.[2] Higher adiponectin levels have been shown to be linked to a lower risk of heart attacks in men and moderately decreased risk of CHD in male diabetic patients.[3,4]

A number of studies have found that niacin has beneficial effects in CVD. A meta-analysis of fourteen trials concluded that niacin significantly reduced major coronary events by 25 per cent, stroke by 26 per cent and cardiovascular events by 27 per cent.[5] The meta-analysis also found that progression of coronary atherosclerosis slowed by 41 per cent in the niacin group. In heart patients, niacin has been shown to reduce total cholesterol levels by 10 per cent, reduce the incidence of non-fatal heart attacks by 27 per cent at the five-year follow-up, and decrease all-cause mortality by 11 per cent at the fifteen-year follow-up.[6]

Niacin used with other cholesterol-lowering drugs has been shown to have additive effects. Niacin used with colestipol in coronary artery bypass patients decreased LDL cholesterol by 43 per cent, increased HDL cholesterol levels by 37 per cent and led to regression of atherosclerosis.[7] Niacin used with clofibrate resulted in a 26 per cent reduction in all-cause mortality and a 36 per cent reduction in CHD deaths after five years of treatment.[8] Niacin used with a statin drug has been shown to reduce LDL cholesterol by 42 per cent, and has led to regression of coronary atheroma and a 90 per cent reduction in markers of atherosclerosis progression in heart patients.[9]

In a study of diabetic and non-diabetic patients with CVD, niacin increased HDL cholesterol by 29 per cent in both groups, decreased LDL cholesterol by 8 per cent in diabetics and 9 per cent in non-diabetics, and decreased triglycerides by 23 per cent in diabetics and 28 per cent in non-diabetics.[10] Glucose levels were modestly increased in both groups, but levels of glycated haemoglobin were unchanged in the diabetic group.

The effect of niacin on serum cholesterol appears to be dose responsive; it is estimated that 1000 mg of niacin lowers total cholesterol by about 5 per cent, 2000 mg lowers total cholesterol by about 10 per cent and 3000 mg lowers total cholesterol by about 16 per cent.[11] For LDL cholesterol, 1000 mg of niacin lowers levels by about 9 per cent, 2000 mg by about 17 per cent and 3000 mg by about 21 per cent. However, doses of 1000 mg or more can cause liver toxicity.

Arthritis

Dr William Kaufman pioneered the use of niacinamide for osteoarthritis in the 1930s.[12] He found that doses of up to 4000 mg a day given in divided doses ten times a day increased joint mobility and reduced pain, stiffness and inflammation after three to four weeks. He recorded his observations over many years of practice, and found that long-term niacinamide treatment was able to maintain joint function for as long as twenty years. However, relapses occurred if patients discontinued their treatment. Dr Kaufman eventually concluded that more frequent dosing using 250 mg of niacinamide was 40–50 per cent more effective than a 500 mg dose used less frequently. Beneficial effects were seen after one to three months. More recently, patients with osteoarthritis given 500 mg niacinamide six times daily were found to have an improvement in global arthritis impact of 29 per cent, increased joint mobility and a reduction of 13 per cent in the use of anti-inflammatory medication.[13]

Schizophrenia

Dr Abram Hoffer pioneered the use of niacin for the treatment of schizophrenia in the 1950s. He formed the theory that schizophrenia was caused by elevated levels of adrenochrome, an oxidised derivative of adrenaline.[14] Dr Hoffer theorised that vitamin B3 might be useful because it had the potential to decrease conversion of noradrenaline to adrenaline and to reconvert adrenochrome to adrenaline in the brain. In a pilot study, 30 acute schizophrenic patients on standard medication were given a placebo, niacinamide or niacin (1 g three times daily for 30 days) and then followed up at one year.[15] Patients who took vitamin B3 during the study were found to have more than double the recovery rate of the placebo group. A subsequent 33-day study used niacin or placebo, and found that significantly more of the patients on niacin improved compared with those on placebo.[15]

After many years of research, Dr Hoffer concluded that niacin is more effective and better tolerated than niacinamide and that acute schizophrenia responds better than the chronic form. He recommended using an initial dose of 1000 mg of niacin three times daily for adults, slowly increasing to 4500–18 000 mg.[15] Such high doses of niacin should only be used under strict medical supervision because of the high risk of adverse effects and toxicity.

REFERENCES

1 Goldberg, A., Alagona, P. Jr, Capuzzi, D.M. et al., Multiple-dose efficacy and safety of an extended-release form of niacin in the management of hyperlipidemia, *Am J Cardiol* (2000), 85(9): 1100–5.

2 Westphal, S. & Luley, C., Preferential increase in high-molecular weight adiponectin after niacin, *Atherosclerosis* (2008), 198(1): 179–83.

3 Pischon, T., Girman, C.J., Hotamisligil, G.S. et al., Plasma adiponectin levels and risk of myocardial infarction in men, *JAMA* (2004), 291(14): 1730–7.

4 Schulze, M.B., Shai, I., Rimm, E.B. et al., Adiponectin and future coronary heart disease events among men with type 2 diabetes, *Diabetes* (2005), 54(2): 534–9.

5 Bruckert, E., Labreuche, J. & Amarenco, P., Meta-analysis of the effect of nicotinic acid alone or in combination on cardiovascular events and atherosclerosis, *Atherosclerosis* (2010), 210(2): 353–61.

6 Canner, P.L., Berge, K.G., Wenger, N.K. et al., Fifteen year mortality in Coronary Drug Project patients: Long-term benefit with niacin, *J Am Coll Cardiol* (1986), 8(6): 1245–55.

7 Blankenhorn, D.H., Nessim, S.A., Johnson, R.L. et al., Beneficial effects of combined colestipol-niacin therapy on coronary atherosclerosis and coronary venous bypass grafts, *JAMA* (1987), 257(23): 3233–40.

8 Carlson, L.A. & Rosenhamer, G., Reduction of mortality in the Stockholm Ischaemic Heart Disease Secondary Prevention Study by combined treatment with clofibrate and nicotinic acid, *Acta Med Scand* (1988), 223: 405–18.

9 Brown, B.G., Zhao, X.Q., Chait, A. et al., Simvastatin and niacin, antioxidant vitamins, or the combination for the prevention of coronary disease, *N Engl J Med* (2001), 345: 1583–92.

10 Elam, M.B., Hunninghake, D.B., Davis, K.B. et al., Effect of niacin on lipid and lipoprotein levels and glycemic control in patients with diabetes and peripheral arterial disease: The ADMIT study—a randomized trial. Arterial Disease Multiple Intervention Trial, *JAMA* (2000), 284(10): 1263–70.

11 Shanes, J.G., A review of the rationale for additional therapeutic interventions to attain lower LDL-C when statin therapy is not enough, *Curr Atheroscler Rep* (2012), 14(1): 33–40.

12 Hoffer, A., Treatment of arthritis by nicotinic acid and nicotinamide, *Can Med Assoc J* (1959), 81: 235–8.

13 Jonas, W.B., Rapoza, C.P. & Blair, W.F., The effect of niacinamide on osteoarthritis: A pilot study, *Inflamm Res* (1996), 45(7): 330–4.

14 Hoffer, A. & Osmond, H., The Adrenochrome Model and schizophrenia 1, *J Nervous Mental Dis* (1959), 128(1): 18–35.

15 Hoffer, A. & Prousky, J., Successful treatment of schizophrenia requires optimal daily doses of vitamin B3, *Altern Med Rev* (2008), 13(4): 287–91.

Therapeutic dose

Oral vitamin B3 may be better absorbed if taken in divided doses. Suggested doses for adults are as follows:

- *Health maintenance:* 10–50 mg daily as niacinamide.
- *Mild deficiency:* 50–100 mg daily as niacinamide.
- *Severe deficiency:* up to 500 mg daily as niacinamide.
- *Cholesterol management:* 1–2 g of niacin two to three times daily (maximum 6 g daily) or 1–2 g daily of slow-release niacin, under medical supervision.
- *Arthritis:* up to 4000 mg daily as niacinamide in divided doses, six to ten times daily.
- *Schizophrenia:* initial dose of 1000 mg niacin three times daily, slowly increasing to 4500–18 000 mg, under medical supervision.

Effects of excess

Niacinamide is well tolerated at doses commonly used, but niacin can cause adverse effects.

Niacin

In almost all patients, niacin supplementation causes vasodilation in the skin, which leads to flushing, itching and a warm or burning sensation mainly affecting the upper body and face that begins about fifteen minutes after the dose and lasts about one hour. This reaction is usually mild, but in some patients it is so intolerable that therapy is discontinued. The 'niacin flush' occurs at relatively low doses of 50–100 mg, but tolerance develops within days of continued use and the flush reduces or disappears. It is believed that flushing is induced by activity of the enzyme COX-1 in immune cells in the skin, which increases production of PGI_2, PGE_2 and PGD_2 and their metabolites. PGD_2 appears to be mainly responsible for skin vasodilation. Levels of these eicosanoids have been shown to decrease as tolerance to niacin develops. The niacin flush can be reduced by use of an antihistamine fifteen minutes prior to a niacin dose or by use of COX-1 inhibitors such as aspirin or non-steroidal anti-inflammatory drugs (ibuprofen, naproxen and indomethacin). A 650 mg dose of aspirin 20–30 minutes prior to taking niacin has been shown to prevent flushing in 90 per cent of patients, but may cause an increased risk of gastrointestinal bleeding. Slow-release niacin products have been developed to minimise the flushing effect.

High-dose niacin use has been associated with stomach upsets, nausea, vomiting and diarrhoea, which may resolve with continued use. Liver toxicity is a more serious adverse effect, which is indicated by increased liver transaminase enzymes in serum, yellowing of the skin and whites of the eyes (jaundice), fatigue and fluid buildup in the abdomen (ascites). Rarely, liver failure may occur. It is recommended that liver function is monitored regularly during niacin therapy. Slow-release niacin products may cause more severe gastrointestinal and liver effects. High-dose niacin has been found to cause a mild increase in insulin resistance in patients with abnormal glucose metabolism. Patients taking niacin may need to have their insulin or oral diabetes medications adjusted.

Adverse reactions can occur at levels of 1 g of niacin daily or more. Most reported adverse reactions have occurred with intakes of 2000–6000 mg per day. A study of high-dose niacin used slow-release and regular, instant-release niacin at doses of 500, 1000, 1500, 2000 and 3000 mg per day for six weeks. There were no adverse reactions at 500 mg a day for either preparation, but doses of 1000 mg daily or more produced gastrointestinal effects in those taking regular niacin and mild liver toxicity in those taking the slow-release form. High doses of the cholesterol-lowering medication simvastatin have been found to increase risk of muscle damage, which may be exacerbated when combined with niacin therapy. It is recommended that no more than 20 mg of simvastatin is taken daily by patients also taking 1 g or more of niacin daily.

Niacinamide

Niacinamide appears to be tolerated better, with fewer adverse effects than niacin. However, it has no effect on blood lipids or cholesterol. Several studies have found no adverse effects for niacinamide intakes of 1000–2900 mg per day. Intakes of more than 3000 mg per day have been associated with liver and gastrointestinal effects, including nausea, dry mouth, stomach upsets, vomiting and diarrhoea.

Supplements

Vitamin B3 is available in Australian supplements as nicotinamide (niacinamide), nicotinamide ascorbate and nicotinic acid (niacin). In Australia, no more than 100 mg of niacin is permitted per dosage unit in non-prescription products. Higher dose niacin products are classed as Schedule 4 (prescription-only) medicines. The dose of niacinamide in products is not restricted.

Vitamin B3 can be produced by bacterial fermentation or by conversion of acetaldehyde and formaldehyde or acrolein and ammonia to 3-picoline and pyridine and then oxidation of 3-picoline or 5-ethyl-2-methylpyridine with nitric acid to form niacin. Alternatively, 3-methylpyridine can be reacted using a vanadium catalyst to form nicotinonitrile, which is then hydrolysed to nicotinamide.

Cautions

High doses of vitamin B3 should only be taken with medical supervision and regular monitoring of liver function. Glucose tolerance should be monitored in patients with diabetes. Because B vitamins work together in many metabolic pathways in the body, it is possible that individual B vitamins taken alone, especially if taken in high doses, may affect the metabolism of other B vitamins, and are not recommended for long-term use unless supervised by a health-care practitioner.

HOW MUCH DO I KNOW?

Choose whether the following statements are true or false. Then review this chapter for the correct answers.

	True (T)	False (F)
1 Vitamin C supports collagen formation in connective tissue.	T	F
2 Key symptoms of beriberi in infants are irritability and tender, painful legs.	T	F
3 Vitamin C helps protect DNA from damage and assists DNA repair.	T	F

	True (T)	False (F)
4 Vitamin B1 supports the citric acid cycle that produces energy in cells.	T	F
5 Loss of appetite, indigestion, weakness, irritability, and depression are key indicators of vitamin B2 deficiency.	T	F
6 Vitamin B1 body levels can be assessed by the amount in whole blood.	T	F
7 Vitamin B2 assists the metabolism of vitamin B3, B6 and folic acid.	T	F
8 Oculo-orogenital syndrome is an indicator of vitamin B3 deficiency.	T	F
9 Vitamin B3 deficiency causes dermatitis, dementia and diarrhoea.	T	F
10 High-dose niacinamide is used to lower serum cholesterol levels.	T	F

FURTHER READING

Braun, L. & Cohen, M., *Herbs & natural supplements: An evidence-based guide*, 3rd ed., Churchill Livingstone Elsevier, New York, 2010.

Gropper, S.S., Smith, J.L. & Groff, J.L., *Advanced nutrition and human metabolism,* 5th ed., Thomson Wadsworth, Belmont, CA, 2009.

Higdon, J., *An evidence-based approach to vitamins and minerals*, Thieme, New York, 2003.

Linus Pauling Institute, Micronutrient Research Center, website, <lpi.oregonstate.edu/infocenter>.

7

Water-soluble vitamins: vitamins B5, B6, B12, folic acid and biotin

VITAMIN B5 (PANTOTHENIC ACID)

VITAMIN B5 STATUS CHECK

1 Do you often get an illness when you are under stress?
2 Do you have a burning feeling in your feet, or have occasional numbness, or 'pins and needles' feelings?
3 Are you frequently tired and irritable?
4 Do you have a poor appetite, indigestion or constipation?

'Yes' answers may indicate inadequate vitamin B5 status. Note that a number of nutritional deficiencies or health disorders can cause similar effects and further investigation is recommended.

FAST FACTS . . . VITAMIN B5

- Vitamin B5 is found in most foods, and especially in royal jelly made by bees.
- It is part of coenzyme A that is essential for energy production in cells.
- It supports the production of fatty acids, ketones, haem, melatonin, eicosanoids, bile salts, vitamin D and steroid hormones.
- A deficiency can cause irritability, unco-operative behaviour, fatigue, apathy, depression, and nervous and digestive system disorders.
- Supplementation may be helpful for acne and stress management.

Vitamin B5, also known as pantothenic acid or pantothenate, is composed of beta-alanine complexed with pantoic acid. It was identified in 1933 by the US biochemist Dr Roger Williams as an essential growth factor for yeast, and was named after the Greek word *pantothen*, meaning 'from everywhere' because of its widespread distribution in biological systems. Its structure was determined in 1939 and it was first synthesised in 1940. In 1947, it was identified as part of the structure of coenzyme A (CoA), which established its essential role in the metabolism of almost all primitive and complex organisms.

Digestion, absorption and transport

Most of the vitamin B5 in food is in the form of CoA, which is hydrolysed by pyrophosphatase and phosphatase enzymes in the digestive tract to 4′-phosphopantetheine (4′-PP), then to pantetheine and finally to pantothenic acid by the enzyme pantetheinase. At low amounts, pantothenic acid is absorbed by a carrier-mediated, sodium-dependent mechanism that also transports biotin and lipoic acid, known as the sodium-dependent multivitamin transport system (SMVT). High amounts are absorbed by diffusion. It is estimated that 40–60 per cent of dietary vitamin B5 is absorbed. Bacteria in the colon can synthesise pantothenic acid, and SMVT has been identified in colon lining cells. However, it is not known whether this is a significant source of vitamin B5 in humans. Pantothenic acid is transported in the bloodstream from intestinal cells (enterocytes) to tissues as free pantothenic acid. A sodium-dependent transporter has been identified in heart, muscle, brain and liver cells, but other tissues are believed to take up pantothenic acid by passive diffusion.

Metabolism, storage and excretion

Inside cells, vitamin B5 is found as pantothenic acid, 4′-PP and pantetheine. Pantothenic acid is converted to CoA in a series of steps requiring ATP and magnesium. The enzyme pantothenate kinase (PanK) converts pantothenic acid to 4′-phosphopantothenate which reacts with the amino acid cysteine to form 4′-PP. 4′-PP is converted to dephospho-CoA and then to CoA. There is no significant storage of vitamin B5 in the body. It is excreted in urine as pantothenic acid.

Functions

Vitamin B5 forms part of the structure of CoA and acyl carrier protein (ACP) that are required for incorporating acetyl and acyl groups, such as acetic, succinic and propionic acids, into molecules. The functions of vitamin B5 include:

- *Energy production.* CoA forms acetyl-CoA and succinyl-CoA, which are key intermediates in the citric acid cycle that oxidises fats, proteins and carbohydrates to produce energy in cells.
- *Production of fatty acids and sterols.* CoA, together with ACP, is essential for fatty acid synthesis. It is part of malonyl-CoA, which is required for making fatty acids, HMG-CoA, which is required for making cholesterol and coenzyme Q10, and acyl-CoA, which is required for making phospholipids for cell membranes and sphingomyelin for the myelin sheath of nerves. CoA supports production of ketones, haem, melatonin, eicosanoids, bile salts, vitamin D and steroid hormones, such as adrenocortical and sex hormones.
- *Acetylation of proteins and sugars.* CoA is required for the incorporation of acetyl and acyl groups into proteins, which helps maintain protein integrity and function. It is required for the function of DNA-binding proteins and for cell division and gene expression. CoA acetylates the amino sugars glucosamine and galactosamine to form N-acetylglucosamine and N-acetylgalactosamine, which may help regulate cell structure and signalling.
- *Nerve function.* CoA maintains the myelin sheath that insulates nerve fibres and supports nerve function by converting choline into the neurotransmitter acetylcholine.
- *Detoxification.* In phase 2 of detoxification, acetyl-CoA and other donor molecules are used to conjugate potentially toxic substances for excretion.
- *Antioxidant activity.* Vitamin B5 increases energy production in cells, which has been shown to increase levels of the antioxidant glutathione.

Dietary sources

Vitamin B5 is found in most foods; good sources include liver, brewer's yeast, egg yolk, meat, poultry, seafood, milk, yoghurt, whole grains, legumes, mushrooms, avocado, broccoli and sweet potatoes. Royal jelly made by bees is a particularly rich source, but should be avoided by asthmatics and people with allergies because it may trigger severe reactions, including anaphylaxis.

The Food Standards Australia New Zealand nutrient database (NUTTAB) at <www.foodstandards.gov.au> provides the amounts found in specific foods.

Factors influencing body status

Vitamin B5 is stable at neutral pH, but is destroyed by heat and alkaline or acidic pH. It is leached out of foods by water processing and cooking methods, and depleted during refining of grains (35–75 per cent lost), freezing (about 10 per cent lost) and canning (about 80 per cent lost). The oral contraceptive pill appears to increase needs, and levels may be depleted in alcoholics because of inadequate intake, diabetics because of increased excretion and people with inflammatory bowel disease because of poor absorption.

Daily requirement

Government recommendations by age and gender (see Table 7.1) can be found in *Nutrient Reference Values for Australia and New Zealand Including Recommended Dietary Intakes*, available at <www.nrv.gov.au>.

Table 7.1 Adequate intake (AI) of vitamin B5 (mg/day)

Age (years)	Female AI	Male AI
1–3	3.5	3.5
4–8	4	4
9–13	4	5
14–18	4	6
19–70	4	6
>70	4	6
Pregnant women		
14–18	5	
19–50	5	
Lactating women		
14–18	6	
19–50	6	

Source: Nutrient Reference Values for Australia and New Zealand Including Recommended Dietary Intakes, National Health and Medical Research Council, Australian Government Department of Health and Ageing, Canberra and Ministry of Health, New Zealand, Wellington, 2006.

Deficiency effects

Unlike some other B vitamins, there is no specific, well-recognised deficiency syndrome associated with vitamin B5, and it is believed that deficiencies are uncommon because it is found in a wide variety of foods. A deficiency is usually linked to generalised malnutrition, and therefore it is difficult to isolate specific effects of inadequate vitamin B5. In animals, an experimental deficiency causes weight loss, fatty liver, elevated serum triglycerides, degeneration of the kidneys and thymus gland, and haemorrhage and destruction of the adrenal glands. Other effects include anaemia, skin rashes, damage to the myelin sheath of nerves, gastrointestinal disorders, stomach ulcers, lung inflammation, greying of fur, low glycogen stores, low blood glucose, reduced endurance, lowered production of antibodies and reproductive failure. Breathing and heart rate become rapid, and convulsions and sudden prostration or coma may result. In animals deprived of CoA for up to nine weeks, levels in tissues remain normal for two to three weeks and then gradually decline to 35–40 per cent of normal.

In humans, defects in the enzyme pantothenate kinase 2 (PANK2), a mitochondrial enzyme required for acetyl-CoA formation, causes the fatal, inherited neurodegenerative disease pantothenate kinase-associated neurodegeneration (PKAN) (formerly known as Hallervorden-Spatz syndrome). Effects include abnormal gait, involuntary muscle contractions, joint disorders, difficulty swallowing and retinitis pigmentosa. Animals lacking PANK2 have shown slowed growth, failure to produce sperm and degeneration of the retina of the eyes.

In severely malnourished prisoners who had been held in Japanese prison camps during World War II, a sensation of burning in the feet was found to respond specifically to vitamin B5 supplementation. Experimentally induced vitamin B5 deficiency in humans causes irritability, uncooperative behaviour, fatigue, apathy, depression, paraesthesia (sensations of numbness, pins and needles or burning) of the hands and feet, indigestion, stomach pain, loss of appetite, constipation, insomnia, postural hypotension (low blood pressure when rising to a standing position), rapid heart rate on exertion, hyperactive deep tendon reflexes and muscle weakness in the hands and feet.

Indicators of inadequate levels may include:

- stress-related disorders
- paraesthesia, especially affecting the hands or feet
- apathy, depression, irritability, insomnia
- poor appetite, stomach discomfort, constipation
- fatigue, listlessness, weak muscles, rapid breathing or heart rate.

Assessment of body status

Assessment of vitamin B5 status is not a common procedure. Whole blood levels are regarded as more reliable than plasma levels; the reference range for whole blood is 1.5–9 μmol/L.[1] Urinary excretion is regarded as an accurate assessment of intake and averages 11.7 μmol/day.[2]

REFERENCES

1 Food and Nutrition Board–Institute of Medicine, *Dietary reference intakes: Thiamin, riboflavin, niacin, vitamin B6, folate, vitamin B12, pantothenic acid, biotin, and choline*, National Academy Press, Washington, DC, 2000.

2 Tarr, J.B., Tamura, T. & Stokstad, E.L., Availability of vitamin B6 and pantothenate in an average American diet in man, *Am J Clin Nutr* (1981), 34(7): 1328–37.

Case reports—vitamin B5 deficiency

- *Three healthy men, 27, 29 and 32 years of age*, took part in a 1954 study of vitamin B5 deficiency induced by the antagonist omega-methylpantothenic acid.[1] After about two weeks of taking the antagonist, they became quarrelsome, sullen, petulant, drowsy and spent a great deal of time in bed. Each subject developed paraesthesia of the hands and feet while at rest, which progressed to a continual state. One subject developed an unpleasant burning sensation of his feet and another developed an abnormal gait and foot drop. The third complained of constant numbness of the hands. All subjects had hyperactive deep tendon reflexes, weakness of the hand muscles and were unable to walk on their toes. Other effects included severely diminished gastric secretions, fast pulse rate, low blood pressure, dizzy spells, increased insulin sensitivity and continual respiratory infections. Vitamin B5 was given after 25 days (4 g daily for six days and then 2 g daily for 24 days) and the antagonist was stopped after 31 days. The nerve symptoms cleared up completely in six days and the motor changes cleared slowly within a month. The infections disappeared and other abnormalities had returned to normal at the end of the study.
- *Six healthy men, 19 to 35 years of age*, took part in a placebo-controlled study of vitamin B5 deficiency in 1958.[2] Two were given a deficient diet, two were given a deficient diet together with a vitamin B5 antagonist and the other two acted as controls. Results were similar to the 1954 study, with deficient subjects experiencing personality changes such as irritability, restlessness and argumentative behaviour, as well as alternate periods of sleepiness and insomnia. They became easily fatigued and developed exercise intolerance, profuse sweating, a staggering gait and poor coordination. They also developed insulin sensitivity, reduced gastric secretions, gastro-oesophageal reflux, a burning sensation in the stomach, loud abdominal rumblings, flatulence, abdominal cramps and episodes of diarrhoea. One subject developed temporary numbness, tingling and burning of the soles of his feet, and those on the antagonist developed numbness of the hands on waking in the morning. Most symptoms appeared at an earlier stage in those on the antagonist. Administration of pantothenic acid (4 g daily) was followed by improvement of the nerve and muscle symptoms, but fatigue and some degree of irritability persisted.

REFERENCES

1 Bean, W.B., Hodges, R.E. & Daum, K., Pantothenic acid deficiency induced in human subjects, *J Clin Invest* (1955), 34(7, Part 1): 1073–84.

2 Hodges, R.E., Ohlson, M.A. & Bean, W.B., Pantothenic acid deficiency in man, *J Clin Invest* (1958), 37(11): 1642–57.

THERAPEUTIC USES OF VITAMIN B5

Dr Roger Williams, who first identified vitamin B5 in 1933, has reported individual cases in which vitamin B5 supplementation improved memory, relieved constipation and prevented hay fever.[1] Because a deficiency causes greying of fur in animals, it has been used to restore hair colour, but there is no evidence that it is effective. Vitamin B5 is popularly used for arthritis, fatigue syndromes and adrenal gland support during stress, and may have therapeutic activity for the following conditions:

Weight loss

Vitamin B5 supplementation was proposed as a weight-loss aid by Hong Kong physician Dr Lit-Hung Leung. The formation of ketones during kilojoule restriction liberates two molecules of CoA, which he theorised was a mechanism to conserve CoA during conditions of increased demand when fatty acids were being broken down for energy. He proposed that vitamin B5 supplementation would maintain adequate CoA and reduce the need for ketone production. Acetyl-CoA would then enter the citric acid directly and produce energy, reducing the formation of ketones, hunger and weakness, thereby reducing the failure rate of people placed on strict diets. Dr Leung studied overweight and obese people on a kilojoule-restricted diet who took a total of 10 g daily of vitamin B5 given in four divided doses.[2] Average weight loss was reported to be 1.2 kg per week. Ketone bodies in urine were either absent or only present in trace amounts, and the subjects did not complain of hunger or weakness. It was found that a maintenance dose of 1–3 g daily, along with continued adherence to a strict diet, was needed to maintain weight loss. No further studies of vitamin B5 and weight loss have been undertaken.

Skin disorders

In cell studies, vitamin B5 has been found to have a strong stimulatory effect on the proliferation of fibroblast skin cells and to be essential for maintaining keratinocyte proliferation and differentiation. Dr Lit-Hung Leung of Hong Kong first proposed that vitamin B5 may be of use in acne in the 1990s, after studying the use of vitamin B5 as a weight-reducing agent and observing that many of the subjects who had acne had a marked reduction in sebum secretion and an overall improvement in their skin condition. He developed the theory that acne is caused by abnormal fatty acid metabolism as a result of inadequate levels of vitamin B5, which results in excess lipids accumulating in sebaceous glands and increased sebum secretion, which in turn provides an environment for rapid growth of *Propionibacterium acnes* bacteria.

Dr Leung treated 100 acne patients with a total of 10 g daily of vitamin B5 given in four divided doses.[3] Subjects also applied a 20 per cent vitamin B5 cream to the affected skin four to six times daily. Facial skin became less oily and there was a decrease in sebum production within a few days, pore size decreased, smaller lesions began to heal, and the rate of new outbreaks reduced. Most subjects with moderate acne found that acne was controlled at eight weeks. Those with severe acne required treatment for six months or longer, and it was noted that some responded more quickly to doses of 15–20 g daily of vitamin B5. Dr Leung found that a maintenance dose of 1–5 g daily was needed to control further outbreaks.

Another study found that patients with acne who took vitamin B5 (2.2 g daily) for eight weeks, together with vitamin B1 (1.5 mg), B2 (1.7 mg), B3 (20 mg), B6 (2 mg), folic acid (400 mcg), vitamin B12 (6 mcg), biotin (300 mcg) and L-carnitine (733.3 mg), had a reduction of more than 56 per cent in the number of lesions and their reported quality of life improved.[4]

D-panthenol (dexpanthenol), a biologically active alcoholic form of vitamin B5, is used topically as an emulsion for skin conditions. It is an effective moisturiser that improves skin hydration and reduces water loss, maintaining softness and elasticity.[5] Dexpanthenol has been shown to relieve skin dryness, roughness, scaling, itching, redness and fissures, to accelerate wound healing, and to have anti-inflammatory activity in sun-exposed skin and skin exposed to radiotherapy. It has been shown to be of benefit for burns, scars, skin transplantation and nappy rash in infants. It has also been shown to reduce skin irritation caused by isotretinoin treatment for acne and, when used as a nasal spray, to relieve rhinitis.

Stress management

Animals deprived of vitamin B5 develop adrenal gland enlargement, haemorrhage, necrosis and reduced resistance to stress. Vitamin B5 supplementation protects adrenal gland function and increases production of anti-stress steroid hormones. It has restored the stress response in animals if given before the adrenal glands are exhausted, and supplementation has been shown to improve resistance to stressful events.[6] Men who were given 10 g of vitamin B5 daily for six weeks were found to have a less pronounced drop in vitamin C levels and white blood cell count after cold-water immersion stress, compared with unsupplemented values.[7]

Elevated serum cholesterol and lipids

Pantethine, the stable disulfate form of pantetheine, is a more metabolically active form of vitamin B5 that improves serum lipid levels, inhibits platelet aggregation and acts as an antioxidant, protecting the lipid carrier apolipoprotein B against peroxidation. Supplemental doses averaging 300 mg three times daily have been found to decrease total serum cholesterol, triglycerides, LDL cholesterol and apolipoprotein B, and increase HDL cholesterol and apolipoprotein A.[8] It appears to be slow-acting, and the best results are observed after four months of daily use. A review of 28 clinical trials found that pantethine supplementation increased HDL cholesterol by 8.4 per cent at four months and decreased LDL cholesterol by 20 per cent and triglycerides by 33 per cent.[9]

REFERENCES

1 Williams, R.J., *Nutrition in a nutshell,* Doubleday, Garden City, NY, 1962.
2 Leung, L.H., Pantothenic acid as a weight-reducing agent: Fasting without hunger, weakness and ketosis, *Med Hypotheses* (1995), 44(5): 403–5.
3 Leung, L.H., Pantothenic acid deficiency as the pathogenesis of acne vulgaris, *Med Hypotheses* (1995), 44: 490–2.
4 Capodice, J.L., Feasibility, tolerability, safety and efficacy of a pantothenic acid based dietary supplement in subjects with mild to moderate facial acne blemishes, *J Cosmetics, Dermatological Sci and Applications* (2012), 1–4.
5 Ebner, F., Heller, A., Rippke, F. & Tausch, I., Topical use of dexpanthenol in skin disorders, *Am J Clin Dermatol* (2002), 3(6): 427–33.
6 Ralli, E.P. & Dumm, M.E., Relation of pantothenic acid to adrenal cortical function, *Vitam Horm* (1953), 11: 133–58.
7 Ralli, E.P., Kuhl, W.J. Jr, Gershberg, H. et al., Effects of vitamin supplementation of the diet on reaction to short-term cold stress in normal young male adults, *Metabolism* (1956), 5(2): 170–96.
8 Horváth, Z. & Vécsei, L., Current medical aspects of pantethine, *Ideggyogy Sz* (2009), 62(7–8): 220–9.
9 McRae, M.P., Treatment of hyperlipoproteinemia with pantethine: A review and analysis of efficacy and tolerability, *Nutr Res* (2005), 25(4): 319–33.

Therapeutic dose

Suggested doses for adults are as follows:

- *Health maintenance:* 10–50 mg daily.
- *Mild deficiency:* 50–100 mg daily.
- *Severe deficiency:* up to 3 g daily.
- *Elevated serum lipids:* as pantethine, 300 mg three times daily; total 900 mg/day.
- *Acne and weight loss:* up to 10 g daily in divided doses.

Effects of excess

Vitamin B5 appears to be non-toxic and well tolerated. Intake in excess of needs is excreted in urine. Doses of 500 and 2000 mg per kg body weight/day in rats and 200–250 mg per kg body weight/day in dogs and monkeys were not associated with adverse effects when given in the diet for six months. In humans, 10 g daily for several weeks or months has not been associated with adverse effects.

Supplements

The permitted forms of vitamin B5 in Australian supplements are pantothenic acid, calcium pantothenate, sodium pantothenate and dexpanthenol. Calcium pantothenate is more stable than pantothenic acid, and is the commonly available oral supplement. Dexpanthenol may be used orally or topically, but is more commonly used in topical preparations, and pantethine is available for topical use only. Calcium pantothenate is produced commercially by reacting pantolactone, beta-alanine and a source of calcium (calcium hydroxide or calcium oxide) in methanol and then removing the residual solvents. Dexpanthenol is made by condensing pantolactone with 3-aminopropanol using methanol and dichloromethane as solvents.

Cautions

Because B vitamins work together in many metabolic pathways in the body, it is possible that individual B vitamins taken alone—especially if taken in high doses—may affect the metabolism of other B vitamins, and this is not recommended in the long term, unless supervised by a health-care practitioner.

VITAMIN B6 (PYRIDOXINE)

VITAMIN B6 STATUS CHECK

1 Do you have numbness, tingling, or pins and needles sensations in your feet or hands?
2 Are you moody, irritable or depressed?
3 Do you have muscle twitches and spasms?
4 Do you have a chronic inflammatory disease?

'Yes' answers may indicate inadequate vitamin B6 status. Note that a number of nutritional deficiencies or health disorders can cause similar effects and further investigation is recommended.

FAST FACTS . . . VITAMIN B6

- Animal foods contain more bioavailable vitamin B6.
- Vitamin B6 is required for amino acid, glycogen and fatty acid metabolism.
- It supports production of the neurotransmitters serotonin, GABA and dopamine.
- A deficiency can cause nerve damage, dermatitis, seizures, fatigue, irritability and depression.
- Supplementation may be helpful for vitamin B6-dependent epilepsy, premenstrual syndrome, nausea and vomiting in pregnancy, diabetes, kidney stones and carpal tunnel syndrome.

Vitamin B6, also called pyridoxine, consists of a pyridine ring with attached hydroxyl, methyl and hydroxymethyl groups. It was discovered in 1934 by Hungarian-born Dr Paul György during his research on vitamin deficiency diseases in England. He identified it as the anti-acrodynia factor because it was able to cure a characteristic form of dermatitis (dermatitis acrodynia) in rats. This factor was isolated in 1938 and found to be a vitamin. It was first synthesised in 1939 and given the name pyridoxine (PN). In 1945, two other natural forms (vitamers) of pyridoxine, pyridoxal (PL) and pyridoxamine (PM), were identified. Each vitamer can be phosphorylated to form pyridoxine 5'-phosphate (PNP), pyridoxal 5'-phosphate (PLP) and pyridoxamine 5'-phosphate (PMP) respectively. Vitamin B6 is the generic term used to refer to all vitamers.

Digestion, absorption and transport

All B6 vitamers are found in food in free forms, and glycated and phosphorylated forms. Pyridoxine, pyridoxal and pyridoxamine are the absorbable forms and phosphorylated forms need to have the phosphate groups removed by phosphatase enzymes, such as zinc-dependent alkaline phosphatase, before absorption. Glycated vitamers can only partially be hydrolysed in the digestive tract and are less bioavailable.

Absorption was believed to be by passive diffusion, but is now thought to be transporter mediated. The mechanism has not been identified. At high levels of intake, absorption may take place by passive diffusion, and phosphorylated vitamers may be absorbed intact by this process. Vitamin B6 can be made by bacteria in the colon and is absorbed into colonocytes by a carrier-mediated process. On average, about 75 per cent of vitamin B6 in food is absorbed but the amount of vitamin B6 absorbed from the colon is unknown. After absorption into enterocytes, pyridoxine, pyridoxal and pyridoxamine are released into the portal vein for delivery to the liver, where they are converted to PLP by FMN-dependent oxidase, a vitamin B2-dependent enzyme, and bound to proteins.

Metabolism, storage and excretion

The liver releases free PLP into the bloodstream for transport to tissues bound to albumin and stores about 5–10 per cent. Phosphatase enzymes in blood remove the phosphate groups from PLP for uptake by cells, which then resynthesise PLP by protein kinase enzymes, trapping vitamin B6 in a bound form that cannot be released from cells. In red blood cells, PLP is bound to haemoglobin. Muscle cells retain relatively large amounts of PLP, which was thought to be a site for body storage, but it now appears that it is a PLP source for use by muscles only. Vitamin B6 is mainly excreted in urine as 4-pyridoxic acid (4-PA).

Functions

The main active form of vitamin B6 in the body is PLP, which is essential for the function of over 140 enzymes. PLP is particularly important for the synthesis, breakdown and interconversion of amino acids. Functions of vitamin B6 include:

- *Amino acid metabolism.* PLP acts as a coenzyme in the formation of amino acids by helping to remove an NH_2 group from one amino acid and transferring it to a keto acid to form a new amino acid, a process called transamination. It is required for the transulfhydration reaction that forms cysteine from methionine and for removal of the hydroxymethyl group from glycine to form serine. It also helps form the amino acids carnitine and taurine.
- *Nerve function.* PLP is required for activity of decarboxylase enzymes that catalyse the formation of amino acid-derived neurotransmitters, such as gamma-amino butyric acid (GABA) produced from glutamate, serotonin produced from 5-hydroxytryptophan, histamine produced from histidine, and dopamine produced from dihydroxyphenylalanine. PLP also helps produce sphingolipid precursors from serine and palmitoyl-CoA.
- *Removal of homocysteine.* Homocysteine (Hcy) is formed during methionine metabolism. Elevated Hcy levels are implicated in CVD, pregnancy complications and cognitive impairment and dementia in later life, and are mainly associated with a folic acid and/or vitamin B12 deficiency, which impairs methionine metabolism. PLP is also important because it is a coenzyme for cystathione synthase and cystathione lyase, the enzymes that remove Hcy by converting it to cystathione and then to cysteine.
- *Haem production.* PLP is a coenzyme that catalyses the formation of haem precursors from glycine and succinyl-CoA, an essential process for formation of the haem required for haemoglobin production.
- *Synthesis of vitamin B3.* PLP is a coenzyme for kynureninase, an enzyme that takes part in the synthesis of niacin from the amino acid tryptophan.
- *Glycogen and fatty acid metabolism.* Glycogen, the stored form of glucose found in muscle cells and the liver, is broken down to glucose by the enzyme glycogen phosphorylase, which is vitamin B6-dependent. PLP is a cofactor for the enzyme delta-6-desaturase, which converts essential fatty acids to other fatty acids, and ultimately to eicosanoids that regulate inflammation.
- *Steroid hormone metabolism.* PLP can reduce tissue sensitivity to steroid hormones by acting to remove the hormone receptor complex from DNA, thereby terminating hormone activity.
- *Antioxidant activity.* PLP assists production of the amino acid cysteine, which is the precursor to the antioxidant glutathione. Vitamin B6 also has direct antioxidant activity by scavenging reactive oxygen and carbonyl species and chelating metals and has a potency similar to carotenes and tocopherols. In cell studies, pyridoxine, pyridoxal and pyridoxamine have been shown to reduce production of superoxide and lipid peroxides.
- *Immunity.* PLP supports T and B lymphocyte proliferation, enhances thymus gland and T lymphocyte activity, and stimulates antibody and interleukin production.

Dietary sources

Vitamin B6 is found in liver, kidneys, heart, poultry, fish, meat, brewer's yeast, whole grains, fortified cereals, legumes, spinach, egg yolk, nuts, seeds, potatoes, bananas and avocadoes. Overall, animal foods are richer sources than vegetables and fruit. Animal foods contain mainly PLP and pyridoxal, with a small amount of PMP; plant foods contain mainly pyridoxine and pyridoxamine, together with their phosphorylated forms, as well as glycated forms of pyridoxine, which are relatively poorly absorbed, having an absorption of only 58 per cent. The main glycated form in plants is pyridoxine-5′-beta-D-glucoside, which can make up 5 to 80 per cent of the total vitamin B6 content.

The Food Standards Australia New Zealand nutrient database (NUTTAB) at <www.foodstandards.gov.au> provides the amounts found in specific foods.

Factors influencing body status

Plant foods contain glycated forms of vitamin B6 that are less well absorbed and animal sources are more bioavailable. Vitamin B6 in food is stable during storage and in acidic environments, but can be broken down by exposure to ultraviolet light and alkaline substances used in food preparation, such as sodium bicarbonate and baking soda. Vitamin B6 is relatively stable to normal cooking temperatures, but is destroyed by high temperature sterilisation of food. Pyridoxine is more stable to heat compared with pyridoxal and pyridoxamine. Refining of grains leads to vitamin B6 losses of 75 to 90 per cent. Vitamin B6 is water soluble and is leached out of food when it is exposed to water during soaking, cooking or processing.

A deficiency of vitamin B2, zinc or magnesium may impair vitamin B6 metabolism, and needs are increased by a high-protein diet and in pregnancy, lactation and the elderly, who have increased breakdown of pyridoxal and PLP. A high alcohol intake impairs vitamin B6 absorption and metabolism. Diuretics that stimulate urine flow increase the loss of vitamin B6 in urine, and central nervous system stimulants—such as the naturally occurring xanthines, which include caffeine, theophylline and theobromine found in coffee, tea, chocolate products, energy drinks and the herb guaraná—have diuretic effects.

People with chronic inflammatory disorders and those on haemodialysis have been found to have lower plasma levels of PLP. In a review of haemodialysis studies, 24–56 per cent of patients were vitamin B6 deficient, and dialysis was found to reduce plasma levels by 28–48 per cent. A number of drugs can reduce body levels, including phenytoin and phenobarbitone (used for epilepsy), theophylline (for asthma), corticosteroids (for inflammation), penicillamine (used to chelate toxic metals), isoniazid (for tuberculosis), cycloserine (an antibiotic) and hydralazine (for elevated blood pressure).

Table 7.2 Recommended dietary intake (RDI) of vitamin B6 (mg/day)

Age (years)	Female RDI	Male RDI
1–3	0.5	0.5
4–8	0.6	0.6
9–13	1.0	1.0
14–18	1.2	1.3
19–50	1.3	1.3
>50	1.5	1.7
Pregnant women		
14–18	1.9	
19–50	1.9	
Lactating women		
14–18	2.0	
19–50	2.0	

Source: Nutrient Reference Values for Australia and New Zealand Including Recommended Dietary Intakes, National Health and Medical Research Council, Australian Government Department of Health and Ageing, Canberra and Ministry of Health, New Zealand, Wellington, 2006.

Daily requirement

Government recommendations by age and gender (see Table 7.2) can be found in *Nutrient Reference Values for Australia and New Zealand Including Recommended Dietary Intakes*, available at <www.nrv.gov.au>.

Deficiency effects

A deficiency of vitamin B6 was thought to be rare, but a large-scale study of vitamin B6 status in the US in 2008 found a surprisingly high incidence of deficiency, as measured by plasma PLP levels—even in those consuming the recommended daily allowance. Those especially at risk included women of reproductive age, women who were current or former users of oral contraceptives, male smokers, and men and women over 65 years of age. Overall, 25 per cent of subjects not taking vitamin supplements were deficient, as were 11 per cent of supplement users.

Early effects of a deficiency are decreased levels of plasma PLP and urinary 4-PA, followed by lowered activity of vitamin B6-dependent enzymes and increased urinary excretion of xanthurenic acid, a by-product of abnormal tryptophan metabolism. In animals, vitamin B6 deficiency causes poor growth and appetite, poor quality of fur and skin, dermatitis, infertility, oedema, weakness, seizures, anaemia and demyelination of nerves. Rats deprived of vitamin B6 have been found to grow at about half the rate of controls, and to have reduced appetite, painful inflammation of the nose, ears, feet and tail, fur loss, weakness, depression and over-grooming behaviour.

In humans, a deficiency is often associated with inadequate vitamin B2 levels because vitamin B2 is required for formation of PLP. A vitamin B6 deficiency can cause hypochromic microcytic anaemia, in which red blood cells are smaller and paler in colour because the haemoglobin content is reduced. It is characterised by abnormal red blood cell production, enlargement of the spleen, and elevated tissue and serum iron levels. Low vitamin B6 impairs immune function by impairing white blood cell production and activity, and reducing production of interleukin–2. A diet inadequate in vitamin B6 has been shown to decrease plasma omega-3 and omega-6 fatty acid concentrations and slightly increase the plasma omega-6:omega-3 ratio, which may increase CVD risk. PLP is a cofactor for the conversion of glyoxylate to glycine, and a deficiency of vitamin B6 can cause glyoxylate conversion to oxalic acid, a component of calcium oxalate kidney stones. Low vitamin B6 status is associated with convulsions in infants that mainly occur between six weeks and four months of age, accompanied by irritability, a piercing cry and sensitivity to noise, and is also associated with convulsions in adults that do not respond to anti-convulsant drugs but respond rapidly to vitamin B6 supplementation.

Indicators of inadequate levels may include:

- peripheral neuropathy—numbness, 'pins and needles' tingling or burning sensations
- dermatitis (similar to that of a vitamin B2 deficiency)—scaly rashes, inflammation of the tongue, cracks and sores at the corners of the mouth or eyes
- epileptic-like seizures
- fatigue, apathy, irritability, depression, mental confusion
- kidney or bladder stones
- joint stiffness, oedema
- lowered immunity
- elevated Hcy levels.

Assessment of body status

The pyridoxine concentration in plasma is not regarded as a good indicator of vitamin B6 status because it reflects recent intake. The concentration of PLP in whole blood has been found to correlate well with overall vitamin B6 status, and is the preferred test. The reference range given by the Biochemistry Department of the Royal Prince Alfred Hospital, Sydney, Australia for PLP levels is 35–110 nmol/L for whole blood and 15–73 nmol/L for plasma. Vitamin B6 status can also be assessed by measuring the increase in activity of the vitamin B6-dependent enzyme erythrocyte glutamic oxaloacetic transaminase (EGOT) in red blood cells after the addition of PLP. Activity co-efficient values greater than 1.8 indicate a deficiency, 1.7–1.8 are marginal and less than 1.7 indicates sufficiency.

A vitamin B6 deficiency impairs the conversion of tryptophan to niacin and leads to elevated xanthurenic and kynurenic acids in urine, which can be measured by a tryptophan load test. After a 2 g oral dose of tryptophan, 24-hour urinary excretion of less than 65 μmol of xanthurenic acid is believed to indicate normal vitamin B6 status. However, this test is not regarded as accurate because it can be affected by other factors, including variations in protein intake, exercise and lean body mass, as well as female hormones and some drugs. Urinary 4-PA levels reflect changes in vitamin B6 intake, rather than body levels, and are not a reliable measure of vitamin B6 status. However, a value greater than 3 μmol/day may indicate an adequate intake.

Case reports—vitamin B6 deficiency

- *Eight patients, 27 to 87 years of age,* were given a vitamin B6 antagonist and developed a range of effects, including scaly, oily, red skin lesions around the eyes, nose and mouth; cracks at the corners of the mouths and eyes; itching, red rashes on arms and legs; and sore, swollen and red mouth and tongue.[1] All effects responded rapidly to administration of 100 mg of pyridoxine daily.
- *A pregnant woman, 30 years of age,* with a history of vitamin B6-dependent seizures in childhood, developed status epilepticus in the fourteenth week of pregnancy.[2] (Status epilepticus is defined as more than 30 minutes of continuous seizure activity or two or more sequential seizures without full recovery of consciousness between seizures.) She did not respond to anti-convulsant drugs, and her blood levels of PLP were found to be low. She was given 100 mg of iv pyridoxine daily and became seizure free within three days. She continued to take pyridoxine throughout her pregnancy and delivered a healthy, full-term infant.
- *An American infant, three months of age,* developed seizures in 1952 after being been fed on formula from birth.[3] The convulsions disappeared when the formula was changed. Over 100 cases of seizures in infants were subsequently identified, all linked to the use of the same formula. The infants' symptoms

included hyper-irritability (particularly sensitivity to noise), diarrhoea, vomiting, projectile vomiting and convulsive seizures lasting from 30 seconds to five minutes, and recurring one to eleven times daily. After considerable research, it was discovered that the original formula had been sterilised at high temperatures, and this process had destroyed the vitamin B6 content. Infants treated with iv pyridoxine had no further symptoms despite continuing on the formula. No further cases were reported after a change in the formulation to include vitamin B6.

- *A man, 78 years of age*, with a history of CVD and diabetes, was admitted to hospital after being diagnosed with a stroke.[4] He developed seizures and was given anti-convulsant therapy with no effect. Plasma PLP was found to be low and he was given 100 mg iv pyridoxine every twelve hours. He became free of seizures within 24 hours.

REFERENCES

1 Mueller, J.F. & Vilter, R.W., Pyridoxine deficiency in human beings induced with desoxypyridoxine, *J Clin Invest* (1950), 29(2): 193–201.

2 Schulze-Bonhage, A., Kurthen, M., Walger, P. & Elger, C.E., Pharmacorefractory status epilepticus due to low vitamin B6 levels during pregnancy, *Epilepsia* (2004), 45(1): 81–4.

3 Nelson, E.M., Association of vitamin B6 deficiency with convulsions in infants, *Public Health Rep* (1956), 71(5): 445–8.

4 Gerlach, A.T., Thomas, S., Stawicki, S.P. et al., Vitamin B6 deficiency: A potential cause of refractory seizures in adults, *J Parenter Enteral Nutr* (2011), 35(2): 272–5.

THERAPEUTIC USES OF VITAMIN B6

The therapeutic actions of vitamin B6 were promoted by Dr John Ellis, a physician and surgeon from Texas, in the 1960s.[1] He developed the theory that low vitamin B6 status was the cause of a characteristic arthritis affecting the hands and upper limbs, causing pain, stiffness and swelling of the fingers and enlargement of the distal finger joints (Heberden's nodes) and often associated with CVD or menopause. He also associated vitamin B6 deficiency with carpal tunnel syndrome, trigger finger, bursitis, paraesthesia, elbow, wrist and shoulder pain, and oedema—particularly puffiness of the backs of the hands. Dr Ellis tested for vitamin B6 deficiency by asking patients to hold their fingers upright and, keeping their wrists and knuckles in a straight line, bend their fingers towards the palm of their hand, bending the finger joints only and not the knuckles. He believed that an inability to touch the palm with the fingertips indicated a deficiency. Dr Ellis found that vitamin B6 supplementation was able to relieve the neuropathy and arthritic symptoms, and resolve generalised oedema, reporting that patients often lost several inches from their waistlines on vitamin B6. Further research is needed to establish the validity of Dr Ellis's theories. Vitamin B6 may have therapeutic activity for the following conditions:

Pyridoxine-dependent epilepsy

Pyridoxine-dependent epilepsy (PDE) can be caused by reduced synthesis or availability of PLP or by increased utilisation or inactivation. It is characterised by seizures that are not controlled with anti-convulsants but respond to large daily supplements of pyridoxine, and is believed to be associated with mutations of the gene ALDH7A1. Electroencephalogram (EEG) findings may be normal, or may range from non-specific slowing to burst suppression pattern, in which periods of normal high brain activity are interrupted by periods of greatly reduced activity.

Typically, PDE causes prolonged seizures and recurrent episodes of status epilepticus, but may also cause partial seizures, generalised seizures, atonic seizures, myoclonic events and infantile spasms, and is often associated with intellectual disability. In newborn infants, irritability, grimacing, crying, fluctuating muscle tone and poor feeding precede the onset of seizures, and some mothers report unusual foetal movements during late pregnancy. Some cases are characterised by seizures beginning at a later age (up to three years), which initially respond to anti-convulsants and then become uncontrollable, and seizures that do not initially respond to vitamin B6 but respond several months later. In older children, PDE can present as tonic-clonic seizures, abnormal behaviour, inconsolable crying, a frightened facial expression, sleep disturbances, loss of consciousness, numbness and visual disorders.

Initial treatment is 100 mg of pyridoxine given intravenously, which relieves the seizure in minutes.[2] The dose can be increased to 500 mg if required for initial seizure control. Less severe cases can be treated with 30 mg per kg body weight/day of oral pyridoxine. Seizures usually cease within a few days of treatment with pyridoxine. In cases of reduced synthesis or availability of PLP, PLP treatment is required rather than pyridoxine.

Pregnancy

Nausea and vomiting

Vitamin B6 supplementation has been shown to be an effective treatment for reducing the severity of pregnancy nausea and vomiting. However, no relationship has been found between vitamin B6 status and the incidence of nausea and vomiting in pregnant women. Women in early pregnancy given 30 mg of vitamin B6 for five days reported a decrease in nausea severity and a trend towards fewer episodes of vomiting.[3] Doses of 10–40 mg of vitamin B6 daily have been found to be effective; larger doses (500 mg daily) have been shown to be well tolerated in early pregnancy, with no adverse effects on foetal development. A study comparing the effectiveness of vitamin B6 and ginger for controlling nausea and vomiting in pregnant women found that ginger was superior.[4]

Anaemia

Healthy pregnant women have been shown to develop low blood levels of iron, ferritin and vitamin B6 by the third trimester, and are at increased risk of anaemia, which may require treatment with both iron and vitamin B6. Anaemic pregnant women with inadequate vitamin B6 levels and resistant to iron therapy have been shown to improve on vitamin B6 supplementation.[5]

Premenstrual syndrome

Vitamin B6 supplementation is popularly used to relieve premenstrual syndrome (PMS). A review of nine trials found that most trials were of low quality but concluded that doses of up to 100 mg/day are likely to be of benefit for premenstrual symptoms and premenstrual depression.[6] A study of magnesium supplementation compared to magnesium combined with vitamin B6 found that the combination of supplements was the most effective for relief of PMS symptoms.[7]

Depression

Clinical depression is associated with abnormal serotonin metabolism, and drugs that act to boost serotonin levels are useful anti-depressants. PLP is required for production of the neurotransmitters serotonin and GABA that moderate mood and pain perception. In animals, a relatively high dose of vitamin B6 (10 mg/kg body weight) has been shown to increase the rate of synthesis of serotonin in the brain.[8] A low plasma level of PLP has been found to be associated with depression,[9] and in one study was found to approximately double the risk.[10] Vitamin B6 has been shown to relieve PMS-related depression and depression related to use of oral contraceptives but there is little evidence for its effectiveness in other types of depression.[11]

Colorectal cancer

A meta-analysis of thirteen studies investigating the role of vitamin B6 in prevention of colorectal cancer found that those with the highest intake of vitamin B6 had a 10 per cent reduced risk and those with the highest blood PLP levels had a 48 per cent reduced risk.[12] The risk was found to decrease by 49 per cent for every 100 pmol/mL increase in blood PLP levels. In experimentally induced colon cancer in animals, a relatively large intake of vitamin B6 was shown to reduce the incidence and number of colon tumours, reduce colon cell proliferation and angiogenesis, and suppress two cancer-promoting genes.[13]

Tardive dyskinesia

Patients with schizophrenia on long-term standard medication are at increased risk of developing the Parkinson-like syndrome tardive dyskinesia, which causes involuntary, repetitive body movements. A study of schizophrenic patients given 1200 mg daily of vitamin B6 for twelve weeks found that Parkinson-like symptoms decreased on average 18.5 points, compared with 1.4 points in patients treated with placebo.[14]

Carpal tunnel syndrome

Vitamin B6 is claimed to relieve the symptoms of carpal tunnel syndrome, in which swelling causes pressure on the median nerve in the wrist, leading to pain, numbness, tingling and weakness in the hand and fingers. Dr John Ellis first developed the theory in the 1960s that carpal tunnel syndrome was associated with vitamin B6 deficiency-associated oedema. Early studies by Ellis on small numbers of patients with carpal tunnel syndrome reported low vitamin B6 status and improvement with vitamin B6 supplementation.[15] Supplementing with 100–300 mg of vitamin B6 daily for twelve weeks was reported to resolve the condition in a number of patients. This research has been criticised for failing to properly identify carpal tunnel syndrome as distinct from a more generalised neuropathy. However, a retrospective study found that people taking 100 mg vitamin B6 twice daily reported better symptom relief than people not on supplementation.[16] Vitamin B6 appears to be particularly helpful for pain relief in carpal tunnel syndrome, but good-quality evidence is lacking.

Lowered immune response

In critically ill patients given daily injections of vitamin B6, plasma PLP increased, as did the total lymphocyte count, and number of T lymphocytes, and T helper and T suppressor cells.[17]

Elevated Hcy levels

Elevated Hcy levels are implicated in CVD, adverse pregnancy outcomes and cognitive impairment and dementia in the elderly, and can be lowered by vitamin B6, vitamin B12 and folic acid supplementation.[18] However, vitamin B12 and folic acid appear to be the main Hcy-lowering agents, and vitamin B6 has not been found to have an additive effect. Lowering Hcy has not been shown to reduce the risk of heart disease, but may reduce stroke incidence and mortality.

High blood pressure (hypertension)

Creating a vitamin B6 deficiency in rats causes hypertension, and is a method used experimentally for blood pressure studies. The mechanism is not well defined, but inadequate vitamin B6 leads to reduced levels of serotonin and GABA, and increased sensitivity of tissues to steroid hormones, which may increase blood pressure. High doses of vitamin B6 given to animals have been shown to prevent spontaneous hypertension, and also hypertension induced by alcohol.[19,20] In humans, a small study found that 5 mg/kg body weight of pyridoxine daily for four weeks reduced systolic and diastolic blood pressure.[21]

Diabetes

In type 1 diabetes, alkaline phosphatase activity is increased and more PLP is dephosphorylated to pyridoxal, which can then leave cells, leading to reduced amounts of intracellular PLP. In cell studies, pyridoxine has been found to restore endothelial cell functions such as migratory ability and resistance to shear stress that are lost when blood glucose is elevated.[22] Vitamin B6—particularly pyridoxamine—may also be useful for preventing some of the adverse effects of poor blood glucose control in diabetic patients. Pyridoxamine has been shown to scavenge toxic carbonyls formed by glucose metabolism, inhibit reactive oxygen species (ROS), and inhibit the reaction of glucose and carbonyl compounds with proteins that irreversibly impairs protein function and causes the formation of glycated haemoglobin (HbA_{1C}) and advanced glycation end-products (AGEs).[23] In animals with diabetes, pyridoxamine has been found to reduce damage to the nervous system and eye tissues.[24]

Kidney stones

Many common types of kidney stones consist of calcium phosphate and calcium oxalate. A vitamin B6 deficiency in animals is associated with increased oxalate in urine and formation of calcium phosphate and calcium oxalate crystals.[25] A large prospective study of women found that those with the highest intake of vitamin B6 (40 mg or more daily) had a 34 per cent reduced risk of stone formation compared with those taking less than 3 mg daily, but this association was not found in men.[26] A small study of patients with a history of recurring calcium oxalate stone formation in the kidneys found that 200 mg of magnesium oxide plus 10 mg of pyridoxine taken for five years prevented stone formation in 83 per cent of subjects.[27]

Chinese restaurant syndrome

Monosodium glutamate (MSG), a flavour enhancer often used in commercial food products and Chinese cuisine, can cause headache, rapid heart beat, palpitations, flushing and nausea in sensitive people, and vitamin B6 supplementation has been shown to prevent sensitivity reactions to MSG in one small study.[28]

Asthma

Patients with asthma on theophylline therapy have been found to have low levels of plasma PLP.[29] A 1975 study reported that 76 asthmatic children given 200 mg/day of pyridoxine had improvement in symptoms and reduced their use of asthma medications.[30]

Childhood behavioural disorders

Autism

Vitamin B6 and magnesium have gained popularity as a treatment for autism after several early studies reported improvements in behavioural markers in autistic children, but it remains a controversial approach. In a study of 33 autistic children given magnesium (6 mg per kg body weight/day) and vitamin B6 (0.6 mg per kg body weight/day), symptoms such as social interaction, communication, stereotyped restricted behaviour and abnormal/delayed functioning improved in 70 per cent of subjects and behavioural measures regressed over several weeks when the supplementation was stopped.[31]

Attention deficit hyperactivity disorder

A study of 40 children with attention deficit hyperactivity disorder (ADHD) given the same doses of magnesium and vitamin B6 as the autistic group (see above) found that hyperactivity and aggressive behaviours were reduced and school attention was improved after two months of supplementation, and behaviour regressed when supplementation was stopped.[32]

REFERENCES

1 Ellis, J.M. & Pamplin, J., *Vitamin B6 therapy: Nature's versatile healer*, Avery, New York, 1999.

2 Gospe, S.M., Pyridoxine-dependent epilepsy, in R.A. Pagon, T.D. Bird, C.R. Dolan et al., eds, *GeneReviews*™ [online], University of Washington, Seattle, 1993, available at <www.ncbi.nlm.nih.gov/books/NBK1486>.

3 Vutyavanich, T., Wongtrangan, S. & Ruangsri, R., Pyridoxine for nausea and vomiting of pregnancy: A randomized, double-blind, placebo-controlled trial, *Obstet Gynecol* (1995), 173 (3 Pt 1): 881–4.

4 Chittumma, P., Kaewkiattikun, K. & Wiriyasiriwach, B., Comparison of the effectiveness of ginger and vitamin B6 for treatment of nausea and vomiting in early pregnancy: A randomized double-blind controlled trial, *J Med Assoc Thai* (2007), 90(1): 15–20.

5 Hisano, M., Suzuki, R., Sago, H. et al., Vitamin B6 deficiency and anemia in pregnancy, *Eur J Clin Nutr* (2010), 64(2): 221–3.

6 Wyatt, K.M., Dimmock, P.W., Jones, P.W., Shaughn O'Brien, P.M., Efficacy of vitamin B-6 in the treatment of premenstrual syndrome: systematic review, *BMJ* (1999), 318(7195): 1375–81.

7 Fathizadeh, N., Ebrahimi, E., Valiani, M. et al., Evaluating the effect of magnesium and magnesium plus vitamin B6 supplement on the severity of premenstrual syndrome, *Iran J Nurs Midwifery Res* (2010), 15(Suppl 1): 401–5.

8 Hartvig, P., Lindner, K.J., Bjurling, P. et al. Pyridoxine effect on synthesis rate of serotonin in the monkey brain measured with positron emission tomography, *J Neural Transm Gen Sect* (1995), 102(2): 91–7.

9 Hvas, A.M., Juul, S., Bech, P. & Nexø, E., Vitamin B6 level is associated with symptoms of depression, *Psychother Psychosom* (2004), 73(6): 340–3.

10 Merete, C., Falcon, L.M. & Tucker, K.L., Vitamin B6 is associated with depressive symptomatology in Massachusetts elders, *J Am Coll Nutr* (2008), 27(3): 421–7.

11 Williams, A.L., Cotter, A., Sabina, A. et al., The role for vitamin B-6 as treatment for depression: A systematic review, *Fam Pract* (2005), 22(5): 532–7.

12 Larsson, S.C., Orsini, N. & Wolk, A., Vitamin B6 and risk of colorectal cancer: A meta-analysis of prospective studies, *JAMA* (2010), 303(11): 1077–83.

13 Komatsu, S., Yanaka, N., Matsubara, K. & Kato, N., Antitumor effect of vitamin B6 and its mechanisms, *Biochim Biophys Acta* (2003), 1647: 127–30.

14 Lerner, V., Miodownik, C., Kaptsan, A. et al., Vitamin B6 treatment for tardive dyskinesia: A randomized, double-blind, placebo-controlled, crossover study, *J Clin Psychiatry* (2007), 68(11): 1648–54.

15 Ellis, J.M., Kishi, T., Azuma, J. & Folkers, K., Vitamin B6 deficiency in patients with a clinical syndrome including the carpal tunnel defect: Biochemical and clinical response to therapy with pyridoxine, *Res Commun Chem Pathol Pharmacol* (1976), 13(4): 743–57.

16 Kasdan, M.L. & Janes, C., Carpal tunnel syndrome and vitamin B6, *Plast Reconstr Surg* (1987), 79(3): 456–62.

17 Cheng, C.H., Chang, S.J., Lee, B.J. et al., Vitamin B6 supplementation increases immune responses in critically ill patients, *Eur J Clin Nutr* (2006), 60(10): 1207–13.

18 Clarke, R. & Armitage, J., Vitamin supplements and cardiovascular risk: Review of the randomized trials of homocysteine-lowering vitamin supplements, *Semin Thromb Hemost* (2000), 26(3): 341–8.

19 Vasdev, S., Ford, C.A. & Parai, S. et al., Dietary vitamin B6 supplementation attenuates hypertension in spontaneously hypertensive rats, *Mol Cell Biochem* (1999), 200(1–2): 155–62.

20 Vasdev, S., Wadhawan, S., Ford, C.A. et al., Dietary vitamin B6 supplementation prevents ethanol-induced hypertension in rats, *Nutr Metab Cardiovasc Dis* (1999), 9(2): 55–63.

21 Aybak, M., Sermet, A., Ayyildiz, M.O, Karakilçik, A.Z. Effect of oral pyridoxine hydrochloride supplementation on arterial blood pressure in patients with essential hypertension, *Arzneimittelforschung* (1995), 45(12): 1271–3.

22 Kelso, B.G., Brower, J.B., Targovnik, J.H. & Caplan, M.R., Pyridoxine restores endothelial cell function in high glucose, *Metab Syndr Relat Disord* (2011), 9(1): 63–8.

23 Voziyan, P.A. & Hudson, B.G., Pyridoxamine: The many virtues of a maillard reaction inhibitor, *Ann NY Acad Sci* (2005), 1043: 807–16.

24 Metz, T.O., Alderson, N.L., Thorpe, S.R. & Baynes, J.W., Pyridoxamine, an inhibitor of advanced glycation and lipoxidation reactions: A novel therapy for treatment of diabetic complications, *Arch Biochem Biophys* (2003), 419(1): 41–9.

25 Di Tommaso, L., Tolomelli, B., Mezzini, R. et al., Renal calcium phosphate and oxalate deposition in prolonged vitamin B6 deficiency: Studies on a rat model of urolithiasis, *BJU Int* (2002), 89(6): 571–5.

26 Curhan, G.C., Willett, W.C., Speizer, F.E., Stampfer, M.J., Intake of vitamins B6 and C and the risk of kidney stones in women, *J Am Soc Nephrol* (1999), 10(4): 840–5.

27 Gershoff, S.N. & Prien, E.L., Effect of daily MgO and vitamin B6 administration to patients with recurring calcium oxalate kidney stones, *Am J Clin Nutr* (1967), 20(5): 393–9.

28 Folkers, K., Shizukuishi, S., Scudder, S.L. et al., Biochemical evidence for a deficiency of vitamin B6 in subjects reacting to monosodium L-glutamate by the Chinese restaurant syndrome, *Biochem Biophys Res Commun* (1981), 100(3): 972–7.

29 Reynolds, R.D. & Natta, C.L., Depressed plasma pyridoxal phosphate concentrations in adult asthmatics, *Am J Clin Nutr* (1985), 41(4): 684–8.

30 Collipp, P.J., Goldzier, S. III, Weiss, N., Soleymani, Y. & Snyder, R., Pyridoxine treatment of childhood bronchial asthma, *Ann Allergy* (1975), 35(2): 93–7.

31 Mousain-Bosc, M., Roche, M., Polge, A. et al., Improvement of neurobehavioral disorders in children supplemented with magnesium-vitamin B6. II. Pervasive developmental disorder-autism, *Magnes Res* (2006), 19(1): 53–62.

32 Mousain-Bosc, M., Roche, M., Polge, A. et al., Improvement of neurobehavioral disorders in children supplemented with magnesium-vitamin B6. I. Attention deficit hyperactivity disorders, *Magnes Res* (2006), 19(1): 46–52.

Therapeutic dose

Oral vitamin B6 may be absorbed better if taken in divided doses. Vitamin B6 supplements may be more effective if taken with a source of vitamin B2, magnesium and zinc, which support vitamin B6 metabolism. Suggested doses for adults are as follows:

- *Health maintenance:* 5–10 mg daily.
- *Mild deficiency:* 10–25 mg daily.
- *Severe deficiency:* up to 200 mg daily or higher short term. Long-term doses greater than 200 mg daily should be supervised by a health-care practitioner.
- *General therapeutic dose range:* 50–100 mg daily or up to 200 mg daily in the short term, reducing to a maintenance dose when symptoms resolve.
- *Pregnancy nausea:* 30–50 mg daily or up to 100 mg daily in the short term as required.
- *PDE:* an initial iv dose of 100 mg of pyridoxine hydrochloride or 30 mg/kg body weight/day orally. In the absence of a clinical response, the dose should be repeated up to a maximum of 500 mg. The initial dose may result in respiratory arrest, and treatment should be given together with respiratory support. For longer-term iv treatment, the dose is 15 to 30 mg/kg body weight/day for infants or up to 200 mg/day for newborns and 500 mg/day for adults. In general, seizures are controlled on 50–100 mg of pyridoxine daily, but the daily dose may need to be doubled for several days during acute illness because of increased risk of seizures. Mothers of a PDE infant are advised to take 50–100 mg daily throughout the last half of any subsequent pregnancies.
- *Genetic dependency conditions:* 200–1000 mg daily for life, with medical supervision.

Effects of excess

All B6 vitamers are well tolerated orally in moderate amounts, but very large doses taken as a single vitamin have been found to be toxic to the nervous system, especially if taken long-term. There is no evidence that moderate amounts of vitamin B6 taken with the full range of other B complex vitamins have caused toxicity, and it may be that the adverse effects of high-dose vitamin B6 are caused by impaired metabolism of other B vitamins or supporting nutrients, such as magnesium; however, evidence for this is lacking.

Daily oral doses of 100 mg of pyridoxine have been taken for periods of three to four years without adverse effects. Higher doses taken long term have caused sensory neuropathy, which was first reported in humans in 1983 when five women and two men aged 20–43 years developed severe sensory neuropathy after taking 2000–6000 mg of pyridoxine daily for two to 40 months. Reported symptoms included numbness, burning pain, tingling, an abnormal gait, poor balance, reduced or absent reflexes, and loss of fine motor control of the hands. Symptoms improve on withdrawal of supplementation, but full recovery may be slow.

Individual responses may differ, and peripheral neuropathy has also been reported at lower doses (500 mg daily or less) if taken for several years. In one report, 60 per cent of women taking an average dose of 117 mg of pyridoxine daily for an average of 2.9 years developed a raised serum vitamin B6 level and neurological symptoms, such as tingling, burning, hypersensitivity to touch, bone pains, muscle weakness and twitches. There was a complete recovery within six months when supplementation was stopped. Conversely, seventeen patients with elevated Hcy in the urine who had been treated with 200–600 mg of pyridoxine daily for 10–24 years underwent extensive neurological examinations, but no evidence of neuropathy was found.

Case report—vitamin B6 toxicity

- *A young woman* developed paraesthesia of the feet, and was found to have sensory nerve damage and elevated blood levels of pyridoxine.[1] She reported that she had read a magazine article on the use of vitamin B6 for PMS, and had taken 1000 mg daily for eighteen months. Her supplementation was stopped, but the numbness and tingling continued to worsen for two to three weeks before a slow improvement. Her symptoms resolved completely over several months.

REFERENCE

1 Barclay, L., A skater with tingling feet, *Medscape Education Family Medicine*, retrieved 20 August 2014 from <www.medscape.org/viewarticle/735293>.

Supplements

The forms of vitamin B6 permitted in Australian supplements are pyridoxine, PLP and pyridoxine hydrochloride, the most common form. Pyridoxine can be produced from the amino acid alanine, which is transformed in several chemical steps to 5-ethoxy-4-methyl-oxazle (EMO). EMO and 2-butene-1,4-diol are reacted to form adducts that are rearranged and hydrolysed with hydrochloric acid to form pyridoxine hydrochloride.

Cautions

Vitamin B6 supplements should not be used in patients with Parkinson's disease who are taking the drug levodopa (L-dopa) because vitamin B6 accelerates the drug's breakdown. Vitamin B6 supplements can cause unusually vivid dreams that may disturb sleep, and are not recommended to be taken in the evening. Because B vitamins work together in many metabolic pathways in the body, it is possible that individual B vitamins taken alone—especially if taken in high doses—may affect the metabolism of other B vitamins, and such a treatment is not recommended for long-term use, unless supervised by a health-care practitioner.

The TGA in Australia requires the following warning statement on vitamin B6 supplements if the product contains more than 50 mg of pyridoxine per recommended daily dose:

'WARNING—this product contains pyridoxine which may be dangerous when used in large amounts or for a long time.'

VITAMIN B12 (COBALAMIN)

VITAMIN B12 STATUS CHECK

1 **Are you pale and tired, and do you get short of breath and feel dizzy frequently?**
2 **Is your tongue smooth and sore, and do you have episodes of diarrhoea?**
3 **Do you get numbness, tingling, 'pins and needles' or burning sensations?**
4 **Do you have a poor memory, and do you get irritable and depressed?**

'Yes' answers may indicate inadequate vitamin B12 status. Note that a number of nutritional deficiencies or health disorders can cause similar effects and further investigation is recommended.

FAST FACTS . . . VITAMIN B12

- **Vitamin B12 is found in liver, kidneys, poultry, meat, fish and particularly shellfish.**
- **It requires the assistance of intrinsic factor and R proteins for absorption.**
- **It supports energy production, and methionine and folic acid metabolism.**
- **A deficiency causes anaemia and nerve damage.**
- **Supplementation may be helpful for the prevention of birth defects in pregnancy, and for mood and neurological disorders.**

Vitamin B12 is made up of a corrin ring with a single cobalt atom in the centre and an attached nucleotide, and was discovered during research into the then fatal blood disorder pernicious anaemia (PA), in which red blood cells fail to develop normally and nerve damage accumulates. US physician George Whipple found that beef liver could stimulate the formation of red blood cells in anaemic dogs, and in the 1920s, Dr George Minot and Dr William Murphy began feeding large amounts of raw or lightly cooked beef liver to their patients with PA and found that about 230 g of liver daily controlled the disease and extended life expectancy beyond two years. US physician William Castle discovered that a substance secreted by the gastric mucosa (intrinsic factor) was essential for the absorption of the anti-PA factor in liver. More potent liver extracts in injectable form were developed for the treatment of PA and, after intensive searching, the anti-PA factor in liver was identified in 1947 and named vitamin B12. The complex structure of this molecule was finally discovered in 1955 by a UK research team, and it was synthesised by bacterial culture soon after and chemically synthesised in 1960. Vitamin B12 injections then became the established treatment for PA.

Cobalamin is a generic name for all forms of vitamin B12, which include hydroxocobalamin (hydroxo-B12), methylcobalamin (methyl-B12), cyanocobalamin (cyano-B12), aquocobalamin (aquo-B12), nitritocobalamin (nitrito-B12) and 5'-deoxyadenosylcobalamin (adenosyl-B12). Methyl-B12 and adenosyl-B12 are the active forms in the body, and can be produced from any of the other forms of B12. Vitamin B12 can only be synthesised by micro-organisms, and it functions in the body as a coenzyme in folic acid and methionine metabolism, and in the citric acid cycle that produces energy in mitochondria.

Digestion, absorption and transport

Vitamin B12 and analogues (non-cobalamin corrinoids), which are substances that have a similar structure but no vitamin B12 activity in the body, are present in foods bound to proteins, and are released by the action of pepsin and hydrochloric acid in the stomach. Free B12 combines in the stomach with a vitamin B12-binding protein (haptocorrin), called R protein, secreted in saliva (see Figure 7.1). In the duodenum, R protein is digested by pancreatic protease

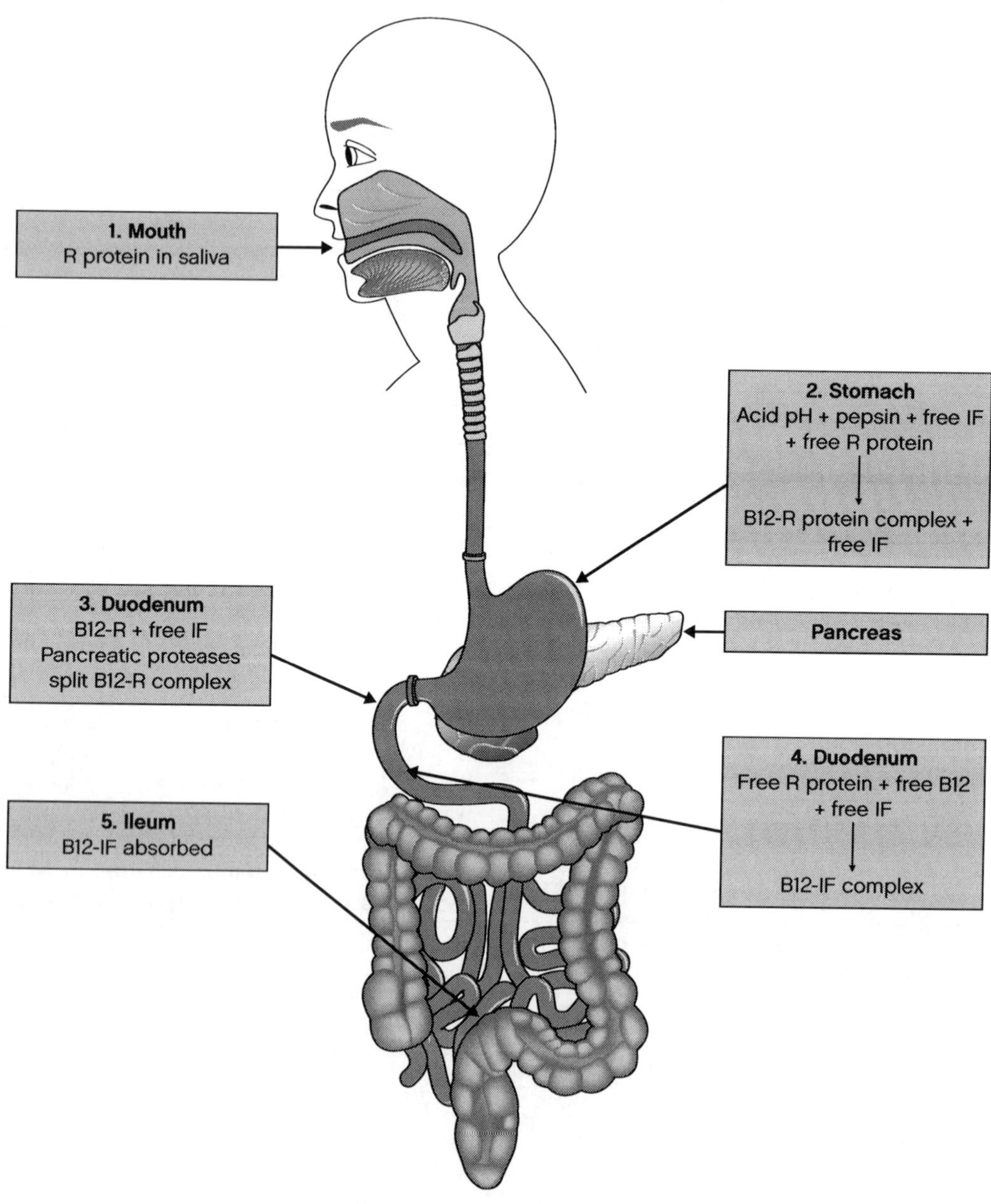

Figure 7.1 Vitamin B12 absorption

enzymes and vitamin B12 is released and binds to intrinsic factor (IF), a gastric glycoprotein produced in the parietal cells of the stomach lining. Binding with IF appears to protect vitamin B12 from enzyme and bacterial activity in the digestive system. The IF-B12 complex binds to receptors (cubulins) in the lower part of the small intestine, and is absorbed into enterocytes by endocytosis (membrane engulfment). Receptor-assisted absorption has a limited capacity, and larger amounts of vitamin B12 are absorbed by passive diffusion, which is rapid but relatively inefficient. It appears that analogues are absorbed in a similar fashion. It is estimated that small amounts of vitamin B12 (0.5 mcg or less) have an absorption of 52 to 97 per cent, whereas a dose of 10 mcg has 16 per cent absorption, and a 50 mcg dose has 3 per cent absorption. Overall, about 11–65 per cent of the amount of vitamin B12 ingested is absorbed.

Vitamin B12 is transported in the bloodstream bound to transport proteins (R proteins) in plasma. Haptocorrin (previously called transcobalamin I and III) carries 70–80 per cent of circulating vitamin B12. Transcobalamin (previously called transcobalamin II) is made in the liver, macrophages and endothelial and intestinal cells, and delivers vitamin B12 and analogues from the digestive tract to the liver and other tissues. It carries 20–30 per cent of circulating vitamin B12 as holotranscobalamin, which is the term used for transcobalamin when it is bound to vitamin B12. The main circulating form of vitamin B12 is methyl-B12, which makes up 60–80 per cent, with smaller amounts of adenosyl-B12 and even smaller amounts of cyano- and hydroxo-B12.

Metabolism, storage and excretion

Receptors for vitamin B12 transport proteins are found in most tissues. In cells, hydroxo-B12 can be converted to methyl-B12 and then to adenosyl-B12. Several years' supply of vitamin B12 (1–5 mg) can be stored in the body, mainly in the liver as adenosyl-B12, and also in the muscles, bones, kidneys, heart, brain and spleen. Vitamin B12 can be excreted in bile bound to R proteins, but there is very little urinary excretion. Non-cobalamin corrinoids are delivered to the liver and excreted in bile.

Vitamin B12 has an enterohepatic circulation, in which vitamin B12 is excreted in bile and reabsorbed in the small intestine, together with vitamin B12 from enterocytes sloughed off as the gut lining is renewed. This helps to maintain body levels and, together with body stores, may provide sufficient vitamin B12 to enable body function for several years or decades of inadequate dietary intake.

Functions

The active forms of vitamin B12 are adenosyl-B12 and methyl-B12, which support the activity of mutase and methyl group transfer enzymes. Vitamin B12 functions include the following.

- *Energy production*. Adenosyl-B12 is required for the enzyme methylmalonyl-CoA mutase, which converts methylmalonyl-CoA to succinyl-CoA in the citric acid cycle in mitochondria.
- *Methionine and folic acid metabolism*. During metabolism of the amino acid methionine, methionine is first converted to S-adenosylmethionine (SAM), then to S-adenosylhomocysteine (SAH), then to homocysteine (Hcy) and finally back to methionine (see Figure 7.2). Methyl-B12 is an essential part of the methionine cycle because it is required for activity of the enzyme methionine synthase, which converts Hcy to methionine. This enzyme works with folic acid to transfer a methyl group from 5-methyl tetrahydrofolate (an inactive form of folic acid) to Hcy, forming active folic acid, methionine and unmethylated vitamin B12.

  Hcy is a nerve and blood vessel toxin implicated in CVD, neurological disorders and pregnancy complications. It can also be removed by conversion to cystathione by an enzyme dependent on vitamin B6. SAM provides methyl groups that play a key role in gene expression, and support the synthesis of hormones, neurotransmitters, the myelin sheath of nerve fibres, cell membrane lipids and proteins.

  Normal activity of the methionine cycle maintains body levels of methionine for protein and glutathione synthesis, reactivates folic acid, produces essential methyl groups and removes potentially toxic Hcy. By reactivating folic acid, vitamin B12 maintains DNA synthesis and cell replication, which is particularly important for normal production of rapidly dividing tissues such as blood cells, the skin and mucous membranes. Without vitamin B12, folic acid becomes trapped in its inactive form and cannot be reactivated.

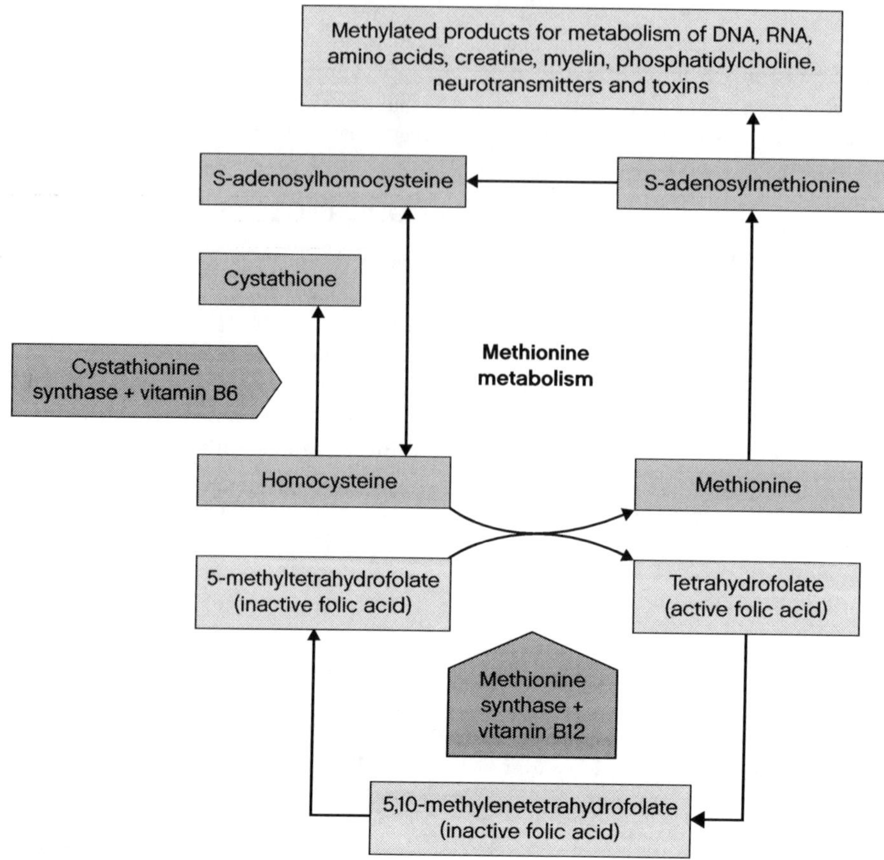

Figure 7.2 Role of vitamin B12 and folic acid in methionine metabolism

Dietary sources

Vitamin B12 is only made by micro-organisms, and is mainly found in animal foods, with small amounts provided by algae as well as plant food that has been fermented or contaminated with bacteria. Ruminant animals have bacteria in the digestive tract that produce vitamin B12, and other animals obtain vitamin B12 from eating animal food or from bacterially contaminated plant food. Sources include liver, kidneys, poultry, meat, fish and particularly shellfish. Mefun (salted fermented salmon kidney eaten in Japan) is a particularly good source of vitamin B12. Dairy products have lower amounts, and egg yolks contain a less well-absorbed form. In Australia, selected soy milks, yeast-based spreads and vegetarian meat substitutes are permitted to be fortified with vitamin B12, and these fortified foods have been shown to have a highly bioavailable form.

In general, amounts in plant foods are very low. Organic plant food grown in manure provides traces of vitamin B12 and tempeh (a fermented soy bean product) has larger amounts but other fermented soy products have trace amounts only. Dried green (*Enteromorpha* spp.) and purple (*Porphyra* spp.) seaweeds (nori and anori) have been found to contain substantial amounts of bioavailable vitamin B12, equivalent to the amount in liver. Other species of algae that were previously thought to be good sources have been found to contain mostly non-cobalamin corrinoids, such as cobamides and cobinamides. It appears that IF, transcobalamin and haptocorrin can bind to these vitamin B12 analogues, but they are either inert or have an inhibiting action on vitamin B12 metabolism and are excreted in bile. Non-cobalamin corrinoids have been included in analyses of algae as active vitamin B12, leading to a greatly over-estimated vitamin B12 content. The blue-green microalgae *Aphanizomenon flos-aquae* appears to contain only inactive analogues, and only about 17 per cent of the corrinoids in the blue-green microalgae spirulina is bioavailable vitamin B12.

The Food Standards Australia New Zealand nutrient database (NUTTAB) at <www.foodstandards.gov.au> provides the amounts found in specific foods.

Factors influencing body status

Vitamin B12 is stable to oxidation and cooking temperatures, but is unstable in acidic or alkaline conditions. It is water-soluble and may be leached out of food by water processing and cooking methods. Low body levels may be caused by malabsorption, inborn errors of metabolism or a strict vegan diet (a diet containing no animal foods). Vegans may show no effects of a vitamin B12-deficient diet for several years, and it is believed that storage and enterohepatic recycling helps to provide at least a subsistence level. Abnormal development of red blood cells is a marker of vitamin B12 deficiency, and many vegans have been shown to have normal red blood cells in spite of low serum vitamin B12, possibly because the ample folic acid provided in most vegan diets enables red blood cell replication even when vitamin B12 levels are low. However, infants of vegan mothers have been shown to develop vitamin B12 deficiency due to the mothers' low vitamin B12 status in pregnancy and inadequate amounts in their breast milk. Children following macrobiotic diets also have been found to have an increased risk of deficiency.

Low vitamin B12 is more common in the elderly, and is usually caused by digestive and absorption dysfunctions, such as inadequate production of hydrochloric acid in the stomach, inflammation of the stomach, over-growth of bacteria, such as *Helicobacter pylori*, in the digestive tract, inadequate pancreatic enzyme production, or autoimmune destruction of the parietal cells in the stomach that produce IF. Gastric surgery and gastric banding for obesity can reduce absorption, with about 10–15 per cent of people who have had a partial gastrectomy becoming deficient in vitamin B12 at about four years post operation. Absorption is also impaired by inflammatory disorders of the small intestine, such as gluten intolerance (coeliac disease) and Crohn's disease.

Bacteria and parasites, such as *Giardia lamblia* and the fish tapeworm *Diphyllobothrium latum*, consume vitamin B12 in the gut. Absorption is impaired by long-term use of anti-diabetic drugs, histamine H_2-receptor antagonists and proton pump inhibitors used to treat gastro-oesophageal reflux. The anaesthetic gas nitrous oxide (laughing gas) inactivates vitamin B12, but is only an issue if used long term. It is used as a dental anaesthetic and as a propellant in some canned foods such as whipped cream. Vitamin B12 deficiency has been observed in people who regularly inhale nitrous oxide from food canisters as a 'party drug', in health professionals who abuse the gas and in people who are exposed in the workplace.

Daily requirement

Government recommendations by age and gender (see Table 7.3) can be found in *Nutrient Reference Values for Australia and New Zealand Including Recommended Dietary Intakes*, available at <www.nrv.gov.au>.

Deficiency effects

In industrialised countries, vitamin B12 deficiency is estimated to affect about 20 per cent of the population overall and 30–40 per cent of sick or institutionalised elderly people. In a deficiency, serum vitamin B12 levels and levels of transcobalamin decrease. Methionine metabolism is impaired, leading to a buildup of Hcy; folic acid metabolism is impaired, causing reduced DNA synthesis and abnormal cell replication; and the conversion of methylmalonyl-CoA to succinyl-CoA is impaired, leading to a buildup of methylmalonic acid (MMA). This results in elevated levels of Hcy and MMA in the blood and urine.

In a vitamin B12 deficiency, and also in a folic acid deficiency, red blood cells fail to develop normally, and are large, immature and unable to carry oxygen effectively (macrocytic (large cell), megaloblastic (immature cell) anaemia). The anaemia is associated with an elevated average red blood cell volume (mean corpuscular volume) and haemoglobin content, and the presence of enlarged, oval-shaped red blood cells and neutrophils with an increased number of nuclear lobes. The total number of both red and white blood cells and platelets may be reduced (pancytopenia), and may lead to reduced immunity. Anaemia symptoms include shortness of breath, fatigue, dizziness, pallor, heart palpitations and irregular heartbeat. If folic acid is amply supplied, blood cell changes may not become evident, and it may be difficult to diagnose a vitamin B12 deficiency until the condition is advanced.

Table 7.3 Recommended dietary intake (RDI) of vitamin B12 (mcg/day)

Age (years)	Female RDI	Male RDI
1–3	0.9	0.9
4–8	1.2	1.2
9–13	1.8	1.8
14–18	2.4	2.4
19–70	2.4	2.4
>70	2.4	2.4
Pregnant women		
14–18	2.6	
19–50	2.6	
Lactating women		
14–18	2.8	
19–50	2.8	

Source: *Nutrient Reference Values for Australia and New Zealand Including Recommended Dietary Intakes*, National Health and Medical Research Council, Australian Government Department of Health and Ageing, Canberra and Ministry of Health, New Zealand, Wellington, 2006.

A vitamin B12 deficiency also damages peripheral nerves, and causes lesions in the cerebrum of the brain and the posterior and lateral columns of the spinal cord (sub-acute combined degeneration). Damage begins in the lower spinal cord and progresses to the cervical spine, the peripheral nerves, optic nerves and brain. Initially, there is loss of myelin, followed by degeneration of axons and death of neurons. Folic acid supplementation can reverse the anaemia of vitamin B12 deficiency, but has no impact on the nerve damage.

Pernicious anaemia

Pernicious anaemia (PA) is an autoimmune disease that damages the parietal cells in the stomach that produce IF, leading to a malabsorption-induced vitamin B12 deficiency and featuring macrocytic, megaloblastic anaemia with digestive disorders and damage to the spinal cord. It may be difficult to detect because the development of symptoms is very slow, and may not be noticed until the condition is advanced. Early symptoms may include weakness, poor concentration, headaches, sore tongue, heart palpitations and chest pain. Some patients with PA develop predominantly nervous system symptoms such as numbness, burning, and pins and needles sensations (paraesthesia), unsteady gait, clumsiness and, in some cases, muscle stiffness (spasticity). Early detection is important because advanced nerve damage is not fully reversible.

There appears to be a genetic factor in PA, because it occurs in close relatives and is more common in people with prematurely greying hair, blue eyes and type A blood group, and is found in association with other autoimmune conditions such as autoimmune thyroid disease, Addison's disease (affecting the adrenal glands), Sjögren's syndrome (dysfunction of the salivary glands and eyes), type 1 diabetes and vitiligo (patchy skin depigmentation).

Indicators of PA may include:

- weight loss, loss of appetite, nausea, vomiting, heartburn, sense of fullness in the abdomen, flatulence, and constipation or several semi-solid bowel movements daily
- anaemia, fatigue, heart palpitations, fast heartbeat, shortness of breath
- lemon-yellow pallor, premature greying/whitening of the hair
- smooth tongue with loss of papillae, redness, burning, soreness of the tongue, beefy and red appearance of the tongue
- paraesthesia, weakness, clumsiness, unsteady gait, loss of balance, poor vision and hearing
- memory loss, irritability, personality changes, delusions, psychosis
- urinary retention
- low-grade fever
- patchy hyperpigmentation of the skin.

In general, most patients with a vitamin B12 deficiency have neurological symptoms—mainly isolated numbness or paraesthesia, gait abnormalities, and abnormal reflexes—and these may precede blood cell abnormalities. Nervous system abnormalities have also been known to develop in people in the low-normal range of serum vitamin B12, and may start with a sensation of cold, numbness or tightness in the tips of the toes and then in the fingertips, and progress to an ascending paraesthesia, limb weakness and ataxia. There is an ascending loss of pinprick, light touch and temperature sensations, and as spinal cord damage progresses, there is poor coordination, loss of position sense, loss of balance and/or paralysis of the legs. The sensations in the feet are sometimes described as feeling as if walking on carpet. Some people develop psychiatric or cognitive symptoms, which may include mood disorders, mental slowness and confusion, poor memory, severe agitation and depression, delusions and paranoid behaviour, visual and auditory hallucinations, and violent maniacal behaviour. The optic nerve may be affected, leading to a progressive dimming of vision. Patients may develop fatigue, dizziness, light-headedness, jaundice, sexual dysfunction, impaired sense of taste and smell, bowel or bladder incontinence and a low-grade fever. Digestive symptoms include heartburn, flatulence, constipation, diarrhoea, loss of appetite and weight loss.

In a study of patients with vitamin B12 deficiency, 74 per cent had neurological symptoms, which included isolated numbness or paraesthesia (33 per cent), gait abnormalities (12 per cent), psychiatric or cognitive symptoms (3 per cent) and visual symptoms (0.5 per cent). About half of the patients had loss of appetite and weight loss, and a third had a low-grade fever. Skin changes include hyperpigmentation of oral mucous membranes, recent scars, palm creases and the backs of the hands and feet, especially around the joints of the fingers and toes. Vitiligo has also been reported.

In infants, a vitamin B12 deficiency may cause apathy, megaloblastic anaemia, hyperpigmentation of the skin, involuntary movements and delayed development. Infants of mothers following a macrobiotic or vegan diet are at increased risk. Infants of mothers following a macrobiotic diet have been found to have reduced psychomotor function, with residual effects in adolescence in spite of dietary improvement in infancy.

In deficient patients, treatment with vitamin B12 leads to a marked sense of wellbeing, and improved alertness and mood. Blood cell abnormalities, elevated Hcy and elevated MMA levels normalise in a few days, and blood cell count increases over six weeks. Nervous symptoms of less than three months' duration are completely reversible within weeks, but more long-standing symptoms are not. Paraesthesia and cognitive function in elderly people may not fully resolve.

Indicators of inadequate levels may include:

- fatigue, pallor, shortness of breath, heart palpitations, dizziness, light-headedness
- shooting pains, sensations of burning, cold, numbness or pins and needles, often beginning in the fingers or toes and ascending
- tight, stiff muscles, muscle weakness, abnormal gait, loss of balance
- insomnia, poor memory and concentration, disorientation, confusion, irritability, depression, dementia, paranoia, delirium, hallucinations, psychosis
- smooth, shiny, sore tongue, abdominal pain, weight loss, constipation, diarrhoea
- dim vision
- jaundice, low-grade fever
- skin pigmentation changes.

Assessment of body status

The vitamin B12 concentration in serum is widely used to assess vitamin B12 status, but reflects recent intakes rather than body stores. It is estimated that using this as a sole measure may miss up to 50 per cent of deficient patients. Many vitamin B12 assays are based on the competitive binding of serum vitamin B12 with reagent IF, and may give false high values when serum containing antibodies that block IF is analysed. Falsely increased values can also be caused by myeloproliferative disorders (over-production of blood cells), liver diseases, kidney diseases, intestinal bacterial overgrowth, congenital transcobalamin deficiency and nitrous oxide exposure. Levels may be normal or even high in patients with alcoholic liver damage—possibly because vitamin B12 storage is impaired.

The reference range given for serum vitamin B12 by the Biochemistry Department of the Royal Prince Alfred Hospital, Sydney, Australia is 150–750 pmol/L. Some researchers believe that the reference range should be adjusted because MMA and Hcy are elevated at levels of 258 pmol/L or less. Other researchers suggest that less than 221 pmol/L may indicate a marginal deficiency. Levels of less than 74 pmol/L are common in patients with pernicious anaemia. Serum holotranscobalamin, which reflects the amount of vitamin B12 available for delivery to cells, may be a more sensitive indicator of status, especially in alcoholics. The reference range is 40–200 pmol/L.

There is an increase in MMA when vitamin B12 is inadequate, and an elevated serum concentration is regarded as a sensitive indicator of even a mild vitamin B12 deficiency; cut-off values vary, but a concentration greater than 0.34 μmol/L may indicate a deficiency. In urine, MMA levels of 300 mg or more over a 24-hour period may indicate a deficiency. Increased plasma Hcy levels are not a specific indicator of vitamin B12 deficiency, as folic acid, vitamin B6 and vitamin B12 are all required for Hcy metabolism. The reference range given by the Royal College of Pathologists of Australasia (RCPA) for plasma Hcy is 5–15 μmol/L.

To test for vitamin B12 malabsorption, the Schilling test was formerly used; this involved taking an oral dose of radioactively labelled vitamin B12 followed by an injection of non-labelled vitamin B12 to load tissues and ensure the oral dose was largely excreted. Urine was collected for 24 hours afterwards to measure the amount of labelled vitamin B12 in urine, with a low amount indicating poor oral absorption. The Schilling test has been replaced by testing for anti-parietal cell and anti-IF antibodies in serum; the presence of antibodies indicates an autoimmune-based malabsorption (PA). Recent vitamin B12 therapy may cause a false positive result for the anti-IF antibody test, and testing should be carried out before treatment is commenced.

The deoxyuridine (dU) suppression test can be used to assess vitamin B12 or folic acid status. It measures the rate of incorporation of thymidine into DNA in leukocytes or bone marrow cells, a process dependent on activity of the folic acid-dependent enzyme thymidylate synthase, after exposure to dU. In normal cells, the rate of incorporation is suppressed by adding dU, but this suppression is inhibited in folic acid-deficient cells and also in vitamin B12-deficient cells because of impaired folic acid activity. An improvement in dU-induced suppression of thymidine incorporation after either folic acid or vitamin B12 exposure indicates that there is a deficiency of the vitamin being tested. This test is used to identify whether vitamin B12 or folic acid deficiency is the cause of megaloblastic anaemia, and is a more reliable indicator than blood concentrations because it can detect subclinical deficiencies in which serum levels of these vitamins are within the normal range. However, it is not routinely used as yet.

Response to treatment can be used to assess vitamin B12 absorption, in which serum vitamin B12 is measured before and after short-term treatment with oral vitamin B12. The amount of increase indicates the level of absorption; if the increase is low, the test is repeated with IF added to the oral dose. A greater rise in serum vitamin B12 after the addition of IF indicates a lack of IF, and no further increase indicates a different type of malabsorption problem which needs further investigation.

Overall, it appears that more than one test should be used to assess vitamin B12 status. It is suggested that a vitamin B12 deficiency should be considered in the following circumstances: if serum vitamin B12 is less than 150 pmol/L and symptoms are present; if serum vitamin B12 levels are less than 150 pmol/L on two occasions; if serum vitamin B12 levels are less than 150 pmol/L and plasma Hcy is greater than 13 μmol/L or serum MMA is greater than 0.4 μmol/L; or if serum holotranscobalamin is less than 35 pmol/L.

Case reports—vitamin B12 deficiency

- *A woman, nineteen years of age*, was investigated for deteriorating vision that had started at age fifteen and had been treated with steroids.[1] She was found to have optic nerve atrophy of both eyes and particularly the left eye, which had severe vision loss. She had a history of low serum vitamin B12 and her presenting serum B12 level was very low (41.32 pmol/L). A diet history revealed that she had not eaten eggs, meat, chicken or seafood for ten years and had rarely eaten these foods as a young child. Her diet was vegetarian and the only animal food included was cheese. She was also a smoker. She was given vitamin B12 and steroid therapy, followed by monthly maintenance B12 treatment, and she also stopped smoking. The vision in her right eye improved slowly, gradually becoming normal. However, the vision loss in her left eye appeared to be permanent.
- *A boy, sixteen years of age*, developed severe personality changes, with irritability, regressive behaviour, apathy, weeping and truancy from school over a twelve-month period.[2] He displayed anxiety during separation from his mother, wept frequently and experienced vague pains, lethargy that alternated with racing thoughts, agitation, irritability, loss of capacity to feel pleasure, and poor memory, concentration, sleep and appetite. He was not able to cope at school, and was frequently absent. He spent long periods on his computer and made frequent purchases online using his parents' credit cards. He reported auditory and visual hallucinations and suicidal thoughts. Investigations revealed inflammation of the tongue, ataxia, rigidity in both shoulders, cog-wheel rigidity in the left elbow, poor coordination and poor balance. Although he was not a vegetarian, he was found to have a low serum

vitamin B12 level (122.5 pmol/L), atrophy of the stomach with the presence of *Helicobacter pylori* and malabsorption of vitamin B12.

He was given the antipsychotic drug risperidone, antibiotics to treat his *H. pylori* infection and intramuscular vitamin B12 injections (500 mcg daily). Within two weeks, no psychotic features were present, his balance had recovered and cerebellar tests were within normal limits. His apathy, weeping, regressive behaviour and truancy had moderated and his serum vitamin B12 had risen to 439 pmol/L. Risperidone was stopped, and he was treated with injections of vitamin B12 monthly for three months. *H. pylori* had been eradicated in his stomach, and he displayed no psychiatric dysfunction during six months of monthly follow-up.

- *A male infant, five months of age*, exclusively breastfed by his vegan mother, developed feeding difficulties, poor weight gain, severe pallor, floppy muscles and excessive sleepiness.[3] His growth was retarded, he had developmental delay, an enlarged liver and spleen and severe pancytopenia. The mother had experienced a normal pregnancy and had taken a multivitamin providing 2.5 mcg of vitamin B12 daily during the second and third trimesters, but had stopped taking this after the birth. The baby's serum vitamin B12 level was 42 pmol/L, and his iron and haemoglobin levels were low but his red blood cells were not megaloblastic—possibly because he was not folic acid-deficient. Brain imaging showed mild dilation of the lateral ventricles with diffuse delayed myelination. He was diagnosed with iron and vitamin B12 deficiency because of the inadequate amounts provided by his mother's breast milk. He was treated with packed red blood cells, vitamin B12 injections (1000 mcg daily for two weeks followed by weekly 1000 mcg injections for six months) and iron supplementation, with rapid improvement in his anaemia. He was weaned at six months, and his diet included green vegetables and fish. However, seven months after the start of therapy, he still showed reduced brain myelination and delayed development of muscle function and language.
- *A man, 72 years of age*, with no history of psychiatric illness, developed apathy, irritability, poor memory and attention span, and began to have psychotic episodes characterised by paranoid thoughts and jealous delusions regarding his wife.[4] He was disoriented, slow in moving and thinking, with poor long-term memory and emotional blunting, and was diagnosed with frontotemporal dementia (dementia due to deterioration of the brain's frontal lobes). He was also found to have peripheral neuropathy, loss of balance and ataxia. His serum vitamin B12 level was 40 pmol/L, and he had macrocytic anaemia, gastric atrophy and elevated plasma Hcy levels. He was then diagnosed with vitamin B12 deficiency-dementia, and was given vitamin B12 injections (1000 mcg three times weekly for 45 days, slowly reducing to 1000 mcg monthly). After one month, his ataxia and cognitive function improved, and his psychotic symptoms disappeared. Serum vitamin B12 and Hcy levels returned to normal over time. Three months after the start of treatment, cognitive function tests were almost normal, and became completely normal at six months.

REFERENCES

1 Gleeson, M.H. & Graves, P.S., Complications of dietary deficiency of vitamin B12 in young Caucasians, *Postgrad Med J* (1974), 50(585): 462–4.

2 Tufan, A.E., Bilici, R., Usta, G. & Erdoğan, A., Mood disorder with mixed, psychotic features due to vitamin B12 deficiency in an adolescent: Case report, *Child Adolesc Psychiatry Ment Health* (2012), 6(1): 25.

3 Guez, S., Chiarelli, G., Menni, F. et al., Severe vitamin B12 deficiency in an exclusively breastfed 5-month-old Italian infant born to a mother receiving multivitamin supplementation during pregnancy, *BMC Pediatr* (2012), 12: 85.

4 Blundo, C., Marin, D. & Ricci, M., Vitamin B12 deficiency associated with symptoms of frontotemporal dementia, *Neurol Sci* (2011), 32(1): 101–5.

THERAPEUTIC USES OF VITAMIN B12

Birth defects

During the third or fourth week of pregnancy, the neural tube of the foetus closes over and eventually forms the infant's spinal cord and brain. Failure of this closure causes neural tube defects (NTDs), such as spina bifida (defects of the spinal cord), anencephaly and encephalocoele (defects of the brain). Folic acid is essential for normal foetal cell replication because it supports DNA synthesis and methylation reactions that have a role in cell signalling and replication, and vitamin B12 is essential to maintain folic acid in its active form.

Public health messages to reduce the risk of NTDs have focused on folic acid because women who take folic acid supplementation for three months prior to conception and during pregnancy have been found to have a greatly reduced incidence of NTDs. Vitamin B12 is now receiving attention because of its supportive role in folic acid metabolism. A meta-analysis of nine trials concluded that low levels of vitamin B12 in pregnancy were associated with a 2.41-fold increased risk of NTDs.[1] Serum vitamin B12 concentrations of less than 185 pmol/L in pregnancy are associated with the highest risk.[2] A serum vitamin B12 level of more than 221 pmol/L is advisable before conception in order to reduce the risk.

Cognitive disorders

Hcy is potentially toxic and is removed by conversion to cystathione or back to methionine, which requires folic acid, vitamin B12 and vitamin B6. In older people, elevated Hcy levels may be associated with cognitive impairment, Alzheimer's disease and diminished sensory and peripheral motor nerve function. A low vitamin B12 status is associated with a 2.3-fold increase in risk of cognitive impairment, high MMA is associated with a 3.5-fold increased risk, low holotranscobalamin is associated with a 4.1-fold increased risk and elevated Hcy is associated with a 4.8-fold increased risk.[3] It is estimated that a doubling of holotranscobalamin levels from 50 to 100 μmol/L reduces the risk of cognitive decline by 30 per cent and a doubling of HCy from 10 to 20 μmol/L or a doubling of MMA from 0.25 to 0.5 μmol/L increases the risk of cognitive decline by 50 per cent.[4] Low or low/normal levels of vitamin B12 are associated with brain atrophy in elderly people, and those with levels in the lowest range have twice the rate of atrophy.[5] Long-term supplementation with 400 mcg of folic acid plus 100 mcg of vitamin B12 in elderly people with depressive symptoms has been shown to improve cognitive function over a two-year period, particularly memory performance.[6] However, not all studies have found positive results. Some types of dementia may be reversible with vitamin B12 therapy but it does not appear to improve cognitive function in people without a pre-existing deficiency.

Depression

Vitamin B12 and folic acid are required for the synthesis of SAM, which provides methyl groups for the production of neurotransmitters that affect mood. SAM, folic acid and vitamin B12 may have anti-depressant activity. Low levels of holotranscobalamin and vitamin B12 have been found to be associated with depression in elderly people.[7] In a prospective study, lower baseline vitamin B12 and folic acid levels and elevated Hcy levels were found to be predictive of the development of depression two to three years later, as was a decline in vitamin B12 levels and an increase in Hcy from baseline.[8]

Cardiovascular disease

Elevated Hcy levels are considered a strong, independent risk factor for CVD, including heart disease, stroke and thrombosis. A review of 30 trials concluded that lowering fasting plasma Hcy by 25 per cent (to about 3 μmol/L) is associated with an 11 per cent reduced risk of ischaemic heart disease and a 19 per cent reduced risk of stroke.[9] Hcy can be lowered by vitamin B12 and folic acid supplementation; folic acid lowers Hcy by 13–25 per cent (according to dose) and vitamin B12 by a further 7 per cent.[10] Although this has not been shown to reduce risk of heart disease, there is some evidence that lowering Hcy may reduce stroke incidence and mortality.[11]

Bone weakness

Low serum vitamin B12 levels appear to be associated with reduced levels of bone metabolism indicators, such as serum alkaline phosphatase and osteocalcin, and there may be an association between serum vitamin B12 concentration and thymidine incorporation into DNA of bone building cells. Elevated Hcy has been found to increase risk of bone fractures. Women with a borderline deficiency of vitamin B12 have been found to have a 4.5-fold increase in risk of osteoporosis and women who are deficient have been found to have a 6.9-fold increased risk.[12] This relationship was not found in men. Elevated Hcy and low vitamin B12 concentrations have been associated with low bone mineral density (as assessed by ultrasound measurement of the heel), high bone turnover and increased fracture risk.[13] Lower levels of serum vitamin B12 have been shown to be associated with more rapid bone loss from the hip in elderly women.[14] The effect of vitamin B12 supplementation on bone density is not known.

Vitiligo

Patients with vitiligo have been found to have elevated Hcy levels and lower vitamin B12 and holotranscobalamin levels than controls. A Hcy level of 15 μmol/L or more and a serum vitamin B12 level of less than 148 μmol/L were found to be significant risk factors, and patients within the lowest range of holotranscobalamin also had an increased risk.[15] Patients with vitiligo were treated with sun exposure and oral folic acid and vitamin B12 supplementation, and nearly two-thirds had no further spread of depigmentation and more than half experienced repigmentation, with total repigmentation in 6 per cent.[16] Supplementation combined with sun exposure was found to improve repigmentation more than either supplementation or sun exposure alone.

Multiple sclerosis

Vitamin B12 deficiency affects myelination of nerve fibres, and multiple sclerosis (MS) features abnormal myelination, indicating that there may be a relationship. MS patients have been found to have lower serum vitamin B12 than control subjects and elevated Hcy levels.[17,18] In a study of 29 patients with MS who were compared with other neurological patients and normal controls, MS patients were found to have lower serum vitamin B12 levels and more macrocytosis.[19] Nine MS patients had serum vitamin B12 levels less than 147 pmol/L and low red blood cell folate levels, and nine MS patients had raised plasma levels of R proteins that were not bound to vitamin B12, including three patients with very high values, indicating abnormal metabolism of vitamin B12. However, the role of vitamin B12 in MS is not well understood, and treatment with vitamin B12 has not been shown to improve the nerve damage of MS.

Hearing disorders

In a study of healthy older women, those with hearing loss were found to have a 38 per cent lower level of serum vitamin B12 and a 31 per cent lower red blood cell folate level than women with normal hearing.[20] A study of patients with tinnitus (noises in the ears) found that 47 per cent were deficient in vitamin B12, and twelve patients given supplementation reported improvements in symptoms.[21] Vitamin B12 injections (1000 mcg daily for seven days and 5000 mcg on day eight) have been shown to improve noise-induced hearing loss in young people.[22]

REFERENCES

1 Wang, Z.P., Shang, X.X. & Zhao, Z.T., Low maternal vitamin B(12) is a risk factor for neural tube defects: a meta-analysis, *J Matern Fetal Neonatal Med* (2012), 25(4): 389–94.

2 Molloy, A.M., Kirke, P.N., Troendle, J.F. et al., Maternal vitamin B12 status and risk of neural tube defects in a population with high neural tube defect prevalence and no folic acid fortification, *Pediatrics* (2009), 123(3): 917–23.

3 Lildballe, D.L., Fedosov, S., Sherliker, P. et al., Association of cognitive impairment with combinations of vitamin B_{12}-related parameters, *Clin Chem* (2011), 57(10): 1436–43.

4 Clarke, R., Birks, J., Nexø, E. et al. Low vitamin B-12 status and risk of cognitive decline in older adults, *Am J Clin Nutr* (2007), 86(5): 1384–91.

5 Vogiatzoglou, A., Refsum, H., Johnston, C. et al., Vitamin B12 status and rate of brain volume loss in community-dwelling elderly, *Neurology* (2008), 71(11): 826–32.

6 Walker, J.G., Batterham, P.J., Mackinnon, A.J. et al., Oral folic acid and vitamin B12 supplementation to prevent cognitive decline in community-dwelling older adults with depressive symptoms—the Beyond Ageing Project: A randomized controlled trial, *Am J Clin Nutr* (2012), 95(1): 194–203.

7 Robinson, D.J., O'Luanaigh, C., Tehee, E. et al., Associations between holotranscobalamin, vitamin B12, homocysteine and depressive symptoms in community-dwelling elders, *Int J Geriatr Psychiatry* (2011), 26(3): 307–13.

8 Kim, J.M., Stewart, R., Kim, S.W. et al., Predictive value of folate, vitamin B12 and homocysteine levels in late-life depression, *Br J Psychiatry* (2008), 192(4): 268–74.

9 Homocysteine Studies Collaboration, Homocysteine and risk of ischemic heart disease and stroke: A meta-analysis, *JAMA* (2002), 288(16): 2015–22.

10 Homocysteine Lowering Trialists' Collaboration, Dose-dependent effects of folic acid on blood concentrations of homocysteine: a meta-analysis of the randomized trials, *Am J Clin Nutr* (2005), 82(4): 806–12.

11 Manolescu, B.N., Oprea, E., Farcasanu, I.C. et al., Homocysteine and vitamin therapy in stroke prevention and treatment: A review, *Acta Biochim Pol* (2010), 57(4): 467–77.

12 Dhonukshe-Rutten, R.A., Lips, M., de Jong, N. et al., Vitamin B12 status is associated with bone mineral content and bone mineral density in frail elderly women but not in men, *J Nutr* (2003), 133(3): 801–7.

13 Dhonukshe-Rutten, R.A., Pluijm, S.M., de Groot, L.C. et al., Homocysteine and vitamin B12 status relate to bone turnover markers, broadband ultrasound attenuation, and fractures in healthy elderly people, *J Bone Miner Res* (2005), 20(6): 921–9.

14 Stone, K.L., Bauer, D.C., Sellmeyer, D., Cummings, S.R., Low serum vitamin B12 levels are associated with increased hip bone loss in older women: a prospective study, *J Clin Endocrinol Metab* (2004), 89(3): 1217–21.

15 Karadag, A.S., Tutal, E., Ertugrul, D.T. et al., Serum holotranscobalamine, vitamin B12, folic acid and homocysteine levels in patients with vitiligo, *Clin Exp Dermatol* (2012), 37(1): 62–4.

16 Juhlin, L. & Olsson, M.J., Improvement of vitiligo after oral treatment with vitamin B12 and folic acid and the importance of sun exposure, *Acta Derm Venereol* (1997), 77(6): 460–2.

17 Nijst, T.Q., Wevers, R.A., Schoonderwaldt, H.C. et al., Vitamin B12 and folate concentrations in serum and cerebrospinal fluid of neurological patients with special reference to multiple sclerosis and dementia, *Neurosurg Psychiatry* (1990), 53(11): 951–4.

18 Vrethem, M., Mattsson, E., Hebelka, H. et al., Increased plasma homocysteine levels without signs of vitamin B12 deficiency in patients with multiple sclerosis assessed by blood and cerebrospinal fluid homocysteine and methylmalonic acid, *Mult Scler* (2003), 9(3): 239–45.

19 Reynolds, E.H., Bottiglieri, T., Laundy, M. et al., Vitamin B12 metabolism in multiple sclerosis, *Arch Neurol* (1992), 49(6): 649–52.

20 Houston, D.K., Johnson, M.A., Nozza, R.J. et al., Age-related hearing loss, vitamin B12, and folate in elderly women, *Am J Clin Nutr* (1999), 69(3): 564–71.

21 Shemesh, Z., Attias, J., Ornan, M. et al., Vitamin B12 deficiency in patients with chronic-tinnitus and noise-induced hearing loss, *Am J Otolaryngol* (1993), 14(2): 94–9.

22 Quaranta, A., Scaringi, A., Bartoli, R. et al., The effects of 'supra-physiological' vitamin B12 administration on temporary threshold shift, *Int J Audiol* (2004), 43(3): 162–5.

Therapeutic dose

Vitamin B12 may be given orally, under the tongue (sublingually), as a nasal spray or gel, or by intramuscular (im) injection. High oral doses have been shown to improve vitamin B12 status as effectively as injections. Vitamin B12 can be absorbed by passive diffusion throughout the entire digestive tract, and sublingual absorption is similar to oral absorption. Nasal spray formulations of vitamin B12 have been found to be absorbed rapidly, and to lead to sustained concentrations in the therapeutic range.

Suggested doses for adults are as follows:

- *Health maintenance:* 5–10 mcg daily (oral) together with dietary sources.
- *Mild deficiency:* 500–1000 mcg daily (oral), and then weekly on improvement.
- *Severe deficiency:* 1000–2000 mcg daily (oral), reducing to 1000 mcg once weekly when the deficiency is

resolved; by im delivery, 1000 mcg twice weekly for two weeks, followed by 1000 mcg once weekly for four weeks, and then 1000 mcg once monthly, changing to 1000 mcg weekly by oral, sublingual or nasal delivery for maintenance dosing.

- *Pernicious anaemia:* as for severe deficiencies until symptoms resolve, then 1000 mcg daily by oral, sublingual or nasal delivery for life.
- *Vegan/macrobiotic diet:* 100–500 mcg daily or weekly.
- *Elderly:* 100–500 mcg daily or weekly.
- *To lower elevated Hcy:* 60–400 mcg daily with 500 mcg folic acid.
- *NTD prevention before and after conception:* 10–50 mcg daily, together with 600 mcg daily of folic acid.
- *After gastric surgery for obesity:* 350 mcg or more daily.

Effects of excess

Vitamin B12 appears to be non-toxic and well tolerated. Intake in excess of needs is excreted in bile. No adverse affects have been reported in individuals receiving up to 4500 mcg daily of cyano-B12 for fourteen days, 2000 mcg daily of cyano-B12 for up to one year or 1000 mcg daily of cyano-B12 for several years.

Supplements

The permitted forms of vitamin B12 in Australian supplements are cyano-B12 and hydroxo-B12, but the cyano form is most commonly used in supplements because of its superior stability. Both forms are bioavailable but cyano-B12 is inactive until the cyano group is removed. Hydroxo-B12 appears to have greater availability to cells and better retention in the body, and can be given at less frequent intervals than cyano-B12. Methyl-B12 is available in some countries as a supplement and appears to have greater retention in the body than cyano-B12.

Vitamin B12 is made commercially by micro-organisms such as *Pseudomonas denitrificans* and *Propionibacterium shermanii*, which make about 100 000 times more vitamin B12 during fermentation than they require for their growth. Random mutations or genetic engineering may be used to obtain species with the highest production capacity. During cultivation, nutrients such as cobalt, glycine, threonine, betaine and choline may be provided to improve yield. After cultivation, pasteurisation is used to inactivate the micro-organisms, and vitamin B12 is then separated, extracted and purified. Cyano-B12 is made by the addition of cyanide or thiocyanate. The cyanide content of cyano-B12 is too small to cause toxic effects in the body, even at high supplementary doses.

Cautions

Vitamin B12 has a specific interrelationship with folic acid, and a high intake of folic acid without adequate vitamin B12 can maintain normal replication of blood cells and prevent the red blood cell changes that are a feature of PA, although the nerve damage caused by low vitamin B12 continues to progress undetected. For this reason, folic acid supplementation should be taken together with vitamin B12, especially in people following vegan or macrobiotic diets, which usually provide large amounts of folate. There is some indication that high doses of vitamin B12 given in a severe deficiency may temporarily increase the requirement of iron and folic acid.

FOLIC ACID

FOLIC ACID STATUS CHECK

1. **Do you get cracks and sores in the corners of your mouth?**
2. **Do you have patches of darkened skin on your face, hands or feet?**
3. **Are you taking the oral contraceptive pill and/or medication for epilepsy?**
4. **Do you rarely eat fresh vegetables?**

'Yes' answers may indicate inadequate folic acid status. Note that a number of nutritional deficiencies or health disorders can cause similar effects and further investigation is recommended.

FAST FACTS . . . FOLIC ACID

- **Folic acid is found in liver, fresh raw vegetables, bean sprouts, whole grains, legumes and orange juice.**
- **It is required for the metabolism of methionine and removal of potentially toxic homocysteine.**
- **It helps produce S-adenosylmethionine, which provides methyl groups for DNA and RNA metabolism and normal cell replication.**

- **A deficiency during pregnancy can lead to neural tube defects in the foetus.**
- **Supplementation is essential in pregnancy, and may also be useful for mood disorders and for reducing elevated homocysteine levels.**

English physician Lucy Wills, working in India in the 1930s, observed macrocytic anaemia in her pregnant patients, and conducted experiments in animals that showed that this type of anaemia was prevented by yeast added to a diet otherwise lacking in B vitamins. Yeast or yeast extract was then found to correct the macrocytic anaemia in her pregnant Indian patients. A nutritional factor in liver, distinct from vitamin B12, was subsequently identified that cured the macrocytic anaemia associated with pernicious anaemia (PA). This factor was shown to be a growth factor for bacteria, and was isolated from spinach in 1941 and named folic acid after *folium*, the Latin word for 'leaf'. Folic acid was found to correct the macrocytic anaemia of PA, but had no effect on the neurological dysfunction, which responded to vitamin B12 therapy.

Folic acid was found to have an important role in cell division and, in the 1960s, folic acid deficiency became known as the major cause of preventable neural tube defects (NTDs) in infants. Consequently, pregnant women were advised to take supplements and, decades later, mandatory food fortification programs were introduced in many countries (including Australia), leading to a dramatic reduction in the incidence of NTDs.

Folate is the generic term for all forms of folic acid. Folic acid (pteroylmonoglutamic acid), used in supplements and in fortified foods, occurs only rarely in food. It consists of a molecule of para-aminobenzoic acid (PABA) linked to a pteridine ring together with one glutamic acid molecule. Food folate is in the form of pteroylpolyglutamates, which contain one to nine additional glutamic acid molecules. In the body and in food, folate is found in various forms, including 5-formyl tetrahydrofolate (5-formyl THF), 10-formyl THF, 5-formimino THF, 5,10 methenyl THF, 5,10-methylene THF and 5-methyl THF. These forms are inter-convertible, except for 5-methyl THF, which cannot convert back to 5,10 methylene THF.

Digestion, absorption and transport

For absorption to take place, the additional glutamate units in food folate must be removed by zinc-dependent pteroylglutamate hydrolase enzymes in the small intestine. This process converts food folate to folic acid, the monoglutamate form. Folic acid from supplements and fortified food is already in the monoglutamate form, and has high bioavailability. Absorption is by an active, carrier-dependent mechanism, with passive diffusion occurring at high levels of intake. In the enterocytes, folic acid is converted to dihydrofolate (DHF) and then to tetrahydrofolate (THF) monoglutamates that are transported to the liver and converted to the polyglutamate forms, which function as coenzymes.

Metabolism, storage and excretion

THF is the active form of folate in the body, and conversion of DHF to THF is dependent on the enzyme DHF reductase. The liver is the main storage site for folate, which is stored mainly as polyglutamate forms of THF and 5-methyl THF. The liver can store 6–14 mg, which is half the total body store; total storage is equivalent to several months' supply.

Folate is released from the liver into the bloodstream as monoglutamates, such as THF, 5-methyl THF and 10-formyl THF, which are transported in free form or bound to folate-binding proteins. Uptake by tissues is via folate receptors, which have been identified in the liver, kidneys and bone marrow. Folate is incorporated into red blood cells during their production, and is not transferred from blood. Once inside cells, folate is converted to the polyglutamate form by the enzyme folylpolyglutamate synthetase to enable its use by enzymes, and to retain it inside the cell. Folate is excreted in bile (about 100 mcg/day), but most of this is reabsorbed in the gut and returned to the liver by the enterohepatic circulation. Folate breakdown products—mainly N-acetyl para-aminobenzoyl glutamate—are excreted in urine.

Functions

Folate coenzymes are involved in one-carbon transfer reactions, which take place during amino acid and DNA metabolism.

Functions of folate include the following:

- *Amino acid metabolism.* Folate is required for the conversion of histidine to glutamic acid, interconversion of serine and glycine, glycine synthesis from choline and the conversion of homocysteine (Hcy) to methionine. During choline metabolism, choline is broken down to form betaine (trimethylglycine), which donates methyl groups to Hcy, generating dimethylglycine (DMG) (see Figure 4.8). DMG is converted to sarcosine and then to glycine, with the support of vitamin B2 and THF, which is converted to the inactive 5,10 methylene form and then to inactive 5-methyl THF.

  During methionine metabolism, a methyl group from 5-methyl THF is transferred to Hcy to form methionine, with the assistance of methyl-B12 and the enzyme methionine synthase (see Figure 7.2). Removal of the methyl group from 5-methyl THF forms THF. Methionine is then converted to S-adenosylmethionine (SAM), then to S-adenosylhomocysteine (SAH), then to Hcy, and finally back to methionine. SAM provides methyl groups that are needed for the metabolism of DNA, RNA, amino acids, neurotransmitters, toxins, creatine (a muscle energy source), myelin (the sheath surrounding nerve fibres) and phosphatidylcholine, an important component of cell membranes. SAM supports synthesis of tetrahydrobiopterin (BH_4), which is a co-factor for phenylalanine, tyrosine and tryptophan metabolism and for production of melatonin and the neurotransmitters adrenaline, histamine, noradrenaline, serotonin and dopamine, which affect mood and behaviour.

  Normal activity of the methionine cycle maintains body levels of methionine for protein and glutathione synthesis, reactivates folic acid, produces essential methyl groups and removes Hcy. Hcy is potentially toxic to nerves and blood vessels, and is implicated in CVD, neurological disorders and adverse pregnancy outcomes. It is removed during the methionine cycle, and also by conversion to cystathione by an enzyme dependent on vitamin B6. If vitamin B12 is inadequate, folic acid becomes trapped in the 5-methyl form, and cannot be converted to other forms for use by coenzymes.
- *Cell replication.* Folate acts as a donor and acceptor of methyl groups required for DNA synthesis and methylation of DNA, RNA and proteins. Folate is required for the synthesis of purine and thymidylate, which support DNA synthesis and repair. Thymidylate is converted to thymidine triphosphate (dTTP), which is essential for DNA synthesis and repair. 10-formyl THF is required for formation of the purine bases guanine and adenine that are building blocks of DNA and RNA. Folate also supports conversion of methionine to SAM, which provides methyl groups for DNA methylation, a process essential for regulation of gene expression, normal cell replication and embryonic development. DNA synthesis and cell replication are particularly important during growth and for normal production of rapidly dividing tissues, such as blood cells, the skin and mucous membranes.

Dietary sources

Folate is found in liver, kidneys, brewer's yeast, fresh raw vegetables and bean sprouts. Green leafy vegetables, such as spinach, cabbage, broccoli, bok choy, choy sum, Brussels sprouts, cauliflower, endive, lettuce and kale, are good sources. Other sources are mushrooms, asparagus, parsnips, peas, avocadoes, bean sprouts, nuts, wheat bran, whole grains, legumes and orange juice. Fermented dairy products contain folate because it is produced by the *Lactobacilli* bacteria used in the fermentation process.

In Australia, there is mandatory fortification of wheat flour for bread-making at a level of 80–180 mcg of folic acid per 100 grams of bread. However, organic bread and bread made from non-wheat cereal flours such as rice, corn or rye are not required to have added folic acid, although it may be added voluntarily. Foods containing added folic acid may also include savoury biscuits, breakfast cereals, pasta, rice, yeast extracts, fruit and vegetable juices, soy drinks and tofu.

The Food Standards Australia New Zealand nutrient database (NUTTAB) at <www.foodstandards.gov.au> provides the amounts found in specific foods.

Factors influencing body status

Bioavailability of food folate averages 50 per cent, whereas folic acid in fortified food is about 85 per cent bioavailable and folic acid supplements taken on an empty stomach have 100 per cent bioavailability. Conjugase inhibitors in legumes, cabbage and oranges impair absorption of folate. In general, food folate is very sensitive to exposure to air, light, heat and room temperature storage, but sensitivity varies according to the type of food. Food harvesting, storage, processing and preparation can cause losses of up to 95 per cent. Folate is water-soluble, and can be leached out of food by water processing and cooking methods. Boiling vegetables has been shown to cause losses of more than 50 per cent, but steaming has little effect.

Folate metabolism requires the presence of vitamins B2, B3, B6, B12 and zinc. B12 deficiency causes folate to become trapped in its inactive form. Absorption of folate is impaired by digestive disorders, alcohol and the cholesterol-lowering drug cholestyramine, and needs are increased during pregnancy, lactation and growth. A deficiency is more common in elderly people, and may be associated with a restricted diet lacking fresh and raw fruit and vegetables. Genetic variations in the gene for 5,10-methylene THF reductase (MTHFR), the enzyme that produces methyl THF, can reduce enzyme activity and impair folate metabolism.

Drugs that impair folate absorption or metabolism include phenytoin and valproic acid (for epilepsy), sulfasalazine (for inflammatory bowel disorders), oral contraceptives, anti-TB drugs, pyrimethamine (for malaria), trimetrexate (for *Pneumocystis carinii* infections), trimethoprim (for bacterial urinary tract infections), triamterene (a potassium-sparing diuretic) and the cancer drugs methotrexate and aminopterin. Non-steroidal anti-inflammatory drugs, including aspirin, ibuprofen and acetaminophen (paracetamol), may have anti-folate activity in large doses. Drugs that are folic acid analogues, which include aminopterin, methotrexate, valproic acid, triamterene and trimethoprim, act by displacing folate from enzymes and blocking DHF reductase reactions. Side-effects mimic severe folate deficiency, and folic acid supplementation can be used to reduce side-effects without reducing drug effectiveness.

Daily requirement

In calculating folate requirements, an adjustment is made for the 50 per cent lower bioavailability of food folate compared with that of folic acid, and the adjusted figures are referred to as dietary folate equivalents (DFEs):

1 mcg of DFE = 1 mcg of food folate
= 0.6 mcg of folic acid from fortified food or as a supplement taken with meals.
= 0.5 mcg of a folic acid supplement taken on an empty stomach.

Government recommendations by age and gender (see Table 7.4) can be found in *Nutrient Reference Values for Australia and New Zealand Including Recommended Dietary Intakes*, available at <www.nrv.gov.au>.

Table 7.4 Recommended dietary intake (RDI) of folate (mcg/day DFE)*

Age (years)	Female RDI	Male RDI
1–3	150	150
4–8	200	200
9–13	300	300
14–18	400	400
19–70	400	400
>70	400	400
Pregnant women		
14–18	600	
19–50	600	
Lactating women		
14–18	500	
19–50	500	

* DFE, dietary folate equivalents: a method of adjusting for the bioavailability of various forms of folate; folic acid from fortified foods and dietary supplements is multiplied by a factor of 1.7 to equate them to the amount of folate available from naturally-occurring folate in foods.

Source: Nutrient Reference Values for Australia and New Zealand Including Recommended Dietary Intakes, National Health and Medical Research Council, Australian Government Department of Health and Ageing, Canberra and Ministry of Health, New Zealand, Wellington, 2006.

Deficiency effects

Folate deficiency is more common in pregnant women, the elderly and alcoholics, and results in reduced DNA synthesis and impairment of cell replication. Effects are more marked in rapidly dividing cells, which include blood cells, the skin and mucous membranes. Inadequate folate intake first leads to a decrease in serum folate concentration, usually within one to three weeks, then to a decrease in red blood cell folate, a rise in Hcy and megaloblastic changes in bone marrow and other tissues with rapidly dividing cells. Blood cells reduce in number and become macrocytic but, as red blood cells live for 120 days, there is no marked abnormality of these cells in the early stages of a deficiency. Eventually, megaloblastic macrocytic anaemia develops, which is characterised by the presence of large immature red blood cells that are fewer in number and do not carry oxygen effectively, and by the presence of hyper-segmented (having more lobes than normal) polymorphonuclear leukocytes (PMNs). Anaemia symptoms include weakness, fatigue, poor concentration, irritability, headache, palpitations and shortness of breath. Associated symptoms may include rapid heartbeat (tachycardia), angina pectoris, heart failure, postural hypotension and lactic acidosis. Vitamin B12 deficiency can also cause macrocytic megaloblastic anaemia because folate becomes trapped in an inactive form and cannot be reactivated.

Abnormal replication of epithelial cells caused by a folate deficiency may cause cracks or sores in the corners of the mouth, inflamed and sore mouth, and a sore tongue that may have a swollen, beefy, red or shiny appearance, initially around the edges and tip. Stomach and intestinal inflammation may cause loss of appetite, indigestion, nausea, vomiting, abdominal pain and diarrhoea. Effects on the skin may include inflammation and patchy hyperpigmentation of the mucous membranes and skin, particularly the face, hands and feet.

A lack of folate in the central nervous system causes reduced SAM production and lower transmethylation activity, which impairs the metabolism of melatonin, adrenaline, histamine, noradrenaline, serotonin and dopamine, as well as the production of membrane phospholipids, and the formation and repair of DNA. Possible effects are mood disorders, depression, insomnia, memory loss and irritability. A modest temperature elevation (to less than 38.9°C) may occur, despite the absence of any infection, which typically falls within 24–48 hours of folic acid treatment and returns to normal within a few days.

In 1962, US physician Dr Victor Herbert self-induced an experimental folate deficiency by eating food that had been boiled three times in large amounts of water and taking supplements of all the water-soluble vitamins except folic acid. He developed megaloblastic anaemia after four and a half months and experienced progressively worsening insomnia and forgetfulness at four months and irritability in the fifth month. These nervous symptoms disappeared within 48 hours after folic acid supplements were introduced, and he noted a marked improvement in mood. He developed abnormal changes in the mucous membranes of his mouth during the experiment, but there was no evidence of abnormalities in the rest of the digestive tract, and food digestion and absorption remained normal.

Some individuals have a genetic predisposition to a folate deficiency because they have inherited a variant of the enzyme MTHFR that is less active and produces lower amounts of methyl THF. This genetic abnormality is associated with a low plasma folate concentration, impaired methionine metabolism and elevated Hcy.

Cerebral folate deficiency syndrome

Cerebral folate deficiency syndrome (CFD) is associated with low levels of 5-methyl THF in the cerebrospinal fluid (CSF), but normal folate levels in plasma and red blood cells. It appears to be caused by decreased transport of folate into the CSF because of binding of autoantibodies to folate receptors. Mitochondrial DNA mutations are common. Symptoms begin at four to six months of age, and include delayed development, slowing of head growth, poor muscle tone, vomiting episodes and ataxia, and may lead to movement disorders, spasticity, speech difficulties, autistic symptoms and epilepsy. Treatment is with folinic acid (5-formyl THF), the immediate precursor to 5,10-methylene THF that is not dependent on activity of the enzyme DHF reductase and does not require the receptor for transport into the CSF.

Pregnancy

Folate requirements increase substantially during pregnancy because of the increased DNA synthesis needed for growth of the foetus, placenta and maternal red blood cells and uterine and breast tissue. When folate intake is inadequate, megaloblastic anaemia may develop in the mother, and cell replication may become abnormal in the foetus.

The neural tube (NT), which becomes the brain and spinal cord, is the first organ to be formed in the foetus, and it begins to form about 21 days after conception—often before a woman is aware of her pregnancy—and is complete by 28 days. A lack of folate at this very early stage of pregnancy impairs cell replication and may lead to a variety of NTDs, including:

- *anencephaly*, a fatal defect involving partial absence of brain tissue
- *meningomyelocoele*, failure of the neural tube to close over, causing the meninges to protrude through the spine—usually in the lumbosacral region. It may be referred to as spina bifida aperta, and is often associated with the Arnold Chiari malformation (a malformation of the cerebellum in the brain)

and hydrocephalus (a buildup of CSF in the brain ventricles)

- *meningocoele*, a less severe variation of the defect that causes meningomyelocoele
- *craniorachischisis*, a fatal defect in which the spinal cord, hindbrain, midbrain and part of the forebrain develop abnormally.

Food-fortification programs and folic acid supplementation have been found to be effective for reducing the occurrence of NTDs.

Severe folate deficiency in pregnant women can lead to severe anaemia, jaundice, upper abdominal pain, red blood cell breakdown (haemolysis) and clotting abnormalities, leading to bleeding from various body orifices. It may mimic HELLP syndrome, which affects pregnant women with pre-eclampsia and is characterised by haemolysis, elevated liver enzymes and low platelet count.

Indicators of inadequate levels may include:

- anaemia, featuring fatigue, weakness, dizziness, breathlessness, palpitations, shortness of breath, pallor, rapid heartbeat
- abnormal cell development, DNA strand breakages and rearrangements
- apathy, withdrawal, lack of motivation, mood swings, dementia, insomnia, anxiety, irritability, memory loss
- cracks or sores in the corners of the mouth, a sore mouth or tongue, inflammatory bowel disorders, diarrhoea, loss of appetite, indigestion
- *pregnant women:* anaemia, jaundice, bleeding, upper abdominal pain, miscarriages, brown patchy skin hyperpigmentation, cracks and sores in the corners of the mouth, abnormal foetal development in early pregnancy, NTDs.

Assessment of body status

Serum folate is an indicator of recent folate intake, and the concentration in red blood cells is a better indicator of long-term intake and body stores. The reference range given by the RCPA is 7–45 nmol/L for serum folate and 360–1400 nmol/L for red blood cell folate. Elevated plasma Hcy, which reflects the inability to convert Hcy to methionine, may indicate a folate, vitamin B12 or vitamin B6 deficiency. The reference range for plasma Hcy is 5–15 μmol/L.

Case reports—folic acid deficiency

- *A girl, thirteen years of age*, developed neurological symptoms, including ataxia, paranoid and suicidal thoughts, paraesthesia in the extremities, intermittent urinary incontinence, impaired writing skills and poor school performance.[1] She had a history of juvenile rheumatoid arthritis, which was treated with naproxen and occasional use of steroids and methotrexate. Her serum folate concentration was found to be normal, but methyl THF in her CSF was low and autoantibodies to the folate receptor were detected. She was then given folinic acid, which led to improvement in her neurological symptoms after three months; two years later, CSF folate was within the normal range on 45 mg daily of folinic acid.
- *A woman, 44 years of age*, developed rapid visual deterioration over a two-week period that was not helped by reading glasses.[2] She was found to have poor colour vision and bilateral central scotomas (spots in the visual field where vision is absent). She was a moderate drinker and smoker, and her diet consisted of a cup of tea with milk and a slice of buttered toast for breakfast, no lunch or a bag of potato crisps, and some meat and potatoes for dinner; other vegetables were eaten rarely. She was found to have low serum and red blood cell folate. She had been diagnosed with low folate levels three years previously, but had not had follow-up tests. She was diagnosed with folate deficient optic neuropathy and was given oral folic acid 5 mg daily long term. She was also advised to reduce her alcohol and tobacco consumption. Her vision had improved at four-week follow-up.
- *A woman, 33 years of age*, with chronic alcoholism, developed acutely progressive 'glove and stocking' polyneuropathy.[3] She was found to have macrocytic anaemia, liver dysfunction and low serum folate. Vitamin B1, B2 and B12 levels were within the normal range. Folic acid supplementation led to a gradual recovery.
- *A group of 335 pregnant women, 15 to 45 years of age*, with megaloblastic anaemia of pregnancy were investigated in 1966.[4] The peak incidence of anaemia was during the four weeks before and after delivery, and the most common accompanying symptoms were cracks and sores in the corners of the mouth, a sore mouth or tongue and loss of appetite. The women were found to have low serum folate

and vitamin B12 levels and a more than two-fold increased risk of stillbirths. Megaloblastic anaemia in these women was associated with multiple births, poor diet, haemolytic anaemia, blood loss during delivery and reduced folate absorption. The anaemia responded to folic acid supplementation, which also normalised vitamin B12 levels.

REFERENCES

1 Koenig, M.K., Perez, M., Rothenberg, S. & Butler, I.J., Juvenile onset central nervous system folate deficiency and rheumatoid arthritis, *J Child Neurol* (2008), 23(1): 106–7.
2 de Silva, P., Jayamanne, G. & Bolton, R., Folic acid deficiency optic neuropathy: A case report, *J Med Case Rep* (2008), 2: 299.
3 Koike, H., Hama, T., Kawagashira, Y. et al., The significance of folate deficiency in alcoholic and nutritional neuropathies: Analysis of a case, *Nutrition* (2012), 28(7–8): 821–4.
4 Giles, C., An account of 335 cases of megaloblastic anaemia of pregnancy and the puerperium, *J Clin Pathol* (1966), 19(1): 1–11.

THERAPEUTIC USES OF FOLIC ACID

Pregnancy

Folate needs are increased during pregnancy and dietary intake may be insufficient to maintain healthy body levels, leading to abnormal cell replication in the foetus. Evidence that folic acid supplementation decreases the risk of NTDs dates back to the 1960s. Low serum and red blood cell folate concentrations in pregnant women are associated with an increased risk of NTDs and a red blood cell folate level of at least 906 nmol/L is considered to reduce the risk.[1] Overall, it is estimated that an adequate intake of folate in the period surrounding conception can prevent 72 per cent of all cases of NTDs.[2] Folic acid may also decrease the risk of cleft lip and palate, club foot and Down syndrome, but more research is needed.

A study evaluating the efficacy of a 4-mg daily dose of folic acid in preventing recurrent NTDs in women who had previously delivered a child with an NTD found that it reduced the rate of recurrence by 72 per cent.[3] A meta-analysis of 41 studies concluded that use of multivitamin supplements containing folic acid provided consistent protection against NTDs, reducing the risk by 33–48 per cent.[4]

In Chile, mandatory wheat flour fortification with folic acid began in 2000 and was shown to increase serum and red blood cell folate levels and reduce the incidence of NTDs by 43 per cent in the absence of supplement use.[5] In Argentina, food fortification led to a decrease of 54 per cent for anencephaly, 33 per cent for encephalocoele and 45 per cent for spina bifida over five years.[5] Canada has reported a 50 per cent reduction in spina bifida since fortification and fortification in the United States decreased the incidence of NTDs by 36 per cent.[5] In Australia, fortification of bread-making flour has led to increased serum and red blood cell concentrations in the population.[6]

Mood and cognitive disorders

Folate is a key component of the methylation cycle, and is required for the synthesis of dopamine, noradrenaline and serotonin, which affect brain function and mood. People with folate deficiency have been found to have a higher risk of depression, to have more severe relapses and to be less likely to respond to anti-depressant drugs. Middle-aged men in the lowest category of dietary folate intake have been found to have a 67 per cent higher risk of depression compared with those in the highest category of intake.[7] Patients with depression have been shown to have a higher prevalence of low serum folate and elevated Hcy levels.[8] Depressed patients with the lowest mean plasma folate concentrations have been found to have more severe symptoms.[9]

Folic acid has been used as a treatment for depression with mixed results. In patients with major depression on lithium therapy, 200 mcg of folic acid daily improved mood symptoms,[10] and another study of patients with depression on fluoxetine therapy found improvements in women taking 500 mcg of folic acid daily.[11] 5-methyl THF has been used successfully in several small studies.[12] 5-methyl THF (50 mg daily) led to an improvement in depressive symptoms in elderly people, in elderly patients with depression and dementia, and in patients with major depression and schizophrenia. Both folic acid and folinic acid have been shown to improve the response to standard anti-depressant therapy. A meta-analysis of eleven trials concluded that there was accumulating evidence that low folate status is associated with depression.[13]

Folate deficiency is relatively common in the elderly, and is linked to an increased risk of dementia.[14] Low folate levels and the MTHFR-variant genotype has been shown to increase dementia risk,[15] and elevated Hcy and the variant MTHFR gene has been associated with schizophrenia.[16] However, a review of trials using folic acid supplementation for dementia patients, with or without vitamin B12, concluded that there was no good evidence of benefits.[17]

Cardiovascular disease

Elevated Hcy levels are associated with folic acid deficiency, and are an independent risk factor for coronary heart disease (CHD). A Hcy level of 5 μmol/L or more increases the risk of CHD 1.6-fold, and low serum folate has been shown to increase the risk of fatal CHD by 69 per cent.[18] Vitamin B6, B12 and folic acid have each been shown to reduce elevated Hcy, with folic acid being the most effective. However, a meta-analysis of trials that used folic acid to lower Hcy concluded that lowering Hcy does not reduce the risk of cardiovascular disease (CVD) overall, but may lead to a small reduction in risk of stroke.[19]

Cancer

In a folate deficiency, the production of SAM from methionine is impaired, which causes impaired DNA synthesis, methylation and repair, and leads to DNA damage and the potential for genetic mutations and abnormal cell development. Moderate to high alcohol intake, which impairs folate metabolism, has been associated with an increased risk of neoplasia (growth of new abnormal tissue).

Folate appears to have a strong protective role in colorectal cancer, with a large number of studies reporting that people with the highest dietary intake of folate or those with the highest blood concentrations have a 40–60 per cent reduced risk of developing colorectal cancer or pre-cancerous adenomatous polyps.[20] Patients with chronic ulcerative colitis on folic acid supplementation have been found to have a 62 per cent lower rate of colonic neoplasia compared with unsupplemented patients.[21]

Folate deficiency induced in cultured skin cells leads to growth arrest and increased levels of DNA damage. In cell studies, a lack of folate in skin cells causes them to become more sensitive to ultraviolet radiation and to have an increased rate of apoptosis and less ability to repair DNA breaks, leading to an increased risk of cancer.[22] The addition of folic acid has been shown to reverse these abnormalities. However, the effectiveness of folic acid supplementation for reducing skin cancer risk in humans has not been established.

There is some evidence for folate's protective role in other cancers, such as neuroblastoma, leukaemia and cancers of the oropharynx, oesophagus, stomach, pancreas, lungs, cervix, ovary and breast.[23] In breast cancer, it appears to be mainly protective in women with a moderate to high intake of alcohol.[24]

The evidence for a protective role in patients with existing cancer is mixed. Some studies have found that folic acid supplementation may stimulate growth of early neoplastic lesions. A meta-analysis of ten clinical trials found that folic acid supplementation was associated with a 7 per cent increased risk of cancer overall, and a meta-analysis of six clinical trials found that supplementation was associated with a 24 per cent increased risk of prostate cancer, but there was no association with other types of cancer.[25]

REFERENCES

1 Tam, C., McKenna, K., Goh, Y.I. et al., Periconceptional folic acid supplementation: A new indication for therapeutic drug monitoring, *Ther Drug Monit* (2009), 31(3): 319–26.

2 Lumley, J., Watson, L., Watson, M. & Bower, C., Periconceptional supplementation with folate and/or multivitamins for preventing neural tube defects, *Cochrane Database Syst Rev* (2001), 3: CD001056.

3 MRC Vitamin Study Research Group, Prevention of neural tube defects: Results of the Medical Research Council Vitamin Study, *Lancet* (1991), 338(8760): 131–7.

4 Goh, Y.I., Bollano, E., Einarson, T.R. & Koren, G., Prenatal multivitamin supplementation and rates of congenital anomalies: A meta-analysis, *J Obstet Gynaecol Can* (2006), 28(8): 680–9.

5 García-Fragoso, L., García-García, I. & Cadilla, C.L., The role of folic acid in the prevention of neural tube defects, in K.L. Narasimhan (ed.), *Neural tube defects: Role of folate, prevention strategies and genetics,* Intech, Dubrovnik, 2012.

6 Brown, R.D., Langshaw, M.R., Uhr, E.J. et al., The impact of mandatory fortification of flour with folic acid on the blood folate levels of an Australian population, *Med J Aust* (2011), 194(2): 65–7.

7 Tolmunen, T., Voutilainen, S., Hintikka, J. et al., Dietary folate and depressive symptoms are associated in middle-aged Finnish men, *J Nutr* (2003), 133(10): 3233–6.

8 Sachdev, P.S., Parslow, R.A., Lux, O. et al., Relationship of homocysteine, folic acid and vitamin B12 with depression in a middle-aged community sample, *Psychol Med* (2005), 35: 529–38.

9 Abou-Saleh, M.T. & Coppen, A., Serum and red blood cell folate in depression, *Acta Psychiatr Scand* (1989), 80(1): 78–82.

10 Coppen, A., Chaudhry, S. & Swade, C., Folic acid enhances lithium prophylaxis, *J Affect Disord* (1986), 10(1): 9–13.

11 Coppen, A. & Bailey, J., Enhancement of the antidepressant action of fluoxetine by folic acid: A randomised, placebo controlled trial, *J Affect Disord* (2000), 60(2): 121–30.

12 Miller, A.L., The methylation, neurotransmitter, and anti-oxidant connections between folate and depression, *Altern Med Rev* (2008), 13(3): 216–26.

13 Gilbody, S., Lightfoot, T. & Sheldon, T., Is low folate a risk factor for depression? A meta-analysis and exploration of heterogeneity, *J Epidemiol Community Health* (2007), 61(7): 631–7.

14 Bottiglieri T., Crellin R. & Reynolds E.H., Folate and neuropsychiatry, In: Bailey LB, ed., *Folate in health and disease*, New York: Marcel Dekker, 1995.

15 Kageyama M., Hiraoka M. & Kagawa Y., Relationship between genetic polymorphism, serum folate and homocysteine in Alzheimer's disease, *Asia Pac J Public Health* (2008), 20, Suppl: 111–17.

16 Nishi A., Numata S., Tajima A. et al., Meta-analyses of blood homocysteine levels for gender and genetic association studies of the MTHFR C677T polymorphism in schizophrenia, *Schizophr Bull* (2014), 40(5): 1154–63.

17 Malouf, M., Grimley, E.J. & Areosa, S.A., Folic acid with or without vitamin B12 for cognition and dementia, *Cochrane Database Syst Rev* (2003), 4: CD004514.

18 Morrison, H.I., Schaubel, D., Desmeules, M. & Wigle, D.T., Serum folate and risk of fatal coronary heart disease, *JAMA* (1996), 275(24): 1893–6.

19 Yang, H.T., Lee, M., Hong, K.S. et al., Efficacy of folic acid supplementation in cardiovascular disease prevention: An updated meta-analysis of randomized controlled trials, *Eur J Intern Med* (2012), 23(8): 745–54.

20 Hubner, R.A. & Houlston, R.S., Folate and colorectal cancer prevention, *Br J Cancer* (2009), 100(2): 233–9.

21 Lashner, B.A., Heidenreich, P.A., Su, G.L. et al., Effect of folate supplementation on the incidence of dysplasia and cancer in chronic ulcerative colitis: A case-control study, *Gastroenterology* (1989), 97(2): 255–9.

22 Williams, J.D. & Jacobson, M.K., Photobiological implications of folate depletion and repletion in cultured human keratinocytes, *J Photochem Photobiol B* (2010), 99(1): 49–61.

23 Mason, J.B., Folate, cancer risk, and the Greek god, Proteus: A tale of two chameleons, *Nutr Rev* (2009), 67(4): 206–12.

24 Larsson, S.C., Giovannucci, E. & Wolk, A., Folate and risk of breast cancer: A meta-analysis, *J Natl Cancer Inst* (2007), 99(1): 64–76.

25 Wien, T.N., Pike, E., Wisløff, T. et al., Cancer risk with folic acid supplements: A systematic review and meta-analysis, *BMJ Open* (2012), 2(1): e000653.

Therapeutic dose

Folic acid should be taken together with a source of vitamin B12. Suggested doses for adults are as follows:

- *Health maintenance:* 400 mcg daily.
- *Mild deficiency:* 1 mg daily.
- *Severe deficiency:* 5 mg daily.
- *Hcy lowering:* up to 5 mg daily.
- *NTD prevention in pregnancy:* at least 600 mcg, taken for at least one month prior to conception and throughout pregnancy. Women who have given birth to an infant with an NTD are recommended to take 4–5 mg daily at least one month prior to conception and throughout pregnancy.
- *Cancer prevention:* 1–5 mg daily.

Effects of excess

Folic acid supplementation given to people with vitamin B12-deficiency anaemia can normalise red blood cells. Masking the anaemia in this way may complicate and delay diagnosis, allowing the neurological damage caused by a lack of vitamin B12 to progress. Studies have found that supplementation with 1 mg/day of folic acid does not appear to mask vitamin B12-deficiency anaemia in the majority of subjects, whereas supplementation with 5 mg/day does. It is advisable that folic acid and vitamin B12 are used as a combination therapy—especially in vegans, who are more likely to be vitamin B12-deficient.

Therapeutic doses used in clinical trials range from 400 mcg to 30 mg daily. Doses greater than 5 mg/day have been associated with mild adverse effects in some individuals, such as skin rash, digestive upsets, irritability and excitability. The safety of folic acid supplementation in patients with existing cancer is not known.

Supplements

Folic acid and calcium folinate are the forms permitted in Australian supplements. Folic acid is produced by chemical synthesis. First, 4-nitrobenzoyl chloride is reacted with monosodium L-glutamate to form N-4-nitrobenzoyl-L-glutamic acid, which undergoes catalytic hydrogenation to form N-4-aminobenzoyl-L-glutamic acid. This is then condensed with 2,4,5-triamino-6-hydroxypyrimidine and 1,1,3-trichloroacetone to form folic acid, which is dispersed into an aqueous solution and spray dried.

Folinic acid (5-formyl THF, also called leucovorin, Fusilev or citrovorum factor) is the immediate precursor to 5,10-methylene THF, and is not dependent on the activity of DHF reductase. It has a bioavailability of 92 per cent. It is produced commercially from folic acid, and is used as calcium or sodium folinate to treat CFD or to reduce gastrointestinal side effects and liver toxicity induced by DHF reductase-inhibiting drugs, such as methotrexate used for cancer, psoriasis and rheumatoid arthritis. Folinic acid may also be used for treating folic acid deficiency anaemia.

Cautions

Folic acid should always be taken with a source of vitamin B12, particularly if the diet is low in animal products. Although folic acid has protective activity against cancer, it has the potential to promote the growth of early neoplastic lesions and should be used with caution in people with a history of abnormal cell growth.

BIOTIN

BIOTIN STATUS CHECK

1 Do you have dry, scaly skin or rashes on your face?
2 Are your nails weak and do they break easily?
3 Is your hair getting thinner?
4 Are you taking medication for epilepsy?

'Yes' answers may indicate inadequate biotin status. Note that a number of nutritional deficiencies or health disorders can cause similar effects and further investigation is recommended.

FAST FACTS . . . BIOTIN

- **Biotin is found in liver, egg yolk, brewer's yeast, grains and legumes.**
- **It is required for the metabolism of amino acids and fatty acids, and for energy production and regulating blood glucose levels.**
- **It has a role in DNA replication and repair, gene expression, and cell growth and development.**
- **A deficiency can lead to dry, scaly skin, rashes around the mouth, nose and eyes, and hair loss.**
- **Supplementation may be useful for diabetes, elevated blood fats, and hair and nail disorders.**

Biotin consists of a ureido and tetrahydrothiophene ring with a valeric acid side chain. In 1901, it was observed that yeast required a factor for growth, named 'bios', which was found to be a mixture of factors, one of which was biotin. In 1927, it was found that animals fed raw egg white developed dermatitis, hair loss and neuromuscular disorders, and liver was found to correct the condition. The protective factor was isolated from egg yolk in 1936 and found to be biotin (previously referred to as vitamin B7 and factor H from the German *Haut*, meaning 'skin'). Its structure was identified in 1942 and it was first synthesised in 1949. Biotin was subsequently found to have an important role as a coenzyme required for the activity of four types of carboxylase enzymes that mediate the binding of bicarbonate to organic acids. It was shown to be essential in the diet, and was classed as a vitamin belonging to the vitamin B group. D-biotin is the natural form that is active in the body.

Digestion, absorption and transport

In food, biotin is bound to proteins or to lysine as biocytin, which is digested by protease enzymes in the digestive tract to yield free biotin, biocytin and biotinyl peptides. In the small intestine, biocytin is hydrolysed by the enzyme biotinidase, and biotinyl peptides are hydrolysed by protein-digesting enzymes to release free biotin. Biotin and biocytin can both be absorbed, and biotin is released from biocytin in the body by the enzyme biotinidase, which is present in plasma and tissues. Absorption is mediated by SMVT that also transports vitamin B5 and lipoic acid. At high levels of intake, absorption is by passive diffusion. Studies of healthy adults have found that oral doses of 2–20 mg are completely absorbed, and half of the oral dose appears in urine within 24 hours as biotin and metabolites. Biotin is synthesised by bacteria in the colon, and can be absorbed, but it appears that insufficient biotin is acquired from this source, making dietary intake essential.

Metabolism, storage and excretion

Biotin is transported in plasma as free biotin and as the protein-bound form, and can be stored in muscles, the liver and the brain. In a deficiency, it appears that levels in the central nervous system are maintained at the expense of liver stores. The enzyme holocarboxylase synthetase attaches biotin to carboxylase enzymes in the mitochondria and cytoplasm of cells to form biotin holocarboxylases, which are the active enzyme forms. These enzymes are eventually broken down to release biocytin and amino acids; biocytin is further broken down by biotinidase to release lysine and free biotin, which can be reused or further catabolised to metabolites and excreted in urine. The main urinary metabolites are bisnorbiotin, tetranorbiotin, biotin sulfoxide and biotin sulfone. Most excretion is via the urine, with very little faecal excretion; the faecal content of biotin is largely derived from unabsorbed biotin produced by colonic bacteria.

Functions

Biotin coenzymes are required for incorporation of bicarbonate into organic acids as a carboxyl group, which takes place during amino acid and fatty acid metabolism, energy production and glucose production. Biotin also plays a role in gene expression.

Functions of biotin include the following:

- *Acetyl-CoA carboxylase (ACC) activity.* Biotin is a coenzyme for ACC1, found in cell cytoplasm and ACC2 in mitochondria. ACC1 converts acetyl-CoA to malonyl-CoA during fatty acid synthesis and ACC2 regulates fatty acid transport into mitochondria.
- *Propionyl-CoA carboxylase (PCC) activity.* Biotin is a coenzyme for PCC, found in cell mitochondria, which takes part in the breakdown of the amino acids isoleucine, valine, methionine and threonine, and also the breakdown of fatty acids with an odd number of carbons (odd chain fatty acids). It converts propionyl-CoA to methylmalonyl-CoA, which is then converted to succinyl-CoA, which takes part in the citric acid cycle of the energy pathway.
- *beta-Methylcrotonyl-CoA carboxylase (beta-MCC) activity.* Biotin is a coenzyme for beta-MCC, found in cell mitochondria, that converts beta-methylcrotonyl-CoA, derived from breakdown of the amino acid leucine, to beta-methylglutaconyl-CoA, which is then converted to acetoacetate and acetyl-CoA that take part in the citric acid cycle.
- *Pyruvate carboxylase activity.* Biotin is a coenzyme for pyruvate carboxylase, found in cell mitochondria, which converts pyruvate to oxaloacetate, which is converted to glucose or enters the citric acid cycle.

- *Gene expression.* About 2000 genes have been identified that are dependent on biotin. It works by attaching to histones, which are DNA-binding proteins in the cell nucleus that take part in the process of gene transcription, a process in which a particular segment of DNA is copied into RNA, and gene translation, in which the RNA copy is used as a blueprint to produce a protein. Biotin has a role in DNA replication and repair, gene expression, and cell growth and development. It promotes the transcription and translation of the gene for glucokinase (GK), an enzyme that acts as a glucose sensor for the pancreas and enhances insulin secretion in response to glucose. There is some evidence that bisnorbiotin also affects gene expression, indicating that biotin catabolites may also have biotin-like functions.
- *Blood glucose regulation.* In cell studies, biotin has been found to enhance insulin secretion, and the expression of genes and signalling pathways that affect pancreatic islet cell function. In animals, biotin supplementation has been shown to have direct effects on pancreatic tissue by increasing the concentration of beta cells. It increases insulin concentrations and improves glucose tolerance.

Dietary sources

Biotin in food originates from synthesis by bacteria, yeasts, moulds, algae and some plants. It is bound to protein or lysine in many foods such as liver, egg yolk, brewer's yeast, soybeans, grains, legumes and nuts.

The Food Standards Australia New Zealand nutrient database (NUTTAB) at <www.foodstandards.gov.au> provides the amounts found in specific foods.

Factors influencing body status

Biotin is relatively heat-stable, and can survive standard cooking temperatures, but it is water-soluble and can be leached out of food by water processing and cooking methods. Absorption of biotin varies with food source, but appears to range from 5 per cent to almost 100 per cent.

A deficiency of magnesium may impair biotin metabolism. Biotin absorption is impaired by digestive disorders, alcohol and epileptic medication, such as phenytoin, primidone and carbamazepine, and its breakdown is increased by pregnancy, cigarette smoking and epileptic drugs. Avidin in raw egg white forms an irreversible bond with biotin that prevents its absorption, and eating raw eggs regularly depletes body levels. Avidin also binds biotin produced by gut bacteria. In food, avidin is broken down by cooking, releasing the biotin for absorption. Vitamin B5 and lipoic acid use the same transporter as biotin for absorption, and high supplemental doses of vitamin B5 may reduce biotin uptake. Antibiotic use may destroy colonic bacteria that produce biotin in the gut. Lower biotin concentrations have been identified in pregnant women, infants who have died of SIDS, alcoholics, patients on kidney dialysis, and patients with inflammatory bowel disease, seborrhoeic dermatitis (scaly skin rashes) and Leiner's disease (a form of seborrhoeic dermatitis in infants).

Daily requirement

Government recommendations by age and gender (see Table 7.5) can be found in *Nutrient Reference Values for Australia and New Zealand Including Recommended Dietary Intakes*, available at <www.nrv.gov.au>.

Table 7.5 Recommended adequate intake (AI) of biotin (mcg/day)

Age (years)	Female AI	Male AI
1–3	8	8
4–8	12	12
9–13	20	20
14–18	25	30
19–70	25	30
>70	25	30
Pregnant women		
14–18	30	
19–50	30	
Lactating women		
14–18	35	
19–50	35	

Source: Nutrient Reference Values for Australia and New Zealand Including Recommended Dietary Intakes, National Health and Medical Research Council, Australian Government Department of Health and Ageing, Canberra and Ministry of Health, New Zealand, Wellington, 2006.

Deficiency effects

Biotin deficiency has been regarded as rare, but recent research indicates that marginal biotin deficiency is not uncommon in pregnancy, protein energy malnutrition and long-term therapy with antibiotics or the anti-convulsants phenytoin, primidone and carbamazepine. Regular consumption of raw eggs causes avidin-induced biotin deficiency ('egg white injury'), and is a standard method of inducing an experimental deficiency. A biotin deficiency leads to reduced activity of carboxylase enzymes, impairment of fatty acid metabolism, energy production and gene expression, and leads to accumulation of odd chain fatty acids and organic acids, such as lactate. A deficiency also promotes elevated blood glucose (hyperglycaemia) by stimulating secretion of the hormone glucagon that elevates blood glucose, and decreasing insulin secretion and sensitivity. In animals, biotin requirement is increased during gestation, and even a marginal deficiency causes a high rate of birth defects, including cleft palate and under-development of the jaw and limbs. The rate of defects increases with the severity of the deficiency until 90 per cent of animals are affected.

Lowered activity of PCC elevates levels of its substrate propionyl-CoA, which is then metabolised by an alternative pathway to 3-hydroxypropionic acid and methylcitrate, which are excreted in urine. Carnitine deficiency may arise due to increased renal excretion as propionyl carnitine. Reduced function of beta-MCC causes elevated beta-methlycrotonyl-CoA, which is then metabolised by an alternative pathway to 3-hydroxyisovaleric acid (3-HIA) and 3-methylcrotonylglycine, which are excreted in urine. Reduced levels of biotin and elevated levels of 3-HIA in urine are used as markers of biotin deficiency.

A biotin deficiency primarily affects the skin, hair, digestive tract and nervous system. The mechanism of action is not fully understood, but may be related to impaired fatty acid metabolism, energy production or gene expression. Symptoms of biotin deficiency appear within three to five weeks of inadequate body levels, and include dry skin, seborrhoeic dermatitis ('cradle cap' in infants), fungal infections, rashes around the eyes, nose, mouth and other body orifices, and hair changes, such as fine, brittle hair, loss of hair colour, thinning hair, partial hair loss or total alopecia. Impaired fatty acid metabolism appears to be responsible for the skin rashes and hair loss because animals with a biotin deficiency do not develop these signs if they are supplemented with omega-6 fatty acids. Digestive tract symptoms include loss of appetite, nausea and vomiting. Neurological symptoms develop about one to two weeks later, and include mild depression, lethargy, sleepiness, hallucinations, muscle pain, hearing loss, increased sensitivity of nerves (hyperaesthesia) and paraesthesia. Loss of taste that responds to high-dose biotin supplementation has been described.

Some individuals have a genetic predisposition to a biotin deficiency because they have lowered activity of the enzyme biotinidase that releases biotin from its bound form, a condition known as multiple carboxylase deficiency. Symptoms may develop in the first weeks of life or up to ten years of age, and include seizures, poor muscle tone, hyperventilation, noisy breathing, apnoea, skin rash, alopecia, conjunctivitis, *Candida* infection, withdrawn behaviour, ataxia and developmental delay. It may be associated with a buildup of beta-hydroxyisovalerate, lactate, beta-methylcrotonylglycine, beta-hydroxypropionate and methyl citrate in urine, acidosis, acidic urine, elevated ammonia in the blood and a deficiency of the amino acid carnitine.

A profound biotinidase deficiency, in which enzyme activity is less than 10 per cent of normal, may result in neurological injury, hearing loss, blindness and death if not diagnosed and treated. In older children, symptoms may include limb weakness, partial paralysis, developmental delay, hearing loss, optic nerve atrophy and recurring infections. A partial biotinidase deficiency (late-onset multiple carboxylase deficiency), in which enzyme activity is 10–30 per cent of normal, causes milder symptoms in early childhood, and may be precipitated by a stress such as an infection.

Multiple carboxylase deficiency symptoms appearing soon after birth are most often caused by reduced activity of the enzyme holocarboxylase synthetase that attaches biotin to apocarboxylases to form activated holocarboxylases. Larger than normal amounts of biotin are required to allow binding to occur. In Australia, blood from newborn infants is routinely screened for holocarboxylase synthetase deficiency. Biotin dependency due to an inherited defect of biotin transport has been described recently.

Biotin deficiency responds to supplementation, which can reverse the biochemical imbalances, hair loss, seizures, low muscle tone and skin rash, and can halt progression of developmental delay, and hearing and vision loss. Skin rashes disappear within a few weeks of treatment, and there is renewed hair growth after one to two months. In infants, poor muscle tone, lethargy and withdrawn behaviour resolve in one to two weeks, followed by improvement in neurological symptoms.

Indicators of inadequate levels may include:

- weak, brittle, splitting nails
- dry skin, seborrhoeic dermatitis, skin rashes, especially around the mouth and other body orifices, fungal infections
- dry hair, weak hair, fading hair colour, thinning hair, hair loss
- muscle pain and weakness, poor muscle tone
- depression, lethargy
- numbness, burning, tingling, 'pins and needles' sensations, nerve sensitivity, hearing loss, vision loss, loss of taste.

Assessment of body status

Serum biotin is not regarded as a good indicator of body status. The serum reference range for adults as reported by the American Medical Association (AMA) is 0.82–2.05 nmol/L. Measurement of urinary biotin and 3-HIA are considered to be early and sensitive indicators of biotin deficiency; the reference range is reported to be 18–77 nmol/day for biotin and 77–195 µmol/day for 3-HIA.[1] Biotinidase and holocarboxylase synthetase deficiencies are diagnosed by testing enzyme activity in serum or analysing DNA to detect common mutations affecting the genes for these enzymes. The reference range for serum biotinidase activity given by the University of California, San Francisco (UCSF) Clinical Laboratories is 3.3–8.7 nmol/mL/min.

REFERENCE

1 Mock N.I., Malik M.I., Stumbo P.J. et al., Increased urinary excretion of 3-hydroxyisovaleric acid and decreased urinary excretion of biotin are sensitive early indicators of decreased biotin status in experimental biotin deficiency, *Am J Clin Nutr* (1997), 65(4): 951–8.

Case reports—biotin deficiency

- *A male infant, three months of age*, presented with a history of five to six convulsive seizures a day, each lasting for five minutes.[1] He was extremely lethargic and sleepy, with a dull, expressionless face, and had difficulty feeding, making eye contact and tracking moving objects, poor muscle tone, thin, sparse scalp hair, a lack of eyebrows and eyelashes, and nappy rash. Three of his siblings had died with similar symptoms. There was a marked increase of 3-HIA, 3-methylcrotonylglycine and methyl citrate in his urine, elevated serum ammonia and lactate, and reduced biotinidase activity, leading to a diagnosis of multiple carboxylase deficiency. The infant was given biotin, 10 mg twice a day, and he became seizure free, more alert and able to feed better within two days. Serum ammonia and lactate levels normalised. Follow-up at five and eight months of age showed dramatic improvement in visual attention and motor activity, and hair growth and psychomotor development normalised.
- *A girl, seven years of age*, was admitted to hospital with suspected brain-stem encephalitis.[2] She had developed mental confusion, could not recognise her parents and siblings, had stopped walking and talking, was unable to swallow, and had frontal headache, continuous vomiting and lethargy. Her parents were distantly related, and she had a sister who had died of a similar condition. On examination, she was found to be drooling and unable to speak, and had severe rigidity in the upper and lower extremities and continuous writhing movements of the limbs (dystonia). Pathological tests could not identify abnormalities. She was given biotin (5 mg/kg body weight/day) and improved dramatically within 24 hours. Within three days, she was discharged as a normal child. Since then, she has twice discontinued her biotin supplements inadvertently, and each time became confused after one month and developed dystonia of the hands that reversed on recommencing supplementation. At age fifteen, she was reported to be an excellent school student, with normal neurology except for a mild stutter.
- *A woman, 62 years of age*, with cirrhosis of the liver, a case reported in 1968, consumed six raw eggs and 1.9 L of skim milk daily for eighteen months, following dietary advice from a physician who was aiming to provide a high intake of essential amino acids for liver regeneration.[3] After a few weeks, she developed loss of appetite, difficulty swallowing and soreness of her tongue and lips, which became fissured and encrusted, and occasionally bled. She became unable to eat regular meals, but persevered in consuming the

raw eggs and skim milk daily, and also took a high-potency multivitamin supplement (lacking in biotin) and several brewer's yeast tablets daily. She was given 100 mcg of vitamin B12 by injection each month. She developed scaly dermatitis, occasional nausea and vomiting, increasing lassitude, malaise, breathlessness on exertion and poor stamina. She had a feeling of pressure in her chest, partially relieved by belching. Mild abdominal swelling had became more severe and she developed swelling of the ankles.

Avidin-induced biotin deficiency was suspected, and she was given intramuscular biotin and multivitamin injections daily while being maintained on her raw eggs and skim milk intake. The condition of her skin, lips and tongue improved within two days, and after four days, her tongue and lips appeared normal and the scaly skin on her arms and the backs of her hands had completely resolved. She was then placed on a regular high-protein diet, given a multivitamin (lacking biotin) and instructed not to eat uncooked eggs. She relapsed three months later, with increasing lassitude, malaise, soreness of the mouth, dry, scaly skin, redness of the palms of the hands and soles of the feet, reddened oral mucosa and tongue, cracked and encrusted lips, mild cracking in the corners of the mouth, and enlargement of the liver and spleen. Another course of daily biotin injections led to a rapid improvement.

REFERENCES

1 Joshi, S.N., Fathalla, M., Koul, R. et al., Biotin responsive seizures and encephalopathy due to biotinidase deficiency, *Neurol India* (2010), 58(2): 323–4.

2 Ozand, P.T., Gascon, G.G., Al Essa, M. et al., Biotin-responsive basal ganglia disease: A novel entity, *Brain* (1998), 121 (Pt 7): 1267–79.

3 Baugh, C.M., Malone, J.H. & Butterworth, C.E. Jr, Human biotin deficiency: A case history of biotin deficiency induced by raw egg consumption in a cirrhotic patient, *Am J Clin Nutr* (1968), 21(2): 173–82.

THERAPEUTIC USES OF BIOTIN

Diabetes

In animals, biotin deficiency impairs pancreatic function and results in impaired glucose tolerance.[1] Patients with type 2 diabetes have been found to have lower blood levels of biotin compared with control subjects, and higher biotin levels are associated with lower fasting blood glucose levels.[2] A small study of patients with type 1 diabetes found that 16 mg of biotin daily reduced blood glucose levels after one week.[2] In another study, biotin supplementation (9 mg daily for one month) decreased fasting blood glucose levels in type 2 diabetics by an average of 45 per cent.[3] Combined biotin and chromium picolinate supplementation in patients with type 2 diabetes (600 mcg chromium and 2 mg biotin for 90 days plus oral anti-diabetic drugs) reduced fasting blood glucose levels, decreased serum triglyceride levels and reduced the concentration of glycated haemoglobin (a marker of red blood cell damage caused by elevated blood glucose).[4]

Elevated plasma triglycerides

Biotin supplementation (15 mg daily for 28 days) was found to lower plasma triglyceride levels in both diabetic and non-diabetic patients with elevated triglyceride levels, but did not affect blood levels of cholesterol, glucose or insulin.[5]

Hair and nail abnormalities

Biotin is popularly used in the treatment of hair loss, and to improve the texture and strength of hair and nails. Biotin is used by veterinarians to improve the health of the hooves and coats of horses and cattle. In human studies, biotin supplements (2.5 mg daily for up to six months) have been found to increase fingernail thickness, and decrease brittleness and splitting.[6]

'Uncombable hair' is a condition in which a child's hair becomes dry, tightly curled, shiny, light-coloured and impossible to comb. It may be familial, and appears from about three months of age. In two children with uncombable hair, as well as brittle fingernails, biotin supplementation (5 mg daily) was reported to normalise the appearance of their hair and nails, although there were no structural changes detected in the hair.[7] The hair remained normal without further biotin at the two-year follow-up. However, nail brittleness required ongoing biotin supplementation.

Two patients receiving long-term total parenteral nutrition (non-oral feeding) are reported to have developed severe hair loss which was related to biotin deficiency. Supplementation with 200 mcg of biotin daily resulted in gradual regrowth of healthy hair.[8] Although biotin deficiency is associated with hair loss, there is no evidence that biotin supplementation can prevent hair loss or restore hair in the absence of a deficiency.

REFERENCES

1 Romero-Navarro, G., Cabrera-Valladares, G., German, M.S. et al., Biotin regulation of pancreatic glucokinase and insulin in primary cultured rat islets and in biotin deficient rats, *Endocrinology* (1999), 140: 4595–600.
2 Coggeshall, J.C., Heggers, J.P., Robson, M.C. & Baker, H., Biotin status and plasma glucose levels in diabetics, *Ann NY Acad Sci* (1985), 447: 389–92.
3 Maebashi, M., Makino, Y., Furukawa, Y., Ohinata, K., Kimura, S. & Takao, S., Therapeutic evaluation of the effect of biotin on hyperglycemia in patients with non-insulin diabetes mellitus, *J Clin Biochem Nutr* (1993), 14: 211–18.
4 Albarracin, C.A., Fuqua, B.C., Evans, J.L. & Goldfine, I.D., Chromium picolinate and biotin combination improves glucose metabolism in treated, uncontrolled overweight to obese patients with type 2 diabetes, *Diabetes Metab Res Rev* (2008), 24(1): 41–51.
5 Revilla-Monsalve, C., Zendejas-Ruiz, I., Islas-Andrade, S. et al., Biotin supplementation reduces plasma triacylglycerol and VLDL in type 2 diabetic patients and in nondiabetic subjects with hypertriglyceridemia, *Biomed Pharmacother* (2006), 60(4): 182–5.
6 Hochman, L.G., Scher, R.K. & Meyerson, M.S., Brittle nails: Response to daily biotin supplementation, *Cutis* (1993), 51(4): 303–5.
7 Boccaletti, V., Zendri, E., Giordano, G. et al., Familial uncombable hair syndrome: Ultrastructural hair study and response to biotin, *Pediatr Dermatol* (2007), 24(3): E14–16.
8 Innis, S.M. & Allardyce, D.B., Possible biotin deficiency in adults receiving long-term total parenteral nutrition, *Am J Clin Nutr* (1983), 37(2): 185–7.

Therapeutic dose

Suggested doses for adults are as follows:

- *Health maintenance:* 25–30 mcg daily.
- *Mild deficiency:* 300 mcg daily.
- *Severe deficiency:* 5–20 mg daily.
- *Biotinidase deficiency:* 5–20 mg daily; up to 100 mg daily may be required in some cases. A daily im injection of 150 mcg has been used.
- *Pregnancy:* the optimum dose is unknown but, due to the lack of toxicity and the high incidence of birth defects caused by marginal biotin deficiency in animals, 30–300 mcg may be required.
- *Hair and nail disorders:* 2.5–5 mg daily.
- *Diabetes:* 9–16 mg daily.
- *Elevated blood fats:* 15 mg daily.

Effects of excess

Doses used in clinical trials range from 2.5–100 mg daily. It appears to be well absorbed and excess is rapidly excreted. Doses greater than 300 mg lead to high biotin levels in the blood, with a corresponding increase in biotin excretion in the urine. No toxicity has been reported in individuals taking 200 mg orally or 20 mg intravenously per day for over six months.

Supplements

The available form in Australian supplements is biotin. Commercial production is carried out by chemical synthesis, starting with fumaric acid and involving a complex series of steps involving bromination, dehydration, acidification, hydrogenation and hydrolysis; this yields nature-identical biotin. Because chemical synthesis is complex and expensive with low yields, efforts are being made to produce biotin by microbial synthesis, but to date the return is low and the quality unstable.

Cautions

Because B vitamins work together in many metabolic pathways in the body, it is possible that individual B vitamins taken alone—especially if taken in high doses—may affect the metabolism of other B vitamins, so such treatment is not recommended in the long term, unless supervised by a health-care practitioner. Biotin supplements should be taken at a separate time from supplements containing vitamin B5 and alpha-lipoic acid because they competitively inhibit biotin absorption.

HOW MUCH DO I KNOW?

Choose whether the following statements are true or false. Then review this chapter for the correct answers.

	True (T)	False (F)
1 Vitamin B5 is part of coenzyme A and supports energy production.	T	F
2 Dexpanthenol is used to treat elevated serum cholesterol and lipids.	T	F
3 Pyridoxamine is a vitamer of vitamin B12.	T	F
4 A vitamin B6 deficiency can lead to convulsions in infants.	T	F
5 Folic acid requires intrinsic factor for absorption.	T	F
6 A vitamin B12 deficiency can lead to a deficiency of biotin.	T	F
7 Folic acid is mainly found in animal foods.	T	F
8 The anaemia of pernicious anaemia responds to folic acid.	T	F
9 Biotin is required for activity of carboxylase enzymes.	T	F
10 Urinary excretion of 3-HIA is a marker of biotin deficiency.	T	F

FURTHER READING

Braun, L. & Cohen, M., *Herbs & natural supplements: An evidence-based guide*, 3rd ed., Churchill Livingstone Elsevier, New York, 2010.

Gropper, S.S., Smith, J.L. & Groff, J.L., *Advanced nutrition and human metabolism*, 5th ed., Thomson Wadsworth, Belmont, CA, 2009.

Higdon, J., *An evidence-based approach to vitamins and minerals*, Thieme, New York, 2003.

Linus Pauling Institute, Micronutrient Research Center, website, available at <lpi.oregonstate.edu/infocenter>.

Part 4
Macrominerals

8

Introduction to minerals and macrominerals: calcium, phosphorus and magnesium

INTRODUCTION TO MINERALS

Minerals are water-soluble elements that exist in the earth's crust. They are released as rocks break down, dissolve in water and are taken up by plant roots. Animals—including humans—obtain minerals from plant food and from eating other animals. In general, animal forms of minerals are better absorbed than those from plants. Although minerals make up just 4 per cent of total body weight, they play a vital role in healthy body function. Unlike vitamins, minerals in food are not affected by heat, light and storage; however, because they are water-soluble, they may be lost by water-processing and cooking methods.

Macrominerals are minerals needed in relatively large amounts in the diet (greater than 100 mg daily) to support body functions; they include phosphorus, calcium, magnesium, potassium, sodium, chloride and sulfur. The amount of individual macrominerals present in the body ranges from 35 g to 1400 g, with the most abundant being calcium, followed by phosphorus, potassium, sulfur, sodium, chloride and magnesium (see Figure 8.1).

Microminerals (trace elements and ultratrace elements) are needed in relatively low amounts (less than 100 mg a day), and body content ranges from less than 1 mg to about 4 g. Trace elements are essential to health, and include iron, zinc, copper, manganese, iodine, selenium, chromium, molybdenum and fluoride. The ultratrace elements, which are present in the body in even smaller quantities than trace elements, include silicon, boron, arsenic, nickel, vanadium and cobalt. Silicon and boron are important for health, but the role of other ultratrace elements is not fully understood.

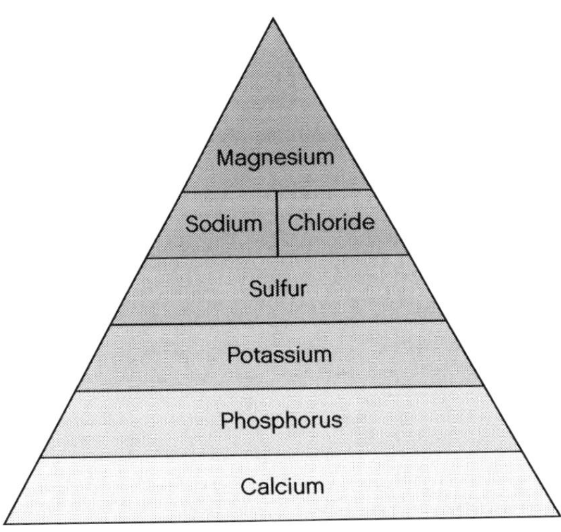

Figure 8.1 Relative body content of macrominerals

Mineral absorption

Minerals in food and water are in the form of compounds (mineral salts) that need to break apart in the gut to release the ionic mineral—for example, the mineral salt sodium chloride breaks down to the positively charged sodium ion (Na^+) and the negatively charged chloride ion (Cl^-). Mineral absorption is affected by the solubility, stability and particle size of the mineral salt. Mineral salts are usually held together by ionic bonds, the strength of which determines the fate of the mineral in the digestive tract. Weak bonds break apart and release mineral ions, and strong bonds do not release the mineral, which is then carried out of the body in faeces. In the diet, most mineral salts have relatively weak bonds, such as calcium lactate and sodium chloride. Hydrochloric acid in the stomach is required to release some mineral ions, in particular iron, zinc, copper and manganese. In general, organic mineral salts, such as lactates and citrates, are more soluble and better absorbed than insoluble inorganic salts, such as oxides and phosphates.

Most mineral ions are positively charged, including calcium^{2+}, magnesium^{2+}, potassium^{+}, sodium^{+}, iron^{2+}, iron^{3+}, zinc^{2+}, copper^{2+}, manganese^{2+} and chromium^{3+}. Positively charged ions (cations) can bind with negatively charged ions (anions) in the gut, which can help or hinder absorption. Useful binding agents include amino acids and soluble mucin, a glycoprotein produced by the lining cells of the digestive tract. Soluble mucin transfers minerals to the mucous membrane lining of the small intestine, where they compete with each other for attachment to binding proteins that allow entry into enterocytes. Minerals with a single positive charge are absorbed better than those with a double positive charge, followed by those with a triple positive charge. At higher than normal levels of intake, mineral ions can be absorbed by passive diffusion, which takes place in the spaces between enterocytes (paracellular absorption).

Mineral bioavailability

Bioavailability has been defined as the percentage of the consumed nutrient that enters the body from the gut and is used for its intended purpose. Dietary mineral absorption is generally poor. Competitive inhibition for binding sites may block absorption, some cations adhere to the negatively charged gut wall and may be lost with epithelial cells when they die off and pass out of the body in faeces, and some may bind strongly to phosphate anions, forming a poorly absorbed complex that is also lost in faeces. Up to 80 per cent of dietary minerals are unabsorbed, but absorption increases considerably in deficiency states.

Mineral chelates

The term 'chelate' (from the Greek word meaning 'claw' and pronounced 'KEY-late') denotes a substance that is able to bind strongly to a mineral. Dietary amino acids, such as aspartate or glycine, and dipeptides from protein-containing foods, if present in the gut at the same time as the mineral ion, can bind with ions to form medium-strength chelates that assist mineral absorption. The mechanism is not well understood, but it may be that mineral-amino acid/dipeptide complexes are absorbed intact or the complex may keep minerals soluble and prevent them from binding to phosphates and passing out of the body. Sodium and potassium, however, can only form weak chelates that do not enhance absorption—for example, sodium bound to glutamic acid (monosodium glutamate).

Mineral amino acid chelates are often used in supplements to improve mineral bioavailability—for example, magnesium amino acid chelate, alternatively called magnesium chelate or chelated magnesium. However, amino acids are bulky and the mineral content of amino acid chelates (referred to as the elemental mineral content) may be relatively low. Therefore, they do not provide a large amount of mineral per tablet/capsule. Mineral amino acid chelates may not be suitable for use in multivitamin and mineral supplements because they may make the tablet too large to swallow and too expensive to be price competitive. In the case of magnesium, the poorly absorbed magnesium oxide form may be used rather than the better-absorbed magnesium amino acid chelate or magnesium citrate. For calcium, calcium carbonate is commonly used instead of the more bioavailable calcium amino acid chelate or calcium citrate because the carbonate form is cheap and provides more elemental calcium. In general, minerals in less well absorbed forms should be taken with meals, as absorption is improved by the presence of stomach acid and the amino acids present in the digestive tract can chelate ionised minerals to enhance uptake.

Some chelates bind minerals so strongly that they become insoluble and therefore cannot be absorbed. Phytate (*myo*-inositol hexaphosphate), a storage compound for phosphorus in whole grains and especially found in wheat bran, seeds and nuts, has six reactive phosphate groups that exert a strong negative charge that binds cations, especially calcium^{2+}, potassium^{+}, magnesium^{2+}, iron^{2+}, iron^{3+} and zinc^{2+}, and inhibits their absorption. Yeast activity during bread-making, as well as long-term fermentation, sprouting or soaking, can break some phytate bonds, as can the enzyme phytase in the small intestine, thereby releasing the minerals for absorption.

Oxalate binds strongly to calcium^{2+}, magnesium^{2+}, iron^{2+} and iron^{3+} and, to a lesser extent, zinc^{2+}, and is found in spinach, beets and beet greens, parsley, coriander, purslane, rhubarb, sorrel, Swiss chard, strawberries, cranberries, wheat bran, amaranth, buckwheat, taro, sweet potato, soy products, legumes, star fruit, dried figs, sesame seeds, sunflower seeds, nuts, cocoa, chocolate and tea. Oxalate-containing foods are particularly poor sources of calcium, magnesium and iron because of very limited absorption; also, any unbound oxalate can bind to these cations in the gut, further reducing mineral bioavailability.

Colloidal minerals

Colloidal minerals are small particles of mineral compounds that remain in suspension rather than sinking when dispersed in water. They are a mixture of clay and water, and can be derived from soils rich in decomposed prehistoric plant life or by grinding and rapid crystallisation. Clay minerals are essentially hydrous aluminium silicates and may contain between 1800 and 4400 parts per million (ppm) of aluminium as well as large amounts of sodium and only very small amounts of other essential minerals and trace elements.

Colloid minerals are poorly absorbed; absorption of silicon from colloidal silica is less than 2 per cent. In chemistry, a colloidal mineral is a mineral with a particle size small enough to keep it suspended in a liquid but large enough to prevent it passing through semi-permeable membranes. Colloidal minerals are insoluble by definition and insoluble forms of minerals are poorly absorbed. The particle size means that they cannot pass through gut membranes intact, and they must ionise in the gut before absorption can take place. Claims that colloidal minerals are well absorbed are unfounded, as are claims that plants absorb minerals from the soil in colloidal form. Colloid mineral particles are too large to enter plant root cells intact, and plants absorb minerals in ionic form.

MACROMINERALS AND BODY pH

Macrominerals leave an acidic or alkaline residue in the body when metabolised. The healthy body has systems that buffer or remove excess acids and alkalis to prevent body pH changing from the healthy neutral range at which body systems can function. The normal pH value for body fluids is 7.35–7.45. A pH value below this range is referred to as acidosis and a pH value above this range is called alkalosis. Body pH is tightly controlled in healthy people, but can change very slightly and temporarily according to mineral intake.

Acid-forming minerals[1]

Sulfur, phosphorus and chloride are regarded as acid-forming minerals, and foods that are relatively high in these minerals are classed as acid-forming. These include meat, fish, chicken, eggs and grains that are high in phosphate and create phosphoric acid residues, as well as animal proteins rich in the sulfur-containing amino acids cysteine and methionine that create sulfuric acid residues. Processed foods and soft drinks may have an acidic effect because phosphates are commonly used as food additives. Salt is 40 per cent sodium and 60 per cent chloride, and 95 per cent of chloride anions are absorbed, causing a net increase in acid load that is independent of the net acid load of the diet.

Foods that contain organic acids and taste acidic, such as citrus fruit that contains citric acid, are not acid-forming because most organic acids can be metabolised completely in the body and produce bicarbonate that is alkaline. Oxalate in foods is potentially acid-forming because the body cannot metabolise this acid completely, but it is poorly absorbed and is unlikely to have much effect on body pH.

Alkaline-forming minerals[1]

Calcium, magnesium, potassium and sodium are regarded as alkaline because they form alkaline residues. In general, fruit, vegetables, nuts and legumes are alkaline-forming. Fruit and vegetables are particularly rich in potassium salts, which form bicarbonate as an end-product and have a neutralising effect on acids. Dairy products contain both acid-forming phosphate and alkaline-forming calcium, and have a slight alkaline effect.

Acid/alkaline diets

Most of the acids in the body are derived from sulfur and phosphate in animal foods and grains, and chloride from salt, and most of the bicarbonate (alkali) is derived from organic anions, such as citrate, provided by the potassium salts in fruit and vegetables. Inadequate fruit and vegetable intake may lead to latent acidosis, which is a slight shift of blood pH in the acid direction, but within the normal range, and a reduction in the total buffering capacity of the blood.

Bone is the largest reserve of alkali in the body, and in acidic conditions, the activity of cells that break down bone (osteoclasts) is increased and the activity of bone-forming cells (osteoblasts) is inhibited and bones release bicarbonate, potassium, sodium, calcium and magnesium to buffer acids.[2] Muscles are broken down to produce ammonia, which is strongly alkaline, and the kidneys increase excretion of acids. The kidneys cannot excrete urine that is more acidic than pH 4.4, and excess acids need to be buffered by forming complexes with minerals, such as potassium, calcium or magnesium, leading to mineral losses in urine. However, the kidneys are not able to excrete all of the acids produced by modern diets, and chronic mild metabolic acidosis may result, in which calcium is lost in urine without a compensatory increase in absorption in the intestine, leading to an overall negative calcium balance.

The outcome of acid–alkali interactions in the body is termed net endogenous acid production (NEAP), and this closely reflects the dietary protein:potassium ratio. Prehistoric diets were high in plant food and wild animal meat, and low in grains, and are believed to have provided higher potassium, lower sodium chloride and more bicarbonate than the average modern diet.[3] The body appears to be designed to handle large loads of bicarbonate and potassium, but not the large net acid loads produced by present-day diets dominated by grains and animal products and low in fruit and vegetables.

A high salt intake has been found to decrease blood pH and deplete bicarbonate, an important acid buffer in plasma, and experimental increases in salt intake have been shown to increase bone resorption and reduce pH by an average of 0.02.[4] Phosphate supplements do not appear to affect acidity. A meta-analysis of twelve studies found that higher phosphate intakes from supplementary sources were associated with decreased urinary calcium and increased calcium retention, irrespective of the calcium content of the diet, and no evidence was found that phosphate supplements contributed to bone demineralisation or to bone calcium excretion.[5]

An acid-forming diet has been shown to increase urinary calcium excretion by an average of 74 per cent, compared with an alkaline-forming diet.[6] Research has shown that acid-forming diets can contribute to osteoporosis, bone fractures, arthritis, loss of muscle mass, kidney stones and reduced growth rates in children.[3] In older people, alkaline-forming diets are associated with greater bone mineral density and less risk of hip fractures, and acid-forming diets are associated with more rapid bone loss and increased risk of hip fractures.[7]

The original valid scientific research on acid and alkaline-forming foods was carried out in the 1910s by Henry Sherman and Alexander Gettler in the United States.[8] They investigated the effects of diets with differing balances of acid-forming and alkaline-forming minerals, and the effect on ammonia metabolism in a human subject, and established that certain foods were acid-forming and others were alkaline-forming. However, the concept was taken over and distorted in the 1930s and 1940s by natural health proponents such as Dr William Hay,[9] who proposed an unnecessarily strict method of eating called 'food combining', which has little scientific basis, and research into Sherman and Gettler's findings lapsed. More recently, interest has been renewed, with researchers investigating the effects of acid-forming diets and supplementation with alkalis on health—particularly bone health.[10]

Researchers have used alkali therapy to improve acid–base balance. Potassium bicarbonate supplementation has been found to improve calcium, phosphate and nitrogen balance, reduce bone resorption and reduce the age-related decline in growth hormone secretion.[3] Potassium citrate has been shown to protect against the adverse effects of sodium chloride on bone by reducing bone resorption and calcium losses in urine.[5] In kidney stone patients, potassium-magnesium citrate has been found to reduce the risk of calcium oxalate stones by 85 per cent over three years.[11] However, alkali therapy should be used with caution because it may cause alkalosis—particularly in people with congestive heart failure and lung or kidney disease, because of impaired ability to regulate pH.

A balance between acid- and alkaline-forming foods is important for health; excess alkalinity is also harmful and acid-forming foods provide important nutrients—particularly protein—and need to be included in the daily diet. Additional intake of alkaline-forming foods has been shown to compensate for the acidic effect of protein foods, and protein provides ammonia that improves the ability of the kidneys to buffer acids in urine.[10] Balancing acid- and alkaline-forming foods does not require extreme or restricted diets, but can be achieved by limiting processed food, soft drinks and salt, and balancing intake of meat, fish, poultry, eggs and grains with fruit, vegetables, nuts, seeds and legumes.

REFERENCES

1 Remer, T., Influence of nutrition on acid-base balance: Metabolic aspects, *Eur J Nutr* (2001), 40(5): 214–20.
2 Bushinsky, D.A., Acid–base imbalance and the skeleton, *Eur J Nutr* (2001), 40(5): 238–44.
3 Frassetto, L., Morris, R.C. Jr, Sellmeyer, D.E. et al., Diet, evolution and aging: The pathophysiologic effects of the post-agricultural inversion of the potassium-to-sodium and base-to-chloride ratios in the human diet, *Eur J Nutr* (2001), 40(5): 200–13.
4 Frings-Meuthen, P., Baecker, N. & Heer, M., Low-grade metabolic acidosis may be the cause of sodium chloride-induced exaggerated bone resorption, *J Bone Miner Res* (2008), 23: 517–24.
5 Fenton, T.R., Lyon, A.W., Eliasziw, M. et al., Phosphate decreases urine calcium and increases calcium balance: A meta-analysis of the osteoporosis acid-ash diet hypothesis, *Nutr J* (2009), 8: 41.
6 Buclin, T., Cosma, M., Appenzeller, M. et al., Diet acids and alkalis influence calcium retention in bone, *Osteoporos Int* (2001), 12(6): 493–9.
7 Sellmeyer, D.E., Stone, K.L., Sebastian, A. et al., A high ratio of dietary animal to vegetable protein increases the rate of bone loss and the risk of fracture in post-menopausal women: Study of Osteoporotic Fractures Research Group, *Am J Clin Nutr* (2001), 73: 118–22.
8 Sherman, H.C. & Gettler, A.O., The balance of acid-forming and base-forming elements in foods, and its relation to ammonia metabolism, *J Biol Chem* (1912), 11: 323–38.
9 Hay, W.H., *Superior health through nutrition*, Health Research, Washington, DC, 1937.
10 Pizzorno, J., Frassetto, L.A. & Katzinger, J., Diet-induced acidosis: Is it real and clinically relevant? *Br J Nutr* (2010), 103(8): 1185–94.
11 Ettinger, B.I., Pak, C.Y., Citron, J.T. et al., Potassium-magnesium citrate is an effective prophylaxis against recurrent calcium oxalate nephrolithiasis, *J Urol* (1997), 158(6): 2069–73.

Hair analysis for assessment of body mineral status

Some naturopaths use scalp hair analysis to assess the body content of minerals. To perform the test, small amounts of hair are cut from different areas of the scalp (usually around the nape area) as close to the scalp as possible, and these are sent to a specialist laboratory for preparation and analysis. Hair is rich in sulfur-containing amino acids that can form stable bonds with minerals. Hair mineral content is a reflection of the concentration of minerals in the hair follicle at the time the hair was formed, minerals present in secretions from sebaceous and apocrine glands that bathe the hair as it emerges through the epidermis, and environmental minerals. In animals, hair mineral content is affected by hair colour, texture, sex, age, season, environment and diet. In particular, dietary intakes of calcium, phosphorus and iron have been found to affect the uptake of other elements in hair.

In general, hair tests are regarded as unreliable for most macrominerals and trace elements. Results are difficult to interpret, and can be affected by hair type, the use of hair shampoos and treatments, and the washing process used by the laboratory. An animal study found that the mineral content of hair that had been exposed to typical treatments used on human hair, such as rinses, sprays, tonics, waving lotions and gels, was very different to the mineral content of untreated hair, and that various commonly used washing procedures did not correct the differences. Washing methods differ between laboratories, and may be responsible for considerable variation in results. When the washing step is omitted, results from different laboratories have been found to be consistent. However, interpretation of the results is inconsistent because of the use of differing reference ranges.

A 2003 report on hair testing by the US Agency for Toxic Substances and Disease Registry (ATSDR) concluded that standardised reference ranges should be established, and identified a number of issues of concern, including difficulties in distinguishing between internal hair mineral content and external mineral contamination, lack of correlation between the mineral content of hair and that of blood and other target tissues, and insufficient understanding of how and to what extent environmental contaminants are incorporated into hair and the relationship of hair mineral content to health effects. Overall, hair tests are considered more reliable for assessing exposure to drugs and potentially toxic elements such as arsenic, cobalt, germanium, lead, lithium, manganese, mercury, nickel and thallium. Hair testing for essential minerals and trace elements should be used as an ancillary, rather than as a primary, diagnostic tool.

CALCIUM

CALCIUM STATUS CHECK

1 **Do you have low bone mineral density or a history of bone fractures?**
2 **Do you often have sore muscles, muscle cramps, spasms or twitches?**
3 **Do you have numbness and tingling around your mouth?**
4 **Do you get anxious, irritable and depressed?**

'Yes' answers may indicate inadequate calcium status. Note that a number of nutritional deficiencies or health disorders can cause similar effects and further investigation is recommended.

FAST FACTS . . . CALCIUM

- **Sources of available calcium include dairy products, fish with bones, calcium-fortified food and drinks and cabbage-family vegetables.**
- **Calcium is part of the structure of bones and teeth.**
- **It supports nerve and muscle function and blood clotting, and helps regulate cell activities.**
- **A deficiency can cause low bone density, osteoporosis, muscle cramps and nervous and digestive disorders.**
- **Supplementation may be helpful for maintaining bone mineral density during ageing, for a healthy pregnancy, to prevent premenstrual syndrome and to protect against colorectal polyps and cancer.**

Calcium has the chemical symbol Ca, and is a naturally occurring mineral found in limestone (calcium carbonate), gypsum (calcium sulfate) and fluorite (calcium fluoride); it makes up about 3 per cent of the earth's crust. It was first isolated by English chemist Sir Humphry Davy in 1808, and the name derives from the Latin *calx* or *calcis* for 'lime' (calcium oxide). Calcium is the most abundant mineral in the human body, comprising about 2 per cent of body weight, 99 per cent of which is in bones and teeth. The remaining 1 per cent is found in the bloodstream, and in intracellular (ICF) and extracellular fluid (ECF).

Digestion, absorption and transport

Calcium is found in foods as various salts, such as calcium lactate and calcium gluconate, most of which can dissolve (solubilise) in the acid medium of the stomach to release calcium cations (Ca^{2+}) that are absorbed in the small intestine. Absorption depends on the ability of the calcium salt to dissolve, and, in insoluble dietary calcium salts, calcium is bound so tightly that calcium cations are not released and the salts are passed through the digestive tract and are excreted in faeces.

At lower levels of intake, absorption of calcium is an active process regulated by calcitriol (1,25-dihydroxycholecalciferol), the active form of vitamin D, which increases calcium uptake from food by stimulating production of the calcium-binding protein calbindin D_{9K} in the enterocytes lining the small intestine. Calbindin D_{9K} binds calcium cations and transports them across the cell interior, from which they are transferred into the bloodstream by the enzyme calcium-ATPase. Calcium is transported in the bloodstream bound to proteins, as free calcium and as calcium sulfate, phosphate, citrate and bicarbonate.

At higher levels of intake, active transport of calcium is inhibited and calcium cations are absorbed paracellularly through the tight junctions between enterocytes in the small intestine by passive diffusion. Paracellular diffusion is also responsible for about 85 per cent of the calcium reabsorbed in the kidneys. In the colon, bacterial activity releases some bound calcium, which is then available for absorption; however, only a small amount of calcium is absorbed in this way. Overall, about 35 per cent of dietary calcium is absorbed when body levels are adequate, which increases to about 75 per cent in deficiency states.

Metabolism, storage and excretion

The extracellular concentration of calcium in the body is about 10 000-fold higher than the concentration of free calcium in the cell interior, and is tightly controlled. The extracellular calcium-sensing receptor (CaR) has been identified in many tissues, and appears to play an important role in regulating calcium levels. When intracellular calcium concentration drops, a stimulus triggers the opening of calcium channels in the cell membrane and calcium ions enter the cell.

Calcium is stored inside cells in a variety of organelles, including the mitochondria, nucleus, sarcoplasmic reticulum, and rough and smooth endoplasmic reticulum. When needed, calcium ions are released from storage organelles and bind to calcium-binding proteins, the most important of which is calmodulin, which can bind four calcium ions per molecule. When bound to calcium, calmodulin undergoes a change to its structural arrangement, which enables it to bind to particular proteins and elicit a specific response. Calcium is also active in cells as free calcium ions. Calcium is removed from the cytosol and the cell by calcium-ATPases and sodium, calcium and potassium exchange systems.

Calcium is secreted in digestive juices, and may be reabsorbed in the same manner as dietary calcium, the unabsorbed portion being excreted in faeces. Bone is the major storage site for calcium. It is excreted in urine, and small amounts may be lost through the skin in sweat.

Regulation of serum calcium

Serum calcium levels are tightly controlled to ensure that calcium levels in ICF and ECF are maintained at a constant level. Bone is the major regulator of calcium in body fluids; calcium is deposited or removed from bone as required, subject to hormonal control.

The parathyroid gland monitors calcium levels in blood and releases parathyroid hormone (PTH) when calcium levels drop. PTH stimulates calcitriol production by the kidneys, which acts on the digestive tract, kidneys and bones. Calcitriol increases blood calcium and phosphate levels by increasing uptake from food, reducing losses in urine and mobilising minerals from bone. In the kidneys, it acts by increasing production of calbindin D_{28K} that enhances calcium reabsorption in kidney tubules. Primarily, calcitriol promotes increased absorption of dietary calcium; however, if calcium intake is too low, bone calcium is then mobilised. PTH also has direct effects on bone by promoting its breakdown to release calcium into the blood. A rise in serum calcium acts to inhibit PTH release, and the thyroid gland releases calcitonin, which strongly inhibits the bone-resorbing activity of osteoclasts. Testosterone, oestrogen, thyroid hormone, growth hormone and pregnancy and lactation hormones also help boost calcium levels by promoting intestinal calcium absorption.

Calcium balance

Calcium balance occurs when body stores of calcium are at an equilibrium over an extended time period, which occurs when growth has ceased in healthy adults. It is calculated by comparing the amount absorbed and the amount excreted, which reflects the mineral status of bone. Positive balance occurs when absorption is greater than losses (when calcium is accumulating in bone during growth) and negative balance occurs when losses are greater than absorption (when bone loss occurs during older age).

Functions

Calcium is a major component of teeth and bones, where it acts as a structural component and a calcium reserve, and is essential for blood clotting, nerve conduction, muscle contraction and cell signalling. Calcium has an alkaline effect on body pH. Intracellular calcium regulates a large number of cell activities, including cell proliferation, differentiation and motility, embryogenesis, eicosanoid formation, inflammation, immune responses, fatty acid oxidation, glycogen metabolism, energy production, gene transcription and cell survival and death. The functions of calcium include the following.

- *Bone formation.* Bone contains a variety of calcium salts, including brushite, octacalcium phosphate, amorphous calcium phosphate, whitlockite and hydroxyapatite. Crystallised calcium compounds—particularly hydroxyapatite, which consists of calcium, phosphate and hydroxyl groups in a lattice-like structure—are major components of teeth and mature bone, where they provide strength and rigidity to the skeleton. Bone is a dynamic structure that is constantly broken down and rebuilt (remodelled) throughout life.

  Bone is formed by osteoblasts, which generate an extracellular matrix consisting of proteins and ground substance to which calcium and other minerals attach and form crystals. Bone is broken down by osteoclasts that release acids and enzymes to break down the matrix, mineral salts and crystallised minerals. Bone serves as a mineral reserve, and calcium and other minerals are mobilised from bones by osteoclast activity as required. When blood levels of calcium drop, calcium released from bones is transferred to the blood and body fluids, and is then available to other tissue cells.

  Bone formation peaks in early adulthood and declines with age. During growth, formation of bone is greater than resorption. In early adulthood, formation is roughly equal to resorption, and resorption overtakes formation in older age. Adequate calcium intake is vital during the period of active bone formation to ensure that accumulation of bone mineral mass is maximised to help protect against the adverse effects of losses in later life.
- *Nerve conduction.* Calcium is involved in the transmission of a nerve impulse from one nerve cell to an adjacent one across the synaptic cleft. When an impulse arrives at the end bulb of a nerve axon, the end bulb membrane becomes more permeable to calcium, which diffuses in and activates enzymes that cause synaptic vesicles containing neurotransmitters to move towards the synaptic cleft. Neurotransmitters are released, diffuse across the cleft and bind to receptors in the postsynaptic nerve membrane, triggering an action potential that travels along the nerve.
- *Muscle function.* Calcium is the main regulatory and signalling molecule in muscle fibres, and is essential for skeletal muscle (voluntary) and cardiac and smooth muscle (involuntary) contractions. In skeletal muscles, calcium is stored in the sarcoplasmic reticulum (SR), where it is bound to the protein calsequestrin. When stimulated by a motor nerve, the surface membrane of a muscle depolarises and this spreads into deeper parts of the muscle fibre, activating the ryanodine receptor that releases calcium from the SR. Calcium then binds to the troponin protein complex and activates the contraction process. When the nerve impulse ceases to act, calcium is returned to the SR by a calcium pump and the muscle relaxes.

  In smooth muscles, contraction occurs when a stimulus causes calcium to enter the cytosol and bind to the protein calmodulin, causing phosphorylation of the light chain of myosin and initiating contraction. The contraction ends when calcium is pumped out of the cytosol and the enzyme myosin phosphatase is activated to dephosphorylate myosin. There are a number of other calcium-binding proteins found in muscle tissue, including parvalbumin, S100 proteins, annexins, sorcin, beta-actinin, calcineurin and calpain, which may be involved in muscle contraction, protein metabolism and muscle cell differentiation and growth.
- *Blood clotting.* Blood clotting is dependent on the sequential activation of blood-clotting proteins (factors), the end result of which is the creation of a tight web of insoluble fibrin that traps blood cells and seals off the site of injury. Calcium takes part in the clotting process by binding to vitamin K-dependent Gla clotting factors, enabling them to bind to phospholipids on the surface of activated blood platelets. Calcium also binds with the enzyme thrombin, and assists the conversion of fibrinogen to fibrin, which creates a mature, functional clot.
- *Cell signalling.* Calcium is a key signalling agent inside every cell, where it acts as a 'second messenger' by relaying signals received by cell membrane receptors to target molecules inside the cell. Damage to the cell membrane allows calcium to enter the cytosol, which is interpreted as a danger signal and triggers calcium-dependent mechanisms that enable membrane repair. Controlled calcium influx and release help to regulate a vast number of cell activities, including cell proliferation, differentiation and motility, embryogenesis, eicosanoid formation, inflammation, immune responses, fatty acid oxidation, glycogen metabolism, energy production, gene transcription and cell survival and death. Calcium is also required for release of the glucose-regulating hormones insulin and glucagon from the pancreas.

Hormone and neurotransmitter signals reaching the cell trigger an increase in intracellular calcium that acts directly on target proteins or via intracellular calcium-binding proteins, several hundred of which have been identified. The primary calcium-binding protein within cells is calmodulin; when bound to calcium, it can bind to and regulate many different cell proteins and affect a wide range of cell functions. Zinc is required for the entry of calcium into cells, and magnesium is required for the binding of calcium to calmodulin. Calmodulin also activates calcineurin, a major regulator of cell functions and an immune booster that stimulates production of the T cell growth factor, interleukin-2. The immunosuppressive drugs cyclosporin A and tacrolimus work by blocking calcineurin function. Disruptions in calcium signalling are a feature of the pathology of a variety of diseases, including Huntington's disease, Alzheimer's disease, cancer, congenital heart failure and diabetes.

Dietary sources

The most bioavailable calcium sources are milk and dairy products, calcium-fortified juices, soy or cereal milks, calcium-processed tofu, fish with bones (such as canned sardines and salmon), snapper, cod, shellfish, prawns, bok choy, Chinese cabbage, broccoli, cauliflower, kale, collards, turnip greens, mustard greens, watercress and sun-dried tomatoes. An Australian study found that calcium in calcium-fortified soy milk has about the same bioavailability as cow's milk calcium. Some mineral waters and domestic water supplies in areas of hard water provide a well-absorbed source of calcium. In Australia, food manufacturers are permitted to voluntarily add calcium to fruit and vegetable juices, fruit and vegetable drinks, fruit cordial, soups and crispbread/cracker-type biscuits.

The Food Standards Australia New Zealand nutrient database (NUTTAB) at <www.foodstandards.gov.au> provides the amounts found in specific foods.

Factors influencing body status

Calcium is water soluble, and may be lost from foods by water-processing and cooking methods. Digestive disorders and inadequate stomach acid may impair absorption, and kidney damage may increase losses in urine. Calcium absorption is reduced by binding to tannins, phosphates and dietary fats in the gut, forming insoluble compounds that are excreted. However, dietary phosphates also have positive effects by reducing calcium excretion in urine. Dietary salt increases urinary excretion of calcium: an extra 2 g of dietary sodium is calculated to increase urinary calcium excretion by an average of 30–40 mg. A predominantly acid-forming diet can lead to losses of calcium from bone and increased urinary excretion. Metabolic alkalosis increases binding of calcium to plasma proteins, and reduces the availability of ionised calcium.

At low levels of intake, calcium absorption depends on calcitriol, and low levels of vitamin D and/or PTH impair absorption. Calcium absorption decreases post-menopause because a lack of oestrogen reduces vitamin D levels. Calcium uptake in the gut may be diminished by an excess of magnesium, iron, zinc and fluoride, which compete for absorption. Conversely, a high calcium intake may deplete levels of these competing minerals. A high phosphorus intake may impair calcium balance, especially if the diet is low in calcium, because, at high levels, phosphorus can form complexes that reduce serum calcium, which stimulates PTH release and mobilises calcium from bones. Adequate magnesium and zinc are required for calcium metabolism. Calcium balance is disturbed in alcoholics because of intestinal malabsorption and low levels of vitamin D, magnesium and albumin, as well as respiratory and metabolic alkalosis and pancreatitis.

Calcium in some plant foods is in a bound form, and is largely unavailable for absorption. It is bound by oxalate, which occurs naturally in spinach, beets, beet greens, parsley, coriander, purslane, rhubarb, sorrel, Swiss chard, strawberries, cranberries, wheat bran, amaranth, buckwheat, taro, sweet potato, soy products, legumes, star fruit, dried figs, sesame seeds, sunflower seeds, nuts, cocoa, chocolate and tea. Only 5 per cent of the calcium from spinach is absorbed, compared with 25–50 per cent from more available food sources. Whole grains, bran, nuts and seeds, and particularly the bran component of cereals, contain phytate, which binds calcium. Soaking, sprouting and bread-making using yeast can release some of the phytate-bound calcium, but has no effect on calcium bound to oxalate.

Dietary lactose, sugars, phosphopeptides and proteins increase calcium absorption. Although protein increases calcium absorption, it also increases calcium losses in urine, and was previously thought to have adverse effects on calcium balance. However, it has been found that about 80 per cent of the excreted calcium is derived from dietary intake rather than bone and, overall, protein has been found to have a positive influence on bone. A high protein intake improves outcomes after hip fracture, and protein supplementation has reduced bone loss in fracture patients. A low protein intake is associated with loss of bone mineral. Because proteins in foods can contribute to acidity, they should be used in balance with alkaline foods to maintain a healthy pH.

Exercise—especially weight-bearing exercise and weight training—increases calcium deposits in bone and a sedentary lifestyle, immobilisation, bed rest or weightlessness (space travel) can lead to bone mineral losses. Some common drugs that have adverse effects on calcium status include proton pump inhibitors, which suppress stomach acid production, and bile acid sequestrants used for lowering elevated serum cholesterol, which may interfere with calcium absorption and increase the loss of calcium in urine. Thiazide and amiloride diuretics can reduce calcium excretion and loop diuretics can increase calcium excretion. Drugs that increase bone resorption and decrease bone formation include Depo-Provera contraceptive injections, anti-epileptic drugs, corticosteroids (anti-inflammatories), unfractionated heparin (a blood thinner) and thiazolidinedione (for diabetes). Other risk factors for bone loss include family history, ageing, menopause, smoking and excessive alcohol intake.

Table 8.1 Recommended dietary intake (RDI) of calcium (mg/day)

Age (years)	Female RDI	Male RDI
1–3	500	500
4–8	700	700
9–13	1000–1300	1000–1300
14–18	1300	1300
19–50	1000	1000
51–70	1300	1000
>70	1300	1300
Pregnant women		
14–18	1300	
19–50	1000	
Lactating women		
14–18	1300	
19–50	1000	

Source: Nutrient Reference Values for Australia and New Zealand Including Recommended Dietary Intakes, National Health and Medical Research Council, Australian Government Department of Health and Ageing, Canberra and Ministry of Health, New Zealand, Wellington, 2006.

Daily requirement

Government recommendations by age and gender (see Table 8.1) can be found in *Nutrient Reference Values for Australia and New Zealand Including Recommended Dietary Intakes*, available at <www.nhmrc.gov.au>.

Deficiency effects

A lack of dietary calcium and inadequate vitamin D are common in Australia; the average intake of calcium in older Australian women is about half the recommended amount. Calcium deficiency is more common in people who avoid dairy foods, and in people following vegan diets, postmenopausal women and younger women whose menstrual cycles have stopped, which may occur in athletes and women with eating disorders.

Because calcium is released from bones when dietary intake is inadequate, blood levels of calcium rarely drop unless there is an underlying metabolic disorder, such as an underactive parathyroid gland, inadequate vitamin D, acute pancreatitis or magnesium deficiency, any of which can impair PTH secretion or function; hyperphosphataemia, in which phosphate binds calcium ions and removes them from the bloodstream; or alkalosis, in which there is increased binding of ionised calcium to albumin.

Low serum calcium (hypocalcaemia) is a common issue in critically ill patients, and occurs when serum calcium is below 2.10 mmol/L or when ionised calcium levels are below 1.16 mmol/L. It can lead to severe, uncontrolled muscle contractions (tetany) because of increased excitability of nerves. Effects include sensations of tingling, numbness or pins and needles (paraesthesia) in the hands and feet and around the mouth, hyperactive deep tendon reflexes, muscle spasms, cramps and twitches in the face or limbs, spasm of the larynx and convulsions. Chvostek's sign (a facial muscle contraction elicited by tapping) or Trousseau's sign (a hand spasm that results from reducing the blood supply in the arm by inflating a blood pressure cuff) may be present. Low calcium affects heart function, causing decreased heart muscle contraction, reduced cardiac output, low blood pressure and disturbance of heart rhythm. Brain function may be impaired, causing anxiety, depression, confusion and psychoses.

More common disorders of calcium balance occur when a low calcium intake, poor absorption of calcium or a vitamin D deficiency leads to elevated PTH secretion (secondary hyperparathyroidism), increased calcitriol production and increased bone resorption. Serum calcium levels are maintained within the normal range by depletion of bone minerals. Apart from its effects on bone, elevated calcitriol appears to trigger the opening of calcium channels in cell membranes, leading to increased calcium ion concentrations inside cells. This rise in calcium in smooth muscle cells increases muscle tone and elevates blood pressure, and also increases fat production and reduces fat breakdown in adipose cells, which may be associated with weight gain. Elevated PTH causes bone weakness and pain, and is also associated with fatigue, lethargy, depression, constipation, heartburn, stomach ulcers, nausea, vomiting, appetite loss and vague abdominal pains. It may increase the risk of kidney stones, pancreatitis, cancers of the colon and the development of brown tumours (benign growths in bones).

Calcium competes for absorption with lead, an environmental pollutant and toxic metal, and inadequate dietary calcium increases lead uptake. Lead impairs brain and nerve function; children under the age of five are more vulnerable to lead toxicity and chronic low-level exposure may lead to irritability, low energy, appetite loss, poor coordination and growth, learning disabilities, behavioural problems and poor school performance.

In children, a calcium deficiency can cause the bone-deforming disorder rickets, in which there are reduced levels of calcified bone (osteomalacia, see Chapter 5: Vitamin D). In adults, osteopenia (low bone mass) develops over time, and may lead to osteoporosis, in which bone minerals are lost and bones become porous, brittle and susceptible to fracture. Osteoporosis is prevalent in most Western societies and hip fractures are the most serious outcome because they may lead to permanent disability and even death. Bone loss begins at an earlier age in women than in men, and accelerates at menopause; women may lose 20–30 per cent of trabecular bone (found in the spine and ends of long bones) and 5–10 per cent of cortical bone (found primarily in the shaft of long bones) between the ages of 50 and 60. Bone loss in men occurs at an older age. Men and women with osteoporosis have increased risk of fracture, and risk increases with age; it is estimated that half of all women and a third of all men over the age of 60 will have a fracture due to osteoporosis.

Osteoporosis may not be detected until the first fracture occurs. Fractures are more common in the hip, spine, wrist, upper arm, ribs or forearm, and can occur from falls or during everyday activities such as bending or lifting. Spinal fractures can cause loss of height, curvature of the upper spine (kyphosis, commonly known as dowager's hump) and postural changes. Osteoporosis is often painless, but may cause dull pain in the bones or muscles, particularly low back pain or neck pain, and may lead to chronic pain. Movements of the affected bones may cause sharper pain and tenderness.

Indicators of inadequate levels of calcium may include:

- *osteoporosis:* low bone mineral density, fractures of the hip, spine, wrist, upper arm, ribs or forearm
- osteomalacia
- backache, aching of long bones
- loss of height, stooped posture, curvature of the upper spine, sway back, protruding abdomen
- muscular soreness, muscle cramps, spasms, twitches
- high or low blood pressure, irregular heart rhythm
- paraesthesia, especially affecting the mouth, throat and limbs
- anxiety, irritability, depression, confusion, psychosis
- *children:* rickets, elevated blood levels of lead leading to irritability, low energy, appetite loss, poor coordination and growth, learning disabilities, behavioural problems and poor school performance.

Assessment of body status

The serum calcium concentration is not regarded as an accurate assessment of body status because it is tightly regulated. The reference range given by the Royal College of Pathologists of Australasia (RCPA) for adults is 2.10–2.60 mmol/L for total calcium, 1.16–1.30 mmol/L for ionised calcium and 2.15–2.60 mmol/L for corrected calcium (an estimate of the total calcium corrected for low albumin concentrations). Chvostek's sign is not regarded as accurate because it is absent in about one-third of patients with hypocalcaemia, and is present in about 10 per cent of people with normal calcium levels. Trousseau's sign is a more sensitive and specific indicator, and is present in 94 per cent of patients with hypocalcaemia and in only 1 per cent of people with normal calcium levels.

Bone mineral density (BMD) can be assessed by a specialised x-ray known as a dual-energy x-ray absorptiometry (DXA or DEXA) scan. The result is expressed as a score that compares a person's BMD with the average BMD of a 30-year-old of the same gender. The World Health Organization (WHO) guidelines for interpreting DXA scores are as follows:

- osteoporosis: less than or equal to –2.5
- osteopenia: –1.0 to –2.5
- normal: greater than –1.0.

Other tests include quantitative computed tomography (QCT) and quantitative ultrasound (QUS). QUS measures BMD at the heel, and is used as an indicator of whole-body BMD. It is convenient to administer, but not as accurate as the DXA scan.

Case reports—calcium deficiency

- *A man, 38 years of age*, developed progressive facial paraesthesia and muscle cramps in the arms and hands after a total thyroidectomy.[1] Chvostek's sign and Trousseau's sign were present, and his total serum calcium level was 1.45 mmol/L, his ionised calcium was 0.84 mmol/L and his PTH level was low, indicating that the operation to remove his thyroid gland had damaged the parathyroid glands. His symptoms resolved with iv calcium gluconate.
- *A young woman, age not reported*, was admitted to a hospital emergency department in a hysterical condition after a car accident in which she had fractured her arm.[2] She complained of paraesthesia around the mouth, and fainted. She was diagnosed with tetany caused by hyperventilation-induced respiratory alkalosis, which had caused a reduction in serum levels of ionised calcium. Correction of the hysterical over-breathing resolved the symptoms.
- *A woman, 43 years of age*, with a long history of Crohn's disease, developed fatigue, weight loss, abdominal colic, muscle cramps and paraesthesia.[2] Positive Chvostek's and Trousseau's signs were found, and her serum calcium, magnesium and potassium were low. She was treated with iv calcium, potassium and magnesium, and was given vitamin D and commenced on tube feeding. On follow-up, her serum electrolyte levels had normalised, her symptoms had improved and she had gained weight.
- *A woman, 65 years of age*, requested an assessment of her osteoporosis risk because of a family history.[3] She had no symptoms apart from a height loss of 5 cm, no history of fractures and was not on medication. Her weight was within the healthy range and she was a non-smoker but drank about four alcoholic drinks daily. A DXA scan resulted in a score of –2.3 at the hip and –2.5 at the spine, and further investigation revealed a vertebral fracture. She was advised to reduce her alcohol intake, and was given drug therapy for osteoporosis with supplementary calcium and vitamin D, and was scheduled for regular monitoring to assess her BMD.
- *A boy, four years of age*, was diagnosed with rickets.[4] He had normal serum levels of vitamin D and high serum levels of calcitriol. He had not been given dairy products of any kind because of allergy, and his diet was low in good sources of calcium. He rapidly improved on an increased calcium intake.

REFERENCES

1 Jesus, J.E. & Landry, A., Images in clinical medicine: Chvostek's and Trousseau's signs, *N Engl J Med* (2012), 367(11): e15.

2 Metheny, N.M., Calcium imbalances. In *Fluid and Electrolyte Balance*, 5th ed., Jones & Bartlett Learning, New York, 2012.

3 Cooper, M., *Clinical Review: Osteoporosis,* GPonline.com, retrieved 20 August 2014 from <www.gponline.com/clinical-review-osteoporosis/rheumatology/osteoporosis-and-bone-disorders/article/1119708>.

4 Davidovits, M., Levy, Y., Avramovitz, T. & Eisenstein, B., Calcium-deficiency rickets in a four-year-old boy with milk allergy, *J Pediatr* (1993), 122(2): 249–51.

THERAPEUTIC USES OF CALCIUM

Bone disorders

Children and adolescents

During pre-pubertal growth, adequate calcium intake, together with exercise, has been found to be important for increasing bone mass, and greater bone mass is associated with lower fracture risk. In children and adolescents, the effects of calcium supplementation studies are conflicting, and a review of nineteen clinical trials concluded that there was evidence for a small improvement in BMD in the upper limbs only, which is unlikely to be of clinical importance.[1]

In children, a calcium deficiency can cause rickets, even when levels of vitamin D are adequate. There is a high prevalence of rickets in children in tropical countries where there is ample sunlight and vitamin D has been used as the primary therapy. However, calcium supplementation, used alone or with vitamin D, has been shown to be superior to vitamin D alone in the treatment of rickets in these children.[2] Case reports of children with rickets from Western countries have found that improving dietary calcium intake normalises serum and urinary calcium levels, and reduces levels of the bone enzyme alkaline phosphatase. Calcified bone volume and indicators of bone mineralisation become normal.

Adults

In Australia, it is estimated that 3.4 per cent of the population have diagnosed osteoporosis and the large majority are women (81.9 per cent) and people over 55 years of age (84 per cent).[3] Overall, a high calcium intake appears to be helpful in preventing osteoporosis. The rate of bone remodelling triples after menopause, and a high calcium intake has been shown to reduce this process to pre-menopause levels and to improve bone strength. Several studies have found that BMD is increased or maintained in mid- to late post-menopausal women who take additional calcium in food or supplements. A research review of 29 clinical trials concluded that calcium supplementation, alone or in combination with vitamin D, is effective in reducing bone loss at the hip and spine in women and men aged 50 years or older.[4] However, vitamin D is required together with calcium for fracture prevention.

Pregnancy

Many women of childbearing age do not have an adequate calcium intake, which may affect maternal and foetal bone. Calcium needs of the foetus are greater in the third trimester, during which it acquires about 350 mg/day.[5] Maternal calcitriol production and calcium absorption increase in line with increased needs, particularly in women with low intakes, but may not be sufficient to supply the total calcium requirement of mother and foetus.

Low calcium intakes during pregnancy stimulate calcitriol secretion, which increases intracellular calcium and smooth muscle contractions, and calcitriol may also have a role in renin release by the kidney. These effects cause constriction of blood vessels, retention of sodium and fluid, elevated blood pressure (pregnancy-induced hypertension, PIH) and increased risk of pre-eclampsia. A review of ten trials of calcium supplementation in pregnant women in developing countries concluded that there was a 45 per cent reduction in risk of PIH in women receiving calcium compared with a placebo.[6] Another comprehensive review of thirteen trials found that the average risk of high blood pressure was reduced by 35 per cent in those receiving calcium supplements and pre-eclampsia risk was reduced by 55 per cent overall and by 64 per cent in women with low calcium intakes at baseline.[7] The reviewers also concluded that calcium supplementation could reduce risk of maternal death or serious illness by 20 per cent and risk of preterm birth by 24 per cent. However, a more recent review of 21 trials found no differences in preterm birth risk and only a slight increase in birth weight.[8] Pregnant women taking 1000 mg of supplemental calcium daily have been shown to have reduced markers of bone turnover in late pregnancy,[9] and high calcium intakes in pregnancy are associated with better bone mass in children at nine years of age.[10]

Colorectal polyps and cancer

The presence of calcium in the colon appears to be protective against colorectal cancer, possibly by binding to potentially toxic bile acids and fatty acids, and forming insoluble soaps that are removed in faeces or by directly acting on the lining of the colon to reduce cell proliferation, stimulate differentiation and induce apoptosis in abnormal cells. People with the highest calcium intake have been shown to have a 22 per cent reduced risk of colorectal cancer, and most of the risk reduction has been achieved with intakes of 700–800 mg/day.[11] Calcium supplementation in patients with a history of adenoma (polyps), a risk factor for colorectal cancer, has resulted in a moderately decreased risk of recurrent adenoma at four years, and a 35 per cent reduced risk in those with advanced adenoma, with the effect persisting for five years after supplementation ceased.[12]

Premenstrual syndrome

It is estimated that 85–90 per cent of premenopausal women experience premenstrual syndrome (PMS) symptoms such as depression, irritability, fatigue, food cravings, abdominal cramps, bloating, breast tenderness, fluid retention and headaches in the luteal phase of the menstrual cycle, about one to two weeks before the onset of menses. Symptoms are mild in most women, but in some may be severe enough to disrupt relationships and daily activities. Calcium and calcium-regulating hormones fluctuate during the menstrual cycle, and some women with PMS have been found to have disturbed calcium metabolism, accompanied by secondary hyperparathyroidism and vitamin D deficiency. PMS may be associated with abnormalities in bone metabolism and reduced bone mass, and it has been suggested that PMS is the clinical manifestation of a calcium deficiency state that becomes overt when ovarian steroid hormones increase during the menstrual cycle.[13] The PMS symptoms of fatigue, depression, anxiety and muscle cramps also occur in hypocalcaemia.

Women with a low intake of calcium have been found to have a 30 per cent higher risk of PMS compared to those with a high intake, and calcium supplementation has led to improvements in fatigue, appetite changes and depression.[14] Calcium supplementation has been found to reduce PMS symptoms overall by 50 per cent.[15] A dietary calcium intake of 1336 mg per day has been found to improve mood, behaviour, pain and fluid retention, and result in an overall 48 per cent reduction in total symptoms by the third treatment cycle.[16]

Antacid activity

Calcium carbonate is popularly used as an over-the-counter antacid by people with gastro-oesophageal reflux disease (GORD), heartburn and gastric ulcers. Common antacids contain about 200 mg of elemental calcium per tablet. Calcium carbonate has been shown to give symptom relief, which was previously thought to be due to its action in neutralising stomach acid. However, more recent research has shown that antacids are primarily active in the oesophagus rather than the stomach. In a study comparing effervescent sodium-potassium bicarbonate solution, chewable antacids and calcium carbonate that was swallowed rather than chewed, it was found that chewable antacids elevated pH within the oesophagus, while the swallowed calcium carbonate had very little effect on oesophageal pH.[17] Only the effervescent sodium-potassium bicarbonate solution was able to elevate gastric pH. It was concluded that chewable antacids relieve acid reflux and related heartburn symptoms by neutralising acid within the oesophagus, rather than in the stomach.

REFERENCES

1 Winzenberg, T.M., Shaw, K., Fryer, J. & Jones, G., Calcium supplementation for improving bone mineral density in children, *Cochrane Database Syst Rev* (2006), 2: CD005119.
2 Thacher, T.D., Fischer, P.R., Pettifor, J.M. et al., A comparison of calcium, vitamin D, or both for nutritional rickets in Nigerian children, *N Engl J Med* (1999), 341(8): 563–8.
3 Australian Institute of Health and Welfare, *A snapshot of osteoporosis in Australia 2011*, AIHW, Canberra, 2011.
4 Tang, B.M., Eslick, G.D., Nowson, C. et al., Use of calcium or calcium in combination with vitamin D supplementation to prevent fractures and bone loss in people aged 50 years and older: A meta-analysis, *Lancet* (2007), 370(9588): 657–66.
5 Hacker, A.N., Fung, E.B. & King, J.C., Role of calcium during pregnancy: Maternal and fetal needs, *Nutr Rev* (2012), 70(7): 397–409.
6 Imdad, A., Jabeen, A. & Bhutta, Z.A., Role of calcium supplementation during pregnancy in reducing risk of developing gestational hypertensive disorders: A meta-analysis of studies from developing countries, *BMC Public Health* (2011), 11 Suppl 3: S18.

7 Hofmeyr, G.J., Lawrie, T.A., Atallah, A.N., Duley, L. & Torloni, M.R., Calcium supplementation during pregnancy for preventing hypertensive disorders and related problems, *Cochrane Database Syst Rev* (2014), 6: CD001059.
8 Buppasiri, P., Lumbiganon, P., Thinkhamrop, J. et al., Calcium supplementation (other than for preventing or treating hypertension) for improving pregnancy and infant outcomes, *Cochrane Database Syst Rev* (2011), 10: CD007079.
9 Janakiraman, V., Ettinger, A., Mercado-Garcia, A. et al., Calcium supplements and bone resorption in pregnancy: A randomized crossover trial, *Am J Prev Med* (2003), 24: 260–4.
10 Cole, Z.A., Gale, C.R., Javaid, M.K. et al., Maternal dietary patterns during pregnancy and childhood bone mass: A longitudinal study, *J Bone Miner Res* (2009), 24: 663–8.
11 Cho, E., Smith-Warner, S.A., Spiegelman, D. et al., Dairy foods, calcium, and colorectal cancer: A pooled analysis of 10 cohort studies, *J Natl Cancer Inst* (2004), 96: 1015–22.
12 Grau, M.V., Baron, J.A., Sandler, R.S. et al., Prolonged effect of calcium supplementation on risk of colorectal adenomas in a randomized trial, *J Natl Cancer Inst* (2007), 99: 129–36.
13 Thys-Jacobs, S., Micronutrients and the premenstrual syndrome: The case for calcium, *J Am Coll Nutr* (2000), 19(2): 220–7.
14 Bertone-Johnson, E.R., Hankinson, S.E., Bendich, A. et al., Calcium and vitamin D intake and risk of incident premenstrual syndrome, *Arch Intern Med* (2005), 165(11): 1246–52.
15 Thys-Jacobs, S., Ceccarelli, S., Bierman, A. et al., Calcium supplementation in premenstrual syndrome, *J Gen Intern Med* (1989), 4: 183–9.
16 Penland, J.G. & Johnson, P.E., Dietary calcium and manganese effects on menstrual cycle symptoms, *Am J Obstet Gynecol* (1993), 168: 1417–23.
17 Robinson, M., Rodriguez-Stanley, S., Miner, P.B. et al., Effects of antacid formulation on postprandial oesophageal acidity in patients with a history of episodic heartburn. *Aliment Pharmacol Ther* (2002), 16(3): 435–43.

Therapeutic dose

Vitamin D status should be assessed and, if required, controlled sun exposure and/or supplementation should be used with calcium supplementation to maximise calcium absorption. Improving dietary intake of calcium should be emphasised. Suggested doses of elemental calcium for adults, in addition to dietary calcium, are as follows:

- *Health maintenance:* 400–800 mg daily.
- *Mild deficiency:* 800 mg daily.
- *Severe deficiency:* 1000–1200 mg daily.
- *Bone disorders:* 1000–1200 mg daily.
- *PMS:* 1000–1200 mg daily.
- *Pregnancy:* 1000–1200 mg daily.
- *Antacids:* Up to 1200 mg daily (equivalent to 3000 mg calcium carbonate).

Effects of excess

Calcium supplements may cause constipation, bloating and flatulence in some people, which may be avoided by administering the supplement in divided doses (a maximum of 500 mg of elemental calcium per dose). The recommended upper level (UL) of calcium intake is 2500 mg/day in children and adults.

Hypercalcaemia

Hypercalcaemia (high serum calcium) occurs when calcium enters the ECF more rapidly than it can be excreted by the kidneys, leading to serum calcium levels rising above 2.6 mmol/L. Hypercalcaemia may be caused by cancer, parathyroid gland or kidney disorders, thiazide diuretics, lithium treatment for mental illness or vitamin D intoxication. It is unlikely to result from standard doses of calcium supplements because body levels are tightly controlled. However, excessively high doses of calcium (an elemental calcium intake of 1600 mg or more daily, which is equal to calcium carbonate intakes of 4000 mg/day or more) have been associated with a form of hypercalcaemia called milk-alkali syndrome (MAS), characterised by hypercalcaemia and metabolic acidosis. In the past, MAS has resulted from a high intake of calcium in the form of antacids and milk, which was a common method of relieving stomach ulcer symptoms. Treatment for this condition is now focused on inhibiting stomach acid production, and MAS has become less common. Most present-day cases occur in female patients taking calcium-containing medications for conditions such as autoimmune disease, organ transplantation, chronic renal failure and osteoporosis.

Hypercalcaemia may cause headache, constipation, elevated cerebrospinal fluid protein, kidney stones, heart dysfunction, high blood pressure, progressive lethargy, drowsiness, mental confusion, muscular weakness, depressed deep-tendon reflexes, convulsions and stupor, and coma may result if serum calcium concentrations rise above 3.5 mmol/L. Mental effects include personality changes, irritability, depression, confusion, poor attention span, poor memory, bizarre behaviour and psychosis. MAS symptoms include hypercalcaemia, hyperphosphataemia (elevated serum phosphate levels), alkalosis, kidney malfunction, and calcium deposits in soft tissue, and may be acute, intermediate or chronic. Chronic MAS may not be fully reversible.

Kidney stones

Dietary calcium does not appear to increase the risk of kidney stones, and does not increase urinary calcium oxalate excretion. In fact, low calcium intake has been found to increase the risk. However, calcium supplementation together with vitamin D has been shown to increase the risk of kidney stones in one study, while another study found that calcium supplements were associated with a small increased risk of kidney stone formation, whereas high dietary calcium was linked to a lower risk.

Prostate cancer

In one study, a high intake of calcium from diet and supplements was associated with risk of prostate cancer. It was not associated with total or non-advanced prostate cancer, but intakes of 1500–1999 mg daily were associated with a higher risk of advanced and fatal prostate cancer, with the most risk being linked to intakes of 2000 mg daily. The lowest risk occurred with intakes of 500–749 mg daily. More research is needed to clarify this risk.

Cardiovascular disease

Calcium deposits in artery walls are a feature of atherosclerosis, a major cause of myocardial infarction (MI, heart attack). Some evidence from research reviews suggests that calcium supplementation, with or without vitamin D, may increase the risk of MI and possibly stroke. However, some individual studies have not found this association and the conclusions of the review have not been universally accepted. More research is needed in this area.

Case reports—calcium excess

- *A pregnant woman, 40 years of age*, developed eclampsia.[1] She was found to have severe hypercalcaemia (corrected calcium level was 4.71 mmol/L) and metabolic alkalosis secondary to MAS. She reported self-medicating with multiple calcium-containing antacid tablets for dyspepsia. Discontinuation of antacid tablets and calcium-lowering treatment led to a full recovery, and her infant was not affected.
- *A man, 81 years of age*, developed lethargy, nausea, disorientation, confusion and sleepiness.[2] He was diagnosed with hypercalcaemia, acute renal failure and metabolic alkalosis, which resolved after treatment. He reported taking about 25 tablets of calcium carbonate every day as self-medication for prevention of osteoporosis.

REFERENCES

1 Metheny, N.M., Calcium imbalances, in *Fluid and Electrolyte Balance*, 5th ed., Jones & Bartlett Learning, New York, 2012.

2 Waked, A., Geara, A. & El-Imad, B., Hypercalcemia, metabolic alkalosis and renal failure secondary to calcium bicarbonate intake for osteoporosis prevention—'modern' milk alkali syndrome: A case report, *Cases J* (2009), 2: 6188.

Supplements

Calcium supplements can be made from powdered rock (especially limestone), seashells, coral, calcium-containing algae (seaweeds), eggshells and oyster shells, which all provide calcium as calcium carbonate. Some types of algae, such as the coralline alga *Corallina officinalis*, secrete calcium carbonate onto the surface of their cells, and are used as calcium supplements. Active Absorbable Algal Calcium (AAA Ca) is a combination of oyster shell and the alga *Cystophyllum fusiforme*, which is reported to be well absorbed and useful for maintaining BMD. Eggshell powder is a source of calcium that has positive effects on bone and cartilage. Bone meal provides calcium phosphate, together with other bone minerals. Natural sources may be contaminated with toxic metals from the environment, and products derived from them should undergo toxicological testing during manufacture.

In Australia, the permitted forms of calcium salts in supplements include calcium amino acid chelate, ascorbate, ascorbate dihydrate, carbonate, citrate, citrate hydrate, diglutamate, gluconate, glycerophosphate, hydrogen phosphate (anhydrous or monophosphate), hydroxide, lactate (anhydrous, gluconate, pentahydrate or trihydrate), orotate, phosphate, phosphate monobasic, sodium caseinate, sodium lactate, succinate and sulfate (dried or anhydrous), as well as microcrystalline hydroxyapatite derived from bone.

The amount of elemental calcium in a specific calcium salt is listed on the product container, and may vary between individual products; the approximate elemental calcium content of some common supplements is shown in Table 8.2.

Calcium supplements are available in tablets, chewable and effervescent formulas, capsules, suspensions and liquids. The most commonly used forms are calcium carbonate and calcium citrate. It is important that calcium tablets are not compacted excessively during manufacture because this may reduce the ability of the tablet to solubilise in the stomach. A method of checking approximate solubility is to soak a tablet in 200 mL vinegar for 30 minutes, stirring at five-minute intervals, by which time the tablet should have disintegrated completely. Absorption of calcium is greatest when taken in individual doses of 500 mg or less, and there is some evidence that taking calcium supplements in the evening may be of benefit to bone by suppressing the rise in bone resorption that occurs naturally while lying down during sleep.

Table 8.2 Elemental calcium content of common supplements

Supplement	Calcium content (%)
Calcium carbonate	40
Calcium phosphate	38
Calcium sulfate	36
Bone meal	31
Oyster shell	28
Microcrystalline hydroxyapatite	24
Dolomite (limestone)	22
Calcium citrate	21
Calcium amino acid chelate	20
Hydroxyapatite	20
Calcium phosphate monobasic	17
Calcium lactate	13
Calcium ascorbate	10
Calcium orotate	10
Calcium gluconate	9

- *Calcium carbonate* is produced from a raw material, usually rock such as limestone or marble, which is heated at high temperatures in the presence of a carbon dioxide-containing gas. This forms calcium carbonate which is then precipitated from solution. Elemental calcium can be obtained by replacing the calcium in calcium carbonate with aluminium in hot, low pressure retorts or by electrolysis of molten calcium chloride.

  Calcium carbonate is the starting material for production of other calcium salts. It is cheaper and contains the most elemental calcium of any of the available mineral salts. However, it is relatively insoluble at a neutral pH and, when taken on an empty stomach, is poorly absorbed by people who do not produce adequate stomach acid, a common problem in the elderly. In these people, it has been shown to be absorbed satisfactorily when taken with a meal. Medications used to treat GORD inhibit stomach acid production and may reduce the absorption of calcium carbonate.

- *Calcium citrate* is produced by the reaction of calcium carbonate, calcium hydroxide or calcium oxide with citric acid in aqueous solution. It is more soluble than calcium carbonate, and is more bioavailable. Calcium absorption from calcium citrate has been found to be 22–27 per cent greater than calcium absorption from calcium carbonate when taken on an empty stomach or with meals. However, it contains less elemental calcium and is more expensive. It is absorbed better than calcium carbonate by people with inadequate stomach acid, and does not have to be taken with meals. It may be the best form of calcium for people on medication for GORD, people with absorption disorders and those with a history of kidney stones because citrate in the urine inhibits calcium oxalate precipitation.
- *Calcium amino acid chelate* is produced by reacting calcium carbonate, calcium hydroxide or calcium oxide with one or more ligands, such as amino acids, protein hydrolysates, polypeptides or dipeptides, in an aqueous environment. Compared with calcium carbonate, it provides less elemental calcium but has been found to have greater bioavailability in humans and has a greater positive effect on BMD in animals.
- *Calcium phosphate* can be extracted from whey derived from milk or from calcium hydroxide from limestone, which is reacted with phosphoric acid. Calcium phosphate supplements appear to be absorbed equally as well as calcium carbonate in animal studies.
- *Calcium ascorbate* is produced by reacting calcium carbonate, calcium hydroxide or calcium oxide with ascorbic acid in an aqueous solution. It provides less elemental calcium than most other calcium salts, and is used primarily as a vitamin C supplement. Calcium appears to have greater bioavailability from calcium ascorbate than from calcium carbonate in animal studies, and bone uptake of calcium has been shown to be higher.
- *Microcrystalline hydroxyapatite (MCH)* is a calcium, phosphate, collagen and peptide supplement derived from bovine bones that also contains other minerals, such as magnesium and zinc. It is purified in the production process to remove contaminants. Although it does not provide as much elemental calcium, hydroxyapatite has been found to have a greater effect on bone growth than calcium carbonate, and a meta-analysis of six clinical trials found that hydroxyapatite is more effective than calcium carbonate in slowing bone loss in patients with osteoporosis.

Cautions

High doses of calcium may reduce the absorption of the following drugs when taken together: bisphosphonates (for bone disorders), the fluoroquinolone and tetracycline classes of antibiotics, levothyroxine (for thyroid function), sotalol (for irregular heart rhythm), phenytoin (for epilepsy) and tiludronate disodium (for Paget's disease). Calcium supplements should be taken two to four hours before or after the drug dose.

Calcium citrate, when taken with aluminium-containing antacids, increases the absorption of aluminium, which is potentially toxic. High doses of calcium may increase the risk of a toxic reaction to the heart drug digoxin. However, low levels of calcium cause digoxin to be ineffective. Taking calcium during treatment with the antibiotic gentamicin may increase the risk of kidney damage, and calcium should not be taken with beta-blockers, calcium-channel blockers or calcipotriene (synthetic calcitriol) without medical advice.

PHOSPHORUS

PHOSPHORUS STATUS CHECK

1. **Do you have low bone mineral density or a history of bone fractures?**
2. **Have your muscles become very weak, and do you have difficulty breathing or swallowing?**
3. **Do you regularly drink alcohol to excess?**
4. **Have you been diagnosed with abnormal heart rhythm or heart failure?**

'Yes' answers may indicate inadequate phosphorus status. Note that a number of nutritional deficiencies or health disorders can cause similar effects and further investigation is recommended.

FAST FACTS . . . PHOSPHORUS

- **Phosphorus is easily absorbed, and is found in animal foods, grains, seeds, nuts and legumes.**
- **Phosphorus is required for carbohydrate metabolism, and energy production and storage.**

- **It supports bone structure, cell structure and function, oxygen release and pH balance.**
- **A deficiency can cause low bone mineral density, osteomalacia and muscle paralysis.**
- **Supplementation may be helpful for the treatment of osteomalacia, osteoporosis or hypophosphataemic rickets.**

Phosphorus has the chemical symbol P, and is a naturally occurring mineral found in the environment as inorganic phosphate compounds such as apatite (calcium phosphate) in rocks. It was first isolated from urine by German alchemist Hennig Brand in 1669 during his quest to turn lead into gold. Its name derives from the Greek *phosphoros*, meaning 'bringing light', because white phosphorus burns when exposed to air and glows in the dark. Phosphorus is the second most abundant mineral in the body: 85 per cent is in bones, 14 per cent in soft tissue and only 1 per cent in body fluids.

Digestion, absorption and metabolism

Phosphorus in food occurs as organic compounds and inorganic phosphates. During digestion, phosphate compounds are solubilised in the stomach by hydrochloric acid and organic forms are hydrolysed by zinc-dependent enzymes to release inorganic phosphate, the absorbed form. Absorption from food ranges from 50–70 per cent, and is higher from animal than plant foods. Phosphorus is absorbed rapidly by passive diffusion, and also by active transport mediated by sodium-dependent phosphate type IIb cotransporters and regulated by calcitriol, the active form of vitamin D. It appears that there is no ceiling for absorption of phosphorus, and blood levels rise rapidly after meals. Absorbed phosphorus is transferred from the small intestine to the ECF and then to the bloodstream. About 70 per cent circulates in the form of organic phosphate, such as phospholipids, and 30 per cent as free monohydrogen and dihydrogen phosphate and inorganic phosphate that is protein bound or bound to sodium, magnesium or calcium.

Metabolism, storage and excretion

Tissues take up phosphorus from the bloodstream mainly via the activity of type III sodium-dependent phosphate cotransporters. Type II sodium phosphate cotransporters are found in the kidneys, intestine, salivary glands, mammary glands and lung, and type I sodium phosphate cotransporters appear to be important for urate handling in the kidneys. Alkalosis and glucose may promote the entry of phosphate into cells. Inside cells, phosphorus is present mainly as part of organic esters of phosphoric acid, including adenosine triphosphate (ATP), 2,3-diphosphoglycerate (2,3-DPG) and cyclic adenosine monophosphate (cAMP). The main storage site is bone, in which it is found as hydroxyapatite. The kidneys are the major regulator of serum levels of phosphorus. Inorganic phosphate in the blood is filtered into kidney tubules and reabsorbed via the type IIa sodium-dependent phosphate cotransporter or excreted in urine. Approximately two-thirds of ingested phosphorus is excreted in urine, and the remainder in faeces.

Regulation of serum phosphate

Phosphate balance is maintained primarily by the bones and kidneys, and regulated by hormones, including parathyroid hormone (PTH), calcitriol and a number of peptides collectively known as phosphatonins. When serum phosphate levels are high, the phosphatonin fibroblast growth factor-23 (FGF-23) is secreted from bone and acts on the kidneys to stimulate rapid removal of phosphate in urine and to reduce calcitriol production, thereby inhibiting active phosphate absorption from food. FGF-23 works with the co-receptor klotho, a transmembrane protein in kidney tubules that binds and activates FGF receptors.

Phosphorus excretion is also stimulated by an increased level of fluid in the body, metabolic acidosis and the hormones PTH, glucocorticoids and calcitonin, and phosphorus excretion is decreased by growth hormone and thyroid hormone. When serum phosphate levels decrease, PTH acts on the kidneys to stimulate calcitriol production, which increases blood calcium and phosphate levels by increasing uptake from food, and mobilising calcium and phosphate from bone. Although PTH reduces calcium losses in urine, it promotes excretion of phosphate and, overall, increases serum calcium levels rather than phosphorus. Positive phosphorus balance (intake greater than excretion) occurs during skeletal growth in childhood and adolescence, and during pregnancy and lactation.

Functions

Phosphorus is important for the structure of bones and cells, energy storage, enzyme and protein activity, oxygen release, detoxification and the buffering of acids and alkalis to maintain a healthy body pH. Phosphorus has an acidic effect on body pH. The functions of phosphorus include:

- *Carbohydrate metabolism and energy production*. Glucose metabolism in cells generates energy, which is contained in molecules such as ATP, which have high-energy phosphate bonds that are broken to release energy as required for cell activities (see Figure 8.2). Creatine phosphate is a source of energy in muscle cells and the brain. During intense but very brief exercise, such as lifting a heavy weight, ATP stores are quickly depleted and creatine phosphate transfers a high-energy phosphate to regenerate ATP.

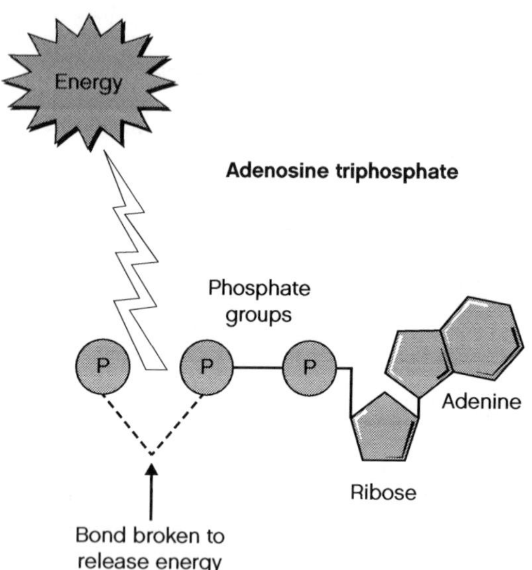

Figure 8.2 Production of energy from adenosine triphosphate

Uridine triphosphate (UTP) is an activator of substrates in metabolic reactions by releasing a phosphate and forming uridine diphosphate (UDP), which is bound to the substrate. UDP-glucose is essential for the conversion of glucose to glycogen and UDP-galactose is required for galactose metabolism. UDP-glucuronate is part of transferase enzymes that add glucuronic acid, derived from glucose, to a wide range of potentially toxic fat-soluble substances, generating products that are more polar and more easily excreted in bile or urine.

- *Bone formation*. Phosphorus is a major structural component of teeth and bones. As calcium phosphate, it is part of hydroxyapatite that forms the crystalline structure of mature bone tissue, providing strength and rigidity to the skeleton and acting as a reserve store of phosphorus that can be mobilised when required to maintain healthy blood levels. Inorganic phosphorus moves in and out of bone mineral by ionic exchange and active bone resorption. Children and adolescents need an adequate calcium and phosphorus intake in order to achieve maximum bone mass in young adulthood and to maintain a healthy BMD in later life.
- *Cell structure and function*. Phosphorus is part of phospholipids that are an integral part of the structure of cell membranes, and the membranes of organelles within cells. It is also part of the structure of the nucleic acids RNA and DNA. As part of cAMP, phosphorus acts as a second messenger in cells. cAMP responds to hormone messages by activating protein kinase enzymes that transfer phosphates from nucleotide triphosphates to proteins to form phosphorylated proteins, which play a key role in most cell activities. In many metabolic reactions, protein and enzyme activation and inhibition are regulated by phosphorylation and dephosphorylation processes. Inositol triphosphate (IP_3) is another phosphate-containing second messenger that acts by triggering calcium release inside cells.
- *Oxygen transfer*. The phosphate compound 2,3-DPG binds to haemoglobin in red blood cells and helps release oxygen to tissues.
- *pH balance*. Phosphates are not important buffers in blood, but have buffering activity inside cells and in urine. In cells, dihydrogen phosphate is able to donate a hydrogen ion (acid), thus lowering pH, and hydrogen phosphate is able to accept a hydrogen ion, thus raising pH. In urine, phosphate is an important buffer that enables excretion of large amounts of hydrogen ions without lowering urinary pH beyond its lower limit (approximately pH 4.4). To alkalise urine, disodium hydrogen phosphate accepts a hydrogen ion and donates a sodium ion (base), raising urinary pH and forming sodium dihydrogen phosphate, which is excreted. The released sodium ion binds with bicarbonate to form sodium bicarbonate, and is reabsorbed into the blood. To acidify urine, sodium dihydrogen phosphate can donate a hydrogen ion and accept a sodium ion, forming disodium hydrogen phosphate, which is excreted.

Dietary sources

Phosphorus is amply supplied in the diet, and a deficiency is not common in healthy people. It is found in grains, seeds, nuts, legumes, meat, fish, chicken, dairy products and eggs. Phosphorus is part of phytate (*myo*-inositol hexaphosphate), a storage compound for phosphorus in grains, bran, seeds and nuts that binds calcium, potassium, magnesium, iron and zinc, and inhibits their absorption in the gut. Wheat bran, wheat germ, brewer's yeast, lecithin and bone meal are rich sources of phosphorus. Phosphorus is also present in cola soft drinks as phosphoric acid, and phosphates are commonly-used food additives. Intake of phosphorus is believed to be increasing because of the increased use of phosphate additives in processed food.

The Food Standards Australia New Zealand nutrient database (NUTTAB) at <www.foodstandards.gov.au> provides the amounts found in specific foods.

Factors influencing body status

Animal foods are richer in bioavailable phosphorus than plant foods. Phosphorus is water soluble, and may be lost from foods by water-processing and cooking methods. Digestive disorders and inadequate stomach acid may impair absorption, and kidney damage may increase losses in urine and lead to a disturbed phosphorus balance.

Phosphate binders such as aluminium hydroxide, calcium carbonate, calcium acetate, lanthanum carbonate, sevelamer and calcium acetate/magnesium carbonate are used to reduce elevated levels of phosphate in chronic kidney disease, and act by decreasing phosphorus absorption. High-dose calcium supplementation can decrease phosphorus absorption; an intake of 1000 to 1500 mg of elemental calcium daily can bind up to 500 mg of phosphorus. Hypercalcaemia increases phosphate losses in urine, whereas hypocalcaemia reduces urinary phosphate losses. A lack of vitamin D may impair active absorption of phosphorus in the gut, and over-activity of PTH increases losses in urine. Other causes of increased urinary losses include an expansion of ECF volume, acute metabolic alkalosis, chronic metabolic acidosis, thiazide diuretics and the disorders X-linked hypophosphataemic rickets, autosomal-dominant hypophosphataemic rickets and tumour-induced osteomalacia. Alcoholics are at risk of impaired phosphorus balance because of intestinal malabsorption; inadequate levels of vitamin D, magnesium and albumin; respiratory and metabolic alkalosis; and pancreatitis. Drugs that increase bone resorption and decrease bone formation (Depo-Provera, anti-epileptic drugs, corticosteroids, unfractionated heparin and thiazolidinedione) may increase the need for phosphate as well as calcium.

Daily requirement

Government recommendations by age and gender (see Table 8.3) can be found in *Nutrient Reference Values for Australia and New Zealand Including Recommended Dietary Intakes*, available at <www.nhmrc.gov.au>.

Table 8.3 Recommended dietary intake (RDI) of phosphorus (mg/day)

Age (years)	Female RDI	Male RDI
1–3	460	460
4–8	500	500
9–13	1250	1250
14–18	1250	1250
19–50	1000	1000
51–70	1000	1000
>70	1000	1000
Pregnant women		
14–18	1250	
19–50	1000	
Lactating women		
14–18	1250	
19–50	1000	

Source: Nutrient Reference Values for Australia and New Zealand Including Recommended Dietary Intakes, National Health and Medical Research Council, Australian Government Department of Health and Ageing, Canberra and Ministry of Health, New Zealand, Wellington, 2006.

Deficiency effects

A low phosphorus intake is not common because of its widespread availability in food, and blood levels are maintained by mobilisation from bones and conservation by the kidneys even when intake is inadequate. Elderly people are more at risk of a low phosphorus intake.

A low serum phosphate level (hypophosphataemia) is rare in healthy people, but can be caused by increased urinary excretion, movement of phosphate into cells—which occurs in critically ill patients—or, rarely, decreased intestinal absorption. Hypophosphataemia may be found in association with chronic alcoholism, diabetic ketoacidosis, chronic ingestion of phosphate-binding antacids, total parenteral nutrition (non-oral feeding) with inadequate phosphate replacement, refeeding after prolonged starvation, use of drugs such as acetazolamide (for glaucoma and epilepsy), foscarnet (for HIV), imatinib and sorafenib (for cancer), and pentamidine (an antibiotic), and in Fanconi syndrome (a kidney disease), hyperparathyroidism or inadequate vitamin D.

If serum phosphorus levels drop, ATP and 2,3-DPG are not produced efficiently, leading to depletion of cellular energy reserves, inadequate oxygenation of tissues, and cell membrane dysfunction and destruction. Glycogen production and bone formation are impaired, and abnormalities of serum magnesium, calcium and potassium levels may occur. Low phosphorus can cause release of calcium from bones and increase losses in urine.

If hypophosphataemia is mild, there may be no symptoms. In more severe hypophosphataemia, the most common symptom is weakness of the skeletal or smooth muscles, which can affect any muscle group and cause a range of symptoms, such as double vision, difficulty speaking and swallowing, and weakness of the large muscle groups of the trunk or extremities. The heart and respiratory muscles may become weak, leading to poor ventricular function, irregular heartbeat, heart failure and difficulty breathing. Muscle tissue may break down (rhabdomyolysis) because ATP is depleted and muscles are unable to maintain membrane integrity—an effect seen more commonly in patients undergoing acute alcohol withdrawal.

Hypophosphataemia may cause impaired mineralisation of bones, leading to bone pain, rickets in children and osteomalacia in adults. However, these bone conditions are more commonly caused by inadequate vitamin D. Bone disorders that are specifically related to hypophosphataemia include X-linked hypophosphataemia (XLH), autosomal-dominant hypophosphataemic rickets (ADHR) and tumour-induced osteomalacia. XLH is the most common form of vitamin D-resistant rickets, and is caused by reduced expression of sodium-phosphate cotransporters in the kidneys, leading to excessive phosphorus losses in urine. XLH is associated with low levels of calcitriol and elevated levels of FGF-23 and alkaline phosphatase (an enzyme involved in bone metabolism).

Other symptoms of hypophosphataemia include loss of appetite, general debility, destruction of red blood cells (haemolytic anaemia), impaired immunity, paraesthesia, ataxia, seizures and mental confusion, and may result in coma and death. Peripheral neuropathy, brain damage and ascending muscle paralysis, similar to Guillain-Barré syndrome, may occur.

Indicators of inadequate levels of phosphorus may include:

- osteomalacia: low BMD, soft bones, bone pain, bone deformities, fractures
- hypophosphataemic rickets in children
- muscle weakness, paralysis, double vision, difficulty speaking and swallowing, breathing difficulties, ataxia
- heart dysfunction, irregular heart rhythm, heart failure
- haemolytic anaemia
- paraesthesia, mental confusion, seizures.

Assessment of body status

Serum phosphate concentration is not regarded as an accurate assessment of body status in healthy people because it is tightly regulated, and abnormal concentrations are usually a result of an underlying health disorder. Urinary phosphate is regulated by PTH as well as by dietary intake, and also may not accurately reflect status. However, an elevated urinary concentration may reflect a high dietary intake or a health issue that is causing excessive losses, and low urinary concentration may indicate a low dietary intake. The reference range given by the RCPA for adults is 0.8–1.5 mmol/L for serum phosphate and 10–40 mmol/day for urine. BMD can be assessed by a DXA scan.

Case reports—phosphorus deficiency

- *A male infant, 22 months of age*, developed generalised oedema, hyperpigmented and hypopigmented skin lesions, abdominal distension, irritability and thin, sparse hair.[1] He had been exclusively breastfed until thirteen months of age and then, because of a history of chronic eczema and suspected milk intolerance, was given a rice 'milk' beverage with very little solid food. The rice drink provided very inadequate amounts of protein and kilojoules. His serum albumin and phosphorus were found to be low. He was diagnosed with severe protein-energy malnutrition and was given gradual refeeding and nutritional supplementation. This was followed by a toddler formula and then a milk-based paediatric nutritional supplement in addition to a regular diet. The child made a total recovery.

- *A woman, 42 years of age*, developed bone pain in the lower extremities over a two-week period.[2] She was found to have severe hypophosphataemia, elevated levels of alkaline phosphatase and calcitriol, microfractures in her bones and indications of osteomalacia. She had a history of duodenal ulcer and had been on long-term treatment with a magnesium-aluminium hydroxide antacid and the drug sucralfate. She recovered completely after withdrawal of the antacids and sucralfate, and short-term treatment with phosphate supplementation.
- *A woman, 49 years of age*, with diabetes, was admitted to intensive care in a coma and with severe ketoacidosis.[3] On treatment, her acidosis and glucose levels improved but her brain dysfunction worsened. She was found to have severe hypophosphataemia (less than 0.20 mmol/L) and prompt phosphate repletion resulted in a progressive and complete recovery.
- *A woman, 34 years of age*, experienced muscle weakness and bone pain, and had a history of multiple fractures of her upper and lower limbs following trivial trauma since she was fourteen years of age.[4] She was found to also have dental caries, spinal and knee deformities and shortening of her left leg. Her serum phosphate and vitamin D levels were low, and alkaline phosphate levels were raised. She was diagnosed with hereditary hypophosphataemic rickets, although no other members of her family were affected. The outcome of treatment was not reported.

REFERENCES

1 Carvalho, N.F., Kenney, R.D., Carrington, P.H. & Hall, D.E., Severe nutritional deficiencies in toddlers resulting from health food milk alternatives, *Pediatrics* (2001), 107(4): E46.

2 Chines, A. & Pacifici, R., Antacid and sucralfate-induced hypophosphatemic osteomalacia: A case report and review of the literature, *Calcif Tissue Int* (1990), 47(5): 291–5.

3 Mégarbane, B., Guerrier, G., Blancher, A. et al., A possible hypophosphatemia-induced, life-threatening encephalopathy in diabetic ketoacidosis: A case report, *Am J Med Sci* (2007), 333(6): 384–6.

4 Baidya, A., Chowdhury, S., Mukhopadhyay, S. & Ghosh, S., Hypophosphatemic rickets: A case of recurrent pathological fractures, *Indian J Endocrinol Metab* (2012), 16(Suppl 2): S402–4.

THERAPEUTIC USES OF PHOSPHORUS

Phosphorus is rarely needed in supplement form because it is readily available from a wide range of foods and is well absorbed. An increased phosphate intake in the diet may be needed in elderly people, who are more likely to have inadequate diets. High-dose phosphate supplementation is primarily used under medical supervision for phosphate replacement therapy in patients with hypophosphataemia, and as a treatment for hypercalcaemia, osteoporosis, Paget's disease (a bone growth disorder), hypophosphataemic rickets, calcium-based kidney stones and diabetic ketoacidosis. Phosphates are also used in enemas as saline laxatives. Phosphates are commonly used for the following:

Bone disorders

Phosphates, in the form of bisphosphonate drugs, are used to improve BMD in osteoporosis and to reduce abnormal bone growth in Paget's disease. Bisphosphonates are prescription medications that are chemically stable analogues of inorganic pyrophosphate, and can be given orally or by infusion. They bind to hydroxyapatite in bone and inhibit osteoclast activity, reducing the breakdown and removal of bone. In osteoporosis, they have been shown to be effective in reducing fracture risk at the spine, hip and other skeletal sites, and are associated with a significant decrease in morbidity and mortality.[1]

In hypophosphataemic rickets, there is a severe loss of urinary phosphate, and medical treatment includes the use of calcitriol, and oral potassium phosphate and sodium acid phosphate, as phosphate replacement therapy. Early treatment can minimise growth impairment, limb deformities and teeth abnormalities, but may not correct the growth deficit, especially when treatment is commenced at a later age.[2]

Laxative activity

Oral or rectal sodium phosphate is used as a medical treatment for constipation and oral sodium phosphate solution (OSPS) is used to evacuate the bowel prior to a colonoscopy.[3]

REFERENCES

1 McClung, M., Harris, S.T., Miller, P.D. et al., Bisphosphonate therapy for osteoporosis: Benefits, risks, and drug holiday, *Am J Med* (2013), 126: 13–20.
2 de Menezes Filho, H., de Castro, L.C. & Damiani, D., Hypophosphatemic rickets and osteomalacia, *Arq Bras Endocrinol Metabol* (2006), 50(4): 802–13.
3 Selby, W., Managing constipation in adults, *Aust Prescr* (2010), 33: 116–19.

Therapeutic dose

Vitamin D status should be assessed and if required, controlled sun exposure and/or supplementation should be used to maximise phosphorus absorption.

Suggested doses of elemental phosphorus for adults are as follows:

- *Health maintenance:* 1000 mg daily from the diet.
- *Mild deficiency:* 1000 mg daily from the diet.
- *Severe deficiency:* medical advice and prescription medication required.
- *Bone disorders:* medical advice and prescription medication required.

Effects of excess

The recommended upper level of intake (UL) for dietary phosphorus is 4000 mg daily for adults, 3500 mg daily in pregnancy and 3000 mg daily for people over 70 years. Phosphate toxicity induced by excessive administration of phosphate salts can lead to low serum calcium and associated symptoms, including tetany, low blood pressure, and tachycardia (fast heart rate), and can be fatal. Bisphosphonate drugs and phosphate salts can lower calcium levels in the body; more common adverse effects of phosphate salts include nausea, vomiting, diarrhoea, dizziness or headache, and reported adverse effects of bisphosphonate drugs include osteonecrosis (bone death) of the jaw, atypical fractures of the femur, atrial fibrillation (heart arrhythmia) and oesophageal cancer.

A higher phosphate intake and lower calcium:phosphorus ratio in the diet has not been found to lower calcium absorption. However, a high phosphorus intake may impair calcium balance—especially if the diet is low in calcium—because, at high levels, phosphorus can form complexes that reduce serum calcium, which stimulates PTH release and mobilises calcium from bones. High dietary phosphorus has been shown to cause bone loss in animals, and the ratio of calcium to phosphorus in the diet appears to be important for bone health. In animal studies, feeding phosphoric acid-containing soft drinks causes increased losses of calcium and phosphorus in urine, and reduced bone mineralisation. Consumption of phosphoric acid-containing soft drinks is associated with low serum calcium levels in postmenopausal women. Dietary phosphorus loading in human studies has caused temporary elevation of serum phosphorus, which is associated with impaired endothelial function in blood vessels and impaired vasodilation. Impaired vasodilation has been shown to be caused by decreased nitric oxide (NO) production in endothelial cells.

High serum phosphorus (hyperphosphataemia)

There is a transient rise in serum phosphate after meals, but sustained hyperphosphataemia is almost always related to kidney disease or genetic factors such as a deficiency of FGF-23, either of which can reduce urinary excretion. Hyperphosphataemia leads to a drop in serum calcium, elevated PTH and calcitriol, defective bone mineralisation, calcium deposits in soft tissue, such as arterial walls and kidney tubules, and the formation of calcium kidney stones. Low serum magnesium, elevated sodium and metabolic acidosis are also associated with hyperphosphataemia.

Elderly patients treated with phosphate-containing laxatives or enemas have developed elevated serum levels of phosphate within an hour, and a decrease in serum calcium levels by twelve hours. In children, phosphate-containing enemas have caused a wide range of complications, including tetany, dehydration, low blood pressure, tachycardia, fever, cardiac arrest and coma.

Cardiovascular calcification

Hyperphosphataemia is regarded as a risk factor for CVD because it promotes calcium phosphate deposits (calcification) in blood vessels, the heart muscle and heart valves. People with chronic kidney disease (CKD) are at considerably increased risk of calcification and CVD. In blood vessels, calcification can take place in the intima muscle layer of arteries, which is associated with atherosclerosis (plaque accumulation), and in the medial muscle layer, which is associated with arteriosclerosis (hardening of the arteries). In general, CKD patients are more at risk of medial muscle calcification, and calcification occurs decades earlier in these patients than in the general population. Vascular calcification is associated with MI, stroke and all-cause and CVD mortality.

In people with normal kidney function, it has also been shown that a serum phosphorus concentration at the higher end of the normal range can be a risk factor for atherosclerosis and carotid intima media thickness (atherosclerosis affecting the medial muscle layer of the carotid artery in the neck), as well as mortality. A study of people without clinically apparent kidney disease or CVD found that each 0.32 mmol/L increase in serum phosphorus concentration was associated with a 31 per cent increased risk of a first major cardiovascular event, and another study found that there was a 27 per cent greater risk of all-cause mortality for each 0.32 mmol/L increase in serum phosphorus.

Kidney damage

Hyperphosphataemia is associated with nephrocalcinosis (calcium phosphate deposits in kidney nephrons), kidney stones and kidney damage, and may progress to kidney failure. A high-phosphate diet has induced nephrocalcinosis in animal studies, and it has been observed in patients given phosphate therapy and calcitriol for treatment of hypophosphataemic rickets. Calcium phosphate deposits can cause long-lasting damage to kidney tubules that may progress to fibrosis and loss of nephrons, and appears to be irreversible.

In people with normal kidney function, hyperphosphataemia, elevated urinary phosphate and nephrocalcinosis can occur following treatment with OSPS as a laxative prior to colonoscopy, and has been termed 'phosphate nephropathy' (PN). In 20 per cent of patients, PN progresses to end-stage renal disease, and variable degrees of CKD may occur in the remainder of patients. Other complications of OSPS include low serum calcium and potassium, elevated sodium and metabolic acidosis. Patients with abnormal gut motility, which boosts phosphate absorption, patients given an excessive dose and patients of advanced age are more at risk of PN following OSPS use.

Premature ageing

In animals, defects in either FGF-23 or klotho cause hyperphosphataemia and a premature ageing syndrome, which can be resolved by reducing blood phosphorus levels. Effects of this premature ageing syndrome in animals include shortened lifespan, growth retardation, under-developed sex organs, thymus, skin and muscle wasting, vascular calcification, osteopenia, pulmonary emphysema, impaired hearing and cognition, and motor neuron degeneration. Elevated phosphorus may promote premature ageing by affecting glucose metabolism, insulin sensitivity and oxidative stress. The effect of hyperphosphataemia on the human ageing process is not known.

Case reports—phosphorus excess

- *A woman, 71 years of age*, developed raised serum creatinine (a breakdown product of muscle creatine) over a ten-week period after use of an OSPS prior to a colonoscopy.[1] A kidney biopsy showed numerous calcium phosphate deposits in her kidney tubules, and her elevated creatinine persisted over twelve months, indicating long-term kidney damage.
- *A man, 79 years of age*, with chronic kidney failure requiring haemodialysis, developed a headache that

persisted for six months.[2] His headache was a dull pain of moderate to severe intensity that was not localised and occurred daily. No obvious cause of the headache was found, and it did not respond to any treatment. A scan of his head revealed calcification in areas of his brain. He was found to have elevated serum phosphorus and PTH and low serum calcium. He was treated with a low-phosphorus diet, phosphate-binding medication, vitamin D and calcium. His serum calcium and phosphate levels normalised and his headache greatly improved, with mild to moderate headaches occurring only occasionally. However, there was no change to the calcification in his brain.

- *A woman, 30 years of age*, developed extreme mental agitation after the onset of carpal (hand) spasm, a tingling sensation in her legs, and numbness around her mouth.[3] Symptoms occurred after her second dose of OSPS before a colonoscopy. She was found to have a positive Chvostek's sign and hyperphosphataemia, hypocalcaemia, low serum potassium (hypokalaemia) and respiratory alkalosis. The excess phosphate from OSPS had formed complexes with calcium, causing acute hypocalcaemic tetany, which was further aggravated by hyperventilation causing acute respiratory alkalosis. Subsequent investigations revealed that she also had type 1 renal tubular acidosis, due to previously undiagnosed Sjögren's syndrome. Her symptoms resolved with iv calcium treatment.

REFERENCES

1 Desmeules, S., Bergeron, M.J. & Isenring, P., Acute phosphate nephropathy and renal failure, *N Engl J Med* (2003), 349(10): 1006–7.

2 Razdan, S., Pandita, K., Chopra, V. & Koul, S., New-onset headache in an elderly man with uremia that improved only after correction of hyperphosphatemia ('uremic headache'): A case report, *J Med Case Rep* (2011), 5: 77.

3 Cho, S.G., Yi, J.H., Han, S.W. & Kim, H.J., Electrolyte imbalances and nephrocalcinosis in acute phosphate poisoning on chronic type 1 renal tubular acidosis due to Sjögren's syndrome, *J Korean Med Sci* (2013), 28(2): 336–9.

Supplements

Phosphorus is rarely used in supplement form, except under medical supervision as a laxative or for specific health conditions. Lecithin is a rich source of organic phosphate compounds, including phosphatidylcholine (PC), phosphatidylethanolamine (PE) and phosphatidylinositol (PI). However, it is ingested in small quantities only, and is not a significant phosphorus source compared with food. Small amounts of phosphorus are found in the following vitamin and mineral supplements: calcium glycerophosphate, hydrogen phosphate and phosphate; ferric glycerophosphate and pyrophosphate; ferrous phosphate; iron phosphate; magnesium glycerophosphate and phosphate; manganese glycerophosphate; potassium glycerophosphate and phosphate; pyridoxal 5'-phosphate; riboflavin sodium phosphate; sodium glycerophosphate and phosphate; and thiamine phosphate acid ester; and also in the supplements creatine phosphate, PC, PE and phosphatidylserine (PS). Mineral salts containing phosphates are produced commercially by combining the mineral with phosphoric acid.

Cautions

High-dose phosphate salts should only be used under medical supervision. Use of high-dose phosphate salts can cause hyperphosphataemia, hypocalcaemia, hypokalaemia, calcium deposits in soft tissue, CVD, kidney damage and other serious and possibly life-threatening side-effects. Phosphate salts can irritate the digestive tract and cause stomach upsets, diarrhoea or constipation, and can bind dietary or supplemental iron and magnesium, and impair absorption of these minerals.

MAGNESIUM

MAGNESIUM STATUS CHECK

1 **Do you have high blood pressure or elevated serum cholesterol?**
2 **Do you have episodes of heart palpitations?**

3 Do you often have muscle weakness, cramps, spasms, tremors, twitches or a feeling of a lump in your throat?
4 Do you feel nervous, tense and irritable, and have mood swings?

'Yes' answers may indicate inadequate magnesium status. Note that a number of nutritional deficiencies or health disorders can cause similar effects and further investigation is recommended.

FAST FACTS . . . MAGNESIUM

- Sources of magnesium include nuts, seeds, legumes and whole grains.
- Magnesium is essential for energy production and storage.
- It acts as a calcium channel blocker.
- A deficiency leads to hyper excitability of nerves and muscles.
- Supplementation may be helpful for a healthy pregnancy, and to protect against cardiovascular disease, diabetes and calcium deposits in soft tissue.

Magnesium has the chemical symbol Mg, and is found in the environment in compounds such as iron-magnesium silicate, magnesite (magnesium carbonate) and dolomite. It makes up about 2.1 per cent of the earth's crust, and is found in mineral water as magnesium sulfate and in sea water as magnesium chloride. The waters of the Dead Sea contain particularly high levels of magnesium chloride.

Magnesium was discovered by Scottish chemist Joseph Black in 1755, and isolated by English chemist Sir Humphry Davy in 1808. In 1831, French scientist Antoine-Alexandre-Brutus Bussy discovered that large amounts of magnesium could be produced by reacting magnesium chloride with potassium. Davy named the element 'magnium', which was later changed to magnesium, a name thought to be derived from Magnesia, a district in Thessaly, Greece.

In plants, magnesium occupies a central position in the chlorophyll molecule and enables photosynthesis, whereas iron occupies the central position in haemoglobin in animals. In the body, 50–60 per cent of magnesium is in bones, 20–25 per cent in soft tissue—especially the muscles, liver and kidneys—and about 1 per cent is in ECF, with 0.3 per cent of total body content in serum.

Digestion, absorption and metabolism

Magnesium is found in foods as various salts that are more soluble and more bioavailable than calcium salts. Magnesium salts solubilise in the acid medium of the stomach to release magnesium cations (Mg^{2+}) that are absorbed in the small intestine. At lower levels of intake, absorption of magnesium is an active process mediated by transient receptor potential cation channel melastatin member 6 (TRPM6) and member 7 (TRPM7). At higher levels of intake, magnesium is absorbed by passive paracellular diffusion, and it is estimated that 80–90 per cent of dietary magnesium is absorbed by this route. Overall, an average of about 40–60 per cent is absorbed, which increases to about 75 per cent if magnesium status is inadequate. If magnesium status is high, absorption is reduced.

After absorption, magnesium is transferred to the bloodstream by a sodium and energy-dependent transporter, and possibly by a calcium-dependent transporter. In plasma, about half the magnesium content is in the form of free magnesium ions, about 33 per cent is bound to proteins, such as albumin and globulins, and about 5 per cent is bound to anions such as citrate and phosphate. Free magnesium in serum has the greatest biological activity and is taken up by cells via the transporter TRPM7.

Metabolism, storage and excretion

Inside cells, about 1–5 per cent of the magnesium content is found as free magnesium ions and the remainder is bound to proteins, negatively charged molecules and ATP. Magnesium is believed to be removed from cells via a sodium–magnesium exchanger and a sodium-independent magnesium transporter, but the exact mechanism is unclear. The major pathway for excretion of magnesium is via the kidneys, with small amounts lost in faeces and sweat. TRPM6 and claudins (magnesium-binding proteins) in kidney tubules may play an important role in magnesium conservation. In normal conditions, about 3–5 per cent of filtered magnesium is lost in urine and the remainder is reabsorbed.

Regulation of serum magnesium

Body concentrations are regulated according to body needs by the kidneys, which increase or reduce urinary excretion, and by the intestines, which increase or reduce absorption. Bones and muscles contain a reserve of magnesium, and bone magnesium can be mobilised to maintain plasma levels. Parathyroid hormone (PTH) helps to maintain serum levels by increasing magnesium conservation by the kidneys, increasing absorption of dietary magnesium and mobilising magnesium from bones. Although vitamin D also enhances magnesium absorption, it does not greatly affect magnesium status because it also enhances excretion. Hormones such as antidiuretic hormone, angiotensin II (a vasoconstrictor) and insulin appear to enhance magnesium accumulation inside cells. Oestrogen increases plasma levels of magnesium by increasing TRPM6 expression.

Functions

Magnesium is essential for the structure or activation of more than 300 enzyme systems. It is part of bones, where it acts as a structural component and a magnesium reserve, and it has a key role in cell function, energy use, muscle and nerve function, and calcium metabolism. Magnesium has an alkaline effect on body pH. The functions of magnesium include the following:

- *Cell function*. In cells, magnesium has a structural role in proteins, polyribosomes, nucleic acids, enzyme complexes and mitochondria. It supports amino acid function, protein synthesis and activity of delta-6-desaturase that takes part in essential fatty acid metabolism. Magnesium is bound to phospholipids in cell membranes, where it has a role in membrane stabilisation, cell adhesion and transport of electrolytes. It has a particular role in regulating potassium concentrations in cells. Magnesium assists nucleic acid synthesis and breakdown, and DNA and RNA transcription, and helps maintain the integrity of DNA. It promotes cell proliferation, cell cycle progression, cell differentiation and cell survival. It also assists the production and function of cAMP, a second messenger that mediates hormone activity in cells.
- *Enzyme function*. In enzyme systems, magnesium can bind to a substrate to enable enzyme activity or directly attach to the enzyme to activate it. Enzymes that are magnesium-dependent include a wide range of kinases, ATPases and cyclases that are essential for normal cell function.
- *Energy production and use*. Magnesium is essential for the formation, storage and use of high-energy compounds. It binds to adenosine diphosphate (ADP) and ATP, and assists in the transfer of phosphate groups and energy release. Magnesium functions in key energy-producing pathways, including glycolysis, the citric acid cycle and the breakdown of fatty acids for use in energy production. Magnesium is required for the production of creatine phosphate, an energy source in muscles, and for the function of the hexose monophosphate shunt, which produces NADPH from NADP. NADPH is required for fatty acid synthesis, cholesterol synthesis, drug detoxification and the production of ribose for nucleotide and nucleic acid synthesis. Magnesium is a cofactor for enzymes required for glucose metabolism, insulin activity and insulin secretion by the pancreas.
- *Calcium metabolism*. Magnesium supports calcium homeostasis because it is required for PTH release, metabolism of vitamin D and sensitivity of target tissues to PTH and calcitriol. Magnesium regulates calcium metabolism by acting as a calcium channel blocker. It controls movement of calcium inside cells by inhibiting inositol triphosphate (IP_3), a messenger chemical that triggers calcium release from storage sites. Magnesium controls calcium movement across cell membranes, and activates the calcium-ATPase pump that removes calcium from cells. It may also bind directly to calcium sites and competitively inhibit calcium-dependent activation. Calcium enables apoptosis and magnesium has an antagonistic effect, promoting cell survival.
- *Cardiovascular function*. Magnesium acts in smooth and cardiac muscles to help regulate vascular tone and stabilise heart rhythm. It regulates movement of ions such as sodium, potassium and calcium across the muscle cell membrane, and regulates the electrical activity of myocardial (heart muscle) cells and the specialised conducting system of the heart. It inhibits calcium release, enhances calcium uptake into the sarcoplasmic reticulum within the muscle cell and stimulates production of the vasodilators prostacyclin and nitric oxide, causing a muscle relaxant effect, vasodilation and a lowering of blood pressure. Magnesium supports blood clotting by regulating calcium and factor IX activity. It has anti-inflammatory effects, improves endothelial function,

inhibits platelet adhesion and aggregation, and helps to regulate cholesterol levels by enhancing breakdown of the enzyme 3-hydroxy-3-methylglutaryl coenzyme A (HMG-CoA) reductase that takes part in cholesterol synthesis. Magnesium supports activity of the enzyme lecithin:cholesterol acyltransferase (LCAT), which lowers LDL cholesterol and triglyceride levels and raises HDL cholesterol.

- *Nerve and muscle function.* Magnesium stabilises nerve axons and increases the threshold of axon stimulation, reducing nerve conduction velocity. It inhibits the entry of calcium into pre-synaptic nerve endings, affecting the release and function of neurotransmitters, suppresses excitatory neurotransmitters such as serotonin and acetylcholine, and stimulates action of the inhibitory, anti-seizure neurotransmitter gamma-aminobutyric acid (GABA). Magnesium may have pain-relieving and anti-seizure effects by blocking the excitatory activity of N-methyl-D-aspartate (NMDA) receptors. Overall, it has a sedative effect on the nervous system. Magnesium also influences muscle contraction and relaxation by its effect on calcium metabolism in muscle cells. It relaxes muscles by inhibiting the release of calcium, and promoting its uptake into the sarcoplasmic reticulum.
- *Bone formation.* Magnesium is part of crystalline bone, together with calcium, phosphate and other minerals, and is also found on the bone surface, where it can readily be mobilised to maintain serum levels. The enzyme alkaline phosphatase, which has a role in bone mineralisation, is dependent on magnesium.
- *Protection against cadmium toxicity.* Cadmium is an environmental and food pollutant, and chronic exposure can lead to kidney and liver damage, osteomalacia, severe bone pain, anaemia and immune dysfunction. It alters gene expression, inhibits DNA repair and apoptosis, and induces oxidative stress, and is classified as a human carcinogen, mainly associated with tumours of the lung, prostate and testes. Cadmium enters cells via the magnesium transporter TRPM7, and the presence of magnesium can block cadmium uptake. Magnesium has been shown to reduce cadmium accumulation in organs, and protect against lipid peroxidation induced by cadmium.

Dietary sources

Magnesium is found in nuts, seeds, whole grains, bran, legumes, soy products, green leafy vegetables, shellfish, cocoa and chocolate. Refined grains such as white rice and white flour products are poor sources. Tap water can be an important source of magnesium, especially mineral water and 'hard' water from domestic water supplies, which can contain up to 30 mg/L of magnesium. It is estimated that hard tap water may provide 6–31 per cent of the daily magnesium requirement.

The Food Standards Australia New Zealand nutrient database (NUTTAB) at <www.foodstandards.gov.au> provides the amounts found in specific foods.

Factors influencing body status

Magnesium is water soluble, and is lost from foods by water-processing and cooking methods. Refining of grains and food processing can deplete magnesium content by up to 85 per cent. Digestive disorders and inadequate stomach acid may impair absorption, and kidney damage may increase losses in urine. Magnesium is bound by phytate in whole grains, bran, nuts and seeds, and is less available for absorption. Soaking, sprouting and bread-making using yeast can release some of the phytate-bound magnesium.

Magnesium can be bound by fats in the digestive tract, forming insoluble compounds that are excreted. Chronic gastrointestinal disorders involving fat mal-absorption cause larger amounts of undigested fats in the gut, and increase the formation of insoluble magnesium compounds. Proton pump inhibitors, used for GORD, decrease magnesium absorption and lead to hypomagnesaemia (low serum magnesium), with esomeprazole having the lowest risk and pantoprazole having the highest risk. Magnesium absorption is inhibited by a high intake of alcohol, calcium, phosphate or zinc, and chronic diarrhoea—which may be caused by Crohn's disease, ulcerative colitis or coeliac disease—leads to excessive losses in faeces. About 19–365 mg/day may be lost in sweat, and strenuous exercise increases urinary and sweat losses. Magnesium absorption declines with age.

Increased urinary excretion of magnesium may occur in chronic kidney disease, phosphate depletion and hypercalcaemia, which can cause greater losses of magnesium than calcium. Loop diuretics cause a marked increase in magnesium excretion, and the increase is greater than that of sodium or calcium, suggesting that loop diuretics may directly inhibit magnesium transport. Thiazide diuretics act in a different part of the kidney tubule, and have less effect on magnesium excretion. Potassium-sparing diuretics appear to help conserve magnesium as well as potassium. Other drugs that increase urinary magnesium losses include digoxin (for heart arrhythmias); cisplatin (for cancer); gentamycin, amphotericin B, pentamidine, foscarnet and aminoglycoside (antibiotics); and cyclosporin and tacrolimus (immune suppressants).

Daily requirement

Government recommendations by age and gender (see Table 8.4) can be found in *Nutrient Reference Values for Australia and New Zealand Including Recommended Dietary Intakes*, available at <www.nhmrc.gov.au>.

Table 8.4 Recommended dietary intake (RDI) of magnesium (mg/day)

Age (years)	Female RDI	Male RDI
1–3	80	80
4–8	130	130
9–13	240	240
14–18	360	410
19–30	310	400
31–70	320	420
>70	320	420
Pregnant women		
14–18	400	
19–30	350	
31–50	360	
Lactating women		
14–18	360	
19–30	310	
31–50	320	

Source: Nutrient Reference Values for Australia and New Zealand Including Recommended Dietary Intakes, National Health and Medical Research Council, Australian Government Department of Health and Ageing, Canberra and Ministry of Health, New Zealand, Wellington, 2006.

Deficiency effects

Magnesium intake appears to be declining in developed countries, due to the increased use of refined grains and processed food. A 1991 Australian dietary survey found that 50 per cent of men and 39 per cent of women have an inadequate magnesium intake. Deficiency is more common in older people, alcoholics and people with malabsorption or kidney disorders.

In healthy people, serum levels are maintained despite low tissue levels, and hypomagnesaemia is likely to reflect the end result of a prolonged deficiency. Hypomagnesaemia may be caused by a redistribution of magnesium across cell membranes, a reduced magnesium intake, reduced intestinal absorption, increased gastrointestinal losses or increased urinary losses. It is relatively common in hospitalised and critically ill patients, and is associated with increased mortality in intensive care patients. It is often associated with other electrolyte abnormalities, occurring in 40 per cent of hypokalaemic (low serum potassium) patients, 30 per cent of hypophosphataemic patients, 23 per cent of hyponatraemic (low serum sodium) patients and 22–32 per cent of hypocalcaemic patients. In hypokalaemia, the potassium depletion cannot be reversed until normal magnesium status is restored.

Magnesium deficiency lowers serum calcium by impairing PTH secretion, stimulating clearance of PTH and increasing tissue resistance to its effect. It also impairs vitamin D metabolism by inhibiting conversion of 25-hydroxycholecalciferol (vitamin D) to the active form calcitriol, stimulating clearance of calcitriol and increasing tissue resistance. Administration of magnesium immediately increases PTH concentration, but it can take several days for the serum calcium concentration to normalise—possibly because calcitriol levels recover more slowly and tissue resistance takes time to resolve.

Magnesium deficiency leads to increased intracellular calcium and sodium, and decreased intracellular potassium. Nerve, heart and muscle functioning becomes abnormal, and glucose metabolism and energy production are impaired. Excitatory neurotransmitters are stimulated, affecting psychological state and behaviour, and tetany develops in muscles because of uncontrolled and prolonged contractions. Contraction of smooth muscles can cause constriction of blood vessels, respiratory passages and the digestive tract, causing high blood pressure, a sensation of chest tightness, a lump in the throat or tight throat, difficulty swallowing, indigestion, diarrhoea or constipation. Blood lipid levels become abnormal, and oxidative stress increases because of increased expression of inducible nitric oxide synthase (iNOS), leading to increased production of nitric oxide. Increased intracellular calcium may activate inflammatory pathways independently of injury or pathogens, and disturbed calcium metabolism may predispose to calcium deposits in soft tissue. Bone formation is inhibited by impairment of calcium and vitamin D metabolism, and PTH release.

Clinical manifestations of hypomagnesaemia may not appear until the deficiency is severe, and may begin insidiously or appear with dramatic suddenness. Symptoms are usually not seen until serum levels drop to 0.5 mmol/L or lower, and may include lack of appetite, nausea, vomiting, lethargy, weakness, paraesthesia, hyperexcitability, agitation, irritability, depression, erratic behaviour, decreased attention span, mental confusion, tremors, muscle cramps, spasms, twitches, seizures and tetany, with positive Chvostek's and Trousseau's signs. The physical signs are largely caused by the associated hypocalcaemia and hypokalaemia.

A magnesium deficiency in animals leads to inflammation and increased production of reactive oxygen species, and has been shown to exacerbate atherosclerosis and vascular damage. In a study of postmenopausal women, a low magnesium diet resulted in abnormal heart rhythm, atrial fibrillation and flutter, decreased serum total cholesterol, decreased red blood cell superoxide dismutase, increased urinary excretion of sodium and potassium and increased serum glucose. Evidence suggests that a magnesium deficiency may play a role in coronary heart disease, congestive heart failure, sudden cardiac death, cardiac arrhythmias (abnormal heart rhythm), high blood pressure, diabetes, osteoporosis and pre-eclampsia/eclampsia (high blood pressure and seizures) in pregnancy. Hypomagnesaemia occurs in up to 90 per cent of cancer patients on chemotherapy with cisplatin, and may be associated with severe pain that does not respond to opiate drugs.

Various mutations in the TRPM6 gene reduce carrier-mediated absorption of magnesium in the small intestine and impair reabsorption in the kidneys. Collectively, these rare disorders are referred to as primary hypomagnesaemia with secondary hypocalcaemia (HSH). HSH affects very young infants, causing generalised convulsions or signs of increased neuromuscular excitability, together with severe hypomagnesaemia, hypocalcaemia and barely detectable PTH levels. Treatment includes iv magnesium, followed by lifelong high-dose oral magnesium supplementation. A variety of other genetic disorders can cause hypomagnesaemia, which may occur together with elevated calcium in the urine, normal calcium in the urine or high calcium in the urine, and hypomagnesaemia is a feature of Bartter syndrome and Gitelman syndrome, in which there is an abnormality of sodium chloride reabsorption in the kidneys.

Indicators of inadequate levels of magnesium may include:

- lethargy, weakness, muscle tremors, spasms, twitches, cramps, seizures
- lack of appetite, nausea, vomiting, tight throat or chest, sensation of a lump in the throat, speech difficulties, difficulty swallowing, indigestion, constipation, diarrhoea
- irregular heart rhythm, heart palpitations, high blood pressure, poor circulation, elevated blood cholesterol
- paraesthesia
- nervous tension, dizziness, hyperexcitability, agitation, aggressiveness, irritability, depression, mood swings, erratic behaviour, decreased attention span, mental confusion
- premenstrual syndrome
- calcium-based kidney and bladder stones, calcium deposits in soft tissues
- bone weakness, fractures, curvature of the spine, osteoporosis.

Assessment of body status

Serum magnesium concentration is not regarded as an accurate indicator of body status because it is tightly regulated and does not reflect total body content. The result may be hard to interpret in acidosis, which causes a shift of magnesium to the extracellular space, and alkalosis, which causes a shift into cells. The reference range given by the RCPA for adults is 0.8–1.0 mmol/L for serum or plasma. Other tests not used routinely include assessment of ionised magnesium (reference range 0.55–0.75 mmol/L), which is difficult to assess accurately, and total magnesium in red blood cells (reference range 1.65–2.65 mmol/L), which does not correlate well with total magnesium status. Patients who have low total magnesium and low albumin may have normal concentrations of ionised magnesium. Trousseau's sign is a good indicator of hypocalcaemia, but may or may not be associated with hypomagnesaemia.

Magnesium wasting via the kidneys can be detected by a 24-hour urine analysis. The reference range for urinary magnesium given by the RCPA for adults is 2.5–8.0 mmol/24 hours, and varies with intake. A high excretion may indicate wasting, and excretion of less than 0.5 mmol/24 hours may indicate a magnesium deficiency. In people with healthy kidneys, a magnesium loading test can be used, in which magnesium is administered intravenously and the amount retained in the body is measured. Increased retention indicates a magnesium deficiency. This test is not used routinely, but appears to be very sensitive, and has been found to correlate well with bone magnesium content.

Case reports—magnesium deficiency

- *A woman, 39 years of age*, developed severe watery diarrhoea and hand spasm after ingesting a handful of magnesium hydroxide tablets.[1] She was found to have hypomagnesaemia and hypocalcaemia, with normal potassium levels. She was treated with calcium gluconate without much response. Her symptoms disappeared spontaneously two days after her diarrhoea subsided. It was concluded that the overdose of magnesium hydroxide caused severe diarrhoea, which led to sudden-onset hypomagnesaemia.
- *A woman, 67 years of age*, developed asymptomatic hypomagnesaemia.[2] She had been taking proton pump inhibitors for GORD for several years, which partially relieved her GORD symptoms. She was found to have a very low level of urinary magnesium but normal serum calcium, phosphorus, potassium and glucose levels, and normal kidney function. Following withdrawal of the proton pump inhibitors, her serum and urinary magnesium levels returned to normal.
- *A man, 37 years of age*, developed fatigue that lasted several weeks.[3] Physical examination revealed a positive Trousseau's sign, and he was found to have hypomagnesaemia and hypocalcaemia as well as increased urinary magnesium. His medical reports revealed a history of hypomagnesaemia and hypocalcaemia associated with convulsions and muscle weakness, which were relieved with regular high-dose magnesium supplements. Genetic analysis revealed mutations of the TRPM6 gene, leading to a diagnosis of HSH. His symptoms resolved on treatment with iv magnesium sulfate, and he was maintained on oral supplementation of 4000 mg of magnesium oxide daily with no return of symptoms.
- *A woman, 40 years of age*, developed weakness, dizziness and paraesthesia in her hands and feet 62 days after a small intestinal bypass operation for obesity.[4] Following the operation, she had lost weight and had developed frequent daily bowel movements. She was found to have a positive Chvostek's and Trousseau's sign, hypocalcaemia, hypomagnesaemia and hypokalaemia, and she was diagnosed with latent tetany due to hypocalcaemia. She was treated with iv calcium gluconate and oral vitamin D, but her serum calcium continued to fall. Her paraesthesia worsened and she was given another dose of iv calcium gluconate with no improvement. A new diagnosis of hypomagnesaemia was made, her calcium supplements were stopped and im injections of magnesium sulfate were commenced. Her symptoms were rapidly relieved and her mineral imbalance was restored to normal within five days.

REFERENCES

1 Joo Suk, O., Paradoxical hypomagnesemia caused by excessive ingestion of magnesium hydroxide, *Am J Emerg Med* (2008), 26(7): 837, e1–2.

2 Furlanetto, T.W. & Faulhaber, G.A., Hypomagnesemia and proton pump inhibitors: Below the tip of the iceberg, *Arch Intern Med* (2011), 171(15): 1391–2.

3 Mallavarapu, R.K. & Peskoe, S.T., Familial hypomagnesemia with secondary hypocalcemia caused by TRPM6 gene mutations, *Am J Kidney Dis* (2008), 51(4): B66.

4 Lipner, A., Symptomatic magnesium deficiency after small-intestinal bypass for obesity, *Br Med J* (1977), 1(6054): 148.

THERAPEUTIC USES OF MAGNESIUM

Magnesium is popularly used for disorders involving hyperexcitability of nerves or muscles, such as nervous tension, and muscle spasms and cramps. It may have therapeutic activity for the following conditions:

Pregnancy

Pre-eclampsia/eclampsia is a serious disorder affecting pregnant women, which features high blood pressure, proteinuria, weight gain and oedema (pre-eclampsia) that may progress to life-threatening seizures (eclampsia). Magnesium has anti-seizure and blood pressure-lowering effects. Intravenous and im magnesium sulfate are widely used as a routine therapy to prevent eclamptic seizures in pregnant women with hypertension. A number of reviews have found that magnesium is more effective than anti-convulsant drugs. A review of fifteen trials concluded that iv magnesium sulfate more than halves the risk of eclampsia and is more effective than diazepam or phenytoin.[1] A review of five clinical trials concluded that magnesium sulfate therapy given to women at risk of preterm birth reduced the risk of cerebral palsy in their infants by 32 per cent, and reduced the risk of substantial gross motor dysfunction in their infants by 39 per cent.[2]

Cardiovascular disease

Magnesium may have protective effects against CVD by improving glucose and insulin metabolism, lowering blood pressure by dilating blood vessels, stabilising heart rhythm, reducing inflammation, blood clotting and platelet aggregation, and improving lipid metabolism and blood lipid profile. An inadequate dietary intake of magnesium has been linked to insulin resistance, metabolic syndrome, type 2 diabetes, high blood pressure and CVD,[3] and low serum magnesium levels are associated with cardiovascular and all-cause mortality, high blood pressure and enlargement of the left ventricle of the heart, which is related to adverse cardiovascular events.[4]

High blood pressure (hypertension)

Low magnesium may lead to abnormal calcium metabolism, increased tone of blood vessels and vaso-spasm, all of which can elevate blood pressure. Some studies have found that patients with hypertension are more likely to have low serum magnesium, and that magnesium supplementation leads to a reduction of blood pressure. However, other studies have not found a relationship. One study found that 400 mg of magnesium oxide daily was able to reduce blood pressure,[5] and another study found that daily intake of 600 mg of magnesium pidolate (magnesium pyro-glutamate, a very soluble form of magnesium) was effective.[6] Reviews of clinical trials have concluded that magnesium supplementation leads to dose-dependent reductions in blood pressure,[7] and enhances the effect of anti-hypertensive drugs.[8] However, a review of twelve trials concluded that magnesium supplementation was related to a small reduction in diastolic blood pressure only.[9] Inconsistencies in research findings may be related to the different forms and doses of magnesium used.

Stroke

A higher magnesium intake has been linked to lower risk of stroke, and has been found to help protect against some risk factors for stroke, such as hypertension, metabolic syndrome and type 2 diabetes. A meta-analysis of seven trials concluded that a higher magnesium intake reduces the risk of stroke, especially ischaemic stroke.[10] Magnesium appears to be neuroprotective in animal models of stroke, with reported reductions in infarct volume (area of damage) of 25–61 per cent.[11] It may act by blocking the NMDA receptor, enhancing cerebral blood flow, inhibiting calcium entry into cells and stimulating cellular energy metabolism. In one study, iv magnesium sulfate given to stroke patients was shown to decrease the number of early deaths.[12] Another study found that magnesium treatment given within twelve hours of stroke onset did not reduce mortality or disability at 90 days, but may have been of benefit for ischaemic lacunar strokes (strokes from circulatory blockage occurring in the deep regions of the brain).[13] A further study found that patients with acute ischaemic stroke treated with magnesium sulfate had a better recovery than patients on placebo.[14] A meta-analysis of eight trials concluded that magnesium sulfate can improve outcomes in patients with acute aneurysmal subarachnoid haemorrhage (rupture of an aneurysm in the brain) but does not decrease mortality.[15]

Atherosclerosis

A magnesium deficiency leads to elevated serum triglycerides and lower levels of protective HDL cholesterol. Magnesium supplementation has been found to lower blood triglycerides and LDL cholesterol and increase HDL cholesterol in patients with high blood pressure and in diabetics.[16,17] Magnesium chloride supplementation taken with a fatty meal has been found to delay and decrease the normal post-meal rise in triglycerides.[18]

It is theorised that magnesium may act like statin drugs to reduce activity of HMG-CoA reductase, the enzyme that converts HMG-CoA to mevalonate and then to cholesterol.[19] By inhibiting HMG-CoA reductase, cholesterol production is reduced, as is mevalonate formation, which leads to improved endothelial function; it also leads to reduced inflammation, and atherosclerotic plaque stabilisation and regression. Statin drugs directly inhibit HMG-CoA reductase activity, whereas magnesium appears to have a controlling function by activating an enzyme that deactivates HMG-CoA reductase.

A higher serum magnesium is associated with lower risk of CHD and lower mortality from CHD.[20,21] Lower serum magnesium levels have been associated with greater intima-media thickness (thickness of the wall of an artery due to cholesterol deposits) and the risk of at least two atherosclerotic plaques in the carotid arteries.[22] In kidney dialysis patients, hypomagnesaemia is associated with increased carotid intima-media thickness and calcification of the peripheral arteries and the mitral valve in the heart.[23,24] Magnesium supplementation has been found to slow down the development of arterial calcification and reduce carotid intima-media thickness in patients with chronic kidney disease.[25]

Heart attack

In a study of acute heart attack (myocardial infarction, MI), iv magnesium sulfate given for five minutes before beginning thrombolytic therapy, followed by a 24-hour infusion, was associated with a 24 per cent decrease in mortality at 28 days, a 25 per cent reduction in left ventricular failure and improved long-term survival.[26] However, magnesium has not been found to be effective in other trials. In patients with a previous MI or CHD, six months of oral magnesium supplementation (365 mg daily as magnesium citrate), together with potassium supplementation, led to improvements in exercise tolerance, exercise-induced chest pain and quality of life.[27]

Arrhythmia

Magnesium may stabilise heart rhythm by blocking calcium influx, reducing sinus node rate firing and slowing conduction through the atrioventricular node. Intravenous magnesium is highly effective in terminating torsades de pointes, a specific form of tachycardia that may trigger ventricular fibrillation (weak, unco-ordinated contractions of the heart ventricles).[28] An increase in serum magnesium has been reported to reduce the frequency of arrhythmias after acute MI,[29] and patients with frequent ventricular arrhythmia have responded to an increased dietary intake of magnesium and potassium.[30] If serum magnesium is low, digoxin therapy can cause arrhythmia, which can be resolved by magnesium administration.[31]

Magnesium sulfate has been recommended for resuscitation of patients with pulseless ventricular fibrillation and ventricular tachycardia when standard drug treatment is ineffective. Low magnesium levels have been associated with an increased incidence of atrial fibrillation (AF) after coronary artery bypass grafting (CABG) and magnesium given to patients for four days after CABG has reduced the incidence of AF.[32,33] However, some studies have not found oral magnesium to be useful. Administration of iv potassium and magnesium has been shown to restore sinus rhythm and improve the success rate of AF patients undergoing cardioversion therapy (a medical technique for converting an erratic heart rate to normal rhythm).[34]

Metabolic syndrome

The metabolic syndrome features a collection of metabolic disorders, including abdominal obesity, high blood pressure, elevated serum triglycerides or reduced HDL cholesterol (dyslipidaemia), insulin resistance and poor blood glucose control. People with metabolic syndrome are at increased risk of CVD and diabetes. A number of studies have found that a low dietary intake of magnesium is associated with increased prevalence of metabolic syndrome. One study found that 65.6 per cent of people with metabolic syndrome had low serum magnesium levels compared with 4.9 per cent of controls, and dyslipidaemia and hypertension were strongly related to low serum magnesium.[35] In people with metabolic syndrome and normal serum magnesium, magnesium supplementation resulted in lower fasting plasma glucose and improved insulin sensitivity, but blood pressure and lipid profile did not change.[36] In people with mild hypertension, magnesium supplementation (600 mg of magnesium pidolate daily) led to reduced total cholesterol, LDL cholesterol and triglyceride levels, increased HDL cholesterol levels and improved insulin sensitivity.[37]

Diabetes

Intracellular magnesium appears to be important for maintaining insulin sensitivity in skeletal muscle and adipose tissue. A higher magnesium intake has been associated with lower fasting glucose and insulin in people with insulin resistance, and trials have found that magnesium supplementation improves both insulin secretion and insulin activity in non-diabetic elderly people.[36,38] In patients with diabetes, plasma levels of magnesium are lower than those of non-diabetic subjects,[39] and higher plasma or red blood cell magnesium levels are associated with lower fasting insulin levels in both diabetic and non-diabetic subjects.[40,41] In animal models of diabetes, magnesium supplementation has been shown to prevent fructose-induced insulin resistance, and to delay the onset of spontaneous type 2 diabetes.[42,43] Several trials have found that magnesium supplementation improves glycaemic control in type 2 diabetes patients, but some trials have found no benefits. A review of nine clinical trials that used an average of 360 mg of magnesium daily concluded that magnesium supplementation for four to sixteen weeks may be effective for reducing plasma fasting glucose levels and raising HDL cholesterol in type 2 diabetic patients.[44]

Premenstrual syndrome

Blood cell levels of magnesium in women with premenstrual syndrome (PMS) have been found to be lower than those of women without PMS.[45] In a group of women with PMS, magnesium pyrrolidone carboxylic acid (providing 360 mg of elemental magnesium) was given daily from the fifteenth day of the menstrual cycle to the onset of menstrual flow and mood changes and depression were found to improve.[46] In women with premenstrual migraine, magnesium supplementation (360 mg daily) during the second half of the menstrual cycle was able to reduce the number of days with a headache.[47] Magnesium oxide (200 mg/day) has relieved symptoms related to premenstrual fluid retention.[48] A review of dietary supplements for PMS concluded that magnesium supplements (200–400 mg daily) may be helpful in relieving PMS symptoms, but the evidence is not as strong as that for calcium supplementation.[49]

Migraine

Migraine is believed to be partly caused by an over-excitable trigeminovascular complex, in which neurons in the trigeminal nerve overreact by releasing neurotransmitters such as serotonin. These neurotransmitters cause an inflammatory response involving vasodilation, mast cell degranulation, increased vascular permeability and swelling, and the transmission of pain signals to the cortex. Serotonin can also induce nausea and vomiting.

Magnesium deficiency is related to several features of migraine, including neurotransmitter release, vasoconstriction, platelet aggregation and cortical spreading depression (CSD), which is a wave of hyperactivity of nerves followed by inhibition. Magnesium deficiency causes substance P release and activation of NMDA receptors, which can trigger CSD and pain. During migraine attacks, patients have been found to have transient hypomagnesaemia and low intracellular magnesium, and some patients have been found to have low magnesium in the cerebrospinal fluid and the brain.[50,51] Magnesium load tests and analyses of ionised serum magnesium have revealed that systemic magnesium deficiencies are more common in migraine patients.[52,53]

Magnesium supplementation (600 mg daily as trimagnesium dicitrate) for twelve weeks has been found to decrease migraine frequency by 41.6 per cent compared with a 15.8 per cent decrease in subjects not on magnesium.[54] The number of migraine days and the amounts of drugs used for symptom relief also decreased in the magnesium group. Another trial using 246 mg of magnesium twice daily showed no benefits.[55] However, diarrhoea occurred in almost half the subjects in this trial, indicating that a more insoluble form of magnesium may have been used that was poorly absorbed. Another study using 600 mg daily of magnesium as magnesium citrate found that it reduced attack frequency and severity, and improved blood flow in the cortex.[56] There are conflicting results from studies using iv magnesium sulfate for pain relief during migraines. One study of fifteen migraine patients found that 1 g of iv magnesium sulfate given over fifteen minutes during an attack was able to stop the pain in thirteen subjects and reduce the pain in two.[57] All accompanying symptoms disappeared in every subject.

Muscle cramps

Magnesium regulates calcium metabolism in muscle cells, and has a muscle-relaxing effect. Although it is popularly used for muscle cramps, there is limited evidence for its efficacy. A study of pregnant women found that magnesium supplementation reduced the frequency and intensity of leg cramps.[58] A trial of magnesium for chronic nocturnal leg cramps (300 mg of magnesium daily given as magnesium citrate for six weeks) found a trend towards fewer cramps, and more of the subjects taking magnesium reported benefits compared with the subjects on placebo.[59] However, other studies have not shown benefits, and a review concluded that there was no good evidence for the use of magnesium for cramps in older people, and that the evidence for pregnancy-related cramps was conflicting.[60]

Osteoporosis

Animal studies show that magnesium deficiency results in bone loss, possibly caused by a substance P-induced release of inflammatory cytokines and impaired metabolism of PTH and calcitriol.[61] A higher magnesium intake has been correlated with greater BMD in elderly caucasians.[62] Serum magnesium was found to be significantly lower in women with osteoporosis than in women with low BMD and women with normal BMD.[63] Magnesium supplementation was associated with reduced bone turnover in healthy young men and osteoporotic women.[64,65] A study of postmenopausal women with low trabecular BMD who took 250–750 mg of magnesium hydroxide daily for six months, followed by 250 mg/day for eighteen months, found that 71 per cent had a 1–8 per cent increase in BMD whereas control subjects experienced decreases in BMD.[66]

Restless legs syndrome

Subjects with restless legs syndrome (RLS) and magnesium deficiency have been found to have neuromuscular hyperexcitability.[67] A small study using magnesium supplementation in patients with mild or moderate insomnia related to RLS or periodic limb movements during sleep found that it decreased the frequency of nocturnal episodes, and improved sleep quality.[68]

Asthma

Inadequate dietary magnesium appears to be linked to the incidence and progression of asthma. Hypomagnesaemia is common in chronic asthmatics, and is associated with more severe asthma and more hospital admissions compared with chronic asthmatics with normal magnesium levels.[69] In children with moderate persistent asthma, oral magnesium supplementation (300 mg daily) helped to reduce bronchial reactivity and allergen-induced skin responses, and improved symptom control.[70] A similar beneficial result was found in a study of adults with mild to moderate asthma, who were given 340 mg of oral magnesium daily in divided doses.[71] Intravenous magnesium sulfate has been used to provide symptom relief in severe acute asthma. In a review of seven trials, asthma patients receiving iv magnesium sulfate during a severe acute attack were found to have improved peak expiratory flow rate and forced expiratory volume (measures of lung function), and reduced hospital admissions.[72]

Soft tissue calcification

Patients with CKD have a greatly increased risk of calcification of blood vessels and CVD. Calcification involves the depositing of calcium phosphate in soft tissue and the formation of hydroxyapatite crystals, and is believed to be caused by alterations in calcium and phosphate balance. Magnesium inhibits calcification by antagonising calcium activity and inhibiting the transformation of calcium phosphate to hydroxyapatite. Low serum magnesium levels have been associated with vascular calcification,[73] and it can be prevented or reduced in animals by dietary magnesium.[74] Patients with end-stage CKD and with peripheral arterial calcification were found to have lower serum magnesium levels than end-stage CKD patients without calcifications, or those in whom calcifications had regressed.[75] Mitral valve calcification in chronic haemodialysis patients is strongly associated with low serum magnesium levels,[76] and is also strongly associated with increased carotid intima media thickness in patients undergoing long-term haemodialysis.[77] In a pilot study of CKD patients on intermittent haemodialysis, long-term use of oral magnesium carbonate used as a phosphate binder was found to slow the rate of arterial calcification.[78]

There is some evidence that magnesium may be protective against calcium oxalate kidney stones. Magnesium can bind oxalate in the digestive tract and decrease oxalate absorption, and it can form complexes with oxalate in urine and decrease supersaturation, the process that drives crystallisation. In a cell study, magnesium was found to reduce deposition of calcium oxalate crystals by 50 per cent.[79] Magnesium supplementation in people with magnesium deficiency has been shown to increase the urinary excretion of citrate, which protects against stone formation.[80] Magnesium potassium citrate has been shown to reduce the recurrence of calcium kidney stones by 90 per cent, having similar efficacy to potassium citrate.[81] However, citrate appears to be the protective factor.

Exercise performance

Strenuous exercise has been shown to increase urinary and sweat magnesium losses, and may increase magnesium requirements by 10–20 per cent.[82] Athletes who need to control their weight may be particularly at risk of low magnesium status. Animals with a marginal magnesium deficiency have reduced exercise capacity and endurance,[83] and postmenopausal women with a marginal deficiency were also found to have impaired exercise performance.[84] Magnesium supplementation or increased dietary intake appears to improve exercise performance in magnesium-deficient athletes, but does not appear to assist performance in athletes who are not deficient.[82]

Depression

Magnesium may help stabilise mood by its effect on neurotransmitter activity, and by blocking NMDA receptors and reducing calcium influx in nerve cells. Patients with major depression appear to have abnormal magnesium metabolism; both high and low magnesium levels have been reported.[85,86] In animals, magnesium supplementation has anti-depressant effects, and it is theorised that anti-depressant drugs act, in part, by increasing nerve cell concentrations of magnesium.[85]

Treatment-resistant depression (TRD) occurs in about 60 per cent of depression cases, and is associated with low magnesium levels in the brain. Cerebrospinal fluid magnesium levels have been found to be low in treatment-resistant suicidal depression, and in patients who have attempted suicide.[87] One study found that magnesium was as effective as the tricyclic anti-depressant imipramine for treating depression in elderly diabetics.[88] Case reports claim recovery from major depression in less than seven days by the use of 125–300 mg of magnesium (as glycinate and taurinate) with each meal and at bedtime.[89] A systematic review of 27 studies concluded that magnesium appears to be effective for the prevention and treatment of depression but more higher quality studies are needed.[90]

Digestive disorders

Magnesium salts, such as magnesium citrate, magnesium hydroxide (milk of magnesia) and magnesium sulfate (Epsom salts), can be used in the short term to treat constipation. As osmotic laxatives, they act by drawing water into the bowel and stimulating bowel movements, which usually occur within a few hours after the dose. A high magnesium and sulfate mineral water (Hépar; Nestlé Waters, Issy-les-Moulineaux, France), 1 L/day, has been found to be more effective for constipation than an equivalent amount of natural water low in minerals.[91] A comparison of oral magnesium sulfate powder, polyethylene glycol electrolyte powder and mannitol for bowel evacuation in constipated patients before colonoscopy found that magnesium sulfate was the most effective and had fewer adverse effects.[92] Magnesium hydroxide has antacid activity, and is used for dyspepsia, gastric ulcers and GORD in combination with aluminium hydroxide, which reduces the laxative effect. At a dose of 800 mg, magnesium hydroxide has been shown to cause an immediate, effective and prolonged antacid action lasting up to 40 minutes.[93]

REFERENCES

1 Duley, L., Gülmezoglu, A.M., Henderson-Smart, D.J. & Chou, D., Magnesium sulphate and other anticonvulsants for women with pre-eclampsia, *Cochrane Database Syst Rev* (2010), 11: CD000025.

2 Doyle, L.W., Crowther, C.A., Middleton, P. et al., Magnesium sulphate for women at risk of pre-term birth for neuroprotection of the fetus, *Cochrane Database of Systematic Reviews* (2009), 1: CD004661.

3 Bo, S. & Pisu, E., Role of dietary magnesium in cardiovascular disease prevention, insulin sensitivity and diabetes, *Curr Opin Lipidol* (2008), 19(1): 50–6.

4 Qu, X., Jin, F., Hao, Y. et al., Magnesium and the risk of cardiovascular events: A meta-analysis of prospective cohort studies, *PLoS One* (2013), 8(3): e57720.

5 Kawano, Y., Matsuoka, H., Takishita, S. & Omae, T., Effects of magnesium supplementation in hypertensive patients: Assessment by office, home, and ambulatory blood pressures, *Hypertension* (1998), 32(2): 260–5.

6 Hatzistavri, L.S., Sarafidis, P.A., Georgianos, P.I.T. et al., Oral magnesium supplementation reduces ambulatory blood pressure in patients with mild hypertension, *Am J Hypertens* (2009), 22(10): 1070–5.

7 Jee, S.H., Miller, E.R. III, Guallar, E. et al., The effect of magnesium supplementation on blood pressure: a meta-analysis of randomized clinical trials, *Am J Hypertens* (2002), 15(8): 691–6.

8 Rosanoff, A., Magnesium supplements may enhance the effect of antihypertensive medications in stage 1 hypertensive subjects, *Magnes Res* (2010), 23: 27–40.

9 Dickinson, H.O., Nicolson, D.J., Campbell, F. et al., Magnesium supplementation for the management of essential hypertension in adults, *Cochrane Database Syst Rev* (2006), 3: CD004640.

10 Larsson, S.C., Orsini, N. & Wolk, A., Dietary magnesium intake and risk of stroke: A meta-analysis of prospective studies, *Am J Clin Nutr* (2012), 95(2): 362–6.

11 Muir, K.W., Magnesium for neuroprotection in ischaemic stroke: rationale for use and evidence of effectiveness, *CNS Drugs* (2001), 15(12): 921–30.

12 Muir, K.W. & Lees, K.R., A randomized, double-blind, placebo-controlled pilot trial of intravenous magnesium sulfate in acute stroke, *Stroke* (1995), 26(7): 1183–8.

13 Muir, K.W., Lees, K.R., Ford, I. & Davis, S., Intravenous Magnesium Efficacy in Stroke (IMAGES) magnesium for acute stroke (Intravenous Magnesium Efficacy in Stroke trial): Randomised controlled trial, *Lancet* (2004), 363(9407): 439–45.

14 Afshari, D., Moradian, N. & Rezaei, M., Evaluation of the intravenous magnesium sulfate effect in clinical improvement of patients with acute ischemic stroke, *Clin Neurol Neurosurg* (2013), 115(4): 400–4.

15 Chen, T. & Carter, B.S., Role of magnesium sulfate in aneurysmal subarachnoid hemorrhage management: A meta-analysis of controlled clinical trials, *Asian J Neurosurg* (2011), 6(1): 26–31.

16 Hadjistavri, L.S., Sarafidis, P.A., Georgianos, P.I. et al., Beneficial effects of oral magnesium supplementation on insulin sensitivity and serum lipid profile, *Med Sci Monit* (2010), 16(6): CR307–12.

17 Corica, F., Allegra, A., Di Benedetto, A. et al., Effects of oral magnesium supplementation on plasma lipid concentrations in patients with non-insulin-dependent diabetes mellitus, *Magnes Res* (1994), 7(1): 43–7.

18 Kishimoto, Y., Tani, M., Uto-Kondo, H. et al., Effects of magnesium on postprandial serum lipid responses in healthy human subjects, *Br J Nutr* (2010), 103(4): 469–72.

19 Rosanoff, A. & Seelig, M.S., Comparison of mechanism and functional effects of magnesium and statin pharmaceuticals, *J Am Coll Nutr* (2004), 23(5): 501S–5S.

20 Liao, F., Folsom, A.R. & Brancati, F.L., Is low magnesium concentration a risk factor for coronary heart disease? The Atherosclerosis Risk in Communities (ARIC) Study, *Am Heart J* (1998), 136(3): 480–90.

21 Ford, E.S., Serum magnesium and ischaemic heart disease: Findings from a national sample of US adults, *Int J Epidemiol* (1999), 28(4): 645–51.

22 Hashimoto, T., Hara, A., Ohkubo, T. et al., Magnesium, ambulatory blood pressure, and carotid artery alteration: The Ohasama study, *Am J Hypertens* (2010), 23(12): 1292–8.

23 Tzanakis, I., Pras, A., Kounali, D. et al., Mitral annular calcification in haemodialysis patients: A possible protective role of magnesium, *Nephrol Dial Transplant* (1997), 12(9): 2036–7.

24 Tzanakis, I., Virvidakis, K., Tsomi, A. et al., Intra- and extracellular magnesium levels and atheromatosis in haemodialysis patients, *Magnes Res* (2004), 17(2): 102–8.

25 Turgut, F., Kanbay, M., Metin, M.R. et al., Magnesium supplementation helps to improve carotid intima media thickness in patients on hemodialysis, *Int Urol Nephrol* (2008), 40: 1075–82.

26 Woods, K.L., Fletcher, S., Roffe, C. & Haider, Y., Intravenous magnesium sulphate in suspected acute myocardial infarction: results of the second Leicester Intravenous Magnesium Intervention Trial (LIMIT-2), *Lancet* (1992), 339(8809): 1553–8.

27 Shechter, M., Bairey Merz, C.N., Stuehlinger, H.G. et al., Effects of oral magnesium therapy on exercise tolerance, exercise-induced chest pain, and quality of life in patients with coronary artery disease, *Am J Cardiol* (2003), 91(5): 517–21.

28 Tzivoni, D., Banai, S., Schuger, C. et al., Treatment of torsade de pointes with magnesium sulfate, *Circulation* (1988), 77(2): 392–7.

29 Abraham, A.S., Rosenmann, D., Kramer, M. et al., Magnesium in the prevention of lethal arrhythmias in acute myocardial infarction, *Arch Intern Med* (1987), 147(4): 753–5.

30 Zehender, M., Meinertz, T., Faber, T. et al., Antiarrhythmic effects of increasing the daily intake of magnesium and potassium in patients with frequent ventricular arrhythmias: Magnesium in Cardiac Arrhythmias (MAGICA), *J Am Coll Cardiol* (1997), 29(5): 1028–34.

31 Cohen, L. & Kitzes, R., Magnesium sulfate and digitalis-toxic arrhythmias, *JAMA* (1983), 249(20): 2808–10.

32 Kaplan, M., Kut, M.S., Icer, U.A. et al., Intravenous magnesium sulfate prophylaxis for atrial fibrillation after coronary artery bypass surgery, *J Thorac Cardiovasc Surg* (2003), 125: 344–52.

33 Fanning, W.J., Thomas, C.S. Jr, Roach, A. et al., Prophylaxis of atrial fibrillation with magnesium sulfate after coronary artery bypass grafting, *Ann Thorac Surg* (1991), 52(3): 529–33.

34 Sultan, A., Steven, D. & Rostock, T., Intravenous administration of magnesium and potassium solution lowers energy levels and increases success rates electrically cardioverting atrial fibrillation, *J Cardiovasc Electrophysiol* (2012), 23(1): 54–9.

35 Guerrero-Romero, F. & Rodríguez-Morán, M., Low serum magnesium levels and metabolic syndrome, *Acta Diabetol* (2002), 39(4): 209–13.

36 Mooren, F.C., Krüger, K., Völker K. et al., Oral magnesium supplementation reduces insulin resistance in non-diabetic subjects: A double-blind, placebo-controlled, randomized trial, *Diabetes Obes Metab* (2011), 13(3): 281–4.

37 Hadjistavri, L.S., Sarafidis, P.A., Georgianos, P.I. et al., Beneficial effects of oral magnesium supplementation on insulin sensitivity and serum lipid profile, *Med Sci Monit* (2010), 16(6): CR307–12.

38 Paolisso, G., Sgambato, S., Gambardella, A. et al., Daily magnesium supplements improve glucose handling in elderly subjects, *Am J Clin Nutr* (1992), 55(6): 1161–7.

39 Resnick, L.M., Altura, B.T., Gupta, R.K. et al., Intracellular and extracellular magnesium depletion in type 2 (non-insulin-dependent) diabetes mellitus, *Diabetologia* (1993), 36(8): 767–70.

40 Rosolová, H., Mayer, O. Jr & Reaven, G.M., Insulin-mediated glucose disposal is decreased in normal subjects with relatively low plasma magnesium concentrations, *Metabolism* (2000), 49(3): 418–20.

41 Ma, J., Folsom, A.R., Melnick, S.L. et al., Associations of serum and dietary magnesium with cardiovascular disease, hypertension, diabetes, insulin, and carotid arterial wall thickness: The ARIC study—Atherosclerosis Risk in Communities Study, *J Clin Epidemiol* (1995), 48(7): 927–40.

42 Balon, T.W., Jasman, A., Scott, S. et al., Dietary magnesium prevents fructose-induced insulin insensitivity in rats, *Hypertension* (1994), 23(6 Pt 2): 1036–9.

43 Balon, T.W., Gu, J.L., Tokuyama, Y. et al., Magnesium supplementation reduces development of diabetes in a rat model of spontaneous NIDDM, *Am J Physiol* (1995), 269(4 Pt 1): E745–52.

44 Song, Y., He, K., Levitan, E.B. et al., Effects of oral magnesium supplementation on glycaemic control in Type 2 diabetes: a meta-analysis of randomized double-blind controlled trials, *Diabet Med* (2006), 23(10): 1050–6.

45 Rosenstein, D.L., Elin, R.J., Hosseini, J.M., Grover, G. & Rubinow, D.R., Magnesium measures across the menstrual cycle in premenstrual syndrome, *Biol Psychiatry* (1994), 35(8): 557–61.

46 Facchinetti, F., Borella, P., Sances, G. et al., Oral magnesium successfully relieves premenstrual mood changes, *Obstet Gynecol* (1991), 78(2): 177–81.

47 Facchinetti, F., Sances, G., Borella, P. et al., Magnesium prophylaxis of menstrual migraine: Effects on intracellular magnesium, *Headache* (1991), 31(5): 298–301.

48 Walker, A.F., De Souza, M.C., Vickers, M.F. et al., Magnesium supplementation alleviates premenstrual symptoms of fluid retention, *J Womens Health* (1998), 7(9): 1157–65.

49 Bendich, A., The potential for dietary supplements to reduce premenstrual syndrome (PMS) symptoms, *J Am Coll Nutr* (2000), 19(1): 3–12.

50 Sarchielli, P., Coata, G., Firenze, C. et al., Serum and salivary magnesium levels in migraine and tension-type headache: Results in a group of adult patients, *Cephalalgia* (1992), 12(1): 21–7.

51 Ramadan, N.M., Halvorson, H., Vande-Linde, A. et al., Low brain magnesium in migraine, *Headache* (1989), 29(7): 416–19.

52 Trauninger, A., Pfund, Z., Koszegi, T. & Czopf, J., Oral magnesium load test in patients with migraine, *Headache* (2002), 42(2): 114–19.

53 Mauskop, A., Altura, B.T., Cracco, R.Q. & Altura, B.M., Deficiency in serum ionized magnesium but not total magnesium in patients with migraines: Possible role of ICa^{2+}/IMg^{2+} ratio, *Headache* (1993), 33(3): 135–8.

54 Peikert, A., Wilimzig, C. & Köhne-Volland, R., Prophylaxis of migraine with oral magnesium: Results from a prospective, multi-center, placebo-controlled and double-blind randomized study, *Cephalalgia* (1996), 16(4): 257–63.

55 Pfaffenrath, V., Wessely, P., Meyer, C. et al., Magnesium in the prophylaxis of migraine: A double-blind placebo-controlled study, *Cephalalgia* (1996), 16(6): 436–40.

56 Köseoglu, E., Talaslioglu, A., Gönül, A.S. & Kula, M., The effects of magnesium prophylaxis in migraine without aura, *Magnes Res* (2008), 21(2): 101–8.

57 Demirkaya, S., Vural, O., Dora, B. & Topçuoğlu, M.A., Efficacy of intravenous magnesium sulfate in the treatment of acute migraine attacs, *Headache* (2001), 41(2): 71–7.

58 Supakatisant, C. & Phupong, V., Oral magnesium for relief in pregnancy-induced leg cramps: A randomised controlled trial, *Matern Child Nutr* (2012), 22 August (epub), doi 10.1111/j.1740-8709.2012.00440.x.

59 Roffe, C., Sills, S., Crome, P. & Jones, P., Randomised, cross-over, placebo controlled trial of magnesium citrate in the treatment of chronic persistent leg cramps, *Med Sci Monit* (2002), 8(5): CR326–30.

60 Garrison, S.R., Allan, G.M. & Sekhon, R.K. et al., Magnesium for skeletal muscle cramps, *Cochrane Database Syst Rev* (2012), 9: CD009402.

61 Rude, R.K. & Gruber, H.E., Magnesium deficiency and osteoporosis: Animal and human observations, *J Nutr Biochem* (2004), 15(12): 710–16.

62 Ryder, K.M., Shorr, R.I., Bush, A.J. et al., Magnesium intake from food and supplements is associated with bone mineral density in healthy older white subjects, *J Am Geriatr Soc* (2005), 53(11): 1875–80.

63 Mutlu, M., Argun, M., Kilic, E. et al. Magnesium, zinc and copper status in osteoporotic, osteopenic and normal post-menopausal women, *J Int Med Res* (2007), 35(5): 692–5.

64 Dimai, H.P., Porta, S., Wirnsberger, G. et al., Daily oral magnesium supplementation suppresses bone turnover in young adult males, *J Clin Endocrinol Metab* (1998), 83(8): 2742–8.

65 Aydin, H., Deyneli, O., Yavuz, D. et al., Short-term oral magnesium supplementation suppresses bone turnover in postmenopausal osteoporotic women, *Biol Trace Elem Res* (2010), 133(2): 136–43.

66 Stendig-Lindberg, G., Tepper, R. & Leichter, I., Trabecular bone density in a two year controlled trial of peroral magnesium in osteoporosis, *Magnes Res* (1993), 6: 155–63.

67 Popoviciu, L., Aşgian B., Delast-Popoviciu, D. et al., Clinical, EEG, electromyographic and polysomnographic studies in restless legs syndrome caused by magnesium deficiency, *Rom J Neurol Psychiatry* (1993), 31(1): 55–61.

68 Hornyak, M., Voderholzer, U., Hohagen, F. et al., Magnesium therapy for periodic leg movements-related insomnia and restless legs syndrome: an open pilot study, *Sleep* (1998), 21(5): 501–5.

69 Alamoudi, O.S., Hypomagnesaemia in chronic, stable asthmatics: Prevalence, correlation with severity and hospitalization, *Eur Respir J* (2000), 16(3): 427–31.

70 Gontijo-Amaral, C., Ribeiro, M.A., Gontijo, L.S. et al., Oral magnesium supplementation in asthmatic children: A double-blind randomized placebo-controlled trial, *Eur J Clin Nutr* (2007), 61(1): 54–60.

71 Kazaks, A.G., Uriu-Adams, J.Y. & Albertson, T.E. et al., Effect of oral magnesium supplementation on measures of airway resistance and subjective assessment of asthma control and quality of life in men and women with mild to moderate asthma: A randomized placebo controlled trial, *J Asthma* (2010), 47(1): 83–92.
72 Rowe, B.H., Bretzlaff, J.A., Bourdon, C. et al., Magnesium sulfate for treating exacerbations of acute asthma in the emergency department, *Cochrane Database Syst Rev* (2000), 2: CD001490.
73 Ishimura, E., Okuno, S., Kitatani, K. et al., Significant association between the presence of peripheral vascular calcification and lower serum magnesium in hemodialysis patients, *Clin Nephrol* (2007), 68(4): 222–7.
74 Gorgels, T.G., Waarsing, J.H., de Wolf, A. et al., Dietary magnesium, not calcium, prevents vascular calcification in a mouse model for pseudoxanthoma elasticum, *J Mol Med (Berl)* (2010), 88(5): 467–75.
75 Meema, H.E., Oreopoulos, D.G. & Rapoport, A., Serum magnesium level and arterial calcification in end-stage renal disease, *Kidney Int* (1987), 32(3): 388–94.
76 Tzanakis, I., Pras, A., Kounali, D. et al., Mitral annular calcification in haemodialysis patients: A possible protective role of magnesium, *Nephrol Dial Transplant* (1997), 12(9): 2036–7.
77 Tzanakis, I., Virvidakis, K., Tsomi, A. et al., Intra- and extracellular magnesium levels and atheromatosis in haemodialysis patients, *Magnes Res* (2004), 17(2): 102–8.
78 Spiegel, D.M. & Farmer, B., Long-term effects of magnesium carbonate on coronary artery calcification and bone mineral density in hemodialysis patients: A pilot study, *Hemodial Int* (2009), 13(4): 453–9.
79 Desmars, J.F. & Tawashi, R., Dissolution and growth of calcium oxalate monohydrate. I. Effect of magnesium and pH, *Biochim Biophys Acta* (1973), 313(2): 256–67.
80 Reungjui, S., Prasongwatana, V., Premgamone, A. et al., Magnesium status of patients with renal stones and its effect on urinary citrate excretion, *BJU Int* (2002), 90(7): 635–9.
81 Ettinger, B., Pak, C.Y., Citron, J.T. et al., Potassium-magnesium citrate is an effective prophylaxis against recurrent calcium oxalate nephrolithiasis, *J Urol* (1997), 158(6): 2069–73.
82 Nielsen, F.H. & Lukaski, H.C., Update on the relationship between magnesium and exercise, *Magnes Res* (2006), 19(3): 180–9.
83 McDonald, R. & Keen, C.L., Iron, zinc and magnesium nutrition and athletic performance, *Sports Med* (1988), 5: 171–84.
84 Lukaski, H.C. & Nielsen, F.H., Dietary magnesium depletion affects metabolic responses during submaximal exercise in postmenopausal women, *J Nutr* (2002), 132: 930–5.
85 Eby, G.A. III & Eby, K.L., Magnesium for treatment-resistant depression: A review and hypothesis, *Med Hypotheses* (2010), 74(4): 649–60.
86 Serefko, A., Szopa, A., Wlaź, P. et al., Magnesium in depression, *Pharmacol Rep* (2013), 65(3): 547–54.
87 Banki, C.M., Vojnik, M., Papp, Z. et al., Cerebrospinal fluid magnesium and calcium related to amine metabolites, diagnosis, and suicide attempts, *Biol Psychiatry* (1985), 20: 163–71.
88 Barragán-Rodríguez, L., Rodríguez-Morán, M. & Guerrero-Romero, F., Efficacy and safety of oral magnesium supplementation in the treatment of depression in the elderly with type 2 diabetes: A randomized, equivalent trial, *Magnes Res* (2008), 21(4): 218–23.
89 Eby, G.A. & Eby, K.L., Rapid recovery from major depression using magnesium treatment, *Med Hypotheses* (2006), 67(2): 362–70.
90 Derom, M.L., Sayón-Orea, C., Martínez-Ortega, J.M. & Martínez-González, M.A., Magnesium and depression: A systematic review, *Nutr Neurosci* (2013), 16(5): 191–206.
91 Dupont, C., Campagne, A. & Constant, F., Efficacy and safety of a magnesium sulfate-rich natural mineral water for patients with functional constipation, *Clin Gastroenterol Hepatol* (2013), 12(8): 1280–7.
92 Tu, T.L. & Kang, M.X., Effective analysis of three kinds of bowel preparation on colonoscopy in patients with constipation, *Mod Med Health* (2011), 10: 1488–9.
93 Passaretti, S., Mazzotti, G., Franzoni, M. & Tittobello, A., Effects of the administration of magnesium hydroxide on gastric acidity in health volunteers, *Minerva Gastroenterol Dietol* (1992), 38(2): 105–8. [Article in Italian]

Therapeutic dose

Improving dietary intake of magnesium should be emphasised. Small frequent doses are better absorbed. Suggested doses of elemental magnesium for adults are as follows:

- *Health maintenance:* 300–400 mg daily.
- *Mild deficiency:* 400 mg daily.
- *Severe deficiency:* 600 mg daily in the short term until symptoms resolve.
- *Magnesium-related disorders:* 400–600 mg daily in the short term until symptoms resolve.

Effects of excess

In people with healthy kidneys, severe side-effects of magnesium supplementation are rare. However, oral magnesium has a laxative action, and can cause abdominal colic and diarrhoea. It is better tolerated when taken in divided doses.

Elevated plasma magnesium (hypermagnesaemia) is more likely to occur with chronic use of magnesium laxatives and in people with kidney disease, elderly people and people given iv magnesium, and may cause nausea, vomiting, a sensation of warmth, flushing, hypotension (low blood pressure), abnormal heartbeat, sleepiness, double vision, slurred speech and weakness. Extremely high plasma magnesium may cause loss of deep tendon reflexes, muscular paralysis, coma and respiratory and cardiac arrest. Hypocalcaemia and hyperkalaemia may aggravate magnesium toxicity. Intravenous calcium gluconate can be used as an antidote, and severe cases may require haemodialysis treatment.

Case reports—magnesium excess

- *A woman, 76 years of age,* with dementia, developed extreme hypotension and unresponsiveness one day after being given 34 g of a magnesium citrate laxative (containing 2.71 g of magnesium) for severe constipation.[1] She developed poor kidney function and an abnormally slow heartbeat that did not respond to medication. Her respiration decreased and she became unconscious and required mechanical ventilation. A scan revealed that her entire colon was filled with faeces, and she was first diagnosed with obstruction of the bowel. Her unresponsiveness and hypotension were attributed to a vasovagal reaction to abdominal pain. Her serum magnesium level was not analysed initially but her condition deteriorated and a diagnosis of hypermagnesaemia was proposed. Blood testing revealed a markedly elevated magnesium level. Haemodialysis was contraindicated because of severe hypotension, and her doctors attempted to clear the residual magnesium from her bowels with an enema and an emergency colonoscopy. Her heart arrhythmia was treated by electrical stimulation. Her doctors admitted that they did not think to use iv calcium. The patient's heart rate normalised and her serum magnesium concentration gradually returned to normal without haemodialysis; her kidney function also normalised and she made a full recovery.
- *A boy, two years of age,* with a history of severe mental retardation, spastic quadriplegia and seizures, was admitted to hospital in cardiopulmonary arrest, not breathing, with no pulse and unresponsive to stimulation.[2] He had been receiving mechanical ventilation via a tracheostomy tube during the night for breathing difficulties, and was fed via a gastrostomy tube. Three weeks before hospitalisation, his mother had begun administering high doses of vitamin and mineral supplements at the recommendation of a private nutritional consultant without his doctor's knowledge. Supplements included magnesium oxide, which the nutritional consultant had recommended for relaxing the boy's muscles and relieving his constipation. Over a three-week period, the boy became drowsy and less able to be aroused, his heart rate slowed, and he was taken to hospital after being found unresponsive, not breathing and with enlarged pupils.

  After successful resuscitation, he was found to have hypermagnesaemia (serum magnesium 8.4 mmol/L), together with low calcium and potassium. His heart rate improved initially after electrical stimulation. He was given haemodialysis, which reduced his serum magnesium level to 3.1 mmol/L, and was followed up with continuous haemofiltration to further reduce the magnesium load. However, the boy died 20 hours after admission because of further deterioration of his heart function.
- *A woman, 61 years of age,* with a past history of chronic constipation and hypertension, developed generalised weakness, body aches and abdominal discomfort over the course of one week.[3] She had been taking thiazide diuretics for hypertension and milk of magnesia for her constipation. On admission

to hospital, she was found to have mild dehydration, and laboratory tests revealed markedly elevated serum magnesium, and low serum phosphate and calcium. She was taken off diuretics and milk of magnesia and rehydrated. Her symptoms improved markedly by the second day, and resolved completely on the third day. Her serum magnesium normalised in three days and she was discharged with instructions to avoid the use of milk of magnesia. Follow-up revealed that all symptoms had completely resolved.

REFERENCES

1 Kontani, M., Hara, A., Ohta, S. & Ikeda, T., Hypermagnesemia induced by massive cathartic ingestion in an elderly woman without pre-existing renal dysfunction, *Intern Med* (2005), 44(5): 448–52.

2 McGuire, J.K., Kulkarni, M.S. & Baden, H.P., Fatal hypermagnesemia in a child treated with megavitamin/megamineral therapy, *Pediatrics* (2000), 105(2): E18.

3 Mazidi, P., Khair, T., Zedudehhali, F. & Petrucelli, O., Symptomatic hypermagnesemia in the absence of renal failure, *Internet J Inter Med* (2009), 9(1).

Supplements

Magnesium can be extracted from sea water by mixing with calcined (thermally decomposed) dolomite or lime (calcium oxide), together with water, to produce an aqueous suspension containing magnesium hydroxide and calcium chloride. Magnesium hydroxide precipitates out of solution, and can be calcined to produce magnesium oxide or treated with hydrochloric acid to form the chloride salt.

In Australia, the permitted forms of magnesium salts in supplements include magnesium amino acid chelate, ascorbate, ascorbate monohydrate, ascorbyl phosphate, aspartate, aspartate anhydrous, aspartate dihydrate, carbonate, carbonate–heavy, carbonate–light, chloride, citrate, diglutamate, gluconate, glycerophosphate, hydroxide, orotate, orotate dihydrate, oxide, oxide–heavy, oxide–light, phosphate, phosphate dibasic, phosphate tribasic, stearate, sulfate (dihydrate, monohydrate or trihydrate) and levocarnitine magnesium citrate.

The amount of elemental magnesium in a specific magnesium salt is listed on the product container and may vary between individual products; the approximate elemental magnesium content of some common salts is shown in Table 8.5.

Table 8.5 Elemental magnesium content of common salts

Salt	Magnesium content (%)
Magnesium oxide	60
Magnesium hydroxide	42
Magnesium carbonate	29
Magnesium citrate	16
Magnesium chloride	12
Magnesium sulfate	10
Magnesium aspartate	8
Magnesium gluconate	5

Magnesium supplements are available in tablets, capsules or suspensions. The most commonly used forms are magnesium oxide, citrate and amino acid chelates. Magnesium oxide is cheap, and provides a lot more elemental magnesium than most other salts. However, inorganic salts, such as magnesium oxide, chloride, sulfate and carbonate, are less bioavailable than organic salts. A cell study found that magnesium oxide was virtually insoluble in water, and only 43 per cent soluble in a hydrochloric acid secretion, whereas magnesium citrate had high solubility even in water (55 per cent), and was substantially more soluble than magnesium oxide in an acid solution.

In an animal study, magnesium absorption from ten magnesium salts was found to vary from 50 to 67 per cent, and organic salts were slightly more available than inorganic salts and had better retention in the body. Magnesium sulfate and magnesium carbonate had the lowest absorption, and magnesium gluconate had the highest bioavailability, with absorption of 66.5 per cent and retention of 48.7 per cent. However, inorganic magnesium salts had an average absorption of 50 per cent and retention of 39 per cent, and were found to be acceptable forms of magnesium supplements. A study of magnesium-deficient animals found that magnesium aspartate (a form of chelated magnesium) was the most effective in resolving the deficiency and had the fastest activity, and magnesium chloride was the most effective of the inorganic magnesium salts.

In humans, magnesium oxide was found to have relatively poor bioavailability (4 per cent absorption), but magnesium chloride, magnesium lactate and magnesium aspartate had a higher and equivalent bioavailability. However, in healthy women, magnesium oxide was found to be better than magnesium citrate for improving intracellular magnesium levels, and total and LDL cholesterol, but both salts had a similar effect in inhibiting platelet aggregation.

Magnesium citrate and magnesium oxide have been shown to be poorly absorbed on an empty stomach, and absorption increases when taken with meals. Magnesium from effervescent tablets has been shown to have better absorption compared with capsules—possibly because dissolving the tablet in water before ingestion improves ionisation—and magnesium absorption from enteric-coated magnesium chloride tablets has been shown to be much less than from standard magnesium acetate tablets.

Magnesium is also available as magnesium 'oil', which is made from magnesium chloride flakes and distilled water and is designed for topical use as a spray for sore muscles. It is not an oil but has an oily feel. It can be made by combining equal parts of magnesium chloride flakes (sold as bath salts) and distilled water and then boiling and stirring until dissolved, after which it is cooled and dispensed into a spray bottle.

Cautions

Oral magnesium has a laxative action, and can cause abdominal colic and diarrhoea. High doses of magnesium should be avoided in people with poor kidney function and the elderly. Magnesium may reduce the absorption of the following drugs when taken together: quinolone antibiotics, bisphosphonates (for bone disorders) and tiludronate disodium (for Paget's disease); magnesium supplements should be taken two to four hours before or after the drug dose. Magnesium hydroxide may increase the absorption of diabetic medications used to control blood sugar levels, and there is some evidence that magnesium-containing antacids reduce the effectiveness of the drug levothyroxine (for thyroid function). Magnesium should not be taken with calcium channel blockers without medical advice.

HOW MUCH DO I KNOW?

Choose whether the following statements are true or false. Then review this chapter for the correct answers.

	True (T)	False (F)
1 Sulfur, phosphorus and chloride are acid-forming minerals.	T	F
2 Minerals can be absorbed in their ionic forms.	T	F
3 Oxalate and phytate in foods enhance mineral absorption.	T	F
4 A low calcium intake leads to reduced levels of parathyroid hormone and calcitriol.	T	F
5 Spinach is a good source of available calcium.	T	F
6 Calcium is part of hydroxyapatite in bone.	T	F
7 A deficiency of phosphorus can cause low bone mineral density, osteomalacia and muscle paralysis.	T	F
8 Calcification of soft tissue results from magnesium overload.	T	F
9 Magnesium regulates nerve and muscle function.	T	F
10 Magnesium may be useful for cardiovascular disease and migraines.	T	F

FURTHER READING

Braun, L. & Cohen, M., *Herbs & natural supplements: An evidence-based guide*, 3rd ed., Churchill Livingstone Elsevier, New York, 2010.

Gropper, S.S., Smith, J.L. & Groff, J.L., *Advanced nutrition and human metabolism*, 5th ed., Thomson Wadsworth, Belmont, CA, 2009.

Higdon, J., *An evidence-based approach to vitamins and minerals*, Thieme, New York, 2003.

Linus Pauling Institute, Micronutrient Research Center, website, available at <lpi.oregonstate.edu/infocenter>.

9

Macrominerals: sodium, potassium, chloride and sulfur

SODIUM

SODIUM STATUS CHECK

1 **Do you have high blood pressure or a family history of high blood pressure?**
2 **Do you eat salted, processed or takeaway foods regularly?**
3 **Do you have poor kidney function?**
4 **Do you drink very little water?**

'Yes' answers may indicate imbalanced sodium status. Note that a number of nutritional deficiencies or health disorders can cause similar effects and further investigation is recommended.

FAST FACTS . . . SODIUM

- **Sodium levels are high in salted, processed and takeaway foods, and most standard diets contain excessive amounts.**
- **Sodium helps maintain water and electrolyte balance.**
- **Sodium is essential for nerve and muscle function, and for maintaining osmotic pressure in extracellular fluid.**
- **A deficiency can cause dehydration, nausea, vomiting, lethargy, weakness, muscle cramps, disorientation and confusion.**
- **Excess may cause elevated blood pressure and cardiovascular disease.**

Sodium is a naturally occurring mineral that makes up about 3 per cent of the earth's crust, and is found in rocks—most commonly as a type of feldspar—and also in the semi-precious gemstone sodalite. It is found as sodium bicarbonate in mineral water, and as sodium chloride in sea water and rock, vegetable and sea salt.

The English chemist Sir Humphry Davy was the first to isolate sodium from electrolysis of sodium hydroxide in 1807. Davy named the element sodium, which is derived from soda, the common name for various forms of sodium salts. Its chemical symbol, Na, is derived from the Latin word *natrium,* meaning 'sodium'.

Sodium is the major extracellular cation in the body, and the concentration is tightly maintained within 135–145 mmol/L. About 5 per cent of body sodium is found within cells and about 50 per cent is in extracellular fluid (ECF), in which it has a vital role in maintaining osmotic pressure across membranes, and in attracting and holding water in the bloodstream to maintain healthy blood volume and blood pressure.

Bones contain 30–40 per cent of total body sodium, in which it is in bone crystals and on the surface of bones for mobilisation as required to maintain healthy ECF levels.

Digestion, absorption and transport

Sodium is found in foods as various salts, particularly as sodium chloride (table salt), which is used widely in food processing and cooking, and as a condiment. Salt is ionised in the stomach to release sodium and chloride ions. Sodium is very soluble, and an average of 98 per cent is absorbed from the diet.

There are three main pathways for sodium absorption in the digestive tract. Sodium and chloride can be absorbed into enterocytes in the small intestine via an energy-dependent sodium/chloride cotransporter (NCC), which exchanges sodium ions for hydrogen ions and chloride ions for bicarbonate ions. Sodium is also taken up by energy-dependent sodium-glucose linked transporters (SGLTs), which also transport glucose, galactose, amino acids, dipeptides, tripeptides, diglycerides, triglycerides and B vitamins. Together with water and other ions, sodium ions also passively diffuse across the wall of the colon via epithelial sodium channels (ENaC). Once absorbed, sodium is moved out of the intestinal cells into the bloodstream by the sodium/potassium-ATPase (Na/K-ATPase) pump.

Metabolism, storage and excretion

Sodium ions in the blood move into the ECF surrounding cells and the Na/K-ATPase pump in cell membranes maintains a higher concentration of sodium ions in the ECF by moving sodium out of cells, and a higher concentration of potassium ions inside the cell by moving potassium into the cell interior. Sodium in bone provides a store that can be mobilised as required. The major pathway for excretion of sodium is via the kidneys, with small amounts lost in sweat. Physical exertion in hot weather can cause marked increases in sweat loss, which stabilises with acclimatisation. Sweat loss is reduced if body levels of sodium are low. About 99.5 per cent of sodium passing through the kidneys is reabsorbed into the bloodstream via NCC and ENaC, together with water, chloride and bicarbonate.

Regulation of sodium and water balance

The sodium:water ratio (osmolality, a measure of the moles of solute per kg of solvent) in ECF is kept under tight control by balancing the intake and excretion of sodium with that of water, because changes in water volume alone will increase or reduce osmolality. If the number of sodium ions increases in the ECF without a change in the amount of water, or when the ECF water volume decreases without a change in the amount of sodium ions, the osmolality of ECF increases. This is detected by the hypothalamus, which produces antidiuretic hormone (ADH), secreted from the posterior pituitary gland, to stimulate retention of water by the kidneys in order to lower osmolality. The hypothalamus also stimulates thirst to increase water intake. If the water amount in ECF increases without a change in sodium content, or if the number of sodium ions reduces with no change in water volume, osmolality decreases. ADH is no longer released and the kidneys get rid of the extra water.

Changes in total body sodium content alter the ECF volume, including plasma volume, which affects blood pressure. Low total body sodium leads to low plasma volume and low blood pressure and triggers reflexes that stimulate the kidneys to increase sodium reabsorption, which normalises blood volume and blood pressure. An increase in total body sodium increases blood volume and blood pressure, which triggers the kidneys to excrete sodium.

A number of sensors in the blood vessels, heart, lungs, liver, kidneys and central nervous system detect changes in ECF volume or osmotic pressure. Intrarenal sensors within the kidney tubules maintain a constant blood flow by causing vasodilation or vasoconstriction, as required.

The system that increases sodium retention includes the following:

- *Aldosterone*. This hormone, produced in the adrenal cortex, stimulates the kidneys to reabsorb sodium and water, thus boosting ECF volume. When sodium intake is high, aldosterone secretion is low, and secretion increases when sodium intake is low or total body sodium levels drop.
- *The renin-angiotensin system*. This system involves release of renin by the kidneys, which acts on angiotensinogen in the bloodstream to produce angiotensin I. This is converted by angiotensin-converting enzyme (ACE)

to the active hormone angiotensin II, which stimulates secretion of aldosterone and ADH, constricts arterioles in the kidneys, boosts sodium reabsorption and stimulates thirst, all of which boost ECF volume and blood pressure. This system is active when perfusion pressure in the kidneys drops during sodium depletion and is inactive when perfusion pressure and sodium levels are adequate.

- *The sympathetic nervous system.* This is stimulated when arterial pressure drops and it acts to enhance renin release, and constrict arterioles in the kidneys in order to reduce sodium and water excretion.
- *Adenosine.* This is a naturally occurring purine nucleoside that is formed from the breakdown of ATP. Adenosine enhances sodium and water retention by affecting kidney blood flow, glomerular filtration rate and renin secretion, and by direct effects on the kidney tubule epithelium.

The system that increases sodium excretion includes the following:

- *Atrial natriuretic peptide (ANP)* and *brain natriuretic peptide (BNP).* ANP is a peptide hormone secreted by cells in the atria of the heart, and BNP is a peptide hormone, first detected in pig brains, secreted by cells in the ventricles of the heart. These hormones are secreted in response to elevated blood pressure and are active when sodium intake is high. They stimulate the kidneys to excrete sodium and water, and reduce renin and aldosterone secretion.
- *Kallikrein.* This is a kidney protease that converts kininogen to kinins that increase sodium and water excretion.
- *Prostaglandins (PGs).* PGs produced in the kidneys have a range of moderating functions on sodium balance, but predominantly stimulate sodium excretion.

Functions

Sodium is essential for maintaining fluid balance and osmotic pressure, transport of substances across cell membranes, nerve transmission and muscle contraction. Sodium has an alkaline effect on body pH. The functions of sodium include:

- *Water and electrolyte balance.* Sodium is an electrolyte (a mineral that carries an electrical charge) that is essential for maintaining water volume and distribution in the body, and osmotic pressure in ECF. Other important electrolytes are calcium, chloride, magnesium, phosphorus and potassium. Sodium helps regulate the body content of potassium, which is excreted by the kidneys when sodium is reabsorbed, and the body content of water and chloride, which are reabsorbed in the kidneys together with sodium.
- *Cell function.* Sodium maintains blood volume and blood pressure to support delivery of nutrients to cells and removal of wastes. The correct ratio of sodium to potassium across cell membranes is essential for maintaining water distribution inside and outside cells and a constant cell volume, which is required for optimum function. Uncontrolled entry of water into cells would lead to cell rupture, and uncontrolled water losses would lead to cell shrinkage and loss of function. The Na/K-ATPase pump uses energy from ATP to simultaneously pump three sodium ions out of the cell and two potassium ions into the cell. It helps control ECF volume and blood pressure in the kidneys, uptake of nutrients in the digestive tract, and nerve and muscle activity. The Na/K-ATPase pump creates an electrochemical gradient across cell membranes, resulting in a relatively negatively charged cell interior. Sodium ions tend to leak into cells via membrane channels because of this gradient, and this helps to transport nutrients such as glucose and amino acids into the cell. Recently, the Na/K-ATPase pump has been found to play a role in cell signalling.
- *Nerve and muscle function.* The different concentrations of sodium and potassium across cell membranes create the resting membrane potential of nerve cells. When stimulated, sodium channels in nerve cell membranes open briefly and sodium enters the interior of the cell, causing depolarisation and generation of an action potential (nerve impulse) that travels along the nerve membrane. Repolarisation occurs when potassium channels open, allowing potassium to leave the cell. Afterwards, the Na/K-ATPase pump restores the resting concentrations of sodium and potassium ions. Nerve impulses arriving at muscle cells trigger calcium release, which then activates the contraction process.
- *Bone structure and mineral reserve.* Sodium is part of the structure of crystalline bone, together with calcium, phosphate, magnesium and other minerals, and can be readily mobilised from the bone surface to maintain serum levels.

Dietary sources

Sodium is naturally found in low levels in many foods, such as seaweed, seafood, meat, nuts, grains, fruit, vegetables and dairy products. Tap water is generally low in sodium, especially in soft water areas. Analyses of tap water in selected areas of Sydney have reported sodium levels of 4.1 to 65.3 mg/L and 4.8 to 12.7 mg/L in selected areas of Melbourne. Bottled mineral waters have widely varying concentrations of sodium, ranging from 1 to 1200 mg/L.

Most standard diets contain excessive levels of sodium. Table salt is 40 per cent sodium (400 mg of sodium per g) and 60 per cent chloride, and a teaspoon of salt (about 5 g) contains about 2 g of sodium. All forms of salt, including vegetable salt, sea salt and rock salt, are predominantly sodium chloride, and foods containing added salt are high in sodium. Most processed food are high in salt. High-salt foods include stock cubes, soy sauce, tomato sauce, breakfast cereals, biscuits, cakes, bread, canned soups and vegetables, salted nuts, processed meats such as sausages, ham, bacon and corned beef, yeast-based spreads, cheese, pizza, savoury snack foods and takeaway foods. Sodium-containing food additives include baking powder (sodium bicarbonate with starch and cream of tartar), baking soda (sodium bicarbonate), sodium nitrite used as a preservative in processed meats and monosodium glutamate (MSG) found in Chinese restaurant meals and processed foods.

A 2013 Australian study found that the adult mean salt intake, as assessed by daily urinary excretion, was 8.9 g/day (3560 mg sodium). In the UK in 2011, the mean estimated salt intake for adults, assessed by urinary excretion, was 8.1 g per day (3240 mg sodium). Men had a mean estimated intake of 9.3 g per day (3720 mg sodium), and women had a mean estimated intake of 6.8 g per day (2720 mg sodium). The US estimated mean daily intake of sodium from all sources for persons aged two years or older during the period 2003 to 2006 was 3614 mg/day.

It is estimated that about 70–75 per cent of total sodium intake comes from processed foods, naturally occurring sodium in unprocessed foods provides about 10–15 per cent and another 10–15 per cent comes from salt used in cooking or added at the table. In Australia, it is estimated that 25 per cent of salt intake comes from bread and bread rolls, 21 per cent from meat and poultry dishes, including processed meat, 17 per cent from cereal products, 8 per cent from savoury sauces and condiments and 5 per cent from cheese. In Australia, foods that have been produced with lower levels of salt than a comparable regular product may be labelled as follows:

- *'Low salt'*, indicating that the food contains no more than 120 mg sodium per 100 mL for liquid food; or 120 mg per 100 g for solid food.
- *'Salt reduced'*, *'Light'* or *'Lite'*, indicating that the food contains at least 25 per cent less sodium than in the same quantity of reference food
- *'No added salt'* or *'Unsalted'*, indicating that the food contains no added sodium compound, including no added salt, and the ingredients of the food contain no added sodium compound, including no added salt.

The Food Standards Australia New Zealand nutrient database (NUTTAB) at <www.foodstandards.gov.au> provides the amounts found in specific foods.

Factors influencing body status

Sodium is water soluble, and is lost from foods by water-processing and cooking methods. Large amounts of fluid ingested in a short space of time can dilute ECF and reduce osmolality, and a high salt intake or a very low fluid intake may increase osmolality. Physical activity can increase sodium losses in sweat, and excess potassium increases sodium losses in urine. An increase in dietary fructose stimulates salt absorption in the small intestine and reabsorption in the kidneys.

In diabetes, elevated glucose exerts an osmotic effect in the kidneys and increases excretion of sodium and water. Elderly diabetics may have inadequate renin and aldosterone secretion, and consequently lose sodium but retain potassium. In older people, the kidneys are less able to regulate the excretion of water and sodium. In cystic fibrosis, there is faulty membrane transport of sodium and chloride, and increased losses in sweat. Endocrine and kidney disorders, fever, vomiting and diarrhoea may cause sodium imbalance. The licorice constituent glycyrrhizin inhibits an enzyme that breaks down cortisol, and the higher cortisol levels cause more stimulation of aldosterone receptors in the kidneys and cause sodium and water retention and potassium loss in urine.

The main drugs that reduce sodium levels are diuretics, which are designed to reduce oedema or high blood pressure by stimulating sodium and water excretion in urine. Thiazide diuretics inhibit sodium and chloride reabsorption in the distal convoluted tubule, and loop diuretics act in the Loop of Henle and have a more powerful effect. Both types of diuretic also lead to potassium losses. Potassium-sparing diuretics antagonise the effects of aldosterone and inhibit reabsorption of sodium in the collecting tubules and duct without loss of potassium. Other drugs that are associated with low sodium levels include psychiatric drugs such as anti-psychotic agents, tricyclic antidepressants, selective serotonin reuptake inhibitors (SSRIs) and serotonin-noradrenaline reuptake inhibitors; ACE inhibitors used for high blood pressure; the diabetic drug chlorpropamide; the anticonvulsant carbamazepine; the anticancer drugs vincristine, vinblastine and cyclophosphamide; and analgesic drugs—especially narcotics—used after surgery. Progesterone increases sodium losses in urine, and non-steroidal anti-inflammatory drugs (NSAIDs), oestrogens and glucocorticoids enhance sodium retention.

Daily requirement

The National Health and Medical Research Council (NHMRC) of Australia recommends that adults eat less than 2300 mg of sodium per day. The NHMRC has also set a suggested dietary target of 1600 mg/day for older, overweight people with elevated blood pressure and for those wishing to maintain low blood pressure over their lifespan.

Government recommendations by age and gender (see Table 9.1) can be found in *Nutrient Reference Values for Australia and New Zealand Including Recommended Dietary Intakes*, available at <www.nhmrc.gov.au>.

Table 9.1 Adequate intake (AI) of sodium (mg/day)

Age (years)	Female AI	Male AI
1–3	200–400	200–400
4–8	300–600	300–600
9–13	400–800	400–800
14–18	460–920	460–920
19–70	460–920	460–920
>70	460–920	460–920
Pregnant women		
14–18	460–920	
19–50	460–920	
Lactating women		
14–18	460–920	
19–50	460–920	

Source: Nutrient Reference Values for Australia and New Zealand Including Recommended Dietary Intakes, National Health and Medical Research Council, Australian Government Department of Health and Ageing, Canberra and Ministry of Health, New Zealand, Wellington, 2006.

Deficiency effects

In the general population, sodium intake is usually adequate or excessive, and a dietary deficiency is an unlikely cause of a low serum sodium concentration (hyponatraemia) because of the tight regulation of serum levels by the kidneys. Hyponatraemia has occurred in infants with diarrhoea who have been given tap water instead of electrolyte replacement fluids and infants fed on very diluted infant formulae. It may occur also in association with the use of certain drugs—primarily diuretics—and in older people and those with various health disorders. It is a relatively common finding in hospital patients, in whom it is usually associated with an excess of water in ECF relative to sodium (hypotonic hyponatraemia), but it can occur as a result of depletion of total body sodium together with a normal amount of water in ECF or a shift of water from cells to the ECF. Hypotonic hyponatraemia is usually caused by a high or normal water intake, together with impaired water excretion in the kidneys and, less commonly, by a very high water intake that overloads the kidneys' ability to excrete it. It can be classified as hypovolaemic (decreased ECF volume), euvolaemic (normal ECF volume) and hypervolaemic (increased ECF volume).

Hypovolaemic hyponatraemia (decreased ECF volume), a state of dehydration, is caused by sodium and water loss, and is associated with diuretic use, especially thiazide diuretics, advanced chronic kidney disease, inadequate aldosterone secretion, burns, vomiting, diarrhoea, haemorrhage, pancreatitis and excessive sweating during extreme physical exertion. A rare type of hypovolaemic hyponatraemia is cerebral salt wasting syndrome, occurring in patients with brain injury and those with subarachnoid haemorrhage (bleeding between the brain surface and the brain lining). It appears to be caused by secretion of BNP. Euvolaemic hyponatraemia (normal ECF volume) is associated with syndrome of inappropriate ADH secretion (SIADH), hypothyroidism, pituitary or adrenal insufficiency and excessive administration of hypotonic fluids post-operatively. Hypervolaemic hyponatraemia (increased ECF volume) is seen in patients with congestive heart failure, nephrotic syndrome (a type of kidney damage) or liver cirrhosis.

Hyponatraemia can be caused by water intoxication, which occurs when a very high water intake exceeds the kidneys' ability to excrete it, causing a fluid overload in the body and a relatively low sodium level in ECF. It is seen in psychiatric disturbances such as schizophrenia, in which compulsive water drinking (primary polydipsia) develops and water consumption may reach 10–15 L/day. It has occurred also in binge drinkers of beer (beer potomania) and in users of the party drug methylenedioxymethamphetamine (MDMA, also known as ecstasy), which, in some people, has been found to trigger SIADH, water intoxication and cerebral oedema when fluid intake is excessive.

In hyponatraemia, water moves from the ECF to the central nervous system, causing swelling of the nerve cells. Mild hyponatraemia may cause loss of appetite, headache, nausea, vomiting and lethargy, and moderate hyponatraemia may lead to personality changes, inappropriate behaviour, delusions, hallucinations, confusion, disorientation, depression, muscle cramps, muscle weakness and ataxia. Mild chronic hyponatraemia may cause no obvious symptoms, but is associated with a reduced bone mass and an increased incidence of falls in elderly people, possibly as a result of impaired brain function and coordination. If hyponatraemia is severe or of rapid onset, it may lead to cerebral oedema and brain stem herniation, signs of which include a fixed, dilated pupil in one eye, drowsiness, involuntary movements, seizures, coma, permanent brain damage and possibly respiratory arrest and death.

Hyponatraemia may be associated with dehydration symptoms such as dry mucous membranes, shrivelled, wrinkled skin (diminished skin turgor), a rapid heartbeat, postural hypotension, heat intolerance, loss of appetite, nausea, a burning sensation in the stomach, constipation, infrequent urination, darker-coloured urine and urinary tract infections. Exercise-induced hyponatraemia has been associated with rhabdomyolysis (destruction of muscle tissue), encephalopathy (brain damage) and death. Hypervolaemic hyponatraemia may cause pulmonary rales (rattling sounds in the lung), a third heart sound (a sound generated by rapid ventricular filling, also called 'gallop rhythms'), distended jugular veins, peripheral oedema and fluid in the abdominal cavity (ascites).

Sodium replacement in hyponatraemia must not be too rapid because there is a risk of central pontine myelinolysis (CPM), in which water is rapidly pulled out of brain cells causing destruction of the myelin sheath covering nerve cells in the pons (the middle of the brainstem) and other parts of the brain. CPM can cause difficulty chewing, swallowing and speaking, and quadriplegia, and may even lead to 'locked-in' syndrome, in which the patient is aware but unable to move or communicate.

Indicators of inadequate levels of sodium may include:

- lethargy, weakness, muscle tremors, spasms, twitches, cramps, ataxia, seizures
- lack of appetite, nausea, vomiting
- personality changes, disorientation, confusion, depression
- dehydration (hypovolaemic hyponatraemia): thirst, headache, fatigue, impaired thinking ability, dry mucous membranes, rapid heartbeat, shrivelled, wrinkled skin, heat intolerance, loss of appetite, nausea, a burning sensation in the stomach, constipation, infrequent urination, darker-coloured urine, urinary tract infections
- irregular heart rhythm, postural hypotension
- fluid retention.

Assessment of body status

Serum sodium concentration does not reflect total body content, but it can be used to indicate abnormal sodium states. The reference range given by the Royal College of Pathologists of Australasia (RCPA) for adults is 135–145 mmol/L for serum or plasma sodium. Hyponatraemia is defined as a serum sodium concentration of less than 135 mmol/L and severe hyponatraemia is defined as a serum sodium concentration of less than 120 mmol/L. Hypernatraemia is defined as a serum sodium level greater than 145 mmol/L. Sodium status also can be assessed by a 24-hour urine analysis. The reference range given by the RCPA for urinary sodium in adults is 75–300 mmol/24 hours and reflects sodium intake.

Case reports—sodium deficiency

- *A girl, 15 years of age*, developed vomiting, dry retching, drowsiness, confusion and seizure-like movements before becoming unconscious and suffering respiratory arrest.[1] Her symptoms occurred some hours after taking the drug ecstasy during a dance party the previous evening. She had apparently remained relatively well for some time after taking the drug, and continued dancing strenuously and drinking large amounts of water before collapsing. She was resuscitated and hospitalised but was pronounced brain dead the following day. During the inquest, it was suggested that she had drunk large amounts of water because of a warning that prolonged dancing without replacing fluids has led to a number of deaths from hyperthermic collapse. Her cause of death was hypoxic encephalopathy caused by cerebral oedema. This had been induced by acute hyponatraemia as a result of water intoxication, secondary to ecstasy ingestion.

- *A woman, 72 years of age*, residing in a nursing home, was taken to hospital because of a sudden change in her mental state.[2] She had a medical history of coronary artery disease and hypertension, and was taking a thiazide diuretic and aspirin. She was found to have decreased skin turgor and postural hypotension, and was disorientated. Her serum sodium was low (110 mmol/L), and had decreased from a level of 135 mmol/L two months before admission. She was treated with intravenous saline solution and her serum sodium level increased to 120 mmol/L after the first 24 hours; her brain function improved gradually over the next three days. Her blood pressure medication was changed and she was discharged in good condition.
- *A woman, 40 years of age*, developed severe anxiety, profuse sweating, tremors, nausea and confusion twelve hours after an uncomplicated rhinoplasty under general anaesthesia.[3] Several hours after discharge, the patient experienced anxiety, which responded poorly to medication. She had a past history of generalised anxiety disorder. During evaluation, she was confused and forgetful, often repeating herself and forgetting to answer simple questions. It was discovered that she had drunk 4 L of water before surgery and 6 L of water during the first few hours after surgery to prevent dehydration, based on the advice of a naturopathic physician. She was found to have low serum sodium and was diagnosed with hyponatraemia due to water intoxication, and treated with fluid restriction and an infusion of saline solution. Her sodium levels normalised overnight and all neurological signs and symptoms resolved.
- *A woman, 34 years of age*, developed symptoms that she believed were caused by dehydration after participating in a half-marathon running event (21 km) during hot weather (33°C).[4] Her training leading up to the event was limited to exercising on a treadmill in an air-conditioned environment once or twice a week (a maximum running distance of 15 km per week). She reported developing nausea and diarrhoea a few days before the race. She drank copious amounts of water before the race, as well as about 4 L of water during the race. Afterwards, she became nauseous and confused, but continued drinking water as she believed she was suffering from dehydration. She was brought to hospital with disorientation, nausea and a sensation of pressure in her chest. She was diagnosed with dehydration/hyponatraemia and given saline treatment. Within five hours, she suffered a grand mal seizure after which she displayed combative behaviour and was given more saline. During several hours of treatment, she produced very little urine, which was highly concentrated. She suffered a second grand mal seizure and developed generalised body aches and elevated creatine phosphokinase and potassium levels, leading to a diagnosis of rhabdomyolysis. Further treatment led to a gradual resolution of symptoms and she was discharged after seven days.

REFERENCES

1 Coroner's report No 2094 (1995), *Reasons for dispensing with inquest in the death of Anna Victoria Wood*. Retrieved 20 August 2014 from <www.erowid.org/chemicals/mdma/mdma_health5.shtml>.

2 Al-Salman, J., Kemp, D. & Randall, D., Hyponatremia, *West J Med* (2002), 176(3): 173–6.

3 Bhananker, S.M., Paek, R. & Vavilala, M.S., Water intoxication and symptomatic hyponatremia after outpatient surgery, *Anesth Analg* (2004), 98(5): 1294–6.

4 Glace, B. & Murphy, C., Severe hyponatremia develops in a runner following a half-marathon, *JAAPA* (2008), 21(6): 27–9.

THERAPEUTIC USES OF SODIUM

Additional sodium is rarely required because intake is usually excessive from the diet. Sodium is used therapeutically for the treatment of hyponatraemia under medical supervision.

Effects of excess

Hypernatraemia occurs when there is a relative excess of sodium to water in ECF, which causes water to move out of neurons and leads to shrinkage of brain cells. In most cases, the thirst response is triggered and water and sodium levels in ECF normalise. If not, the brain tries to adapt in the short term by shifts in sodium and potassium, and in the longer term by accumulating organic osmolytes, such as *myo*-inositol, glutamine and glutamate, within cells. Hypernatraemia can cause dehydration signs and symptoms, such as thirst, low ECF volume, postural hypotension, tachycardia (rapid heartbeat), dry mouth and abnormal skin turgor, as well as change of consciousness, lethargy, neuromuscular irritability, weakness, seizures and coma. It can result in brain haemorrhage and clots, including venous sinus thrombosis, a condition in which a blood clot forms in the dural venous sinuses that drain blood from the brain. Older patients may not show marked symptoms until sodium concentration exceeds 160 mmol/L. An acute, sudden rise in sodium levels can lead to vascular rupture, brain haemorrhage, permanent brain damage or death. Correction of hypernatraemia needs to be slow in order to avoid brain damage.

Hypernatraemia more commonly affects infants, the elderly and hospitalised patients. It can be caused by low body water content caused by inadequate fluid intake, increased water losses, defects in the thirst mechanism or inadequate ADH. Hypernatraemia can also be caused by a high sodium intake or excessive sodium reabsorption in the kidneys because of abnormally high aldosterone levels. Marked hypernatraemia can be induced by the administration of hypertonic sodium-containing solutions, which may be used to treat metabolic acidosis or as an emetic or gargle. However, this normalises rapidly in patients with healthy kidney function.

In elderly patients, hypernatraemia can be caused by reduced fluid intake, an impaired sense of thirst (hypodipsia), medication use, vomiting or diarrhoea. Elderly people have impaired kidney function, which limits the ability to excrete sodium, and many of the medications they use are a source of sodium. Soluble (effervescent) paracetamol, such as Panadol Rapid Soluble, is routinely given to elderly patients as an analgesic, and each tablet contains 425.5 mg sodium; eight tablets a day will provide about 3400 mg of sodium or 8.7 g of salt, which is well above the recommended intake. Antacids and laxatives commonly used by the elderly may also contain considerable amounts of sodium.

Hypernatraemia may develop in infants who are fed formula that has not been properly diluted, and in breastfed infants with feeding difficulties. Symptoms may occur at about eight to ten days of age, and include weight loss, lethargy, excessive crying, low urine output, lack of bowel movements, changes in brain cell osmolality and cerebral oedema, with fullness of the anterior fontanelle that may disguise the underlying dehydration. It may lead to seizures, brain haemorrhages and clots, brain damage and death.

Increased water losses in urine are caused by loop diuretics, hyperglycaemia, the use of mannitol as a diuretic, increased urea excretion from a high-protein diet or kidney disease. More rarely, water losses can be caused by inadequate ADH or abnormal thirst sensations. Inadequate ADH (diabetes insipidus) features the passing of copious amounts of dilute urine and the need to drink large amounts of water. Hypernatraemia does not develop if water intake is high enough to compensate. Thirst is regulated by osmoreceptors in the hypothalamus that are sensitive to changes in the osmotic pressure of body fluids, and a defect in these osmoreceptors causes adipsic hypernatraemia, in which there is a lack of thirst in spite of an increase in osmotic pressure.

Water can be lost from the body as a result of heavy sweating, vomiting or diarrhoea. Transient hypernatraemia can develop after vigorous exercise because the breakdown of glycogen into smaller, more osmotically active molecules, such as lactate, increases osmolality of cells and causes water movement into cells. The plasma sodium concentration returns to normal shortly after the exercise ceases.

An excessive sodium intake is unlikely to cause hypernatraemia in healthy people, but is associated with high blood pressure and a number of cardiovascular diseases (CVD), especially heart disease and stroke, and a high sodium concentration in urine causes increased urinary calcium and is associated with osteoporosis and calcium-based kidney stones.

SODIUM AND BLOOD PRESSURE

Blood pressure (BP) is assessed by measuring systolic BP, the pressure exerted on artery walls when the heart contracts, and diastolic BP, the pressure exerted when the heart is relaxed, and is measured in millimetres of mercury (Hg), which was used in the original BP measuring instruments. Elevated BP (hypertension) is considered a major risk for CVD, especially heart attack and stroke. A systolic BP greater than 115 mmHg is estimated to contribute to almost half of all coronary heart disease (CHD) cases and 62 per cent of all stroke cases.[1]

It is well accepted that populations with higher salt intakes have higher rates of BP. Native populations such as the Yanomami Indians in the Amazon region of Brazil, who live a 'Stone Age' existence, have a very low sodium intake (about one-twentieth of the intake of developed nations) and a high potassium intake, and have low BP that does not increase with ageing.[2] Modern diets are much higher in salt and much lower in potassium than primitive diets because processed foods have replaced fresh fruit and vegetables. A high potassium intake leads to sodium losses in urine and a potassium deficiency may be a contributing factor to sodium excess.

The current salt intake in developed countries ranges from 9–12 g daily and reducing intake to 5–6 g/day lowers BP in people with high BP and those with normal BP.[3] A further reduction to 3–4 g of salt daily has an even greater effect. A high salt intake has been shown to be associated with left ventricular hypertrophy (LVH), independent of BP, and elevated BP and LVH are important risk factors for heart failure. In heart failure patients, a high salt intake aggravates salt and fluid retention, and exacerbates heart failure symptoms and disease progression.

The mechanisms by which a high dietary salt intake causes elevated BP are poorly understood. When sodium is given as sodium chloride, the blood pressure response is greater than when the same amount of sodium is administered in non-chloride forms, indicating that sodium chloride is specifically responsible for much of the effect on BP. Key factors contributing to sodium-induced hypertension include ENaC, the renin-angiotensin system, endogenous digitalis-like factor (EDLF), oxidative stress and the sympathetic nervous system.[4] It is suggested that a high salt intake induces secretion of EDLFs, such as endogenous ouabain (EO), by the brain and adrenal glands that inhibit Na/K-ATPase activity. EO appears to act both centrally and peripherally to constrict blood vessels and elevate BP.

The Dietary Approaches to Stop Hypertension (DASH) diet is rich in fruit, vegetables, whole grains, low-fat dairy products, poultry, fish, nuts, seeds and beans, and low in fat, red meat, refined carbohydrates and sugar-containing beverages. The DASH diet has been shown to be effective for reducing BP, reducing blood cholesterol and homocysteine levels, and enhancing the effects of BP medication.[5] Further reductions in sodium in the DASH diet have been shown to cause greater effects on BP. Lowering sodium to 1500 mg daily lowered BP by twice as much as an intake of 2400 mg.[6] The DASH diet combined with a sodium intake of 1500 mg daily led to a BP reduction of 8.9/4.5 mmHg overall (an average of 7.1/3.7 mmHg reduction in subjects with normal BP and 11.5/5.7 mmHg reduction in subjects with high BP).[6] A meta-analysis of six studies found that the DASH diet can reduce the risk of CVD by 20 per cent, coronary heart disease (CHD) by 21 per cent, stroke by 19 per cent and heart failure by 29 per cent.[7] Another study found that subjects with the best adherence to a DASH diet were found to have a reduced risk of kidney stones; the risk was reduced by 45 per cent in men, by 42 per cent in older women and by 40 per cent in younger women.[8]

A research review found that BP increases with higher sodium, alcohol and protein intakes, and decreases with higher potassium, calcium and magnesium intakes.[9] It concluded that the best strategy for lowering BP appears to be moderate salt restriction (6–7 g of sodium chloride daily) together with anti-hypertensive drug therapy and the DASH diet. A World Health Organization (WHO) report concluded that reducing sodium intake reduces systolic and diastolic BP in adults and children, independent of baseline sodium intake, and reduces the risk of CVD, stroke and CHD in adults.[1] Based on the evidence, reducing sodium intake to less than 2 g/day was found to be more effective for lowering BP than consuming higher amounts. Therefore, the WHO recommends reducing sodium intake to less than 2 g/day (5 g/day sodium chloride).

Recommendations for reducing salt intake for populations are controversial because not all individuals have changes in BP after changes in sodium chloride intake, and it appears that some individuals are salt sensitive and some are not (salt resistant). Salt sensitivity may be defined as either a reduction in BP in response to a lower salt intake or a rise in BP in response to sodium loading. Patients with elevated BP appear to be more salt sensitive than people with normal BP.[10] A study of salt sensitivity found that 26 per cent of the subjects with normal BP were salt sensitive and 58 per cent were resistant, and 51 per cent of those with high BP were salt sensitive and 33 per cent were resistant.[11] Salt sensitivity has been associated with genetic factors, altered kidney function, lower levels of plasma aldosterone and ANP, lower renin activity, abnormalities of intracellular sodium, calcium and magnesium concentrations, and alterations in extracellular pH and bicarbonate.[11] Age has been found to be related to salt sensitivity in many studies, and salt-sensitive individuals have been found to have a greater rise in BP over time than those who are salt resistant.[12] Insulin resistance is associated with high BP because insulin can promote sodium reabsorption in the kidneys, and it is suggested that elevated insulin levels may be involved in salt sensitivity.[13] Potassium appears to play an important role, and potassium supplementation during sodium loading reduces the effect of sodium on BP.[14]

It appears that extreme reductions in sodium intake (0.46 to 0.69 g/day) are not necessary, and have been associated with insulin resistance and increases in serum total and LDL cholesterol concentrations.[15] However, modest sodium reduction (1.7 g/day) does not appear to affect serum cholesterol. As dietary intake of sodium from standard diets is far greater than physiological needs, and potassium intake is often inadequate, moderating salt intake and increasing potassium intake is recommended, especially for protecting against elevated BP and CVD.

REFERENCES

1 World Health Organization, *Guideline: Sodium intake for adults and children*, WHO, Geneva, 2012.

2 Takahashi, H., Yoshika, M., Komiyama, Y. & Nishimura, M., The central mechanism underlying hypertension: a review of the roles of sodium ions, epithelial sodium channels, the renin-angiotensin-aldosterone system, oxidative stress and endogenous digitalis in the brain, *Hypertens Res* (2011), 34(11): 1147–60.

3 He, F.J., Burnier, M. & Macgregor, G.A., Nutrition in cardiovascular disease: Salt in hypertension and heart failure, *Eur Heart J* (2011), 32(24): 3073–80.

4 Blaustein, M.P., Leenen, F.H., Chen, L. et al., How NaCl raises blood pressure: A new paradigm for the pathogenesis of salt-dependent hypertension, *Am J Physiol Heart Circ Physiol* (2012), 302(5): H1031–49.

5 Craddick, S.R., Elmer, P.J., Obarzanek, E. et al., The DASH diet and blood pressure, *Curr Atheroscler Rep* (2003), 5(6): 484–91.

6 Sacks, F.M., Svetkey, L.P., Vollmer, W.M. et al., Effects on blood pressure of reduced dietary sodium and the Dietary Approaches to Stop Hypertension (DASH) diet, *N Engl J Med* (2001), 344: 3–10.

7 Salehi-Abargouei, A., Maghsoudi, Z., Shirani, F. & Azadbakht, L., Effects of Dietary Approaches to Stop Hypertension (DASH)-style diet on fatal or nonfatal cardiovascular diseases-Incidence: A systematic review and meta-analysis on observational prospective studies, *Nutrition* (2013), 29(4): 611–18.

8 Taylor, E.N., Fung, T.T. & Curhan, G.C., DASH-style diet associates with reduced risk for kidney stones, *J Am Soc Nephrol* (2009), 20(10): 2253–9.

9 Suter, P.M., Sierro, C. & Vetter, W., Nutritional factors in the control of blood pressure and hypertension, *Nutr Clin Care* (2002), 5(1): 9–19.

10 Weinberger, M.H., Salt sensitivity of blood pressure in humans, *Hypertension* (1996), 27(3 Pt 2): 481–90.

11 Weinberger, M.H., Miller, J.Z., Luft, F.C. et al., Definitions and characteristics of sodium sensitivity and blood pressure resistance, *Hypertension* (1986), 8(suppl II): II-127–34.

12 Rodriquez, B.L., Labarthe, D.R., Huang, B. & Lopez-Gomez, J., Rise of blood pressure with age, *Hypertension* (1994), 24: 779–85.

13 Rocchini, A.P., The relationship of sodium sensitivity to insulin resistance, *Am J Med Sci* (1994), 307(suppl 1): S75–80.

14 Weinberger, M.H., Luft, F.C., Bloch, R. et al., The blood pressure-raising effects of high dietary sodium intake: racial differences and the role of potassium, *J Am Coll Nutr* (1982), 1: 139–48.

15 Food and Nutrition Board, *Dietary reference intakes for water, potassium, sodium, chloride, and sulfate*, National Academies Press, Washington, DC, 2005.

Case reports—sodium excess

- *An infant girl, two weeks of age*, developed an eye infection, sneezing, coughing, irritability and an increasing reluctance to breastfeed.[1] Her mother had experienced difficulties breastfeeding, and had required considerable assistance from the lactation nurse while in hospital after the birth. However, the mother and infant had been discharged after two days with no homecare nurse follow-up. On examination, the infant was extremely lethargic, very hypotonic (floppy) and had a weak cry and a wasted appearance. The infant was found to have hypernatraemia and severe dehydration, and was rehydrated slowly, which corrected the hypernatraemia. On follow-up over two and a half years, her development was assessed as normal or advanced, and there was no evidence of any residual effects.
- *A man, 89 years of age*, with mental confusion, cancer of the prostate gland, spinal metastases and impaired kidney function, was given soluble paracetamol (1 g four times daily) for back pain.[2] Ten days later, his serum sodium concentration had increased from 142 mmol/L to 165 mmol/L. He was treated with aggressive fluid resuscitation for dehydration, but the hypernatraemia failed to improve until the soluble paracetamol was slowly withdrawn, 21 days after he began taking it. However, his health deteriorated severely because of sepsis of unknown origin and worsening kidney function, and he died at 30 days.
- *A man, 41 years of age*, consumed a concentrated salt water mixture containing 70–90 g of salt (about a third of a cup of salt) that was intended for gargling.[3] He developed seizures and hypernatraemia (serum sodium 209 mmol/L). He was treated with hypotonic fluids but failed to recover, and died three days later.

REFERENCES

1 Clarke, T.A., Markarian, M., Griswold, W. & Mendoza, S., Hypernatremic dehydration resulting from inadequate breastfeeding, *Pediatrics* (1979), 63: 931–2.

2 Siau, K. & Khanna, A., Hypernatremia secondary to soluble paracetamol use in an elderly man: A case report, *Cases J* (2009), 2: 6707.

3 Moder, K.G. & Hurley, D.L., Fatal hypernatremia from exogenous salt intake: Report of a case and review of the literature, *Mayo Clin Proc* (1990), 65(12): 1587–94.

Supplements

Sodium is not required as a supplement because it is amply supplied in the diet. Sodium chloride appears to be the main sodium salt linked to adverse health outcomes, and intake should be restricted. Small amounts of sodium are found in supplements such as sodium ascorbate, which provides about 116 mg/g of sodium, and are not likely to be of concern in the context of a low-salt diet.

POTASSIUM

POTASSIUM STATUS CHECK

1 **Do you have high blood pressure, or a family history of high blood pressure?**
2 **Is your diet low in fruit and vegetables?**
3 **Is most of your food cooked or processed?**
4 **Do you become tired easily, and do you have weak muscles?**

'Yes' answers may indicate inadequate potassium status. Note that a number of nutritional deficiencies or health disorders can cause similar effects and further investigation is recommended.

FAST FACTS . . . POTASSIUM

- **Potassium is found in fruit, vegetables and juices.**
- **It helps maintain water and electrolyte balance.**
- **It is essential for maintaining pH balance, osmotic pressure, nerve transmission and muscle contraction.**
- **A deficiency can cause nerve and muscle dysfunction.**
- **Increasing potassium intake and reducing sodium intake may reduce the risk of high blood pressure and cardiovascular disease.**

Potassium is a naturally occurring mineral that makes up 2.6 per cent of the earth's crust, where it is found in feldspar, clay and salt beds, and is part of seawater, mainly as potassium chloride. It was first isolated in 1807 by Sir Humphry Davy from electrolysis of potassium hydroxide, and named after the English word 'potash', meaning pot ashes obtained from the burning of plant material. Its chemical symbol is K, derived from the Latin word *kalium*, which comes from the Arabic word for 'plant ashes'.

Potassium is the major intracellular cation in the body, especially found in muscles and bones. About 95–98 per cent of the body content is found within cells, three-quarters of which is in muscle cells, and the concentration is tightly maintained. Potassium has a vital role, together with sodium, in maintaining electrolyte balance and osmotic pressure across membranes. Potassium on the surface of bones can be mobilised as required to maintain healthy levels inside cells.

Digestion, absorption and transport

Potassium is found in foods as various salts, mainly as potassium citrate and malate, with smaller amounts of potassium chloride, galacturonate, oxalate and tartrate. Potassium is very soluble, and over 90 per cent of dietary intake is absorbed. Most potassium salts, except for potassium oxalate and tartrate, ionise readily in the stomach to release potassium ions. Potassium is also a component of digestive secretions. The absorption mechanism is not well understood, but appears to take place in the small intestine, possibly by passive diffusion through membrane channels, and in the colon by apical membrane channels or by the hydrogen/potassium-ATPase (H/K-ATPase) pump, which exchanges a hydrogen ion for a potassium ion. Potassium may be secreted or absorbed in the colon according to body needs.

Metabolism, storage and excretion

Once absorbed, potassium moves out of intestinal cells into the bloodstream through potassium channels, and is taken up by tissues and pumped into cells by the Na/K-ATPase pump in cell membranes. This pump is responsible for maintaining a higher concentration of potassium ions inside cells, and a higher concentration of sodium ions outside cells.

The major pathway for potassium removal from the body is via the kidneys, and the main site of potassium secretion is the cortical collecting duct. About 85–90 per cent of secreted potassium is reabsorbed, and the rest is excreted in urine. Sweat losses are generally low, but increase during heavy exercise—especially in hot environments. The colon can also excrete potassium via apical BK channels, leading to losses in faeces.

Regulation of potassium balance

Potassium levels are kept under tight control, and are regulated mainly by kidney absorption or excretion. Excretion in the kidneys increases or reduces in line with changes in intake. An increased potassium concentration stimulates Na/K-ATPase in the kidneys, which moves potassium into the tubules for excretion. Increased sodium and water in the distal tubules of the kidneys also stimulate Na/K-ATPase and increase tubular flow, leading to potassium being washed out in urine. If there is a sudden increase in the amount of potassium entering the body, potassium can be moved rapidly into muscles and the liver via Na/K-ATPase in order to maintain low levels in ECF. This process is enhanced by insulin release after a meal, and by the release of catecholamines (dopamine, noradrenaline and adrenaline), which occurs after exercise.

Hormones that increase potassium losses in urine include aldosterone, the renin-angiotensin system, ADH and glucocorticoids. Aldosterone is the major regulator of potassium levels. It is released when plasma levels of potassium increase, and acts at the collecting duct of the kidney to increase reabsorption of sodium, which simultaneously causes excretion of potassium. The collecting duct can also actively reabsorb potassium via activity of H/K-ATPase. Aldosterone also enhances potassium secretion into the colon when potassium levels are elevated.

Functions

Together with sodium, potassium is essential for maintaining electrolyte and pH balance, osmotic pressure, nerve transmission and muscle contraction. Potassium helps to maintain bone mineral density, and acts as a cofactor for enzymes that trigger insulin release, metabolise carbohydrates, synthesise proteins and phosphorylate creatine to provide an energy source for muscles.

The functions of potassium include:

- *Electrolyte and pH balance.* A higher concentration of potassium inside cells and a higher concentration of sodium outside cells is essential for maintaining osmotic pressure across cell membranes. In fruit and vegetables, potassium is bound to organic anions, such as citrate, that are converted in the body to bicarbonate which buffers acids. Potassium bicarbonate buffers sulfate ions derived from protein metabolism to maintain a healthy body pH. Bone surfaces are rich in potassium relative to calcium and, in conditions of acidosis, potassium ions are released in larger amounts than calcium ions to buffer acidity.
- *Nerve and muscle function.* The difference in concentrations of sodium and potassium across cell membranes creates the resting membrane potential of nerve cells. Sodium influx generates a nerve impulse, and potassium efflux causes repolarisation. The resting concentrations of sodium and potassium ions are restored by the Na/K-ATPase pump. By working together with sodium to generate nerve impulses, potassium enables nerve stimulation of muscles. Potassium has vasodilating effects in the smooth muscles of blood vessels, increasing blood flow.
- *Bone mineral density (BMD).* The ECF in bone has higher concentrations of potassium and sodium, and lower concentrations of calcium and phosphorus, compared with bone crystals or plasma. Potassium in ECF in bone and potassium on bone surfaces can buffer acids and protect bone minerals. Potassium maintains BMD by stabilising pH, which reduces calcium losses from bone and in urine.
- *Gastric acid secretion.* Healthy gastric acid secretion requires a sufficient concentration of potassium ions in the lumen. Secretion of hydrogen ions in the stomach is dependent on the H/K-ATPase pump, which moves hydrogen ions into the lumen of the stomach in exchange for potassium ions.

Dietary sources

Potassium is found in fruit and vegetables, dried fruit, fruit and vegetable juices, molasses, treacle, whole grains, nuts, legumes, vegetable cooking water, vegetable soups, seaweed, meat, poultry, fish, dairy products, coffee and tea. Good sources include avocadoes, green leafy vegetables, potatoes, bananas, melons and orange juice. Fruit and vegetables have a greater buffering effect in the body than other potassium sources by providing potassium bound to organic anions, which form bicarbonate during metabolism.

Bottled mineral waters have widely varying concentrations of potassium, ranging from 0.5 mg/L to more than 20 mg/L. However, this is insignificant when compared to potassium intake from food—for example, one banana (120 g) contains about 415 mg. Many food additives used in food processing, such as preservatives and acidity regulators, are potassium salts. Potassium chloride is available as a salt substitute, and these products may provide about 500 mg of potassium per gram.

The Food Standards Australia New Zealand nutrient database (NUTTAB) at <www.foodstandards.gov.au> provides the amounts found in specific foods.

Factors influencing body status

Potassium is water soluble, and is lost from foods by water processing and cooking methods. Boiling and soaking lead to leaching of potassium, and it is estimated that about half of the potassium content of flour is lost during the refining process. Endocrine disorders affecting potassium, sodium and water balance, and vomiting and diarrhoea, may cause potassium imbalance. Potassium can be lost in sweat during prolonged intense exercise, and excess intake of caffeine and stimulants can increase losses in urine. Colonic excretion of potassium appears to be increased in patients with end-stage kidney disease, severe ulcerative colitis, secretory-type rectal villous adenoma (a type of bowel polyp) and laxative abuse.

Potassium is lost in urine in kidney disorders such as chronic kidney failure or renal tubular acidosis, in which the kidneys fail to reabsorb sufficient bicarbonate or fail to excrete sufficient hydrogen ions. Overproduction of aldosterone in adrenal gland disorders, as well as Bartter syndrome and Gitelman syndrome, in which there is an abnormality of sodium chloride reabsorption in the kidneys, increase urinary losses.

A magnesium deficiency reduces Na/K-ATPase activity and enhances aldosterone secretion, and leads to potassium losses in urine and faeces. Potassium levels in the body are closely related to sodium levels, but the amount of sodium in the diet does not appear to stimulate potassium excretion until sodium intake rises above 6900 mg/day. Potassium moves into cells from the bloodstream under the influence of insulin and catecholamines. If insulin production is inadequate, potassium levels in plasma may increase. Acidosis enhances potassium retention and alkalosis enhances potassium excretion. In acidosis, the elevated concentration of hydrogen ions outside cells causes them to move into cells, which results in potassium moving out of cells to maintain electroneutrality. Alkalosis and hyperglycaemia result in the movement of potassium into cells.

The main drugs that reduce potassium levels are diuretics, such as thiazide and loop diuretics, which promote potassium excretion by the kidneys. However, potassium-sparing diuretics inhibit reabsorption of sodium in the collecting tubules and duct without loss of potassium. Other drugs that are associated with low potassium levels include laxatives, corticosteroids, the antifungal drugs amphotericin B and fluconazole, antacids, insulin and the asthma drug theophylline. The licorice constituent glycyrrhizin causes sodium retention and potassium loss in urine.

In digoxin toxicity, the Na/K-ATPase pump is inhibited and serum potassium levels may increase. Low serum potassium increases the risk of digoxin toxicity. The blood-thinning drug heparin is a potent inhibitor of aldosterone production and may elevate serum potassium. Other drugs that may increase potassium levels include ACE inhibitors, angiotensin receptor blockers and beta-adrenergic antagonists (used for high BP), non-steroidal anti-inflammatory drugs (NSAIDs), cyclosporin and tacrolimus (immune suppressants), trimethoprim and pentamidine (antibiotics), amiloride and triamterene (potassium-sparing diuretics) and spironolactone (an aldosterone antagonist used for oedema).

Daily requirement

Government recommendations by age and gender (see Table 9.2) can be found in *Nutrient Reference Values for Australia and New Zealand Including Recommended Dietary Intakes*, available at <www.nhmrc.gov.au>.

Table 9.2 Adequate intake (AI) of potassium (mg/day)

Age (years)	Female AI	Male AI
1–3	2000	2000
4–8	2300	2300
9–13	2500	3000
14–18	2600	3600
19–70	2800	3800
>70	2800	3800
Pregnant women		
14–18	2800	
19–50	2800	
Lactating women		
14–18	3200	
19–50	3200	

Source: Nutrient Reference Values for Australia and New Zealand Including Recommended Dietary Intakes, National Health and Medical Research Council, Australian Government Department of Health and Ageing, Canberra and Ministry of Health, New Zealand, Wellington, 2006.

Deficiency effects

Potassium is abundant in fruit and vegetables, and serum levels are tightly regulated by the kidneys. However, the kidneys, which readily excrete excess potassium, are less efficient at conserving potassium when dietary intake is inadequate. A diet low in fruit and vegetables is inadequate in both potassium and bicarbonate precursors, and minerals in bone are withdrawn to neutralise acidity, causing demineralisation of bone and increased calcium and reduced citrate in urine. Inadequate potassium in the diet is associated with salt sensitivity, elevated BP, stroke, kidney stones, low BMD and osteoporosis.

A low level of serum potassium (hypokalaemia) is most commonly caused by excessive losses in urine or a redistribution of potassium in the body, but may also result from an inadequate intake or increased losses in faeces. Hypokalaemia is commonly associated with hypomagnesaemia. Inadequate magnesium causes potassium losses in urine, and leads to hypokalaemia that does not respond to potassium therapy and can only be corrected by restoring normal magnesium levels. Hypokalaemia is the most common electrolyte abnormality encountered in hospitals, and is more common in the elderly, in people with kidney disease, diabetic acidosis or burn injuries, and as a consequence of heavy sweating, vomiting, diarrhoea or use of thiazide or loop diuretics. Diuretic therapy, diarrhoea and chronic laxative abuse are the most common causes in elderly people.

Hypokalaemia has wide-ranging effects that are primarily apparent as nerve and muscle dysfunction. Mild hypokalaemia may have no obvious symptoms, or may cause irregular heart rhythm, muscle weakness, fatigue, leg cramps, constipation, elevated calcium in urine (hypercalciuria) and glucose intolerance. Cardiovascular effects include electrocardiographic (ECG) changes, rapid irregular heart rhythm, ventricular tachycardia, ventricular fibrillation, low BP and heart muscle damage. Muscle damage and rhabdomyolysis may result because of reduced glycogen production. Nervous system effects include weakness, ascending flaccid paralysis, breathing difficulties, muscle pain, tenderness, cramps and tetany. Effects on the brain include lethargy, apathy, depression, acute memory loss, disorientation and confusion.

In the kidneys, urine output increases, ammonia production increases and metabolic alkalosis is promoted by increased bicarbonate reabsorption and increased chloride excretion. In the digestive tract, there is decreased gastric acid secretion and decreased motility of the intestines, leading to constipation and obstruction (paralytic ileus). Endocrine effects include increased renin secretion and decreased aldosterone and insulin release. Severe hypokalaemia may lead to sudden death from cardiac arrest.

Periodic paralysis related to hypokalaemia may occur because of a genetic disorder or in association with thyrotoxicosis (over-activity of the thyroid gland). Familial hypokalaemic periodic paralysis (FHPP) is a rare genetic disorder more commonly seen in men, which is caused by a rapid shift of potassium into the muscles. It features episodes of flaccid paralysis affecting the limbs and trunk, but rarely affecting the facial and respiratory muscles. It usually starts in childhood or adolescence, and occurs while asleep, causing weakness or paralysis and abnormal heart rhythm. Episodes occur on average every four to six weeks, and last several hours or several days. They may be triggered by strenuous exercise, adrenaline, a high carbohydrate or sodium intake, hypothermia, or administration of glucose, insulin or glucagon. Correcting the hypokalaemia relieves the symptoms. Thyrotoxic periodic paralysis (ThPP) primarily affects Asian populations, particularly males aged 30 or older. It has the same features as FHPP, and is reversed by correcting the abnormally high thyroid hormone level.

Indicators of inadequate levels of potassium may include:

- lethargy, weakness, muscle paralysis mainly affecting the limbs and trunk, muscle pain, cramps
- irregular heart rhythm, low BP
- indigestion, constipation
- apathy, depression, memory loss, disorientation, confusion.

Assessment of body status

Serum or plasma potassium concentration does not reflect total body content, but can indicate abnormal potassium states. The reference range given by the RCPA for adults is 3.4–4.5 mmol/L for plasma and 3.8–4.9 mmol/L for serum. Mild hypokalaemia is defined as a serum potassium concentration of 3.0–3.5 mmol/L, moderate as 2.5–3.0 mmol/L and severe as less than 2.5 mmol/L. Mild hyperkalaemia (elevated serum potassium) is defined as a serum potassium concentration of 5.0–5.9 mmol/L, moderate as 6.0–6.4 mmol/L and severe as equal to or more than 6.5 mmol/L. Potassium status can be assessed also by a 24-hour faecal or urine analysis. The reference range for adults given by the RCPA for potassium in faeces is less than 5 mmol/24 hours, and 40–100 mmol/24 hours for potassium in urine.

Case reports—potassium deficiency

- *A man, 29 years of age*, developed sudden-onset paralysis during sleep, and woke in the night unable to move his limbs.[1] He reported several previous episodes of waking up with a racing heart. On examination, he was found to have an elevated heart rate, high BP and flaccid paralysis of all limbs, including the hips and shoulders. His serum potassium was 1.6 mmol/L and intravenous (iv) potassium reversed his symptoms in two hours. Further testing revealed an underlying hyperthyroid condition, and he was diagnosed with ThPP.
- *A man, 76 years of age*, developed muscular weakness that progressed to paralysis involving all his limbs.[2] His serum potassium was found to be 1.8 mmol/L, and he had metabolic alkalosis and hypernatraemia. He was treated with iv potassium and then oral supplementation and potassium-sparing diuretics. His muscle symptoms improved as his serum potassium rose, but potassium did not reach normal levels. On further investigation, he reported drinking tea flavoured with about 100 g of natural licorice root every day for three years. The licorice root was found to contain 2.3 per cent glycyrrhizin, and his estimated intake was 2.3 g daily. One week after stopping licorice tea, his serum potassium was still

low despite potassium supplementation. After two weeks, his serum potassium and BP had returned to normal and he had lost 4 kg of body weight. It was concluded that improvement was slow because glycyrrhizin is widely distributed in the body, has a long half-life and a considerable amount of the glycyrrhizin excreted in bile is reabsorbed and recirculated.

- *A man, 44 years of age*, developed sudden onset of muscle weakness after returning home from an evening of kangaroo shooting.[3] He had difficulty moving and standing, and the weakness was progressive. On examination, he was found to have generalised muscle weakness, which progressed to breathing difficulties requiring artificial ventilation. His serum potassium level was 1.4 mmol/L, his urinary potassium was elevated and he had osmotic diuresis (excessive urine output caused by a high level of solutes). His serum potassium normalised in 24 hours with iv fluid treatment, and he regained muscle strength. It was discovered subsequently that he had been in the habit of drinking approximately 4 L of a cola drink on most days for the last three years and up to 10 L when he went kangaroo shooting at night. During this time, he had experienced frequent urination. He ceased his cola consumption and his serum potassium remained normal; he had no further episodes of muscle weakness. It was concluded that the high sugar intake from the cola drink caused osmotic diuresis and potassium loss, which was not replaced by dietary intake. This condition was aggravated by the caffeine content of the drink, which blocks adenosine receptors in the kidneys and causes excessive urination.

REFERENCES

1 Soule, B.R. & Simone, N.L., Hypokalemic periodic paralysis: A case report and review of the literature, *Cases J* (2008), 1(1): 256.

2 Lin, S.H., Yang, S.S., Chau, T. & Halperin, M.L., An unusual cause of hypokalemic paralysis: Chronic licorice ingestion, *Am J Med Sci* (2003), 325(3): 153–6.

3 Mudge, D.W. & Johnson, D.W., Coca-Cola and kangaroos, *Lancet* (2004), 364(9440): 1190.

THERAPEUTIC USES OF POTASSIUM

Cardiovascular disease and high blood pressure

Potassium is believed to stimulate Na/K-ATPase in vascular smooth muscle cells and adrenergic nerves, and enhance endothelium-dependent relaxation, causing vasodilation and lowering BP. BP appears to be more closely associated with the sodium:potassium ratio than intake of either electrolyte alone. Lower potassium intake has been associated with elevated BP and stroke, and a higher intake appears to be protective. A meta-analysis of 22 trials concluded that increased potassium intake (3510–4680 mg/day) can reduce systolic BP by 3.49 mmHg and diastolic BP by 1.96 mmHg and reduce the risk of stroke by 24 per cent.[1] Potassium appears to be more effective in reducing BP at higher levels of sodium consumption, and the largest benefit was found when sodium intake was more than 4000 mg/day, which is a common level of intake in many populations. Potassium chloride and potassium bicarbonate have been found to improve endothelial and arterial function, reduce left ventricular mass and improve left ventricular function in people with mildly elevated BP on a relatively low-salt and high-potassium diet.[2] Potassium-induced reduction in BP lowers the incidence of stroke, coronary heart disease, myocardial infarction (heart attack) and other cardiovascular events.[3] Increasing consumption of potassium to 4700 mg per day has been predicted to lower the incidence of future CVD, with estimated decreases of 8–15 per cent for stroke and 6–11 per cent for heart attacks.[3]

Bone mineral density

Consumption of a standard Western diet is associated with chronic, low-grade metabolic acidosis. During metabolic acidosis, small decreases in pH lead to increased activity of osteoclasts that break down bone, and a more alkaline pH, induced by diet or supplements, leads to positive effects on calcium balance and bone metabolism. Potassium is an alkaline mineral, and a higher potassium intake has been associated with improved bone metabolism in elderly women.[4]

However, fruit and vegetables have a stronger alkaline effect than other potassium foods because they provide both potassium and bicarbonate. Evidence shows that intake of fruit and vegetables provides a consistent beneficial effect on indices of bone health in young boys and girls, premenopausal, perimenopausal and postmenopausal women, and elderly people.[5] A study found that increasing fruit and vegetable intake from 3.6 to 9.5 servings daily decreased urinary calcium excretion from 157 to 110 mg/day.[6]

In people with mildly elevated BP on a relatively low-salt and high-potassium diet, potassium bicarbonate supplementation decreased urinary calcium excretion, improved the calcium:creatinine ratio and decreased levels of plasma beta-C-terminal telopeptide (beta-CTx), a marker of degradation of mature type I collagen that indicates that bone is being broken down.[2] A study of older men and women found that supplementation with potassium citrate (2340 or 3510 mg/day) completely neutralised dietary acidity at six months, and reduced serum beta-CTx and urinary calcium excretion compared with a placebo.[7] Parathyroid hormone levels decreased and net calcium balance improved in the group on the higher potassium intake. In healthy elderly people without osteoporosis, treatment with potassium citrate (6480 mg/day) for two years, together with calcium and vitamin D, resulted in a significant increase in BMD and improved bone micro-architecture.[8] The separate effects of potassium chloride, potassium bicarbonate, sodium chloride and sodium bicarbonate (90 mmol/day) were studied in a small number of subjects on a fixed diet.[9] Both potassium salts reduced calcium excretion, with potassium bicarbonate having the greatest effect and potassium chloride also reduced the fasting urinary calcium:creatinine ratio. Sodium bicarbonate had no effect on calcium excretion, and sodium chloride increased calcium excretion.

Glucose tolerance

Potassium is important for insulin function, and a low potassium intake leading to low body levels is associated with reduced glucose metabolism, reduced insulin release and impaired glucose tolerance.[10] A high potassium intake is associated with a lower risk of developing type 2 diabetes in women,[11] and a lower serum potassium level is an independent predictor of development of diabetes.[12] In a study of people with high BP, subjects with higher serum potassium levels had a lower prevalence of pre-diabetes and newly diagnosed diabetes.[13] A study of people on thiazide diuretics found that diuretic-induced potassium losses were associated with the development of glucose intolerance, but there was no change in glucose tolerance when potassium levels were maintained by supplementation.[14]

Kidney stones

Calcium kidney stones, commonly made up of calcium oxalate or calcium phosphate, are associated with hypercalciuria, and potassium citrate supplementation has been shown to decrease calciuria.[9] Citrate and alkalis are protective against stone formation by decreasing urinary saturation of calcium oxalate and inhibiting its spontaneous nucleation. Potassium citrate or magnesium potassium citrate supplementation have been found to reduce the rate of stone recurrence, and increase the clearance rate and dissolution of stone fragments.[15] A study of stone-forming patients with low citrate in the urine found that potassium citrate supplementation (3240 or 6480 mg/day) taken for three years increased urinary citrate and pH, and reduced stone formation from an average of 1.2 stones per patient per year to 0.1 stones per patient year, which was a significantly lower rate of stone formation than the placebo group.[16] A study of patients after shockwave lithotripsy (SWL) for calcium oxalate kidney stones found that patients whose stones were cleared had no recurrence of stone formation in the twelve month period afterwards if taking potassium citrate (4200 mg/day), whereas control patients had a recurrence rate of 28.5 per cent.[17] Patients with residual stone fragments after SWL had a recurrence rate of 12.5 per cent on potassium citrate, compared with a rate of 44.5 per cent in controls. Potassium citrate has also been found to prevent kidney stones in epileptic children on ketogenic diets for seizure control.[18]

REFERENCES

1 Aburto, N.J., Hanson, S., Gutierrez, H. et al., Effect of increased potassium intake on cardiovascular risk factors and disease: Systematic review and meta-analyses, *BMJ* (2013), 346: f1378.

2 He, F.J., Marciniak, M., Carney, C. et al., Effects of potassium chloride and potassium bicarbonate on endothelial function, cardiovascular risk factors, and bone turnover in mild hypertensives, *Hypertension* (2010), 55: 681–8.
3 Houston, M.C., The importance of potassium in managing hypertension, *Curr Hypertens Rep* (2011), 13(4): 309–17.
4 Zhu, K., Devine, A. & Prince, R.L., The effects of high potassium consumption on bone mineral density in a prospective cohort study of elderly postmenopausal women, *Osteoporos Int* (2009), 20(2): 335–40.
5 Lanham-New, S.A., The balance of bone health: Tipping the scales in favor of potassium-rich, bicarbonate-rich foods, *J Nutr* (2008), 138(1): 172S–7S.
6 Appel, L.J., Moore, T.J., Obarzanek, E. et al., A clinical trial of the effects of dietary patterns on blood pressure. DASH Collaborative Research Group, *N Engl J Med* (1997), 336(16): 1117–24.
7 Moseley, K.F., Weaver, C.M., Appel, L. et al., Potassium citrate supplementation results in sustained improvement in calcium balance in older men and women, *J Bone Miner Res* (2013), 28(3): 497–504.
8 Jehle, S., Hulter, H.N. & Krapf, R., Effect of potassium citrate on bone density, microarchitecture, and fracture risk in healthy older adults without osteoporosis: A randomized controlled trial, *J Clin Endocrinol Metab* (2013), 98(1): 207–17.
9 Lemann, J. Jr, Pleuss, J.A., Gray, R.W. & Hoffmann, R.G., Potassium administration reduces and potassium deprivation increases urinary calcium excretion in healthy adults [corrected], *Kidney Int* (1991), 39(5): 973–83.
10 Rowe, J.W., Tobin, J.D., Rosa, R.M. & Andres, R., Effect of experimental potassium deficiency on glucose and insulin metabolism, *Metabolism* (1980), 29(6): 498–502.
11 Colditz, G.A., Manson, J.E., Stampfer, M.J. et al., Diet and risk of clinical diabetes in women, *Am J Clin Nutr* (1992), 55: 1018–23.
12 Chatterjee, R., Yeh, H.C., Shafi, T. et al., Serum and dietary potassium and risk of incident type 2 diabetes mellitus: The Atherosclerosis Risk in Communities (ARIC) study, *Arch Intern Med* (2010), 170(19): 1745–51.
13 Meisinger, C., Stöckl, D., Rückert, I.M. et al., Serum potassium is associated with prediabetes and newly diagnosed diabetes in hypertensive adults from the general population: The KORA F4-study, *Diabetologia* (2013), 56(3): 484–91.
14 Helderman, J.H., Elahi, D., Andersen, D.K. et al., Prevention of the glucose intolerance of thiazide diuretics by maintenance of body potassium, *Diabetes* (1983), 32(2): 106–11.
15 Caudarella, R. & Vescini, F., Urinary citrate and renal stone disease: The preventive role of alkali citrate treatment, *Arch Ital Urol Androl* (2009), 81(3): 182–7.
16 Barcelo, P., Wuhl, O., Servitge, E. et al., Randomized double-blind study of potassium citrate in idiopathic hypocitraturic calcium nephrolithiasis, *J Urol* (1993), 150(6): 1761–4.
17 Soygür, T., Akbay, A. & Küpeli, S., Effect of potassium citrate therapy on stone recurrence and residual fragments after shockwave lithotripsy in lower caliceal calcium oxalate urolithiasis: A randomized controlled trial, *J Endourol* (2002), 16(3): 149–52.
18 McNally, M.A., Pyzik, P.L., Rubenstein, J.E., Hamdy, R.F. & Kossoff, E.H., Empiric use of potassium citrate reduces kidney-stone incidence with the ketogenic diet, *Pediatrics* (2009), 124(2): e300–4.

Effects of excess

Excess potassium is excreted in urine and faeces, and hyperkalaemia is more commonly related to kidney or adrenal dysfunction, use of certain drugs such as ACE inhibitors for high BP and metabolic disorders such as acidosis, in which potassium in ECF increases and excretion in the kidneys is reduced. In conditions of blood cell breakdown, potassium is released into the circulation but does not reflect the true underlying serum potassium level (pseudohyperkalaemia). A high intake of potassium-rich foods is very unlikely to cause hyperkalaemia in healthy people, but it may result from excessive intake of potassium supplements and potassium-based salt substitutes. Older people and infants are more at risk of adverse effects of a high potassium intake.

Hyperkalaemia is a serious condition requiring immediate treatment because of the high risk of sudden death. Mild hyperkalaemia may have no obvious symptoms. Excess potassium causes depolarisation of cell membranes, slows electrical conduction in the heart and decreases the duration of the action potential, causing characteristic ECG changes and abnormal heart rhythm, and may result in ventricular fibrillation and cardiac arrest. The risk of cardiac arrest increases when serum potassium is over 6 mmol/L, and the risk increases considerably at levels above 8 mmol/L—particularly if the increase is rapid. Excess potassium causes reduced renin secretion, and increased aldosterone and insulin release. In the kidneys, sodium is lost in urine, bicarbonate reabsorption is reduced and production of ammonia decreases, leading to mild metabolic acidosis. Effects of hyperkalaemia include paraesthesia, muscle weakness, flaccid paralysis, breathing difficulties and absence of deep tendon reflexes.

Hyperkalaemic periodic paralysis (HYPP) is a rare genetic condition that causes a rise in plasma potassium (up to 8.0 mmol/L), accompanied by episodes of muscular weakness and paralysis. It usually begins in early childhood, and episodes may occur daily or a few times per year but are usually shorter (lasting one to two hours), more frequent and less severe than the hypokalaemic form. Heart rhythm abnormalities are uncommon, and the respiratory and throat muscles are usually not affected. In some cases, potassium levels are normal during attacks. Episodes may be triggered by a high potassium intake, glucocorticoids, hypothermia, fasting, alcohol and during the recovery phase after strenuous exercise. Between episodes, patients often experience muscle spasms, stiffness or difficulty relaxing their muscles (myotonia).

No adverse effects have been reported in small trials of older subjects given 2340 mg of potassium as potassium chloride for four weeks or in younger adult subjects given 1900 mg potassium for fifteen weeks. However, potassium chloride supplements have been associated with a bitter or metallic taste or aftertaste, heartburn, nausea, abdominal pain and diarrhoea, as well as ulceration of the digestive tract, which has been associated with the use of standard-release and slow-release potassium chloride tablets. Patients at higher risk of digestive lesions from potassium chloride tablets include the elderly and the immobile, patients with scleroderma, diabetes, enlargement of the heart, oesophageal stricture, impaired motility of the digestive tract and bowel pockets (diverticulosis), and those who have had a mitral valve replacement.

Case reports—potassium excess

- *A male infant, two months of age,* was given three doses of 1500 mg potassium chloride with breast milk over one and a half days as a treatment for colic, the mother having followed information given by the American nutrition writer Adelle Davis.[1,2] A few hours after the third dose, the infant became listless, turned blue and stopped breathing, and was rushed to a hospital. His serum potassium level was found to be 10 mmol/L, and remained elevated despite treatment. The baby died 28 hours after admission. The parents successfully sued the author's estate, the publisher and the manufacturer of the potassium product, and the book was withdrawn, revised and reissued in 1982.
- *A man, 26 years of age,* was found unconscious at home in bed after an evening of drinking alcohol and taking cocaine.[3] He was found to have a low oxygen concentration (hypoxia), reduced breathing rate, metabolic acidosis, low BP, abnormal heart rhythm and a serum potassium level of 8.9 mmol/L. He was diagnosed with cocaine-induced rhabdomyolysis, causing kidney failure and hyperkalaemia, and was placed in intensive care on mechanical ventilation. He was given insulin and dextrose to treat the hyperkalaemia, followed by cardioversion to restore his heart rhythm. His heart rhythm normalised when his serum potassium levels decreased to 5.1 mmol/L. However, his hypoxia rapidly deteriorated due to pulmonary oedema. He continued to require ventilation, and was placed on intermittent haemodialysis. Two weeks later, after discharge from intensive care, he had a grand mal seizure. It was concluded that earlier, more vigorous treatment of his hyperkalaemia might have improved his heart dysfunction and reduced the severity of his multi-organ failure. The patient's longer-term outcome was not reported.

- *A woman, 66 years of age*, with a history of obesity, type 2 diabetes, hypertension, elevated serum cholesterol, gout, anxiety and chronic kidney disease, developed nausea, vomiting and progressive malaise over several hours.[4] She was found to have rapid breathing and a slow heartbeat (bradycardia), and was experiencing episodes of cardiac arrest (asystole). She was taking multiple medications for her health disorders, and the only change in her routine was the consumption of about 200 g of dulse (seaweed) the previous day. Her serum potassium level was found to be 8.6 mmol/L, and she was diagnosed with hyperkalaemia secondary to kidney failure, triggered by ingesting a high mineral load from dulse. Treatment of hyperkalaemia and cessation of her gout, diabetic and BP medication resulted in normalisation of her serum potassium and heart rhythm within a few hours. She remained stable and was discharged seven days after admission.
- *A man, 65 years of age*, with a history of coronary artery disease, hypertension, chronic kidney failure, stroke and diabetes, and on multiple medications, developed generalised chest and body pain, low back pain, severe limb pain and weakness, and difficulty walking.[5] He reported blurred vision, shortness of breath and dizziness. He was found to have irregular heart rhythm, low BP and breathing rate, and hypoxia. He collapsed and became unresponsive within two hours of admission to hospital, failed to respond to resuscitation and was pronounced dead. His serum potassium was found to be 8.2 mmol/L, but the result did not come through until the time of his collapse. An autopsy showed severe heart disease, cirrhosis and fluid in the abdominal cavity. The patient's family sued the attending medical staff for malpractice for waiting for laboratory results before instituting treating for hyperkalaemia, but it was concluded by the review panel that medical staff did not breach the standard of care.

REFERENCES

1 Davis, A., *Let's have healthy children*, 3rd ed., Harcourt Brace Jovanovich, New York, 1972.

2 Barrett, S.B., The legacy of Adelle Davis, QuackWatch, retrieved 20 August 2014 from <www.quackwatch.com/04ConsumerEducation/davis.html>.

3 Siddiqui, F., Slater, R. & Ashraf, S., Life threatening hyperkalemia following cocaine ingestion: A case report, *Cases J* (2009), 2: 7355.

4 McGrath, B.M., Harmon, J.P. & Bishop, G., Palmaria palmata (dulse) as an unusual maritime aetiology of hyperkalemia in a patient with chronic renal failure: A case report, *J Med Case Rep* (2010), 4: 301.

5 Sullivan, W.P. & Dalsey, W.C., Hyperkalemia case review, retrieved 20 August 2014 from <www.acep.org/WorkArea/DownloadAsset.aspx%3fid=41168>.

Supplements

Potassium is not often required in supplement form because it is readily obtainable from fruit and vegetables, which provide much greater amounts than can be obtained from most over-the-counter supplements. Almost all commercial potassium is extracted from potassium chloride deposits found in salt basins, salt lakes and natural brines. Extraction is followed by milling, washing, screening, flotation, crystallisation, refining and drying. Potassium chloride is reacted with various acids, such as ascorbic, aspartic, orotic, phosphoric, sulfuric or citric acid, to obtain other potassium salts.

In Australia, the permitted forms of potassium salts in supplements include potassium ascorbate, ascorbate dihydrate (primarily sources of vitamin C), aspartate, aspartate monohydrate, aspartate dihydrate, citrate, hydroxycitrate, gluconate, glycerophosphate, iodide (primarily a source of iodine), orotate, phosphate (dibasic, monobasic, tribasic) and sulfate. Potassium supplements are available as tablets, slow-release and effervescent formulations. The approximate elemental potassium content of some common salts is shown in Table 9.3.

Potassium bicarbonate is used for the treatment of potassium depletion in metabolic acidosis, and is available on prescription as effervescent tablets for the prevention or treatment of hypokalaemia.

Table 9.3 Elemental potassium content of common salts

Salt	Potassium content (%)
Potassium chloride	52
Potassium sulfate	40
Potassium bicarbonate	39
Potassium citrate	38
Potassium iodide	30
Potassium aspartate	20
Potassium orotate	20

Cautions

Potassium supplements should be used with caution, and high doses should be used only on medical advice and under medical supervision. Potassium supplements, potassium chloride salt substitutes and high-potassium foods should be avoided in people taking potassium-sparing diuretics. Potassium supplements or potassium chloride salt substitutes should not be used by patients with organ dysfunction, chronic kidney failure, heart disease, acidosis, acute dehydration or adrenal insufficiency. Patients with health disorders should seek advice from a health-care practitioner before taking potassium supplements. Potassium chloride tablets should not be used because of their potential to cause ulceration of the digestive tract.

CHLORIDE

CHLORIDE STATUS CHECK

1 Are you taking diuretic drugs?
2 Do you have a very low-salt diet?
3 Do you have poor kidney function?
4 Do you have chronic diarrhoea?

'Yes' answers may indicate inadequate chloride status. Note that a number of nutritional deficiencies or health disorders can cause similar effects and further investigation is recommended.

FAST FACTS . . . CHLORIDE

- Chloride is a component of salt as sodium chloride, and high levels are found in salted, processed and takeaway foods.
- Chloride is an electrolyte, and helps maintain pH balance in the body.
- Chloride is essential for muscle and nerve function, epithelial tissue function, digestion, carbon dioxide transport and cell function.
- A deficiency can cause metabolic alkalosis, digestive disorders, nerve and muscle dysfunction, abnormal heart rhythm and mental confusion.
- Excess may cause metabolic acidosis, dehydration symptoms, headache, nausea, vomiting, weakness, nerve and muscle dysfunction, and an accelerated heart and breathing rate.

Chlorine is a greenish-yellow gas that is not found in its free form in nature but rather as chloride mineral salts, sodium chloride being the most common. Sea water and salt lakes are rich sources of sodium chloride. Chlorine gas was discovered by the Swedish chemist Carl Scheele in 1774. It has the chemical symbol Cl, and was established as an element by Sir Humphrey Davy in 1810 and named after the Greek word *chloros*, meaning 'green'. In the body, about 88 per cent of total body chloride is in ECF and about 12 per cent is inside cells. Cerebrospinal fluid and gastrointestinal secretions are rich in chloride. It is the major anion in the body, and plays an important role in maintenance of osmotic pressure and electrolytic balance.

Digestion, absorption and transport

Chloride is found in food as various chloride salts, particularly sodium chloride, which is ionised in the stomach to release sodium and chloride ions. Chloride ions are readily absorbed into enterocytes with sodium via an energy-dependent sodium/chloride cotransporter (NCC) that exchanges sodium ions for hydrogen ions and chloride ions for bicarbonate ions. Chloride is absorbed also by passive paracellular diffusion following sodium uptake by sodium-glucose transporters (SGLT), or by cation-chloride cotransporters, which allow chloride ions to follow cations (mainly sodium and potassium) across cell membranes. In general, chloride accompanies sodium in the body.

Metabolism, storage and excretion

In tissues, a number of chloride channels and transporters allow movement of chloride across cell membranes, including cystic fibrosis transmembrane conductance regulators (CFTR), calcium-activated chloride channels, voltage-gated chloride channels and chlorine/hydrogen antiporters. Chloride is primarily excreted by the kidneys. Most (99 per cent) of the filtered chloride in kidneys is reabsorbed, either by passive diffusion or by active transport accompanied by passive diffusion of sodium or potassium. Digestive secretions are rich in chloride, which is largely reabsorbed. Chloride can be lost in sweat with sodium, but losses are small unless sweating is pronounced.

Chloride and bicarbonate are the main anions in the body, and a deficiency of one will lead to an increase in the other in order to preserve electrical neutrality. Chloride levels are regulated primarily through sodium regulation, and changes in chloride usually reflect changes in sodium, except in acid–base disorders in which changes in chloride are independent.

Functions

The movement of chloride across cell membranes helps control electrical excitability of muscles and nerves, secretion of salt and water by epithelial tissues, stomach acid production, carbon dioxide transport, maintenance of cell volume and the function of intracellular organelles. Chloride also appears to act as a second messenger in cells by binding to and regulating the function of a variety of proteins. The functions of chloride include the following:

- *Electrolyte and pH balance.* Chloride anions help balance cations to maintain electrical neutrality. To maintain pH balance, the kidneys excrete chloride or bicarbonate. If pH decreases, chloride ions are excreted by the kidneys in exchange for bicarbonate, and if pH increases, chloride is retained and bicarbonate is excreted.
- *Carbon dioxide transport.* Chloride ions in red blood cells help transport carbon dioxide from cells to the lungs. Carbon dioxide is taken up by red blood cells, and combines with water to form carbonic acid via the action of the zinc-dependent enzyme carbonic anhydrase. Carbonic acid then dissociates to form bicarbonate ions and hydrogen ions. Bicarbonate ions diffuse into blood plasma and chloride ions diffuse into red blood cells to take their place (the chloride shift) to counteract any potential changes in the acid–base balance.
- *Production of epithelial secretions.* In epithelial cells, the movement of chloride ions across membranes enables secretion of water and production of normal mucus, sweat, saliva, tears and digestive enzymes. Chloride anions move through CFTR channels in epithelial cells, and mutations in the gene for this channel cause the excessively thick secretions characteristic of cystic fibrosis.
- *Digestive function.* Digestion of food is dependent on chloride, which is the main electrolyte driving fluid secretion into the lumen of the intestine. About 8 L a day of fluid is secreted into the digestive tract, most of which is reabsorbed. Intestinal epithelial cells secrete chloride ions into the intestinal lumen via CFTR. Accumulation of chloride anions in the lumen creates an electrical potential that attracts sodium, pulling it into the lumen, with the net result of secretion of sodium chloride. The presence of sodium chloride causes osmotic pressure that attracts water into the lumen, which digestive enzymes use to break down food molecules.

  In the salivary glands, acinar cells secrete sodium chloride-rich fluid, and the cells of the salivary duct absorb most of the sodium and chloride via the epithelial sodium channel (ENaC) and secrete potassium and bicarbonate into saliva. In the stomach, apical chloride channels in parietal cells in the stomach lining secrete chloride and hydrogen ions are secreted by H/K-ATPase. Hydrogen and chloride combine to form the hydrochloric acid needed to initiate digestion. Histamine, gastrin and acetylcholine regulate chloride secretion and acid production. In the pancreas, acinar cells secrete a small amount of sodium chloride-rich fluid into the pancreatic duct, which reabsorbs the chloride and secretes bicarbonate by a chloride/bicarbonate exchanger, together with fluid. This process provides bicarbonate that is secreted in pancreatic juice to solubilise large molecules and neutralise stomach acid to provide an optimum pH for the function of intestinal digestive enzymes.
- *Cell function.* Chloride channels play an important role in controlling cellular pH and volume. Chloride and bicarbonate help regulate pH inside cells by moving into or out of cells through chloride

channels and exchangers. Cells regulate their volume when there is a decrease in osmotic pressure in ECF (hypotonicity) that may lead to water entering the cell, causing swelling and bursting, and an increase of osmotic pressure (hypertonicity) that may lead to loss of water from the cell, causing cell shrinkage and loss of function. If the ECF becomes hypotonic, cells can release solutes by opening swelling-activated potassium and chloride channels and, when the ECF is hypertonic, cells can take up sodium and chloride by the activation of sodium/hydrogen and chloride/bicarbonate exchangers. Chloride channels and transporters also help control the volume of organelles inside the cell, maintain their electrical neutrality and move anionic substrates, such as phosphate and sulfate, out of organelles.

- *Nerve and muscle function.* Chloride channels help regulate membrane electrical excitability. The inhibiting neurotransmitters glycine and GABA act by opening chloride channels and moving chloride into the nerve cell, which inhibits nerve activity. Chloride channels appear to regulate muscle activity in smooth and skeletal muscles.
- *Immune function.* Chloride is important in epithelial tissue for secretion of mucus that acts as a barrier to invasion by pathogens. CFTR chloride channels are found in neutrophils, macrophages, monocytes, dendritic cells and lymphocytes. In macrophages, they appear to have a role in antigen presentation, activity of toll-like receptor 4 (a protein that enables recognition of pathogens), bactericidal activity, phagocytosis, production of pro-inflammatory cytokines and removal of dead cells.

Dietary sources

Chloride is found in eggs, meat, seafood, seaweed, olives, rye, tomatoes, lettuce, celery, table salt (sodium chloride, which contains 600 mg/g of chloride), and foods with added salt. It is also found in food additives and salt substitutes. In Australia, permitted food additives that contain chloride include potassium chloride (508), calcium chloride (509), ammonium chloride (510), magnesium chloride (511) and stannous chloride (512). However, these provide small amounts of chloride, the main input coming from salt intake.

The Food Standards Australia New Zealand nutrient database (NUTTAB) provides the amounts found in specific foods. See <www.foodstandards.gov.au>.

Factors influencing body status

Chloride can be lost from the body in the same way as sodium. A low intake of chloride is uncommon, but may occur in people on very low-salt diets. Losses can occur with loss of body fluids through sweating, wounds or burns, or with loss of digestive secretions through prolonged or severe vomiting or diarrhoea. Chloride losses in urine may be caused by osmotic diuresis, adrenal insufficiency and kidney diseases such as interstitial nephritis, chronic renal failure and post-obstructive diuresis. Low chloride levels may also be associated with nasogastric suctioning, acid–base imbalances, endocrine disorders, bowel polyps and cystic fibrosis.

Drugs that affect sodium levels also affect chloride levels; these include loop and thiazide diuretics, laxatives, bicarbonate antacids and corticosteroids. Diuretics impair the reabsorption of chloride and sodium in the kidneys, and cause greater loss of chloride than bicarbonate. Carbonic anhydrase inhibitors, which impair the activity of the enzyme carbonic anhydrase, cause loss of potassium and bicarbonate in urine and retention of chloride, and are used as diuretics or for the treatment of glaucoma, seizures, gastric and duodenal ulcers and osteoporosis. Elderly patients are particularly at risk of low chloride levels because of medication use, reduced kidney function and vomiting and diarrhoea episodes.

Daily requirement

There are no government recommendations for chloride in *Nutrient Reference Values for Australia and New Zealand Including Recommended Dietary Intakes*, available at <www.nhmrc.gov.au>. The USA Dietary Reference Intakes are given in Table 9.4.

Deficiency effects

A chloride deficiency is rare, but may be caused by a low intake, losses from the gut, kidney or skin, or impaired chloride metabolism. Most diets supply ample chloride in the form of salt, but very low-salt diets may lead to a deficiency. Impaired chloride transport in the body is associated with a range of diseases, including epilepsy, myotonia, lysosomal storage disease (accumulation of undigested or partially digested macromolecules in cells), deafness, kidney stones and osteopetrosis (increased bone

Table 9.4 Adequate intake (AI) of chloride (mg/day)

Age (years)	Female AI	Male AI
1–3	1500	1500
4–8	1900	1900
9–13	2300	2300
14–18	2300	2300
19–50	2300	2300
51–70	2000	2000
>70	1800	1800
Pregnant women		
14–18	2300	
19–50	2300	
Lactating women		
14–18	2300	
19–50	2300	

Source: National Research Council, *Dietary Reference Intakes: The Essential Guide to Nutrient Requirements,* National Academies Press, Washington, DC, 2006.

mass and fragility). Genetic diseases associated with low chloride levels include cystic fibrosis (chloride losses through the skin), congenital chloride-losing diarrhoea (inability to reabsorb chloride in the gut), Bartter syndrome and Gitelman syndrome (impaired salt and chloride absorption in the kidney), and congenital adrenal hyperplasia (increased sodium and chloride losses in urine).

Inadequate chloride levels may impair immune defence, nerve and muscle function and the production of mucus and digestive secretions. A chloride deficiency causes an increase in bicarbonate in order to maintain electrical neutrality, which may lead to metabolic alkalosis. Chloride-responsive alkalosis is due to loss of hydrogen ions (acid) and chloride-containing ECF. Chloride-resistant alkalosis results from excessive secretion of mineralocorticoid hormones, which causes increased bicarbonate reabsorption.

Low serum chloride (hypochloraemia) can be caused by the loss of chloride from ECF or the addition of water to ECF. Excess water in ECF can cause a dilutional hyponatraemia and hypochloraemia, but total body chloride is not deficient and ECF volume is increased. Loss of chloride from ECF is associated with reduced ECF volume and increased potassium and sodium losses in urine, and may result in metabolic alkalosis. Urinary chloride and sodium are characteristically low. However, levels of these ions in urine may be increased if hypochloraemia is due to kidney malfunction.

Symptoms of hypochloraemic alkalosis include dehydration symptoms, muscle weakness, loss of reflexes, paraesthesia, headache, spasms of the hands or feet, twitches, convulsions, tetany, tachycardia, low BP, low breathing rate, cyanosis, loss of appetite, dizziness, confusion, irritability, restlessness, aggressiveness, apathy and lethargy, and may result in coma and death if severe. Infants inadvertently fed a chloride-deficient formula developed loss of appetite, weakness and failure to thrive.

Indicators of inadequate levels of chloride may include:

- lethargy, weakness, paraesthesia, muscle spasms, twitches, seizures
- tachycardia, low BP
- loss of appetite, digestive disorders
- apathy, confusion, irritability, restlessness, aggressiveness
- slow breathing rate.

Assessment of body status

Serum chloride concentration does not always indicate total body content because extra fluid in ECF can be a cause of hypochloraemia. However, hypochloraemia with reduced ECF volume and alkalosis usually indicates a chloride deficiency. The reference range for serum or plasma chloride given by the RCPA for adults is 95–110 mmol/L. Chloride status can also be assessed by a 24-hour urine analysis, which is useful for the differential diagnosis of persistent metabolic alkalosis. The reference range given by the RCPA for urinary chloride in adults is 100–250 mmol/24 hours, and reflects chloride intake. Metabolic alkalosis together with a urinary chloride level of less than 10 mmol/L indicates chloride deficiency caused by gut or sweat losses. Chloride levels in sweat can be assessed in suspected cystic fibrosis. The reference range given by the RCPA for chloride in sweat in children is less than 40 mmol/L. Levels greater than 60 mmol/L indicate cystic fibrosis.

Case reports—chloride deficiency

- *A group of 141 infants, less than one year of age*, developed hypochloraemic metabolic alkalosis after being fed on an infant formula deficient in chloride in 1978 and 1979.[1] They were also found to have hypokalaemia, hyponatraemia, hyperaldosteronism, elevated plasma renin activity, elevated serum calcium and phosphate, as well as increased urinary calcium and magnesium and absence of urinary chloride. Their symptoms included loss of appetite, weakness, lethargy, poor growth and failure to thrive. The biochemical abnormalities and symptoms reversed following dietary supplementation with either sodium or potassium chloride.
- *A man, 36 years of age*, had recurring episodes of severe nausea and vomiting, and a compulsion to take hot showers almost continually.[2] He was found to have acute kidney impairment and hypochloraemic, hyponatraemic dehydration with metabolic alkalosis. He reported having used marijuana regularly since high school, and was diagnosed with cannabinoid hyperemesis (vomiting) syndrome, which results from chronic cannabis use and features severe vomiting and compulsive bathing. His symptoms resolved when marijuana was discontinued.
- *A woman, 26 years of age*, developed weakness and lassitude over several months.[3] She was found to have severe alkalosis, hypokalaemia and very low urinary chloride (5 mmol/L). No cause for the abnormalities could be found, and she denied a history of vomiting or diarrhoea. Further investigations found some oral signs of chronic vomiting episodes and, as all other causes were ruled out, it was concluded that she was suffering from a loss of chloride from the digestive tract due to bulimia (self-induced vomiting). She denied having bulimia, refused counselling and eventually left the hospital without the issue being resolved.

REFERENCES

1 Malloy, M.H., Graubard, B., Moss, H. et al., Hypochloremic metabolic alkalosis from ingestion of a chloride-deficient infant formula: Outcome 9 and 10 years later, *Pediatrics* (1991), 87(6): 811–22.

2 Abodunde, O.A., Nakda, J., Nweke, N. & Veera, R.L., Cannabinoid hyperemesis syndrome presenting with recurrent acute renal failure, *J Med Cases* (2012), 4(3): 173–5.

3 Woywodt, A., Herrmann, A., Eisenberger, U. et al., The tell-tale urinary chloride, *Nephrol Dial Transplant* (2001), 16(5): 1066–8.

Effects of excess

Excessive intake of chloride as sodium chloride is associated with increased risk of high BP. Elevated serum chloride (hyperchloraemia) is associated with hypernatraemia, and may be caused by loss of body water due to sweating, fevers or inadequate water intake, or the use of hypotonic fluids or sodium chloride-containing fluids. Hyperchloraemia causes low plasma bicarbonate levels and metabolic acidosis, which is most commonly caused by bicarbonate loss from the digestive tract, renal tubular acidosis, drug-induced hyperkalaemia, early renal failure or administration of acids. Hyperchloraemia may occur also in hyperparathyroidism, diabetes insipidus, respiratory alkalosis, hyperadrenocorticism (excess cortisol production) and due to the use of drugs such as carbonic anhydrase inhibitors.

Symptoms of hyperchloraemic acidosis include dehydration symptoms, headache, nausea, vomiting, weakness, lethargy, increased breathing rate, breathlessness, mental confusion, stupor and tachycardia, which may lead to ventricular fibrillation and heart failure with pulmonary oedema. Chronic acidosis may lead to calcium imbalance and bone loss. Renal tubular acidosis is associated with increased risk of kidney stones.

Case reports—chloride excess

- *A boy, 4 years of age*, developed unsteadiness while walking, drowsiness, dizziness, lethargy and watery diarrhoea.[1] On investigation, he was found to have poor muscle development, abdominal distension, poor coordination and irritability. Laboratory tests showed hyponatraemia, hypokalaemia and hyperchloraemic metabolic acidosis. His serum chloride was 122 mmol/L. His history revealed that he had experienced episodes of diarrhoea from the age of two years that were diagnosed as irritable bowel syndrome and controlled with a low-fibre diet and lactose-free milk. Blood tests for gluten intolerance (coeliac disease) were negative at two and four years. The boy had experienced four similar episodes previously after eating large amounts of bread, cakes or pizza. Each time, his symptoms had resolved in hospital within two days but the hyperchloraemic metabolic acidosis persisted. Investigation of his intestine revealed damage consistent with coeliac disease, and his symptoms were attributed to a coeliac crisis caused by exposure to large amounts of gluten. He was placed on a gluten-free diet and improved progressively.

- *A man, 29 years of age*, developed severe muscular weakness.[2] He was found to have hyperchloraemic metabolic acidosis, hypokalaemia, rhabdomyolysis and impaired kidney function. He was given potassium chloride and alkaline salts, and his kidney function, serum potassium and acid–base status normalised within five days, but his muscle strength did not improve and he became unresponsive. After several days, he regained consciousness but had no feeling in his skin from the neck down, and was quadriplegic. His history revealed that he had been a habitual glue-sniffer for eight years, and his condition was diagnosed as toluene intoxication. He had experienced a similar episode of muscle weakness five months earlier, but had recovered after treatment and had continued glue sniffing. On this second occasion, he did not recover and, after twelve months, was still quadriplegic and only able to communicate by blinking or head shaking.
- *A woman, 71 years of age*, developed lethargy, nausea and diarrhoea lasting for three weeks.[3] On admission to hospital, she was found to have dehydration and hyperkalaemic, hyperchloraemic metabolic acidosis. Her serum chloride was 114 mmol/L. She had a medical history of hypertension, congestive heart failure, atrial fibrillation, chronic obstructive pulmonary disease and gout, and was on numerous medications, including diuretics. The potassium-sparing diuretic spironolactone had been introduced one month prior to admission. She was diagnosed with an adverse reaction to spironolactone, which has been associated with the renal tubular acidosis, hyperkalaemia, hyperchloraemia and dehydration. She was withdrawn from spironolactone, and treated with fluids and medication to reduce her elevated potassium levels. However, her acidosis was still present at discharge, and she was readmitted eighteen days later with the same symptoms. Again, her acidosis persisted despite treatment but was normal at follow-up several months later.

REFERENCES

1 Oba, J., Escobar, A.M., Schvartsman, B.G. & Gherpelli, J.L., Celiac crisis with ataxia in a child, *Clinics (Sao Paulo)* (2011), 66(1): 173–5.

2 Hong, J.J., Lin, J.L., Wu, M.S. et al., A chronic glue sniffer with hyperchloraemia metabolic acidosis, rhabdomyolysis, irreversible quadriplegia, central pontine myelinolysis, and hypothyroidism, *Nephrol Dial Transplant* (1996), 11(9): 1848–9.

3 Khan, S.A., Singh, S.C. & Cymet, T.C., Type 4 renal tubular acidosis induced by spironolactone, *Hosp Physician* (2001), 37(11): 63–5.

Supplements

Chloride is not required as a supplement because it is amply supplied in the diet. Chloride is available as a component of some mineral salts that may be used as supplements—for example, chromic chloride, ferric chloride, ferrous chloride, magnesium chloride, manganese chloride, sodium chloride and zinc chloride—but these are not commonly used in mineral supplements. Chloride is also part of hydrochloride in supplements such as betaine hydrochloride, used as a buffered source of hydrochloric acid to support stomach function, and thiamine hydrochloride, a common form of vitamin B1 supplement.

Cautions

Sodium chloride appears to be the main sodium salt linked to adverse health outcomes, and intake should be restricted. Potassium chloride tablets should be avoided because they have the potential to damage the lining of the digestive tract.

SULFATE

SULFATE STATUS CHECK

1 Do you eat a low-protein diet?
2 Do you have a vegan (no animal food) diet based mainly on legumes, fruit and vegetables?
3 Do you have osteoarthritis?
4 Do you take pain-relieving medication, and are you regularly exposed to environmental pollutants?

'Yes' answers may indicate inadequate sulfate status. Note that a number of nutritional deficiencies or health disorders can cause similar effects and further investigation is recommended.

FAST FACTS . . . SULFATE

- Sulfate is a component of sulfur-containing amino acids, and is found in cabbage and onion family foods.
- Sulfate is important for phase II detoxification of unwanted or potentially toxic compounds.
- It is essential for connective tissue and myelin formation, hormone function, digestion, cholesterol and iron metabolism, and antioxidant protection.
- Deficiency effects are not well understood, but may include digestive disorders, a buildup of toxins, and growth, connective tissue, hormone and neurological abnormalities.
- Elevated serum levels may occur in chronic kidney failure, and lead to abnormal calcium metabolism.

Sulfate is derived from the element sulfur, which is a yellow crystalline solid that occurs in nature as the pure element or as sulfide and sulfate mineral salts in rocks, salts and sediments in the seabed. Most forms of environmental sulfur are harmless, but the gases sulfur dioxide and hydrogen sulfide are toxic. Plants take up sulfur that has been dissolved in water, and animals obtain sulfur from eating plants and other animals. Sulfur has the chemical symbol S, and was named after the Latin word *sulphurium*, known historically as brimstone (burning stone). Over time, the official spelling was changed from 'sulphur' to 'sulfur'. The French scientist Antoine Lavoisier helped to establish that sulfur was an element in 1777. Inorganic sulfate is the fourth most abundant anion in the body but, in the past, has been regarded as an inert substance. Its main functions have been considered to be as part of cysteine, methionine and taurine, the sulfur-containing amino acids (SAAs) in proteins. SAAs contain sulfhydryl (thiol) groups that consist of a sulfur atom bonded to a hydrogen atom. However, evidence is accumulating that sulfate is an important anion involved in many physiological processes in the body, referred to as sulfonation (also called sulfation) reactions.

Digestion, absorption and excretion

Sulfate is found in food and water, and is also formed from oxidation of SAAs in the body, which provides most of the body's requirement. Sulfite from the diet is readily oxidised in food or in the digestive tract by sulfite oxidase (SOX) to form sulfate. Dietary sulfate appears to be rapidly and almost completely absorbed. Absorption in the small intestine is via a sodium-dependent sulfate cotransporter (NaS-1) and a sulfate anion exchanger. Transport of sulfate from enterocytes to the ECF appears to be mediated by a sulfate/chloride exchanger and sulfate in ECF enters cells via NaS-1 for use in sulfonation reactions.

Metabolism, storage and excretion

SAAs such as cysteine can be broken down to produce sulfite ions, which are further oxidised to inorganic sulfate ions by the enzyme SOX. Sulfate is incorporated into glutathione, an important antioxidant that also acts as a storage form of sulfate. In order to take part in sulfonation reactions in the body, inorganic sulfate must be activated by incorporation into the universal sulfate donor 3'-phosphoadenosine-5'-phosphosulfate (PAPS) by the enzyme PAPS synthetase. A sulfonate group can then be transferred from PAPS by sulfotransferase enzymes (SULTs) to biological molecules during sulfonation reactions, which alter the configuration and activity of the molecule. The main pathway for sulfate excretion is in urine. About 80–95 per cent of filtered sulfate in the kidneys is reabsorbed by NaS-1 and a sulfate/oxalate/bicarbonate anion exchanger (Sat-1).

Functions

Sulfonation processes in the body are vital for normal metabolism, and are dependent on the availability of inorganic sulfate. Sulfonation affects a wide range of substances, including glycoproteins, glycolipids, cholesterol, hormones and peptides. The addition of a sulfate group to a molecule creates a negative charge that can induce a change in shape and solubility, and promote interactions with ions, thereby having a major influence on the molecule's function and activity. Sulfur-containing compounds include acetyl-CoA, the skin pigment melanin, insulin, thiamin, biotin and alpha-lipoic acid. The functions of sulfate include the following:

- *Detoxification.* Detoxification involves phase I and phase II reactions—primarily in the liver—that change unwanted or potentially toxic fat-soluble compounds to water-soluble excretable forms. Both xenobiotics (foreign chemicals) and endogenous substances (substances made in the body) undergo detoxification, including drugs, toxins, alcohol, toxic metals, steroid hormones, catecholamines (dopamine, adrenaline and noradrenaline), fat-soluble vitamins, bilirubin, bile acids, neurotransmitters, fatty acids and eicosanoids. Sulfate conjugation is an important step in phase II detoxification pathways, involving the transfer of sulfonate from PAPs to the substrate by SULT enzymes to produce a highly water-soluble sulfuric acid ester that can be excreted in urine. However, there is a relatively low concentration of PAPS in the body, which limits its capacity for detoxification. In general, sulfate conjugation is a high-affinity but low-capacity pathway of conjugation, whereas glucuronic acid conjugation is a low-affinity but high-capacity pathway. In some cases, sulfate conjugation can increase the toxicity of xenobiotics because certain sulfate conjugates are chemically unstable and break down to form potent reactive molecules.
- *Formation of connective tissue.* Glycosaminoglycans (GAGs), previously called mucopolysaccharides, are long polysaccharide chains that are found on cell surfaces and, together with a protein core, form the proteoglycans that are the ground substance in the extracellular matrix of connective tissue. Chondroitin sulfate, dermatan sulfate, heparin, heparan sulfate and keratan sulfate are sulfate-containing GAGs. Another GAG, hyaluronic acid, is not sulfonated. On cell surfaces, GAGs assist cell function by binding to growth factors, enzymes and cell surface receptors and transmitting messages into the cell (cell signalling).

  Chondroitin sulfate is the most abundant GAG in the body, and is found in bone, heart valves and cartilage. It is an important structural component of joint cartilage, acting to hold water and lubricate and protect the bone surfaces. Dermatan sulfate is found in the skin, blood vessels, heart valves, tendons and lungs. It is the major GAG in skin, and also plays a role in cell growth, differentiation, morphogenesis (shaping) and cell migration. Heparin is found in mast cell granules, where it enables storage of histamine, proteases and inflammatory mediators. Heparan sulfate is a GAG that is found in connective tissue and on cell surfaces. Heparan sulfate proteoglycans on cell surfaces bind numerous growth factors, proteases, cytokines and, in liver cells, chylomicron remnants to enable their removal from the bloodstream. Keratan sulfate is found in bones, cartilage, the brain and the cornea of the eye, together with chondroitin sulfate. It has a structural role in cartilage in joints, and works like chondroitin sulfate to hold water and provide lubrication. It appears to promote hydration of the cornea and scar formation in the brain after injury. Sulfatase enzymes play important roles in the breakdown of sulfonated GAGs and glycolipids in cell lysosomes, and in remodelling sulfonated GAGs in the connective tissue matrix.
- *Formation of cholesterol sulfate.* Cholesterol sulfate is a major sterol sulfate in the bloodstream, and is also found in seminal fluid, sperm, skin, hair, nails, the aorta, adrenal glands, the liver and the kidneys. It stabilises cell membranes, and appears to be an important regulatory molecule involved in cell signalling, cell adhesion, blood clotting, sperm development and skin growth. By activating protein kinase C, cholesterol sulfate modulates membrane structure, regulates gene transcription, mediates immune responses, regulates cell growth and may also desensitise membrane receptors.

  Cholesterol sulfate can block cholesterol synthesis in skin cells by inhibiting the enzyme HMG-CoA reductase and can block the formation of cholesterol esters by inhibiting the enzyme lecithin:cholesterol acyltransferase (LCAT). It also appears to promote fatty acid synthesis and platelet aggregation, and its role in atherosclerosis is not yet understood.

- *Formation of bile.* Bile acids are secreted into bile in the form of conjugates with glycine or the SAA taurine, and they act to solubilise dietary lipids, enhancing their digestion and absorption.
- *Glycoprotein and glycolipid function.* The addition of a sulfonate group to a carbohydrate attached to a lipid (glycolipid) or protein (glycoprotein) changes the carbohydrate into a unique recognition site for a specific receptor or carbohydrate-binding protein. Glycoproteins that are sulfonated include sulfomucins found in the mucous layer that covers the epithelial linings of the body and lubricates and protects the epithelium.

  The two main forms of sulfonated glycolipids (sulfoglycolipids) in the body are sulfatides (glycosphingolipid sulfate, also called cerebroside sulfate) and seminolipids. Sulfatides are abundant in the myelin sheath of nerves, and are essential for myelin development, maintenance and function. Seminolipids are glycerolipids found in sperm-producing cells that appear to be important for normal sperm production. Sulfoglycolipids are found also in the kidneys and intestine, and interact with extracellular matrix proteins, cellular adhesion receptors, blood clotting systems and micro-organisms.
- *Hormone and peptide function.* Many proteins secreted by cells, such as hormones and peptides, are modified by sulfonation of their tyrosine component before secretion, which appears to affect their ability to be processed by the cell and their function in the body. Sulfonation is important for the activity of thyroid-stimulating hormone and the production and metabolism of thyroid hormones. Sulfonation of tyrosine in cholecystokinin (a digestion stimulating hormone) increases its potency 250-fold. However, the peptide angiotensin II is 30 times less potent in increasing blood pressure when sulfonated. Sulfonation extends the lifespan and decreases the biological activity of steroid hormones by inhibiting their ability to bind to receptors. Steroid sulfates are the major form of steroids supplied to foetal tissues during pregnancy. A large proportion of the catecholamines in the circulation are sulfonated, which extends their half-life from about three minutes to about three hours.
- *Antioxidant protection.* Thiol (SH) groups can act as intracellular antioxidants through enzymatic reactions and by directly scavenging free radicals. Thiol antioxidants include the glutathione system (glutathione and the enzymes glutathione reductase and glutathione peroxidase), dihydrolipoic acid (DHLA), formed from alpha-lipoic acid, and thioredoxin. The glutathione system is the most important thiol system in cells, helping to maintain proteins and thiols in a reduced state and protecting cells from free radicals, drugs and heavy metals. Glutathione and glutathione peroxidase also inhibit production of prostaglandins derived from arachidonic acid metabolism, and may have anti-inflammatory effects.
- *Iron metabolism.* Inorganic sulfate combines with iron to form iron-sulfur (Fe-S) clusters that can bind electron-rich substrates for enzymes, accept or donate electrons and stabilise proteins. They are required for the function of proteins involved in the electron transport chain in mitochondria that produces energy and for regulatory sensing and DNA repair.

Dietary sources

Sulfate is found in SAAs in eggs (egg white protein is about 8 per cent SAAs), chicken, fish and beef proteins (about 5 per cent SAA) and dairy proteins (about 4 per cent SAAs). In general, plant proteins provide less than 4 per cent SAAs. Legumes are particularly low in SAAs, but grains and seeds have higher amounts. Sulfur compounds are found in the *Allium* food family (garlic, onions, scallions, shallots, leeks and chives) and the *Brassica* food family (cruciferous vegetables including bok choy, cabbage, Chinese cabbage, broccoli, Brussels sprouts, cauliflower, collard greens, watercress, kale, kohlrabi, mustard, rutabaga, turnip, radish, horseradish and wasabi). These compounds provide inorganic sulfate that may have a sparing effect on SAAs, allowing them to be used for protein synthesis rather than for provision of inorganic sulfate for sulfonation reactions.

The Food Standards Australia New Zealand nutrient database (NUTTAB) at <www.foodstandards.gov.au> provides the amounts of sulfate and SAAs found in specific foods.

Only a limited number of mineral waters provide sulfates; amounts range from negligible to more than 1000 mg sulfate/L. Australian drinking water guidelines state that levels greater than 500 mg/L in drinking water are not recommended because they may have laxative effects. Tap water sulfate levels for Melbourne, Victoria, range from 0.9 to 21.5 mg/L and those for Sydney, New South Wales from 1–16 mg/L. A 2004 WHO report did not formulate guidelines for the level of sulfate in drinking water because of the absence of adverse effects. However, the report concluded that sulfate can affect water taste and has a laxative effect at concentrations of 1000–1200 mg/L, but does not lead to diarrhoea, dehydration or weight loss.

Sulfite salts are used as preservatives, mainly in sausages, dried fruit, fruit products, pickles, relishes, fruit juice, cordial and wine, and must be declared on the label if the food contains 10 mg/kg or more because they can cause hypersensitivity reactions. Sulfites may also be used in the processing of some food ingredients, including beet sugar, corn sweeteners, food starches and gelatin. In Australia, permitted food additives that are sulfur salts include sulfur dioxide (220), sodium sulfite (221), sodium bisulfite (222), sodium metabisulfite (223), potassium metabisulfite (224), potassium sulfite (225) and potassium bisulfite (228).

Factors influencing body status

An inadequate intake of SAAs or a low-protein diet may reduce the amount of inorganic sulfate available for sulfonation reactions. A diet deficient in protein or overnight fasting can halve serum sulfate levels in animals. In humans, a high-protein meal has been shown to increase serum sulfate levels dramatically. Inadequate production of stomach acid or other digestive disorders may reduce digestion and absorption of SAAs.

Exposure to xenobiotics that are detoxified by sulfate conjugation may increase the need for sulfate; pain-relieving drugs such as aspirin and paracetamol have been found to deplete PAPS and sulfate levels in the body. Exposure to heavy metals, such as mercury, cadmium and lead, inhibits NaS-1 activity. Hyperthyroidism is associated with elevated serum sulfate levels, and hypothyroidism is associated with reduced expression of NaS-1 and decreased serum sulfate. Vitamin D and the thyroid hormone tri-iodothyronine (T3) help to regulate NaS-1 activity, and a deficiency of vitamin D or hypothyroidism may cause impaired uptake of sulfate by cells and increased losses in urine. Caffeine enhances urinary losses, and serum sulfate levels decline in women after menopause—possibly because of increased urinary losses.

Daily requirement

There are no Australian or New Zealand government recommendations for inorganic sulfate intake. The sulfate compounds found in *Allium* and *Brassica* foods are not regarded as essential nutrients. The recommendations for protein intake (see Table 2.7) found in *Nutrient Reference Values for Australia and New Zealand Including Recommended Dietary Intakes* available at <www.nhmrc.gov.au> are intended to provide adequate amounts of SAAs.

Deficiency effects

A sulfate deficiency is unlikely unless the diet is deficient in protein or SAAs. Vegetarian diets are more likely to be low in SAAs, and the amount of sulfur compounds provided by *Allium* and *Brassica* vegetables appears to be insufficient to supply the body's needs for inorganic sulfate. In spite of the importance of sulfonation reactions, sulfate levels are rarely assessed in clinical practice, and the consequences of insufficient inorganic sulfate are not well understood. A lack of inorganic sulfate results in abnormal sulfonation of sulfoconjugates, and may impair phase II detoxification, hormone and digestive function, myelin production and production of GAGs in connective tissue. Low serum sulfate (hyposulfataemia) may lead to reduced amounts of sulfomucins in intestinal mucus, which may impair intestinal barrier function and increase the risk of infections and toxin-induced colitis.

Reduced sulfonation of GAGs in cartilage may contribute to osteoarthritis. Cell studies have found that a reduction in sulfate concentration results in a reduction in GAG synthesis. In animals, paracetamol (acetaminophen) administration has been found to lower serum sulfate levels and reduce the GAG content of cartilage. In humans, serum sulfate has been found to correspond with sulfate levels in synovial fluid in joints, and glucosamine sulfate—a popular arthritis treatment—has been shown to elevate serum sulfate concentrations. It has been proposed that the sulfate component of glucosamine is largely responsible for the therapeutic effect.

Some autistic children have reduced serum levels of sulfate and elevated urinary losses, and a theory has been proposed that autism may be caused by insufficient supply of cholesterol sulfate to the infant during gestation and after birth. The diastrophic dysplasia sulfate transporter protein transports extracellular sulfate into cartilage cells (chondrocytes), and mutations in the gene for this transporter are associated with four types of human inherited osteochondrodysplasia disorders (dwarfism). In these conditions, there is reduced sulfonation of cartilage, and abnormal bone and cartilage growth. Other conditions in which there is abnormal sulfate metabolism or transport include metachromatic leukodystrophy (accumulation of sulfatides in cells) and disorders involving abnormal GAG metabolism (mucopolysaccharidoses), such as Hunter's syndrome, Morquio's syndrome, Maroteaux–Lamy syndrome and multiple sulfohydrolase deficiency (buildup of GAGs in the body). The genetic disorder multiple sulfatase deficiency features growth retardation, skeletal abnormalities, neurological defects and early mortality.

In an animal study, inactivation of NaS-1, the main sulfate transporter in the body, caused increased urinary losses of sulfate and hyposulfataemia, reduced growth, reduced fertility in females, liver enlargement and seizures. Serum levels of insulin-like growth factor were lower, and bile acids were higher, than in normal animals. However, the homeostasis of other ions such as phosphate, calcium, sodium, potassium and chloride was not affected. Other studies have found that animals lacking NaS-1 have reduced circulating steroid levels, increased urinary steroid excretion, reduced mucosal barrier defence against bacterial infection, enhanced growth of experimentally induced tumours and greater susceptibility to liver damage and experimentally induced colitis. Animals lacking Sat-1 develop elevated serum levels of oxalate, increased oxalate in urine and calcium oxalate kidney stones, as well as hyposulfataemia and increased sulfate losses in urine. Vitamin D-deficient animals develop hyposulfataemia, increased urinary losses of sulfate and abnormal sulfate metabolism that is corrected by vitamin D supplementation. It is theorised that impaired sulfate metabolism in vitamin D deficiency may contribute to the abnormalities observed in rickets and osteomalacia.

Assessment of body status

Serum sulfate concentration is rarely measured in clinical practice. The reference range for serum sulfate given by the American Medical Association is 310–990 μmol/L. Sulfate status can also be assessed by a 24-hour urine analysis, which is used more often as a method of measuring protein adequacy rather than sulfate status. The reference range given by the US Mayo Medical Laboratories (Mayo Clinic) for urinary sulfate in adults is 7–47 mmol/24 hours.

Effects of excess

Elevated serum sulfate (hypersulfataemia) is rare in healthy people, even when protein intake is high, but it is common in chronic renal failure (CRF), in which levels may exceed 2.5 mmol/L. An increase in ECF sulfate leads to increased calcium excretion and chronic hypersulfataemia may contribute to the abnormal calcium metabolism seen in patients with CRF, which leads to renal osteodystrophy (loss of calcium from bones caused by inability of the kidneys to maintain calcium levels). Sulfate has been associated with an increase in body acidity and reduced osmolality of body fluids.

Supplements

If protein intake is adequate, the diet should provide sufficient sulfate. *Brassica* and *Allium* foods can be used to increase intake of inorganic sulfate. Sulfate is available as various mineral salt supplements such as calcium sulfate, calcium sulfate anhydrous, chondroitin sulfate, cupric sulfate (anhydrous, monohydrate, pentahydrate), ferrous sulfate, glucosamine sulfate, magnesium sulfate (monohydrate, dihydrate, trihydrate), manganese sulfate, manganese sulfate monohydrate, potassium sulfate, S-adenosylmethionine (SAM or SAMe), sodium sulfate, sodium sulfate anhydrous and zinc sulfate (monohydrate, hexahydrate). Sulfate is also part of the supplements thiamine hydrochloride, biotin and alpha-lipoic acid. Magnesium sulfate (Epsom salts) is used as a laxative.

Cautions

Magnesium sulfate is absorbed less well than other sulfate salts, and causes loose stools or diarrhoea. Sulfite food additives can cause sensitivity reactions, particularly in asthmatics, and have been associated with asthma attacks, urticaria (hives), angio-oedema (swelling), nausea, abdominal pain, diarrhoea, seizures and anaphylaxis, which may be life-threatening.

HOW MUCH DO I KNOW?

Choose whether the following statements are true or false. Then review this chapter for the correct answers.

	True (T)	False (F)
1 Sodium helps maintain water and electrolyte balance.	T	F
2 Sodium is the major intracellular cation in the body.	T	F
3 It is recommended that adults ingest less than 2300 mg of sodium/day.	T	F
4 Potassium may be useful for protection against cardiovascular disease.	T	F
5 Potassium is very insoluble and is not easily absorbed.	T	F
6 Potassium-sparing diuretics can cause hypokalaemia.	T	F
7 Chloride ions in red blood cells help transport carbon dioxide from cells to the lungs.	T	F
8 Chloride is required for secretion of digestive juices.	T	F
9 A lack of inorganic sulfate may impair detoxification and connective tissue formation.	T	F
10 Sulfur-containing compounds include acetyl-CoA, melanin, insulin and thiamin.	T	F

FURTHER READING

Braun, L. & Cohen, M., *Herbs & natural supplements: An evidence-based guide*, 3rd ed., Churchill Livingstone Elsevier, New York, 2010.

Gropper, S.S., Smith, J.L. & Groff, J.L., *Advanced nutrition and human metabolism*, 5th ed., Thomson Wadsworth, Belmont, CA, 2009.

Higdon, J., *An evidence-based approach to vitamins and minerals*, Thieme, New York, 2003.

Linus Pauling Institute, Micronutrient Research Center, website, available at <lpi.oregonstate.edu/ infocenter>.

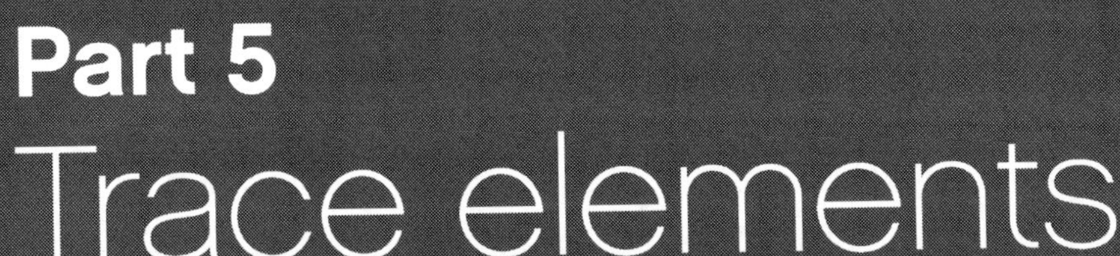

Part 5
Trace elements

10

Introduction to microminerals and trace elements: iron and zinc

INTRODUCTION TO MICROMINERALS

Microminerals include trace elements and ultratrace elements, and are needed in relatively low amounts (less than 100 mg a day). They are present in the body in amounts less than 0.01 per cent of body weight. The amount of microminerals present in the body ranges from less than 1 mg to about 4 g. Trace elements that are acknowledged to be essential to health include iron, zinc, copper, manganese, iodine, selenium, chromium and molybdenum. Fluoride is regarded as possibly essential because of its role in the health of bones and teeth. The ultratrace elements are present in the body in even smaller quantities than trace elements, and are required in amounts of 1 mg/day or less. They include boron and silicon, which may be essential nutrients, as well as aluminium, arsenic, cobalt, germanium, lithium, nickel, rubidium, tin and vanadium, which have physiological activity in the body but are not regarded as essential. It is possible that several of the ultratrace elements may be more important in human nutrition than is currently believed.

As with macrominerals, microminerals are found in the earth's crust, and are released as rocks break down, dissolve in water and are taken up by plant roots and transferred to animals when plants are eaten. They are not affected by heat, light and storage but, as they are water soluble, they may be lost from food by water processing and cooking methods. The most abundant micromineral in the body is iron, followed by zinc and then copper (see Figure 10.1). There are smaller, roughly equal amounts of manganese, iodine and selenium, followed by chromium. The body content of molybdenum, fluoride and the ultratrace elements is not well established.

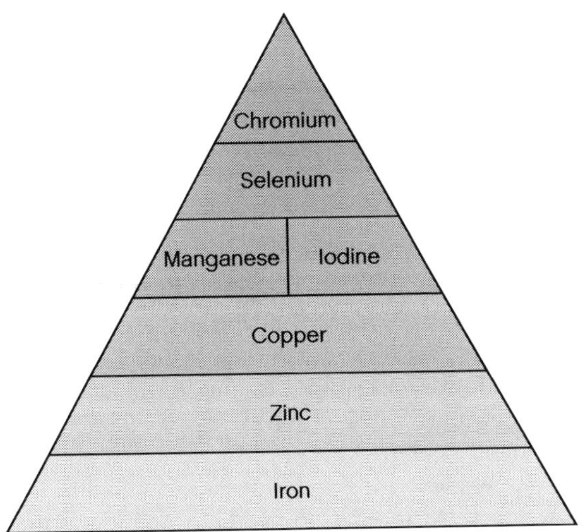

Figure 10.1 Relative body content of the main trace elements

TRACE ELEMENTS

Iron

IRON STATUS CHECK

1 Do you get tired easily, and do you get breathless and have heart palpitations when you exercise?
2 Do you have a pale appearance and pale mucous membranes around your eyes?
3 Do you get cravings to eat ice or non-food items?
4 Do you have an unpleasant, irritable feeling in your legs when at rest, and do you feel the need to move them?

'Yes' answers may indicate inadequate iron status. Note that a number of nutritional deficiencies or health disorders can cause similar effects and further investigation is recommended.

FAST FACTS . . . IRON

- The most available sources of iron include red meat, organ meats, seafood and poultry.
- Iron is required for haemoglobin and red blood cell production and oxygen delivery to tissues.
- It supports energy production, immune function, detoxification and metabolism.
- A deficiency can cause anaemia, which is associated with fatigue, irritability, pallor, muscle weakness, breathlessness on exertion, reduced work performance and endurance, and lowered immunity.
- Supplementation may be helpful for restless legs syndrome (RLS), heart failure, cognitive function and breath-holding episodes in children.

Iron is a naturally occurring mineral that makes up about 5 per cent of the earth's crust, in which it is found as various iron oxides, such as the minerals hematite and magnetite. The metal iron was first used by humans around 1200 BCE, the start of the Iron Age, and iron salts were used as medicine by the ancient Greeks. Iron was discovered in the blood in 1713, and it was used as a medicine to treat chlorosis, the name given to a common disorder causing paleness and weakness that affected young women at that time, now identified as anaemia.

The chemical symbol for iron, Fe, derives from the Latin word *ferrum*, meaning 'iron', and the word iron appears to be derived from the Anglo-Saxon word *iron* or *iren*. In biological systems, iron exists mainly in two valency states: the reduced ferrous (Fe^{2+}) form at acidic pH and the oxidised ferric (Fe^{3+}) form at neutral or alkaline pH. Iron can accept and donate electrons, and is essential for all living organisms because it plays an important role in electron transport, oxygen transport and DNA synthesis, as well as photosynthesis and respiration in plants. Most of the iron in the human body is in haemoglobin (Hb) in red blood cells, myoglobin (Mb) in muscles and within macrophages in the reticuloendothelial system. The remaining body iron is in iron stores, which are primarily in the liver as ferritin, in blood as transferrin (TF) and in iron-containing enzymes. Ferritin and phytoferritin from plants consist of a protein cage, in the centre of which are thousands of ferric ions linked by oxygen atoms. Iron is tightly controlled in the body, and almost all is bound to proteins because iron readily takes part in redox reactions (chemical reactions involving a transfer of electrons that changes the oxidation state of atoms), and free iron is a potent generator of damaging reactive oxygen species (ROS).

Digestion, absorption and transport

If body levels of iron are adequate, about 1–2 mg of iron is absorbed from the diet daily. Animal foods provide haem iron (ferrous iron surrounded by a porphyrin ring) as part of Hb and Mb, as well as ferritin and the non-haem form, and plant foods provide only non-haem iron, which is mainly ferric iron. Legumes and grains contain ferric iron in the form of phytoferritin, which is the plant form of ferritin.

Hb and Mb from food are hydrolysed in the digestive tract by protease enzymes to remove the globin component, forming haem iron, which is soluble and can be absorbed intact, assisted by the presence of amino acids and dipeptides derived from globin. Haem iron is well absorbed compared with non-haem iron. The method of uptake of haem iron by enterocytes in the gut wall is not well understood, but may occur via binding to receptors and endocytosis (engulfing of substances by the cell membrane) and/or via direct transport by either or both of the recently discovered haem transporters, proton-coupled folate transporter

(PCFT), also called haem carrier protein 1 (HCP1), and feline leukaemia virus subgroup C receptor (FLVCR). After endocytosis, haem is broken down inside the cell—possibly by the enzyme haem oxygenase 2—to release ferrous iron, which joins the non-haem iron pool in the enterocyte.

Unlike haem iron, the amount of non-haem iron absorbed varies according to the presence in the gut of inhibitors or enhancers of absorption. Overall, absorption is low. Non-haem iron must be released from the binding proteins in food by protease enzymes in the stomach and intestine before absorption, and requires the presence of hydrochloric acid in the stomach to increase its solubility. In the alkaline environment of the small intestine, non-haem ferric iron can form ferric hydroxide, which is insoluble and has low absorption. The absorption of ferric iron can be enhanced by its conversion to the ferrous form by the enzyme duodenal cytochrome B, which appears to use vitamin C as the electron donor.

The divalent metal transporter 1 (DMT1) facilitates uptake of non-haem ferrous iron in the gut, as well as the uptake of other minerals and toxic metals. Ferric iron is absorbed via an integrin-mobilferrin (IM) pathway not shared by other trace elements. Ferritin and phytoferritin appear to be absorbed intact via a specific absorption mechanism in enterocytes involving endocytosis, after which the protein cage is digested to release the iron into the intracellular iron pool. Lactoferrin, an iron-binding protein in milk, appears to be absorbed intact via a specific lactoferrin receptor and a similar method of endocytosis.

Once inside enterocytes, iron (originating from haem or non-haem iron) can be used by mitochondria in energy-production pathways, transferred to the bloodstream for delivery to other body tissues or stored as ferric iron in ferritin deposits. In the cytoplasm, ferric iron-IM complexes combine with flavin mono-oxygenase, beta-2 microglobulin and DMT1 in the cell interior to form paraferritin, a large protein complex that converts ferric iron to ferrous iron for transport out of the cell. Ferrous iron is transferred to the bloodstream by ferroportin 1 (FPN1), where it is oxidised by the copper-containing protein hephaestin to the ferric form in order to bind to TF, the main transporting protein in blood. Ceruloplasmin (CP), a copper-containing protein in plasma, is also involved in the conversion of ferrous iron to ferric iron during binding to TF. Intact haem may be transported from the enterocyte to the blood stream by FLVCR, where it binds to the plasma protein haemopexin.

TF is made up of a glycoprotein core that can bind one or two atoms of ferric iron. A molecule of TF containing two atoms of iron is referred to as fully saturated. In normal conditions, about one-third of the TF in the circulation is saturated. Cells can take up iron from TF when it binds to TF receptor 1 (TfR1) on the cell surface, and is taken into the cell interior by endocytosis. Fully saturated TF has a greater affinity for the receptor than less saturated forms. The iron in endosomes is released in the cell interior and transferred to the cell cytoplasm by DMT1, and either stored as ferritin or used within the cell. The TF glycoprotein and the TfR return to the cell surface for reuse. TfR1 is found in all cell membranes, and a second TF receptor (TfR2) is found mainly in liver cells and in tissue cells that produce red blood cells. TfR1 production is regulated by the amount of iron within the cell, whereas TfR2 production is regulated by the amount of TF that is saturated.

Zinc transporters (ZIPs) also have a role in the cellular uptake of iron as well as zinc and manganese. The ZIP14 transporter is involved in iron uptake in the liver, and also transports zinc, manganese and cadmium. It appears to have a role in iron uptake from TF and uptake of non-TF bound iron (NTBI), which builds up in iron overload when the iron-carrying capacity of TF is exceeded. The ZIP8 transporter appears to play a role in iron metabolism in the placenta, pancreas, lung and other organs. It may contribute to NTBI uptake during iron overload.

Metabolism, storage and excretion

Iron is stored in cells as insoluble ferritin in the cytoplasm, mainly in the liver, which contains about 25 per cent of total body iron, as well as in bone marrow and the spleen. On average, each ferritin molecule stores about 2000 iron atoms. Ferritin contains ferric iron in a crystalline structure as the mineral ferrihydrite, which can be converted to soluble ferrous iron and released when required. In the liver, ferrous iron released from ferritin can be transferred to the bloodstream via FPN1, with the assistance of CP, for use by other tissues. Small ferritin stores have also been discovered in the cell nucleus and mitochondria, in which they may act as protective iron scavengers. The function of serum ferritin is not well understood, but it may act as an iron scavenger or transporter. When ferritin capacity in cells is reached, iron can be stored also as haemosiderin, a breakdown product of ferritin, in iron-rich lysosomes (siderosomes) found mainly in macrophages. This storage form of iron cannot be released readily for use by the cell. In the brain, iron is also found in neuromelanin, which may act as an iron-storage molecule or bind iron in order to protect the brain from iron-induced oxidation.

The body has no pathway for excreting excess iron, and body iron is conserved by recycling. Red blood cells that have reached the end of their lifespan are engulfed by macrophages and the iron is released into the bloodstream for reuse. If red blood cells break down prematurely (haemolysis), free Hb binds to haptoglobin, a liver-derived protein in plasma, and free haem binds to haemopexin, both of which are taken up by macrophages and the iron recycled. Small amounts of iron are lost daily in sweat, urine and hair and skin cells when they are shed. Iron stored in enterocytes is lost in faeces when enterocytes die off and are shed into the gut. Losses also occur during haemorrhages and menstruation.

Regulation of body levels

In the absence of a pathway for excretion, iron levels are maintained largely by changes in the amount of iron absorbed from the diet and control of the release of iron into plasma from macrophages, liver stores and the diet. Absorption of dietary iron increases as ferritin stores decrease, and reduces when stores are adequate.

Hepcidin, a circulating peptide produced by the liver, is the major regulator of plasma iron levels, acting to inhibit iron metabolism. It decreases production of DMT1 in enterocytes, and binds to FPN1 and removes it from the cell surface, thereby reducing uptake and movement of dietary iron from enterocytes and liver cells into the bloodstream and reducing release of recycled red blood cell iron from macrophages. The liver produces more hepcidin when iron levels are high and in inflammation and infection, and reduces production when iron levels are low and in conditions of inadequate oxygenation of tissues (hypoxia). FPN1 can also be regulated independently by hypoxia-inducible factors and iron regulatory proteins (IRPs).

IRP1 and IRP2 sense the amount of iron inside cells and bind to specific regions of messenger RNA (mRNA) called iron-responsive elements (IREs), thereby regulating expression of iron metabolism genes. If iron is low, IRPs act to stabilise TfR mRNA and inhibit the translation of ferritin mRNA, which leads to less movement of iron into storage and increased iron uptake because of more TfRs on the cell membrane. Overall, these changes enhance iron availability in the cell. If iron is adequate, IRP2 is broken down and IRP1 does not bind to IREs, but binds an iron-sulfur compound (Fe-S cluster), and functions as an aconitase enzyme to convert citrate to isocitrate in the citric acid cycle of the energy pathway. IRPs affect enterocytes as they mature, and there is a lag time of one to two days before changes in absorption take effect.

Functions

The active forms of iron in the body are iron-containing haem proteins (Hb and Mb), haem-containing enzymes (cytochromes, catalases, peroxidases and myeloperoxidase), enzymes that contain Fe-S clusters and other iron-containing enzymes such as ribonucleotide reductase. Fe-S clusters usually contain four iron and four inorganic sulfur atoms, and can readily accept or donate electrons; they are found in dehydrogenase, oxidase, hydroxylase and aconitase enzymes. Iron is essential for oxygen transport and storage, energy production, immunity, detoxification and the function of enzymes involved in the metabolism of proteins, neurotransmitters and nucleotides. The functions of iron include the following:

- *Oxygen transport.* In its ferrous form, iron is part of the haem molecule in Hb in red blood cells that transports oxygen around the body. One molecule of Hb has four haem groups and can bind four oxygen molecules. About 25 mg of iron is required each day for Hb synthesis during production of red blood cells. When oxygen diffuses through lung tissue into red blood cells, it binds loosely to haem iron to form oxyHb, which has a bright red colour. The oxygenated red blood cells circulate around the body, and oxygen is transferred from oxyHb to tissues, forming deoxyHb, which is dark purple in colour. Simultaneously, deoxyHb can bind some of the carbon dioxide produced in body tissues and carry it to the lungs, where it is exhaled.
- *Oxygen supply in muscles.* Mb acts as an oxygen carrier and reserve supply in cardiac and oxidative skeletal muscle. Each molecule of Mb contains one haem group. Mb takes up oxygen from red blood cells, and helps transfer it to mitochondria when energy demands are increased, and provides a store of oxygen for use when oxygen supply is limited. It also appears to scavenge ROS by-products of the electron transport chain in mitochondria in cardiac and skeletal muscle.

- *Energy production*. Iron is an integral part of the electron transport chain in mitochondria that produces energy. Electron transport is facilitated by flavoproteins containing Fe-S complexes, haem-containing cytochromes and the iron-containing non-haem enzymes NADH dehydrogenase and succinate dehydrogenase. The Fe-S-containing enzyme aconitase converts citrate to isocitrate in the citric acid cycle.
- *Immune function*. During an immune response, iron is required for T lymphocyte proliferation, the bactericidal activity of macrophages and the production of myeloperoxidase, an iron-containing enzyme that produces ROS in order to destroy pathogens.
- *Detoxification and antioxidant activity.* Iron-containing cytochromes belonging to the P450 family are essential for the breakdown of foreign substances (xenobiotics) and unwanted metabolites during phase 1 of detoxification and the haem-containing enzymes catalase and peroxidase act as important scavengers for the ROS hydrogen peroxide. The Fe-S-containing enzyme aldehyde oxidase takes part in detoxification of drugs and alcohol by converting aldehydes to carboxylic acids during phase 1 reactions. The enzyme xanthine oxidase contains Fe-S clusters, vitamin B2 as flavin adenine dinucleotide (FAD) and molybdenum, and is part of the xanthine oxidoreductase (XOR) system. It is involved in the production of superoxide, and the breakdown of purine nucleotides to form uric acid. The XOR system appears to be important for detoxification and generation of protective ROS during immune reactions.
- *Amino acid metabolism*. The iron-containing enzymes phenylalanine hydroxylase, tyrosine hydroxylase and tryptophan hydroxylase are required for the production of the hormones adrenaline and noradrenaline, the neurotransmitters dopamine and serotonin and the skin pigment melanin. In connective tissue, iron is required, together with vitamin C, for the activity of the enzymes prolyl hydroxylase and lysyl hydroxylase that form collagen.
- *Sulfate metabolism*. The haem enzyme sulfite oxidase converts dietary sulfites to sulfates in the gut prior to absorption.
- *Cell metabolism and replication*. The haem enzyme thyroid peroxidase is required for incorporation of iodine into thyroid hormones that regulate the metabolic activity of cells. Iron is required for the activity of ribonucleotide reductase, an enzyme essential for DNA synthesis during cell replication. The haem enzyme tryptophan 2,3-dioxygenase is required for tryptophan conversion to the pyridine nucleotide NAD that is essential for many metabolic pathways, including energy production and DNA stability and repair.

Dietary sources

Haem iron, mainly in the form of Hb and Mb, is found in animal meats—especially red meat and organ meats—as well as fish, shellfish and poultry, and is more bioavailable, with an absorption of 20–30 per cent. It is not affected by absorption-inhibiting factors present in the diet. Non-haem iron is the major form of iron in most diets, and can make up 90–95 per cent of total daily iron intake. It is found in eggs and plant foods, such as whole grains, bran, legumes, dried fruit, nuts, seeds and dark-green vegetables such as spinach, broccoli and kale. There are only small amounts of iron (non-haem) in dairy products. Legumes and grains contain iron in the form of ferritin, which appears to be readily absorbed. Food cooked in iron cookware provides an additional source of iron.

In many plant foods, iron is bound to insoluble proteins, phytates, oxalates and phosphates and is relatively poorly absorbed overall. Absorption ranges from 2–10 per cent, depending on the balance between iron absorption inhibitors and iron absorption enhancers, such as ascorbic acid (vitamin C), present in the diet. The seaweed species *Ulva*, *Sargassum*, *Porphyra* and *Gracilariopsis* are good sources of ascorbic acid and bioavailable iron. According to the World Health Organization (WHO), mixed diets that contain generous amounts of meat and/or food rich in ascorbic acid have the highest iron bioavailability, and diets based on cereals and/or tubers with negligible amounts of meat and ascorbic acid-containing food have the lowest bioavailability.

In Australia, all cow's milk infant formulas are fortified with iron, and food manufacturers are permitted to voluntarily add iron (up to 25 per cent of the RDI) to bread, breakfast cereals, cereal flours, pasta, extracts of meat, vegetables or yeast, orange juice, vegetarian meat substitutes, formulated beverages, formulated meal replacements, formulated supplementary foods, infant foods and formulated supplementary sports foods. Iron salts permitted for use in food fortification in Australia are ferric ammonium citrate, ferric ammonium phosphate, ferric citrate, ferric hydroxide, ferric phosphate, ferric pyrophosphate, ferric sodium edetate (not permitted in breakfast cereals or supplementary foods for young children), ferric sulfate, ferrous carbonate, ferrous citrate, ferrous fumarate, ferrous gluconate, ferrous lactate, ferrous succinate, ferrous sulfate and ferrum reductum (reduced iron). Iron compounds with superior bioavailability include ferrous sulfate, ferrous fumarate, ferric pyrophosphate and electrolytic iron powder, and are recommended by the WHO for fortifying food.

The Food Standards Australia New Zealand nutrient database (NUTTAB) at <www.foodstandards.gov.au> provides the amounts found in specific foods.

Factors influencing body status

Iron absorption increases when ferritin stores are low, and reduces when stores are adequate. Overall, it is estimated that, in people with no iron stores, iron bioavailability from mixed diets is 14–18 per cent and bioavailability from vegetarian diets is 5–12 per cent. Haem iron absorption is relatively stable, and more efficient than non-haem iron. Its absorption is enhanced by amino acids and peptides that maintain it in a soluble state. Ferritin in legumes is relatively well absorbed compared with other plant sources of iron.

Plant iron absorption is limited because ferric iron is bound by phytate (*myo*-inositol hexaphosphate) in grains, legumes, nuts and seeds, especially whole grains and bran. Phytate can be broken down by prolonged soaking, sprouting or using yeast as a leavening agent when baking bread. In general, vegetarian and whole-food diets provide less absorbable iron. Premenopausal women have been found to absorb 3.5 times more non-haem iron and about six times more total iron from a non-vegetarian diet than from a lacto-ovo-vegetarian diet (plant foods plus eggs and dairy) containing similar amounts of iron.

Ferric iron in the digestive tract can be bound by polyphenols, such as tannins, that reduce absorption. Beverages containing polyphenols such as red wine, tea, coffee, cocoa and many herbal teas have a strong inhibiting effect when taken with meals. Beverages containing 20–50 mg of total polyphenols per serving have been found to reduce non-haem iron absorption from a bread meal by 50–70 per cent, and beverages containing 100–400 mg total polyphenols per serving reduce iron absorption by 60–90 per cent. Absorption of non-haem iron from a bread meal was found to be reduced 84 per cent by peppermint tea, 73 per cent by pennyroyal tea, 71 per cent by cocoa, 59 per cent by vervain tea, 52 per cent by lime flower tea and 47 per cent by camomile tea. In comparable quantities, black tea polyphenols have a more inhibiting effect than herbal tea or wine polyphenols. A cup of tea with a bread meal reduces iron absorption by 79–94 per cent and drinking green tea with a pasta meal reduces iron absorption by 26 per cent. After a mixed meal, 150 mL of strong black tea drunk within an hour of eating reduces iron absorption by 75–80 per cent, although enhancers such as ascorbic acid partially compensate for this effect. The addition of milk to tea has little effect.

Coffee reduces iron absorption from a hamburger meal by up to 39 per cent, a cup of drip coffee ingested with a test meal reduces absorption by up to 72 per cent and instant coffee reduces absorption by up to 81 per cent. Doubling the strength of instant coffee reduces absorption by up to 91 per cent. On average, a cup of coffee drunk within one hour of a meal inhibits iron absorption by about 60 per cent. The inhibition does not appear to be affected by the presence of caffeine or milk.

Calcium and dairy protein have been shown to inhibit iron absorption in single meal studies, but the effect is less important in studies of multiple meals. In Asia, consumption of betel leaves has a potent inhibiting effect on iron absorption. Iron may be bound by oxalate in some foods such as spinach, beets and beet greens, parsley, purslane, rhubarb, sorrel, Swiss chard, strawberries, cranberries, wheat bran, amaranth, soy products, nuts, cocoa and tea, but the effect on iron absorption appears to be minor. Soy protein was thought to decrease iron absorption, but is now believed to have little effect. Meat, fish and poultry enhance non-haem iron absorption from plant foods eaten at the same meal, but milk and egg protein inhibit iron absorption. Egg yolk contains phosvitin, a highly phosphorylated protein that chelates iron and forms insoluble phosvitin-iron complexes, and casein and whey proteins found in milk bind iron and reduce its absorption.

Non-haem iron absorption is enhanced by the presence of reducing substances, such as acids, that convert iron to the ferrous form in the gut. Reducing substances include stomach acid, ascorbic acid, citric, tartaric and malic acids found in fruit, and lactic acid found in yoghurt, cheese, soy sauce and fermented foods. The most significant enhancer is ascorbic acid, which can partially counteract the inhibiting effects of phytates, polyphenols, calcium and milk proteins, and may increase absorption by up to six-fold in people with low iron stores. The addition of 50 mg of ascorbic acid to a meal can increase iron absorption three- to six-fold. An antioxidant food additive derived from ascorbic acid, erythorbic acid (additive number 315), appears to be almost twice as effective as ascorbic acid in enhancing non-haem iron absorption.

Alcohol has been found to increase serum iron and ferritin levels. Vitamin A is required for red blood cell production and the release of iron from ferritin stores. In one study, vitamin A and beta-carotene appeared to reduce the inhibitory effect of phytates on non-haem iron absorption; providing vitamin A together with a cereal increased iron absorption three-fold for rice, 2.4-fold for wheat and 1.8-fold for corn, and beta-carotene increased absorption almost three-fold for each of the three cereals. However, another study found that vitamin A had no effect on iron absorption. A deficiency of copper, molybdenum, sulfate or vitamin B2 may impair iron metabolism.

Iron demand is increased during times of rapid growth such as infancy, childhood, adolescence and pregnancy. Athletes may have an increased need for iron because of increased red blood cell production and inadequate intake associated with high-carbohydrate sports diets, as well as losses in sweat and the premature breakdown of red blood cells that occurs with strenuous activity. Iron is lost with blood loss that may occur because of trauma, blood donations, frequent nose bleeds, digestive tract ulcers, long-term use of aspirin, inflammatory bowel diseases and menstruation.

Non-haem iron uptake is reduced by stomach acid depletion associated with ageing and long-term use of antacid or proton pump inhibitors, which decrease stomach acid concentrations. Inadequate production of stomach acid inhibits iron absorption by about 50 per cent. Inflammatory bowel disease, parasites, gastric surgery, coeliac disease and stomach infection with *Helicobacter pylori* may reduce iron absorption.

Daily requirement

Australian and New Zealand government recommendations by age and gender (see Table 10.1) can be found in *Nutrient Reference Values for Australia and New Zealand Including Recommended Dietary Intakes*, available at <www.nhmrc.gov.au>.

Table 10.1 Recommended dietary intake (RDI) of iron (mg/day)

Age (years)	Female RDI	Male RDI
1–3	9	9
4–8	10	10
9–13	8	8
14–18	15	11
19–50	18	8
51–70	8	8
>70	8	8
Pregnant women		
14–18	27	
19–50	27	
Lactating women		
14–18	10	
19–50	9	

Source: Nutrient Reference Values for Australia and New Zealand Including Recommended Dietary Intakes, National Health and Medical Research Council, Australian Government Department of Health and Ageing, Canberra and Ministry of Health, New Zealand, Wellington, 2006.

Deficiency effects

Iron deficiency is the most common and widespread nutritional disorder in the world. It is more common in preterm or low birth weight infants, weaning infants, preschool children, adolescents and pregnant women because of increased demands; vegetarians and vegans because of lower iron absorption; and menstruating women because of increased losses. A persistent and unexplained iron deficiency commonly accompanies undiagnosed coeliac disease (gluten intolerance).

The WHO has estimated that 30–40 per cent of preschool children in developed countries are iron deficient, and the prevalence of anaemia among pregnant women is about 20 per cent. A UK survey in 1994 found that 90 per cent of menstruating and 34 per cent of non-menstruating women had inadequate iron intakes. A 2010 report by the UK Scientific Advisory Committee on Nutrition on iron and health found that children aged eighteen months to three and a half years, girls aged eleven to eighteen years and women aged nineteen to 49 years were most at risk of inadequate iron intakes. The prevalence of iron deficiency in the US, 2003–06, was 14 per cent for children aged one to two years, 4 per cent for children aged three to five years, and 9 per cent for teenage girls and menstruating women.

The prevalence of iron deficiency in Australia is not clear. However, a 2008 Australian study of adults found that 10.6 per cent of women aged less than 50 years were iron deficient, as were 2.8 per cent of women aged 50 and over and 0.3 per cent of men. The WHO has estimated that, in Australia, 8 per cent of preschool children, 12 per cent of pregnant women and 15 per cent of non-pregnant women of reproductive age have anaemia, most commonly related to iron deficiency.

When iron intake is inadequate, iron is released from ferritin stores to supply tissue requirements, and absorption of dietary iron increases. If dietary iron is not sufficient to supply body needs, iron depletion develops, in which ferritin stores are slowly used up, leading to reduced serum ferritin and a reduction in circulating TF saturation. Iron transport and functions may be unchanged at this stage. When iron stores are depleted, iron deficiency develops, which impairs red blood cell production and increases the amount of protoporphyrin (a precursor to Hb) in red blood cells.

In animals, iron deficiency affects neurotransmitter synthesis and metabolism, mitochondrial function, brain iron deposition, protein synthesis, and electron transport and redox reactions. Early effects of iron deficiency in humans include fatigue, irritability, headaches, depression, reduced exercise tolerance and increased susceptibility to infections. If the deficiency continues, iron deficiency anaemia develops. It appears that iron deficiency impairs brain function before the onset of anaemia, causing behavioural and cognitive impairment that is more pronounced in children and adolescents.

Iron deficiency anaemia

In iron deficiency anaemia (IDA), there is exhaustion of iron stores, low serum ferritin, low TF saturation, reduced serum iron concentration and increased total iron binding capacity (TIBC). It is a microcytic, hypochromic anaemia, in which reduced Hb concentration in red blood cells and reduced red blood cell volume cause red blood cells to appear pale and smaller than normal. The plasma membranes of some iron-deficient red blood cells become abnormally rigid, forming small, stiff, misshapen cells (poikilocytes) that are cleared by the reticuloendothelial system. A high platelet count (thrombocytosis) is common.

Some people with iron deficiency or IDA may have no obvious symptoms, or have only vague symptoms that are not recognised. The abnormalities of red blood cells lead to impaired tissue oxygen delivery and impaired energy production, causing a pale appearance, pale mucous membranes, vertigo and light-headedness. A lack of Mb and intracellular iron in skeletal muscles impairs energy production, which causes muscle weakness and limits exercise performance and endurance. Exercise may induce palpitations, a fast heart rate (tachycardia) and breathlessness. Inadequate thyroid hormone production may cause a lowered body temperature and sensation of coldness.

The high-turnover cells of the skin, nails and digestive tract may develop changes linked to IDA. Digestive tract changes include painful cracks at the corners of the mouth (cheilosis) and inflammation of the tongue (glossitis), with swelling, a burning sensation and flattened papillae, giving the tongue a smooth and shiny appearance. The stomach lining may atrophy, impairing digestion. A rare outcome of IDA is Plummer-Vinson syndrome, which features the formation of small, thin, web-like growths of tissue in the oesophagus, causing problems with swallowing. Some people with IDA develop a craving for eating unusual substances (pica), such as ice or icy drinks (pagophagia), clay (geophagia), dry pasta (amylophagia), paper, paint, chalk, laundry starch, paste, cigarette butts, hair, lead or foam rubber, or a craving for chewing rubber bands. Clay and starch can bind iron in the digestive tract and exacerbate the iron deficiency.

In IDA, the skin may be paler, inelastic and itchy, and there is an increased risk of bacterial and fungal infections, such as impetigo, boils and thrush (candidiasis). Nails may develop thick, length-wise ridges or transverse depressions, and become softer, brittle and curved upwards at the edges into a spoon shape (koilonychia). Hair may thin out and become dry, brittle and dull. The whites of the eyes may become paler or bluish in colour, and the conjunctiva of the eyes may have a pale appearance.

Iron deficiency in the brain may impair neurotransmitter and motor nerve functions. Restless legs syndrome (RLS), the compulsion to move the legs when at rest, is associated with IDA, and may respond to improved intake of iron. Iron deficiency increases susceptibility to infections. It reduces oxygen delivery and energy production in immune cells and tissues, and impairs the activity of ribonucleotide reductase, leading to reduced DNA synthesis. This may depress the immune response by reducing proliferation of immune cells such as T lymphocytes and neutrophils. Inadequate iron also may impair production of leukocyte-generated hydroxyl free radicals that destroy pathogens. Iron deficiency can have adverse effects on the heart, leading to left ventricular enlargement, impaired blood flow and heart failure.

Pregnant women

During an entire pregnancy, about 600 mg of iron is required to support the mother's increase in red blood cell production and a further 300 mg is needed by the foetus. The demand for iron increases steadily from about 0.8 mg daily in the first ten weeks of gestation to 7.5 mg daily in the last ten weeks. Iron deficiency in pregnancy may affect maternal morbidity, foetal and infant development and pregnancy outcomes. It may be linked to an increased risk of preterm delivery, low birth weight infants, placental abruption (detachment of the placenta) and increased maternal blood loss during birth. A lack of iron in early pregnancy has been shown to cause an imbalance of neural precursor cells, which may affect the infant's brain development after birth. Untreated iron deficiency or IDA in the third trimester strongly predisposes to iron deficiency or IDA in the mother after the birth, and may cause emotional imbalances and fatigue, affecting her ability to bond with and care for her baby. Iron-deficient pregnant women may have reduced immunity, pale skin, lips and nails, poor concentration and memory, irritability, weakness, fatigue, dizziness, heart palpitations and shortness of breath, especially on exertion such as walking up stairs. Pica, especially for ice, is a strong indicator of iron deficiency in pregnancy.

It has been shown that 40 mg of ferrous iron daily from eighteen weeks of gestation prevents iron deficiency in 90 per cent of pregnant women, and prevents IDA in 95 per cent of pregnant women. However, some researchers do not recommend the general use of iron supplementation in pregnancy because it may impair absorption of other trace elements and increase oxidative stress. It has been suggested that serum ferritin should be used to indicate whether a supplement is necessary.

Infants and children

About 80 per cent of the iron present in a newborn infant is acquired during the third trimester of pregnancy. The ability to accumulate iron is impaired in preterm infants and in infants of mothers with IDA, diabetes or maternal hypertension with intrauterine growth restriction. Infants only have about 10 per cent of the adult iron concentration in their brains at birth, which rises to about 50 per cent at the age of ten years and reaches normal levels between the ages of twenty and 30 years. At birth, iron stores last for four to six months, and the requirement for iron increases dramatically from the fourth month because of depletion of body stores and rapid growth. In full-term newborn infants, delaying the clamping of the umbilical cord for at least two minutes following birth improves the infant's iron status. Preterm breastfed infants are at higher risk of iron deficiency, whereas formula-fed preterm infants may be able to obtain enough iron from the formula to prevent a deficiency. However, it is estimated that 14 per cent of preterm infants develop iron deficiency between four and eight months of age, despite the use of iron-containing formulas.

The risk of IDA in infants is greatest from age six months to two years, and is related to poor iron stores at birth, exclusive breastfeeding for longer than six months, using cow's milk rather than formula prior to twelve months of age, and excessive drinking of cow's milk that leads to a lower intake of solid food. Iron deficiency in infants and children may cause lowered immunity and retarded growth and development, and has been associated with febrile seizures and increased body levels of the toxic metals cadmium and lead. Lead is a developmental neurotoxin, interfering with neurotransmission and cellular migration in the central nervous system (CNS) and impairing the ability of nerve synapses to adapt to stimuli (synaptic plasticity), an ability that is important for learning and memory. Lead can cause neurotoxicity even at very low blood concentrations, and also inhibits enzymes that synthesise haem, contributing to anaemia. It shares an absorption pathway with iron, and a lack of iron allows more lead to be absorbed. Children can absorb up to 50 per cent of ingested lead compared with 5 per cent in adults. Children with IDA have increased lead concentrations, and iron supplementation may lower blood lead levels in children with and without IDA.

Iron deficiency impairs energy metabolism in nerve cells, the metabolism of neurotransmitters, myelination of nerve fibres and memory function. Iron deficiency in infants and children is associated with behavioural and cognitive impairment, and early iron deficiency may lead to irreversible damage to brain cells. The developing hippocampus in the brain, which is responsible for learning and memory, is particularly affected. Infants with IDA have lower mental and motor function scores and behavioural abnormalities, and children with iron deficiency or IDA may have fatigue, listlessness, apathy, restlessness, attention deficit hyperactivity disorder (ADHD), irritability and impaired growth, cognitive intellectual and language development, memory, concentration, learning ability and school performance. Severe, chronic IDA in infancy may cause long-term brain, developmental and behavioural effects that may not be reversible with iron supplementation.

Athletes

An apparent anaemia occurring in athletes (sports anaemia) is related to a short-term expansion of plasma volume induced by increased aerobic fitness, and is not a true anaemia. However, athletes are at increased risk of iron deficiency because of the greater amount of iron needed to support an increased number of red blood cells, increased iron losses caused by sweating, gastrointestinal tract bleeding and impact haemolysis, and reduced intake caused by restrictive diets, such as high carbohydrate or weight-control diets.

Athletes—particularly elite-level females competing in endurance sports—commonly develop depletion of iron stores and early functional iron deficiency, which may impair exercise performance. Functional iron deficiency occurs when there is insufficient iron incorporation into red blood cell precursors, in spite of apparently adequate iron stores. Even a mild functional iron deficiency can reduce maximum oxygen uptake, aerobic efficiency and endurance. In a study of adolescent and adult female athletes, 25–36 per cent were found to be iron deficient, and this increased to 70 per cent during the athletic season. Increased hepcidin levels have been reported in athletes in some studies—possibly because of exercise-induced inflammation, which may contribute to functional iron deficiency. However, other studies have reported that exercise has a lowering effect on hepcidin levels.

In some studies, iron supplementation has been found to improve physical performance in athletes and previously untrained subjects with an existing iron deficiency, but other studies report no effects on performance. High-dose iron supplements should be used with caution in athletes because of the risks of increased oxidative stress and the potential for iron overload in athletes with a genetic predisposition.

Indicators of inadequate levels of iron may include:

- *early effects:* fatigue, irritability, headaches, depression, reduced exercise tolerance, increased susceptibility to infections
- pale, inelastic and itchy skin, pale mucous membranes, pale conjunctiva, bacterial and fungal skin infections
- muscle weakness, reduced work performance and endurance, restless legs
- vertigo, light-headedness, heart palpitations, tachycardia, breathlessness, especially on exertion
- lowered immunity, lowered body temperature, sensation of coldness
- pale or bluish whites of the eyes, cheilosis, glossitis, smooth, shiny tongue, atrophy of the stomach, Plummer-Vinson syndrome
- *pica:* craving for ice, icy drinks, clay, dried pasta, paper, paint, chalk, laundry starch, paste, cigarette butts, hair, lead, foam rubber, chewing rubber bands
- *nails:* thick length-wise ridges or transverse depressions, soft, brittle, spoon-shaped
- *hair:* thinning, dry, brittle, dull
- *pregnancy:* preterm delivery, low birth weight infants, placental abruption, increased maternal blood loss during birth
- *children:* increased lead levels, fatigue, listlessness, apathy, febrile seizures, restlessness, irritability, ADHD, impaired growth and cognitive and intellectual development, poor memory, concentration, learning ability and school performance.

Assessment of body status

Measurement of Hb in red blood cells is a commonly used screening test for IDA. There are several other causes of low Hb apart from iron deficiency, and a diagnosis of IDA can be confirmed only by the presence of low Hb together with other abnormal measures of iron status, such as low serum ferritin. Determining the concentration of Hb in red blood cells is a more sensitive and direct indicator of IDA than haematocrit, which is a measure of the percentage of red blood cells in whole blood. The reference range given by the Royal College of Pathologists of Australasia (RCPA) for Hb concentration is 135–195 g/L for cord blood in a newborn infant, 95–135 g/L for an infant aged three to six months, 105–135 g/L for a child aged one year, 105–140 g/L for a child aged three to six years, 115–145 g/L for a child aged ten to twelve years, 115–165 g/L for a woman and 130–180 g/L for a man. Anaemia in children has been defined by the RCPA as a Hb concentration of less than 90 g/L at two months of age; 95 g/L at two to six months; 105 g/L at six to 24 months; 115 g/L at two to eleven years; 120 g/L for girls over twelve years; and 130 g/L for boys over twelve years. In pregnancy, anaemia has been defined by the British Committee for Standards in Haematology as an Hb level less than 110 g/L in the first trimester, less than 105 g/L in the second and third trimesters and less than 100 g/L after the birth.

Several measures of iron status, including TF saturation, and serum iron, TF and ferritin, need to be used together in order to get a true picture of iron status. In general, iron deficiency features elevated serum TF, low TF saturation, low serum iron and low serum ferritin. A low level of serum iron together with a raised level of serum TF is very strong evidence of iron deficiency. The reference ranges given by the RCPA are 6.0–35.0 μmol/L for serum iron concentration, 2.0–3.6 g/L for serum TF and 16–45 per cent for TF saturation. TF saturation reflects the percentage of TF that is carrying iron and is the ratio of serum iron to TIBC, multiplied by 100. TIBC is elevated in iron deficiency but is lowered by anaemia of chronic disease, and is a less sensitive test than serum ferritin. A TF saturation greater than 45 per cent, together with a serum ferritin greater than 250 mcg/L for a premenopausal woman or greater than 300 mcg/L for a postmenopausal woman or man, indicates iron overload.

Serum ferritin concentration reflects the total amount of storage iron, and higher levels indicate higher stores of iron. A concentration of 1 mcg/L is equivalent to approximately 8 mg of stored iron. Serum ferritin is the only measure that can indicate normal, deficient or excess iron status. The reference range given by the RCPA for serum ferritin in adults is 15–200 mcg/L for premenopausal women and 30–300 mcg/L for men; levels progressively change over time to male levels in women after menopause.

Serum ferritin may be normal or raised during an acute phase response, which occurs in infection, inflammation, liver disease or cancer, even when iron stores are low. Patients with an acute phase response have reduced plasma iron and TF, and raised serum ferritin. An acute phase response can be detected by measuring C-reactive protein (CRP) in serum. The reference range given by the RCPA for serum CRP is less than 5 mg/L.

The soluble TF receptor concentration in plasma reflects the body's demand for iron, and this will increase in iron deficiency, IDA, haemolytic anaemia and disorders of red blood cell production, such as thalassaemia and megaloblastic anaemia. The reference measure given by Austin Pathology, Melbourne, Australia for plasma soluble TF receptor concentration in adults is less than 1.55 mg/L. TF receptor levels are less affected by an acute phase response than serum ferritin, and can indicate the severity of iron deficiency.

Microcytic anaemia is most often caused by IDA, and is diagnosed by a mean corpuscular volume (MCV) of red blood cells of less than 80 femtolitres (fL). However, it is not specific to IDA, and must be used with other measures of iron status. The first stage of iron deficiency is generally characterised by low serum ferritin concentrations and early functional iron deficiency; the second stage features increased serum TF receptors and reduced TF saturation; and the third stage features below-normal Hb concentrations and reduced MCV.

Case reports—iron deficiency

- *A woman, 21 years of age*, had a two-year history of a strong craving for ice, eating two to three trays of ice and two to three bags of crushed ice a day.[1] She was in the habit of scratching ice off her freezer to eat in the early hours of the morning. She did not have fatigue or breathlessness, but on examination, she was found to have pallor, pale conjunctiva and a smooth, shiny, painful tongue. She was found to have microcytic hypochromic anaemia, and blood tests showed that she was iron deficient. She was given supplementary iron, which led to improvement of her symptoms in two weeks and complete disappearance of her ice craving in one month.
- *A man, 62 years of age*, developed bleeding bowel polyps, and was found to have blood abnormalities characteristic of iron deficiency.[2] He reported a craving for drinking icy cold water. He was in the habit of putting his bottled water in the freezer, and drinking three or four bottles daily. His polyps were removed and he was given iron therapy. His craving for icy water lessened within two months.
- *A boy, three years of age*, developed inattention, hyperactivity and impulsivity at school and home.[3] His parents reported that he was continually moving about, had difficulty going to sleep, was restless during sleep and was not able to pay attention, listen, wait his turn or play quietly. At kindergarten, he could not pay attention, frequently interrupted others, and had difficulty finishing his activities and sitting still when required. His mother's pregnancy and delivery had been normal, as had his physical and neurological development since birth. No obvious cause could be found for his symptoms and he was diagnosed with ADHD. Blood tests later revealed that his serum ferritin was low, and he was placed on iron therapy, which

gradually raised his serum ferritin to normal values over a period of eight months. There was a steady improvement in his symptoms, and at eight months his behaviour was described as transformed. He was less hyperactive, more attentive, less impulsive and slept better, although he still had difficulties with frustration. At kindergarten, he was more organised in his activities, more attentive, and less forgetful and impulsive. His relationships with other children improved markedly.

- *A boy, 15 years of age*, developed fatigue, pallor and progressive difficulty swallowing over a one-year period.[4] He had difficulty swallowing solid foods, and was underweight and small for his age. He did not eat any meat or meat products, and had no pica. Blood tests revealed he had IDA, and examination of his throat found a web blocking the cervical oesophagus, which was removed by balloon dilation. He was given iron therapy, and his fatigue and difficulty swallowing disappeared at one month, together with an improvement in measures of his iron status. At six months follow-up, he was reported to be in good health with no problems swallowing his food.
- *A woman, 25 years of age*, was found to have IDA after blood tests were undertaken to determine the cause of a stomach upset.[5] The only associated symptom she reported was mild exercise intolerance. She was not vegetarian, and her diet seemed well balanced. She reported having a history of heavy menstrual bleeding, and this was presumed to be the cause of her IDA. Iron supplementation reversed the anaemia for two years, but it returned when the supplement was discontinued. After this time, the anaemia returned in spite of iron supplementation. She was then given treatment to relieve her heavy menstruation, together with iron supplements, but her anaemia worsened. After five years of iron treatment, her diet was carefully reviewed, and it was discovered that she was in the habit of drinking about 1.5 litres of tea daily with no other liquids. She took her iron supplement with a large cup of tea each day. She stopped drinking tea and her iron status normalised five months later.

REFERENCES

1 Osman, Y.M., Wali, Y.A. & Osman, O.M., Craving for ice and iron-deficiency anemia: A case series from Oman, *Pediatr Hematol Oncol* (2005), 22(2): 127–31.

2 Khan, Y. & Tisman, G., Pica in iron deficiency: A case series, *J Med Case Rep* (2010), 4: 86.

3 Konofal, E., Cortese, S., Lecendreux, M. et al., Effectiveness of iron supplementation in a young child with attention-deficit/hyperactivity disorder, *Pediatrics* (2005), 116(5): e732–4.

4 Dinler, G., Tander, B., Kalayci, A.G. & Rizalar, R., Plummer-Vinson syndrome in a 15-year-old boy, *Turk J Pediatr* (2009), 51(4): 384–6.

5 Gabrielli, G.B. & De Sandre, G., Excessive tea consumption can inhibit the efficacy of oral iron treatment in iron-deficiency anemia, *Haematologica* (1995), 80(6): 518–20.

THERAPEUTIC USES OF IRON

Iron is used primarily for the prevention and treatment of iron deficiency and IDA, and also may have therapeutic activity for the following conditions:

Restless legs syndrome

Restless legs syndrome (RLS) is the compulsion to move the legs when at rest, especially while lying in bed at night. It is associated with iron deficiency and IDA, and may respond to improved intake of iron. Pregnant women, people with IDA or end-stage renal disease, and children with ADHD have a higher prevalence of RLS. It has been estimated that 11–27 per cent of pregnant women experience RLS during pregnancy, most often in the third trimester, although it usually disappears after the birth.[1] It is theorised that iron transport from blood to the CNS is impaired in RLS, and iron deficiency may impair dopamine neurotransmitter functions in the brain, affecting control of movement.[2] The amount of iron in the blood varies through a 24-hour day, and drops to about half at night when RLS symptoms are more severe.[3] The level of iron in cerebrospinal fluid has been shown to be 65 per cent lower in people with RLS, and the level of TF 300 per cent higher than controls,[4] and lower iron uptake and storage have been found in the substantia nigra, the part of the brain that controls movement.[5] Lower serum ferritin (less than 50 mcg/L) has been associated with greater RLS severity and decreased sleep quality.[6]

A study of iron supplementation in RLS patients with low serum ferritin found that 325 mg of ferrous sulfate twice daily for three months increased serum ferritin and improved symptoms of RLS.[7] Iron supplementation has been found to improve motor and sensory symptoms, and also improve sleep, sleepiness, depression, fatigue and quality of life in RLS patients.[8] However, a systematic review of six trials concluded that there was insufficient evidence to support the role of iron in the treatment of RLS.[9]

Breath-holding attacks in children

Breath-holding attacks (BHA) affect approximately 5 per cent of apparently healthy children, and are most common from the age of six months to six years, particularly from six months to eighteen months. They are induced by an emotional stress, during which the child holds his/her breath, becomes pale or blue and may lose consciousness and have convulsive movements. Most children with BHA have several attacks per week, and many have two to five attacks per day. Although the cause of BHA is not clear, it appears to be aggravated by IDA, possibly because inadequate Hb leads to decreased oxygen-carrying capacity that may lead to rapid loss of oxygen in brain tissues. In addition, iron-deficient children are more irritable, and may have more extreme responses to stressful events.

Low Hb levels are associated with BHA, and iron supplementation has been shown to reduce or eliminate episodes.[10,11,12] Children with IDA and BHA have responded to iron supplementation before the anaemia has been corrected, and it appears that iron deficiency is a key factor, with or without anaemia. However, children with apparently normal iron status have also responded to iron supplementation for BHA. It may be that, in sub-clinical or very mild iron depletion, most iron-dependent body functions are maintained at the expense of neurotransmitter production. A meta-analysis of two trials of iron supplementation concluded that 5 mg/kg/day of elemental iron for sixteen weeks appears to be useful in reducing the frequency and severity of BHA, particularly in children with IDA but also in children with normal or low normal Hb levels.[13]

Heart failure

Iron deficiency is common in patients with heart failure, and is associated with a poor prognosis; it has been found to be an independent predictor of death or urgent heart transplantation.[14] Heart failure involves generalised inflammation that features an increased immune response, overactive immune cells and high levels of pro-inflammatory mediators. Inflammation stimulates hepcidin production, which impairs iron metabolism and may lead to a functional iron deficiency in heart failure patients.

Intravenous (iv) iron treatment in patients with IDA, heart failure and impaired renal function has improved their functional status, exercise capacity and quality of life.[15] Intravenous iron has improved exercise tolerance and heart failure symptoms in patients with iron deficiency or IDA, with greater improvements in patients with IDA.[16] Long-term therapy with iv iron and erythropoietin (a hormone that stimulates red blood cell production) in heart failure patients has led to improvements in cardiac and kidney function, a marked reduction in the need for diuretics and a reduction in hospitalisations of 91.9 per cent.[17] Intravenous iron given to heart failure patients with iron deficiency or IDA for six months was associated with rapid improvements across the whole clinical spectrum of heart failure.[18] A meta-analysis of four trials concluded that iv iron therapy is safe in heart failure and is associated with improved quality of life, reduced hospitalisation, and increased exercise capacity.[19]

Cognitive function

Decreased iron stores in the brain may impair the activity of iron-dependent enzymes that metabolise the neurotransmitters dopamine, serotonin and noradrenaline. Iron supplementation has been shown to improve memory, attention, mood and energy in people with IDA before any change in Hb.[20] Non-anaemic iron-deficient teenage girls given 260 mg elemental iron daily as ferrous sulfate for eight weeks showed improvements in verbal learning and memory.[21] Children with ADHD who were iron deficient but not anaemic showed improvements in overall symptoms, hyperactivity, impulsiveness and inattention after supplementation with 80 mg of iron as ferrous sulfate for twelve weeks.[22] An Australian study of premenopausal women found that a history of iron deficiency within the previous two years was associated with a lower score for cognitive and physical function and vitality,[23] and a follow-up study of premenopausal Australian women who were iron deficient found that increasing iron intake by diet or supplements resulted in improved mental health and decreased fatigue.[24]

A systematic review of fourteen studies of infants, children and adolescents concluded that iron supplementation may have a modest beneficial effect on cognition and psychomotor outcomes in anaemic infants and children if continued for at least two months.[25] A meta-analysis of fourteen studies of anaemic children older than six years, adolescents and women concluded that there is some evidence that iron supplementation improves attention and concentration in adolescents and women, irrespective of baseline iron status, and improves IQ in women and children who were anaemic at baseline.[26]

REFERENCES

1 Manconi, M., Govoni, V., De Vito, A. et al., Pregnancy as a risk factor for restless legs syndrome, *Sleep Med* (2004), 5(3): 305–8.

2 Allen, R., Dopamine and iron in the pathophysiology of restless legs syndrome (RLS), *Sleep Med* (2004), 5(4): 385–91.

3 Scales, W.E., Vander, A.J., Brown, M.B. & Kluger, M.J., Human circadian rhythms in temperature, trace metals, and blood variables, *J Appl Physiol* (1988), 65: 1840–6.

4 Earley, C.J., Connor, J.R., Beard, J.L. et al., Abnormalities in CSF concentrations of ferritin and transferrin in restless legs syndrome, *Neurology* (2000), 54: 1698–1700.

5 Allen, R.P. & Earley, C.J., Restless legs syndrome: A review of clinical and pathophysiologic features, *J Clin Neurophysiol* (2001), 18(2): 128–47.

6 Sun, E.R., Chen, C.A., Ho, G. et al., Iron and the restless legs syndrome, *Sleep* (1998), 21(4): 371–7.

7 Wang, J., O'Reilly, B., Venkataraman, R. et al., Efficacy of oral iron in patients with restless legs syndrome and a low-normal ferritin: A randomized, double-blind, placebo-controlled study, *Sleep Med* (2009), 10(9): 973–5.

8 Cuellar, N.G., Hanlon, A. & Ratcliffe, S.J., The relationship with iron and health outcomes in persons with restless legs syndrome, *Clin Nurs Res* (2011), 20(2): 144–61.

9 Trotti, L.M., Bhadriraju, S. & Becker, L.A., Iron for restless legs syndrome, *Cochrane Database Syst Rev* (2012), 5: CD007834.

10 Daoud, A.S., Batieha, A., Al-Sheyyab, M. et al., Effectiveness of iron therapy on breath-holding spells, *J Pediatr* (1997), 130: 547–50.

11 Mocan, H., Yildiran, A., Orhan, F. et al., Breath holding spells in 91 children and response to treatment with iron, *Arch Dis Child* (1999), 81: 261–2.

12 Bhatia, M.S., Singhal, P.K., Dhar, N.K. et al., Breath holding spells: An analysis of 50 cases, *Indian Pediatr* (1990), 27: 1073–9.

13 Zehetner, A.A., Orr, N., Buckmaster, A. et al., Iron supplementation for breath-holding attacks in children, *Cochrane Database Syst Rev* (2010), 5: CD008132.

14 Macdougall, I.C., Canaud, B., de Francisco, A.L. et al., Beyond the cardiorenal anaemia syndrome: Recognizing the role of iron deficiency, *Eur J Heart Fail* (2012), 14(8): 882–6.

15 Jankowska, E.A., von Haehling, S., Anker, S.D. et al., Iron deficiency and heart failure: Diagnostic dilemmas and therapeutic perspectives, *Eur Heart J* (2013), 34(11): 816–29.

16 Okonko, D.O., Grzeslo, A., Witkowski, T. et al., Effect of intravenous iron sucrose on exercise tolerance in anemic and nonanemic patients with symptomatic chronic heart failure and iron deficiency FERRIC-HF: A randomized, controlled, observer-blinded trial, *J Am Coll Cardiol* (2008), 51(2): 103–12.

17 Silverberg, D.S., Wexler, D., Blum, M. et al., The use of subcutaneous erythropoietin and intravenous iron for the treatment of the anemia of severe, resistant congestive heart failure improves cardiac and renal function and functional cardiac class, and markedly reduces hospitalisations, *J Am Coll Cardiol* (2000), 35(7): 1737–44.

18 Anker, S.D., Comin Colet, J., Filippatos, G. et al., Ferric carboxymaltose in patients with heart failure and iron deficiency, *N Engl J Med* (2009), 361: 2436–48.
19 Avni, T., Leibovici, L. & Gafter-Gvili, A., Iron supplementation for the treatment of chronic heart failure and iron deficiency: Systematic review and meta-analysis, *Eur J Heart Fail* (2012), 14(4): 423–9.
20 Yehuda, S. & Youdim, M.B.H., Brain iron: A lesson from animal models, *Am J Clin Nutr* (1989), 50: 618–29.
21 Bruner, A.B., Joffe, A., Duggan, A.K. et al., Randomised study of cognitive effects of iron supplementation in non-anaemic iron-deficient adolescent girls, *Lancet* (1996), 348(9033): 992–6.
22 Konofal, E., Lecendreux, M., Arnulf, I. & Mouren, M.C., Iron deficiency in children with attention-deficit/hyperactivity disorder, *Arch Pediatr Adolesc Med* (2004), 158(12): 1113–15.
23 Patterson, A.J., Brown, W.J., Powers, J.R. & Roberts, D.C., Iron deficiency, general health and fatigue: Results from the Australian Longitudinal Study on Women's Health, *Qual Life Res* (2000), 9(5): 491–7.
24 Patterson, A.J., Brown, W.J. & Roberts, D.C., Dietary and supplement treatment of iron deficiency results in improvements in general health and fatigue in Australian women of childbearing age, *J Am Coll Nutr* (2001), 20(4): 337–42.
25 Hermoso, M., Vucic, V., Vollhardt, C. et al., The effect of iron on cognitive development and function in infants, children and adolescents: A systematic review, *Ann Nutr Metab* (2011), 59(2–4): 154–65.
26 Falkingham, M., Abdelhamid, A., Curtis, P. et al., The effects of oral iron supplementation on cognition in older children and adults: A systematic review and meta-analysis, *Nutr J* (2010), 9: 4–5.

Therapeutic dose

Iron is a potential oxidant and generator of ROS that are damaging to body tissues. For this reason, iron exists mainly in bound forms in the body, and levels are tightly regulated. High-dose, long-term use of iron supplements has the potential to overload binding proteins and lead to free iron accumulation and organ damage. However, this is unlikely unless there is a genetic abnormality that affects iron regulation.

In all cases of iron deficiency, intake of food containing haem iron should be increased, a source of vitamin C should be taken with each meal and drinking tea or coffee within two hours of meals should be avoided. Supplements are rarely required by men or postmenopausal women unless there is an inadequate dietary intake or an underlying health condition causing a higher requirement than can be obtained from the diet. High-dose supplements should be used with caution and under supervision by a health-care practitioner who is able to monitor iron status. They should be taken in divided doses, and discontinued when the iron deficiency has been rectified.

In IDA, effective iron replacement therapy should stimulate red blood cell production within 72 hours, and result in a rise in Hb concentration of about 1 g/L per day, equivalent to about 20 g/L every three weeks, but this varies between individuals. Once the Hb concentration is within the normal range, iron supplementation should continue for about three months in order to replenish iron stores. Failure to respond may indicate faulty absorption or an underlying health disorder, such as coeliac disease, that should be investigated.

Suggested doses of elemental iron (ferrous iron) are as follows:

- *Health maintenance:* ensure adequate intake of haem iron foods; take a source of vitamin C with meals containing non-haem iron.
- *Mild deficiency:* adults—30–60 mg daily; infants and children—1–2 mg/kg/day (a maximum of 15 mg/day).
- *Severe deficiency/IDA:* adults—100–200 mg daily, continue treatment for 3–6 months after normalisation of Hb; infants and children—3–6 mg of elemental iron/kg/day (approx. 25–60 mg/day),

continue treatment for 2–3 months after normalisation of Hb; pregnancy—100–200 mg daily.

- *Prevention of iron deficiency in pregnancy:* 40 mg daily from eighteen weeks of gestation until delivery; or 30–40 mg daily if serum ferritin is 31–70 mcg/L; 60–80 mg daily if serum ferritin is less than 31 mcg/L; 100 mg daily if serum ferritin is less than 15 mcg/L.
- *Preterm, exclusively breastfed infants:* 2 mg/kg/day from one month to twelve months of age.
- *Exclusively breastfed infants:* 1 mg/kg/day from four months of age, continuing until iron-containing foods have been introduced.
- *Restless legs syndrome with iron deficiency:* adults—100–200 mg daily until deficiency is corrected.
- *Cognitive and behavioural disorders in children with iron deficiency:* 30–60 mg daily until deficiency is corrected.
- *BHA in children:* 5 mg/kg/day for sixteen weeks.

Effects of excess

In healthy individuals, iron overload is unlikely to result from dietary or supplemental intake, as absorption is reduced when iron stores are replete. However, toxicity can result from the acute ingestion of a large quantity of high-dose iron supplements, and may be fatal in young children. Iron supplements may irritate the digestive tract, and are associated with a high incidence of relatively mild side-effects, which include nausea, constipation, black-coloured faeces, diarrhoea, dizziness, abdominal discomfort, fatigue and headaches. It has been estimated that 20 per cent of patients who start taking iron supplements discontinue them because of side-effects. These may be reduced by dividing the dose, taking the supplement with a meal and vitamin C or at night, or using an alternative form of iron, such as iron amino acid chelate, which may be better tolerated.

Acute iron toxicity in children

Iron poisoning is the most common cause of overdose deaths in children less than six years of age. More than 30 mg of elemental iron per kg body weight is toxic in children, and a fatal dose is typically more than 250 mg/kg. However, doses as low as 60 mg/kg have resulted in death. Initial effects of iron poisoning include irritation of the digestive tract causing vomiting, diarrhoea, abdominal pain and gastrointestinal haemorrhage, which may progress to shock, coma, seizures and death, or may resolve within six hours. This is followed 12–48 hours after ingestion by a buildup of iron in cells, leading to organ damage, multi-organ failure and possibly death. Acute liver failure is common, and gastrointestinal stricture (narrowing) may develop later as a consequence of the corrosive effects of large amounts of iron.

Genetic iron overload disorders

Certain genetic mutations can lead to primary iron overload disorders. Type 1, the most common form, is associated with mutations in the HFE gene on chromosome 6 (hereditary haemochromatosis, or HH); type 2 (juvenile haemochromatosis) has mutations in the HJV gene (sub-type A) on chromosome 1 and the HAMP gene (sub-type B) on chromosome 19; type 3 has mutations in the TfR2 gene on chromosome 3; and type 4 has mutations affecting the FPN1 gene on chromosome 2. Secondary iron overload may develop as a result of repeated blood transfusions, which are used frequently for the treatment of various anaemias, such as thalassaemia major.

HH occurs in individuals with a genetic mutation that prevents the ability to regulate iron absorption. It involves inadequate production of hepcidin, which results in dietary or supplemental iron being absorbed at a rate two to three times greater than normal in spite of high body levels. Over time, it can lead to overload of the body's storage capacity and iron deposits, in the form of haemosiderin, accumulating in cells in body tissues, such as the liver, heart, pancreas, pituitary gland, joints and skin. Iron buildup in organs causes oxidation damage, fibrosis and loss of function. Iron overload in HH also increases the production and activity of suppressor T cells, decreases the production and activity of helper T cells, impairs the generation of cytotoxic T cells and alters immunoglobulin secretion, causing reduced ability to control cancer cells and pathogens. An increased amount of unbound iron supports replication of bacteria and viruses.

HH is the most common genetic disease in Caucasian races, especially in people with a northern European or Celtic background, but not all people with the genetic mutation develop HH. It is most often associated with people who have both forms of the HFE gene pair carrying the C282Y mutation (homozygous), which occurs in about one in 200 Caucasians. Most people with HH develop the first symptoms between the ages of 30 and 60 years. Iron overload is 24-times more common in men than women because iron losses in menstruation and increased demand for iron in pregnancy delay the onset of the condition in women.

There may be no symptoms until HH is advanced, or symptoms may be vague and difficult to diagnose. Gene testing is indicated if a first-degree relative has been diagnosed with HH and/or if serum ferritin and TF saturation are elevated on more than one occasion; the serum ferritin level is the most useful monitoring tool. Effects of iron overload may include lethargy, weakness, joint pain, swelling and tenderness, loss of libido, impotence, upper abdominal discomfort, enlarged liver and grey/bronze skin pigmentation. Advanced HH is associated with osteoporosis, cirrhosis of the liver, liver cancer, cardiomyopathy, heart rhythm abnormalities, diabetes and testicular atrophy.

Treatment of HH is by regular blood removal (venesection), the frequency of which is adjusted according to serum ferritin levels and TF saturation. Initially, one or two venesections are undertaken per week until the excess iron stores are depleted (serum ferritin less than 50 mcg/L), followed by one venesection every three to four months in the long term to keep levels within the normal range, which may take many months or even years. Losing too much blood too rapidly by venesection can lead to iron avidity, in which there is a normal to low serum ferritin with elevated TF saturation, and excessive venesection can cause IDA. A serum ferritin range of 25–75 mcg/L may be optimal to avoid either IDA or iron overload. Vitamin B12 and folate supplements are useful to support red blood cell production during the venesection process. Patients who do not tolerate venesection because of anaemia, cardiovascular instability or poor vascular access can be given the iron-chelating agent desferrioxamine, which is given by injection and forms water soluble complexes with iron that can then be excreted in urine.

Dietary modification is generally unnecessary in HH, but large amounts of red meat, organ meats and iron supplementation should be avoided. Alcohol should be avoided initially to reduce stress on the liver, and tea or coffee taken with meals containing non-haem iron can help to reduce iron absorption. Vitamin C is an important protective antioxidant in HH but should not be taken with meals because it enhances non-haem iron uptake.

Iron overload in the brain

Iron is widely distributed in the brain and accumulates progressively during ageing and in neurodegenerative diseases such as Alzheimer's disease (AD), Parkinson's disease (PD) and Huntington's disease (HD). Friedreich's ataxia, neuroferritinopathy, pantothenate kinase-associated neurodegeneration (PKAN) (formerly known as Hallervorden-Spatz syndrome) and aceruloplasminaemia are genetic disorders affecting iron metabolism that also cause iron buildup in the brain. In younger people, the largest amounts of iron in the brain are in myelin-producing oligodendrocytes, whereas most of the iron in the brain in older people is in the microglia (macrophage cells) and astrocytes (support cells) of the cortex, cerebellum, hippocampus, basal ganglia and amygdala. Mitochondrial malfunction associated with ageing may reduce Fe-S cluster synthesis, and lead to activation of DMT1 and decreased activity of FPN1, causing iron accumulation. During ageing, iron in the brain is partially converted from ferritin, a stable and soluble form, to haemosiderin and other derivatives that are more reactive. Excessive amounts of intracellular reactive iron increase oxidative stress, which causes lipid peroxidation, DNA abnormalities, protein misfolding and aggregation, and nerve cell dysfunction and death. Iron accumulation in microglia might trigger inflammatory activity and contribute to AD and PD. Although iron builds up in the brain in AD and PD, the level of iron is relatively low, and nerve damage might involve a combination of iron and other toxins. However, it has not yet been established whether the iron accumulation is a cause or consequence of neurodegeneration. Iron deposits are difficult to remove from the brain and the effect of iron removal on neurodegeneration is not clear.

AD features the accumulation of amyloid-beta peptide, which impairs nerve cell and synapse activity, and interacts with signalling pathways to cause hyperphosphorylation of tau, a microtubule-associated protein. This leads to the accumulation of toxic forms of tau and the formation of neurofibrillary tangles (NFTs). Amyloid-beta is damaging because it has the ability to reduce metal ions by transferring electrons to oxygen, generating hydrogen peroxide that produces hydroxyl radicals. Amyloid-beta plaques have toxic effects on nerve cell synapses, block protein breakdown, inhibit mitochondrial activity, alter intracellular calcium levels and stimulate inflammatory reactions. Imbalances of several minerals, including calcium, copper, zinc and iron, are implicated in AD. Iron metabolism appears to be abnormal in AD, and iron accumulates around amyloid-beta plaques and NFTs. It is not clear whether amyloid-beta plaques are a cause of brain damage, or are generated to bind iron in an attempt to protect nerve cells. Mutation of the HFE gene has been found in AD patients, and may contribute to iron overload in the brain.

PD is characterised by the loss of the dopaminergic nerve cells in the substantia nigra and the deposition of intracellular inclusion bodies (Lewy bodies). Although the role of iron in PD is not clear, the amount of reactive iron bound to neuromelanin increases in the substantia nigra during the course of the disease, possibly causing oxidative damage to dopaminergic nerve cells.

HD is a genetic disorder characterised by progressive worsening of motor, cognitive and psychiatric functions caused by an abnormal Huntington protein that destroys nerves in the striatum and cerebral cortex. Iron accumulation in HD may be a consequence rather than a cause of the death of nerve cells.

Iron overload in pregnancy

Pregnant women who are not iron deficient should use iron supplements cautiously. High levels of Hb, haematocrit and ferritin in pregnancy are associated with an increased risk of low birth weight, preterm delivery and pre-eclampsia. Iron supplements and increased iron stores are associated with elevated risk of gestational diabetes and increased oxidative stress in pregnancy, and iron supplementation in pregnant women with normal Hb levels in the second trimester is associated with a low birth weight infant and maternal hypertension.

Iron and cardiovascular disease

It has been proposed that elevated iron stores are associated with increased risk of cardiovascular disease (CVD) and coronary heart disease (CHD). Iron can enhance oxidation, and high iron and a lack of antioxidants may be contributing factors. However, iron is found in the body in a bound state that is less likely to have oxidant effects. The vast majority of epidemiological studies have found no association between serum ferritin and risk of developing CHD. Some studies suggest that a high intake of haem iron (a high meat diet) is associated with increased risk of CVD, but this may be due to other factors, such as saturated fat in meat, salt and nitrite preservatives in processed meat or an unbalanced diet of meat without an adequate intake of fruit and vegetables.

Case reports—iron excess

- *A boy, 18 months of age*, died after consuming an estimated 30–40 tablets of a pregnancy supplement, each of which contained 60 mg of elemental iron as ferrous sulfate.[1] The tablets were in an uncapped bottle on a table.
- *A woman, 68 years of age*, developed weakness and sought medical advice.[2] It was discovered that she had been advised by a doctor fifteen years earlier to take a ferrous sulfate supplement containing 100 mg of iron daily for anaemia, which she had continued doing ever since. Physical examination revealed moderate arthritis of the finger and knee joints, and mild generalised hyperpigmentation. Her TF saturation was 11 per cent and her Hb level was below normal, but her serum ferritin was 2100 mcg/L. She was found to have spherocytosis (abnormally shaped red blood cells), which was the cause of her anaemia. She had gastric atrophy, markedly increased iron in macrophages and iron deposits in the liver, but no fibrosis or cirrhosis. Family history was negative for anaemia, haemochromatosis or iron overload, and genetic tests revealed that she did not have HH. Iron supplements were discontinued and she was treated successfully with venesection to remove the excess iron. Her iron status remained normal without venesection over the next six years.
- *A woman, 72 years of age*, developed loose stools, progressive weakness, weight loss and leg swelling.[2] She reported taking 105 mg of iron daily as ferrous gluconate for the previous 35 years, as prescribed by a doctor for low-grade anaemia. She was found to have markedly increased iron in macrophages, liver enlargement and iron deposits in the liver. Her TF saturation was 83 per cent and her serum ferritin was 1947 mcg/L. Family history was negative for anaemia, haemochromatosis or iron overload, and genetic tests revealed that she did not have HH. Investigation of her digestive tract revealed coeliac disease, and a gluten-free diet reversed her bowel symptoms and weight loss. Iron supplements were discontinued, and she was treated with venesection to remove the excess iron. Six years later, her TF saturation was 47 per cent and her serum ferritin was 457 mcg/L.

- *A man, 39 years of age*, developed progressive pain and tenderness in both hands and intermittent swelling of the metacarpal–phalangeal joints over a six-month period.[3] He had no family history of arthritis and no other abnormalities were detected, except for markedly elevated serum iron and serum ferritin (2318 mcg/L) and a TF saturation of 96 per cent. Genetic studies confirmed that he had HH, and he was treated with venesection.
- *A man, 57 years of age*, developed decreased appetite, nausea and continuous abdominal pain, as well as fatigue and weight loss.[4] Initial investigations could not find a cause of his symptoms. Subsequent laboratory tests found that he had TF over-saturation (greater than 100 per cent), markedly elevated serum ferritin (2282 mcg/L) and low testosterone levels. He was found to have extensive iron deposits in the liver and pituitary gland, and some iron deposits in his pancreas. An iron-induced pituitary gland dysfunction appeared to be the cause of his low testosterone levels. Genetic tests revealed he had HH, and he was treated with testosterone and venesection.

REFERENCES

1 Centers for Disease Control and Prevention (CDC), Toddler deaths resulting from ingestion of iron supplements—Los Angeles, 1992–1993, *MMWR Morb Mortal Wkly Rep* (1993), 42(6): 111–13.

2 Barton, J.C., Lee, P.L., West, C. & Bottomley, S.S., Iron overload and prolonged ingestion of iron supplements: Clinical features and mutation analysis of hemochromatosis-associated genes in four cases, *Am J Hematol* (2006), 81(10): 760–7.

3 Wimalawansa, S.M. & Alsamkari, R., Unusual presentation of hemochromatosis as isolated metacarpophalangeal joint osteoarthritis: A case report, *Hand (NY)* (2011), 6(3): 329–32.

4 Wlazlo, N., Peters, W. & Bravenboer, B., Hypogonadism in a patient with mild hereditary haemochromatosis, *Neth J Med* (2012), 70(7): 318–20.

Supplements

Iron supplements are available in standard tablets, capsules and liquids, as well as enteric-coated controlled-release tablets and capsules. Controlled-release formulations appear to have fewer digestive side-effects but, in some people, may not release iron in the optimum part of the intestine for absorption. Iron supplements should be taken with vitamin C to maximise absorption, and with folic acid and vitamin B12 to support red blood cell production. In Australia, iron supplements are required to have child-proof packaging if they contain more than 5 mg of elemental iron in each dosage unit for a solid formulation, and if they contain more than 250 mg of elemental iron in total for a liquid formulation.

The permitted forms of iron salts in oral supplements in Australia include ferric ammonium citrate, ferric chloride anhydrous, ferric chloride hexahydrate, ferric glycerophosphate, ferric pyrophosphate, ferrous carbonate, ferrous chloride, ferrous fumarate, ferrous gluconate, ferrous gluconate dihydrate, ferrous lactate, ferrous phosphate, ferrous succinate, ferrous sulfate, ferrous sulfate–dried, iron amino acid chelate and iron phosphate. Ferrous salts and amino acid chelates are preferred because they more bioavailable; commonly used ferrous salts are ferrous sulfate, ferrous gluconate and ferrous fumarate. The amount of elemental iron in a specific iron salt is listed on the product container, and may vary between individual products; the approximate elemental iron content of some common salts is shown in Table 10.2.

Table 10.2 Elemental iron content of common salts

Salt	Iron content (%)
Ferrous sulfate, dried	32.5
Ferrous fumarate	33.0
Ferrous sulfate	20.0
Iron amino acid chelate	20.0
Ferrous gluconate	12.0

- *Ferrous sulfate* is the least expensive and most commonly used iron supplement. It is highly soluble, and can be produced commercially by the action of sulfuric acid on ferrous oxide (extracted from the environment) or by the oxidation of pyrites followed by leaching and treatment with scrap iron. It can also be obtained as a by-product of pickling of steel or the manufacture of titanium dioxide.

- *Ferrous gluconate* is highly soluble, but is lower in elemental iron than ferrous sulfate and fumarate. It can be prepared commercially from barium gluconate and iron sulfate, by a reaction involving calcium gluconate and ferrous sulfate or by a reaction involving ferrous carbonate and gluconic acid (from fermentation of glucose).
- *Ferrous fumarate* is less soluble in water than ferrous sulfate and gluconate, but is soluble in stomach acid. It can be produced commercially by a reaction involving ferrous sulfate, fumaric acid and ammonium.
- *Iron amino acid chelate* is produced by reacting ferrous oxide with one or more ligands, such as amino acids, protein hydrolysates, polypeptides or dipeptides, in an aqueous environment. Compared with ferrous sulfate, it provides less elemental iron but has been found to have two to six times greater bioavailability and fewer digestive side-effects. In adolescents with IDA, 30 mg of iron from an iron amino acid chelate supplement (ferrous bisglycinate chelate) was found to be as effective as 120 mg of iron in the form of ferrous sulfate.

Cautions

Parents should be made aware of the dangers of unintentional iron consumption by children, and should be advised to keep all iron-containing products out of reach of children at all times. Multivitamin and mineral supplements and low-dose iron supplements are not recommended for the treatment of IDA, as the iron content is low and absorption may be reduced by competition with other trace elements in multivitamins. Because of their much higher bioavailability, iron amino acid chelates should be used in lower doses than other forms of iron supplements.

High-dose iron may reduce zinc absorption, and may reduce the absorption of the following drugs when taken together: bisphosphonates (for bone disorders), the fluoroquinolone and tetracycline classes of antibiotics, levothyroxine (for thyroid function), levodopa (for PD), methyldopa (for high BP), mycophenolate mofetil (for immune suppression) and penicillamine (a metal chelator). Iron supplements should be taken two to four hours before or after the drug dose.

Zinc

ZINC STATUS CHECK

1. Do you have a poor sense of taste and/or smell?
2. Do you often get skin rashes or skin infections?
3. Do you have smelly feet or a strong body odour?
4. Do you have a poor appetite, poor digestion and/or bowel problems?

'Yes' answers may indicate inadequate zinc status. Note that a number of nutritional deficiencies or health disorders can cause similar effects and further investigation is recommended.

FAST FACTS . . . ZINC

- The most available sources of zinc include shellfish, seafood, red meat, organ meats and poultry.
- Zinc is required for cell growth and development, immunity and antioxidant protection.
- It supports brain and nerve function, detoxification, digestion and reproductive functions.
- A deficiency can cause infections, skin rashes, diarrhoea, loss of appetite and sense of taste, digestive disorders, and impaired male sexual development at puberty.
- Supplementation may be helpful for diarrhoea and pneumonia prevention in under-nourished children, vision disorders, cancer prevention, diabetes, bowel disorders, sensory nerve and brain disorders, anorexia nervosa and the treatment of elevated copper levels.

Zinc is a naturally occurring mineral that is found in soil and seawater as various zinc salts, such as zinc sulfide, zinc silicate and zinc oxide. Zinc ores were used to make brass in ancient times, and its name is reported to be derived from an old German word, *zinke*, meaning 'pointed', in reference to the shape of zinc crystals. The German chemist Andreas Marggraf is believed to have first isolated zinc in 1746. It has the chemical symbol Zn, and Zn^{2+} is the most common ionic form. Its importance for human health was established in 1960 by the biochemist Ananda Prasad, who discovered that impaired sexual maturation and dwarfism in Middle Eastern males was related to a zinc deficiency caused by a diet based around phytate-containing unleavened bread.

Zinc is one of the most important trace elements in biological systems, in which it functions within cells as part of enzymes (metalloenzymes) and proteins. Many zinc proteins function as transcription factors (proteins that bind to specific DNA sequences and regulate the transfer of genetic information from DNA to messenger RNA). Zinc has the ability to form strong but flexible bonds with organic molecules; however, unlike iron and copper, it does not have redox properties, and therefore does not promote oxidation in the body. About 90 per cent of zinc in the body is in skeletal muscles and bones, in which turnover is slow, and the remaining 10 per cent is metabolically very active and sensitive to changes in dietary intake.

Digestion, absorption and transport

Zinc is found in food bound to proteins and nucleic acids. During digestion, protease and nuclease enzymes release zinc from food, and the presence of hydrochloric acid in the stomach increases its solubility. Zinc uptake is increased by binding to ligands such as picolinic acid, citric acid, prostaglandins and dietary peptides and amino acids, particularly histidine and cysteine, and possibly lysine and glycine. Picolinic acid is made in the liver and kidneys from the amino acid tryptophan, stored in the pancreas and secreted during digestion. It appears to bind to many trace elements, including zinc, chromium, manganese, copper, iron and molybdenum, to enhance their absorption.

To date, 24 zinc transporters have been identified, and these are divided into two main classes: the ten members of the SLC39 (ZIP) family and the fourteen members of the SLC30 (ZnT) family. ZIP transporters increase zinc levels in cell cytoplasm by moving zinc into cells from extracellular fluid (ECF) and from intracellular vesicles into the cytoplasm, and ZnT transporters decrease zinc levels in cell cytoplasm by exporting zinc from cells to ECF and moving it into intracellular vesicles from the cytoplasm. At normal dietary levels (intakes below about 9 mg/day), zinc is absorbed into enterocytes by an active carrier-mediated process involving ZIP4, which transports zinc exclusively. At higher levels of intake, zinc is absorbed by passive diffusion. The divalent metal transporter 1 (DMT1) also appears to facilitate uptake of zinc in the gut, as well as the uptake of iron, other minerals and toxic metals.

Inside enterocytes, zinc can be used within the cell, stored bound to proteins or transferred to the bloodstream. Transfer to the bloodstream appears to be via the ZnT1 transporter. About 70 per cent of zinc in blood is bound to albumin, and the remainder is bound to TF, alpha-2-macroglobulin and immunoglobulin G. Albumin-bound zinc is the main form of zinc that is delivered to tissues, where it is taken up by various ZIP transporters for use by cells. About 40 per cent of the zinc content in the cell is in the nucleus, and about half is in the cytosol and membranes. Transport of zinc within cells is via ZIP and ZnT transporters.

Metabolism, storage and excretion

In most tissue cells, zinc binds to cysteine-rich thionein proteins to form metallothioneins (MTs), which have antioxidant activity and act as a zinc reserve and transporter. MTs can also bind copper, cadmium and mercury. Although MTs have a higher affinity for copper and cadmium than for zinc, they are usually found bound to zinc in the body; one MT molecule can bind up to seven zinc ions. Increased zinc or heavy metal levels in cells triggers activity of the metal-response element-binding transcription factor-1 (MTF-1), which binds to sections of genes called metal response elements (MREs) to promote production of thionein. MTs are found in the body in four forms—MT1 and MT2 being the most common—and they act to move zinc through cells and release it to zinc-requiring proteins. The highest concentrations of MTs are found in the liver, kidney, intestine and pancreas. Zinc can be released from MTs by nitric oxide (NO) activity, and by protease enzymes in cell lysosomes.

There is no specific storage depot for zinc in the body. MTs may act as a small intracellular store of zinc in most tissues. The zinc concentration in bones and muscles is preserved in a deficiency, but zinc can be mobilised from other zinc-containing proteins and enzymes. Zinc is lost primarily by excretion in faeces, which contain dietary zinc that has not been absorbed and endogenous zinc, which includes zinc that has been excreted in bile, pancreatic and intestinal mucosal secretions and zinc in intestinal lining cells that have been shed. The kidneys can also excrete small amounts of zinc in urine, and small amounts are lost in sweat and hair, and in semen during ejaculation.

Regulation of body levels

Zinc in plasma, ECF, the liver, pancreas, kidneys and intestines comprises about 10 per cent of body zinc and makes up a rapidly exchangeable pool of zinc and has a turnover of about 12.5 days. Skeletal muscle and bone makes up a slowly exchangeable pool, and comprises about 90 per cent of body zinc, with a turnover of about 300 days. Zinc balance in the body is largely regulated by adjusting the amount of zinc excreted by the digestive tract to the amount absorbed. Excretion in urine also can be altered in response to severe overload or deficiency.

Changes in MT and transporter expression regulate total body zinc, as well as the zinc concentration in organs and tissues. A high level of zinc in the gut stimulates production of intestinal MTs, which hold zinc in enterocytes and limit its transfer into the circulation. In a zinc deficiency, MTs may act to reduce losses in digestive secretions. ZIP14 is found in the liver and appears to facilitate uptake of zinc and iron, especially in response to acute inflammation and infection. During infection, interleukin-1 increases thionein production in the liver and zinc is moved from the plasma to liver MTs to reduce its availability to pathogens; the amount of MTs in the liver can increase as much as 100-fold within two to four hours.

ZIP4 expression in enterocytes can be down-regulated to reduce absorption of zinc or up-regulated to increase absorption. The ZIP5 transporter, found in enterocyte cell membranes adjacent to the bloodstream, appears to take up zinc from the blood, possibly to supply zinc to these cells for their own use in a deficiency or as a pathway for excretion of excess zinc in faeces. It has been suggested that ZIP5 may communicate body zinc status to enterocytes to control ZIP4 expression. ZIP8 enhances zinc uptake in immune cells during an immune response and plays an important role in zinc uptake in the foetus during pregnancy, and in newborn infants.

The expression of the ZnT1 transporter in enterocytes is regulated by the amount of dietary zinc, and appears to control the movement of zinc from enterocytes to the blood. ZnT2 and ZnT4 in enterocytes are involved in the movement of zinc in endosomes, possibly regulating intracellular movement of zinc. ZnT4 is also involved in the secretion of zinc in breast milk during lactation. ZnT3 is found in the synaptic vesicles in some types of nerve cells. ZnT5 helps regulate zinc balance in the pancreas, ZnT6 in the brain and ZnT7 in the prostate gland, and they appear to be involved in zinc uptake in the Golgi apparatus, the protein-processing centre in cells. ZnT8 is associated with the secretory granules of pancreatic beta cells that produce insulin.

In a zinc deficiency, ZIP4 expression becomes more widespread in the villi that line the small intestine, in order to maximise zinc absorption, and ZIP5 is broken down to reduce uptake of zinc into enterocytes from the bloodstream. ZnT1 in the liver increases in order to move more zinc into the circulation for transport to tissues.

Functions

Body cells contain genes that encode for over 3000 zinc proteins, 1000 of which are enzymes in which zinc is required for enzyme activity, with the remainder being proteins in which zinc has a structural and stabilising role. Zinc enzymes identified to date include hydrolases, ligases, transferases, oxidoreductases and lyases/isomerases; zinc proteins include transcription factors, signalling proteins, transport/storage proteins, proteins with structural zinc sites, proteins involved in DNA repair, replication and translation, zinc finger proteins and other proteins of unknown function. The functions of zinc include the following:

- *Cell metabolism, replication and growth.* About half of all DNA-binding domains in gene transcription factors contain 'zinc fingers', which are sections of the protein that require the binding of zinc to maintain their structural integrity and function. Zinc finger proteins are also part of receptors in cell nuclei that interact with steroid hormones to affect gene expression. Zinc finger proteins are involved in signal transduction, gene expression and cell differentiation, proliferation and adhesion. Krüppel-like factors (KLFs) are members of the zinc finger family of transcription factors that have recently been found to be critical regulators of key physiological functions, including production of red blood cells, cardiac remodelling, fat and glucose synthesis, maintenance of stem cells and the epithelial barrier, cell proliferation, endothelial function, skeletal and smooth muscle development, monocyte activation, intestinal and conjunctival goblet cell development, retinal nerve regeneration and lung development in newborn infants. Zinc-dependent enzymes, such as DNA and RNA polymerases, kinases, nucleases, transferases, phosphorylases and transcriptases, help control normal DNA replication and cell proliferation, differentiation and suppression of transformation to malignant cell forms.

Zinc is required for the entry of calcium into cells. It preserves cell function and lifespan by preventing oxidative damage and damage induced by toxins, thereby suppressing the activation of caspase enzymes that trigger apoptosis. Zinc protects and stabilises cell proteins and membranes, DNA, cell organelles and the cytoskeleton (microtubules and microfilaments that provide form and structure to cells). Zinc is required for autophagy (self-digestion), the process by which long-lived cytosolic proteins and organelles are broken down and recycled in lysosomes. Autophagy is important for adaptation to changing environmental conditions, cellular remodelling during development and differentiation, defence against pathogens and cell lifespan.

- *Tissue regeneration.* Matrix metalloproteinases (MMPs) are a family of zinc-dependent enzymes that break down components of the extracellular matrix, such as basement membrane, collagen, proteoglycans, fibronectin and laminin, and have an important role in connective tissue remodelling and tissue repair. MMPs interact with various cytokines and chemokines, the basic messengers of the immune system, to support cell proliferation, migration, differentiation, apoptosis, bone growth and remodelling, blood vessel growth (angiogenesis), immunity, wound healing, embryonic development and the breakdown of fibrin in blood clots. MMPs enhance removal of dead tissue and keratinocyte migration during wound repair. MMP expression is low in healthy tissue, but is elevated when tissue is disrupted because of injury or disease or during pregnancy. Abnormal MMP activity is associated with disorders such as rheumatoid arthritis, osteoarthritis, atherosclerosis, tumour growth and metastasis, and fibrosis.
- *Immune function.* Zinc is essential for the activity of cells that are part of the innate immune system (the first response phase of an immune reaction), such as natural killer (NK) cells, dendritic cells, macrophages, neutrophils, mast cells and granulocytes. Zinc is needed for DNA synthesis, RNA transcription, cell division and cell activation in immune cells, and is an essential component of thymulin, a thymus gland hormone involved in maturation and differentiation of thymus-derived immune cells (T cells). Zinc supports production of the cytokines interleukin-2 (IL-2), which promotes proliferation of T and B lymphocytes, IL-12, generated by stimulated monocytes/macrophages, interferon-gamma (IFN-gamma), secreted by T cells and NK cells, and tumour necrosis factor-alpha (TNF-alpha), which suppresses tumour growth. IFN-gamma and IL-12 play a key role in enabling monocytes/macrophages to destroy parasites, viruses and bacteria by engulfment (phagocytosis).

  Zinc promotes immune signalling and tumour suppression, and functions as an antioxidant to stabilise membranes of body cells during an immune response. Both zinc and MTs are needed for the development, maturation and function of natural killer T cells (NKT cells), which are cytotoxic and also act as a link between the innate immune system and the adaptive immune system (the second phase response that generates antibodies). The zinc transporters ZIP6, ZIP8 and ZIP14 are part of signalling pathways that direct the innate and adaptive immune responses. Activation of nuclear factor kappaB (NF-kappaB) in monocytes induces expression of the gene for the zinc transporter ZIP8, which increases uptake of zinc from the bloodstream. Induction of ZIP8 is essential to immune activation and prevents excessive inflammation associated with the immune response.
- *Antioxidant, anti-inflammatory and detoxifying activity.* Zinc supports the integrity of protein sulfhydryl (SH) groups that are involved in the regulation of ROS levels and stabilises the structure of the copper and zinc-containing antioxidant enzymes superoxide dismutase 1 (SOD1), found in cell cytoplasm, and superoxide dismutase 3 (SOD3), found in the extracellular compartment. SODs remove superoxide radicals that can react with NO to form peroxynitrite, leading to lipid peroxidation, inactivation of enzymes and other proteins, activation of MMPs and cell damage. SODs convert superoxide radicals to oxygen and hydrogen peroxide, which is subsequently broken down by catalases and glutathione peroxidase. If SOD1 and SOD3 are low in zinc, the copper component becomes more reactive and the enzymes scavenge less superoxide, becoming pro-oxidants rather than antioxidants.

  Zinc maintains tissue concentrations of MTs, powerful free radical scavengers that inhibit free radical reactions stimulated by iron and copper. The presence of ROS or pathogens activate NF-kappaB, which stimulates production of many cytokines, chemokines, immune receptors and cell surface adhesion molecules involved in the inflammatory process. By decreasing ROS, zinc helps to suppress inflammation. Zinc also helps regulate oxidation and inflammation by enhancing the absorption of protective fatty acids and fat-soluble nutrients, such as vitamin E, and the metabolism of essential fatty acids and their incorporation into cell membrane phospholipids. Zinc may help to protect the liver against toxic chemicals by inducing MT production and by its antioxidant activity.

- *Brain and nerve function*. Zinc-containing nerve cells form a complex network that interconnects most of the cerebral cortices and limbic structures. Zinc modulates synaptic transmission, oxidation, cell signalling, nerve cell proliferation and differentiation, and cell survival. Zinc can activate extracellular signal-regulated kinase (ERK) pathways in nerve cells that help control cell proliferation, differentiation and survival, and the synaptic plasticity (adaptability) that is responsible for learning and memory. Zinc appears to protect the blood–brain barrier against oxidative stress, which helps to maintain normal brain function. During foetal development, zinc regulates many stages of nervous system development, including nerve cell proliferation, survival and differentiation.

  MTs store and distribute zinc in the nervous system, and protect nerve cells from damage. MTs expressed in astrocytes following CNS injury may have both neuroprotective and neurodegenerative properties, and may be essential for recovery. In the CNS, free zinc is found in pre-synaptic vesicles of axons of nerve cells that use glutamate as a neurotransmitter (glutamatergic neurons) and helps control the balance between excitation and inhibition in the brain. Zinc is transported into presynaptic vesicles by the zinc transporter ZnT3, which is expressed exclusively in the brain. During glutamatergic nerve activation, both glutamate and zinc are released into the synaptic cleft, and zinc may act to modulate the activity of glutamate receptors on the postsynaptic membrane that are involved in nerve impulse transmission.
- *Bone metabolism*. The zinc enzyme alkaline phosphatase, found in bones and the liver, removes clusters of oxygen and phosphate groups from other molecules. In bone, it appears to increase the amount of inorganic phosphate, which promotes bone mineralisation, and to decrease the amount of extracellular pyrophosphate, which inhibits mineralisation. Zinc also may regulate bone cell formation by stimulating collagen and osteocalcin production, increasing the proliferation and differentiation of osteoblasts (bone-building cells) and inhibiting the differentiation of osteoclasts (bone-resorbing cells). Zinc activates the enzymes aminoacyl-tRNA synthetases, each of which transfers the code for a specific amino acid to transfer RNA (tRNA), which is an essential step in protein production in osteoblasts. It also influences the activity of the calcium-regulating hormones calcitriol and parathyroid hormone (PTH), and inhibits PTH-induced bone resorption. Zinc appears to inhibit mitochondrial aconitase activity, leading to the accumulation of citrate that plays a role in osteoblast activity. Zinc is also required for the activity of collagenase, a member of the family of MMPs involved in collagen turnover in bone that is essential for bone resorption and remodelling.
- *Digestion*. Zinc plays an important role in maintaining the integrity of the intestinal barrier that comprises epithelial cells, and apical junction complexes that link cells and the surrounding connective tissue. An increase in intestinal permeability is associated with the development of autoimmune and inflammatory diseases, such as food allergies, inflammatory bowel disease and coeliac disease. Zinc protects barrier function, possibly by its protective antioxidant activity, by its role in maintaining the expression of junction proteins and by protecting against damage caused by the inflammatory cytokine TNF-alpha. Zinc interacts with TNF-alpha to promote cell survival by modulating gene expression of transcription factors and signalling proteins. Paneth cells in the small intestine secrete antimicrobial defensin peptides together with zinc, which appears to assist their function.

  Zinc is important for maintaining the structural integrity of pancreatic acinar cells that produce and secrete digestive enzymes, and is required for the activity of the protein-digesting enzymes carboxypeptidase A, produced by the pancreas, and aminopeptidase, produced by the small intestine. Zinc supports iron absorption by increasing expression of the iron transporter DMT1, and it is required for activity of the enzyme polyglutamate hydrolase that removes glutamate groups from dietary folate to form folic acid, the absorbable monoglutamate form. Zinc is required for the supply of bile phospholipids to enterocytes to enable formation of the chylomicrons that transport dietary lipids and lipid-soluble nutrients from the gut to the tissues.

- *Appetite and taste sensitivity.* Animal studies have found that zinc induces expression of the appetite-stimulating peptides orexin and neuropeptide Y in the hypothalamus. Zinc also appears to mediate activity of the hormone leptin that regulates eating behaviour. Zinc is required for activity of gustin (carbonic anhydrase VI), which is secreted by the salivary glands and regulates taste sensations. Gustin may act as a growth factor that promotes the growth and development of taste buds on the tongue. Decreased secretion of salivary gustin has been associated with reduced or distorted taste and smell function.
- *Alcohol and retinol metabolism.* The zinc-containing enzyme alcohol dehydrogenase is essential for the conversion of alcohol to aldehyde in the liver, and the zinc-dependent enzyme retinol dehydrogenase is essential for the conversion of retinol to retinal during vitamin A metabolism in the intestine, liver, testes and the retina of the eye. Zinc is also required for vitamin A absorption, synthesis of retinol-binding protein for retinol transport, retinol mobilisation within cells and in the liver, and tissue utilisation. It supports dark adaptation and night vision by facilitating conversion of retinol to retinal, the production of opsin in the eyes and transmission of visual images to the brain.
- *Blood glucose regulation.* Zinc has a role in insulin signalling, activation of insulin receptors and blood glucose regulation. Insulin is stored bound to zinc in pancreatic beta cells, and secreted together with zinc ions. Secreted zinc appears to inhibit secretion of the insulin antagonist glucagon. Zinc acts like insulin to enhance glucose transport, stimulate glucose uptake and fat production in fat cells, increase glycogen synthesis and inhibit glucose production and fat breakdown. Zinc is required for the activity of insulin-degrading enzyme (IDE) that breaks down insulin and glucagon to terminate their activity. This enzyme has a higher affinity for insulin, and may help to prevent blood glucose from dropping too low.
- *Hormone function.* Zinc finger proteins are part of receptors in cell nuclei that interact with retinoic acid, vitamin D, thyroid hormone, glucocorticoids and sex hormones to affect gene transcription. Zinc is required for the secretion of growth hormone from the pituitary gland and for production of insulin-like growth factor 1 (IGF-1), both of which stimulate growth and development. Zinc is part of thyroid hormone transcription factors required for production of thyroid hormones, which maintain the body's metabolic rate.
- *Reproductive function.* Zinc finger proteins are found in the nuclear receptors for steroid hormones, and the metabolism of androgens, oestrogens and progesterone is zinc-dependent. Zinc also plays a role in prostaglandin pathways that regulate conception, maintenance of pregnancy and initiation of birth contractions. Zinc has an important antioxidant role in male reproductive organ function, fertility and growth and development during puberty. The testes, prostate and epididymis in men require a high zinc concentration to maintain production and secretion of testosterone, and to promote development and viability of spermatocytes. Zinc is needed for DNA condensation and packaging in spermatids during development, and it may prolong the lifespan of sperm after ejaculation.

  Seminal fluid produced by the prostate gland contains a high level of zinc, which appears to play a role in sperm release and motility. The transporter ZIP1 transfers zinc from the bloodstream to the prostate gland, and ZIP2 and ZIP3 retain zinc in prostate cells. The prostate gland has extremely high levels of citrate—approximately three- to ten-fold higher than in other soft tissues—but the role of citrate in prostate gland function is not well established. Zinc is responsible for the accumulation of citrate by inhibiting mitochondrial aconitase in the citric acid cycle; this leads to reduced energy production, which may play a role in suppressing cell proliferation.
- *Red blood cell production and function.* The zinc-dependent enzyme delta-aminolaevulinic acid dehydratase in bone marrow is required for the formation of porphobilinogen, which is a precursor to haem. The zinc-dependent enzyme carbonic anhydrase, found in red blood cells and the kidneys, catalyses the reaction of carbon dioxide and water to form bicarbonate and hydrogen ions, a process that helps to remove carbon dioxide from tissues and maintain pH balance in the body.
- *Methionine metabolism.* During methionine metabolism, the zinc-dependent enzyme betaine-homocysteine S-methyltransferase (BHMT) removes potentially

toxic homocysteine by using betaine as the methyl donor for the conversion of homocysteine to methionine. Zinc is also required for activity of the enzyme cobalamin-dependent methionine synthase, which transfers a methyl group from 5-methyl tetrahydrofolate to homocysteine to form methionine. By these actions, zinc supports the generation of methyl donors that are needed to make DNA, RNA, hormones, neurotransmitters, the myelin sheath of nerve fibres, cell membrane lipids and proteins.

Dietary sources

Food sources of zinc are similar to sources of iron. Good sources of bioavailable zinc include shellfish, such as oysters, mussels, crab and lobster, as well as organ meats, red meat, chicken, liver, eggs, milk, cheese and brewer's yeast. Shellfish are exceptionally rich in zinc, with 100 g of oysters supplying about 48 mg. Overall, animal sources are more bioavailable because zinc in many plant foods, such as bran, whole grains, legumes, seeds and nuts, is bound by phytate that inhibits absorption. It has been found that approximately twice as much zinc is absorbed from a non-vegetarian or high-meat diet compared with a diet based on rice and wheat flour. Bioavailability from phytate-containing foods can be improved by baking with yeast, fermentation, sprouting or prolonged soaking. Fruit and refined grain products are not good zinc sources. Overall, the amount of zinc absorbed from the diet averages 33 per cent, and absorption varies according to zinc status.

In Australia, food manufacturers are permitted to voluntarily add zinc to breakfast cereals, cereal products, plant-based milk and dairy food substitutes, and meat substitutes. Zinc salts used in fortification include zinc sulfate, chloride, gluconate, oxide and stearate. Zinc oxide is less soluble, but is commonly used in foods and appears to be equivalent in bioavailability to the more soluble form, zinc sulfate—possibly because its solubility is increased by stomach acid.

The Food Standards Australia New Zealand nutrient database (NUTTAB) at <www.foodstandards.gov.au> provides the amounts found in specific foods.

Factors influencing body status

Zinc absorption increases when zinc intake is inadequate, and reduces when intake is adequate. Zinc absorption increases due to increased needs during infancy, pregnancy and lactation. Up-regulation of absorption appears to occur within four weeks of commencing a low-zinc diet, and absorption can reach 90 per cent initially during severe restriction. The main inhibitor of zinc absorption is phytate, and reducing the phytate content of plant foods has been shown to increase absorption. Soy-based infant formula has very low zinc bioavailability compared with cow's milk formula and breast milk, but bioavailability improves when phytate is removed. Zinc absorption has been found to be 25 per cent lower on a high-phytate diet (phytate:zinc molar ratio of 15) compared with a low-phytate diet (phytate:zinc molar ratio of 4). A phytate:zinc molar ratio of no more than 10 has been recommended to ensure adequate zinc bioavailability. At a phytate:zinc molar ratio greater than 15, zinc absorption does not increase, even though the diet is low in zinc. The average dietary phytate:zinc molar ratio reported for standard Western diets is about 8, but this rises to about 15 or higher for vegetarian diets. High ratios are found in predominantly vegetarian cultures around the world, where zinc deficiencies are common. Other inhibitors of zinc absorption include unabsorbed fat in the digestive tract, stomach surgery for weight loss and disorders of the liver, gall bladder, pancreas or small intestine, such as Crohn's disease and coeliac disease. Inadequate production of stomach acid and the use of proton pump-inhibiting drugs (PPIs), which inhibit stomach acid production, reduce zinc absorption. Patients taking PPIs have been shown to have 28 per cent lower plasma levels of zinc.

As the amount of protein in a meal increases, zinc absorption increases, apparently because amino acids released from dietary protein bind to zinc and improve its solubility. Tryptophan, histidine, methionine, proline and cysteine, as well as organic acids, such as citric acid in citrus fruits, lactic acid in cultured milk products, malic acid in apples and tartaric acid in grapes, have been found to enhance zinc absorption. The digestibility of a protein also affects zinc absorption. Casein in cow's milk products has been shown to impair zinc absorption by releasing calcium phosphopeptides during digestion that bind zinc, but absorption is enhanced by whey proteins. Zinc in breast milk has markedly higher bioavailability compared with cow's milk because of the higher digestibility of breast milk protein. Animal protein has been found to help counteract the inhibitory effect of phytate on zinc absorption, possibly by supplying binding amino acids. In contrast to iron, polyphenol-rich beverages, tea extract, red grape juice, tannic acid, tartaric acid and quercitin have been shown to bind zinc and increase its absorption.

Calcium has the potential to form insoluble complexes with phytate and zinc that are poorly absorbed, but the interaction is complex and the effect on zinc absorption from a meal is not well understood. Long-term use of calcium supplements has been found to have no effect on zinc status. High-dose iron can impair zinc absorption if taken together, but iron in the amounts found in foods is unlikely to cause such an effect. Long-term iron supplementation does not appear to impair zinc status. The toxic metal cadmium impairs zinc uptake and body status; cadmium accumulation and toxicity are increased by a low zinc intake, and a higher zinc intake is protective.

Low zinc levels may be associated with surgery, burns, major trauma, diabetes, alcoholism, cirrhosis, kidney failure, haemolytic anaemia and chronic blood loss from hookworm and other intestinal parasites. Excessive losses in sweating may be a factor in zinc deficiency-induced dwarfism. The diuretic amiloride increases body levels of zinc, ACE inhibitors (for elevated blood pressure) decrease zinc levels, and the cancer drug cisplatin, thiazide diuretics and the iron chelator desferrioxamine increase zinc losses in urine.

Table 10.3 Recommended dietary intake (RDI) of zinc (mg/day)

Age (years)	Female RDI	Male RDI
1–3	3	3
4–8	4	4
9–13	6	6
14–18	7	13
19–70	8	14
>70	8	14
Pregnant women		
14–18	10	
19–50	11	
Lactating women		
14–18	11	
19–50	12	

Source: Nutrient Reference Values for Australia and New Zealand Including Recommended Dietary Intakes, National Health and Medical Research Council, Australian Government Department of Health and Ageing, Canberra and Ministry of Health, New Zealand, Wellington, 2006.

Daily requirement

Australian and New Zealand government recommendations by age and gender (see Table 10.3) can be found in *Nutrient Reference Values for Australia and New Zealand Including Recommended Dietary Intakes*, available at <www.nhmrc.gov.au>.

Deficiency effects

Dietary zinc intakes and serum zinc concentrations have been shown to be lower in populations in developing countries, where vegetarian diets are standard. The WHO has estimated that the global prevalence of zinc deficiency is 31 per cent of the population, and ranges from 4–73 per cent across sub-regions, with Africa, the Eastern Mediterranean and Southeast Asia having the highest prevalence. There is little data on zinc deficiency in Australia, but one survey of Australian adults found that daily zinc intakes were marginal, with 67 per cent of men and 85 per cent of women below recommended levels. The 2007 Australian National Children's Nutrition and Physical Activity Survey found that 29 per cent of boys aged 14–16 years had inadequate zinc intakes. In Australasia, groups believed to be at risk of zinc deficiency are preschool children, adolescents (especially those of Pacific Islander and Aboriginal backgrounds), elderly people in institutions and possibly people with diabetes. A severe zinc deficiency is most commonly associated with the genetic disorder acrodermatitis enteropathica, but has also occurred in patients receiving total parenteral nutrition (non-oral feeding) lacking zinc, and in patients receiving penicillamine chelation therapy.

An inadequate zinc intake causes a marked reduction of losses in faeces within two days and, if intake is severely low, urinary losses also reduce. If these changes are not sufficient to re-establish zinc balance, signalling changes cause shifts in tissue zinc distribution. Zinc is mobilised from the rapidly exchangeable zinc pool in the body, which becomes depleted over several weeks and leads to multiple effects on body function. Because zinc has a role in so many metabolic pathways in the body, zinc deficiency can affect almost any tissue or organ system, and may not be easy to identify. Zinc deficiency often accompanies iron deficiency because dietary sources are very similar.

In experimental animals, low-zinc diets cause poor growth, skin lesions, sparse and rough fur, and a cyclical pattern of food intake that features alternating periods of eating and lack of appetite, averaging 3.5 days each. When not eating, the animals' muscles break down and nutrients, including zinc, are released. This eating pattern appears to extend survival. Zinc deficiency in animals leads to reduced expression of genes that encode proteins involved in eating behaviour, growth regulation, amino acid metabolism, xenobiotic and alcohol metabolism, the stress response, intracellular trafficking and signal transduction pathways. The availability of lipids and lipid-soluble nutrients is impaired because of decreased chylomicron formation, which leads to reduced lipid transport from the gut to the tissues. There is a decrease in essential fatty acids in membrane phospholipids. The expression of genes encoding for lipid synthesis increases, and the expression of genes encoding for lipid breakdown and mobilisation reduces, which results in the accumulation of fat in the liver.

Zinc deficiency in humans was first identified in 1958 by Ananda Prasad when a 21-year-old male patient in Iran was investigated for dwarfism, under-developed sex organs (hypogonadism), an enlarged spleen, rough and dry skin, mental lethargy, clay-eating pica and iron deficiency anaemia. It was discovered that his diet consisted of only unleavened bread, and he consumed 0.5 kg of clay daily. Subsequently, many other similar cases in male adolescents were identified in the Middle East. Replacement of iron or addition of animal protein were not able to reverse the growth retardation or hypogonadism, which could only be reversed by zinc supplementation. It was subsequently discovered that zinc deficiency impairs the entry of calcium into cells, which may impair cell proliferation and growth, and also decreases activity of the epiphyseal growth plate that is responsible for lengthwise bone growth. Prasad reported that the adolescents began to develop a moustache, beard and armpit hair within three weeks of zinc supplementation, their genitalia became completely normal within six months, and they gained about 12–15 cm in height within one year. These findings led to the establishment of zinc as an essential nutrient.

An early symptom of a subclinical zinc deficiency may be impaired sense of taste and/or smell, which can be reversed by zinc supplementation over several months. Features of a zinc deficiency include reduced immunity leading to increased susceptibility to infection, impaired taste sensitivity, loss of appetite, photophobia, skin rashes, psoriasis-like skin lesions, poor wound healing, reduced testosterone and sperm formation in men and decreased clearance of alcohol by the liver. The retina appears to be more sensitive to a lack of dietary zinc than the liver. Eye abnormalities, possibly related to impaired retinol metabolism, include inflammation of the eyelids, photophobia, conjunctivitis, corneal opacities and cataracts. Mental symptoms include irritability, depression, nervousness and restlessness. Pica can be associated with either an iron or a zinc deficiency.

Skin changes in zinc deficiency include redness, thickening, dryness, cracks and fissures at the corners of the mouth, and scaly plaques that can develop into blisters or pustules. Offensive body or foot odour may develop. Secondary bacterial and fungal infections are common, especially around the nails. Nails may become thinner and develop inflammation or infections of the cuticle, white marks or white transverse bands, or transverse indentations. A lack of zinc impairs connective tissue metabolism, and may be associated with the development of stretch marks, and joint pain and inflammation.

An experimental diet deficient in zinc was given to adults for five to six weeks and resulted in sore throats, facial rashes, mouth ulcers, rashes in the scrotal region and fungal infections of the feet, all of which reversed within six days of zinc repletion. Acute zinc deficiency has resulted in loss of appetite after two to three days, lost of taste, irritability, aggressiveness, depression, sleepiness, cognitive and memory disorders, tremors, gait abnormalities and slurred speech. Men on experimental zinc-deficient diets for four to nine weeks developed diarrhoea, sore throat, headaches, insomnia, bad dreams, dizziness, defective hair growth, reduced libido, reduced sense of taste, itchiness of the ear canals and skin problems, ranging from mild patches of dry skin to acne severe enough to require medical treatment. There was evidence of decreased cell turnover, mucosal cell changes, hair bulb alterations, decreases in the number of red and white blood cells, impaired activity of some enzymes and decreased absorption of folate.

A low zinc intake is associated with elevated body levels of copper and vice versa. Low serum zinc and increased copper has been found in pregnant women and women taking oral contraceptives, and in patients with acute infections, cancer, cardiovascular disease, kidney disease, schizophrenia, acromegaly (excess secretion of growth hormone caused by a tumour of the pituitary gland) and Addison's disease (chronic adrenal insufficiency).

The effects of zinc deficiency in infants may include skin rashes, diarrhoea, failure to thrive, irritability and inconsolable crying. Avoidance of eye contact has been reported. In children, zinc deficiency is related to higher illness and mortality rates, and impaired growth and development, and a sub-clinical zinc deficiency has been associated with growth retardation in apparently healthy infants and young children in many countries around the world. A WHO review of eleven studies concluded that zinc deficiency in children aged less than five years increases the risk of diarrhoeal disease 1.28-fold, pneumonia 1.52-fold and malaria 1.56-fold. A low intake of zinc and low serum zinc has been associated with poor cognition and impaired taste perception in adolescent girls. Adolescent boys who are zinc deficient have short stature and impaired growth of sex organs at puberty, as identified by Prasad.

Immune effects

Serum levels of zinc decrease rapidly during infections, which may be the body's method of preventing pathogens from accessing zinc for replication. Zinc deficiency impairs multiple aspects of immune function, including barrier and non-specific immunity, production and activity of immune cells, and the function of immune mediators such as glucocorticoids, thymulin and cytokines, and is associated with many types of infections. Zinc deficiency reduces the production of the cytokines IL-2 and IFN-gamma, and also production of IL-12 by macrophages, leading to impaired phagocytosis.

In animals, experimental zinc deficiency decreases resistance to a range of bacterial, viral, fungal and parasitic infections, and leads to atrophy of the thymus gland and lymphoid tissue, a decrease in spleen cell numbers, a decreased response to antigens and an inability to generate a cytotoxic T cell response to tumours. Cytokine production, phagocyte activity, the production and function of T and B cells and the ability to respond to pathogens are severely disrupted. A marginal zinc deficiency has been shown to increase oxidative stress, reduce the ability to detoxify xenobiotics, impair DNA integrity and increase DNA damage in blood cells, which are reversed by zinc repletion.

Reproductive effects

It has been estimated that 82 per cent of pregnant women around the world have inadequate intakes of zinc. In female animals, zinc deficiency causes impaired synthesis and secretion of follicle-stimulating hormone and luteinising hormone, abnormal ovarian development, disruption of the oestrous cycle, spontaneous abortion, pre-eclampsia and toxaemia, a prolonged gestation period or preterm birth, retarded growth of the foetus, foetal malformations including neural tube defects (NTDs), birth complications, stillbirths and low birth weight infants. Pregnant women with acrodermatitis enteropathica (a genetic disorder of zinc absorption) have an elevated risk of death of the foetus or of having an infant with an NTD. Infants born with NTDs have been found to have low serum zinc, which may impair folic acid absorption and metabolism and the generation of methyl donors required for gene expression and DNA metabolism. Zinc is required for alcohol metabolism, and may protect against foetal alcohol syndrome, in which excess alcohol in pregnancy causes low birth weight, facial abnormalities and reduced IQ in the infant. Alcohol can trigger an acute phase response that causes an increased sequestering of zinc in the mother's liver, reducing its availability to the foetus. In animals, the ability of alcohol to cause birth defects is increased in zinc deficiency, and is reduced when animals are given supplementary zinc.

Zinc deficiency reduces circulating testosterone concentrations, thereby contributing to male reproductive dysfunction. In male animals, zinc deficiency leads to decreased luteinising hormone and testosterone concentrations, altered steroid metabolism in the liver, and a reduced number of androgen receptors and an increased number of oestrogen receptors. These changes are associated with impaired sperm formation, viability and motility, and sperm defects. Studies from the Middle East have confirmed the essential role of zinc in the growth and development of male sexual organs at puberty. A low-zinc diet decreases serum testosterone concentrations in young men and zinc supplementation for six months almost doubled serum testosterone in marginally zinc-deficient elderly men. Experimental zinc deficiency in men leads to a decreased sperm count, which returns to normal six to twelve months after zinc supplementation. Marginal zinc deficiency in animals increases oxidative stress in the prostate gland that leads to DNA damage, and marginal zinc deficiency in men has been associated with impaired function of the testes, which may lead to infertility.

Digestive effects

It is estimated that zinc deficiency causes about 14.5 per cent of all taste disorders. Zinc deficiency in animals leads to reduced appetite, and oral zinc supplementation rapidly stimulates food intake. In humans, a low zinc intake is associated with a reduced ability to taste salt, which commonly occurs with ageing. Taste disorders and impaired salivary secretions causing dry mouth have been found in patients with zinc deficiency, which are reversed by zinc supplementation taken for six months.

In animals, a very low-zinc diet decreases the amount of zinc in the pancreas within two days, and decreases activity of polyglutamate hydrolase, required for dietary folate absorption, by more than 50 per cent. In humans, polyglutamate hydrolase production also decreases in zinc deficiency, as does the activity of enzymes required for protein digestion.

Zinc deficiency has adverse effects on the integrity of the intestinal barrier by causing breakdown of tight junction proteins, inflammation, increased protein leakage from blood vessels and increased gut permeability (leaky gut), especially when oxidative stress is increased during infections or chronic alcohol intake. Even a marginal zinc deficiency aggravates the adverse effect of alcohol on the intestinal barrier. A leaky gut may contribute to food allergies and intolerances, coeliac disease, Crohn's disease, liver damage in alcoholic liver disease and the development of endotoxaemia (the presence of bacterial toxins in the bloodstream).

Blood glucose effects

Zinc is important for pancreatic function, and decreased serum zinc concentrations are associated with decreased SOD and MT levels and chronic pancreatitis. Dysfunction of the zinc transporter ZnT8 has been associated with impaired blood glucose control. Inadequate zinc reduces insulin secretion and function, and a severe deficiency induces elevated blood glucose (hyperglycaemia) and elevated insulin levels (hyperinsulinaemia).

Brain and nervous system effects

Zinc is essential for normal brain development. Decreased zinc in nerve cells may cause cell cycle arrest and apoptosis. Severe zinc deficiency during pregnancy can lead to defects of the brain, spinal cord, eye and olfactory tract in the foetus, and a mild deficiency can impair nerve transmission, cell signalling, growth and development of nerve cells, neuronal migration, differentiation and apoptosis, and can have long-term effects on the function of the nervous system of the offspring, leading to behavioural and cognitive disorders. Zinc deficiency increases ROS that damage nerve cells, and reduces production of new nerve cells during development and in adulthood that may be important for learning and memory.

Visual effects

A zinc deficiency impairs vitamin A metabolism in the eyes, and may lead to inflammation of the eyelids, photophobia, poor dark adaptation, night blindness, conjunctivitis, corneal opacities, cataracts and macular degeneration (loss of central vision).

Genetic disorders affecting zinc status

In lactating women, the zinc transporter ZnT2 is essential for the secretion of zinc into breast milk, and rare mutations of the gene for ZnT2 have resulted in a more than 75 per cent reduction in the amount of zinc in the mothers' breast milk, leading to zinc deficiency in their infants while being fully breastfed.

The main genetic disorder affecting zinc metabolism is acrodermatitis enteropathica (AE). AE is caused by severe impairment of zinc absorption due to a mutation of the gene that codes for ZIP4, and was a fatal condition until the 1970s when zinc supplementation was introduced as therapy. It often presents during infancy after weaning from breast milk to formula or cereal, and is characterised by severe progressive dermatitis, diarrhoea, hair loss, mental disturbances and frequent infections. Red and inflamed patches of dry and scaly skin that become crusted, blistered and pus-filled develop initially around the mouth and progress to involve the face, extremities and genital and anal regions. Eye abnormalities may occur, and include inflammation of the eyelids, photophobia, conjunctivitis, corneal opacities and cataracts. On zinc supplementation (about 1–2 mg/kg body weight/day), diarrhoea usually resolves within 24 hours and skin lesions heal within one to two weeks. Zinc supplementation must be continued for life.

Indicators of inadequate levels of zinc may include:

- impaired sense of taste and/or smell, reduced ability to taste salt
- sore throat, mouth ulcers, itchiness of the ear canals
- impaired salivary secretions, poor digestion, loss of appetite, leaky gut, digestive tract inflammation, irritable bowel syndrome, diarrhoea, pancreatitis, pica, food allergies and intolerances
- *skin:* rashes, particularly affecting the face and genital region, cracks and fissures at the corners of the mouth, redness, thickening and dryness of the skin, psoriasis-like skin lesions, scaly plaques, blisters or pustules, bacterial and fungal skin infections, stretch marks, poor wound healing, offensive body or foot odour
- *nails:* white marks or white transverse bands, transverse depressions, weak nails, infections
- *hair:* thinning, dry
- *eyes:* inflammation of the eyelids, photophobia, poor dark adaptation, night blindness, conjunctivitis, corneal opacities, cataracts, macular degeneration
- poor immunity, increased susceptibility to infection
- elevated blood glucose, elevated insulin levels
- headaches, insomnia, bad dreams, dizziness, irritability, nervousness, restlessness, poor memory
- reduced ability to detoxify alcohol and drugs, fatty liver, liver damage
- elevated copper levels
- *pregnancy:* spontaneous abortion, pre-eclampsia, toxaemia, a prolonged gestation period or preterm birth, retarded growth of the foetus, NTDs/foetal malformations of the brain, spinal cord, eye and olfactory tract, birth complications, stillbirths, low birth weight infants
- *infants:* skin rashes, diarrhoea, failure to thrive, irritability, inconsolable crying
- *children/adolescents:* poor growth, poor appetite, failure to thrive, diarrhoea, impaired development of male sexual organs at puberty, behavioural and cognitive disorders, poor learning ability, reduced resistance to infections
- *men:* reduced testosterone, impaired sperm formation, impaired viability and motility of sperm, sperm defects, reduced libido, infertility, prostate gland disorders.

Assessment of body status

Serum or plasma zinc concentrations are commonly used to assess zinc status. However, zinc in the bloodstream is tightly controlled, even with varying dietary intake, and a decrease occurs only when zinc depletion is severe or prolonged. The reference range given by the RCPA for plasma or serum zinc is 12–20 μmol/L. Plasma zinc varies throughout the day, with higher levels in the morning, and zinc is redistributed to tissues during endotoxaemia, tissue injury, infection, cancer, acute stress, steroid use, oral contraceptive use and after meals. Plasma volume expansion because of pregnancy or water overload can cause a drop in plasma zinc. Measurements of proteins that are elevated in response to tissue injury or infection can be used to help interpret the cause of low plasma zinc levels.

Urinary zinc can also be measured, but is not regarded as a good reflection of body levels. The reference range given by the RCPA is 8–11 μmol/24 hours. High urinary zinc, together with low serum zinc, may be caused by liver cirrhosis, cancer or increased breakdown of body tissues. High urinary zinc with normal or elevated serum zinc may reflect the use of high-dose zinc supplements, and low urinary zinc with low serum zinc may indicate inadequate intake.

The zinc taste test is used by some naturopaths to assess zinc status. A 10 mL dose of a dilute zinc sulfate solution is held in the mouth for five to ten seconds and the taste sensation is noted. A severe zinc deficiency is indicated if it tastes like plain water during the entire time period, a mild deficiency if it tastes slightly dry, furry or metallic after several seconds, a marginal deficiency if a strong but not unpleasant taste develops after several seconds and no deficiency if a very strong or metallic taste is noted immediately, which may be very unpleasant. The zinc solution may be spat out or swallowed after the test. It is recommended that patients not eat, drink, smoke or chew gum for 30 minutes before the test. Some studies have shown a correlation between the taste test and zinc levels in sweat and serum, but at present there is insufficient evidence for the accuracy of the test for assessing body zinc levels.

Case reports—zinc deficiency

- *A female infant, nine months of age*, developed a rash that did not respond to topical steroids or oral antibiotics.[1] She also had a four-week history of watery diarrhoea, had lost 1.5 kg in weight and was irritable. She was found to have large areas of red, thin, scaly papules around her mouth and perineum, and on her cheeks, elbows and knees. She had very low serum zinc (3.21 μmol/L), and genetic testing confirmed that she had AE. She was given oral zinc sulfate, which led to rapid healing of the skin lesions and alleviation of the diarrhoea.

- *A woman, 37 years of age*, reported having experienced a loss of smell and taste during the previous twelve months, as well as heavy menstrual periods, chronic fatigue and listlessness.[2] She reported an overwhelming desire to eat toilet tissue, and would frequently wake at night and dash to her bathroom to eat it. Her diet consisted mainly of carbohydrates. She was found to have iron deficiency and low serum zinc (4.28 μmol/L), and was treated with 24 mg of elemental zinc twice daily and 300 mg of ferrous sulfate three times daily. Her ability to taste and smell normalised within a week, at which time her serum zinc level had increased to 14.54 μmol/L, and her energy level and sense of wellbeing improved. Her symptoms reversed after one month of supplementation, and her iron and zinc levels returned to normal.
- *A woman, 37 years of age*, with lifelong epilepsy and cognitive impairment, developed a non-itchy, brownish-red, scaly rash on one hand that was unresponsive to topical steroids.[3] She also had a *Candida* infection around her mouth, a rash on the vulva and a non-healing sore on her right foot. She had been treated long term with phenobarbitone, carbamazepine and phenytoin for epilepsy, but had been changed to high-dose sodium valproate two years previously. The change of medication had induced vomiting, weight loss of 25.4 kg, hair loss and dry skin. After seven months, she was changed to phenytoin but the weight loss continued, together with a poor sense of taste, refusal of food, vomiting and alternating diarrhoea and constipation. Her serum zinc concentration was found to be 8.2 μmol/L, and she was given oral zinc sulfate supplementation. All signs and symptoms responded within two weeks and there was no relapse despite continuing treatment of her epilepsy with phenytoin and carbamazepine.
- *A girl, two years of age*, developed a poor appetite from the age of eighteen months and began to attempt to eat metallic objects, such as aluminium foil and keys and, to a lesser extent, her own hair.[4] She was in the habit of gnawing at the metal strips on the edge of carpets. She was found to have poor growth, a marked silver discolouration of her teeth caused by her pica, a normal Hb level and low hair zinc. She was given a zinc sulfate supplement and her pica disappeared in three days. Her hair zinc, appetite and food intake improved, and she gained height and weight.

REFERENCES

1 Ashkenazi-Hoffnung, L., Bilavsky, E. & Amir, J., Acrodermatitis enteropathica in a 9 month old infant, *Isr Med Assoc J* (2011), 13(4): 258.

2 Chisholm, J.C. Jr & Martin, H.I., Hypozincemia, ageusia, dysosmia, and toilet tissue pica, *J Natl Med Assoc* (1981), 73(2): 163–4.

3 Lewis-Jones, M.S., Evans, S. & Culshaw, M.A., Cutaneous manifestations of zinc deficiency during treatment with anticonvulsants, *Br Med J (Clin Res Ed)* (1985), 290(6468): 603–4.

4 Hambidge, K.M. & Silverman, A., Pica with rapid improvement after dietary zinc supplementation, *Arch Dis Child* (1973), 48(7): 567–8.

THERAPEUTIC USES OF ZINC

Childhood diarrhoea and pneumonia

Diarrhoea and pneumonia are major causes of morbidity and mortality in children in developing countries, causing almost two million deaths each year, and mostly affecting those under two years of age.[1] Zinc deficiency is also prevalent in these countries, and supplementation has been found to reduce the duration and severity of diarrhoeal episodes and reduce the risk of subsequent infections for two to three months.[2] Zinc may exert protective effects via enhancing the integrity of the digestive tract and enhancing immunity, but the exact mechanism is not clear. The WHO recommends the use of low concentration oral rehydration salts and routine use of zinc supplementation in at-risk children; ten to fourteen days of 10 mg elemental zinc daily is recommended for those under six months of age and 20 mg/day for children older than six months.[1]

It is estimated that daily zinc supplementation for all children under twelve months of age in zinc-deficient populations can reduce the incidence of diarrhoea by 11–23 per cent and, overall, zinc supplements are estimated to reduce childhood deaths from diarrhoea by 13 per cent.[3] A systematic review of 26 trials concluded that zinc supplementation may shorten the duration of acute diarrhoea by about 20 per cent and by 15–30 per cent in persistent diarrhoea.[4] Higher doses of zinc led to greater reductions in duration of diarrhoea. Another systematic review found that zinc supplementation may shorten the duration of acute diarrhoea by about ten hours in children older than six months and reduce the duration of acute diarrhoea by about 27 hours in children with signs of moderate malnutrition.[5] However, zinc has not been found to be an effective treatment for acute diarrhoea in children under six months of age.

Zinc supplements also may be protective against pneumonia in zinc-deficient populations. A review of six trials found that zinc supplementation was able to reduce the incidence of pneumonia by 13 per cent and prevalence by 41 per cent in children from two to 59 months of age.[6]

Age-related macular degeneration

Age-related macular degeneration (ARMD) is degeneration of the macula lutea in the retina of the eyes that gradually reduces the ability to see objects in sharp focus in the central field of vision, and is the major cause of blindness in older adults in Western countries. ARMD is classified as non-exudative (dry) ARMD, featuring accumulation of cellular debris (drusen) caused by photo-oxidative damage and depigmentation of the retinal pigment epithelium, and exudative (wet) ARMD, featuring overgrowth of blood vessels in the retina and accumulation of scar tissue. In Australia, it is estimated that approximately 12 per cent of people over 50 years of age have some form of macular degeneration and 2 per cent have late-stage ARMD.[7] More than 14 per cent of people aged over 80 years have vision loss or blindness caused by ARMD.

In animals, zinc oxide has been shown to be effective in preventing damage to the retina of the eyes when exposed to intense visible light for several hours.[8] It was particularly effective when given before light exposure and in high doses. Animals given zinc had higher zinc levels in serum and retinal pigment epithelium, changes in gene expression in the retina and evidence of reduced oxidation damage.

The use of nutrients for the treatment of ARMD has been investigated in the Age-Related Eye Disease Study (AREDS) that began in 1992.[9] There were four treatment groups: zinc, 80 mg/day as zinc oxide with 2 mg copper as cupric oxide; antioxidants (500 mg vitamin C, 400 IU vitamin E, 15 mg beta-carotene); zinc plus antioxidants; or placebo. After an average of 6.3 years of supplementation, there was a 28 per cent reduction in the risk of developing advanced ARMD in the group taking antioxidants with zinc, a 25 per cent reduction in the zinc-only group and a 20 per cent reduction in the antioxidants-only group compared with the placebo group. A significant reduction in risk of moderate visual acuity loss occurred only in the antioxidants plus zinc group. A ten-year follow-up report from AREDS found that subjects on the AREDS supplementation had a 34 per cent reduced risk of developing advanced ARMD overall, and a 40 per cent reduced risk of developing advanced wet ARMD compared with placebo.[10] However, there was no reduction in risk of developing the advanced form of dry ARMD. Supplementation was associated with a 29 per cent reduction in risk of developing moderate vision loss. In addition, mortality was reduced in participants taking zinc, especially death from circulatory diseases.

Cancer

Zinc has multiple protective roles against cancer and exposure of cancer cells to zinc leads to growth arrest and death.[11] Cancer patients have been found to have increased total serum copper levels and elevated serum copper:zinc ratio compared with control subjects.[12] Zinc deficiency is associated with increased risk of some cancers, such as prostate, lung, oesophageal and oral cancers and abnormal zinc transporter activity and abnormal levels of intracellular zinc are implicated in the development of cancer.[13] Some cancer cells accumulate zinc and others are depleted in zinc; breast and lung cancer cells have higher zinc levels compared with normal tissue, whereas ovarian and prostate cancer cells have lower zinc levels.

The inability to accumulate zinc and citrate is a key characteristic of prostate malignancy, and occurs early in cancer development.[14] ZIP1 gene expression is inhibited in prostate cancer cells, leading to a decrease in the ZIP1 transporter protein that transfers zinc from the bloodstream to cells; levels of zinc in prostate cancer tissue are about 85 per cent lower than in normal prostate tissue.[15] Because zinc has anti-tumour activity and is toxic to prostate cancer cells, it is believed that these cells silence ZIP1 gene expression in order to deplete cellular zinc.

In contrast to the established finding that the presence of zinc in prostate tissue is protective against cancer, epidemiological studies of zinc intake and prostate cancer have shown mixed results. Zinc intake has been reported to have no effect, preventive effects or adverse effects in prostate cancer. One study found that high-dose zinc (more than 100 mg/day) or long-term supplementation use was associated with a small increased risk of advanced prostate cancer.[16] In contrast, another study found that long-term zinc supplementation was associated with reduced risk of advanced prostate cancer.[17] The results are difficult to interpret and, at present, the relationship between dietary or supplemental zinc intake and the risk of prostate cancer is not clear.

Benign prostatic hyperplasia

Benign prostatic hyperplasia (BPH), enlargement of the prostate gland, develops in men with ageing, and is estimated to affect more than 90 per cent of men at some point in their life, and often leads to urination difficulties.[18] Zinc is essential for testosterone metabolism, and is especially high in the prostate gland, where it increases citrate levels and inhibits cell proliferation. The mean zinc content of prostate tissue in BPH has been shown to be 61 per cent lower than in normal tissue.[19]

The enzyme 5-alpha reductase (type 2) converts testosterone to dihydrotestosterone (DHT), which is primarily responsible for prostate gland overgrowth. Inhibitors of 5-alpha reductase reduce prostate size, mainly by reducing production of vascular-derived endothelial growth factor and inducing apoptosis. In a study of human BPH tissue, low concentrations of zinc increased activity of 5-alpha reductase but higher concentrations inhibited its activity.[20] In cell studies, zinc treatment inhibits the growth of BPH cells, mostly due to zinc-induced apoptosis, but does not inhibit growth of normal prostate cells.[21] The effect of zinc supplementation in the prevention and treatment of BPH has not been established.

Sickle cell anaemia

The genetic disorder sickle cell anaemia is caused by an abnormal form of haemoglobin (haemoglobin S) that causes red blood cells to develop a sickle, or crescent, shape instead of the normal biconcave disc shape. Sickle cells are stiff and sticky, and can block blood flow and increase the risk of infections. Zinc levels in plasma and red blood cells of patients with sickle cell anaemia have been found to be lower, and urinary zinc excretion higher, than in control subjects.[22] Zinc supplementation has been shown to increase growth rate in children with sickle cell anaemia, and long-term zinc sulfate supplementation has been found to reduce the number of sickle cell crises and reduce the total number of clinical infections.[23]

Inflammatory bowel disorders

Inflammatory bowel disease tissue has been found to have increased production of ROS and reactive nitrogen species (RNS) that are associated with inflammatory activity. Decreased levels and lower activity of Cu/Zn SOD have been reported in inflammatory bowel disease tissue. A small study of patients with severe active Crohn's disease or ulcerative colitis found that treatment with bovine Cu/Zn SOD led to remission in more than 80 per cent of cases.[24]

Zinc deficiency is associated with a damaged epithelial barrier and dysfunction of the innate immune system that occurs in inflammatory bowel diseases such as Crohn's disease and ulcerative colitis. In cell studies, exposure to zinc stimulates repair of tight junctions in gut tissue.[25] Zinc supplementation has been shown to prevent gut leakiness in a number of diseases, including Crohn's disease and experimental colitis.[26,27] In Crohn's disease patients in remission, zinc supplementation (110 mg of zinc sulfate three times daily for eight weeks) has been found to reduce gut permeability and may reduce the risk of relapse.[27]

Skin disorders

Zinc may be helpful for the treatment of acne vulgaris, nappy rash, seborrhoeic dermatitis, dandruff, psoriasis, viral warts, herpes infections and chronic skin ulcers. Oral and topical zinc has been used for acne, and has been found to decrease sebum production and have antibacterial and anti-inflammatory effects. In acne patients, zinc sulfate (600 mg daily for twelve weeks) resulted in a decrease in the number of papules, infiltrates and cysts in 58 per cent, and an increase in serum retinol levels.[28] In inflammatory acne, 30 mg/day of elemental zinc as zinc gluconate was found to reduce inflammation.[29] Zinc sulfate (135 mg elemental zinc/day), alone and in combination with vitamin

A (300 000 IU/day), was compared with vitamin A alone or placebo for acne therapy.[30] Zinc treatment led to significant improvement in twelve weeks; the combination of vitamin A and zinc did not have a greater effect than zinc alone. A comparison of zinc and antibiotic treatment for acne found that both were effective, but antibiotic therapy was superior.[31]

Zinc has been used successfully for the treatment of viral warts. Twenty-three patients with multiple warts were found to have low serum zinc and were given oral zinc sulfate at a dose of 10 mg/kg body weight daily (up to 600 mg day), resulting in increased serum zinc and complete clearance of warts in twenty patients after two months.[32] In fourteen patients, warts completely cleared after one month.

Nappy rash and slow hair growth has been associated with reduced hair zinc in infants. Newborn infants given 10 mg of zinc daily for four months were found to have a reduced incidence of nappy rash.[33] In cell studies, zinc exposure has been found to inactivate various forms of herpes simplex viruses.[34] Patients with recurring episodes of herpes simplex skin infections treated with topical applications of a solution containing 4 per cent zinc sulfate in water had complete resolution of pain, tingling and burning within the first 24 hours and lesions formed crusts within one to three days.[35] Zinc has been proposed as a useful treatment for vitiligo because it is required for production of zinc alpha 2-glycoprotein (ZAG), which has multiple roles in the body including regulation of melanin production.[36]

Zinc is essential for wound healing because it supports cell proliferation and MMP activity that enhances removal of dead tissue and keratinocyte migration during wound repair. Zinc has antibacterial and anti-inflammatory effects, and a low zinc status impairs wound healing in animals. Topical zinc oxide has been found to promote cleansing and re-epithelialisation in leg ulcers, and to reduce the risk of infections and deterioration.[37]

Autism and attention deficit hyperactivity disorder

Zinc deficiency, an abnormally high copper:zinc ratio and copper, lead and mercury toxicity have been detected in infants with autistic spectrum disorders (ASD), and it has been suggested that zinc deficiency leading to toxic metal accumulation may play an important role in autism.[38,39] Lower zinc tissue levels have also been found in children with ADHD, and one trial reported improvement of symptoms on zinc supplementation (150 mg zinc sulfate daily for twelve weeks).[40] However, the findings of this trial are inconclusive because it was carried out in Turkey, where zinc deficiency is common and the excessively high dose led to many subjects failing to complete the study.

Depression

In animals, zinc deficiency has been associated with the development of depressive-like symptoms, such as behavioural despair and anxiety,[41] and low zinc status has been associated with high depression scores in humans.[42] A review of four trials found that zinc supplementation used together with anti-depressant drugs lowers symptom scores in patients with depression and in those who are resistant to anti-depressants.[43] There is conflicting evidence about the effectiveness of zinc supplementation for the prevention of depression.

Alzheimer's disease

A zinc imbalance caused by alterations in the expression of the zinc transporters ZnT1, ZnT4 and ZnT6 in the brain is a feature of preclinical and early-stage Alzheimer's disease (AD).[44] Ageing is associated with decreased brain levels of ZnT3, the transporter that concentrates zinc in the presynaptic vesicles of nerves, and this decrease is more severe in AD. A lack of synaptic zinc is associated with a reduced level of synaptic proteins that are important for memory and learning. In AD, zinc increases the aggregation and precipitation of amyloid-beta, especially in areas where ZnT3 is expressed. Plaques of amyloid-beta accumulate zinc, and it has been suggested that this trapping of zinc by amyloid-beta impairs the availability of zinc for cell metabolism and causes adverse effects on brain function. A deficiency of zinc impairs activity of IDE that can break down amyloid-beta as well as insulin. Drugs aimed at improving zinc balance in AD have shown benefits, and metal-protein attenuation compounds (MPACs) that act to remove zinc from amyloid-beta and relocate it to areas where it is needed have been trialled; however, results to date have been negative.[45]

The role of zinc supplementation in AD is unclear. Zinc initiates amyloid-beta deposition, but this may be a protective mechanism against oxidative stress and the neurotoxicity it causes. Zinc also reduces copper toxicity that is implicated in AD. In an animal model of

AD, zinc supplementation has been found to maintain mitochondrial function, reduce hyperphosphorylation of tau, reduce amyloid-beta accumulation in the hippocampus and prevent cognitive and mitochondrial impairment. There is some preliminary evidence that zinc supplementation may be of benefit in humans with AD. A slow-release form of zinc (150 mg/day) used for six months in patients with mild to moderate AD was reported to stabilise cognitive function in older patients.[46] Zinc supplementation (50 mg three times daily as zinc aspartate), given iv and orally for three to twelve months, was reported to improve memory, understanding, communication and social contact in a small number of patients with AD.[47] However, there is insufficient evidence to establish the role of zinc supplementation conclusively.

Wilson's disease

Wilson's disease is a genetic disorder in which the body is unable to excrete excess copper, leading to accumulation of free copper and liver and brain damage. Zinc is useful because it can block copper absorption by stimulating production of MTs, which have a higher affinity for copper than zinc. Copper bound to MTs remains trapped in enterocytes, and is lost when cells are shed in faeces, reducing body load. In treatment, the chelating agents trientine and penicillamine are used initially, and zinc is more often used for maintenance therapy. Zinc therapy appears to be more successful in cases of nerve damage, and may not be as effective in patients with liver impairment, who require additional chelation therapy.[48,49]

Diabetes

Zinc has insulin-like and anti-diabetic effects in cell cultures and animal models of type 1 and type 2 diabetes.[50] Markedly increased urinary zinc excretion is a feature of diabetes.[50] Zinc protects pancreatic beta cells from cytokine-induced destruction, which occurs in both type 1 and type 2 diabetes.[51] Zinc deficiency in animals causes reduced ability to secrete insulin in response to a glucose load,[52] and zinc supplementation has been found to improve carbohydrate and lipid metabolism, and prevent or improve diabetes in animal models.[53] Both zinc and MTs protect cells against increased oxidative stress that occurs in diabetes and contributes to diabetic complications.[54]

The zinc transporter ZnT8 has been identified in pancreatic islets, in which it supplies zinc to beta cells that secrete insulin.[55] Expression of ZnT8 protects beta cells from apoptosis related to zinc depletion. Mutations in the gene for this zinc transporter are associated with glucose intolerance and type 2 diabetes. In type 1 diabetes, ZnT8 is targeted by autoantibodies. The inflammatory cytokine interleukin-1 beta (IL-1β) suppresses ZnT8 expression in beta cells, impairs glucose-stimulated insulin release and is involved in islet cell destruction in type 1 and type 2 diabetes. Zinc helps to reduce the production of inflammatory cytokines that lead to beta cell death.

An Australian study found that a higher total dietary zinc intake and high zinc:iron ratio are associated with lower risk of type 2 diabetes in women.[56] Zinc supplementation in animals and humans has been shown to improve blood glucose control in type 1 and type 2 diabetes. A review of twelve studies comparing the effects of zinc supplementation on fasting blood glucose in patients with type 2 diabetes found that it was associated with lower levels of fasting and post-meal blood glucose, and lower levels of glycated haemoglobin (HbA_{1C}), a marker of glucose control.[57] A review of eight studies comparing the effects of zinc supplementation on cholesterol levels in patients with type 2 diabetes found that zinc was associated with lower total cholesterol and LDL cholesterol.[57] Zinc supplementation has also resulted in reduced blood pressure[57] and, in an animal model of type 1 diabetes, protection of the aorta against oxidative damage that leads to inflammation, fibrosis and increased wall thickness.[58]

Anorexia nervosa

A zinc deficiency adversely affects neurotransmitters and leptin production, and leads to loss of appetite in animals.[59] Zinc deficiency and anorexia nervosa (AN) have similar symptoms, such as loss of appetite, poor growth, weight loss, skin abnormalities, cessation of menstruation and depression. Zinc absorption is impaired in AN, and about half of AN patients may be zinc deficient.[60]

Zinc supplementation has been shown to improve weight gain in AN patients in a number of studies. A study using 45–90 mg of zinc daily as zinc sulfate in twenty patients with AN found that none lost weight and seventeen patients increased their body weight by more than 15 per cent over eight to 56 months, with one patient gaining 24 per cent after three months and one gaining 57 per cent after 24 months.[61] Menstruation was restored in thirteen patients after one to seventeen months of zinc supplementation. Another study found that 50 mg of elemental zinc daily decreased depression and anxiety in AN patients.[62] A study of 35 women with AN found that 14 mg of zinc daily as zinc gluconate increased weight twice as rapidly compared to those on placebo and it has been suggested that 14 mg of elemental zinc daily for two months should be standard therapy in patients with AN.[63]

Tinnitus

Some patients with tinnitus (ringing or noises in the ears) have been found to be low in zinc, and zinc supplementation (34–68 mg daily for over two weeks) has been found to elevate serum zinc and improve tinnitus symptoms in these patients.[64] Severity of tinnitus was improved in another study in patients given 50 mg of zinc for two months.[65] However, other studies have reported that zinc supplementation is not effective.

Colds

A comprehensive review that included thirteen therapeutic trials and two preventive trials investigating the use of zinc supplementation for the common cold concluded that zinc given within 24 hours of symptom onset reduces the duration and severity of the common cold in otherwise healthy people, and that supplementation for at least five months reduces cold incidence, school absenteeism and prescription of antibiotics in children.[66] Zinc lozenges at doses of more than 75 mg daily have been found to reduce the duration of a cold but may cause loss of taste sensations.[67]

REFERENCES

1 World Health Organization, *The treatment of diarrhoea: A manual for physicians and other senior health workers*, WHO, Geneva, 2005.
2 WHO/UNICEF, Joint Statement, *Clinical management of acute diarrhea*, WHO, Geneva, 2004.
3 Penny, M.E., Zinc supplementation in public health, *Ann Nutr Metab* (2013), 62(Suppl 1): 31–42.
4 Patel, A., Mamtani, M., Dibley, M.J. et al., Therapeutic value of zinc supplementation in acute and persistent diarrhea: A systematic review, *PLoS One* (2010), 28: 5(4): e10386.
5 Lazzerini, M. & Ronfani L., Oral zinc for treating diarrhoea in children, *Cochrane Database Syst Rev* (2013), 1: CD005436.
6 Lassi, Z.S., Haider, B.A. & Bhutta, Z.A., Zinc supplementation for the prevention of pneumonia in children aged 2 months to 59 months, *Cochrane Database Syst Rev* (2010), 12: CD005978.
7 Macular Degeneration Foundation, *Macular degeneration: Facts and figures,* available at <www.mdfoundation.com.au/resources/1/facts-figures_2012.pdf>.
8 Organisciak, D., Wong, P., Rapp, C. et al., Light-induced retinal degeneration is prevented by zinc, a component in the age-related eye disease study formulation, *Photochem Photobiol* (2012), 88(6): 1396–407.
9 Age-Related Eye Disease Study Research Group, A randomized, placebo-controlled, clinical trial of high-dose supplementation with vitamins C and E, beta carotene, and zinc for age-related macular degeneration and vision loss: AREDS report no. 8, *Arch Ophthalmol* (2001), 119(10): 1417–36.
10 Chew, E.Y., Clemons, T.E., Agrón, E. et al., Age-Related Eye Disease Study Research Group, Long-term effects of vitamins C and E, β-carotene and zinc on age-related macular degeneration: AREDS Report No. 35, *Ophthalmology* (2013), 10 April, pii: S0161-6420(13)00036-5.
11 Kriedt, C.L., Baldassare, J., Shah, M. & Klein, C., Zinc functions as a cytotoxic agent for prostate cancer cells independent of culture and growth conditions, *J Exp Ther Oncol* (2010), 8(4): 287–95.
12 Zowczak, M., Iskra, M., Torliński, L. & Cofta, S., Analysis of serum copper and zinc concentrations in cancer patients, *Biol Trace Elem Res* (2001), 82(1–3): 1–8.
13 Prasad, A.S., Beck, F.W., Snell, D.C. & Kucuk, O., Zinc in cancer prevention, *Nutr Cancer* (2009), 61(6): 879–87.

14 Costello, L.C. & Franklin, R.B., The clinical relevance of the metabolism of prostate cancer; zinc and tumor suppression: Connecting the dots, *Mol Cancer* (2006), 5: 17.

15 Zaichick, V.Y., Sviridova T.V. & Zaichick S.V., Zinc in the human prostate gland: normal, hyperplastic and cancerous, *Int Urol Nephrol* (1997), 29(5): 565–74.

16 Leitzmann, M.F., Stampfer, M.J., Wu, K. et al., Zinc supplement use and risk of prostate cancer, *J Natl Cancer Inst* (2003), 95(13): 1004–7.

17 Gonzalez, A., Peters, U., Lampe, J.W. & White E., Zinc intake from supplements and diet and prostate cancer, *Nutr Cancer* (2009), 61(2): 206–15.

18 Monash Institute of Reproduction and Development, Australia, *Monash Institute News* (2004), 25 (September), available at <www.monashinstitute.org/assets/media/minews/2004–09.pdf>.

19 Christudoss, P., Selvakumar, R., Fleming, J.J. & Gopalakrishnan, G., Zinc status of patients with benign prostatic hyperplasia and prostate carcinoma, *Indian J Urol* (2011), 27(1): 14–18.

20 Leake, A., Chisholm, G.D. & Habib, F.K., The effect of zinc on the 5 alpha-reduction of testosterone by the hyperplastic human prostate gland, *J Steroid Biochem* (1984), 20(2): 651–5.

21 Feng, P., Li, T.L., Guan, Z.X. et al., Direct effect of zinc on mitochondrial apoptogenesis in prostate cells, *Prostate* (2002), 52(4): 311–18.

22 Prasad, A.S., Schoomaker, E.B., Ortega, J. et al., Zinc deficiency in sickle cell disease, *Clin Chem* (1975), 21(4): 582–7.

23 Swe, K.M., Abas, A.B., Bhardwaj, A. et al., Zinc supplements for treating thalassaemia and sickle cell disease, *Cochrane Database Syst Rev* (2013), 6: CD009415.

24 Emerit, J., Pelletier, S., Tosoni-Verlignue, D. & Mollet, M., Phase II trial of copper zinc superoxide dismutase (CuZnSOD) in treatment of Crohn's disease, *Free Radic Biol Med* (1989), 7(2): 145–9.

25 Wang, X., Valenzano, M.C., Mercado, J.M. et al., Zinc supplementation modifies tight junctions and alters barrier function of CACO-2 human intestinal epithelial layers, *Dig Dis Sci* (2013), 58(1): 77–87.

26 Sturniolo, G.C., Fries, W., Mazzon, E., Di Leo, V., Barollo, M. et al., Effect of zinc supplementation on intestinal permeability in experimental colitis, *J Lab Clin Med* (2002), 139: 311–15.

27 Sturniolo, G.C., Di Leo, V., Ferronato, A. et al., Zinc supplementation tightens 'leaky gut' in Crohn's disease, *Inflamm Bowel Dis* (2001), 7(2): 94–8.

28 Brandt, S., The clinical effects of zinc as a topical or oral agent on the clinical response and pathophysiologic mechanisms of acne: A systematic review of the literature, *J Drugs Dermat* (2013), 12(5): 542–5.

29 Dreno, B., Amblard, P., Agache, P. et al., Low doses of zinc gluconate for inflammatory acne, *Acta Derm Venereol* (1989), 69(6): 541–3.

30 Michaëlsson, G., Juhlin, L. & Vahlquist, A., Effects of oral zinc and vitamin A in acne, *Arch Dermatol* (1977), 113(1): 31–6.

31 Dreno, B., Moyse, D., Alirezai, M. et al., Multicenter randomized comparative double-blind controlled clinical trial of the safety and efficacy of zinc gluconate versus minocycline hydrochloride in the treatment of inflammatory acne vulgaris, *Dermatology* (2001), 203: 135–40.

32 Al-Gurairi, F.T., Al-Waiz, M. & Sharquie, K.E., Oral zinc sulphate in the treatment of recalcitrant viral warts: Randomized placebo-controlled clinical trial, *Br J Dermatol* (2002), 146(3): 423–31.

33 Collipp, P.J., Effect of oral zinc supplements on diaper rash in normal infants, *J Med Assoc Ga* (1989), 78(9): 621–3.

34 Arens, M. & Travis, S., Zinc salts inactivate clinical isolates of herpes simplex virus in vitro, *J Clin Microbiol* (2000), 38(5): 1758–62.

35 Wahba, A., Topical application of zinc-solutions: A new treatment for herpes simplex infections of the skin? *Acta Derm Venereol* (1980), 60(2): 175–7.

36 Bagherani, N., The newest hypothesis about vitiligo: Most of the suggested pathogeneses of vitiligo can be attributed to lack of one factor, zinc-α2-glycoprotein, *ISRN Dermatol* (2012): 405268.
37 Agren, M.S., Studies on zinc in wound healing, *Acta Derm Venereol Suppl (Stockh)* (1990), 154: 1–36.
38 Lakshmi Priya, M.D. & Geetha, A., Level of trace elements (copper, zinc, magnesium and selenium) and toxic elements (lead and mercury) in the hair and nails of children with autism, *Biol Trace Elem Res* (2011), 142(2): 148–58.
39 Faber, S., Zinn, G.M., Kern, J.C. & Kingston, H.M., The plasma zinc/serum copper ratio as a biomarker in children with autism spectrum disorders, *Biomarkers* (2009), 14(3): 171–80.
40 Arnold, L.E. & DiSilvestro, R.A., Zinc in attention-deficit/hyperactivity disorder, *J Child Adolesc Psychopharmacol* (2005), 15(4): 619–27.
41 Tassabehji, N.M., Corniola, R.S., Alshingiti, A. & Levenson, C.W., Zinc deficiency induces depression-like symptoms in adult rats, *Physiol Behav* (2008), 95(3): 365–9.
42 Maes, M., D'Haese, P.C., Scharpé, S. et al., Hypozincemia in depression, *J Affect Disord* (1994), 31(2): 135–40.
43 Lai, J., Moxey, A., Nowak, G. et al., The efficacy of zinc supplementation in depression: systematic review of randomised controlled trials, *J Affect Disord* (2012), 136(1–2): e31–9.
44 Watt, N.T., Whitehouse, I.J. & Hooper, N.M., The role of zinc in Alzheimer's disease, *Int J Alzheimers Dis* (2010): 971021.
45 Sampson, E.L., Jenagaratnam, L. & McShane, R., Metal protein attenuating compounds for the treatment of Alzheimer's dementia, *Cochrane Database Syst Rev* (2014), 2: CD005380.
46 Brewer, G.J., Copper excess, zinc deficiency, and cognition loss in Alzheimer's disease, *Biofactors* (2012), 38(2): 107–13.
47 Constantinidis, J., Treatment of Alzheimer's disease by zinc compounds, *Drug Development Res* (1992), 27(1): 1–14.
48 Linn, F.H.H., Houwen, R.H.J., van Hatten, J. et al., Long-term exclusive zinc monotherapy in symptomatic Wilson disease: Experience in 17 patients, *Hepatology* (2009), 50: 1442–52.
49 Weiss, K.H., Gotthardt, D.N., Klemm, D. et al., Zinc monotherapy is not as effective as chelating agents in treatment of Wilson disease, *Gastroenterology* (2011), 140(4): 1189–98.
50 Chausmer, A.B., Zinc, insulin and diabetes, *J Am Coll Nutr* (1998), 17(2): 109–15.
51 Ohly, P., Dohle, C., Abel, J. et al., Zinc sulphate induces metallothionein in pancreatic islets of mice and protects against diabetes induced by multiple low doses of streptozotocin, *Diabetologia* (2000), 43(8): 1020–30.
52 Faure, P., Roussel, A., Coudray, C. et al., Zinc and insulin sensitivity, *Biol Trace Elem Res* (1992), 32: 305–10.
53 Vardatsikos, G., Pandey, N.R. & Srivastava, A.K., Insulino-mimetic and anti-diabetic effects of zinc, *J Inorg Biochem* (2013), 120: 8–17.
54 Prasad, A.S., Zinc in human health: Effect of zinc on immune cells, *Mol Med* (2008), 14(5–6): 353–7.
55 Kawasaki, E., ZnT8 and type 1 diabetes, *Endocr J* (2012), 59(7): 531–7.
56 Vashum, K.P., McEvoy, M., Shi, Z. et al., Is dietary zinc protective for type 2 diabetes? Results from the Australian longitudinal study on women's health, *BMC Endocr Disord* (2013), 13(1): 40.
57 Jayawardena, R., Ranasinghe, P., Galappatthy, P. et al., Effects of zinc supplementation on diabetes mellitus: A systematic review and meta-analysis, *Diabetol Metab Syndr* (2012), 4(1): 13.
58 Miao, X., Wang, Y., Sun, J. et al., Zinc protects against diabetes-induced pathogenic changes in the aorta: Roles of metallothionein and nuclear factor (erythroid-derived 2)-like 2, *Cardiovasc Diabetol* (2013), 12: 54.
59 Shay, N.F. & Mangian, H.F., Neurobiology of zinc-influenced eating behavior, *J Nutr* (2000), 130(5S Suppl): 1493S–9S.

60 Humphries, L., Vivian, B., Stuart, M. & McClain, C.J., Zinc deficiency and eating disorders, *J Clin Psychiatry* (1989), 50(12): 456–9.
61 Safai-Kutti, S., Oral zinc supplementation in anorexia nervosa, *Acta Psychiatr Scand Suppl* (1990), 361: 14–17.
62 Katz, R.L., Keen, C.L., Litt, I.F. et al., Zinc deficiency in anorexia nervosa, *J Adolesc Health Care* (1987), 8(5): 400–6.
63 Birmingham, C.L. & Gritzner, S., How does zinc supplementation benefit anorexia nervosa? *Eat Weight Disord* (2006), 11(4): e109–11.
64 Ochi, K., Ohashi, T., Kinoshita, H. et al., [The serum zinc level in patients with tinnitus and the effect of zinc treatment]. *Nihon Jibiinkoka Gakkai Kaiho* (1997), 100(9): 915–19 [Article in Japanese].
65 Arda, H.N., Tuncel, U., Akdogan, O. & Ozluoglu, L.N., The role of zinc in the treatment of tinnitus, *Otol Neurotol* (2003), 24(1): 86–9.
66 Singh, M. & Das, R.R., Zinc for the common cold, *Cochrane Database Syst Rev* (2011), 2: CD001364.
67 Eby, G.A. III, Zinc lozenges as cure for the common cold: A review and hypothesis, *Med Hypotheses* (2010), 74(3): 482–92.

Therapeutic dose

Zinc deficiency may accompany iron deficiency, and additional iron supplementation may be required. Zinc and copper need to be in balance in the body, and copper supplementation is recommended if high doses of zinc (more than 40 mg daily) are given long term. The optimal ratio of zinc to copper appears to be 5:1. High-dose supplementation (more than 20 mg elemental zinc daily) is not required for general health purposes.

Suggested doses of elemental zinc for adults are as follows:

- *Health maintenance:* 10–15 mg daily.
- *Mild deficiency:* 15–20 mg daily for at least six months.
- *Severe deficiency:* 50 mg or more daily for about six months, reducing as serum zinc levels normalise.
- *AE:* 1–2 mg/kg body weight of zinc daily for life.
- *General therapeutic dose:* 20–50 mg daily.
- *Acute diarrhoea or pneumonia protection in malnourished children less than six months:* 10 mg daily.
- *Acute diarrhoea or pneumonia protection in malnourished children six to 36 months:* 20 mg daily.
- *Prevention of ARMD:* 80 mg with 2 mg copper daily in combination with antioxidants.
- *Treatment of colds, acute infections:* 20–50 mg oral zinc daily, short-term only.
- *ADHD in children:* 20–50 mg daily, reducing when symptoms improve.

Effects of excess

High-dose zinc supplements should be mainly used in the short term, except in AE, where lifelong supplementation is required. In animal toxicity studies, zinc acetate was the most likely to cause adverse effects at high doses, followed by zinc nitrate, zinc chloride and zinc sulfate. A dose equivalent to about 27 g of zinc daily given to humans has caused deaths in animals. A one-off dose of 450 mg of zinc sulfate has caused a hot taste, dry mouth, nausea, vomiting, stomach and abdominal pain, and diarrhoea in humans. Extremely high doses (about 86 mg zinc/kg/day) were reported to cause lethargy, light-headedness and staggering in one patient. However, a high dietary intake from the richest source, shellfish, does not appear to cause adverse responses.

In clinical trials, up to 600 mg of zinc sulfate (about 138 mg of elemental zinc) has been taken daily in divided doses for several months without any reported adverse effects. However, a prolonged daily intake of high-dose zinc has been associated with suppressed immunity, decreased HDL cholesterol levels, increased risk of kidney stones and urinary tract infections, and hypochromic microcytic anaemia. Plasma LDL cholesterol, total cholesterol and triglycerides are not affected by an intake of up to 150 mg of zinc daily. In AREDS patients, 80 mg of zinc daily for several years appeared to increase the risk of urinary tract infections, especially in women, and may have increased the risk of kidney stones in men.

A long-term high intake of zinc may decrease absorption of copper and iron, leading to deficiencies. Decreased copper status may inhibit the transport of iron and result in anaemia. Prolonged intake of 100 mg or more of zinc daily has been shown to cause a copper deficiency, which can be reversed by reducing zinc and increasing copper intake to restore balance. A high zinc intake (140 mg/day) inhibits absorption of calcium if calcium intake is low (230 mg/day) but this inhibition does not occur if zinc intake is lower (100 mg/day). In general, long-term intake of up to 40 mg elemental zinc daily in adults is unlikely to cause adverse effects. In children, supplementation with 5–20 mg of zinc daily for up to one year has not caused adverse effects.

In animals, excessively high levels of zinc prior to and/or during gestation have led to foetal resorption, reduced foetal weight, altered tissue concentrations of foetal iron and copper, and reduced growth in the offspring. However, zinc sulfate (0.3 mg zinc/kg/day) taken by pregnant women during the last two trimesters did not cause any adverse reproductive effects.

Intranasal zinc sprays are not recommended because they have been found to damage olfactory cells in the nose and cause loss of the ability to smell. When used topically, zinc chloride is caustic and can cause severe skin irritation, zinc sulfate is less irritating and zinc oxide, which is commonly used in topical applications, does not have adverse effects.

Case reports—zinc excess

- *A woman, nineteen years of age,* developed anaemia and severely low levels of neutrophils (neutropenia).[1] She had been taking about 121.25 mg of zinc daily for more than five years as part of her treatment for the genetic movement disorder Hallervorden–Spatz syndrome. Her daily intake of copper was 2 mg. She was found to be markedly anaemic and had elevated serum zinc and low serum copper and ceruloplasmin levels. She was diagnosed with zinc-induced copper deficiency, and zinc therapy was discontinued. At eight months follow-up, her anaemia had reversed and her trace element levels had normalised.
- *A man, 57 years of age,* developed numbness and tingling in his toes, which progressed to involve his legs, hands and lower torso.[2] He had episodes of bladder incontinence, difficulty holding objects, keeping his balance and walking, and had frequent falls. He was diagnosed with macrocytic anaemia, and vitamin B12 deficiency was suspected. However, his serum B12 concentration was normal, and symptoms did not improve on B12 treatment. Further questioning revealed that the patient had worn dentures for ten years and he was in the habit of using excessive amounts of denture adhesive, which contains zinc. His serum zinc concentration was elevated (21.7 μmol/L) and his copper concentration was very low. The patient was diagnosed with copper deficiency myeloneuropathy caused by zinc toxicity from his denture adhesive. He was given cupric sulfate (2 mg/day) intravenously for five days, followed by long-term oral copper gluconate supplementation (2 mg/day), and his denture cream was changed. At follow-up two months later, the patient's anaemia had reversed, his copper concentration was normal and his zinc concentration remained slightly increased. He reported considerable improvement of his paraesthesia and incontinence symptoms.
- *A woman, 22 years of age,* developed abdominal pain, nausea, vomiting, loss of appetite and peripheral oedema.[3] She had not menstruated for more than a year. Her only reported medications were over-the-counter zinc gluconate, B-complex vitamins and a multivitamin supplement. She was diagnosed with pyelonephritis (kidney infection), but no cause could be found. She also was found to have microcytic hypochromic anaemia. She improved on antibiotic and diuretic therapy, and was discharged but returned two weeks later with severe fatigue, breathlessness on exertion, abdominal pain and a persistent, throbbing, diffuse headache. She was hospitalised and given antibiotic therapy. During further questioning, she reported taking 2000 mg of zinc gluconate daily (40 × 50 mg tablets, equivalent to about 280 mg of elemental zinc) for over twelve months for acne and oily skin. When her acne was worse, she took an additional two to three 100 mg tablets of zinc gluconate a day. She was also taking between eight and 30 B complex tablets and one multivitamin daily. It was then discovered that she had a high serum zinc and low serum copper concentration, and was diagnosed with zinc-induced copper deficiency. Her supplements were discontinued, and she was placed on a high-copper diet. At follow-up, she reported improvement in her stamina and general wellbeing, but her kidney symptoms returned after four weeks, her serum copper remained low and serum zinc remained elevated. The outcome is unknown because she did not return for further consultations.

REFERENCES

1 Irving, J.A., Mattman, A., Lockitch, G. et al., Element of caution: a case of reversible cytopenias associated with excessive zinc supplementation, *CMAJ* (2003), 169(2): 129–31.
2 Sommerville, R.B. & Baloh, R.H., Anemia, paresthesias, and gait ataxia in a 57-year-old denture wearer, *Clin Chem* (2011), 57(8): 1103–6.
3 Hein, M.S., Copper deficiency anemia and nephrosis in zinc-toxicity: A case report, *S D J Med* (2003), 56(4): 143–7.

Supplements

Zinc supplements are available in tablets, capsules, powders and liquids. The permitted forms of zinc salts in oral supplements in Australia include zinc amino acid chelate, ascorbate, chloride, citrate, citrate dihydrate, citrate trihydrate, gluconate, oxide, succinate, sulfate, sulfate hexahydrate and sulfate monohydrate. The forms of zinc used in most clinical trials in humans include zinc sulfate, acetate, gluconate and amino acid chelate. Zinc sulfate and chloride are very soluble, and zinc oxide is very insoluble and depends on the presence of stomach acid for absorption. Inadequate stomach acid production has been shown to reduce zinc absorption from zinc oxide by 82 per cent. Zinc methionine, a zinc amino acid chelate, was found to have twice the availability of zinc sulfate in an animal study when consumed with corn, soybeans or soy isolate. Water solutions of zinc are well absorbed, with absorption ranging from about 46 per cent to about 73 per cent according to dose. The approximate absorption of zinc from aqueous solutions taken on an empty stomach is 60 per cent for a 5 mg dose, 50 per cent for a 10 mg dose and 40 per cent for a 15 mg dose. In general, zinc supplements are better absorbed if taken in divided doses.

The amount of elemental zinc in a specific zinc salt is listed on the product container and may vary between individual products; the approximate elemental zinc content of some common salts is shown in Table 10.4.

- *Zinc oxide* is the least expensive form of supplementary zinc, contains the most elemental zinc and is more stable when used as a food additive. It is absorbed well in people with normal levels of stomach acid. In the French Process production method, zinc is melted, vaporised and processed in an oxidation chamber to produce the oxide form. Zinc oxide is used in mineral supplements, animal feeds and in topical preparations for skin care, such as sun screens, ointments, creams and powders.
- *Zinc sulfate* is more soluble but lower in elemental zinc than zinc oxide, and is a commonly used form of zinc in supplements and clinical trials. It can be prepared commercially from the reaction of sulfuric acid with zinc oxide.
- *Zinc gluconate* is a bioavailable form of zinc that contains less elemental zinc than zinc sulfate. It is prepared commercially by the reaction of gluconic acid derived from glucose with zinc oxide.
- *Zinc amino acid chelate* has a low zinc content but is a well-absorbed form of zinc that is produced by chelation of zinc from zinc oxide with an amino acid derived from acid hydrolysis of a protein source, such as soy bean. Zinc bisglycinate has been found to have about 43 per cent higher bioavailability than zinc gluconate.

Cautions

Long-term high-dose zinc (greater than 40 mg daily) may decrease copper absorption, and should be used with copper supplementation. Zinc nasal sprays damage the sense of smell and should not be used, and chewable zinc lozenges may impair taste sensations.

Table 10.4 Elemental zinc content of common salts

Salt	Zinc content (%)
Zinc oxide	80
Zinc chloride	48
Zinc succinate	36
Zinc citrate	31
Zinc sulfate	23
Zinc ascorbate	15
Zinc gluconate	14
Zinc amino acid chelate	10

Iron supplements and phytates, found in grains and legumes, can inhibit zinc absorption, and should be ingested at least two hours apart from zinc supplements. Zinc may antagonise the action of immunosuppressant drugs and may increase the effect of cisplatin (a cancer drug). High-dose zinc may reduce the absorption of the following drugs when taken together: the fluoroquinolone and tetracycline classes of antibiotics, penicillamine (a metal chelator), bisphosphonates (for osteoporosis) and non-steroidal anti-inflammatory drugs (NSAIDs). Zinc supplements should be taken two to four hours before or after the drug dose.

HOW MUCH DO I KNOW?

Choose whether the following statements are true or false. Then review this chapter for the correct answers.

	True (T)	False (F)
1 Iron is the most abundant micromineral in the body.	T	F
2 Haem iron is poorly absorbed.	T	F
3 Transferrin is a zinc transporter.	T	F
4 Iron deficiency anaemia can cause a craving for eating ice.	T	F
5 People with restless legs may respond to iron supplementation.	T	F
6 ZIP4 is a transporter that facilitates iron uptake in the digestive tract.	T	F
7 Zinc fingers are involved in gene expression.	T	F
8 Zinc maintains the integrity of the intestinal barrier.	T	F
9 Phytate in food can reduce absorption of zinc.	T	F
10 Zinc is essential for growth and the development of sex organs in males at puberty.	T	F

FURTHER READING

Braun, L. & Cohen, M., *Herbs & natural supplements: An evidence-based guide*, 3rd ed., Churchill Livingstone Elsevier, New York, 2010.

Gropper, S.S., Smith, J.L. & Groff, J.L., *Advanced nutrition and human metabolism*, 5th ed., Thomson Wadsworth, Belmont, CA, 2009.

Higdon, J., *An evidence-based approach to vitamins and minerals*, Thieme, New York, 2003.

Linus Pauling Institute, Micronutrient Research Center, website, available at <lpi.oregonstate.edu/infocenter>.

11

Trace elements: copper, manganese and iodine

COPPER

COPPER STATUS CHECK

1 Do you have loose, wrinkled, pale skin and coarse, tangled hair that is extremely difficult to manage?
2 Do you have hypermobile joints or bones that fracture easily?
3 Do you have chronic anaemia or elevated blood pressure, serum cholesterol and blood fats?
4 Do you have numbness, pins and needles, or tingling in your arms and/or legs?

'Yes' answers may indicate inadequate copper status. Note that a number of nutritional deficiencies or health disorders can cause similar effects and further investigation is recommended.

FAST FACTS . . . COPPER

- Good sources of copper include shellfish, organ meats, whole grains, legumes, nuts, potatoes, dark-green leafy vegetables, dried fruit, cocoa, chocolate, black pepper and yeast.
- Copper is required for energy production, iron metabolism, connective tissue integrity, blood clotting, nerve and brain function, and antioxidant protection.
- A deficiency can cause weak connective tissue, defective melanin production, liver damage, anaemia, cardiovascular disorders, impaired glucose tolerance, inflammation and lowered immunity.
- Menkes disease is a genetic copper deficiency disorder and Wilson's disease is a genetic copper toxicity disorder.

Copper is a naturally occurring mineral that is found in the environment as various copper salts, mainly as chalcopyrite (a sulfide of copper and iron), and also as bornite, covellite and chalcocite. Copper was discovered in about 9000 BCE in the Middle East, and was the first metal used by early humans because it was easily shaped into tools.

Copper (cuprum) derives its name from the Latin *aes Cyprium*, meaning 'metal of Cyprus', because the island of Cyprus was an important source of copper. It has the chemical symbol Cu, and is found in biological systems in two forms: cuprous (Cu^{+}) and cupric (Cu^{2+}), which is the most common ionic form. Copper was a common medicine used throughout history for various disorders, including infections, wound healing, and skin and eye diseases. It was established as an essential trace element in 1928, when it was discovered that a copper-deficient diet in rats led to impaired production of red blood cells. Nineteenth-century Italian and French physicians found that copper sulfate was an effective treatment for iron-deficiency anaemia that did not respond to iron supplementation, and in 1885, the French physician Luton reported using copper acetate for the treatment of arthritis.

Copper forms tight bonds with proteins, and has a higher affinity for proteins than that of most other metals. Because copper has the ability to exist in two oxidation states, copper-containing proteins can take part in redox reactions in the body, and are essential for cellular respiration, free radical defence, melanin synthesis, connective tissue formation and iron metabolism. Copper has the potential to act as an oxidant and generate damaging reactive oxygen species (ROS), and protein binding is a protective mechanism that reduces copper toxicity. The highest concentrations of copper are found in the brain, kidneys, liver and heart.

Digestion, absorption and transport

Copper is found in food bound to amino acids. During digestion, pepsin and other protease enzymes release copper, and the presence of hydrochloric acid in the stomach increases its solubility. Copper uptake is believed to be increased by binding to ligands, such as the amino acids histidine, cysteine, methionine and lysine, as well as picolinic acid present in digestive juices. At low dietary levels, copper is absorbed into enterocytes as the cuprous form by an active carrier-mediated process involving the copper transporter 1 (CTR1) and possibly the divalent metal transporter 1 (DMT1). At higher levels of intake, copper is absorbed by passive diffusion.

In enterocytes, copper is passed into the bloodstream by the action of the copper exporter P-type ATPase 7A (ATP7A), and binds mainly to the serum proteins albumin and alpha-2-macroglobulin for transport to the liver and other tissues. A small amount is transported in association with the protein transcuprein, and the amino acids histidine and cysteine.

Metabolism, storage and excretion

In the liver, copper is taken up via CTR1, and is rapidly bound to proteins to protect cells against copper-induced oxidation. Copper can be either stored in liver cells as metallothioneins (MTs), transferred to chaperone proteins for delivery to a variety of essential copper proteins, incorporated into ceruloplasmin (CP), the major copper transporter in the bloodstream, and secreted back into the circulation, or excreted in bile. The liver copper exporter ATP7B, also found in the kidneys, mammary glands, brain and eyes, is required for the production of CP and the excretion of copper into bile.

Copper in the blood is taken up by tissue cells by the activity of CTR1, with the assistance of ascorbic acid, which reduces cupric copper to the cuprous form. It is rapidly bound to glutathione and transferred to MTs or other copper-binding proteins. Copper bound to MTs can be carried by the transporter CTR2 into intracellular vesicles for temporary storage. A variety of transporters, exporters and chaperone proteins are involved in copper metabolism within cells. The copper exporter ATP7A, in conjunction with chaperone proteins such as the copper transport proteins ATOX1, CCS2 and COX17, transfers copper from the cytosol to the secretory pathway of the Golgi apparatus for incorporation into various copper-dependent enzymes.

There is limited storage of copper in the body. Most of the body's stores are in the liver in the form of copper proteins, chaperones and MTs, and there is a small intracellular store in most other tissues. Copper is excreted mainly in bile, some of which is reabsorbed in the digestive tract; the remainder is excreted in faeces. Small amounts of copper are excreted in urine and trace amounts are lost in sweat, skin cells, hair, nails and semen, and during menstruation. Daily copper losses are estimated to be 1.3 mg in adults.

Regulation of body levels

In cells, copper levels are regulated by the copper exporters ATP7A and ATP7B, which actively transport copper out of cells. They are normally found in the trans-Golgi network (TGN), but when copper levels rise, they move to intracellular vesicles located near cell membranes and facilitate export of copper from the cell. When copper levels return to normal, these exporters return to the TGN. Two chaperones, copper metabolism MURR1 domain (COMMD1) and clusterin, appear to interact to down-regulate ATP7A and ATP7B.

The liver is the major regulator of total body copper status. ATP7B triggers excretion of copper in bile when copper levels rise, and excretion is reduced when copper levels are low. Changes in absorption also regulate copper levels; absorption of copper increases or decreases according to the amount in the diet. In response to a low copper diet, CTR1 levels in the intestinal wall increase in order to increase absorption and CTR1 is broken down if copper intake is high.

Functions

Copper is an essential cofactor for about twelve enzymes in which copper is bound to specific amino acid residues in an active site. Copper enzymes include cytochrome c oxidase, used in mitochondrial electron transfer; copper and zinc-containing superoxide dismutases (SOD1 and SOD3), used for quenching the superoxide radical; dopamine beta-monooxygenase, used for conversion of the neurotransmitter dopamine to noradrenaline; lysyl oxidase, used for cross-linking elastin and collagen in connective tissue; peptidylglycine alpha-amidating monooxygenase (PAM), used to activate neuropeptides; CP and hephaestin, used for iron transport and metabolism; and amine oxidases and diamine oxidases, used for the breakdown of amines such as neurotransmitters, histamine and xenobiotics. Like zinc, copper binds to transcription factors and modulates gene expression. The functions of copper include the following:

- *Energy production.* In the electron transport chain in mitochondria, the copper enzyme cytochrome c oxidase receives electrons from cytochrome c and passes them to oxygen to form water. This process is required for creating the difference in proton electrochemical potential across the mitochondrial membrane that drives energy (ATP) production.
- *Antioxidant protection.* Copper is part of the enzymes SOD1, found in cell cytoplasm, and SOD3, found in extracellular compartments, that are important antioxidants. They react with superoxide radicals, produced as a by-product of cellular metabolism, to form oxygen and hydrogen peroxide, which is broken down by catalases and the glutathione system. Copper is an essential component in this reaction and cannot be replaced by any other metal. SOD1 has also been found to have a regulating role in energy pathways and the immune response. SOD3 is produced and secreted by vascular smooth muscle cells and fibroblasts, and appears to protect the heart and blood vessels from oxidative damage. The copper chaperone ATOX1 has recently been found to have antioxidant properties. MTs have antioxidant activity because their multiple sulfhydryl groups can interact with ROS and they can sequester copper and prevent it from acting as a pro-oxidant.
- *Connective tissue integrity.* Lysyl oxidase is a copper-dependent enzyme that oxidises the lysyl residues of collagen and elastin in the extracellular matrix of connective tissue. This enables the formation of cross-links that resist breakdown by proteolytic enzymes and provide strength to connective tissue in body structures such as bones, tendons, ligaments, joints, blood vessels and the skin. In addition, four lysyl oxidase-like (LOXL) proteins have been identified that have a role in the regulation of cell processes such as chemotactic responses, cell proliferation and tumour cell invasion and metastasis.
- *Wound healing.* During wound healing, glycyl-L-histidyl-L-lysine (GHK), a growth-modulating tripeptide that complexes with copper, reduces oxidative damage to tissue after injury and activates tissue remodelling. Copper stimulates the formation of new blood vessels in the area of damage (angiogenesis), and enhances the expression of integrin, a regulator of cell signalling, cell cycle and cell shape and motility. It also stabilises fibronectin, a cell-adhesion glycoprotein found in the extracellular matrix that assists healing, and is essential for activity of lysyl oxidase that assists matrix remodelling.
- *Iron metabolism.* In enterocytes, the copper-containing oxidase hephaestin, in conjunction with CP, oxidises ferrous iron to the ferric form to enable it to bind to the iron transport protein transferrin. CP assists ferroportin 1-mediated mobilisation of iron from the liver. Another copper-containing oxidase, zyklopen, assists transport of iron across the placenta during pregnancy. Copper also plays an essential role in the production of haem and protoporphyrin for red blood cell formation, and maintaining the lifespan of red blood cells.
- *Nerve and hormone function, skin pigmentation.* Copper helps support energy production, and provides antioxidant protection in the nervous and endocrine systems. Specific copper-rich sites in the nervous system include the basal ganglia, hippocampus,

cerebellum, synaptic membranes and the cell bodies of cortical pyramidal and cerebellar granule neurons. The enzyme tyrosinase is a copper-containing oxidase that converts tyrosine to L-dopa, the precursor of dopamine, and helps produce pigments such as melanins in the skin. Dopamine beta-monooxygenase is a copper-containing enzyme that works with vitamin C to convert dopamine to the neurotransmitter noradrenaline that plays a major role in alertness, arousal, the stress response and reward-motivated behaviour, and also has anti-inflammatory activity and helps control motor functions and the release of several hormones.

Copper modulates transmission of nerve impulses from cell to cell via synapses by binding to voltage-gated calcium channels that are essential for synaptic nerve transmission, binding to receptors for the inhibitory neurotransmitter gamma-aminobutyric acid (GABA), and binding to N-methyl-D-aspartate (NMDA) receptors that are important for controlling synaptic plasticity and memory function. Copper appears to be essential for the formation and repair of myelin, the insulating sheath around nerve cell axons that facilitates nerve transmission, and for the production of enkephalins that elevate mood and provide pain relief.

The copper enzyme PAM activates and stabilises peptides in the nervous and endocrine systems by adding an alpha-amide group, a process called amidation. Peptide hormones that require amidation include calcitonin, that helps regulate calcium levels: gastrin, that stimulates stomach acid secretion; and cholecystokinin, that stimulates release of bile and pancreatic secretions.

- *Detoxification.* Copper amine and diamine oxidases help break down amines to aldehydes and play an important role in the breakdown of histamine, neurotransmitters and xenobiotics.
- *Immune function.* CP levels increase in inflammation and infections in order to deliver copper to sites of immune activity. Copper has antimicrobial properties because it can induce oxidation and disrupt the protein structure of pathogens. It supports macrophage activity by assisting in the generation of the respiratory burst of free radicals that kills micro-organisms. The mechanism is not well understood, but it appears that copper enters vesicles in the cytoplasm of phagocytes, and it may be that the presence of copper enhances conversion of hydrogen peroxide, produced by SOD, to the highly reactive and destructive hydroxyl radical.
- *Blood clotting.* Blood clotting is dependent on the sequential activation of blood-clotting proteins (factors), and factor V and factor VIII contain copper, which appears to enhance their activity.

Dietary sources

Good sources of copper include shellfish such as oysters, mussels, crab and lobster, organ meats, whole grains, legumes, nuts, potatoes, dark-green leafy vegetables, dried fruit, cocoa, chocolate, black pepper and yeast. Dairy products are poor sources. Bioavailability is higher from animal sources, but the copper content of a vegetarian diet is generally higher and, overall, vegetarian diets lead to greater copper intake. Copper can be bound by phytate, but evidence suggests that this is not a significant inhibitor of absorption. In general, copper levels in Australian water supplies average 0.8 mg/L.

The Food Standards Australia New Zealand nutrient database (NUTTAB) at <www.foodstandards.gov.au> provides the amounts found in specific foods.

Factors influencing body status

Absorption of copper is considerably greater than for most other trace elements, ranging from 20–70 per cent, and varies according to body status. Absorption increases if copper status is inadequate, during pregnancy and in cancer. In lactating animals, a large amount of copper is diverted to breast tissue rather than the liver and kidneys, particularly in the early stages of lactation. An infant's absorption of copper from breast milk averages 60 per cent, but averages only 15 per cent from cow's milk.

High amounts of zinc, iron, molybdenum, lead or cadmium reduce copper absorption by either competing for transport pathways or increasing MTs in the intestine that bind copper, with zinc and cadmium having the most potent inhibiting effect. However, iron supplements do not appear to inhibit copper absorption. The effect of calcium is unclear, with some studies showing reduced copper absorption and others showing increased absorption. Antacid medication and fructose intake impair copper absorption.

Copper can leach out of copper cookware and household utensils, and increase levels in food. Enhancers of copper absorption include sulfur-containing amino acids, such as histidine, methionine, cysteine and glutathione, and acids that increase copper solubility, such as stomach acid, and the organic acids citric, lactic, malic and acetic acid. Some studies have indicated that vitamin C (ascorbic acid) may impair copper absorption, but a study of healthy young men living in a controlled environment found that copper absorption, copper retention, total serum copper and CP levels were not affected by changes in vitamin C intake. However, 650 mg daily of vitamin C decreased the oxidase activity of serum CP by an average of 21 per cent. The relevance of this to health is not known. A lack of vitamin C may impair the copper-dependent conversion of dopamine to noradrenaline.

Copper levels reduce considerably after gastric surgery for obesity. Drugs that may reduce copper levels include the calcium channel blocker nifedipine (used for angina and high blood pressure), allopurinol (used for gout) and the metal chelator penicillamine (used for copper toxicity and rheumatoid arthritis). Serum copper levels are considerably elevated in response to inflammation and infections, and the use of oral contraceptives and female hormone replacement therapy (HRT) may also increase serum levels.

Table 11.1 Adequate intake (AI) of copper (mg/day)

Age (years)	Female AI	Male AI
1–3	0.7	0.7
4–8	1	1
9–13	1.1	1.3
14–18	1.1	1.5
19–70	1.2	1.7
>70	1.2	1.7
Pregnant women		
14–18	1.2	
19–50	1.3	
Lactating women		
14–18	1.4	
19–50	1.5	

Source: Nutrient Reference Values for Australia and New Zealand Including Recommended Dietary Intakes, National Health and Medical Research Council, Australian Government Department of Health and Ageing, Canberra and Ministry of Health, New Zealand, Wellington, 2006.

Daily requirement

Australian and New Zealand government recommendations by age and gender (see Table 11.1) can be found in *Nutrient Reference Values for Australia and New Zealand Including Recommended Dietary Intakes*, available at <www.nhmrc.gov.au>.

Deficiency effects

Copper deficiency was first identified in farm animals, in which it causes osteoporosis, anaemia, neutropenia (decreased levels of neutrophils), rupture of the arteries, and lesions and demyelination of the spinal cord. In animal studies, treatment with the copper chelator cuprizone kills mature myelin-producing oligodendrocytes and demyelinates nerve axons. When cuprizone is withdrawn, remyelination occurs. Cardiovascular effects in animals include fissures and rupture of the aorta, atherosclerotic changes in artery walls, heart enlargement and rupture, clots in the coronary arteries and heart attacks. In sheep, copper deficiency causes paralysis of the hind legs ('swayback'), reduced elastin in lung tissue, lack of pigmentation of wool and 'steely wool', which is a loss of crimp and a coarse texture. Severe copper deficiency in animals lacking the gene for CTR1 has been shown to be lethal. Effects include decreased SOD activity, elevated serum cholesterol, triglycerides and uric acid, glucose intolerance, reduced haemoglobin levels, heart rhythm abnormalities and sudden death due to heart rupture.

Copper deficiency is rarely diagnosed in humans and severe deficiency is rare, but marginal or unrecognised deficiencies may exist. Deficiencies may occur after gastric surgery for obesity or after penicillamine chelation therapy; in preterm infants because of insufficient liver stores; in people on parenteral (non-oral) nutrition that is inadequate in copper; in people with severe malabsorption disorders such as coeliac or Crohn's disease; in kidney disorders, in which copper losses are increased; or following long-term, high-dose zinc supplementation.

The average intake of copper by women of childbearing age is believed to be lower than the adequate intake, and marginal deficiencies may occur in pregnancy. Inadequate copper status in pregnancy can lead to spontaneous abortion, prolonged pregnancy, premature rupture of the foetal and placental membranes, and brain abnormalities and connective tissue defects in infants. Infants of women who took metal-chelating drugs during pregnancy have been born with loose, wrinkled skin, hypermobile joints, fragile veins and many soft tissue abnormalities.

In adults, copper deficiency appears to affect the liver, and the nervous and cardiovascular systems, in particular. It has been associated with anaemia, impaired neurological function, bone malformations, low bone mineral density, spontaneous fractures, impaired melanin production, joint and skin abnormalities, lowered immunity, abnormal blood lipids and cardiovascular disease (CVD). In a study of experimentally induced copper deficiency in humans, low copper caused a marked lowering of plasma enkephalins, which rapidly returned to normal when copper was supplied. Some subjects developed serious heart abnormalities, including heart attacks, rapid heartbeat and heart block, and had to be removed from the study. Other human studies have found that low copper is associated with decreased immune response, altered blood clotting, impaired bone metabolism and increased markers of oxidation.

Bone effects

Copper is required for the connective tissue enzyme lysyl oxidase that forms mature collagen in bone and other tissues. Infants with low copper levels develop bone changes that are similar to those of scurvy, including sub-periosteal bleeding (bleeding under the surface membrane of bone), low bone density and multiple spontaneous bone fractures that may be misdiagnosed as child abuse. Enlargement of the costochondral junctions is similar to the effects of rickets. The growth plates of long bones show abnormalities, which include concavity, flaring, irregularities, spur formation and fractures at spur sites. Commonly affected bones include the lower femur, the upper tibia, the lower tibia and the distal radius and ulna. Low copper may be associated with osteoporosis in older adults.

Blood cell effects

Copper deficiency causes hypochromic, normocytic or macrocytic anaemia that does not respond to iron or vitamin B12 therapy. It features decreased haemoglobin, haematocrit and red blood cell count, and elevated serum erythropoietin (a bone marrow-stimulating hormone). Bone marrow abnormalities include the presence of vacuoles in myeloid precursor cells, iron granules in plasma cells, a decrease in granulocyte precursors and immature red blood cells containing iron around the nuclei (ring sideroblasts).

In a recent nationwide study in Scotland, sixteen patients were identified with copper deficiency. In fifteen patients, the initial signs were anaemia, neutropenia, and decreased levels of platelets (thrombocytopenia). Twelve patients had neurological impairment, including progressive walking difficulties and paraesthesia. Investigations revealed abnormalities of the subcortical white matter and spinal cord, and atrophy of the cerebrum and cerebellum. Copper supplementation was effective in reversing the blood abnormalities in all but one patient. However, only 25 per cent had improved neurological function on copper replacement, 33 per cent deteriorated and 42 per cent had no change.

Cardiovascular effects

Copper deficiency is a possible contributing factor to CVD. The effects of a deficiency include high blood pressure, elevated uric acid levels, impaired glucose tolerance, oxidative damage, inflammation, anaemia, reduced blood clotting and adverse effects on the heart and blood vessels, leading to structural weakness and impaired energy production and function. In animals, a low-copper diet has been found to cause inflammation, elevated serum cholesterol and triglycerides, heart enlargement, heart attacks, aortic fissures and rupture, thickening and loss of elasticity of the wall of the aorta and haemorrhages in the walls of the carotid, coronary and thoracic arteries. Fructose feeding markedly enhances the adverse effects of a low-copper diet in animals. 'Falling disease' in farm animals, in which animals drop dead suddenly, is caused by cardiac fibrosis (the replacement of atrophied heart muscle cells with connective tissue) and is the end result of copper deficiency.

Patients with ischaemic heart disease have been found to have decreased levels of copper in the heart and leukocytes, and decreased activity of some copper-dependent enzymes. Experimental marginally low copper diets in humans have led to increased serum cholesterol and triglycerides, elevated blood pressure, abnormal electrocardiograms (ECGs) and impaired glucose tolerance in some studies. However, other human studies of the effect of copper on serum lipids have shown conflicting results.

Liver effects

A low copper intake is associated with abnormal fat metabolism in the liver, and may be implicated in non-alcoholic fatty liver disease (NAFLD) and non-alcoholic steatohepatitis (NASH). In patients with NAFLD, a lower concentration of copper in the liver is associated with more severe fat accumulation. In animals, copper deficiency leads to increased fat synthesis and iron deposits in the liver, increased lipid peroxidation, metabolic syndrome and liver damage and fat accumulation, which are exacerbated markedly by fructose feeding. Fructose also inhibits the increase in the CTR1 transporter in the gut that is the normal response to copper deficiency. Copper supplementation has been shown to improve NAFLD in an animal study.

Glucose metabolism effects

Copper deficiency in animals leads to altered carbohydrate metabolism, reduced glucose tolerance, reduced insulin secretion, insulin resistance and increases in early and advanced glycation end-products (AGEs), indicators of protein damage.

Neurological effects

A key feature of copper deficiency is neurological dysfunction, such as copper deficiency myelopathy (CDM), a recently identified copper-deficiency syndrome that has very similar features to sub-acute combined degeneration of the spinal cord seen in vitamin B12 deficiency, including bone marrow changes and neurodegenerative symptoms. CDM most frequently appears in middle-aged or older people, particularly women, and may be misdiagnosed as motor neurone disease, sideroblastic anaemia or myelodysplastic syndrome. Patients with CDM have low serum and urinary copper and low CP levels and may have anaemia, leucopenia, polyneuropathy, a spastic ataxic gait, over-active reflexes and sensory loss in the extremities. CDM may be associated with elevated serum zinc. Copper supplementation can prevent further neurological deterioration, but may not reverse the condition completely. It is recommended that copper deficiency be considered in the diagnosis of disorders such as multiple sclerosis, sub-acute combined degeneration of the spinal cord, optic myeloneuropathy, post-gastric reduction surgery neuropathy or, in other cases of myelopathy, optic neuropathy or polyneuropathy associated with a low copper intake or excessive zinc supplementation.

Genetic disorders causing copper deficiency

Menkes disease

Menkes disease (MD) is a genetic disorder of copper metabolism, mainly affecting male infants, that is caused by mutations of the gene for ATP7A. It leads to severe illness and, in most cases, death in early childhood. It was identified as a copper deficiency disease by Dr David Danks in the 1970s at the Royal Children's Hospital in Melbourne, Australia, who noted the similarity between MD and copper deficiency in animals. In MD, infants may be born with spontaneous fractures and haemorrhages affecting the skull, and then develop prolonged jaundice, hypothermia, hypoglycaemia, feeding difficulties, vomiting, diarrhoea, floppiness, sunken chest, umbilical and inguinal hernias and failure to thrive. An early and striking feature of MD is abnormal appearance of the hair ('kinky' hair). Hair is sparse, dull, lacks pigment and forms kinks and tangles that have the appearance of steel wool. Infants may have pale, loose, dry skin, a misshapen skull, a small jaw, pudgy cheeks and an expressionless appearance. Psychomotor development begins to regress at two to four months of age. Therapy-resistant seizures, spasticity, osteoporosis, fractures, hypermobile joints, dermatitis, weakness of the extremities, drowsiness and lethargy develop. The disease may progress to include blindness, subdural haematoma and respiratory failure, and may end in death by the age of three years due to infection, haemorrhages or neurological dysfunction. Subcutaneous injections of copper may relieve some of the symptoms but may not extend lifespan beyond childhood.

Occipital horn syndrome

Occipital horn syndrome (OHS) is the mildest form of MD, and is characterised by connective tissue defects and the appearance of occipital horns, which are symmetrical, downward-pointing outgrowths of the occipital bone. Symptoms in infants are similar to MD, such as wrinkled, loose skin, hernias, hypothermia, jaundice, floppiness and feeding problems. Diarrhoea and recurrent urinary tract infections are common. OHS also features low IQ, poor muscle tone, spinal and skeletal defects, hypermobile joints and facial abnormalities, including a long, thin face, drooping eyes and a large nose and ears. Hair may be coarse and dull. Orthostatic (postural) hypotension, varicose veins and aneurysms of the arteries may occur. Because of its milder presentation, it is usually not diagnosed until five to ten years of age. Treatment is similar to MD and lifespan is usually much longer.

Aceruloplasminaemia

Aceruloplasminaemia is a lack of circulating CP because of a mutation of the CP gene. This leads to impaired iron metabolism, but does not appear to affect copper metabolism. It causes a buildup of iron in tissues, especially the liver, pancreas, retina and central nervous system, and leads to tissue and organ damage. Aceruloplasminaemia is associated with diabetes, degeneration of retinal pigment, involuntary muscle movements, cerebellar ataxia and dementia.

ATP7A-related motor neuropathy

Mutations in the gene for ATP7A have been associated with a form of distal hereditary motor neuropathy that causes abnormal ATP7A activity, affecting motor neuron functions specifically. It features lower motor neuron weakness and muscular atrophy, leading to hand and foot deformities.

Indicators of inadequate levels of copper may include:

- anaemia, leukopenia, neutropenia, decreased haemoglobin, haematocrit and red blood cell count and elevated serum erythropoietin levels, bone marrow abnormalities
- loss of pigmentation of the hair or skin, dermatitis, loose wrinkled skin, coarse tangled 'kinky' hair
- liver damage, fat and iron accumulation in the liver
- brain atrophy, demyelination of nerve fibres, spinal cord lesions, ataxia, optic nerve damage, overactive reflexes, sensory loss in the extremities
- low bone mineral density, spontaneous fractures, osteoporosis, hypermobile joints
- heart attacks, rapid heartbeat, heart enlargement, heart block, aortic aneurysm, haemorrhages, coronary artery thrombosis, high blood pressure, elevated serum cholesterol, triglycerides and uric acid, reduced blood clotting, abnormal ECG
- impaired glucose tolerance, reduced insulin secretion, insulin resistance, increase in AGEs
- lowered immunity, infections, inflammation
- *pregnancy:* spontaneous abortion, prolonged pregnancy, premature rupture of the foetal and placental membranes
- *infants:* brain defects, loose and wrinkled skin, hypermobile joints, pale and tangled hair, fragile veins, prolonged jaundice, hypothermia, hypoglycaemia, feeding difficulties, vomiting, diarrhoea, floppiness, sunken chest, umbilical and inguinal hernias, failure to thrive, seizures, spasticity, bone changes that resemble scurvy or rickets, spontaneous fractures, hypermobile joints, dermatitis, weakness of the extremities, drowsiness, lethargy.

Assessment of body status

Serum or plasma copper concentrations are commonly used to assess copper status, but are difficult to interpret and may not reflect the activity of copper-dependent enzymes in cells. The reference range given by the Royal College of Pathologists of Australasia (RCPA) for plasma or serum copper is 13–22 μmol/L. Low plasma copper is regarded as a good indicator of a moderate to severe deficiency. However, plasma/serum copper may be normal or increased even when copper in tissues is low. Various factors can cause an increase in serum copper, including the acute phase response to infection and inflammation, pregnancy and hormonal disorders, some cancers and smoking. The reference range for the concentration of free copper (copper not bound to proteins) in serum is less than 1.6 μmol/L. Higher levels may indicate a copper toxicity syndrome, such as Wilson's disease.

About 70–80 per cent of plasma copper is associated with CP, and CP levels can be used as a measure of copper status. CP levels decline in a copper deficiency and copper supplementation causes an increase in CP only in people who are moderately or severely copper deficient. However, CP responses are variable in people with marginal deficiencies. The reference range given by the RCPA for plasma or serum CP is 150–450 mg/L.

The level and activity of copper-containing enzymes in blood cells may be better indicators of metabolically active copper and copper stores. However, a review of methods of copper assessment found that measurement of erythrocyte SOD activity was not reliable and that, overall, there was insufficient evidence about the reliability of using copper-containing enzymes as a measure of copper status.

Urinary copper can also be measured, but is not regarded as a good reflection of body levels. However, increased urinary copper may indicate Wilson's disease. The reference range given by the RCPA is less than 1.2 μmol/24 hours. An amount greater than 25 μmol/24 hours indicates possible Wilson's disease.

Case reports—copper deficiency

- *A male infant, two months of age,* with poor muscle tone, lethargy and seizures, was admitted to hospital.[1] He had first been seen when he was eleven days old because of floppiness, red, flaking skin and sparse, brittle hair, but was discharged without diagnosis.

At two months, the skin redness had improved but the hair abnormalities persisted. Examination revealed a severe hypotonia with normal tendon reflexes, lethargy, loose skin and kinky hair. He was found to have epilepsy, brain haemorrhages, spurs on the long bones, metaphyseal widening and wormian bones (extra bone pieces within sutures in the cranium). His serum copper and CP were low. Genetic testing revealed mutations in the ATP7A gene, and he was diagnosed with Menkes disease. He was given subcutaneous copper histidine therapy with no improvement. He died from respiratory failure at the age of two years.

- *A man, 44 years of age*, had experienced generalised fatigue, chronic diarrhoea and tingling and numbness in the lower extremities for six months.[2] He was found to have low leukocyte and haemoglobin levels, and his bone marrow showed ringed sideroblasts and vacuoles in the cytoplasm of red blood cell precursors. He was diagnosed with possible myelodysplasia (a malignant bone marrow disorder) and given blood transfusions and growth factor support, but did not respond. Chemotherapy with a demethylating agent was considered. At that point, an external consultant recommended investigating his copper levels, and he was found to have very low serum copper and CP. He was treated with 2.5 mg intravenous (iv) copper chloride daily for fourteen days. His leukocyte and haemoglobin levels increased, and his bone marrow, serum copper and CP normalised. His fatigue improved considerably and there was some improvement in his paraesthesia. No cause could be found for his copper deficiency.
- *A woman, 38 years of age*, developed progressive fatigue and severe shortness of breath.[3] She became breathless on the slightest exertion. She had been given a Roux-en-Y gastric bypass procedure for obesity sixteen years earlier, and since then had a history of frequent upper respiratory tract infections, urinary tract infections and yeast infections. Blood tests revealed leukopenia and signs of megaloblastic anaemia, and she was given blood transfusions. Further investigations discovered that she had become clumsy during the past two years and that her legs fell asleep easily, she felt unbalanced and she could not walk in the dark or on uneven ground. She had also developed shooting pains in her legs, and tingling and numbness in her arms and legs. A bone marrow biopsy showed the presence of vacuoles in red blood cell precursors and ringed sideroblasts. Her doctors could not identify a cause, and she was eventually screened for heavy metal toxicity, which revealed severely low serum copper levels and abnormally high serum zinc. She was given copper iv for two days, which improved the anaemia and leukopenia. She was then prescribed multivitamins and 6 mg of oral copper daily. Two months later, her anaemia and leukopenia had resolved. Her paraesthesia symptoms were still present but had not progressed.

REFERENCES

1 Galve, J., Vicente, A., González-Enseñat, M.A. et al., Neonatal erythroderma as a first manifestation of Menkes disease, *Pediatrics* (2012), 130(1): e239–42.

2 Sharma, V.R., Copper deficiency: Clinical review of an obscure imitator, *J Med Sci* (2012), 32(1): 1–7.

3 Khambatta, S., Nguyen, D.L. & Wittich, C.M., 38-year-old woman with increasing fatigue and dyspnea, *Mayo Clin Proc* (2010), 85(4): 392–5.

THERAPEUTIC USES OF COPPER

Copper is used primarily for the prevention and treatment of copper deficiency or zinc overload. Oral copper supplementation is ineffective for MD because there is impaired transport of copper from the intestine to tissues. Intravenous or subcutaneous copper histidine appears to be the most effective treatment, but must begin as early as possible, preferably within the first two weeks of life. A case of MD diagnosed before birth was treated with copper histidine (900 mcg per dose), administered directly to the foetus by intramuscular injection, which was effective in increasing serum copper and CP, and daily copper histidine therapy (250 mcg subcutaneously twice daily) was given immediately after birth.[1] However, the infant showed floppiness, developmental delay and ECG abnormalities, and died of respiratory failure at five and a half months of age. Genetic testing revealed a genetic mutation leading to a complete absence of ATP7A. Infants with partially functional ATP7A respond better and some live up to the age of thirteen years or more.

Copper complexes are currently being investigated for use as drugs that can act as antimicrobial, antiviral, anti-inflammatory and anti-tumour agents, enzyme inhibitors or nucleases.[2] Copper complexes of non-steroidal anti-inflammatory drugs (NSAIDs) have been found to have enhanced anti-inflammatory and anti-ulcer activity, and less gastrointestinal toxicity compared with standard NSAIDs. Copper complexes show promise as antimicrobials for HIV or H1N1 viruses (swine flu) and antibiotic-resistant bacteria. Binary Cu^{2+} chelate complexes may be useful in cancer therapy because they are able to trigger cell apoptosis or inhibit enzyme activity.[2] Ternary Cu^{2+} complexes have shown anti-inflammatory, antibacterial and anticancer activity against various cell lines. These copper complexes have the ability to destroy cells directly by causing dysfunction and cleavage of proteins and DNA, as well as indirectly by producing destructive ROS.

Copper bracelets are popularly used for arthritis, and there are subjective reports of improvements in symptoms. Copper metal as powder applied to the skin has been found to oxidise and penetrate the stratum corneum after forming an ion pair with skin exudates.[3] However, one study found that copper bracelets were generally ineffective for managing pain, stiffness and physical function in osteoarthritis patients.[4] The effectiveness of copper skin patches is yet to be determined.

REFERENCES

1 Haddad, M.R., Macri, C.J., Holmes, C.S. et al., In utero copper treatment for Menkes disease associated with a severe ATP7A mutation, *Mol Genet Metab* (2012), 107(1–2): 222–8.

2 Iakovidis, I., Delimaris, I. & Piperakis, S.M., Copper and its complexes in medicine: A biochemical approach, *Mol Biol Int* (2011): 594529.

3 Hostýnek, J.J., Dreher, F. & Maibach, H.I., Human stratum corneum penetration by copper: In vivo study after occlusive and semi-occlusive application of the metal as powder, *Food Chem Toxicol* (2006), 44(9): 1539–43.

4 Richmond, S.J., Brown, S.R., Campion, P.D. et al., Therapeutic effects of magnetic and copper bracelets in osteoarthritis: A randomised placebo-controlled crossover trial, *Complement Ther Med* (2009), 17(5–6): 249–56.

Therapeutic dose

Zinc and copper need to be in balance in the body, and copper supplementation is recommended if high doses of zinc (more than 40 mg daily) are given long term. The optimal ratio of zinc to copper appears to be 5:1. Suggested doses of elemental copper for adults are as follows:

- *Health maintenance:* 1–2 mg daily.
- *Mild deficiency:* 2 mg daily.
- *Severe deficiency:* iv copper supplementation followed by oral doses of 2 mg or more daily, reducing as serum copper and CP levels normalise.
- *MD/OHS:* 500 mcg daily delivered subcutaneously for life.
- *General therapeutic dose:* 2 mg daily.

Effects of excess

Copper toxicity can cause jaundice, weakness, tremors, loss of appetite and haemolytic crisis, leading to liver, kidney and brain damage. Liver damage appears to be the most common effect. In animals, chronic intake of copper sulfate in amounts greater than 100 times the daily requirement has caused inflammation, necrosis and liver damage. Other studies report damage to the kidneys.

In clinical trials, 2 mg of elemental copper is a standard dose, and is not associated with adverse effects. Short-term doses of 4–10 mg of copper daily and 0.14–0.17 mg copper/kg body weight/day taken for several months have not been associated with adverse effects on the liver in adults. High one-off doses of copper cause salivation, a metallic taste, upper abdominal pain, nausea, vomiting and diarrhoea, and can be fatal.

According to the World Health Organization (WHO), the fatal oral dose of copper salts is about 200 mg/kg body weight. The WHO has advised that the safe upper level of copper in drinking water is 2 mg/L. A daily intake greater than 4.8 mg of copper from drinking water may cause gastric irritation.

Chronic exposure to excess copper is associated with liver damage in children, but this is less common in adults. In children, copper toxicity is associated with Indian childhood cirrhosis (ICC) and childhood idiopathic chronic toxicosis (ICT), both of which may involve predisposing genetic factors. ICC involves massive copper overload in the liver, and has been caused by feeding infants animal milk that has been stored or heated in copper or brass containers, causing the milk to have 50–100 times more copper than breast milk. ICT involves liver damage attributed to copper overload in the water supply, or the use of copper utensils to prepare or store infant foods.

Wilson's disease

Wilson's disease is an inherited disease of abnormal copper metabolism caused by a variety of mutations in the gene for ATP7B. There is impaired excretion of copper in bile and a deficiency of serum CP, which lead to elevated amounts of free copper in the bloodstream and in tissues. Previously, Wilson's disease was regarded as a copper overload condition, but it now appears that excess levels of free copper are the main cause of the pathology. Free copper damages the liver, the brain and the cornea of the eyes, and liver damage commonly leads to acute hepatitis, chronic active hepatitis, cirrhosis and acute liver failure. Effects usually become apparent after seven years of age, and include chronic liver disease, neurological or psychiatric dysfunction, kidney malfunction and abnormalities of the eyes, blood and bones. Effects on the nervous system include speech difficulties, tremor, twitches, involuntary muscle movements, seizures, ataxia, drooling, Parkinsonism and eye movement abnormalities. Cognitive impairment may lead to impulsivity, promiscuity, impaired social judgement, apathy, decreased attention span, mood swings, slowness of thinking, poor ability to plan and make decisions, personality changes and memory loss.

Patients with Wilson's disease may develop copper deposits in the cornea, known as Kayser-Fleischer (KF) rings, which appear as partial or complete brown or brownish-green rings around the outer section of the iris of the eye. Other effects of copper toxicity include kidney stones, gallstones, osteoporosis, osteomalacia, arthritis, joint pain, scanty or absent menstruation, heart fibrosis, inflammation of the heart muscle, postural hypertension and pancreatic dysfunction.

Although copper levels are high in tissues in Wilson's disease, serum concentrations of copper and CP are low, and copper excretion in urine is increased. Dietary copper restriction has little effect on the course of the disease. Treatment of Wilson's disease often involves copper-chelating agents such as penicillamine, trientine or thiomolybdate, and high-dose oral zinc supplementation (40–50 mg/day). Zinc induces MTs that bind copper in the mucosa of the gut, and lead to its excretion in faeces. However, chelation therapy appears to aggravate copper intoxication and cause a worsening of symptoms. A newer approach uses high-dose zinc as the sole therapy in order to normalise free copper concentrations. In patients with neurological effects, it is important that treatment begins promptly after diagnosis because a delay of one month or more is associated with a poorer outcome and some degree of permanent disability.

Coronary heart disease

Because of the ability of copper to enhance oxidation, high copper levels have been suggested as a possible risk factor for coronary heart disease (CHD). Serum copper and CP levels are higher in patients with CHD, but this appears to be caused by the acute phase response that occurs in all inflammatory disorders. CHD is associated with copper deficiency rather than excess, and there is no evidence of higher rates of CHD in patients with Wilson's disease.

Alzheimer's disease

Disruption of copper homeostasis and an increase in free copper is considered to be a factor in Alzheimer's disease (AD). Increased levels of free copper have been found in parts of the brain most affected by AD. Proteins involved in AD pathology, such as amyloid precursor protein, amyloid-beta and tau, are copper-binding proteins with key roles in brain metal regulation. Mutations of ATP7B have been identified as a risk factor for AD, and AD has similar neurological features to Wilson's disease, which is also associated with an increase in free copper.

According to the metal hypothesis of AD, the interaction of amyloid-beta with specific metals—especially copper—promotes the aggregation of amyloid-beta and neurotoxicity. Amyloid-beta can bind copper and zinc but, in conditions of acidosis, copper completely displaces zinc. Treatment with copper and iron chelators has been shown to inhibit the toxic effect of amyloid-beta on nerve cells, whereas replacing copper and iron restores toxicity.

Prion diseases

Prion diseases are caused by a change in the normal prion protein (PrPC) in the brain to an infectious, toxic form (PrPSc) that disrupts nerve function, leading to a range of neurodegenerative disorders referred to as transmissible spongiform encephalopathies (TSEs), of which the best known is 'mad cow' disease. The role of PrPC in the brain is not clear, and it has been suggested that it may act as a copper-binding transport protein. In animals, copper binding to PrPC increases its conversion to PrPSc, and copper chelation delays the onset of prion disease. The role of copper in prion diseases has yet to be established.

Case reports—copper excess

- *A man, 26 years of age*, took 30 mg of copper daily for 30 months and then 60 mg daily for another twelve months because he believed it was a performance enhancer.[1] He developed acute liver failure and required an emergency liver transplant, which had a successful outcome.
- *A boy, 16 years of age*, developed involuntary snake-like movements of his tongue over a six-week period.[2] The movements did not interfere with swallowing or speech, and were not present during sleep. He also developed a flapping-like motion of his hands, sudden jumping movements of his legs, and tilting movements of his neck and torso. No cause could be found after thorough examination and blood testing. His CP and copper levels were low, and his urinary copper excretion was normal. Challenge with the copper-chelating agent penicillamine considerably increased his urinary copper excretion, but it was lower than the cut-off level for diagnosis of Wilson's disease. His symptoms worsened after this challenge. Genetic testing for Wilson's disease was negative, and there were no other indications of Wilson's disease. However, copper toxicity was suspected, and he was given oral zinc gluconate (50 mg three times daily). Eight weeks later, his involuntary movements had disappeared, although his copper and CP levels had not yet normalised.
- *A woman, eighteen years of age*, developed slight rigidity of both arms and KF rings in the irises of both eyes.[3] Her urinary copper concentration was about three times higher than normal, her serum copper and CP concentrations were in the low-normal range and her free copper was elevated. She was diagnosed with Wilson's disease, and was given 200 mg of zinc sulfate three times daily, providing a total of 135 mg daily of elemental zinc. Her free serum copper and urinary copper concentrations normalised and her signs and symptoms resolved.
- *A woman, nineteen years of age*, developed haemolytic anaemia and acute liver failure that required liver transplantation, but a donor organ was not available.[3] While on the transplant waiting list, it was found that she had a high concentration of urinary copper and elevated free copper in her serum. She was diagnosed with Wilson's disease and given a total of 135 mg daily of elemental zinc as zinc sulfate. She made a rapid recovery and was removed from the transplant waiting list.

REFERENCES

1 O'Donohue, J., Reid, M., Varghese, A. et al., A case of adult chronic copper self-intoxication resulting in cirrhosis, *Eur J Med Res* (1999), 4(6): 252.
2 Goez, H.R., Jacob, F.D. & Yager, J.Y., Lingual dyskinesia and tics: A novel presentation of copper-metabolism disorder, *Pediatrics* (2011), 127(2): e505–8.
3 Hoogenraad, T.U., Paradigm shift in treatment of Wilson's disease: Zinc therapy now treatment of choice, *Brain Dev* (2006), 28(3): 141–6.

Supplements

Copper is available in multivitamin and mineral supplements in tablets and capsules, but is not often used as a single supplement. The permitted forms of copper salts in oral supplements in Australia include copper gluconate, cupric citrate, cupric citrate hemipentahydrate, cupric oxide, cupric sulfate anhydrous, cupric sulfate monohydrate and cupric sulfate pentahydrate. The maximum permitted amount of copper per daily dose in a supplement product is regulated as follows:

- *copper gluconate:* a maximum of 5 mg elemental copper
- *cupric citrate, cupric citrate hemipentahydrate:* a maximum of 750 mcg elemental copper
- *cupric oxide, cupric sulfate anhydrous, cupric sulfate monohydrate, cupric sulfate pentahydrate:* no restriction.

In animals, most forms of copper salts are highly bioavailable. However, cupric oxide has less than 40 per cent of the bioavailability of copper chloride in sheep, and has virtually zero bioavailability in chicks and pigs. Copper amino acids and copper proteinate have been reported to have better absorption than cupric sulfate. The amount of elemental copper in a specific copper salt is listed on the product container, and may vary between individual products. The approximate elemental copper content of some common salts is shown in Table 11.2.

Table 11.2 Elemental copper content of common salts

Salt	Copper content (%)
Copper oxide	80
Cupric sulfate	40
Cupric citrate	37
Copper gluconate	14

- *Cupric oxide* has a high concentration of copper and is acid soluble, but appears to be largely unavailable for absorption from the gut and is not recommended as a supplement. It can be commercially manufactured by pyrolysis of copper nitrate or copper carbonate or by the addition of hydroxide to a copper salt solution and subsequent dehydration.
- *Copper gluconate* is relatively low in copper, but is water soluble and well absorbed. It is more stable than cupric sulfate and is prepared commercially by the reaction of gluconic acid derived from glucose with cupric oxide.
- *Cupric sulfate* is relatively high in elemental copper, is soluble in water and is less expensive than copper gluconate. It can be prepared commercially from the reaction of sulfuric acid with cupric oxide.
- *Cupric citrate* has slightly less elemental copper than cupric sulfate, and is insoluble in water but soluble in acids. It can be produced by reacting copper sulfate with trisodium citrate or by reacting copper ethanoate with citric acid.

Cautions

Zinc supplements can inhibit copper absorption, and should be taken at least two hours apart from copper supplements. The contraceptive pill, hormone replacement therapy for menopausal women and cimetidine, used for ulcers and gastro-oesophageal reflux, can increase blood levels of copper. The effect of this is not clear, but it may be prudent to avoid copper supplementation in excess of the AI if taking these medications. Copper may increase the activity of NSAIDs. Penicillamine, used as a metal chelator and for rheumatoid arthritis, and allopurinol, used for gout, can reduce copper levels. High-dose copper can reduce the absorption of fluoroquinolone antibiotics when taken together; copper supplements should be taken two to four hours before or after the drug dose.

MANGANESE

MANGANESE STATUS CHECK

1 Do you have joint or bone deformities?
2 Do you have abnormally low serum cholesterol?
3 Has your hair lost pigmentation?
4 Do you have scaly, blistery skin rashes?

'Yes' answers may indicate inadequate manganese status. Note that a number of nutritional deficiencies or health disorders can cause similar effects and further investigation is recommended.

FAST FACTS . . . MANGANESE

- **Good sources of manganese include whole grains, wheat germ, bran, legumes, tofu, leafy vegetables, dried fruit, pineapple, chocolate, cinnamon, nuts, seeds and beverages such as coffee, wine and tea.**
- **Manganese is essential for antioxidant protection in mitochondria and the integrity of connective tissue, including joint cartilage, ligaments, tendons and bones.**

- **It plays a role in immune function, amino acid, lipid and carbohydrate metabolism, cholesterol synthesis, regulation of blood glucose, energy production, reproduction and blood clotting.**
- **Deficiency is rare, but can cause weak connective tissue, bone and joint deformities, skin rashes, loss of hair pigmentation and low serum cholesterol.**
- **Long-term exposure to high levels of manganese causes severe, irreversible neurological damage.**

Manganese is a naturally occurring mineral that is found in the environment as various mineral ores, such as pyrolusite (manganese dioxide), rhodochrosite (manganese carbonate) and manganite (manganese oxide hydroxide). It has been used throughout history, in prehistoric times as a pigment for cave paintings and later for making colourless glass. It was first isolated in 1774 by Swedish mineralogist Johan Gottlieb Gahn by heating manganese dioxide with charcoal.

Manganese is believed to derive its name from the Latin *magnes*, meaning 'magnet', because it came from the same region of Magnesia in Greece where magnesium was found. It has the chemical symbol Mn, and is found in biological systems in two forms, Mn^{2+} and Mn^{3+}. Manganese acts as an enzyme activator, and also has a structural role in enzymes in the body, but it can be replaced by magnesium or other minerals in most reactions. It does not act as an oxidant in the body but, in the form of Mn^{3+}, is a good electron acceptor, which enables it to act as a potent antioxidant. The highest concentrations of manganese are found in the pancreas, liver, kidneys and bones.

Digestion, absorption and transport

The digestion, absorption and transport of manganese is not well understood. It is assumed that manganese is bound to amino acids in food, and released by proteases during digestion. Manganese is taken up by enterocytes by active transport via the divalent metal transporter 1 (DMT1) and by passive diffusion. It is transported in the bloodstream as Mn^{2+} bound to alpha-2-macroglobulin and albumin, and a small amount is present as manganese citrate. Some Mn^{2+} is oxidised to Mn^{3+}, possibly by ceruloplasmin, and transported bound to the iron-carrying protein transferrin, or possibly to a specific transmanganin protein.

Cells take up Mn^{2+} from the bloodstream by a variety of metal transporters that may include DMT1, ZIP8, ZIP14, the transferrin receptor (TfR), a manganese citrate transporter and calcium channels. There appears to be competition between manganese and other minerals, such as iron and magnesium, for uptake by cells. Transferrin-bound manganese appears to be taken up by tissues other than the liver. It is believed that the transferrin-Mn^{3+} complex binds to TfR on the cell surface, triggering formation of endosomes that move the complex into the cell where manganese is released as Mn^{2+} by DMT1. Alternatively, Mn^{2+} may be released from the transferrin-Mn^{3+} complex at the cell membrane and transported into the cell independently of transferrin. Manganese crosses the blood–brain barrier by facilitated diffusion, and also by active transport via DMT1, ZIP8 and transferrin, and can accumulate in the brain.

Metabolism, storage and excretion

Intracellular manganese is found mainly in cell mitochondria and nuclei as manganese proteins. It forms tight complexes with other substances, and there is little free manganese in the body. Mn^{2+} is readily transferred to the liver and rapidly excreted in bile, with only a small amount reabsorbed from the gut. There does not appear to be a body store of manganese. There are some losses of manganese in sweat and skin cells, but very little is excreted in urine.

Regulation of body levels

Manganese levels are regulated mainly by changes in the liver excretion of manganese in bile, which is increased when body levels are high and reduced when body levels are low. Also, absorption is increased or decreased according to body status.

Functions

Manganese is an activator of enzymes that include oxidoreductases, transferases, hydrolases, lyases, isomerases and ligases, and is a structural component of the enzymes arginase, glutamine synthetase, phosphoenolpyruvate carboxykinase (PEPCK) and manganese-containing superoxide dismutase (SOD2). Manganese acts as a second messenger in cells by stimulating cyclic adenosine monophosphate (cAMP), and may regulate calcium metabolism. It plays a role in amino acid, lipid and carbohydrate metabolism, antioxidant protection, immune function, cholesterol synthesis, regulation of blood glucose, energy production, reproduction, and connective tissue and bone formation, and works with vitamin K to support blood clotting. The functions of manganese include the following:

- *Connective tissue formation.* Manganese is essential for activating glycosyltransferase and xylosyltransferase enzymes that help produce glycoproteins and glycosaminoglycans (GAGs), which are part of proteoglycans in the extracellular matrix of connective tissue. In this reaction, manganese cannot be replaced by any other mineral. Proteoglycans are required for the integrity of bones, joint cartilage, ligaments, tendons, blood vessels and the skin. Manganese also activates the enzyme prolidase, which breaks down proline-containing components of collagen to form iminodipeptides; these are then broken down into amino acids that can be reused to form collagen for connective tissue maintenance and repair, and wound healing.
- *Antioxidant protection and regulation of cell proliferation.* Manganese is part of the enzyme SOD2 found in cell mitochondria, which is important for protecting mitochondria from superoxide radicals produced by lipid oxidation. SOD2 and mitochondria-generated ROS are believed to be essential for regulating cell division, and a lack of SOD2 leads to abnormal cell proliferation. Manganese plays a role in gene transcription by activating RNA polymerase required for RNA synthesis.
- *Glucose synthesis.* Glucose can be made in the body from non-carbohydrate sources by the action of the manganese-containing enzymes PEPCK and pyruvate carboxylase.
- *Amino acid and neurotransmitter metabolism.* Manganese is part of glutamine synthetase, the enzyme that produces glutamine from glutamate and ammonia. Glutamine forms part of proteins, and is a source of nitrogen for production of nucleotides and non-essential amino acids, including GABA. Glutamine plays a role in immune responses, regulation of pH balance in the kidneys, cell signalling, gene expression and formation of the antioxidant glutathione, and can be used as a substrate for energy production. GABA is an inhibitory neurotransmitter that has a sedative, anti-convulsant effect. Manganese can activate the enzyme catechol-O-methyltransferase (COMT), which helps to break down the catecholamine neurotransmitters dopamine, adrenaline and noradrenaline.
- *Detoxification of ammonia.* In the liver, the manganese-containing enzyme arginase is one of the enzymes of the urea cycle, which detoxifies ammonia by converting arginine to ornithine and urea.
- *Reproductive function.* Manganese supports healthy male and female reproductive functions by its protective antioxidant activity as SOD2.

Dietary sources

Good sources of manganese include whole grains, wheat germ, bran, legumes, tofu, leafy vegetables, dried fruit, pineapple, chocolate, cinnamon, nuts, seeds and beverages such as coffee, wine and tea. There is some manganese in shellfish but, in general, animal foods are poor sources, and vegetarian diets generally supply a greater amount of manganese. It is estimated that the average Australian dietary intake is 5.53 mg/day for men and 2.96 mg/day for women and the average New Zealand intake is estimated to be 4.33 mg/day. However, only about 1–14 per cent of dietary manganese is absorbed, with average absorption estimated to be less than 5 per cent.

Australian drinking water guidelines recommend that tap water should contain no more than 0.5 mg/L of manganese because higher levels may cause manganese toxicity. No more than 0.1 mg/L is preferable for aesthetic reasons; above this level, manganese gives an undesirable taste and can stain plumbing and laundry. In Australia, domestic water supplies commonly have manganese levels of less than 0.01 mg/L.

The Food Standards Australia New Zealand nutrient database (NUTTAB) at <www.foodstandards.gov.au> provides the amounts found in specific foods.

Factors influencing body status

Absorption of manganese is poor and varies according to body status. Absorption is inhibited by non-haem iron, which competes with manganese for uptake in the gut. Other inhibitors may include copper, calcium, magnesium, phosphorus, fibre, phytate, oxalate and tannins. Absorption is increased by citrate and the amino acid histidine. Chronic use of anti-psychotic medication may increase body levels of manganese. In animals, oral resveratrol (a natural constituent of red wine) has been shown to specifically increase SOD2 levels 6-fold and the activity of SOD2 14-fold, which may be one of the mechanisms by which resveratrol exerts its protective effects in the body. The action of manganese on the breakdown of dopamine is inhibited by ascorbic acid, dehydroascorbic acid and vitamin B1.

Daily requirement

Australian and New Zealand government recommendations by age and gender (see Table 11.3) can be found in *Nutrient Reference Values for Australia and New Zealand Including Recommended Dietary Intakes*, available at <www.nhmrc.gov.au>.

Table 11.3 Adequate intake (AI) of manganese (mg/day)

Age (years)	Female AI	Male AI
1–3	2.0	2.0
4–8	2.5	2.5
9–13	2.5	3.0
14–18	3.0	3.5
19–70	5.0	5.5
>70	5.0	5.5
Pregnant women		
14–18	5.0	
19–50	5.0	
Lactating women		
14–18	5.0	
19–50	5.0	

Source: Nutrient Reference Values for Australia and New Zealand Including Recommended Dietary Intakes, National Health and Medical Research Council, Australian Government Department of Health and Ageing, Canberra and Ministry of Health, New Zealand, Wellington, 2006.

Deficiency effects

Manganese deficiency is believed to be rare in humans. In animals, manganese deficiency is associated with depressed SOD2 activity, impaired growth, reproduction and glucose tolerance, altered lipid and carbohydrate metabolism, and abnormalities of bones and connective tissue, such as enlarged joints, slipped tendons, deformed legs with thickened and shortened long bones, and lameness. Experimental deficiency in animals is also associated with testicular degeneration, depigmentation of hair and seizures. Reduced levels of serum HDL cholesterol and HDL apoE have been reported.

Lower concentrations of SOD2 have been implicated in cancer in animals and humans. Tumour cells have very low or absent SOD2 activity, and increased amounts have been shown to be protective against cancer. It is suggested that the gene for SOD2 is a tumour suppressor gene. Animals with no SOD2 in the brain developed severe gait abnormalities and seizures, and were found to have cortical lesions similar to spongiform encephalopathy (prion disease).

In humans, low dietary manganese or low blood and tissue manganese have been associated with osteoporosis, diabetes, atherosclerosis, impaired wound healing and cataracts. Abnormal manganese metabolism may play a role in epilepsy, maple syrup urine disease, phenylketonuria (PKU), amyotrophic lateral sclerosis (ALS, or motor neurone disease) and acromegaly. It has been suggested that manganese deficiency may be associated with Mseleni joint disease, which is endemic in northern Zululand, South Africa. This disease affects most joints—especially the hip—and features displacement of the hip socket and hip dysplasia.

Experimental manganese deficiency was induced in young men fed a purified diet containing 0.01 mg/day of manganese for 10 days and 0.11 mg/day for 30 days. Effects included a scaly, blistery skin rash on the upper torso, reduced serum cholesterol, increased serum calcium and phosphorus concentrations and increased serum alkaline phosphatase activity. Women on a low-manganese diet (less than 1 mg/day) developed altered mood and increased pain during the premenstrual phase of their menstrual cycle. A four-month study of vitamin K deficiency inadvertently induced a manganese deficiency in one male subject. Symptoms included low serum cholesterol levels, scaly dermatitis, hair depigmentation and reduced vitamin K-dependent clotting proteins. Vitamin K supplementation did not reverse the symptoms, which gradually cleared after the end of the experimental diet.

Indicators of inadequate levels of manganese may include:

- bone and joint abnormalities
- loss of pigmentation of the hair
- skin rashes
- impaired glucose tolerance
- low serum cholesterol.

Assessment of body status

Whole-blood manganese is used to assess manganese status, but it is not a reliable indicator because of the relatively short half-life of manganese in the bloodstream. It is used mainly to screen for manganese toxicity but is a better indicator of recent exposure, rather than past exposure. The reference range given by the RCPA for blood manganese is 140–220 nmol/L. Magnetic resonance imaging (MRI) also can detect manganese overload in the brain and reflect recent exposure. Urine levels do not vary with changes in intake, and do not appear to be useful indicators of manganese status.

THERAPEUTIC USES OF MANGANESE

There is very little good evidence that manganese supplementation is useful for health disorders. However, preliminary studies show that it may have potential in osteoporosis, arthritis and diabetes.

Osteoporosis

In female animals without ovaries, manganese supplementation has slowed loss of bone[1] and increased bone mineral density and bone formation.[2]

Arthritis

An animal study found that the local application of SOD2 applied every two days reduced swelling and slowed bone destruction in arthritis, whereas Cu/Zn SOD had no effect.[3] Chondrocytes from osteoarthritic cartilage have been found to have higher intracellular ROS and lower levels of SOD2 in mitochondria.[4] Patients with rheumatoid arthritis have been found to have lower SOD2 levels and lower activity of arginase in synovial fluid in arthritic cartilage, but normal serum levels of SOD2 and normal serum arginase activity.[5]

Diabetes

In animals with diabetes, manganese supplementation has reduced expression of the inflammatory intercellular adhesion molecule 1 (ICAM-1) in artery walls and reduced ROS independently of SOD2.[6] These effects may reduce the risk of endothelial dysfunction—a key factor in atherosclerosis—in diabetes. In animals fed a high-fat diet and supplemented with manganese, serum insulin levels increased and glucose tolerance improved to a level similar to that of animals on a standard diet.[7]

Tardive dyskinesia

Increased free radical levels and decreased SOD2 activity have been found in psychiatric patients who develop the Parkinson's-like condition tardive dyskinesia (TD) on anti-psychotic medication. A study found that schizophrenic patients with a gene for SOD2 that caused it to have increased activity had lower risk of TD.[8] In a small number of psychiatric patients with TD, it was reported that manganese supplementation resulted in complete reversal of symptoms or improvement in all but one subject.[9]

REFERENCE

1 Rico, H., Gómez-Raso, N., Revilla, M. et al., Effects on bone loss of manganese alone or with copper supplement in ovariectomized rats: A morphometric and densitomeric study, *Eur J Obstet Gynecol Reprod Biol* (2000), 90(1): 97–101.

2 Bae, Y.J. & Kim, M.H., Manganese supplementation improves mineral density of the spine and femur and serum osteocalcin in rats, *Biol Trace Elem Res* (2008), 124(1): 28–34.

3 Shingu, M., Takahashi, S., Ito, M., Hamamatu, N. et al., Anti-inflammatory effects of recombinant human manganese superoxide dismutase on adjuvant arthritis in rats, *Rheumatol Int* (1994), 14(2): 77–81.

4 Ruiz-Romero, C., Calamia, V., Mateos, J. et al., Mitochondrial dysregulation of osteoarthritic human articular chondrocytes analyzed by proteomics: A decrease in mitochondrial superoxide dismutase points to a redox imbalance, *Mol Cell Proteomics* (2009), 8(1): 172–89.

5 Sarban, S., Isikan, U.E., Kocabey, Y. & Kocyigit, A., Relationship between synovial fluid and plasma manganese, arginase, and nitric oxide in patients with rheumatoid arthritis, *Biol Trace Elem Res* (2007), 115(2): 97–106.

6 Burlet, E. & Jain, S.K., Manganese supplementation reduces high glucose-induced monocyte adhesion to endothelial cells and endothelial dysfunction in Zucker diabetic fatty rats, *J Biol Chem* (2013), 288(9): 6409–16.
7 Lee, S.H., Jouihan, H.A., Cooksey, R.C. et al., Manganese supplementation protects against diet-induced diabetes in wild type mice by enhancing insulin secretion, *Endocrinology* (2013), 154(3): 1029–38.
8 Hori, H., Ohmori, O., Shinkai, T. et al., Manganese superoxide dismutase gene polymorphism and schizophrenia: Relation to tardive dyskinesia, *Neuropsychopharmacology* (2000), 23(2): 170–7.
9 Kunin, R.A., Manganese and niacin in the treatment of drug-induced dyskinesias, *J Orthomolecular Psych* (1976), 5(1): 4–27.

Therapeutic dose

Manganese is rarely required in supplement form because it is amply supplied in the diet. In the absence of evidence of widespread deficiencies, and because of its potential toxicity, it is recommended that total manganese intake is restricted to the adequate intake amount of 5 mg daily.

Effects of excess

Oral doses of manganese up to 10 mg daily in healthy people have not been associated with adverse effects. Excess manganese can accumulate in the brain, especially the basal ganglia, and cause nerve dysfunction that leads to cognitive, psychiatric and movement abnormalities (manganism). Because of its poor absorption, oral intake of manganese from food is unlikely to cause adverse effects, but high levels in water may be a cause for concern. People with impaired ability to excrete manganese in bile are at higher risk of developing manganism.

Manganese can enter the brain from the nose, from the blood via the blood–brain barrier, and from the blood via the cerebral spinal fluid. Manganism more commonly results from industrial exposure to manganese fumes, and miners, welders, smelters, workers in ferro-alloy plants and dry-cell battery workers are at higher risk. Manganese is a component of tobacco smoke, and it is added to unleaded petrol as an anti-knock agent in the form of methylcyclopentadienyl manganese tricarbonyl (MMT), which is combusted to a number of inorganic manganese species, such as manganese sulfate, phosphate or silicate, about 12–16 per cent of which reaches the atmosphere in vehicle exhaust emissions. Airborne manganese can travel to the olfactory bulb in the brain via the nose, and is taken up by the lungs more readily than ingested forms are taken up by the gut.

Inhaled manganese causes respiratory effects, including cough, bronchitis, inflammation of the alveoli in the lungs and impaired lung function. Brain dysfunction in manganism appears to be due to manganese-induced activation of nerve cell apoptosis, accumulation of glutamate and dysfunction of dopaminergic neurons in the nigrostriatal pathway that controls motor functions. The initial symptoms may include weakness, loss of appetite, palpitations, headache, memory loss, nervousness, irritability, intellectual deficits, mood changes, compulsive behaviour, impotence, loss of libido, muscle pain in the lower limbs, heaviness or stiffness of the legs, increased muscle tone and reduced response speed. Affected people may speak slowly without tone or inflection, and have a dull and emotionless facial expression and slow, clumsy limb movements. This may progress to Parkinson's disease (PD)-like symptoms, such as a staggering gait, tremor, generalised slowness of movement and rigidity; however, unlike PD, it does not involve degeneration of mid-brain dopaminergic neurons, and L-dopa is not an effective therapy. Manganism features a less frequent resting tremor, more frequent muscle spasms and a tendency to fall backwards, which differentiate it from PD.

Typical signs and symptoms of manganism include apathy, psychosis, a mask-like face, soft speech, rigid limbs, tremors affecting the mouth, tongue and hands, difficulty writing or drawing—particularly drawing circles—very small handwriting, muscle spasms, gait disturbance, a cock-like walk (a high-stepping gait, strutting on the toes with flexed elbows and erect spine), slurred speech, salivation, sweating and lack of balance. Manganese psychosis may present as nervousness, irritability, aggressiveness, destructiveness and bizarre behaviour such as involuntary spasmodic laughter or crying, and bouts of singing, dancing or running.

Manganese concentrations may return to normal after several months once the environmental exposure ceases, and symptoms may stabilise or improve to some extent, but they are generally not fully reversible.

Manganese has also been associated with ALS, which features degeneration of motor neurons in the spinal cord, brain and brainstem. People with ALS have been found to have higher manganese concentrations in the spinal cord than control subjects, which may be a cause of neurological damage.

High levels of manganese in drinking water have been associated with mild neurological dysfunction in children, such as poor memory and learning ability, low IQ and hyperactive behaviour. In Eastern Europe and Russia, young people who regularly inject the psycho-stimulant drug methcathinone (ephedrone, or 'Russian cocktail') have been found to develop a form of PD. Methcathinone is a form of ephedrine that has been oxidised using potassium permanganate and acetic acid, and large amounts of manganese accumulate in the body after multiple injections. Blood levels of manganese in addicts can reach 36 404–54 606 nmol/L. Another manganese-containing street drug, known as 'basuco' or 'bazooka', is associated with neurological damage. It is made from the dried residue of cocaine base, and is contaminated with manganese carbonate used in the preparation of the drug and the petrol used to leach out cocaine from coca leaves.

Genetic manganese toxicity

A recently discovered mutation of the gene for solute carrier family 30, member 10 (SLC30A10), previously thought to be a zinc transporter, is linked to manganese overload in the liver and brain. It causes walking difficulties, muscle spasms, impairment of fine motor movements and liver cirrhosis in children, and PD-like symptoms, liver enlargement and elevated manganese levels in adults.

Case reports—manganese excess

- *A girl, six years of age,* developed mood changes and pica, and became withdrawn and less verbal, with repetitive stuttered speech and impaired balance, coordination and fine motor skills.[1] She became unable to stand independently or walk, tended to fall backwards and developed a high-stepping 'cock-like' walk. She was found to have severe manganese neurotoxicity, severe iron deficiency and elevated cobalt and red blood cell levels (polycythaemia). Her blood manganese level was 723 nmol/L. It was suspected that ingestion of well water high in manganese during time spent at the family's summer cottage, together with a high dietary intake of manganese, was the cause of her symptoms. However, other family members were not affected, despite having elevated manganese levels. Although the cause was never defined, it may be that lack of dietary iron—a competitor of manganese absorption—caused increased uptake of manganese. She was treated for iron deficiency and polycythaemia, given chelation therapy and put on a manganese-free diet. There was partial improvement of her neurological symptoms and, at the age of ten years, she was able to walk 40 m unaided. However, she needed a wheelchair for extra mobility.
- *A man, 50 years of age,* developed muscle weakness, dizziness, abdominal pain, nausea and diarrhoea after ingesting Epsom salts as part of a liver-cleansing diet.[2] It was discovered that the manufacturer of the Epsom salts had used manganese sulfate by mistake instead of magnesium sulfate. The patient died and 33 other people taking the same batch of product developed similar symptoms, but were treated successfully.
- *A group of 23 methcathinone users* in Latvia developed gait abnormalities, difficulty walking—especially when walking backwards—falling episodes, soft, slow speech, impassive face, slow movement and very small handwriting, but no apparent cognitive impairment.[3] One patient was unable to speak and one required a wheelchair. Symptoms appeared after an average of nearly six years of using the drug. They were found to have elevated blood manganese and brain damage consistent with manganese toxicity. No patient had liver failure, a condition that may predispose to manganese toxicity. Some patients had ceased drug use several years ago, and had markedly lower blood manganese levels and less severe brain abnormalities, but they had no substantial improvements in gait or speech after drug cessation. The patients did not respond to L-dopa or chelation therapy.
- *A man, 44 years of age,* developed progressively more severe headaches, irritability, insomnia and lethargy after working as an arc welder for 23 years, welding railroad track made of manganese-steel alloy.[4] He subsequently developed progressive confusion, poor memory, impaired cognition, paranoid thoughts, weakness of the right leg, slurred speech, sweating

and an inability to perform routine tasks. He had elevated blood manganese, and brain MRI revealed changes consistent with manganese toxicity. He stopped work and was given chelation treatment, which decreased his blood manganese. His MRI normalised at six months. However, there was no improvement in his neurological symptoms, and he was unable to function independently.

REFERENCES

1 Sahni, V., Léger, Y., Panaro, L. et al., Case report: a metabolic disorder presenting as pediatric manganism, *Environ Health Perspect* (2007), 115(12): 1776–9.

2 Sánchez, B., Casalots-Casado, J., Quintana, S. et al., Fatal manganese intoxication due to an error in the elaboration of Epsom salts for a liver cleansing diet, *Forensic Sci Int* (2012), 223(1–3): e1–4.

3 Stepens, A., Logina, I., Liguts, V. et al., A Parkinsonian syndrome in methcathinone users and the role of manganese, *N Engl J Med* (2008), 358(10): 1009–17.

4 Nelson, K., Golnick, J., Korn, T. & Angle, C., Manganese encephalopathy: Utility of early magnetic resonance imaging, *Br J Ind Med* (1993), 50(6): 510–13.

Supplements

Manganese is available in multivitamin and mineral supplements in tablets and capsules, but is not often used as a single supplement. The permitted forms of manganese salts in oral supplements in Australia include manganese amino acid chelate, aspartate, chloride, gluconate, glycerophosphate, oxide, sulfate and sulfate monohydrate. The most soluble and bioavailable forms appear to be manganese amino chelate and manganese aspartate. Manganese sulfate and manganese chloride have slightly less bioavailability, and manganese oxide has low bioavailability. The amount of elemental manganese in a specific manganese salt is listed on the product container, and may vary between individual products. The approximate elemental manganese content of some common salts is shown in Table 11.4.

Table 11.4 Elemental manganese content of common salts

Salt	Manganese content (%)
Manganese oxide	60
Manganese chloride	44
Manganese sulfate	30
Manganese aspartate	17
Manganese gluconate	11
Manganese amino acid chelate	10

- *Manganese oxide* has the highest concentration of manganese, but is relatively poorly absorbed. It occurs in nature as the rare mineral manganosite, and can be produced commercially by heating manganese carbonate in the absence of air or by passing hydrogen or carbon monoxide over manganese dioxide.
- *Manganese chloride* has a high content of elemental manganese, and is relatively well absorbed. It is produced by reacting manganese oxide with hydrochloric acid.
- *Manganese sulfate* has a moderate content of elemental manganese, and is relatively well absorbed. It is produced by reacting manganese oxide with sulfuric acid.
- *Manganese aspartate* has a relatively low content of elemental manganese but is a well-absorbed form. It is produced by reacting manganese carbonate or chloride with the amino acid aspartic acid.
- *Manganese amino acid chelate* has a low content of elemental manganese but is a well-absorbed form. It is produced by reacting manganese sulfate, carbonate or chloride with two or more amino acids derived from hydrolysis of soybean protein.

Cautions

Manganese supplements should be used with caution; doses greater than 5 mg daily are not recommended long-term. Manganese supplements may inhibit iron absorption and should be taken at least two hours apart from iron supplements. High-dose manganese may reduce the absorption of the fluoroquinolone and tetracycline classes of antibiotics; manganese supplements should be taken two to four hours before or after the drug dose.

IODINE

IODINE STATUS CHECK

1 Do you feel the cold intensely?
2 Do you gain weight very easily?
3 Is your face puffy and dull looking?
4 Do you feel lethargic and mentally sluggish?

'Yes' answers may indicate inadequate iodine status. Note that a number of nutritional deficiencies or health disorders can cause similar effects and further investigation is recommended.

FAST FACTS . . . IODINE

- Good sources of iodine include iodised salt, bread, seaweed and seafood.
- Iodine is essential for healthy thyroid function.
- It plays a role in maintaining a healthy metabolic rate and has antioxidant, anticancer and antimicrobial activity.
- A deficiency can cause goitre, slow metabolic rate, weight gain, sensation of coldness, fluid retention and mental and physical sluggishness.
- Excess iodine can disrupt thyroid function.

Iodine is a naturally occurring mineral found in the environment and especially in sea water, which contains about 50–60 mcg/L, mainly as sodium and potassium iodides. Iodine is given off from sea water into the atmosphere and deposited with rainfall in coastal soils. It has a strong affinity for soil, and only small amounts are taken up by plants; plant levels range from 10–1000 mcg/kg dry weight. Plants grown in inland areas and in regions that have undergone glaciation, flooding or erosion that removes surface soil contain very little iodine. Iodine deficiency is a significant health issue in many inland and mountainous regions around the world.

Iodine-containing substances, such as seaweeds, have been used throughout history as antiseptics for wounds. Iodine was first isolated in 1811 from seaweed ash by French chemist Bernard Courtois. The nineteenth-century French physician Jean Guillaume Auguste Lugol developed an iodine solution (Lugol's solution) for the treatment of tuberculosis (TB). Although not effective for TB, it was later used as an effective treatment for thyroid disorders, and is still in use today as an antiseptic.

Iodine has the chemical symbol I, and was named after the Greek word *iodes*, meaning 'purple', the colour of iodine gas. Iodine is found in biological systems as inorganic iodides and iodates, inorganic diatomic iodine (molecular iodine) (I_2) and organic monoatomic iodine (I). In the body, iodine concentrates in the thyroid gland, and is incorporated into the thyroid hormones responsible for regulating the metabolic rate of cells. Other body tissues that take up iodine are the ovaries, placenta, cervix, mammary glands, kidneys, skin, salivary glands, lacrimal glands, gastric mucosa and the choroid plexus in the brain, which produces cerebrospinal fluid.

Digestion, absorption and transport

Iodine in food is bound to amino acids or is present as free iodate and iodide. Iodide is released from amino acids during digestion, and iodate is reduced to iodide by glutathione. Some forms of bound iodine are absorbed intact, but absorption is lower than for iodide. Iodide is taken up by enterocytes via the sodium/iodide symporter (NIS), a protein that transports two sodium ions and one iodide ion across cell membranes using the sodium gradient maintained by Na/K-ATPase. Iodine is transferred to the bloodstream and circulates as free iodide, which is taken up by the thyroid gland and other tissues via NIS.

Metabolism, storage and excretion

The thyroid gland consists of multiple follicles, the inner space of which (lumen) is filled with colloid and lined by follicular cells (thyrocytes). Colloid consists of the glycoprotein thyroglobulin (Tg), which is made by thyrocytes. The thyroid gland traps about 60 mcg of iodine daily if no deficiency exists, which is sufficient to maintain thyroid hormone synthesis and balance daily losses. Iodide entering thyrocytes is transferred to the lumen by pendrin, a chloride-iodide transporter protein, and oxidised to iodine by the haem-dependent enzyme thyroperoxidase (TPO) using hydrogen peroxide. Iodine then undergoes organification by binding to tyrosine residues of Tg to form Tg-3-monoiodotyrosine (Tg-MIT) and

Tg-3,5-diiodotyrosine (Tg-DIT). Tg-MIT and Tg-DIT are combined by TPO to form Tg-3,5,3'-triiodothyronine (Tg-T3) and some reverse T3 (Tg-rT3), an inactive form. Two molecules of DIT are combined by TPO to form Tg-3,5,3',5'-tetraiodothyronine (Tg-T4). The iodinated forms of Tg (Tg-T3, Tg-rT3 and Tg-T4) are stored in thyroid follicle colloid for several months. When required, iodinated Tg is transferred to thyrocytes via endocytosis and hydrolysed in lysosomes to form triiodothyronine (T3) and thyroxine (T4), the active forms of thyroid hormones that are released to the blood. T4 makes up about 90 per cent of released thyroid hormones and T3 makes up about 10 per cent.

T3 and T4 are transported in the bloodstream by binding to thyroxine-binding globulin, which carries about 75 per cent of total thyroid hormones; transthyretin, which carries about 20 per cent; albumin, which carries about 5 per cent; and a small amount is transported as free T3 and T4, which are believed to be the forms most readily taken up by cells. Some T4 is converted to T3 by the liver. Plasma contains about 50 times more T4 than T3, but T3 is 3.3 times more potent. Specific thyroid hormone transporters in cell membranes include monocarboxylate transporter 8 (MCT8), MCT10 and organic anion-transporting polypeptide 1C1 (OATP1C1). In cells, thyroid hormones, particularly T3, bind to the zinc finger-containing thyroid receptors (TRs) TR alpha and TR beta, and induce gene expression, increasing mRNA and protein synthesis.

Within some tissues, such as the liver, kidneys, pituitary gland, brain, mammary glands and brown adipose tissue, selenium-containing type 1 or type 2 iodothyronine deiodinase enzymes (D1 and D2) generate T3 from T4. D1 is found mainly in breast tissue during pregnancy and lactation, whereas D2 is found in a variety of tissues. Selenium-containing type 3 iodothyronine deiodinase (D3) inactivates T3 and T4.

Iodine from broken-down thyroid hormones can be reused to make new thyroid hormones. The main storage site for iodine is the thyroid gland, which stores iodine in the form of iodinated Tg. More than 90 per cent of ingested iodine is excreted by the kidneys, with the amount varying according to dietary intake. A small proportion of body iodine is lost in faeces and sweat.

Regulation of body levels

Absorption of iodine increases when body levels are low and decreases when levels are adequate. Levels of T3 and T4 in plasma are monitored by the hypothalamus, which releases thyrotropin-releasing hormone (TRH) when plasma levels drop. TRH stimulates the anterior pituitary gland to release thyroid-stimulating hormone (TSH), which induces expression of NIS in the thyroid gland, allowing it to trap more circulating iodides, and stimulates breakdown of Tg and synthesis and release of T3. When plasma levels of thyroid hormones are high, the hypothalamus releases the hormone somatostatin, which blocks release of TRH.

The thyroid gland also has a self-regulating mechanism. Iodine can react with double bonds on lipids to form iodolipids, such as iodoaldehydes and iodolactones, which regulate thyroid cell metabolism. Delta-iodolactone, an iodinated arachidonic acid derivative, is an iodolipid that inhibits thyroid cell proliferation and gland growth.

Deiodinases play a role in regulating thyroid hormone levels in cells. If the thyroid gland is underactive or is iodine deficient, the T3-producing enzyme D2 is upregulated, while levels of the inactivating enzyme D3 are decreased. If the thyroid gland is overactive, high levels of T4 inactivate D2 and excess T3 rapidly induces expression of D3. During pregnancy, maternal plasma T3 passes to the foetus, in which it is necessary for normal development and growth. D3 is highly expressed in the placenta, the endometrium and in many embryonic tissues and maintains free T3 levels almost ten-fold lower in the foetus than in maternal plasma.

Functions

Iodine's main function is as part of thyroid hormones which, overall, have a stimulating effect on cell activities. They act to increase basal metabolic rate, oxygen consumption, heat production, growth and development. Thyroid hormones also function at the plasma membrane, in cytoplasm and in mitochondria, and play a role in regulating ion transport systems, cell proliferation and mitochondrial gene transcription. Iodine may also function as an antioxidant and immune system regulator, and a detoxifying, anticancer and antimicrobial agent. The functions of iodine include the following:

- *Cell metabolism, growth and development.* Iodine is incorporated into the thyroid hormones T3 and T4, which control cell metabolism. T3 binding to nuclear receptors modifies the expression of numerous genes involved in metabolism, detoxification, signal transduction, cellular adhesion and migration, and cell proliferation and has a stimulating effect on protein production in the cell. Respiratory proteins are increased, energy production, oxygen consumption and heat production increase and bone growth is stimulated. Thyroid hormones increase the synthesis and secretion of growth hormone and growth factors. T3 is essential during pregnancy for normal growth of the foetus and foetal nervous system development, and after birth for linear growth and maturation of the infant's nervous system.

- *Carbohydrate metabolism.* Thyroid hormones increase absorption of glucose in the gut, increase insulin secretion and the uptake of glucose by cells, and stimulate glucose synthesis (gluconeogenesis) and glycolysis, the first step in glucose breakdown in the energy cycle.
- *Lipid and cholesterol metabolism.* Thyroid hormones increase the breakdown of stored fat in adipose tissue, increase the level of free fatty acids in plasma, stimulate oxidation of fats and regulate serum cholesterol levels. Sterol regulatory element-binding protein 2 (SREBP-2) is regulated by thyroid hormone; it acts to reduce gene expression of LDL cholesterol receptors when cell levels of cholesterol rise, thereby reducing uptake of LDL cholesterol by cells. Lack of iodine stimulates TSH, which appears to boost cholesterol synthesis in the liver by stimulating expression of the enzyme HMG-CoA reductase independently of thyroid hormone.
- *Circulation.* Thyroid hormones increase the number of receptors for catecholamine hormones, which increase heart rate, cardiac output, stroke volume and peripheral vasodilation, leading to warm, moist skin.
- *Antioxidant protection.* Inorganic iodine has antioxidant activity in the seaweed kelp, where it has been shown to neutralise hydrogen peroxide, a cell-damaging oxidant. In the thyroid gland, hydrogen peroxide is produced by the enzyme dual oxidase 2 (DUOX2), which oxidises NADPH to generate superoxide radicals that are rapidly converted to hydrogen peroxide by SODs. The enzyme TPO uses hydrogen peroxide to generate iodine from iodide during the process of making thyroid hormones, thereby reducing levels of hydrogen peroxide. Low iodide concentrations stimulate production of hydrogen peroxide and high levels inhibit it.

  Iodine can react with double bonds on lipids to form iodolipids, such as iodoaldehydes and iodolactones, which provide protection from ROS. Sodium iodide added to human serum has been shown to increase the total antioxidant capacity, possibly by acting as an electron donor or by activating other antioxidant enzymes. Sodium iodide, at a concentration of 15 μM in serum, was only slightly less effective in increasing total antioxidant capacity than an ascorbic acid concentration of 50 μM.
- *Skin integrity.* TRs have been detected in many skin cells, including epidermal keratinocytes, skin fibroblasts, hair arrector pili muscle cells, other smooth muscle cells, sebaceous gland cells, vascular endothelial cells, Schwann cells and hair follicle cells. The exact function of T3 in the skin is not well established, but it appears to have a growth-regulating role in various skin cells.
- *Detoxification.* Iodine appears to boost the activity of enzymes such as cytochrome P450, which are involved in detoxifying metabolites and xenobiotics (foreign or unwanted substances) in the liver.
- *Anticancer activity.* Iodine appears to act by a variety of mechanisms to suppress abnormal cell replication. In cancer cells, oxidised iodine can trigger apoptosis directly via mitochondrial pathways and indirectly through iodolipids that activate peroxisome proliferator-activated receptor gamma (PPAR-gamma), a transcription factor that triggers apoptotic or differentiation pathways. However, exposure to iodine does not trigger apoptosis in normal cells.
- *Antimicrobial activity.* Iodine is an effective antiseptic, and is the only agent that is consistently active against Gram positive and Gram negative bacteria, drug-resistant bacteria, spores, amoebic cysts, fungi, protozoa, yeasts and viruses. Contact with free I_2 destroys microbes by inhibiting protein synthesis, disrupting electron transport, denaturing DNA or destabilising membranes, and does not lead to the development of microbial resistance.

Dietary sources

Dietary iodine is rapidly and almost completely absorbed. Good sources of iodine include iodised salt, bread, seaweed such as kelp, nori and wakame, and seafood, including shellfish and fish. Other sources include eggs, dairy foods and meat. Seaweeds are particularly rich sources, containing about 0.5–0.8 mg/g of iodine, and intake of iodine from traditional Japanese diets averages 2–3 mg/day. Levels in land plants are much lower (about 0.001 mg/g), and are unreliable because their iodine content depends on the amount in the soil in which they are grown. In the past, milk was an important source of iodine because it contained trace amounts of iodophors used to disinfect equipment but these are no longer used.

Iodised salt contains potassium or sodium iodate or iodide, providing 25–65 mcg/g (mean 44 mcg/g) of iodine. Non-iodised salt, sea salt, rock salt and vegetable salts are mainly sodium chloride, and contain less than 2 mcg of iodine per gram unless fortified with iodine. Iodised salt is rarely used in commercially manufactured foods. In Australia in October 2009, due to concern about inadequate iodine intake, legislation was introduced to make it mandatory to use iodised salt in bread making. Organic bread, bread with no added salt and bread mixes for home baking are not required to contain iodised salt. The iodine salts permitted for food fortification in Australia and New Zealand are sodium iodate, potassium iodate, sodium iodide and potassium iodide. Iodates are more stable and are more commonly used.

Other sources of iodine include kelp supplements and the food additives aquamin, a red seaweed-derived source of iodine; carrageenan (additive 407), a polysaccharide derived from red seaweed, and erythrosine (additive 127), a red colouring agent used in preserved (maraschino) cherries, icings and frostings. Iodine is in water-purification tablets, some types of contrast media used with medical imaging procedures and some drugs, including amiodarone (for arrhythmias), cough and cold medications, and the topical antiseptic povidone-iodine.

The Food Standards Australia New Zealand nutrient database (NUTTAB) at <www.foodstandards.gov.au> provides the amounts found in specific foods.

Factors influencing body status

Iodine intake needs to be kept within relatively narrow limits because a low iodine intake may lead to thyroid gland underactivity and enlargement (goitre), and a high intake may suppress thyroid function or trigger hyperactivity. Many people are unaware of the importance of using iodised salt, and people who are health-conscious have minimised salt intake overall, including intake of iodised salt, in order to reduce the risk of elevated blood pressure. Although iodised salt must now be used in bread-making, people on low-carbohydrate diets and those with coeliac disease (gluten intolerance) are unlikely to eat enough bread to benefit from this initiative. People who choose organic bread or bread with no added salt, and those who make their own bread, will also not benefit.

Natural plant compounds with the potential to impair thyroid function are called goitrogens because they impair thyroid metabolism and promote goitre formation. Goitrogens include glucosinolates, cyanogenic glucosides and thiocyanates that inhibit uptake of iodine by the thyroid gland. Glucosinolates are present in cruciferous (cabbage-family) vegetables, such as cabbage, kale, cauliflower, broccoli, rutabaga, turnips, Brussels sprouts, mustard greens and rapeseed (canola seed), and cyanogenic glucosides are found in lima beans, linseed, sorghum, maize, millet, cassava, bamboo shoots and sweet potato. Thiocyanates are found in tobacco smoke, antibiotics, pesticides and herbicides, and are also formed in the body during metabolism of glucosinolates.

The isoflavones genistein and daidzein, found in soy beans, chick peas and red clover, inhibit TPO activity, and may depress thyroid function if large amounts are eaten and iodine intake is low. Adequate iodine protects against the adverse effects. Millet contains high amounts of the flavonoids apigenin and luteolin, which reduce the organification and secretion of thyroid hormones. In general, food flavonoids are present in small amounts, and have limited absorption, and goitrogens are broken down by cooking. Overall, most of these thyroid inhibitors are not believed to affect people with healthy thyroid function, and are only of concern in people with existing thyroid disorders.

Environmental pollutants, many of which contaminate food and water, can impair thyroid function. These include perchlorate found in rocket fuel and used in manufacturing; phthalates found in plastics; polychlorinated biphenyls (PCBs) used in electrical equipment manufacturing; polyaromatic hydrocarbons (PAHs) from bushfires, charred meat and burning fossil fuels; bisphenol A (BPA), found in plastic food and drink containers; organochlorine pesticides used in farming; dioxins, a by-product of bushfires, incineration of wastes, smelting, chlorine bleaching of wood pulp and pesticide manufacture; hexachlorobenzene, a fungicide previously used on seed grains; triclosan, an antibacterial found in soaps; polybrominated diphenyl ethers (PBDEs), flame retardants; and ultraviolet filters in sunscreens. The effects on the thyroid of exposure to multiple pollutants is not yet well understood.

In pregnancy, iodine demand is increased because of an increased production of thyroid hormones, greater losses of iodine in urine and transfer of iodine to the foetus. At the beginning of the second trimester, thyroid hormone concentrations are 30–100 per cent higher than pre-pregnancy levels. Low levels of selenium may reduce deiodinase activity, and low iron may impair the function of TPO. Low vitamin A reduces expression of the gene for TSH in the anterior pituitary gland. Drugs that may affect thyroid hormone function include amiodarone, used for heart arrhythmias, which contains iodine; lithium, used for psychiatric disorders, which inhibits formation of thyroid hormones, and may lead to hypothyroidism; glucocorticoids, used for inflammation, which reduce the release of TSH; interferon alpha, used for cancer or hepatitis, which can cause thyroiditis; and tyrosine kinase inhibitors, used for cancer, which can cause hypo- or hyperthyroidism.

Daily requirement

Australian and New Zealand government recommendations by age and gender (see Table 11.5) can be found in *Nutrient Reference Values for Australia and New Zealand Including Recommended Dietary Intakes*, available at <www.nhmrc.gov.au>.

Table 11.5 Recommended dietary intake (RDI) of iodine (mcg/day)

Age (years)	Female RDI	Male RDI
1–3	90	90
4–8	90	90
9–13	120	120
14–18	150	150
19–70	150	150
>70	150	150
Pregnant women		
14–18	220	
19–50	220	
Lactating women		
14–18	270	
19–50	270	

Source: Nutrient Reference Values for Australia and New Zealand Including Recommended Dietary Intakes, National Health and Medical Research Council, Australian Government Department of Health and Ageing, Canberra and Ministry of Health, New Zealand, Wellington, 2006.

The National Health and Medical Research Council (NHMRC) of Australia recommends that all women who are pregnant, considering pregnancy or breastfeeding should take an iodine supplement providing 150 mcg/day.

Deficiency effects

Iodine deficiency is prevalent in inland and mountainous regions around the world, such as the Himalayas, the European Alps, the Pyrenees and the Andes. It has been estimated that about 1.88 billion people worldwide had insufficient iodine intakes in 2011, including 241 million school children. Infants and children are at most risk of the adverse effects of iodine deficiency. In general, soils throughout New Zealand are low in iodine. In Australia, the mountainous areas of northern and eastern Tasmania, the Atherton Tablelands of north Queensland, the Great Dividing Range in New South Wales, the plains surrounding Canberra, the eastern region of Victoria and the Adelaide Hills are low-iodine regions.

In Australia, inadequate iodine intake was common across all population groups prior to the introduction of mandatory use of iodised salt for bread-making. A 2008 survey found that 43 per cent of Australians did not get enough iodine, and 70 per cent of women of child-bearing age and about 10 per cent of children aged two to three years were iodine deficient. Women generally had lower intakes than men, and more than half of girls aged fourteen years or more had inadequate status. Children in Victoria, New South Wales and Tasmania were more likely to be mildly iodine deficient. Pregnant women in Australia have consistently been found to have low iodine status, and surveys have shown that 19–58 per cent have very low status. The iodine status of Australian women has improved since the mandatory use of iodised salt in bread-making was introduced, but supplementation is still required during pregnancy.

New Zealand has a very low iodine environment and goitre was endemic in the early 1900s. The introduction of iodised salt helped to correct the problem but iodine status has again declined and surveys of children and pregnant women have revealed widespread low iodine status. The mandatory use of iodised salt for bread making is expected to help improve iodine status.

Iodine deficiency disorders (IDD) is the term used to describe the effects of iodine deficiency on growth and development. A lack of iodine causes thyroid hormone production to diminish and triggers release of TSH, which boosts growth of the thyroid gland in an attempt to make more thyroid hormones. This may appear as a swelling in the base of the neck (goitre) or as nodules in the thyroid gland. If the gland enlarges enough to make sufficient thyroid hormones, but does not develop nodules, it is referred to as diffuse non-toxic goitre, simple goitre or colloid goitre. This is the most common outcome of long-term iodine deficiency, and a geographic region where the goitre incidence is greater than 5 per cent of the population is referred to as an 'endemic goitre' region. If the extra thyroid tissue is not effective in maintaining adequate levels of thyroid hormones, symptoms of an underactive thyroid will appear. Goitre can also be due to an autoimmune attack on the thyroid, which can be detected by the presence of antibodies to TPO and Tg.

Thyroid nodules and goitre are more common with age, and especially affect women. A goitre may press on the trachea and the oesophagus, and cause discomfort, shortness of breath, a high-pitched wheezing sound when breathing (stridor), difficulty swallowing, cough and a hoarse voice. Thyroid nodules may haemorrhage, leading to a sudden increase in thyroid size and tenderness.

Underactivity of the thyroid gland (hypothyroidism) is the most common hormone deficiency disorder, and more often affects women. It leads to a generalised slowing down of metabolism, energy production and heat generation (myxoedema), the effects of which include weight gain, feeling cold even in warm temperatures, fatigue, muscle weakness, drowsiness and fluid retention (oedema), which appears as puffiness of the face, eyelids, shins, hands and feet, and is non-pitting (finger indentation does not persist after pressing the affected area). There may be a dull, expressionless facial appearance, pallor, dry and brittle hair, thin and brittle nails, coarse, thin, scaly skin and loss of hair. Cardiovascular effects include a slow pulse, low blood pressure, elevated serum cholesterol, enlarged heart, pleural effusion, pericarditis, congestive heart failure and increased risk of CVD. Other effects include stiff and tender joints, particularly in the hands, feet and knees, reduced immunity, excessive menstrual bleeding, reduced fertility, ataxia and hearing loss. Effects on brain function include apathy, mental confusion, mood swings, memory loss, depression and psychosis. Mild to moderate iodine deficiency is associated with a higher risk of more aggressive sub-types of thyroid cancer.

Myxoedema coma (myxoedema crisis) may occur in older patients with long-standing hypothyroidism, and can be precipitated by hypothermia, hypoglycaemia, infection, trauma, haemorrhage or a change of medication. It causes sudden mental deterioration and seizures, but only rarely leads to coma. It is fatal in 60–70 per cent of untreated patients and 20–25 per cent of treated patients.

Subclinical hypothyroidism involves elevated TSH levels, and is estimated to occur in 4–20 per cent of the adult population. It may progress to overt hypothyroidism over time. There may be no obvious effects, or there may be mild effects similar to those of hypothyroidism. Subclinical hypothyroidism is associated with diastolic hypertension, isolated diastolic dysfunction (a decline in the ability of heart ventricles to fill with blood), abnormal blood lipids, insulin resistance, weight gain and increased risk of CVD.

Pregnancy

Thyroid hormones are needed for general growth and development of the foetus, and particularly for nervous system development, including neural migration, differentiation, myelinisation, nerve transmission and the formation of nerve synapses. The requirement for iodine increases considerably during pregnancy because of the increased production of thyroid hormones, and iodine deficiency may occur in women with borderline iodine status, as well as in those with existing deficiencies. Maternal transfer of T4 to the foetus is important throughout pregnancy because the thyroid gland of the foetus does not fully mature until late pregnancy and after birth. Early gestation is a critical time because the foetus is not able to produce any thyroid hormones prior to weeks twelve to fourteen.

Inadequate iodine intake in pregnancy may lead to hypothyroidism, which can cause increased risk of miscarriage, pre-eclampsia, placental abruption, foetal death, stillbirths, preterm birth and low birth weight. Development of the brain and nervous system in the foetus is impaired, especially if maternal production of thyroid hormones is inadequate during the first twelve weeks of pregnancy. Hypothyroidism in pregnancy is associated with autoimmune reactions; thyroid autoantibodies are detected in about 50 per cent of pregnant women with subclinical hypothyroidism and in 80 per cent of women with clinical hypothyroidism. Iodine supplementation throughout the entire pregnancy for women with severe iodine deficiency improves foetal outcomes, and supplementation of women with mild iodine deficiency appears to be beneficial for the neurocognitive development of their infants.

Infants and children

A severe deficiency of thyroid hormones during pregnancy can lead to pronounced and irreversible physical and mental impairment (cretinism) in the infant. Infants with cretinism may have hypothermia, slow heart rate, prolonged jaundice, an umbilical hernia, a hoarse cry, strabismus (squint), puffiness of the face, coarse, flat features, an under-developed jaw, thickened, dry skin, sparse hair, constipation, sleepiness and feeding difficulties. Effects in children include abnormal bone development, poor growth, dwarfism, muscle spasticity, deafness, inability to talk (mutism), a low IQ and delayed sexual maturation. Some cretins have a goitre and some have thyroid atrophy with extremely low serum levels of T4 and T3 and extremely high TSH levels. Neurological abnormalities predominate in some (neurological cretinism), and other symptoms of hypothyroidism predominate in others (myxoedematous or hypothyroid cretinism).

Endemic cretinism is present in a geographical region if there is a prevalence of 1–10 per cent in the population. Cretinism is extremely rare in Australia and New Zealand, and is found mainly in Central Africa, South and Latin America, Asia, Southeast Asia and the highlands of Papua New Guinea. Less severe neurological abnormalities in infants and children ('subcretin' or 'cretinoid') are also common in these regions.

Milder forms of hypothyroidism are common in many countries worldwide. If present at birth, it is associated with poor growth and impaired intellectual or psychomotor development in early childhood. Affected children may have a lower IQ, poor concentration and learning ability, poor school performance and behaviour problems such as attention deficit hyperactivity disorder (ADHD). Mild, subclinical developmental impairments can occur in infants and children of mothers whose thyroid hormone levels during pregnancy were in the low-normal range. A mild iodine deficiency has been found to be associated with altered neurological development in children aged three to ten years, and a severe iodine deficiency is estimated to lead to a mean reduction of 12.45 IQ points. Iodine supplementation has been shown to improve perceptual reasoning in children with a mild iodine deficiency, indicating that even mild deficiencies impair intellectual potential. Subclinical hypothyroidism in children and adolescents may lead to an abnormal blood lipid profile that is associated with increased risk of atherosclerosis. Iodine supplementation in moderately iodine-deficient children has been shown to improve blood lipids and reduce insulin levels.

Elderly

Subclinical hypothyroidism is relatively common in elderly people, especially women, and the effects are often regarded as normal signs of ageing. Signs and symptoms include hoarse voice, deepening of the voice, puffy eyes, abnormal blood lipids and a worsening of existing conditions such as dry skin, feeling cold, fatigue, weak muscles, muscle cramps, constipation, depression, slow thinking, poor memory and difficulty doing mathematical calculations.

Indicators of inadequate levels of iodine may include the following:

- *Hypothyroidism:* goitre, hoarse voice, difficulty swallowing or breathing, cough, puffiness of the face, eyelids, hands, shins or feet, weight gain, feeling cold, dull, expressionless face, fatigue, muscle weakness, drowsiness, dry hair, thickened dry skin, hair loss, stiff and tender joints, slow pulse, low blood pressure, enlarged heart, congestive heart failure, elevated serum cholesterol, reduced immunity, excessive menstrual bleeding, reduced fertility, hearing loss, apathy, mental confusion, memory loss, mood swings, depression.
- *Infants:* prolonged jaundice, umbilical hernia, hoarse cry, strabismus, puffiness of the face, coarse flat features, underdeveloped jaw, thickened dry skin, sparse hair, constipation, sleepiness, feeding difficulties.
- *Children and adolescents:* abnormal bone development, poor growth, dwarfism, muscle spasticity, deafness, mutism, low IQ, delayed sexual maturation, abnormal blood lipids, poor concentration and learning ability, poor school performance, behavioural disorders.
- *Elderly:* hoarse voice, deepening of the voice, puffy eyes, dry skin, feeling cold, fatigue, weak muscles, muscle cramps, constipation, depression, slow thinking, poor memory, difficulty doing mathematical calculations.

Assessment of body status

Mean urinary iodine concentration (MUIC) is used for assessing iodine status in populations because it is a measure of recent intake. The WHO considers that the iodine status of a population is optimal if the MUIC ranges from 100–200 mcg/L, and excessive if it exceeds 300 mcg/L. Excretion of 100 mcg/L reflects a dietary intake of 150 mcg/day. Mild iodine deficiency exists when the MUIC is 50–100 mcg/L. In pregnancy, iodine levels are inadequate if the MUIC is less than 150 mcg/L; adequate if it is 150–249 mcg/L; more than adequate if it is 250–500 mcg/L; and excessive if it is more than 500 mcg/L.

The serum Tg concentration is raised in iodine deficiency, and declines when iodine intake increases. It has been used to monitor the response to improved iodine intake in populations. The reference range given by the RCPA for serum Tg is less than 38 μg/L. In individuals, this test is used mainly for follow-up monitoring after surgery for thyroid cancer.

Methods used for assessing iodine status of an individual include measuring urinary iodine, thyroid volume, serum thyroxine and serum TSH. The amount of iodine excreted in urine over a 24-hour period or the amount of iodine excreted per gram of creatinine can be tested. Urinary excretion can vary widely, and is not a reliable reflection of iodine status; several urine tests are preferred to increase the accuracy of the result. Thyroid volume is assessed by ultrasound, and enlargement indicates a long-term significant iodine deficiency but it is not a sensitive measure of recent iodine intake.

Serum levels of thyroxine and TSH are good indicators of iodine status in individuals with moderate to severe deficiency. The reference range given by the RCPA for free serum thyroxine is 10–25 pmol/L, and the reference range for serum TSH is 0.4–5.0 mIU/L (milli-international units per litre). In overt hypothyroidism, there is elevated TSH with low free thyroxine levels, and in subclinical hypothyroidism, there is high TSH with normal or borderline free thyroxine levels. TSH is used as an initial test for patients with goitre, together with testing for antibodies against TPO (anti-TPO) and Tg (anti-Tg).

The basal body temperature test can be used as an indicator of thyroid function. A non-digital thermometer is used to take the temperature under the arm first thing in the morning after waking, while still in bed and before moving about, on three consecutive mornings. The thermometer should be kept in place for ten minutes and then the temperature should be recorded. If the three readings are below 36.6°C (97.8°F), hypothyroidism is a possibility and should be investigated further.

Case reports—iodine deficiency

- *A male infant, seven and a half months of age*, was investigated for severe failure to thrive, lack of appetite, developmental delay, poor muscle tone, lethargy, severe bone weakness and a visible goitre.[1] He was found to have a markedly increased serum TSH, and low free thyroxine and carnitine levels. His father was a lactovegetarian and his mother was a strict vegan. The infant had been exclusively breastfed until the age of 2.5 months, but was then weaned onto a cow's milk formula because he was not gaining weight. However, he developed eczema and was then changed to a home-prepared mixture of almond extract in water. He also ate cereals and some fruit but his appetite was poor. His diet contained no vitamin B12 and was especially deficient in kilojoules, calcium, iron, iodine, vitamin D and the amino acids lysine, leucine and threonine. The parents adamantly refused to change his diet or use carnitine supplementation, but permitted the use of iodine supplementation (50 mcg/day). Six days later, thyroid function had normalised, the goitre had reduced in size and there was some improvement in muscle tone. Iodine supplementation was stopped by the parents after three weeks against medical advice. At ten months of age, body weight and growth had improved but poor muscle tone persisted, and carnitine supplementation was again refused despite warnings that low carnitine could lead to heart damage.
- *A boy, four years of age*, was investigated for short stature.[2] He had been fed cow's milk formula for six months and then solid food. At two years of age, he had a poor appetite and constipation, and his height and weight were below normal. A dietitian advised the use of soy milk as a replacement for cow's milk but he then developed diarrhoea. A naturopath diagnosed him with allergies to cow's milk, dairy products, goat's milk, eggs, chocolate, sugar, food additives, fish, beef, lamb and pork, and these items were removed from his diet, after which his growth rate deteriorated. His mother then sought medical advice and he was found to have elevated serum TSH and low levels of free thyroxine and urinary iodine. His restricted diet provided an average iodine intake of only 40 mcg/day. He was placed on a normal diet that included cow's milk, together with iodine supplementation (40 mcg/day). His thyroid function normalised in four weeks, he became more lively and active, and he no longer had diarrhoea or allergic

symptoms. His iodine supplement was discontinued and, at eight weeks, his thyroid remained normal and he had gained height and weight.

- *A woman, 34 years of age*, developed cold intolerance, constipation and fatigue.[3] She was found to have an enlarged thyroid gland, elevated serum TSH, low serum free thyroxine and very low urinary iodine. She had no personal or family history of thyroid disease. She had avoided salt for several years to reduce her risk of high blood pressure, and she rarely ate fish or dairy products. She was advised to use iodised salt in food and to eat seafood. Two months later, she reported improvement in her symptoms, her thyroid gland had reduced in size and her thyroid function tests had normalised.

REFERENCES

1 Kanaka, C., Schütz, B. & Zuppinger, K.A., Risks of alternative nutrition in infancy: A case report of severe iodine and carnitine deficiency, *Eur J Pediatr* (1992), 151(10): 786–8.

2 Labib, M., Gama, R., Wright, J., Marks, V. & Robins, D., Dietary maladvice as a cause of hypothyroidism and short stature, *BMJ* (1989), 298(6668): 232–3.

3 Nyenwe, E.A. & Dagogo-Jack, S., Iodine deficiency disorders in the iodine-replete environment, *Am J Med Sci* (2009), 337(1): 37–40.

THERAPEUTIC USES OF IODINE

Cancer

Iodine appears to have anticancer activity in tissues that are able to take up iodine. Iodine is incorporated into iodolactones, which may play a role in regulating proliferation in the thyroid, prostate and mammary glands. Delta-iodolactone appears to be a particularly potent tumour inhibitor. Molecular iodine (I_2) is selectively accumulated by breast tissue and, in animal and human studies, iodine supplementation, if given as molecular I_2 or iodide, suppresses the growth of both benign and cancerous growths in cells that have TPO activity.[1] Iodine levels have been found to be lower in human breast cancer tissue than in surrounding normal tissue[2] and additional iodine, as I_2, potassium iodide or the seaweeds wakame or mekabu, has been found to induce apoptosis in human breast cancer tissue.[3] In animals, Lugol's solution has suppressed the development of mammary tumours.[4] Loss of TRs and alterations in TR genes are features of cancer tissue, and inducing the expression of TR beta1 in liver cancer and breast cancer cells in animals has been shown to reduce tumour growth and have a potent inhibitory effect on tumour invasiveness, blood vessel leakage and metastasis.[5] A meta-analysis of 28 trials concluded that women with goitre, anti-thyroid antibodies or autoimmune thyroiditis have more than twice the risk of breast cancer.[6]

Higher iodine intake is associated with a lower risk of breast cancer in some studies.[7,8] Intake of the seaweed gim (*Porphyra* sp.) by Korean women is associated with decreased risk of breast cancer.[9] Iodine appears to reduce the risk of developing thyroid cancer after exposure to radioactive iodine (^{131}I) in childhood. The radiation leak caused by the Chernobyl nuclear power plant accident in Russia in April 1986 led to a large increase in the incidence of childhood thyroid cancer.[10] The risk of radiation-induced thyroid cancer was found to be three times higher in iodine-deficient areas, and administration of potassium iodide was found to reduce this risk by 66 per cent.[10]

Benign breast disease

In a study of women with benign breast disease, the overall prevalence of hypothyroidism was 23.2 per cent.[11] The rate of hypothyroidism and the mean serum TSH concentration were significantly higher among patients with nipple discharge than among those with breast pain (mastalgia) or breast lumps. Thyroxine replacement alleviated symptoms in 83 per cent of the hypothyroid women.

In fibrocystic breast disease (FBD), characterised by the development of microcysts, fibrosis, overgrowth of epithelial tissue and painful lumpy breasts, I_2 has been found to be superior to other forms of iodine. In a study comparing sodium iodide, protein-bound iodine and I_2, 74 per cent of women given 0.08 mg I_2/kg body weight had disappearance of microcysts within five months, 40 per cent of women taking protein-bound iodine had clinical improvement and 70 per cent of women given sodium iodide had clinical improvement, but with a high rate of side effects.[12]

Infections

Free I_2 has potent antimicrobial activity. Iodophor solutions, such as polyvinylpyrrolidone I_2 complex (povidone-iodine, PVP-I), are complexes that deliver free I_2, and have improved stability and less toxicity than regular iodine solutions. They are commonly used as topical antiseptics. Prior to surgery, topical application of a PVP-I solution is used routinely to reduce bacterial load around the surgical site.

It has been suggested that PVP-I might delay wound healing, based on studies on cultured fibroblasts in which PVP-I was shown to reduce the migration and proliferation of fibroblasts.[13] It has also been proposed that topical iodine treatment may affect thyroid function. However, a review of the use of iodine antiseptics concluded that there was no evidence of a higher risk of adverse effects related to PVP-I compared with other antiseptics, and that available evidence suggests that iodine is an effective antiseptic agent that does not disrupt thyroid function or delay the wound-healing process.[14]

Potassium iodide and supersaturated potassium iodide (SSKI) are used orally for the treatment of inflammatory skin diseases such as panniculitis and neutrophilic dermatoses, as well as fungal skin diseases such as some types of sporotrichosis.[15] SSKI contains 1000 mg of potassium iodide per mL of solution, each drop providing about 50 mg of iodine.

REFERENCES

1 Aceves, C., Anguiano, B. & Delgado, G., The extrathyronine actions of iodine as antioxidant, apoptotic, and differentiation factor in various tissues, *Thyroid* (2013), 23(8): 938–46.

2 Kilbane, M.T., Ajjan, R.A., Weetman, A.P. et al., Tissue iodine content and serum-mediated 125I uptake-blocking activity in breast cancer, *J Clin Endocrinol Metab* (2000), 85(3): 1245–50.

3 Funahashi, H., Imai, T., Mase, T. et al., Seaweed prevents breast cancer? *Jpn J Cancer Res* (2001), 92(5): 483–7.

4 Funahashi, H., Imai, T., Tanaka, Y. et al., Suppressive effect of iodine on DMBA-induced breast tumor growth in the rat, *J Surg Oncol* (1996), 61(3): 209–13.

5 Martínez-Iglesias, O., Garcia-Silva, S., Tenbaum, S.P. et al., Thyroid hormone receptor beta1 acts as a potent suppressor of tumor invasiveness and metastasis, *Cancer Res* (2009), 69(2): 501–9.

6 Hardefeldt, P.J., Eslick, G.D. & Edirimanne, S., Benign thyroid disease is associated with breast cancer: A meta-analysis, *Breast Cancer Res Treat* (2012), 133(3): 1169–77.

7 Parkin, D.M., Pisani, P. & Ferlay, J., Global cancer statistics, *CA Cancer J Clin* (1999), 49: 33–64.

8 Belfiore, A., La Rosa, G.L., La Porta, G.A. et al., Cancer risk in patients with cold thyroid nodules: Relevance of iodine intake, sex, age and multinodularity, *Am J Med* (1992), 93: 363–9.

9 Yang, Y.J., Nam, S.J., Kong, G. & Kim, M.K., A case-control study on seaweed consumption and the risk of breast cancer, *Br J Nutr* (2010), 103(9): 1345–53.

10 Cardis, E., Kesminiene, A., Ivanov, V. et al., Risk of thyroid cancer after exposure to 131I in childhood, *J Natl Cancer Inst* (2005), 97(10): 724–32.

11 Bhargav, P.R., Mishra, A., Agarwal, G. et al., Prevalence of hypothyroidism in benign breast disorders and effect of thyroxine replacement on the clinical outcome, *World J Surg* (2009), 33(10): 2087–93.

12 Ghent, W.R., Eskin, B.A., Low, D.A. & Hill, L.P., Iodine replacement in fibrocystic disease of the breast, *Can J Surg* (1993), 36(5): 453–60.

13 Thomas, G.W., Rael, L.T., Bar-Or, R. et al., Mechanisms of delayed wound healing by commonly used antiseptics, *J Trauma Acute Care Surg* (2009), 66(1): 82–91.

14 Vermeulen, H., Westerbos, S.J. & Ubbink. D.T., Benefit and harm of iodine in wound care: A systematic review, *J Hosp Infect* (2010), 76(3): 191–9.

15 Hassan, I. & Keen, A., Potassium iodide in dermatology, *Indian J Dermatol Venereol Leprol* (2012), 78: 390–3.

Therapeutic dose

Iodine in supplement form should be used cautiously and, because of its potential toxicity, it is recommended that doses are restricted to RDI amounts. There is no evidence that higher doses are of benefit for maintaining thyroid function in healthy individuals. High-dose iodine supplementation for the treatment of thyroid disorders should be used only under medical supervision.

In countries with endemic goitre and endemic cretinism, iodised oil is given orally or by intramuscular injection once yearly. Oral administration is more common because it is simpler to administer. Treatment is directed towards women of childbearing age, pregnant women and children. The standard dose for adults is 400 mg iodine/year, 100 mg/year for infants up to six months of age and 200 mg/year for children seven to 24 months of age. In these regions, iodine can also be given orally as potassium iodide in drops or tablets in a dose sufficient to increase total intake (from food and the supplement) to the recommended daily amount. The standard oral dose of potassium iodide for school-age children is 30 mg once monthly or 8 mg twice weekly.

Effects of excess

Acute iodine toxicity can cause vomiting, diarrhoea, metabolic acidosis, cardiovascular disturbances, cyanosis, seizures, stupor, delirium, collapse and coma. Treatment with iodine-containing drugs or the use of iodine as a radiographic contrast media—or, rarely, the use of topical iodine—may cause sensitivity reactions, such as swelling of the salivary glands (iodide mumps), acne-like inflamed skin eruptions (iododerma) or fever (iodide fever).

The NHMRC of Australia has stated that the safe upper limit (UL) of iodine intake for adults is 1.1 mg daily. However, Japanese populations have an average intake of 2–3 mg/day, and some studies have used 3–6 mg of molecular iodine daily for up to five years in people without existing thyroid disorders and found no disturbance of thyroid function. People with existing thyroid disorders or with a long history of iodine deficiency are more likely to have adverse effects from high iodine intakes, and may have effects at intakes below the UL.

Large doses of iodine may disrupt thyroid function and potentially lead to hypothyroidism, autoimmune thyroiditis, hyperthyroidism (thyrotoxicosis) or increased risk of papillary thyroid cancer. Large amounts of iodine may also cause temporary hypothyroidism (Wolff-Chaikoff effect) due to inhibition of iodine organification and decreased production of thyroid hormones. The effect usually reverses in about two days, even if iodine intake remains high, because there is a decrease in NIS, which reduces transport of iodine into the thyroid.

The frequency of thyroiditis has been found to increase in endemic goitre regions after iodine replacement. Excess dietary iodine has been associated with goitre and thyroid dysfunction in children, which responds to reduction in iodine intake. In China, long-term high intake is associated with a small increase in subclinical hypothyroidism and autoimmune thyroiditis, and modestly increased rates of hypothyroidism and hyperthyroidism have been reported in Denmark after correction of mild to moderate iodine deficiencies.

In Korea, lactating mothers traditionally consume brown seaweed (*Undaria pinnatifida*) soup during the early period after birth to increase breast milk supply, and their iodine intake is estimated to be more than 2 mg/day. This leads to high iodine levels in breast milk, and has been found to trigger hypothyroidism in some infants, which usually reverses when the seaweed intake is ceased.

Autoimmune thyroid disease

Autoimmune thyroid disease (AITD) includes Graves' disease (GD) and chronic autoimmune thyroiditis (CAT), also known as Hashimoto's thyroiditis. These disorders are more common in areas where iodine intake is adequate and increases in AITD correlate with increases in dietary iodine. In CAT, the TSH receptor antibody (TRAb) binds to TSH receptors and blocks TSH activity, leading to thyroid gland damage and atrophy and hypothyroidism. In GD, TRAb binding increases thyroid hormone production and causes overgrowth of thyroid tissue and hyperthyroidism. Autoantibodies to Tg and TPO are also present.

The role of excess iodine in AITD is not well understood, but it may act by increasing the iodine content of Tg, thereby increasing its ability to trigger immune reactions, by stimulating the activity of lymphocytes that have been primed by thyroid-specific antigens, by enhancing the antigen-presenting capabilities of macrophages or by causing genetically predisposed normal thyrocytes to convert to antigen-presenting thyrocytes.

Case reports—iodine excess

- *An Australian woman, 36 years of age,* was found to have a mildly elevated serum TSH concentration during screening for in vitro fertilisation.[1] She had no thyroid antibodies, but very high iodine levels in her urine (4445 mcg/L). It was discovered that she had been drinking a brand of soy milk that contained the seaweed kombu (kelp), and testing revealed that the milk contained 25 000 mcg/L of iodine. Her TSH returned to normal when she stopped drinking the milk.
- *A Korean woman living in Australia* consumed soup made with dried seaweed during pregnancy and after birth.[2] Her infant had a normal TSH level shortly after birth, but then developed jaundice and was found to have elevated serum TSH, low serum levels of free thyroxine and elevated urinary iodine at three weeks of age. The infant was given short-term thyroxine and thyroid functions normalised after the mother stopped using seaweed soup. Two seaweed samples were tested and found to contain 291 mcg/g and 424 mcg/g of iodine.
- *A Japanese man, 63 years of age,* developed general malaise, loss of appetite, weight loss, diarrhoea and constipation.[3] He seemed to be depressed, and had a myxoedematous appearance. His thyroid gland was slightly enlarged, his serum levels of free T3 and thyroxine were low and he had a markedly elevated serum TSH. It was revealed that he had a long history of throat discomfort and, over more than ten years, was in the habit of gargling with a povidone-iodine solution three to five times daily. The patient was reluctant to stop gargling, so he was changed to a non-iodine gargling solution. Twelve days after stopping gargling with povidone-iodine, his serum levels of free T3 and thyroxine increased and there was a rapid decrease in serum TSH. However, his TSH rose again after he began taking large amounts of kelp in the belief that the iodine in it would be good for him. His TSH dropped after he was convinced to discontinue taking excessive amounts of kelp.
- *A woman, 72 years of age,* developed symptoms of hyperthyroidism that included weight loss despite a normal appetite, excessive sweating, fatigue and the passing of several soft stools a day.[4] She had no personal or family history of thyroid disorders. Testing revealed an enlarged thyroid and elevated levels of T3, thyroxine and TSH. It was found that she had been taking four to six tablets of kelp daily for a year, with each tablet providing 700 mcg of iodine. Her total daily iodine intake was 2.8–4.2 mg. After stopping the kelp tablets, her symptoms cleared, she gained weight and her thyroid gland decreased in size. Six months later, her serum thyroid hormones and TSH had returned to normal.

REFERENCES

1 Crawford, B.A., Cowell, C.T., Emder, P.J. et al., Iodine toxicity from soy milk and seaweed ingestion is associated with serious thyroid dysfunction, *Med J Aust* (2010), 193(7): 413–15.

2 Emder, P.J. & Jack, M.M., Iodine-induced neonatal hypothyroidism secondary to maternal seaweed consumption: A common practice in some Asian cultures to promote breast milk supply, *J Paediatr Child Health* (2011), 47(10): 750–2.

3 Sato, K, Ohmori. T., Shiratori, K. et al., Povidone iodine-induced overt hypothyroidism in a patient with prolonged habitual gargling: Urinary excretion of iodine after gargling in normal subjects, *Intern Med* (2007), 46(7): 391–5.

4 Shilo, S. & Hirsch, H.J., Iodine-induced hyperthyroidism in a patient with a normal thyroid gland, *Postgrad Med J* (1986), 62(729): 661–2.

Supplements

Iodine is obtained from brine containing natural gas and salt, and is extracted together with natural gas. The salt concentration in brine is almost the same as that of sea water, but the iodine concentration is almost 2000 times higher. Iodine is extracted from brine by a vaporisation process or an ion-exchange resin process. The permitted form of iodine in oral supplements in Australia is potassium iodide, available in tablets, capsules and liquids. Iodine-containing seaweeds approved for use as oral supplements include the blue-green microalgae spirulina (*Arthrospira platensis*, *Arthrospira maxima*), the green microalgae *Chlorella* spp., the red algae *Alsidium helminthochorton*,

Chondrus crispus (Irish moss), *Gelidium amansii*, *Gigartina mamillosa* and *Iridophycus flaccidum*, and the brown algae *Alaria esculenta* (winged kelp), *Ascophyllum nodosum*, *Fucus vesiculosus* (kelp), *Laminaria* spp. (kelp), *Macrocystis pyrifera* (giant kelp) and *Sargassum* spp.

Iodine is highly bioavailable, and there is little difference in bioavailability between various forms of iodine salts or seaweeds. The amount of elemental iodine in a specific iodine salt is listed on the product container, and may vary between individual products. The approximate elemental iodine content of some common salts is shown in Table 11.6.

Table 11.6 Elemental iodine content of common salts

Salt	Iodine content (%)
Sodium iodide	85.0
Potassium iodide	76.5
Sodium iodate	64.0
Potassium iodate	59.5

- *Sodium iodide* contains the most elemental iodine, and is produced by reacting iodine with sodium hydroxide.
- *Potassium iodide* is produced by reacting iodine with potassium hydroxide.
- *Sodium iodate* is produced by reacting sodium hydroxide with iodic acid.
- *Potassium iodate* is produced by reacting iodic acid with potassium hydroxide.
- *Lugol's solution* consists of 5 per cent iodine and 10 per cent potassium iodide in purified water. One drop provides 6.3 mg of iodine. It should not be used long term as an iodine supplement because it may lead to iodine toxicity.
- *Iodoral* is a tablet form of Lugol's solution; it provides 12.5 mg iodine per tablet, equivalent to two drops of the solution. It should not be used long term as an iodine supplement because it may lead to iodine toxicity.
- *Iodised oil* is made by esterification of the unsaturated fatty acids in seed or vegetable oils and the addition of iodine to the double bonds. It is used as a once-yearly supplement in countries with endemic goitre and endemic cretinism.

Cautions

Iodine supplements should be used with caution and doses greater than the RDI are not recommended in the long term, especially in people with a history of thyroid dysfunction. Iodine supplements should not be taken together with the iodine-containing drug amiodarone because of possible toxicity. High-dose iodine supplements should not be used in hyperthyroidism or hypothyroidism except under medical supervision.

HOW MUCH DO I KNOW?

Choose whether the following statements are true or false. Then review this chapter for the correct answers.

		True (T)	False (F)
1	Copper is found in shellfish and whole grains.	T	F
2	Copper is required for connective tissue integrity and iron metabolism.	T	F
3	Bone and joint abnormalities can occur in a copper deficiency.	T	F
4	Manganese is part of thyroid hormones.	T	F
5	A Parkinson's disease-like disorder is caused by iodine overload.	T	F
6	Manganese balance is regulated by changes in excretion in bile.	T	F

7	Wilson's disease is caused by iodine excess.	T	F
8	Thyroid hormone T4 is more potent than T3.	T	F
9	Iodine has anticancer and antiseptic activity.	T	F
10	The RDI for iodine in pregnancy is 220 mcg/day.	T	F

FURTHER READING

Braun, L. & Cohen, M., *Herbs & natural supplements: An evidence-based guide*, 3rd ed., Churchill Livingstone Elsevier, New York, 2010.

Gropper, S.S., Smith, J.L. & Groff, J.L., *Advanced nutrition and human metabolism*, 5th ed., Thomson Wadsworth, Belmont, CA, 2009.

Higdon, J., *An evidence-based approach to vitamins and minerals*, Thieme, New York, 2003.

Linus Pauling Institute, Micronutrient Research Center, available at <lpi.oregonstate.edu/infocenter>.

12

Trace elements: selenium, chromium, molybdenum and fluorine, and ultratrace elements: boron and silicon

TRACE ELEMENTS

Selenium

> **SELENIUM STATUS CHECK**
>
> 1 Do you have an underactive thyroid gland?
> 2 Do you have cancer or a history of cancer?
> 3 Do you have a chronic inflammatory disorder?
> 4 Do you have weak heart muscle function or cardiomyopathy?
>
> 'Yes' answers may indicate inadequate selenium status. Note that a number of nutritional deficiencies or health disorders can cause similar effects and further investigation is recommended.

> **FAST FACTS . . . SELENIUM**
>
> - Good sources of selenium include Brazil nuts, high-selenium yeast, brewer's yeast, cashew nuts, garlic, onion, wheat, broccoli, cabbage, tomatoes, mushrooms, liver, kidneys, meat, eggs and seafood.
> - Selenium is essential for antioxidant protection.
> - It is important for maintaining redox balance, and has anti-inflammatory, anticancer, immune-stimulating and detoxifying activity.
> - A deficiency can cause impaired muscle function, cardiomyopathy, degenerative joint disease and diseases related to oxidative stress.
> - There is a relatively narrow margin between beneficial effects and toxicity; excess selenium can cause abnormalities of skin, nails and teeth, hair loss and dysfunction of the nervous system.

Selenium is present in the environment as elemental selenium, selenides, selenites and selenates, often in association with sulfur-containing minerals. The concentration in soil varies widely according to geographic region, ranging from 5 to 1.2 million mcg/kg, and is higher in soils of more recent volcanic origin. High-selenium soils are found in the Northern Great Plains of North America (which extend from northern Nebraska to areas of southern Canada), some areas of Venezuela and parts of China. Australian soils have a moderate selenium content and New Zealand soils have a very low content; selenium fortification of fertilisers for cereal crops and importation of Australian wheat have improved selenium levels in the New Zealand population. Selenium is available for uptake by plants in alkaline soils, but is bound in acidic soils by iron and aluminium. Plants release selenium into the air as hydrogen selenide, elemental selenium, selenites and selenates.

Selenium was discovered in 1817 by Swedish chemists Jöns Berzelius and Johan Gottlieb Gahn, who initially believed it to be the element tellurium. Tellurium was named after Telles, the Roman goddess of the earth, and selenium was therefore named after Selene, the Greek goddess of the moon. It has the chemical symbol Se, and can exist in four oxidation states: selenide (Se^{2-}), elemental selenium (Se), selenite (Se^{4+}) and selenate (Se^{6+}). It is classed as a metalloid; it can behave as a metal by donating electrons during a chemical reaction and behave as a non-metal by accepting electrons. It has similar chemical properties to sulfur in biological systems, and can be incorporated into the amino acids methionine and cysteine to form selenomethionine and selenocysteine. Cells are genetically designed to incorporate selenocysteine into certain body proteins (selenoproteins) and, although it has long been believed that only twenty amino acids are needed by the body for making structural proteins, selenocysteine is of such importance that it is now considered to be the 21st amino acid. Selenoproteins are found throughout the body, including the kidneys, liver, spleen, pancreas, heart, brain, lungs, bones and skeletal muscles. Some are known to be important for antioxidant protection, redox reactions and thyroid hormone metabolism, but the functions of many selenoproteins are still unknown.

Digestion, absorption and transport

Selenium is present in food as organic selenomethionine, selenocysteine, selenoneine, Se-methylselenocysteine and gamma-glutamyl-Se-methylselenocysteine. Plants may also contain inorganic sodium selenate. Protease enzymes, with the assistance of hydrochloric acid in the stomach, digest selenoproteins, and selenomethionine and selenocysteine are transported into enterocytes by amino acid transporters. The absorption pathways of other forms of dietary selenium have not been well established, but may involve the SLC26 multifunctional anion exchanger family that transports chloride, sulfate, bicarbonate, formate, oxalate and hydroxyl ions. Absorbed forms of selenium are converted to selenide in enterocytes; it is then incorporated into proteins as selenocysteine. Selenoproteins are transported in the bloodstream in association with lipid-carrying alpha and beta globulins found in very low-density and low-density lipoproteins, and delivered to the liver, which produces selenoprotein P (SePP), encoded by the SEPP1 gene. SePP is the major selenium transporter in plasma and the main regulator of selenium status in the body. It is also produced in the brain, kidneys, heart and lungs, and may be important for maintaining selenium levels in these tissues in deficiency states. Selenium transport to the thyroid gland appears to occur by a SePP-independent transport mechanism. Uptake of selenium from SePP by tissue cells is believed to be via the apolipoprotein E receptor 2 (apoER2) and the megalin receptor that are part of the low-density lipoprotein receptor family.

Metabolism, storage and excretion

In cells, selenomethionine can be used for production of proteins, stored with other amino acids, converted to selenocysteine or converted by the enzyme gamma-lyase to methylselenol and then to selenide. Selenocysteine can be broken down by the enzyme beta-lyase to release free selenium, which can be converted to selenide. Gamma-glutamyl-Se-methylselenocysteine is first converted to Se-methylselenocysteine and then to methylselenol by beta-lyase and is either metabolised to selenide or excreted. Inorganic forms of selenium can also be metabolised to selenide. Selenide is converted by the enzyme selenophosphate synthetase to selenophosphate, which is then used to make selenocysteine and selenoproteins.

Selenium from broken-down selenoproteins and excess selenium are converted to selenide and methylated for excretion; about half is excreted in urine and about half is excreted in faeces. Urinary excretion reflects dietary intake: 50–60 per cent of dietary intake is excreted each day. At low or normal levels of intake, selenium is excreted in urine as the selenosugar 1beta-methylseleno-N-acetyl-D-galactosamine. At higher levels of intake, it is excreted in urine mainly as trimethylselenium. Dimethylselenide can be excreted via the skin and lungs, which can cause garlic-smelling breath.

Functions

Selenium's role in the body is not fully understood. Seventeen selenoprotein gene families have been identified, some with multiple genes with similar functions. The best-characterised selenoproteins are glutathione peroxidase, thioredoxin reductase, iodothyronine deiodinase and selenophosphate synthetase. Other selenoproteins include SePP and selenoprotein (SeP) 15, H, I, K, M, N, O, R, S, T, V and W. There are also two proteins that bind selenium: selenium-binding protein 1 (SeBP1) and 2 (SeBP2).

Selenoproteins appear to function mainly as enzymes involved in antioxidant protection, immune function, pancreatic function, detoxification and DNA repair. Selenium has similar functions to vitamin E in the body, and vitamin E can modulate the effects of selenium deficiency in animals. The functions of selenium include:

- *Antioxidant activity, redox balance.* Glutathione peroxidase (GPx) enzymes are among the most important antioxidant enzymes in the body. Five GPx enzymes are selenoproteins, namely cytosolic GPx (GPx1), gastrointestinal-specific GPx (GPx2), plasma GPx (GPx3), phospholipid hydroperoxide GPx (GPx4) and GPx6. GPxs remove damaging hydrogen peroxide and organic hydroperoxides formed by superoxide dismutases during the process of scavenging superoxide radicals. GPx1 is the main form found in cell cytoplasm, GPx2 protects the gut from ingested lipid hydroperoxides, GPx3 protects blood lipids, GPx4 protects spermatozoa and GPx6 protects the developing embryo and the olfactory epithelium in the nose. Selenomethionine and selenocysteine can also bind metals and inhibit damage to DNA.

  Oxidation-reduction (redox) status is an important regulator of cell metabolism. Thioredoxin reductase (TrxR) enzymes are flavoprotein oxidoreductases that contain selenocysteine at their active site. They are part of the thioredoxin (Trx) system in cells, consisting of Trx, TrxR and NADPH, that helps maintain redox balance. There are three types of TrxR enzymes: cytosolic TrxR1, mitochondrial TrxR2 and testes-specific Trx-glutathione reductase (TrxGR). TrxR1 and 2 are present in many body tissues, and act to convert oxidised Trx to its reduced active form, which, in turn, reduces oxidised cysteine residues on cellular proteins. The Trx system plays an important role in antioxidant defence, cellular redox balance, gene transcription, DNA synthesis and repair, protein repair, cell proliferation, apoptosis, immunity, redox-regulated signalling, calcium metabolism and regeneration of vitamin C, alpha-lipoic acid and coenzyme Q10 to their active forms. TrxR also plays a role in metabolising various selenium compounds, and helps regulate selenoprotein synthesis.

  Other selenoproteins also have an antioxidant role. SePP may remove peroxynitrite radicals that can damage DNA and lipids. SePK is an antioxidant in heart tissue and also may act in skeletal muscle, the pancreas, the liver and the placenta. SePR assists the repair of proteins that have been damaged by oxidation, and SePS has anti-inflammatory activity that protects cells from the damaging consequences of endoplasmic reticulum stress. SePN and SePW appear to protect muscle tissue, but their role is not well understood.
- *Thyroid hormone function.* Selenium-containing type 1 or type 2 iodothyronine deiodinase enzymes (D1 and D2) are found in tissues such as the liver, kidneys, pituitary gland, brain, mammary glands and brown adipose tissue. These enzymes are essential for the conversion of thyroxine (T4) to the more potent form (T3), and are important for thyroid hormone activity, which maintains the body's metabolic rate. Selenium-containing type 3 iodothyronine deiodinase (D3) inactivates T3 and T4, which helps regulate thyroid hormone levels in tissues.
- *Detoxification.* Selenium may induce expression of genes related to phase II detoxification enzymes. Selenium supplementation in animals without selenium deficiency has been shown to protect against the toxicity of various chemical carcinogens, including 3-methyl-4-dimethyl-aminoazobenzene, 2-acetylaminofluorene, diethylnitrosamine, aflatoxin, 7,12-dimethylbenz[a]anthracene, benzopyrene and 3-methylcholanthrene. Selenium interacts with toxic elements, such as arsenic, mercury, cadmium, thallium and, to a limited extent, silver, reducing their toxicity by forming inert metal selenide complexes.

  Methylmercury (MeHg) is a highly specific, irreversible inhibitor of selenium-dependent enzymes. Selenium, as selenide, is protective because it breaks down MeHg to the less toxic form, inorganic mercury. In animals, mercury exposure causes nerve damage and death if dietary selenium is low, but less serious effects if dietary selenium is adequate and no effects if dietary selenium is high. Selenoneine, found in fish such as tuna, accelerates the excretion and demethylation of MeHg.

  Selenium is protective against arsenic, a pro-oxidant and human carcinogen (cancer-causing agent). Selenium and arsenic are antagonistic, and have been shown to detoxify each other when given together. Selenium may reduce chronic arsenic accumulation and protect against arsenic-related skin lesions that are common in regions of the world where there is arsenic contamination of the water supply.

- *Anticancer activity.* Selenium has anticancer activity by inducing expression of glutathione S-transferases (GSTs) that assist detoxification of carcinogens and by influencing antioxidant defence, cell cycle regulation, DNA and protein repair, immune surveillance, apoptosis, cancer cell migration and angiogenesis (growth of new blood vessels). The active forms of selenium that are protective against cancer may be methylated selenium compounds, particularly methylselenol. Methylselenol has been shown to selectively destroy abnormal cells by increasing formation of reactive oxygen species (ROS), inducing DNA damage, triggering apoptosis and inhibiting angiogenesis. Key selenoproteins that have anticancer activity include GPx1, GPx4, SeP15, SePP and TrxR1. SeP15, located in the endoplasmic reticulum in cells, helps regulate protein folding, and may have antioxidant and anticancer activity. SePP also may have anticancer effects through its role in detoxification and cell growth regulation.
- *Immune activity.* Selenoproteins influence both innate and adaptive immune responses by reducing oxidative stress and balancing redox reactions in immune cells. Selenium has a role in the production of interferon-gamma and other cytokines, T cell and T helper cell proliferation and differentiation, lymphocyte toxicity, natural killer (NK) cell activity, antibody responses and immunoglobulin (Ig) G and IgM concentrations. It supports thyroid hormone activity, which stimulates development and function of T cells and stimulates GPx1 activity in neutrophils, which protects them from the free radicals that are produced in the respiratory burst. Selenium has anti-viral activity, and can boost the immune response to antiviral vaccines. GPx1 appears to prevent the mutation of viruses to more pathogenic forms.
- *Anti-inflammatory activity.* The presence of free radicals enhances expression of inflammatory genes, and the antioxidant activity of selenoproteins reduces inflammation. Selenoproteins help to turn off inflammation by increasing production of eicosanoids such as prostacyclin that inhibit inflammation, and by reducing expression of the inflammatory cytokine nuclear factor kappa-B (NF-kappaB). Selenium also reduces inflammation by removing hydrogen peroxide that activates the p38 mitogen-activated protein kinase (p38MAPK) pathway of cell signalling. This pathway leads to expression of high levels of cyclooxygenase 2 (COX-2) and increased production of inflammatory eicosanoids.
- *Male fertility.* Selenium is important for testosterone synthesis, sperm viability and motility and male fertility. Spermatozoa contain a high concentration of selenium, which is required for antioxidant protection and normal sperm development. GPx4 is concentrated in the mid-piece of spermatozoa, where it stabilises the integrity of the sperm flagella and enhances sperm motility.

Dietary sources

Brazil nuts are a particularly good source of selenium if grown in selenium-rich soil, and average 920 mcg of selenium per 100 g. The selenium content is reported to vary widely, ranging from 0.4–158.4 mcg/g. Consumption of two Brazil nuts daily has been shown to be as effective in raising plasma selenium concentration and GPx activity as the consumption of 100 mcg of a selenomethionine supplement. Brazil nuts are known to accumulate radioactive elements, such as strontium, radium and barium, at levels up to 1000 times greater than in other foods. However, the total amount of radioactive elements is very low, and unlikely to have health effects. Because the selenium level is unpredictable and selenium is toxic in high doses, it is advisable to limit the consumption of Brazil nuts.

Other sources of selenium include high-selenium yeast, brewer's yeast, cashew nuts, garlic, onion, wheat, broccoli, cabbage, tomatoes, mushrooms, liver, kidneys, meat, eggs and seafood. High-selenium yeast may contain 1000–3000 mcg/g. Wheat is a major source if soil selenium content is adequate because it is a large component of most Western diets. In Australia, wheat products such as bread and cereals are the major sources of selenium, and the selenium content of Australian meat is relatively high compared with other countries.

Some plants are able to accumulate large amounts of selenium from soil. The best selenium accumulators are milkvetch plants (*Astragalus* sp. *Fabaceae*), which can contain up to 3000 mg/kg. *Astragalus membranaceus*, commonly used as a medicinal herb for boosting immunity, is not a selenium accumulator. Other high accumulators include some daisy family plants (*Oonopsis*, *Xylorhiza* and *Machaeranthera*) and a brassica family species, prince's plume (*Stanleya*), which may contain up to 800 mg selenium/kg. Lower selenium accumulators include some plants of the sunflower family (*Aster*, *Grindelia*, *Gutierrezia*), some saltbush family plants (*Atriplex*), some figwort family plants (*Castillaja*) and some sandalwood family plants (*Comandra*), which may contain 25–100 mg selenium/kg. Plants containing more than 5 mg/kg are toxic to grazing animals.

Most of the selenium in food is in the form of organic selenium compounds, such as selenomethionine and selenocysteine, which are highly bioavailable. Absorption averages 90–95 per cent. Onions and garlic contain the selenium compound gamma-glutamyl-Se-methylselenocysteine and broccoli contains Se-methylselenocysteine. In some plants, including beets, cabbage and garlic, about half the selenium content is in the form of selenate, which is equally well absorbed. Absorption of selenite averages more than 80 per cent, but elemental selenium is poorly absorbed. Selenoneine in tuna appears to be less well absorbed than selenite, whereas absorption of selenium from other seafoods is high.

The Food Standards Australia New Zealand nutrient database (NUTTAB) at <www.foodstandards.gov.au> provides the amounts found in specific foods.

Factors influencing body status

Organic forms of selenium have greater bioavailability than inorganic selenium, and are better retained in the body. Mercury, phytates, guar gum and a high sulfur intake reduce dietary selenium absorption. Vitamin C decreases the uptake of selenite by reducing it to elemental selenium, which is poorly absorbed. However, this interaction occurs only when both are taken on an empty stomach with no other nutrients, and is therefore unlikely to impair selenite uptake from food. Protein and vitamins A, C and E appear to increase the absorption of food selenium.

A deficiency of methionine may lead to the incorporation of selenomethionine into structural proteins, which may reduce the amount of selenomethionine available for the production of selenoproteins. Lack of vitamin B12 impairs the methylation and excretion of selenium because of a lack of production of the methyl donor S-adenosylmethionine, which is B12 dependent. Low iron and copper impair GPx synthesis, and low copper impairs deiodinase enzyme activity. Lead depletes selenium in tissues by competitive binding to sulfhydryl groups in proteins. Drugs that may lower selenium levels in the body include cisplatin (for cancer), clozapine (for psychiatric disorders), corticosteroids (for inflammation) and valproic acid (for epilepsy and psychiatric disorders).

Daily requirement

Australian and New Zealand government recommendations by age and gender (see Table 12.1) can be found in *Nutrient Reference Values for Australia and New Zealand Including Recommended Dietary Intakes*, available at <www.nhmrc.gov.au>.

Table 12.1 Recommended dietary intake (RDI) and upper level of intake (UL) of selenium (mcg/day)

Age (years)	Female RDI	Male RDI	UL
1–3	25	25	90
4–8	30	30	150
9–13	50	50	280
14–18	60	70	400
19–70	60	70	400
>70	60	70	400
Pregnant women			
14–18	65		400
19–50	65		400
Lactating women			
14–18	75		400
19–50	75		400

Source: Nutrient Reference Values for Australia and New Zealand Including Recommended Dietary Intakes, National Health and Medical Research Council, Australian Government Department of Health and Ageing, Canberra and Ministry of Health, New Zealand, Wellington, 2006.

Deficiency effects

Selenium levels have declined in many countries over the last few decades. A 2004 Australian study found that body levels of selenium have dropped by 20 per cent since the 1970s, and over a third of people were below the required level. In New Zealand, deficiencies were widespread but selenium intake has improved in recent decades as a consequence of selenium fertilisers and the importation of Australian wheat.

In animals, low selenium is associated with white muscle disease in sheep, goats, cattle and horses. Affected lambs have heart and skeletal muscle weakness, tremors, a stiff, stilted gait and an arched back, and become unable to walk, dying within a few days. Muscles show paleness, white patches or flecks. Other conditions that may be associated with low selenium in sheep are scouring, poor growth, poor wool production and impaired reproduction in ewes, with death of the foetus at about 35 days gestation.

In humans, low selenium is associated with impaired immunity and thyroid hormone function, decreased antioxidant protection, muscle weakness and cardiomyopathy. Selenium deficiency has been observed in people on long-term total parenteral nutrition (TPN, non-oral feeding), in patients after gastric bypass surgery for obesity and in children placed on a ketogenic diet (a high fat, moderate protein, very low carbohydrate diet that induces ketosis) for the treatment of intractable seizures.

Very low selenium status is associated with Keshan disease, an endemic cardiomyopathy found in the Keshan district of northeast China, and endemic sudden cardiac death in Yunnan, China is strongly associated with low SePP and GPx levels. Keshan disease causes multifocal necrosis and the replacement of muscle tissue in the heart with fibrous tissue, resulting in acute or chronic heart failure. Selenium supplementation, as sodium selenite, has been used effectively to prevent and reverse the condition in children at high risk, but the role of selenium was not well understood. It has since been found that levels of antibodies against Coxsackie virus are higher in the serum of Keshan disease patients than in normal subjects. Animals fed grains grown in the Keshan district and infected with Coxsackie virus develop severe heart pathology, but animals fed grains from selenium-replete areas and infected with the same virus develop only a mild form of heart pathology. Lack of selenium has been found to convert the virus into a more pathogenic form, and it appears that Keshan disease may be an outcome of selenium deficiency-induced susceptibility to infection and increased viral virulence.

In South America, low selenium is implicated in cardiomyopathy and heart failure occurring in people infected with the protozoa *Trypanosoma cruzi* (Chagas disease). Patients with low selenium status are more at risk of heart complications. The degenerative joint disorder Kashin-Beck disease (KBD) affects children and adults, and is endemic in rural areas of the world which are selenium deficient, such as eastern Siberia, northern Korea, central China and Tibet. In some villages, 60–90 per cent of children are affected. It causes destruction of bone and cartilage in joints and severe, symmetrical joint deformities, especially of the ankles, wrists, knees and elbows. Effects include joint enlargement, morning stiffness, pain, restriction of movement, shortened fingers and, more rarely, dwarfism. The cause is obscure but it may be related to selenium deficiency and associated immune suppression, and the presence of mycotoxins (toxins produced by moulds and fungi). An alternative theory is that a combined selenium and iodine deficiency may be involved.

People with KBD have been found to live in villages with fungal contamination of cereals and to have low body levels of selenium. Trichothecene (T-2) toxins, produced by the fungal organism *Fusarium* sp., inhibit protein synthesis, and can impair joint cartilage metabolism and cause joint abnormalities in animals. Selenium has been shown to protect chondrocytes from T-2 toxicity, possibly by increasing GPx activity. Animals genetically unable to make selenoproteins in joint tissue develop growth retardation, abnormal bone growth and destruction of joint cartilage. Selenium supplementation has been reported to be effective in some, but not all, areas with KBD. Provision of cereals imported from non-KBD areas, together with selenium supplements, appears to be a more effective treatment and has led to a greatly decreased prevalence of KBD.

Indicators of inadequate levels of selenium may include:

- impaired thyroid hormone function, hypothyroidism
- impaired immunity, increased severity of viral infections
- weak muscles, abnormal muscle function, cardiac muscle weakness, cardiomyopathy.
- degenerative joint diseases
- disorders related to oxidative stress, such as inflammatory diseases, diseases of ageing, chronic degenerative diseases, fatigue syndromes, auto-immune diseases, liver damage and alcohol-induced diseases, lung damage, male infertility, cancer.

Assessment of body status

Urinary excretion of selenium varies widely according to dietary intake, and reflects recent intake, not long-term status. It has been suggested that total dietary intake of selenium can be estimated by doubling the amount of daily excretion. Daily excretion of less than

10 mcg indicates an inadequate selenium intake and more than 35 mcg indicates excessive intake.

More commonly, selenium status is assessed by measuring the amount in plasma/serum, whole blood or red blood cells, and sometimes by measuring the amount in hair and nails. Plasma or serum selenium is believed to reflect short-term status and red blood cell/whole blood selenium is believed to reflect longer-term status. The reference range given by the Royal College of Pathologists of Australasia (RCPA) for plasma selenium is 0.75–1.35 μmol/L and 1.1–2.5 μmol/L for whole blood selenium. Toenail selenium may reflect long-term status, as may hair selenium, but hair levels can be affected by selenium-containing shampoos. However, tissue levels may not reflect activity of selenoproteins because, if selenomethionine intake is high, it is non-specifically incorporated into proteins as selenomethionine in the place of methionine, and will lead to elevated tissue levels.

Selenoprotein activity can be assessed by measuring plasma and red blood cell GPx activity because it drops rapidly in animals fed a selenium-deficient diet. However, GPx activity plateaus when blood selenium levels are greater than 1.27 μmol/L. Platelet GPx appears to respond more quickly to selenium supplementation, and can be used as a marker of response to treatment. A study of a US population found that SePP concentration was the best plasma biomarker for assessing optimal expression of all selenoproteins. It was concluded that 75 mcg/day of selenium as selenomethionine would allow full expression of selenoproteins.

Case reports—selenium deficiency

- *A male infant, fifteen months of age*, from Saudi Arabia, with a history of chronic diarrhoea and asthma, developed failure to thrive, a fever lasting six months, loss of weight and respiratory distress.[1] He was found to have dilated cardiomyopathy and congestive heart failure. Medication relieved his symptoms, but did not address the cause. He was found to have very low serum selenium (0.12 μmol/L). He was given selenium supplementation (2 mcg/kg/day), together with drugs for heart failure. He responded to treatment after three to four months, with weight gain and improvement in his cardiac function, skin, hair, appetite and general health. Cardiac function normalised, and his serum selenium increased to 1.19 μmol/L. The cause was not determined but it was suspected that the dependence of Saudi Arabians on imported processed food may have contributed to the infant's selenium deficiency.
- *A woman, 28 years of age*, with a seven-year history of anorexia nervosa treated with intermittent parenteral nutrition, developed generalised fatigue and was placed on TPN for one month.[2] She then developed proximal muscle pain and weakness in her limbs, and had difficulty walking or standing up. Her serum creatine kinase, an indicator of muscle breakdown, was found to be very high, her serum selenium concentration was very low (0.17 μmol/L) and her GPx concentration was reduced. Muscle biopsy revealed pale muscles that were severely atrophied. She was placed on an oral diet, and her muscle pain improved within a few days. Her serum creatine kinase concentration gradually decreased and was normal in one month and she was able to walk unassisted and stand up from a chair in two months. Serum selenium and GPx also improved. It was concluded that TPN provided inadequate selenium, leading to a human form of 'white muscle disease'.
- *A woman, 39 years of age*, who had undergone gastric bypass surgery seven years previously, developed a change in her mental status and generalised weakness.[3] She was found to have low blood pressure, and was in mild respiratory distress. After two days in hospital, she developed respiratory and circulatory collapse requiring endotracheal intubation and mechanical ventilation. Her left ventricular ejection fraction was less than 20 per cent, indicating impaired heart function. She was found to have low serum selenium (0.37 μmol/L) and was given selenium supplementation, which improved her heart function and increased her ejection fraction to 55 per cent.
- *A boy, five years of age*, who had been placed on a ketogenic diet to control his intractable seizures, developed acute cardiomyopathy and ventricular tachycardia (rapid beating of the heart ventricles).[4] He was found to have markedly low serum selenium despite a normal selenium level before starting the diet. The ketogenic diet was stopped and he was given supplementary selenium, which led to a rapid improvement in his heart function.

REFERENCES

1 Al-Matary, A., Hussain, M. & Ali, J., Selenium: A brief review and a case report of selenium responsive cardiomyopathy, *BMC Pediatr* (2013), 13: 39.

2 Ishihara, H., Kanda, F., Matsushita, T. et al., White muscle disease in humans: Myopathy caused by selenium deficiency in anorexia nervosa under long term total parenteral nutrition, *J Neurol Neurosurg Psychiatry* (1999), 67(6): 829–30.

3 Huseini, M., Raza, N., Still, C. & Komar, M., Selenium deficiency causing cardiomyopathy in a patient with gastric bypass surgery, Poster 1292, presented at 77th Annual Scientific Meeting of the American College of Gastroenterology (ACG), 2012, retrieved 20 August 2014 from <http://d2j7fjepcxuj0a.cloudfront.net/wp-content/uploads/2012/10/ACG2012_Poster 1292.pdf>.

4 Sirikonda, N.S., Patten, W.D., Phillips, J.R. & Mullett, C.J., Ketogenic diet: Rapid onset of selenium deficiency-induced cardiac decompensation, *Pediatr Cardiol* (2012), 33(5): 834–8.

THERAPEUTIC USES OF SELENIUM

Cancer

Selenium appears to be protective against some types of cancers, including lung, bladder, colorectal, liver, oesophageal, gastric cardia, thyroid and prostate cancers. A number of studies have found that people with lower plasma selenium concentrations have a higher risk of cancer, especially gastrointestinal and prostate cancers, than those with higher levels.[1] Selenium-enriched yeast supplements have reduced cancer incidence and mortality in men with a low plasma selenium concentration at baseline, but subjects with higher baseline plasma selenium had a non-significant trend towards increased cancer incidence.[2] A meta-analysis of studies of selenium supplementation concluded that it was associated with reduced cancer incidence in men but not women.[3]

A meta-analysis of 20 trials of selenium supplementation concluded that it was associated with a 25–60 per cent reduction in risk of gastrointestinal cancers, such as oesophageal, gastric, small intestine, colorectal, pancreatic, liver and biliary tract cancers.[4] In China, table salt fortified with 15 ppm of sodium selenite was used in a large population for over eight years, and resulted in a 35 per cent decreased incidence of primary liver cancer compared with a population not using selenium-fortified salt.[5] A trial of selenium supplementation (200 mcg/day) given as high-selenium yeast in patients with a history of skin cancer found that there was a 25 per cent reduction in total cancer incidence and reductions in total cancer mortality and the incidence of lung, colorectal and prostate cancers.[2] However, there was an increase in non-melanoma skin cancers. A small sub-group of subjects from this trial was given high-selenium yeast providing 400 mcg a day of selenium, and had greater increases in serum selenium levels than subjects taking 200 mcg of selenium; however, the higher dose was not more effective in reducing total cancer risk.[6]

Low serum selenium levels are associated with a greater risk of prostate cancer,[7] and a meta-analysis of sixteen trials concluded that selenium intake reduced the relative risk of prostate cancer by about 30 per cent.[8] However, the large-scale Selenium and Vitamin E Cancer Prevention Trial (SELECT) in 2009 did not show a reduction in prostate cancer risk in relatively healthy men who took 200 mcg a day of selenomethionine for over five years.[9] There is some evidence that selenium may be more effective in protecting against aggressive prostate cancer and its progression.[10] Several studies have found that selenium supplementation may protect against the toxicity of radiotherapy and chemotherapy, and reduce the risk of side-effects, especially during cisplatin treatment.[10]

To date, the evidence for benefits of selenium supplementation on cancer risk is conflicting, and the optimal form of selenium supplement for reducing cancer risk is not known. It is possible that genetic factors play a role. Mutations in genes for SePP, GPx1, GPx4 and SeP15 have been associated with increased risk of many cancers, and variants of the gene for GPx4 have been associated with increased mortality in patients with breast cancer.[10]

Overall, it appears that there is a relatively narrow range of benefit in terms of selenium intake, blood levels and anticancer effects. It has been suggested that a plasma/serum selenium concentration of 1.52–1.91 μmol/L may be protective, a level that can be achieved by an intake of 100–150 mcg of selenium a day.[10] Serum levels greater than 2.03 μmol/L may possibly increase the risk of some types of cancer.[10]

Asthma

Asthma patients have been found to have lower serum selenium concentrations and higher indicators of oxidative stress.[11] However, inflammatory disorders are known to lead to decreased serum selenium levels; therefore, the relationship with selenium is difficult to interpret. Animal studies suggest that dietary selenium can have a marked influence on allergic asthma by modulating immune responses.[12] Some studies in humans have found that lower selenium status is associated with poorer lung function and higher incidence, prevalence and severity of asthma, but other studies have not found such a link.[13] A meta-analysis of 62 studies of nutrient intake and the risk of developing asthma concluded that selenium intake has not been shown to be of benefit in reducing risk.[14] However, there is some evidence to indicate that higher maternal selenium levels during pregnancy may have a protective effect against wheezing in the infant.[15] Selenium supplementation was found to significantly decrease use of corticosteroid drugs in one study of corticoid-dependent asthmatics, but this result has not been replicated in other studies.[16]

Cardiovascular disease

Selenium deficiency can impair heart function, and a meta-analysis of 25 studies found that low selenium status was associated with increased risk of coronary heart disease but the evidence was not of sufficient quality to draw firm conclusions.[17] One study found that a plasma selenium concentration of less than 0.57 μmol/L was associated with an increased risk of ischaemic heart disease and myocardial infarction (MI, heart attack) and a two- to three-fold increase in cardiovascular disease (CVD) mortality,[18] but other studies are conflicting. Low serum selenium has been associated with a 3.7-fold increased risk of stroke mortality.[19] Selenium may be protective in people with low selenium status but does not appear to be protective in people with adequate status.

Brain disorders

The importance of selenium to the brain is indicated by the fact that the brain retains selenium even when intake is inadequate. Selenoproteins protect against nerve damage caused by oxidative stress, which is implicated in disorders such as Alzheimer's disease (AD) and Parkinson's disease (PD). AD is associated with oxidative stress, build-up of amyloid-beta in the brain and deterioration of the cholinergic system. SePP is a key selenoprotein in brain tissue that increases with ageing, and deletion of the gene for SePP impairs learning and memory functions in animals. SePP has been found in AD plaques and neurofibrillary tangles, in which it may have an antioxidant role. Selenium supplementation has been shown to decrease toxicity of amyloid-beta peptide.[20] A review of research related to selenium and AD concluded that selenium has a decisive role in the pathogenesis of AD at the molecular level, but there is no consistent clinical evidence that selenium supplementation is of benefit for AD treatment.[21] However, there is some evidence of an association between selenium status and cognitive function.

PD involves loss of dopamine-releasing nerve cells in the substantia nigra of the brain, which impairs movement. In animal models of PD, selenium deficiency is associated with increased damage to dopaminergic neurons, and selenium supplementation has been shown to have protective activity and to enhance GPx activity.[22] In older people, low serum selenium is associated with decreased performance on tests of coordination.[23] People with PD have been found to have 63 per cent lower serum selenium than normal subjects, and about half the normal level of glutathione in the substantia nigra in the brain, which may lead to impaired GPx activity and oxidation damage.[24] The level of GPx4 and SePP has also been found to be lower in the substantia nigra in people with PD compared with controls.[25] The effect of selenium supplementation in AD and PD is unknown.

Immune disorders

Selenium supplementation boosts immune responses, including proliferation of activated T cells and NK cell activity.[26] Oxidative stress is a consequence of selenium deficiency, and is associated with impaired immune responses and the rapid mutation of benign variants of RNA viruses to more pathogenic forms that are consistent and long-lived.[27] If selenium-deficient hosts are supplemented with dietary selenium, viral mutation rates reduce and immunocompetence improves. People with low selenium status given 50 mcg and 100 mcg daily of sodium selenite, and challenged with an oral, live, attenuated polio virus, were able to clear the virus more rapidly than control subjects.[28]

Human immunodeficiency virus type 1 (HIV-1) infected drug users with low plasma selenium have been found to have a three-fold higher risk of developing mycobacterial disease—especially tuberculosis—than those with higher plasma selenium.[29] Selenium deficiency has been associated with decreased survival in people with HIV-1,[30] and supplementation with 200 mcg per day has been shown to increase CD4 count, suppress viral replication and decrease hospital admissions and the percentage of admissions due to infection.[31,32]

Selenium supplementation has been found to be protective in autoimmune thyroiditis. A meta-analysis concluded that supplementation with 80 mcg or 200 mcg daily of sodium selenite or selenomethionine is effective in lowering thyroid peroxidase autoantibodies in Hashimoto's disease, improving the structure of the thyroid gland and improving mood and general wellbeing.[33] In Graves' disease (GD), selenium supplementation appears to improve quality of life, reduce eye involvement and have a beneficial effect on mild cases of the associated inflammatory eye disorder, orbitopathy.[34] Higher serum selenium has been associated with remission of GD.[35] Selenium supplementation in pregnant women has been shown to decrease the risk of postpartum thyroiditis and hypothyroidism developing after the birth.[36]

REFERENCES

1 Willett, W.C., Polk, B.F., Morris, J.S. et al., Prediagnostic serum selenium and risk of cancer, *Lancet* (1983), 2(8342): 130–4.

2 Duffield-Lillico, A.J., Reid, M.E., Turnbull, B.W. et al., Baseline characteristics and the effect of selenium supplementation on cancer incidence in a randomized clinical trial: A summary report of the Nutritional Prevention of Cancer Trial, *Cancer Epidemiol Biomarkers Prev* (2002), 11(7): 630–9.

3 Bardia, A., Tleyjeh, I.M., Cerhan, J.R. et al., Efficacy of antioxidant supplementation in reducing primary cancer incidence and mortality: Systematic review and meta-analysis, *Mayo Clin Proc* (2008), 83(1): 23–34.

4 Bjelakovic, G., Nikolova, D., Simonetti, R.G. & Gluud, C., Antioxidant supplements for preventing gastrointestinal cancers, *Cochrane Database Syst Rev* (2008), 3: CD004183.

5 Yu, S.Y., Zhu, Y.J. & Li, W.G., Protective role of selenium against hepatitis B virus and primary liver cancer in Qidong, *Biol Trace Elem Res* (1997), 56(1): 117–24.

6 Reid, M.E., Duffield-Lillico, A.J., Slate, E. et al., The nutritional prevention of cancer: 400 mcg per day selenium treatment, *Nutr Cancer* (2008), 60(2): 155–63.

7 Vogt, T.M., Ziegler, R.G., Graubard, B.I. et al., Serum selenium and risk of prostate cancer in U.S. blacks and whites, *Int J Cancer* (2003), 103(5): 664–70.

8 Etminan, M., FitzGerald, J.M., Gleave, M. & Chambers, K., Intake of selenium in the prevention of prostate cancer: a systematic review and meta-analysis, *Cancer Causes Control* (2005), 16(9): 1125–31.

9 Lippman, S.M., Klein, E.A., Goodman, P.J. et al., Effect of selenium and vitamin E on risk of prostate cancer and other cancers: The Selenium and Vitamin E Cancer Prevention Trial (SELECT), *JAMA* (2009), 301(1): 39–51.

10 Fairweather-Tait, S.J., Bao, Y., Broadley, M.R. et al., Selenium in human health and disease, *Antioxid Redox Signal* (2011), 14(7): 1337–83.

11 Guo, C.H., Liu, P.J., Hsia, S. et al., Role of certain trace minerals in oxidative stress, inflammation, CD4/CD8 lymphocyte ratios and lung function in asthmatic patients, *Ann Clin Biochem* (2011), 48(Pt 4): 344–51.

12 Hoffmann, P.R. & Berry, M.J., The influence of selenium on immune responses, *Mol Nutr Food Res* (2008), 52(11): 1273–80.

13 Norton, R.L. & Hoffmann, P.R., Selenium and asthma, *Mol Aspects Med* (2012), 33(1): 98–106.

14 Nurmatov, U., Devereux, G. & Sheikh, A., Nutrients and foods for the primary prevention of asthma and allergy: systematic review and meta-analysis, *J Allergy Clin Immunol* (2011), 127(3): 724–33.

15 Devereux, G., McNeill, G., Newman, G. et al., Early childhood wheezing symptoms in relation to plasma selenium in pregnant mothers and neonates, *Clin Exp Allergy* (2007), 37(7): 1000–8.

16 Gazdik, F., Kadrabova, J. & Gazdikova, K., Decreased consumption of corticosteroids after selenium supplementation in corticoid-dependent asthmatics, *Bratisl Lek Listy* (2002), 103(1): 22–5.

17 Flores-Mateo, G., Navas-Acien, A., Pastor-Barriuso, R. & Guallar, E., Selenium and coronary heart disease: A meta-analysis, *Am J Clin Nutr* (2006), 84(4): 762–73.

18 Salonen, J.T., Alfthan, G., Huttunen, J.K. et al., Association between cardiovascular death and myocardial infarction and serum selenium in a matched-pair longitudinal study, *Lancet* (1982), 2(8291): 175–9.

19 Virtamo, J., Valkeila, E., Alfthan, G. et al., Serum selenium and the risk of coronary heart disease and stroke, *Am J Epidemiol* (1985), 122(2): 276–82.

20 Gwon, A.R., Park, J.S., Park, J.H. et al., Selenium attenuates A beta production and A beta-induced neuronal death, *Neurosci Lett* (2010), 469(3): 391–5.

21 Loef, M., Schrauzer, G.N. & Walach, H., Selenium and Alzheimer's disease: A systematic review, *J Alzheimers Dis* (2011), 26(1): 81–104.

22 Zafar, K.S., Siddiqui, A., Sayeed, I. et al., Dose-dependent protective effect of selenium in rat model of Parkinson's disease: Neurobehavioral and neurochemical evidences, *J Neurochem* (2003), 84(3): 438–46.

23 Shahar, A., Patel, K.V., Semba, R.D. et al., Plasma selenium is positively related to performance in neurological tasks assessing coordination and motor speed, *Mov Disord* (2010), 25(12): 1909–15.

24 Zeevalk, G.D., Razmpour, R. & Bernard, L.P., Glutathione and Parkinson's disease: Is this the elephant in the room?, *Biomed Pharmacother* (2008), 62(4): 236–49.

25 Bellinger, F.P., Raman, A.V., Rueli, R.H. et al., Changes in selenoprotein P in substantia nigra and putamen in Parkinson's disease, *J Parkinsons Dis* (2012), 2(2): 115–26.

26 Rayman, M.P., Selenium and human health, *Lancet* (2012), 379(9822): 1256–68.

27 Harthill, M., Review: Micronutrient selenium deficiency influences evolution of some viral infectious diseases, *Biol Trace Elem Res* (2011), 143(3): 1325–36.

28 Broome, C.S., McArdle, F., Kyle, J.A. et al., An increase in selenium intake improves immune function and poliovirus handling in adults with marginal selenium status, *Am J Clin Nutr* (2004), 80(1): 154–62.

29 Shor-Posner, G., Miguez, M.J., Pineda, L.M.R. et al., Impact of selenium status on the pathogenesis of mycobacterial disease in HIV-1-infected drug users during the era of highly active antiretroviral therapy, *J Acquir Immune Defic Syndr* (2002), 29(2): 169–73.

30 Baum, M.K., Shor-Posner, G., Lai, S. et al., High risk of HIV-related mortality is associated with selenium deficiency, *J Acquir Immune Defic Syndr Hum Retrovirol* (1997), 15(5): 3704.

31 Hurwitz, B.E., Klaus, J.R., Llabre, M.M. et al., Suppression of human immunodeficiency virus type 1 viral load with selenium supplementation: A randomized controlled trial, *Arch Intern Med* (2007), 167(2): 148–54.

32 Burbano, X., Miguez-Burbano, M.J., McCollister, K. et al., Impact of a selenium chemoprevention clinical trial on hospital admissions of HIV-infected participants, *HIV Clin Trials* (2002), 3(6): 483–91.

33 Toulis, K.A., Anastasilakis, A.D., Tzellos, T.G. et al., Selenium supplementation in the treatment of Hashimoto's thyroiditis: A systematic review and a meta-analysis, *Thyroid* (2010), 20(10): 1163–73.

34 Marcocci, C., Kahaly, G.J., Krassas, G.E. et al., European Group on Graves' Orbitopathy, Selenium and the course of mild Graves' orbitopathy, *N Engl J Med* (2011), 364(20): 1920–31.
35 Wertenbruch, T., Willenberg, H.S., Sagert, C. et al., Serum selenium levels in patients with remission and relapse of Graves' disease, *Med Chem* (2007), 3(3): 281–4.
36 Negro, R., Greco, G., Mangieri, T. et al., The influence of selenium supplementation on postpartum thyroid status in pregnant women with thyroid peroxidase autoantibodies, *J Clin Endocrinol Metab* (2007), 92(4): 1263–8.

Therapeutic dose

Selenium has protective effects, but has the potential to cause toxicity, and the margin between health benefits and adverse effects is relatively narrow. Most clinical trials have used 200 mcg of selenium daily, and there is no evidence that higher doses provide additional benefits. For health maintenance or therapeutic purposes, the total daily dose should be restricted to no more than 200 mcg/day.

Effects of excess

Selenite, selenate and selenomethionine forms of selenium have similar acute toxicity in animals, but organic selenium (selenomethionine) has lower chronic toxicity than inorganic selenite and selenate. Selenate is the least toxic of the inorganic forms. The toxicity of selenite is enhanced by vitamin B12 deficiency. The mechanism of selenium toxicity is not well understood, but may be due to glutathione depletion, inhibition of protein synthesis, impairment of sulfur-dependent reactions or the formation of metabolites, such as hydrogen selenide, which undergo redox cycling to produce ROS that cause DNA strand breaks.

Acute selenium toxicity in humans causes excessive salivation, vomiting, diarrhoea, hair loss, fatigue, restlessness, spasms, tachycardia, pulmonary oedema, toxic cardiomyopathy and garlic-smelling breath due to the excretion of volatile selenium metabolites. It may lead to severe shock, which may result from decreased heart function and lowered peripheral vascular resistance. Stupor, respiratory depression and death can occur within hours.

Selenium toxicity is cumulative. Farm animals grazing on selenium accumulator plants may develop 'blind staggers' due to chronic selenium poisoning (selenosis), which features respiratory distress, restlessness, blindness, staggering, head pressing, loss of appetite, excessive salivation, abdominal pain, watery diarrhoea, convulsions, paralysis and death.

Key symptoms of selenosis in humans are abnormalities of the hair, nails and skin, including very brittle hair that breaks off easily at the scalp, lack of pigment in new hair regrowth and the development of an intensely itchy scalp rash. There are fluid effusions and discolouration of the nail bed. Nails become brittle, with white or red ridges that can be either transverse or longitudinal; the thumb is usually involved first, and infections around the nail bed and loss of nails may occur. The skin becomes red and swollen, with blistering, eruptions and a yellowish discolouration, and skin lesions are slow to heal. Other effects include loss of appetite, headaches, dizziness, mottled and decayed teeth, and neurological disturbances, such as numbness, burning or tingling sensations (paraesthesia), pain, overactive reflexes, convulsions and paralysis.

In China, endemic selenosis has occurred in villages where the daily intake of selenium was 5000 mcg, causing a mortality rate of 50 per cent. Most affected people recovered after evacuation from the area and a change of diet. People living in areas of China with an intake of 750 mcg/day of selenium have been reported to show no overt signs of selenosis, and the average intake in areas with endemic selenosis was 3000–6000 mcg/day. Selenosis has not been observed in regions of the United States that have high selenium intakes (up to 724 mcg/day). Amazonian Indians eating a traditional diet have been found to have median plasma selenium levels of 1.71 μmol/L (range 0.68–11.6 μmol/L) without any signs or symptoms of selenosis.

Acute selenium poisoning appears to occur at a dose of 500 mcg/kg body weight or higher. In human volunteers, selenium supplementation of 200 mcg/day taken for ten years did not result in selenosis. Doses of up to 388 mcg selenium/day for shorter periods have not caused obvious adverse effects. The no observed adverse effect level (NOAEL) of selenium is estimated to be 850 mcg/day, and an intake of 910 mcg/day or more may lead to toxicity. Decreases in the concentration of glutathione in blood have been reported at dietary intakes exceeding 750–850 mcg/day. The European Safety Authority states that no selenosis has been observed at intakes of 240–1510 mcg/day. The recommended upper limit (UL) of intake in Australia and New Zealand is 400 mcg/day for adults.

Selenium has been found to have insulin-like activity, improve glucose metabolism and protect against diabetes in some studies. However, other studies have found an association between high plasma selenium levels and increased risk of type 2 diabetes, hyperglycaemia and dyslipidaemia. A study of people supplemented with selenium (200 mcg/day as high-selenium yeast), and followed up for an average of 7.7 years, found that supplementation was associated with increased risk of type 2 diabetes, mainly in those with high selenium levels at baseline. Another study found that 200 mcg selenium per day as selenomethionine had no effect on risk of type 2 diabetes after an average follow-up of 5.5 years.

If selenium is implicated in diabetes, it may be because excess selenium increases GPx1 activity, which interferes with insulin signalling. Animals over-expressing GPx1 develop hyperglycaemia, hyperinsulinaemia and insulin resistance. Alternatively, high plasma selenium levels may be caused by abnormal carbohydrate metabolism. Elevated serum glucose up-regulates expression of glucose synthesising enzymes in the liver and peroxisomal proliferator-activated receptor gamma coactivator 1-alpha (PGC1α), which aggravates hyperglycaemia. PGC1α also increases SePP production, leading to elevated serum selenium. More research is needed to clarify the effects of selenium on diabetes risk.

Case reports—selenium excess

- *An Australian man, 75 years of age,* became concerned about having prostate cancer after a test showed he had an elevated prostate-specific antigen (PSA) level.[1] After researching on the internet, he purchased a total of 200 g of sodium selenite as powder and tablets from two separate pharmacies for oral supplementation, and took a 10 g dose. Three and a half hours later, he developed abdominal pain, vomiting and diarrhoea, and was admitted to hospital. He was found to have poor tissue perfusion, low blood pressure, abnormal heart function, acidosis, low serum potassium and an extremely high serum selenium level (68.0 μmol/L). In spite of treatment, he developed ventricular tachycardia, his low potassium and acidosis worsened and he went into cardiac arrest and died six hours after the selenium dose.
- *A man, 46 years of age,* developed intermittent episodes of profuse watery diarrhoea, vomiting, abdominal pain and weight loss over the course of four weeks.[2] On admission to hospital, he was found to have strong garlic-smelling breath and his hair had begun to fall out. Investigations did not reveal a cause, but he improved in hospital and was discharged. He was readmitted two weeks later with a return of his symptoms. He had also developed a purple-red discolouration at the base of his fingernails and toenails, and was dehydrated and mildly jaundiced. Further investigations could not find a cause. He recovered in hospital and went home, but was readmitted two days later when his symptoms returned. Deliberate poisoning was suspected, but was dismissed by the man as highly unlikely. He was tested for arsenic and thallium poisoning, with negative results. He returned home and did not return to the hospital until three months later, reporting that he had become seriously ill and bed-ridden, at which time his girlfriend, who had been living with him, left him. He recovered his health after this and claimed that his girlfriend had been poisoning him, and had defrauded him of a large sum of money. Subsequent investigation discovered that his girlfriend had purchased large quantities of gun blue, a lubricant solution containing selenious acid, nitric acid and copper nitrate, at a local gun shop, and it was suspected that she had attempted to poison him with it. However, there was no evidence, as his body fluids had not been retained by the hospital.
- *A group of people in the US* ingested a liquid multivitamin and mineral supplement purchased from a chiropractor, and developed symptoms of gastrointestinal illness and hair loss.[3] The chiropractor advised that the dose of the supplement should be doubled, after which their symptoms worsened and they developed discolouration of their nail beds. Investigation of the product by health authorities revealed that it was labelled as containing 200 mcg of selenium per 30 mL as sodium selenite, but it actually contained about 200 times more (40 800 mcg of selenium per 30 mL). The excess selenium content of the product was found to be caused by an employee error at one of the ingredient suppliers. The product was recalled and 201 cases of poisoning were investigated. Serum selenium concentrations at symptom onset ranged from 4.08 to 19.05 μmol/L. It was found that the main symptoms were diarrhoea,

fatigue, hair loss, joint pain, nail discolouration or brittleness, nausea, headache, smelly breath and skin eruptions, with some symptoms persisting for 90 days or more after stopping the supplement. Hair loss ranged from 10–100 per cent of scalp hair. All the affected people recovered over time.

REFERENCES

1 See, K.A., Lavercombe, P.S., Dillon, J. & Ginsberg, R., Accidental death from acute selenium poisoning, *Med J Aust* (2006), 185(7): 388–9.

2 Ruta, D.A. & Haider, S., Attempted murder by selenium poisoning, *BMJ* (1989), 299(6694): 316–17.

3 MacFarquhar, J.K., Broussard, D.L. & Melstrom, P. et al., Acute selenium toxicity associated with a dietary supplement, *Arch Intern Med* (2010), 170(3): 256–61.

Supplements

Selenium is a by-product of the refining of certain metals, particularly copper. It is found in insoluble by-products—'slimes'—that consist of 5–25 per cent selenium. Selenium dioxide is extracted from slimes by soda ash roasting or sulfuric acid roasting, and then mixed with water and acidified to form selenious acid. Selenious acid is reacted with sulfur dioxide to give elemental selenium.

Selenium is available as tablets, capsules and powders. The forms of selenium permitted in oral supplements in Australia are selenocysteine, selenomethionine, sodium selenate, sodium selenite, sodium selenite pentahydrate and high-selenium yeast. The Therapeutic Goods Administration of Australia (TGA) restricts the amount of selenium in oral supplements to no more than 26 mcg of selenium per maximum recommended daily dose (MRDD) for organic forms of selenium and to no more than 52 mcg of selenium per MRDD for inorganic forms. For products that contain both inorganic and organic selenium, the sum of the organic selenium amount and half of the inorganic selenium amount must equal 26 mcg or less per MRDD.

In clinical trials, selenium has been given mainly as inorganic sodium selenite, organic selenomethionine or selenium-enriched yeast. Organic selenium is more bioavailable than inorganic selenium. The amount of elemental selenium in a specific selenium source is listed on the product container, and may vary between individual products; the approximate elemental selenium content of some common forms is shown in Table 12.2.

- *Sodium selenite* can be prepared by reacting selenious acid, formed from selenium dioxide and water, with sodium hydroxide.

Table 12.2 Elemental selenium content of common forms

Form	Selenium content (%)
Sodium selenite	46
Sodium selenate	43
High-selenium yeast (as selenomethionine)	Up to 0.3

- *Sodium selenate* can be produced from sodium selenite or by reacting selenic acid, formed by oxidising selenious acid with hydrogen peroxide, with sodium carbonate.
- *High-selenium yeast* is made by aerobic fermentation of the yeast *Saccharomyces cerevisiae* (brewer's yeast) in a selenium-enriched medium, which produces selenomethionine that is incorporated into yeast proteins or is bound to macromolecules in yeast cell walls.
- *Selenium sulfide* is an ingredient in anti-dandruff shampoos that can cause allergic reactions, but topical selenium is poorly absorbed and does not contribute to selenosis. It is not suitable for oral use because it is carcinogenic and has been found to cause liver tumours in animals.

Cautions

Selenium supplements should be used with caution, and doses greater than the RDI are not recommended in the long term. Selenium supplements should not be taken together with anticoagulant drugs, as they may increase the risk of bleeding by prolonging clotting time. This effect appears to be related to increased prostacyclin formation. The TGA requires the following advisory statement on the labels of all supplements that contain selenium:

'This product contains selenium which is toxic in high doses. A daily dose of 150 micrograms for adults of selenium from dietary supplements should not be exceeded.'

Chromium

CHROMIUM STATUS CHECK

1. **Do you have a family history of diabetes and cardiovascular disease?**
2. **Do you have glucose intolerance, insulin resistance or diabetes?**
3. **Do you have atherosclerosis?**
4. **Do you have a high-sugar or high-refined carbohydrate diet?**

'Yes' answers may indicate inadequate chromium status. Note that a number of nutritional deficiencies or health disorders can cause similar effects and further investigation is recommended.

FAST FACTS . . . CHROMIUM

- **Good sources of chromium include brewer's yeast, egg yolks, organ meats, meat, poultry, shellfish, cheese, whole grains, mushrooms, broccoli, molasses, black pepper, thyme, spices, grape juice, tea, wine and beer.**
- **Chromium is important for insulin function and blood glucose regulation.**
- **It is important for carbohydrate, lipid, cholesterol and protein metabolism, and may have antioxidant, anti-inflammatory and gene-regulating activity.**
- **A deficiency can cause impaired glucose tolerance, and is implicated in cardiovascular disease and atherosclerosis.**
- **Chromium VI is a toxic form of chromium.**

Chromium is a metal found in the environment in rocks, soil and water; the richest concentration is in chromite ore (iron chromium oxide). It exists in five oxidation states, the most common of which are chromium metal, trivalent chromium (chromium III) and hexavalent chromium (chromium VI). Trivalent chromium is the most common form in nature; it is relatively non-toxic, and is the most stable and physiologically important form. Hexavalent chromium is derived from the oxidation of trivalent chromium, and is a potentially toxic form used for industrial purposes. Elemental chromium is not absorbed and has no nutritional value.

Chromium was discovered by the French chemist Nicolas-Louis Vauquelin in 1798. It has the chemical symbol Cr, and was named after the Greek word *chroma*, meaning 'colour', because many of its compounds are highly coloured. Chromium has been considered an essential nutrient, but this has recently been disputed because it does not have a clearly defined biochemical function or deficiency state. Unlike other essential minerals, a lack of chromium has not been shown to cause death or interrupt the life-cycle. However, pharmacological amounts of chromium can have health benefits, and it may be a conditionally essential nutrient. In the body, chromium is predominantly found in the liver, pancreas, kidneys, muscles, spleen, heart and bones.

Chromium's most well-defined role is in enhancing insulin activity, and it may be beneficial for improving glucose tolerance in diabetes. In the 1970s, it was proposed that a compound in brewer's yeast called glucose tolerance factor (GTF), consisting of chromium, vitamin B3 and the amino acids glutamic acid, glycine and cysteine, was essential for utilisation of the hormone insulin that moves glucose from the bloodstream into insulin-sensitive tissues. More recently, a low molecular weight chromium-binding substance has been identified in brewer's yeast that consists of glutamic acid, glycine, cysteine, nicotinic acid (vitamin B3) and chromium; a high-molecular weight chromium-binding substance has also been identified. Although brewer's yeast is a good source of organic chromium, the importance of GTF has not been proven. More recent research shows that the active form of chromium that influences insulin activity is chromodulin, a chromium and amino acid complex made in the body. Some researchers believe that GTF is a decomposition product of chromodulin, or an artefact formed during attempts to isolate the active compound from yeast.

Digestion, absorption and transport

Chromium in food is in the form of inorganic compounds or organic complexes, which are more bioavailable. The mechanism of absorption is not well understood, but it appears that inorganic trivalent chromium is absorbed by passive diffusion. It is transported in the bloodstream bound to transferrin, the main transporter. If large amounts of chromium are ingested, it can also bind to albumin, gamma and beta globulins and lipoproteins. It is believed that tissues take up transferrin-bound chromium by binding to the transferrin receptor, and the complex is taken into the cell interior by endocytosis. Chromium is taken up by insulin-sensitive cells when blood glucose rises and insulin is released.

Metabolism, storage and excretion

Inside cells, chromium is released in the acidic pH of the endosome, and binds to low-molecular weight chromium-binding substance (LMWCr), also called apochromodulin, which mainly consists of the amino acids glutamic acid, glycine, aspartic acid and cysteine. LMWCr can take up four chromic ions; binding chromium converts it to holochromodulin, usually called chromodulin.

Chromium is stored in the kidneys, liver, muscles, spleen, heart, pancreas and bones, and may be stored together with ferric iron. It is excreted in urine as chromodulin, and a small amount is eliminated in hair, skin cells and sweat. Chromium in faeces is mainly the unabsorbed portion from the diet.

Functions

The main role of chromium in the body appears to be enhancement of insulin activity as chromodulin. By its effect on insulin, chromium affects glucose, lipid, cholesterol, protein, muscle and bone metabolism. Other possible functions of chromium include modulating gene activity, and antioxidant and anti-inflammatory activity. The functions of chromium include:

- *Insulin activity and carbohydrate metabolism.* Increased glucose concentration in the bloodstream triggers release of insulin, which acts to promote uptake of glucose and chromium into insulin-sensitive cells. Insulin binds to the insulin receptor in cell membranes, causing conformational change that transfers phosphate groups (autophosphorylates) to tyrosine residues on the receptor, turning the receptor into an active tyrosine kinase enzyme. Chromodulin binds to the activated receptor and increases tyrosine kinase activity eight-fold, which enhances the cell's sensitivity to insulin. Insulin binding to the receptor ultimately leads to the translocation of glucose transporter 4 (GLUT4) vesicles from the cytoplasm to the cell surface, where they transport glucose into the cell. Chromodulin may also promote glucose uptake by inhibiting the enzyme phosphotyrosine phosphatase that inactivates tyrosine kinase. The end result of chromodulin activity is increased glucose uptake, oxidation and glycogen synthesis. When the level of insulin in blood decreases, chromodulin is removed from cells.
- *Insulin metabolism.* Chromium supports the activity of insulin in cells. Insulin enhances glycogen accumulation in the liver and production of fatty acids, which are exported as lipoproteins. Fat cells take up fatty acids from lipoproteins and use them to form triglycerides. Insulin also inhibits breakdown of triglycerides in fat tissue by inhibiting the enzyme lipase that breaks them down to release fatty acids. The overall effect of insulin is to encourage fat synthesis and storage. The activity of the enzyme HMG-CoA reductase, an initiator of cholesterol production, is controlled by the cholesterol concentration in cells and the cyclic adenosine monophosphate (cAMP) signalling pathway. Insulin leads to a decrease in cAMP, which leads to activation of cholesterol synthesis. Insulin promotes the uptake of amino acids and stimulates protein synthesis, causing a growth-promoting (anabolic) effect on body tissues, including muscles. Insulin helps to maintain bone density by reducing the ability of parathyroid hormone to activate protein kinase C in osteoblasts, thereby reducing mobilisation of calcium from bone. Insulin also promotes collagen production by osteoblasts and may enhance bone growth.
- *Antioxidant and anti-inflammatory activity.* In cell studies, chromium has been found to reduce oxidative stress, inhibit protein glycation and lipid peroxidation, and inhibit the release of pro-inflammatory cytokines when glucose is elevated. Chromium chloride, chromium histidinate and chromium picolinate have shown protective antioxidant effects in cell cultures exposed to hydrogen peroxide-induced oxidative stress. In animals, chromium supplementation reduces levels of the inflammatory cytokines TNF-alpha, interleukin-6 (IL-6) and C-reactive protein, and reduces lipid levels and oxidative stress. One animal study found that supplementary chromium acetate and niacin-bound chromium had antioxidant effects in the liver and kidneys, chromium picolinate had antioxidant effects in the liver but not the kidneys and chromium chloride had no antioxidant effects.

- *Gene expression.* Chromium has an affinity for nucleic acids that is stronger than that of other metal ions, and may have a role in DNA structure and gene expression. Chromium is concentrated in cell nuclei, and has been shown to bind to chromatin and increase RNA synthesis in cell studies.

Dietary sources

Good sources of chromium include brewers' yeast, egg yolks, organ meats, meat, poultry, shellfish, cheese, whole grains, mushrooms, broccoli, molasses, black pepper, thyme, spices, grape juice, tea, wine and beer. Traces of chromium can dissolve out of stainless steel cookware into acidic foods.

Chromium absorption is generally low, ranging from 0.4–2 per cent. Organic chromium is absorbed better than inorganic chromium. It has been shown that the percentage of chromium absorbed decreases as the dietary level increases and plateaus at 0.5 per cent at an intake of 40 mcg/day or more.

The Food Standards Australia New Zealand nutrient database (NUTTAB) at <www.foodstandards.gov.au> provides the amounts found in specific foods.

Factors influencing body status

Chromium absorption is increased by amino acids, picolinic acid, oxalates, vitamin B3 and vitamin C. Picolinic acid is a metabolite of the amino acid tryptophan that is present in digestive juice. Non-steroidal anti-inflammatory drugs that block the formation of prostaglandins may increase the absorption of chromium. Absorption of inorganic chromium is reduced by a neutral or alkaline environment in which chromium reacts with hydroxyl ions and precipitates. Other factors that reduce absorption include antacids, phytates, ageing and high dietary iron or zinc, which compete with chromium for uptake. Urinary excretion of chromium is increased by a high-sugar or refined-carbohydrate diet, as well as by stress. When under stress, secretion of cortisol increases, which increases blood glucose concentration and reduces glucose utilisation by tissues. Increased blood glucose levels stimulate the mobilisation of chromium from the blood to the tissues and enhance its excretion in urine. Vitamin B3 may have a role in chromium metabolism. Chromium needs are increased in diabetes, chronic inflammatory diseases, infections, pregnancy and lactation, and in athletes and people taking corticosteroid drugs.

Daily requirement

Australian and New Zealand government recommendations by age and gender (see Table 12.3) can be found in *Nutrient Reference Values for Australia and New Zealand Including Recommended Dietary Intakes*, available at <www.nhmrc.gov.au>.

Table 12.3 Recommended adequate intake (AI) of chromium (mcg/day)

Age (years)	Female AI	Male AI
1–3	11	11
4–8	15	15
9–13	21	25
14–18	24	35
19–70	25	35
>70	25	35
Pregnant women		
14–18	30	
19–50	30	
Lactating women		
14–18	45	
19–50	45	

Source: Nutrient Reference Values for Australia and New Zealand Including Recommended Dietary Intakes, National Health and Medical Research Council, Australian Government Department of Health and Ageing, Canberra and Ministry of Health, New Zealand, Wellington, 2006.

Deficiency effects

It is believed that chromium deficiency is very rare but, as the effects are not well defined, unrecognised deficiencies may exist. Deficiencies may be more common in impaired glucose tolerance and diabetes, during pregnancy, lactation and stress, and in athletes, people taking corticosteroids and those who eat a high-sugar or high refined-carbohydrate diet. In animals, experimentally induced chromium deficiency leads to reduced glucose tolerance despite normal insulin levels, impaired growth, elevated serum cholesterol and triglycerides, increased incidence of atherosclerosis, corneal lesions and decreased fertility and sperm count. There are few reports of chromium deficiencies in humans, and most are associated with long-term TPN. Effects include glucose intolerance, elevated plasma fatty acids, encephalopathy (brain dysfunction) and peripheral neuropathy. Early case reports are difficult to evaluate, as measurements of serum chromium levels were unreliable in the past. The main effect of chromium deficiency appears to be dysfunction of glucose metabolism.

Indicators of inadequate levels of chromium may include:

- glucose intolerance, insulin resistance, diabetes
- CVD, atherosclerosis
- peripheral neuropathy
- decreased male fertility.

Assessment of body status

Chromium status is difficult to assess accurately. Serum levels do not reflect tissue stores, and urinary levels reflect recent intake rather than long-term status. Hair chromium has been used in population studies, but does not appear to be a reliable marker of chromium status in individuals. Toenail chromium levels have been used as a measure in some clinical trials. Recently, urinary chromium response to an insulin challenge has been proposed as an indicator of chromium status, but was not found to be reliable in an animal study. Whole blood may be a better indicator than serum levels, especially for chromium toxicity. The reference range given by the Biochemistry Department of the Royal Prince Alfred Hospital, Sydney, Australia for whole blood chromium is 6–26 nmol/L. Chromium deficiency can be diagnosed by an improvement in a glucose tolerance test after chromium supplementation. However, this test is time-consuming, and is not performed routinely.

Case reports—chromium deficiency

- *A woman, 40 years of age*, on TPN providing 2 mcg chromium/day for three and a half years, developed unexplained weight loss, peripheral neuropathy, impaired glucose tolerance and elevation of plasma free fatty acids.[1] She was given 250 mcg of chromium daily in the TPN solution for two weeks followed by a maintenance dose of 20 mcg/day and her symptoms reversed.
- *A woman, 63 years of age*, on TPN providing 6 mcg chromium/day for six and a half months, developed glucose intolerance with no history of diabetes or evidence of an infection.[2] Her plasma chromium level was low, and supplemental chromium chloride (200 mcg/day) iv for fourteen days reversed the condition.
- *A woman, 45 years of age*, on TPN, developed severe glucose intolerance, weight loss and a confused state (encephalopathy) after five months.[3] Serum chromium levels were in the low-normal range. Supplementation of 150 mcg chromium/day iv reversed her glucose intolerance, reduced her insulin requirements and resulted in weight gain and the disappearance of encephalopathy.
- *A man, 40 years of age*, on TPN developed peripheral neuropathy and glucose intolerance.[4] His serum chromium was elevated. He was given 250 mcg chromium chloride for two weeks, and his symptoms reversed four days later and nerve conduction studies normalised within three weeks.

REFERENCES

1 Jeejeebhoy, K.N., Chu, R.C., Marliss, E.B. et al., Chromium deficiency, glucose intolerance, and neuropathy reversed by chromium supplementation, in a patient receiving long-term total parenteral nutrition, *Am J Clin Nutr* (1977), 30(4): 531–8.

2 Brown, R.O., Forloines-Lynn, S., Cross, R.E. & Heizer, W.D., Chromium deficiency after long-term total parenteral nutrition, *Dig Dis Sci* (1986), 31(6): 661–4.

3 Freund, H., Atamian, S. & Fischer, J.E., Chromium deficiency during total parenteral nutrition, *JAMA* (1979), 241(5): 496–8.

4 Verhage, A.H., Cheong, W.K. & Jeejeebhoy, K.N., Neurologic symptoms due to possible chromium deficiency in long-term parenteral nutrition that closely mimic metronidazole-induced syndromes, *J Parenter Enteral Nutr* (1996), 20(2): 123–7.

THERAPEUTIC USES OF CHROMIUM

There is no reliable evidence that chromium supplements promote muscle building or weight-loss. Chromium supplementation may be useful for the following conditions:

Glucose intolerance, insulin resistance, diabetes

Chromium does not appear to have an effect on glucose metabolism or insulin function in people with normal blood glucose handling. A number of studies have reported that chromium has beneficial effects in diabetes, but the evidence is conflicting. Diabetic patients have been found to have lower serum chromium levels and elevated urinary chromium.[1] Some trials of patients with type 1, type 2, gestational and steroid-induced diabetes have shown that chromium can improve glucose and insulin metabolism.[2] Some studies reporting negative results have used poorly absorbed inorganic chromium or doses less than 250 mcg/day, which are regarded as too low to be effective.

A meta-analysis of seven clinical trials concluded that chromium supplementation significantly reduces fasting blood glucose, but there was no benefit on blood lipids and glycated haemoglobin (HbA_{1C}).[3] A meta-analysis of six trials using oral chromium picolinate in diabetes concluded that it was effective for moderately lowering HbA_{1C}, fasting blood glucose, two-hour postprandial (post-meal) blood glucose and fasting insulin levels, but has no effect on blood lipids.[4] In fourteen hospitalised patients with profound insulin resistance and uncontrolled hyperglycaemia, iv chromium was shown to decrease insulin needs and improve glucose control at twelve and 24 hours compared with baseline values, and may be a potential new therapy for this condition.[5]

Polycystic ovarian syndrome (PCOS) features lack of ovulation, elevated male hormones and insulin resistance. In a small study of women with PCOS, chromium picolinate, providing 1000 mcg chromium/day, led to a 38 per cent mean improvement in glucose disposal rate.[6] Another study found that chromium picolinate (200 mcg/day) improved glucose tolerance but did not affect ovulation or reproductive hormones.[7]

Cardiovascular disease

In animals, a chromium-deficient diet leads to increased blood lipid levels and atherosclerosis and chromium supplementation has led to a decreased total cholesterol:HDL cholesterol ratio.[8] An animal study has reported a reduction in blood pressure after chromium supplementation.[9] A small number of human studies have found that chromium supplementation increases HDL cholesterol and decreases total cholesterol, LDL cholesterol and triglycerides, but the evidence for the benefit of chromium supplementation is conflicting and, overall, chromium does not appear to affect serum lipids and cholesterol in non-diabetics.[10] However, there is some evidence that chromium may be associated with risk of CVD. Diabetic patients and patients with diabetes and CVD have been found to have lower toenail chromium than healthy control subjects.[11] A study of toenail chromium levels found that the risk for MI was reduced in men with levels in the highest range, but only in subjects with greater body mass index (BMI).[12]

Bone mineral density

In one study, chromium picolinate was found to reduce urinary excretion of hydroxyproline and calcium in postmenopausal women, which may indicate a reduced rate of bone resorption.[13] Another study of postmenopausal women found that chromium picolinate lowered insulin and blood glucose levels, reduced calcium excretion and raised serum levels of dehydroepiandrosterone (DHEA), a hormone that may play a role in preserving bone mineral density.[14]

Depression

There are a very small number of case reports that suggest chromium supplementation improves the response to antidepressant medication, and leads to remission of symptoms.[15]

REFERENCES

1 Morris, B.W., MacNeil, S., Hardisty, C.A., et al., Chromium homeostasis in patients with type II (NIDDM) diabetes, *J Trace Elem Med Biol* (1999), 13(1): 57–61.

2 Cefalu, W.T., & Hu, F.B., Role of chromium in human health and in diabetes, *Diabetes Care* (2004), 27(11): 2741–51.
3 Abdollahi, M., Farshchi, A., Nikfar, S. & Seyedifar, M., Effect of chromium on glucose and lipid profiles in patients with type 2 diabetes: A meta-analysis review of randomized trials, *J Pharm Sci* (2013), 16(1): 99–114.
4 Patal, P.C., Cardino, M.T. & Jimeno, C.A., A meta-analysis on the effect of chromium picolinate on glucose and lipid profiles among patients with type 2 diabetes mellitus, *Consultant* (2010), 48(1): 32–7.
5 Drake, T.C., Rudser, K.D., Seaquist, E.R. & Saeed, A., Chromium infusion in hospitalized patients with severe insulin resistance: A retrospective analysis, *Endocr Pract* (2012), 18(3): 394–8.
6 Lydic, M.L., McNurlan, M., Bembo, S. et al., Chromium picolinate improves insulin sensitivity in obese subjects with polycystic ovary syndrome, *Fertil Steril* (2006), 86(1): 243–6.
7 Lucidi, R.S., Thyer, A.C., Easton, C.A. et al., Effect of chromium supplementation on insulin resistance and ovarian and menstrual cyclicity in women with polycystic ovary syndrome, *Fertil Steril* (2005), 84(6): 1755–7.
8 Wallach, S., Clinical and biochemical aspects of chromium deficiency, *J Am Coll Nutr* (1985), 4(1): 107–20.
9 Preuss, H.G., Grojec, P.L., Lieberman, S. & Anderson, R.A., Effects of different chromium compounds on blood pressure and lipid peroxidation in spontaneously hypertensive rats, *Clin Nephrol* (1997), 47(5): 325–30.
10 Balk, E.M., Tatsioni, A., Lichtenstein, A.H. et al., Effect of chromium supplementation on glucose metabolism and lipids: A systematic review of randomized controlled trials, *Diabetes Care* (2007), 30(8): 2154–63.
11 Rajpathak, S., Rimm, E.B., Li, T. et al., Lower toenail chromium in men with diabetes and cardiovascular disease compared with healthy men, *Diab Care* (2004), 27: 2211–16.
12 Rimm, E.B., Guallar, E., Giovannucci, E. et al., Toenail chromium levels and risk of coronary heart disease among normal and overweight men, paper presented at the American Heart Association 42nd Annual Conference on Cardiovascular Disease, Epidemiology and Prevention, 23–26 April 2002, Honolulu.
13 McCarty, M., Anabolic effects of insulin on bone suggest a role for chromium picolinate in preservation of bone density, *Med Hypotheses* (1995), 45(3): 241–6.
14 Evans, G. et al., Chromium picolinate decreases calcium excretion and increases dehydroepiandrosterone (DHEA) in postmenopausal women, *FASEB J* (1995), 9: A449.
15 McLeod, M.N., Gaynes, B.N. & Golden, R.N., Chromium potentiation of antidepressant pharmacotherapy for dysthymic disorder in 5 patients, *J Clin Psychiatry* (1999), 60(4): 237–40.

Therapeutic dose

There is limited information on the optimal therapeutic dose of chromium, but it appears that the effective dose in diabetes is more than 250 mcg/day.

Effects of excess

Chromium VI is an environmental pollutant that is highly toxic by ingestion and inhalation, and is mutagenic. Skin contact can cause dermatitis and lesions. It has 100-fold greater toxicity than chromium III because of its high water solubility, mobility and easy reduction. It is absorbed more efficiently than chromium III but absorption appears to be less than 5 per cent. When ingested, some chromium VI can be reduced to chromium III in the gut, which has lower absorption than chromium VI, and this limits toxicity from oral intake. Inhaled chromium VI can be reduced to chromium III in the body by vitamin C and glutathione. Chromium III has limited entry to cells but, once inside cells, all forms of chromium can only be removed slowly. Unlike chromium III, chromium VI readily crosses cell membranes using sulfate transporters, and can accumulate inside cells, where it is reduced to chromium III which can enter the nucleus and form covalent bonds with DNA, causing DNA damage. Inhalation of chromium VI damages the respiratory tract and lungs, and inhalation or oral exposure may damage the liver, kidneys and the gastrointestinal and immune systems, and have carcinogenic effects.

Chromium III rarely causes adverse effects unless consumed in very large amounts. Excess chromium may interfere with iron uptake and metabolism, and supplementation may lead to an excessive lowering of blood glucose in diabetics on medication. In animals given up to 750 mg/kg body weight/day, chromium levels increased in the kidneys and liver, but there were no significant adverse effects. Chromium nicotinate has been used at levels of 200 to 800 mcg/day for periods of about two months with no reported adverse effects, and chromium chloride and niacin-bound chromium supplementation of up to 1000 mcg/day is generally considered to be without risk.

Chromium picolinate has been associated with adverse effects. Unlike other forms of chromium, chromium picolinate moves from the bloodstream into cells intact, and then dissociates, and toxicity may be related to accumulation of intracellular chromium III ions or accumulation of picolinic acid. It has been associated with enhanced production of hydroxyl radicals, depletion of antioxidant enzymes, DNA damage and mutagenesis. Comparative cell studies of chromium picolinate and niacin-bound chromium have shown that chromium picolinate produces a greater amount of oxidative stress and DNA damage, and the picolinic acid component is believed to be largely responsible. In animals, it has been found to cause oxidative damage to lipids and DNA. However, in a short-term study, animals given 33, 250 or 2000 mg/kg of chromium picolinate, equivalent to 4.1, 30.8 and 246 mg/kg of chromium, showed no evidence of chromosomal damage in their bone marrow cells. Chromium picolinate has been implicated in a variety of adverse effects, including kidney and liver dysfunction, skin blisters and pustules, anaemia, haemolysis, tissue oedema and nerve damage. Many of the proposed adverse effects in humans are based on case reports in which chromium picolinate has not been proven to be the causative factor. In 2004, the UK Committee on Mutagenicity of Chemicals in Food, Consumer Products and the Environment reviewed the evidence, and concluded that the balance of the evidence suggested that chromium picolinate was not genotoxic, and that its use should not be restricted.

Case reports—chromium excess

- *A woman, 33 years of age*, developed weight loss, anaemia, thrombocytopaenia (low platelets), haemolysis (red blood cell destruction), liver dysfunction and kidney failure.[1] It was discovered that she had taken 1200–2400 mcg/day of chromium picolinate for the previous four to five months for weight loss. Her plasma chromium concentration was two to three times higher than normal, and no other causes of her pathology were discovered. Her chromium intake was stopped, and she was treated with blood product transfusions and haemodialysis. Her haemolysis stabilised, and her liver and kidney function improved. One year later, all laboratory values were within normal limits.
- *A woman, 24 years of age*, developed muscle cramps, which were diagnosed as rhabdomyolysis (muscle destruction).[2] It was discovered that she had been taking 1200 mcg/day of chromium picolinate for two days, together with more than 30 other supplements. After stopping all her supplements for three days, her muscle damage reversed, but she was left with some residual kidney dysfunction.

REFERENCES

1 Cerulli, J., Grabe, D.W., Gauthier, I. et al., Chromium picolinate toxicity, *Ann Pharmacother* (1998), 32(4): 428–31.

2 Martin, W.R. & Fuller, R.E., Suspected chromium picolinate-induced rhabdomyolysis, *Pharmacotherapy* (1998), 18(4): 860–2.

Supplements

Chromium is produced commercially mainly by aluminothermic production. In this process, chromite ore is roasted with soda and lime to form sodium chromate, from which chromic oxide is produced. This is then mixed with powdered aluminium, barium peroxide and magnesium powder and ignited, causing oxygen from chromic oxide to react with aluminium to produce aluminium oxide and molten chromium metal.

Chromium is available as tablets and capsules, and is found mainly in multivitamin and mineral formulations. The forms of chromium permitted in oral supplements in Australia are chromic chloride (chromium chloride), chromium nicotinate (niacin-bound chromium) and chromium picolinate. All forms of chromium supplements have low absorption, averaging less than 1 per cent.

The amount of elemental chromium in a specific chromium source is listed on the product container, and may vary between individual products. The approximate elemental chromium content of some common forms is shown in Table 12.4.

Table 12.4 Elemental chromium content of common forms

Form	Chromium content (%)
Chromium chloride	33
Chromium picolinate	13
Chromium nicotinate	12

- *Chromium chloride* can be produced by reacting chromic oxide with hydrochloric acid and then alcohol. It is an inorganic form of chromium that is less bioavailable than other forms.
- *Chromium nicotinate* can be produced from niacin (nicotinic acid, vitamin B3) and chromium chloride hexahydrate. Vitamin B3 appears to be important for chromium metabolism, and chromium nicotinate has been shown to have 3.2- to 8.4-fold higher body retention than chromium chloride or chromium picolinate in animals. A study of healthy older people found that chromium nicotinate supplementation led to a 7 per cent decrease in fasting glucose, whereas chromium and nicotinic acid supplements given separately had no effect.
- *Chromium picolinate* can be produced by reacting chromium chloride hexahydrate with picolinic acid. It is relatively well absorbed, and may lead to chromium accumulation in tissues.

Cautions

Chromium may lower blood glucose levels, and people on diabetic medication or insulin may need to reduce their medication dose. Chromium may decrease the absorption of the drug levothyroxine (used for hypothyroidism); chromium supplements should be taken two to four hours before or after the drug dose. Chromium picolinate has been associated with adverse effects and should not be used in high doses.

Molybdenum

MOLYBDENUM STATUS CHECK

1 Do you have reduced serum and urinary uric acid levels?
2 Do you have elevated xanthines in your urine?
3 Do you have sensitivity reactions to sulfite food additives?
4 Do you get nasal congestion and/or skin flushing after drinking alcohol?

'Yes' answers may indicate inadequate molybdenum status. Note that a number of nutritional deficiencies or health disorders can cause similar effects and further investigation is recommended.

FAST FACTS . . . MOLYBDENUM

- Good sources of molybdenum include legumes, grains, nuts, liver and kidneys.
- Molybdenum is important for purine breakdown, detoxification of drugs and xenobiotics, sulfite metabolism and lactation.
- It may have potential for the treatment of sulfite sensitivity, Wilson's disease, cancer and atherosclerosis.
- A deficiency can cause elevated xanthines in urine, sulfite accumulation and reduced uric acid levels.
- Excess molybdenum is unlikely, but may be associated with reduced copper status, elevated uric acid levels and gout in susceptible people.

Molybdenum is a metal found in the environment mainly as molybdenite and also as wulfenite, ferrimolybdate, jordisite and powellite. Plants take up molybdenum from soil as the molybdate ion (Mo^{6+}), which they require for nitrogen fixation, nitrate reduction and growth. In ancient times, molybdenite, lead, galena, graphite and some other substances were collectively known by the Greek word *molybdos*, meaning 'lead-like'. In 1768, the Swedish scientist Carl Scheele came to the conclusion that molybdenite was a sulfide compound of an as yet unidentified element, and the element molybdenum was isolated by his colleague Peter Hjelm in 1782. It has the chemical symbol Mo.

In living organisms, molybdenum is usually bound to oxygen or sulfur, and is an essential constituent of some enzymes that catalyse the transfer of an oxygen atom to or from a substrate. Each reaction—either reduction or oxidation—involves the transfer of two electrons, thereby causing a change in the oxidation state of the molybdenum atom from Mo^{4+} to Mo^{6+} or vice versa. In animals, molybdenum is concentrated in the liver, kidneys, bones and adrenal glands, and is required for the metabolism of sulfites, aldehydes, purines and xanthines.

Digestion, absorption and transport

Molybdenum in food is efficiently absorbed, but the mechanism of digestion and absorption is not well established. It appears that it is absorbed as the molybdate ion and mechanisms may include passive diffusion, sulfur transporters or a specific transporter—possibly molybdate transporter type 2 (MOT2), which has been identified in animals. There does not appear to be an upper ceiling of absorption. Molybdenum may be transported in the bloodstream as molybdate or bound to the plasma protein alpha-2-macroglobulin. It is found in cells mainly bound to protein; protein-bound molybdenum makes up about 83–97 per cent of the total molybdenum in red blood cells.

Metabolism, storage and excretion

Molybdenum is an essential cofactor for certain enzymes, in which it is not directly attached to the active site of the enzyme but is complexed within a specific compound, molybdopterin, which forms the molybdenum cofactor (Moco). The formation of Moco requires iron and copper. There is little storage of molybdenum in the body, and most tissue molybdenum appears to be associated with molybdoenzymes. Absorption of molybdenum is high, and increases with increased intake. Molybdenum is rapidly excreted in urine, and body status is regulated primarily by urinary excretion. Urinary excretion is a direct reflection of the dietary molybdenum intake; about 60 per cent of dietary intake is excreted when intake is low, and more than 90 per cent when intake is high. At low intakes, there is increased transfer of molybdenum from plasma to tissues, which conserves body molybdenum and reduces urinary excretion. Little molybdenum is excreted in faeces.

Functions

Molybdenum is essential for the activity of four enzymes that catalyse redox reactions. These are aldehyde oxidase, sulfite oxidase, xanthine oxidoreductase (also known as xanthine dehydrogenase and xanthine oxidase) and the more recently discovered mitochondrial amidoxime reducing component (mARC). The functions of molybdenum include the following:

- *Purine breakdown, formation of uric acid.* Molybdenum is a cofactor for the enzyme xanthine oxidoreductase (XOR), which contains flavin adenine dinucleotide (FAD), molybdenum and an iron-sulfur centre in the active site. XOR exists in two interchangeable forms, xanthine dehydrogenase (XDH), which prefers NAD^+ as the substrate, and xanthine oxidase (XO), which prefers O_2. XDH predominates in normal conditions in tissues. XOR breaks down heterocyclic nitrogen compounds, such as the purines and pyrimidines that are part of the structure of DNA, by converting hypoxanthine to xanthine and then to uric acid, which is excreted in urine.
- *Immune activity.* XOR stimulates white blood cell activity in infections, and destroys pathogens by reducing oxygen and promoting the formation of the superoxide radical and hydrogen peroxide. It stimulates inflammation that is part of the immune response to tissue damage, and is active in epithelial tissues, bile and throughout the digestive tract. XOR activity is associated with oedema, sepsis syndrome and post-ischaemic reperfusion injury (damage caused by restoration of blood supply to tissue after a blockage). XOR also produces uric acid, which has protective antioxidant activity but only acts as an antioxidant in a watery environment, and can become a pro-oxidant in a lipid environment by reacting with other radicals and causing damage to blood and membrane lipids.
- *Detoxification activity.* Molybdenum is a cofactor for the enzyme aldehyde oxidase (AO), which contains FAD, molybdenum and an iron-sulfur centre in the active site. AO catalyses the breakdown of a number of aldehydes, including acetaldehyde, produced by alcohol metabolism and by yeast organisms such as *Candida*. Acetaldehyde is a major cause of alcohol-induced tissue damage; it impairs mitochondrial function and reacts with amino, hydroxyl and sulfhydryl groups to impair protein and enzyme structure. Acetaldehyde stimulates the release of signalling molecules that trigger alcohol intolerance

reactions, such as vasodilation, facial flushing, irregular heartbeat and raised blood pressure.

AO also helps to break down nitrogenous heterocyclic xenobiotics, including nicotine, and some drugs, including some anticancer drugs, anti-malarial drugs, prolintane (a stimulant), azapetine (a vasodilator), hydralazine (for elevated blood pressure) and aciclovir (for herpes virus infections). Some anticancer prodrugs that require activation in the body are activated by AO. AO also catalyses the metabolism of monoamine neurotransmitters and the vitamin A metabolite retinaldehyde, the vitamin B6 metabolite pyridoxal and the vitamin B3 metabolite N1-methylnicotinamide. XOR takes part in detoxification by breaking down the xanthine stimulants theophylline, found mainly in tea, and caffeine, found in tea, coffee and cocoa.

- *Sulfite metabolism.* Molybdenum is a cofactor for the enzyme sulfite oxidase (SOX), which converts sulfite to sulfate; it is then either excreted in urine or reused to make sulfur-containing proteins and lipids, and connective tissue glycosaminoglycans.
- *Drug activation and detoxification, function of mARC.* Two mARC proteins have been identified in mammals, mARC1 and mARC2. They work with the electron transport proteins NADH-cytochrome b5 reductase and cytochrome b5 in mitochondrial and endoplasmic reticulum membranes to reduce N-hydroxylated compounds. They play a major role in drug metabolism, especially in the activation of amidoxime-prodrugs and the detoxification of N-hydroxylated xenobiotics. mARC proteins may also help to protect DNA from the incorporation of toxic N-hydroxylated base analogues by converting them into the correct purine or pyrimidine bases.
- *Lactation.* XOR is needed for the secretion of fat globules during breast milk production in lactation. It also reacts with oxygen to release hydrogen peroxide that has antibacterial properties, and may help to protect the infant from gut infections.
- *Glucocorticoid metabolism.* Molybdenum appears to interact with the glucocorticoid receptor complex, and to inhibit its activation; it may play a similar role in other steroid hormone receptors.

Dietary sources

Molybdenum is found in almost all foods in trace amounts as soluble molybdates. Good sources of molybdenum include legumes, grains, nuts, liver and kidneys. Overall, plants are richer than animal foods—except for organ meats—but the content in plants varies according to the soil in which they are grown. Plants take up molybdenum more efficiently from neutral or alkaline soils. Molybdenum absorption from food ranges from 88–93 per cent, and increases as intake increases.

The Food Standards Australia New Zealand nutrient database (NUTTAB) at <www.foodstandards.gov.au> provides the amounts found in specific foods.

Factors influencing body status

A high silicon intake reduces molybdenum uptake and a high sulfate intake may decrease molybdenum absorption through competitive inhibition. A lack of iron or copper impairs production of Moco. In the body, menadione (vitamin K3), methadone (a heroin substitute), chlorpromazine (an anti-psychotic drug), anti-histamines (for hay fever) and oestradiol (a female hormone) inhibit AO activity, and the gout medication allopurinol inhibits XOR activity. Many plant flavonoids, such as isovanillin, baicalein, apigenin, chrysin, luteolin, isorhamnetin, kaempferol, myricetin and quercetin, impair XOR and AO function, and most have more potent inhibiting activity on AO. Kidney dysfunction may reduce the ability to excrete molybdenum in urine. People with chronic *Candida* (thrush) infections, and those taking prescription or non-prescription drugs or drinking excess alcohol, may have increased needs for molybdenum.

Daily requirement

Australian and New Zealand government recommendations by age and gender (see Table 12.5) can be found in *Nutrient Reference Values for Australia and New Zealand Including Recommended Dietary Intakes*, available at <www.nhmrc.gov.au>.

Deficiency effects

Low dietary molybdenum can lead to low urinary and serum uric acid concentrations, elevated xanthines in urine, impaired sulfur-containing amino acid metabolism and sulfite accumulation, and may be associated with impaired breakdown of drugs and intolerance to sulfite food additives and alcohol. Because molybdenum is widespread in food, it has not been possible to induce a recognisable deficiency syndrome in animals. Molybdenum deficiency appears to be extremely rare in humans, and has been observed

Table 12.5 Recommended dietary intake (RDI) of molybdenum (mcg/day)

Age (years)	Female RDI	Male RDI
1–3	17	17
4–8	22	22
9–13	34	34
14–18	43	43
19–70	45	45
>70	45	45
Pregnant women		
14–18	50	
19–50	50	
Lactating women		
14–18	50	
19–50	50	

Source: Nutrient Reference Values for Australia and New Zealand Including Recommended Dietary Intakes, National Health and Medical Research Council, Australian Government Department of Health and Ageing, Canberra and Ministry of Health, New Zealand, Wellington, 2006.

mainly in individuals with a genetic disorder affecting molybdenum-dependent enzymes.

Genetic disorders affecting molybdenum-dependent enzymes

Genetic disorders resulting in a deficiency of SOX, XOR or AO have been reported. Genetic dysfunction of XOR is marked by excessive excretion of xanthine in urine (xanthinuria), often accompanied by low serum levels of uric acid. It may be caused by a non-functional or unstable XOR, a defect in the molybdopterin sulfurase gene required for incorporation of sulfur in the molybdenum centres of XOR and AO, leading to inactivity of both enzymes, or by a defect in the gene for Moco and consequent inactivity of XOR, AO and SOX (molybdenum cofactor deficiency, MoCD). MoCD causes progressive neurological damage associated with sulfite accumulation and usually leads to death within the first year of life. In a world first in 2009, Monash Children's Hospital in Melbourne, Australia, successfully treated a week-old infant girl known as Baby Z with injections of the experimental drug cyclic pyranopterin monophosphate (cPMP), a precursor of Moco. Her elevated sulfite levels were restored to normal in three days and her symptoms improved markedly, but she has residual brain damage as a result of her excessive sulfite levels prior to treatment. Since then, there have been reports of other infants with MoCD responding to cPMP treatment.

Indicators of inadequate levels of molybdenum may include:

- reduced serum and urinary uric acid levels
- xanthinuria
- sulfite accumulation, leading to progressive neurological damage
- sulfite sensitivity: wheezing, shortness of breath, itchy skin rashes
- alcohol intolerance: nasal congestion, flushing, irregular heartbeat, elevated blood pressure.

Assessment of body status

Plasma molybdenum concentrations appears to reflect longer-term molybdenum intake, and 24-hour urinary excretion appears to reflect recent intake. The reference range given by the Mayo Medical Laboratories in the United States for serum molybdenum is 0.3–2.0 ng/mL, and the reference range for urinary molybdenum is 22–173 mcg/24-hour urine. Serum molybdenum less than 0.3 ng/mL or urinary molybdenum less than 20 mcg/24-hour urine indicates a potential deficiency. However, testing for molybdenum deficiency is rarely performed because of the absence of evidence for deficiencies in humans. Molybdenum assessment is used more commonly in patients on TPN or people with molybdenum-based joint prostheses. Serum concentrations greater than 10 ng/mL indicate significant wear of the replacement joint and release of metals into the body.

Case reports—molybdenum deficiency

- *A newborn female infant* developed persistent episodes of tonic seizures 24 hours after birth, which were controlled with drug therapy.[1] At two months of age, she was found to have underdevelopment of the brain, facial abnormalities, rigidity of the muscles, overactive reflexes and severe feeding difficulties. Genetic testing revealed MoCD. At twelve months of age, she had severe psychomotor delay, no language development, no head control, inability to roll over and her severe feeding difficulties persisted, leading to aspiration pneumonia on several occasions.

- *A boy, five years of age*, was investigated for poor growth, rigid muscles, poor vision, inability to sit without support and inability to talk and to follow or grasp objects.[2] He was found to have brain atrophy, low serum uric acid and elevated urinary S-sulfocysteine and xanthine. He was diagnosed with MoCD, but no treatment was available at the time and his abnormalities persisted when last seen at eight years of age.
- *A man, 24 years of age*, with Crohn's disease who was on TPN for eighteen months developed rapid heartbeat, rapid breathing, severe headaches, night blindness, nausea and vomiting, followed by lethargy, disorientation, severe oedema and coma.[3] He was found to have elevated plasma methionine and low serum uric acid, as well as elevated thiosulfate and low uric acid and sulfate in his urine, indicating impaired activity of XOR and SOX. There was no molybdenum in his TPN solution and ammonium molybdate, 300 mcg daily, was added, resulting in reversal of his symptoms and biochemical abnormalities.

REFERENCES

1 Fathalla, W.M., Mohamed, K.A. & Ahmed, E., Molybdenum cofactor deficiency: Report of a new case and literature review, *Ibnosina J Med Biomed Sci* (2010), 2(3), retrieved 20 September 2014 from <http://journals.sfu.ca/ijmbs/index.php/ijmbs/article/view/81>.

2 Ngu, L.H., Afroze, B., Chen, B.C. et al., Molybdenum cofactor deficiency in a Malaysian child, *Singapore Med J* (2009), 50(10): e365–7.

3 Abumrad, N.N., Schneider, A.J., Steel, D. & Rogers, L.S., Amino acid intolerance during prolonged total parenteral nutrition reversed by molybdate therapy, *Am J Clin Nutr* (1981), 34: 2551–9.

THERAPEUTIC USES OF MOLYBDENUM

Sulfite sensitivity

Sulfites, such as sulfur dioxide and the sodium and potassium salts of bisulfite, sulfite and metabisulfite, are widely used as preservatives in foods and drinks, including meat, fish, salads, dried fruit and vegetables, pickled and vinegar-containing foods, fruit-based drinks, beer, wine and pharmaceuticals. In Australia, the food additives numbered 220–228 are sulfite additives. Most reactions to sulfites are mild and include hay fever-like reactions, wheezing and hives.[1] More severe symptoms occur in asthmatics, such as bronchoconstriction, wheezing, shortness of breath and, rarely, anaphylaxis. Anecdotal and case report evidence suggests that supplementary molybdenum may improve tolerance to sulfites and relieve asthmatic symptoms. Two severe asthma cases treated with iv molybdenum were reported to have improved sulfite metabolism and a reduction in asthma symptoms.[2]

Wilson's disease

Wilson's disease is a genetic disorder in which the body is unable to excrete excess copper and levels of free copper accumulate. Tetrathiomolybdate (TM) has been developed as an alternative to copper-lowering drugs for patients with neurological disorders associated with Wilson's disease.[3] It works by complexing with copper and dietary proteins to reduce copper absorption and complexing with copper and plasma proteins to reduce uptake by cells. TM has been shown to halt copper-induced neurological deterioration more effectively than the chelating agents penicillamine and trientine.[3]

Cancer

Low molybdenum in soil can lead to the accumulation of potentially cancer-causing nitrosamines in plants, and was believed to be related to the high incidence of stomach and oesophageal cancer in Linxian, China. However, supplementation with 30 mcg of molybdenum daily as high-molybdenum yeast, given with 120 mg of vitamin C, did not reduce the cancer incidence, but supplementation with selenium, vitamin E and beta-carotene was effective in reducing cancer mortality.[4]

TM and ATN-224 (choline tetrathiomolybdate), a second-generation analogue of TM, have been found to be potent inhibitors of tumour angiogenesis and tumour metastasis, possibly by suppressing NF-kappaB signalling, a key pathway in the development of cancer.[5] Studies in cancer patients have found that TM is associated with halting cancer progression. TM sensitises ovarian cancer cells to chemotherapeutic drugs,[6] has maintained remission in breast cancer patients at high risk of relapse[7] and is a potent suppressor of head and neck tumour metastasis[8] and malignant lung mesothelioma progression after surgery.[9] In contrast, TM was not able to delay cancer progression in men with hormone-refractory prostate cancer.[10]

Atherosclerosis

Copper chelation by TM has been shown to inhibit some types of acute inflammatory responses. Mice deficient in apolipoprotein E are at increased risk of atherosclerosis and TM has been shown to reduce the development of atherosclerotic lesions in the entire aorta by 25 per cent and in the descending aorta by 45 per cent in these animals.[11] TM was found to decrease several markers of inflammation in the animals but had no effect on serum levels of oxidised LDL.

REFERENCES

1 Lester, M.R., Sulfite sensitivity: significance in human health, *J Am Coll Nutr* (1995), 14(3): 229–32.
2 [No author listed], Molybdenum monograph, *Altern Med Rev* (2005), 10(4): 156–61.
3 Brewer, G.J., Neurologically presenting Wilson's disease: Epidemiology, pathophysiology and treatment, *CNS Drugs* (2005), 19(3): 185–92.
4 Blot, W.J., Li, J.Y., Taylor, P.R. et al., Nutrition intervention trials in Linxian, China: Supplementation with specific vitamin/mineral combinations, cancer incidence, and disease-specific mortality in the general population, *J Natl Cancer Inst* (1993), 85(18): 1483–92.
5 Brewer, G.J., Copper lowering therapy with tetrathiomolybdate as an antiangiogenic strategy in cancer, *Curr Cancer Drug Targets* (2005), 5(3): 195–202.
6 Kim, K.K., Lange, T.S., Singh, R.K. et al., Tetrathiomolybdate sensitizes ovarian cancer cells to anticancer drugs doxorubicin, fenretinide, 5-fluorouracil and mitomycin C, *BMC Cancer* (2012), 12: 147.
7 Jain, S., Cohen, J., Ward, M.M. et al., Tetrathiomolybdate-associated copper depletion decreases circulating endothelial progenitor cells in women with breast cancer at high risk of relapse, *Ann Oncol* (2013), 24(6): 1491–8.
8 Kumar, P., Yadav, A., Patel, S.N. et al., Tetrathiomolybdate inhibits head and neck cancer metastasis by decreasing tumor cell motility, invasiveness and by promoting tumor cell anoikis, *Mol Cancer* (2010), 9: 206.
9 Pass, H.I., Brewer, G.J., Dick, R. et al., A phase II trial of tetrathiomolybdate after surgery for malignant mesothelioma: Final results, *Ann Thorac Surg* (2008), 86(2): 383–9, discussion at 390.
10 Henry, N.L., Dunn, R., Merjaver, S. et al., Phase II trial of copper depletion with tetrathiomolybdate as an antiangiogenesis strategy in patients with hormone-refractory prostate cancer, *Oncology* (2006), 71(3–4): 168–75.
11 Wei, H., Zhang, W.J., McMillen, T.S. et al., Copper chelation by tetrathiomolybdate inhibits vascular inflammation and atherosclerotic lesion development in apolipoprotein E-deficient mice, *Atherosclerosis* (2012), 223(2): 306–13.

Therapeutic dose

There is limited information on the optimal therapeutic dose of molybdenum; doses of 50–6000 mcg daily have been used. Doses greater than 2 mg daily are not recommended because of the potential to elevate uric acid levels. The effective dose of TM appears to be 120–150 mg daily.

Effects of excess

Animals are more sensitive than humans to a high molybdenum intake, and can develop molybdenum toxicity (molybdenosis or teart), in which copper status is impaired, leading to anaemia, loss of appetite, diarrhoea, joint and bone abnormalities, coat discolouration and death. Hexavalent molybdenum (sodium molybdate) has been associated with toxicity when given to animals in high doses. Symptoms include anaemia, anorexia, loss of weight, hair loss and abnormalities of the skin and bones. Trivalent molybdenum (molybdenite) appears to be far less toxic in animals. In general, TM is well tolerated, but may cause copper deficiency, anaemia and neutropenia in high doses.

There is little information available on the toxicity of oral molybdenum in humans, but toxicity is believed to be rare because it is excreted readily in urine. The Australian and New Zealand recommended upper level (UL) of intake is 2 mg/day for most age groups. No adverse effects were reported in healthy young men given 22–1490 mcg/day of molybdenum for 24 days.

Excess molybdenum may cause reduced copper status, increased uric acid production and impaired uric acid excretion, causing gout in susceptible people. A population study in an area of Armenia with high levels of molybdenum in the soil found that intake of 10–15 mg of molybdenum daily was associated with elevated molybdenum levels in blood and urine, and gout-like symptoms, such as joint pain in the hands, feet and knees; gout-like symptoms also occurred in a population exposed to 1–2 mg/daily. In India, a high incidence of knock-knees in certain regions is thought to have been related to low calcium intake, and an increased amount of molybdenum in the staple food, sorghum; the daily intake of molybdenum was estimated to be 1.5 mg. It is believed that the excess molybdenum caused a copper deficiency that impaired bone formation. Occupational exposure to molybdenum is associated with weakness, fatigue, headaches, dizziness, irritability, lack of appetite, stomach pain, joint and muscle pain, weight loss, hand tremors, sweating and red, moist skin.

Case report—molybdenum toxicity

- *A male health practitioner, aged in his late thirties*, was advised by a colleague to take a molybdenum supplement to overcome his allergy to the perfume of his patients.[1] He began taking 300 mcg daily, and increased his intake gradually to 700–800 mcg daily. After seven days, he developed anxiety and agitation; after fourteen days, he became mildly psychotic and experienced visual and auditory hallucinations and an intense craving for salt. He stopped taking molybdenum after eighteen days, but continued to have severe psychosis with strong audio and visual hallucinations, insomnia, intense craving for salt, diarrhoea and painful, cold extremities. On day 22, he developed seizures, and he attempted suicide during a psychotic episode on day 24. His condition could not be controlled with medication. His wife raised the possibility of molybdenum toxicity, but this was ignored despite blood tests revealing elevated molybdenum. He continued to deteriorate, and became confined to a wheelchair with ongoing seizures and psychosis. Eventually, it was decided to use chelation therapy for metal intoxication, which stopped his seizures after two hours. His psychosis resolved after four chelation treatments, but he became severely depressed. Investigations revealed low testosterone levels and damage to the frontal cortex of his brain. A year after taking molybdenum, he was found to have an impaired ability to make decisions, learning disability, major depression and post-traumatic stress disorder, and was unable to return to his profession.

REFERENCE

1 Momcilović, B., A case report of acute human molybdenum toxicity from a dietary molybdenum supplement—a new member of the 'Lucor metallicum' family, *Arh Hig Rada Toksikol* (1999), 50(3): 289–97.

Supplements

Molybdenum is available as tablets and capsules, and is found mainly in multivitamin and mineral formulations, and liver support and detoxification products. Molybdenum is commercially extracted by separating molybdenum disulfide from the molybdenum-containing ore, and roasting it in air, which produces a roasted molybdenite concentrate.

The forms of molybdenum permitted in oral supplements in Australia are molybdenum trioxide and high-molybdenum yeast. The TGA in Australia restricts the maximum daily dose of molybdenum from molybdenum trioxide to 125 mcg and to 62.5 mcg from high-molybdenum yeast. Bioavailability of molybdenum is generally high, and molybdenum supplements appear to have greater bioavailability than food-bound molybdenum. More water-soluble molybdenum compounds, such as molybdenum trioxide and calcium molybdate, are better absorbed than insoluble forms such as molybdenum disulfide. Molybdenum trioxide and sodium molybdate are strong eye and skin irritants, and are not recommended for topical use.

The amount of elemental molybdenum in a specific molybdenum source is listed on the product container, and may vary between individual products; the approximate elemental molybdenum content of some common forms is shown in Table 12.6.

Table 12.6 Elemental molybdenum content of common forms

Form	Molybdenum content (%)
Molybdenum trioxide	67.0
High-molybdenum yeast	0.2

- *Molybdenum trioxide* can be produced from roasted molybdenite concentrate by sublimation (directly converting the solid phase to the gas phase) or by dissolving the concentrate in an alkaline medium and converting the resulting ammonium molybdate to molybdenum trioxide by high-temperature processing (calcination).
- *High-molybdenum yeast* can be produced by growing the yeast organism *Saccharomyces cerevisiae* in the presence of a natural substrate and sodium molybdate. During growth, molybdenum becomes incorporated into cells. The yeast is killed and enzymes are used to break down the cell walls to release the contents, which are then spray dried.

Cautions

Molybdenum may reduce copper levels and elevate uric acid levels if used in high doses. People with a history of gout should restrict molybdenum intake to the RDI amount.

Fluoride

FLUORIDE STATUS CHECK

1 **Do you live in a low-fluoride region?**
2 **Do you have a lot of tooth decay and many fillings?**

'Yes' answers may indicate a benefit from improved fluoride status.

FAST FACTS . . . FLUORIDE

- **Good sources of fluoride include fluoridated tap water, tea, seaweeds, grains and fish with bones, such as canned sardines, anchovies and salmon.**
- **Fluoride protects against tooth decay by improving the resistance of tooth enamel to demineralisation, enhancing remineralisation and acting as an antimicrobial in the mouth.**
- **It increases bone density, but reduces bone strength and quality, and may increase the risk of fractures.**
- **There are no known effects of fluoride deficiency in humans.**
- **Excess fluoride is associated with dental and skeletal fluorosis, and may have adverse effects on thyroid function and children's neurological development.**

The element fluorine is a gas, but it occurs in the environment and living organisms bound to various compounds as fluoride. Rocks and soils contain fluoride as fluorspar, fluorapatite and cryolite. The element fluorine was discovered by the English chemist Sir Humphry Davy in 1813, and isolated by the French chemist Henri Moissan in 1886. It was named after the Latin *fluere*, meaning 'to flow' from the use of fluorspar (calcium fluoride) as a flux in metallurgy. It has the chemical symbol F.

Fluoride compounds, such as calcium fluoride, occur naturally in small amounts in drinking water and food. In the 1930s and 1940s, a low fluoride intake was found to be linked to tooth decay. Subsequently, it was found that the natural level of fluoride in most water sources in Australia and New Zealand was insufficient to protect teeth, and fluoride was added to drinking water in most urban areas. Fluoride does not appear to have an essential role in human growth and development, but it is considered an essential trace element because of its effects on teeth, and possibly bones.

Digestion, absorption and transport

Fluoride in aqueous solutions, such as in fluoridated water, is converted into hydrogen fluoride (HF) in the presence of stomach acid, and is rapidly absorbed in the stomach. Fluoride in food is bound to proteins, and needs to be released by protease enzymes in the digestive tract before absorption. Fluoride absorption in the stomach appears to occur via passive diffusion, and absorption in the intestine may occur via a carrier-mediated process, possibly by a F^{-}-H^{+} cotransporter or F^{-}-OH^{-} exchangers. Fluoride absorption increases as intake increases.

Fluoride is transported in the bloodstream as ionic fluoride, HF, or as fat-soluble fluorocompounds, and is distributed throughout the body, with the greatest amount retained in calcium-rich tissues, such as bones and teeth. Fluoride is taken up by cells as HF following a pH gradient from the more acidic to the more alkaline compartment.

Metabolism, storage and excretion

In bone, fluoride is located in the hydration shells on bone crystallites, from which it can readily be exchanged with ions in the surrounding extracellular fluid, and it is also found in association with hydroxyapatite in crystalline bone, from which it can be slowly mobilised during bone resorption and remodelling. Fluoride is incorporated into the hydroxyapatite of tooth enamel and dentin only during the development phase, but is not essential for tooth development. Fluoride is excreted mainly in urine, and excretion increases with increases in urinary pH. About 10–20 per cent of ingested fluoride is excreted in faeces, and small amounts are lost in sweat.

Functions

Fluoride does not have an identified role in tissues other than bones and teeth, and is not metabolised. The functions of fluoride include:

- *Structure of bones.* Fluoride has been shown to stimulate proliferation of osteoblasts and increase mineral deposition in bone. Fluoride entering bones results in partial substitution of fluoride for hydroxyl groups of hydroxyapatite, forming fluoroapatite, which is more stable and more compact, and leads to increased density and hardness but may reduce mechanical strength, causing brittle bones. Fluoride alters bone crystal structure, and can delay bone mineralisation. In trabecular bone, volume and thickness are increased, but trabecular connectivity does not improve, resulting in reduced bone quality.
- *Structure of teeth.* Dental enamel consists mainly of minerals, particularly hydroxyapatite crystals, which combine to form enamel prisms interspersed with fluid. During tooth development, fluoride can be exchanged with the hydroxyl groups of hydroxyapatite to form fluoroapatite, which is incorporated into developing dental enamel. The development of tooth enamel is completed between the ages of two to twelve months for deciduous teeth and by the age of seven to eight years for permanent teeth, except in the third molars, in which it is completed by the age of twelve to sixteen years. The fluoride concentration in enamel is a reflection of the amount taken up during tooth formation. In contrast, dentin and skeletal bone can accumulate fluoride throughout life, in proportion to the amount absorbed.

  In mature teeth, only the surface layers of enamel are affected by the fluoride concentration in the mouth. Fluoride enters the intercrystalline fluid, and can be exchanged with the hydroxyl groups of hydroxyapatite on the outer surface of tooth enamel to form fluoroapatite, which protects enamel from dissolution (tooth decay, caries) induced by a fall in pH due to acid production by oral bacteria. Fluoride also combines with calcium from saliva and enamel surfaces to form calcium fluoride, which deposits on the tooth surface and releases protective fluoride ions when oral pH drops. Fluoride promotes the remineralisation of tooth enamel in areas that have been demineralised by acids.
- *Antimicrobial activity.* Fluoride has been shown to impair the metabolism of oral bacteria by forming HF that enters bacterial cells and dissociates, causing acidification, inhibition of enzyme activity and increased permeability of the bacterial cell membrane.

Dietary sources

Fluoride is found in fluoridated tap water, tea, seaweeds, grains and fish with bones, such as canned sardines, anchovies and salmon. Tea contains relatively high levels of fluoride, especially the mature tea leaves used in brick tea, which may contain two to four times more fluoride than black or green leaf tea. Consumption of brick tea is associated with fluoride toxicity in some countries. The use of polytetrafluoroethylene-coated (Teflon) cookware may increase the fluoride content of food. Absorption from food averages 50–80 per cent.

In Australia, naturally occurring fluoride levels in water are generally very low (less than 0.1 mg/L). Higher concentrations are often associated with underground sources. In a large survey of groundwater boreholes in central Australia, half of the bores tested contained more than 1.5 mg/L of fluoride and several had levels of 3–9 mg/L.

Many countries around the world add fluoride to drinking water supplies to reduce the incidence of caries. About 90 per cent of drinking water in Australia is fluoridated, as is about 85 per cent of New Zealand drinking water, and fluoridation has been carried out for more than 30 years in many areas. The maximum level of added fluoride permitted in Australian and New Zealand drinking water is 1 mg/L (1 part per million, or ppm). Sodium fluoride, sodium fluorosilicate and fluorosilicic acid are used to fluoridate water because they are rapidly and almost completely absorbed, whereas poorly soluble fluoride compounds, such as calcium fluoride, magnesium fluoride, aluminium fluoride and fluoride compounds in food, are less well absorbed.

The Food Standards Australia New Zealand nutrient database (NUTTAB) at <www.foodstandards.gov.au> provides the amounts found in specific foods.

Factors influencing body status

The amount of fluoride retained in the body varies with age. Infants retain about 80–90 per cent of absorbed fluoride, and adults retain about 60 per cent. About 40 per cent of absorbed fluoride is retained in bones and teeth in adults, and about 55 per cent in young children. Inadequate stomach acid and bile salt production impair fluoride absorption, and absorption is reduced by magnesium, phosphorus and aluminium, which form insoluble complexes with fluoride. Calcium from food impairs absorption, but calcium from supplements does not. Fluoride absorption from milk, milk-based infant formula and other calcium-rich foods can be as low as 25 per cent. Soluble fluorides, such as sodium fluoride, are more easily absorbed (90–97 per cent absorption) compared with less soluble salts such as calcium fluoride (62 per cent absorption). Kidney dysfunction may reduce fluoride excretion, and lead to elevated levels in the body. A high intake of tea may lead to elevated body levels of fluoride.

Daily requirement

Australian and New Zealand government recommendations by age and gender (see Table 12.7) can be found in *Nutrient Reference Values for Australia and New Zealand Including Recommended Dietary Intakes*, available at <www.nhmrc.gov.au>.

Table 12.7 Adequate intake (AI) of fluoride (mg/day)

Age (years)	Female AI	Male AI
1–3	0.7	0.7
4–8	1.0	1.0
9–13	2.0	2.0
14–18	3.0	3.0
19–70	3.0	4.0
>70	3.0	4.0
Pregnant women		
14–18	3.0	
19–50	3.0	
Lactating women		
14–18	3.0	
19–50	3.0	

Source: Nutrient Reference Values for Australia and New Zealand Including Recommended Dietary Intakes, National Health and Medical Research Council, Australian Government Department of Health and Ageing, Canberra and Ministry of Health, New Zealand, Wellington, 2006.

Deficiency effects

In animals, fluoride deficiency leads to poor growth, infertility and anaemia, but fluoride deficiency has not been identified in humans. The development of caries is not regarded as a sign of fluoride deficiency. One study of infants from an area with low fluoride in drinking water reported that there was a higher rate of growth and weight gain in those given a fluoride supplement (0.25 mg/day from birth), compared with infants not receiving fluoride; however, no causal relationship has been established.

Assessment of body status

Markers of recent fluoride intake include the amount in blood, bone surface, saliva, breast milk, sweat and urine, and markers of longer-term fluoride status include the amounts in bones, teeth, nails and hair. The reference range given by the Mayo Medical Laboratories in the United States for serum fluoride is 0.0–4.0 μmol/L. People using fluoridated water typically have plasma fluoride levels of 1–4 μmol/L, compared with less than 1 μmol/L in those not using fluoridated water. Plasma fluoride values greater than 4 μmol/L indicate excessive exposure.

THERAPEUTIC USES OF FLUORIDE

Dental caries

Caries are estimated to effect 60–90 per cent of schoolchildren, and the vast majority of adults in industrialised countries worldwide.[1] It is caused by demineralisation of the tooth surface by acids produced by the action of micro-organisms in dental plaque on fermentable carbohydrates. Ingested fluoride protects against dental caries by its incorporation into teeth during all stages of tooth formation, and by its presence in saliva where it protects the outer surfaces of teeth and inhibits bacterial activity.[2] Fluoride in solution around the teeth is more effective in inhibiting demineralisation than fluoride incorporated into enamel, and has much greater protective activity.

The existing body of evidence strongly suggests that water fluoridation is beneficial for reducing dental caries in children. Systematic reviews have concluded that more children exposed to fluoridated water are free of caries compared with those not exposed, and water fluoridation leads to a reduction in the number of teeth affected by caries.[3]

Topical fluoride agents include stannous fluoride, sodium fluoride and amine/potassium fluoride mouth rinses, gels, pastes and varnish. Stannous fluoride appears to have more potent antimicrobial activity than sodium fluoride, and has been shown to protect against caries, plaque, gingivitis, tooth hypersensitivity and bad breath.[4] However, it may lead to reversible staining of the teeth. Topical gels and varnishes provide a temporary layer of fluoride on the enamel surface, which is released in an acidic environment to impair bacterial metabolism and assist remineralisation of enamel. A review of 75 studies found that fluoride toothpastes with concentrations of 1000 ppm (1000 mg/kg) and above prevented caries in children and adolescents compared with non-fluoridated toothpaste.[5] A review of seventeen studies found that topical fluoride treatments were moderately effective in adults at higher risk of caries.[6] Organic amine fluorides are a newer form of topical fluoride treatment that have been shown to be superior to inorganic fluorides, such as sodium fluoride, for protection against caries because they lead to a marked increase in enamel hardness when compared with sodium fluoride.[7]

Because of concerns about fluoride causing dental fluorosis (discolouration of the teeth), low-fluoride toothpastes (containing less than 600 ppm fluoride) have been developed for use by preschool children. However, a review of five clinical trials in pre-schoolers found that low-fluoride toothpastes increased the risk of caries in primary teeth by 13 per cent, and did not decrease the risk of tooth mottling in permanent teeth, and concluded that there was no evidence to support their use.[8]

Dental hypersensitivity

Stannous fluoride (0.717 per cent solution) applied directly to the sensitive area of the teeth for one minute and allowed to remain for three to five minutes, with an additional one minute if needed, is reported to have an immediate and noticeable desensitising effect, which is maintained for several months afterwards.[9] Application of 0.4 per cent stannous fluoride solution has more gradual effects, and requires approximately two to four weeks of continuous treatment to be effective.[9]

Gingivitis

Gingivitis is irritation, redness and swelling of the gums, and is often associated with bleeding. It may lead to more serious gum disease (periodontitis) and eventual tooth loss. Use of 0.454 per cent stannous fluoride toothpaste has led to a 50–74 per cent reduction in bleeding sites in patients with gingivitis, with nearly half having no bleeding or only one site of bleeding after three months of use.[10]

Breath odour

A meta-analysis of four studies that investigated patients with bad breath, as measured by the presence of volatile sulfur compounds, found that 0.454 per cent stannous fluoride toothpaste improved breath odour compared with a control toothpaste (0.243 per cent sodium fluoride).[11]

Osteoporosis

Osteoporosis is loss of bone mineral density that occurs during ageing, and especially in women after menopause. A meta-analysis of eleven studies that used fluoride for postmenopausal osteoporosis concluded that fluoride can increase bone mineral density at the lumbar spine but does not result in a reduction of vertebral fractures and increasing the dose of fluoride does not protect against vertebral fractures and can increase the risk of non-vertebral fracture and gastrointestinal side-effects.[12]

Otosclerosis

Otosclerosis is abnormal bone growth in the middle ear that can cause tinnitus (ringing in the ears), dizziness and progressive hearing loss. Low-fluoride regions have been found to have a higher incidence of otosclerosis.[13] Fluoride may have therapeutic effects by inhibiting the activity of proteolytic enzymes, reducing bone resorption, changing active bone lesions to more dense inactive lesions and increasing new bone formation. Several case-control studies and a clinical trial of the use of sodium fluoride in otosclerosis patients found less deterioration in hearing after two years in the treatment group.[14]

REFERENCES

1 European Food Safety Authority (EFSA), EFSA Panel on Dietetic Products, Nutrition, and Allergies (NDA), Scientific Opinion on Dietary Reference Values for fluoride, *EFSA J* (2013), 11(8): 3332.

2 Buzalaf, M.A., Pessan, J.P., Honório, H.M. & ten Cate, J.M., Mechanisms of action of fluoride for caries control, *Monogr Oral Sci* (2011), 22: 97–114.

3 Australian Government National Health and Medical Research Council, *A systematic review of the efficacy and safety of fluoridation; Part A: Review of methodology and results*, Australian Government, Canberra, 2007.

4 Makin, S.A., Stannous fluoride dentifrices, *Am J Dent* (2013), 26 Spec No A: 3A–9A.

5 Walsh, T., Worthington, H.V., Glenny, A.M. et al., Fluoride toothpastes of different concentrations for preventing dental caries in children and adolescents, *Cochrane Database Syst Rev* (2010), 1: CD007868.

6 Gibson, G., Jurasic, M.M., Wehler, C.J. & Jones, J.A., Supplemental fluoride use for moderate and high caries risk adults: a systematic review, *J Public Health Dent* (2011), 71(3): 171–84.

7 Priyadarshini, S., Raghu, R., Shetty, A., Gautham, P.M., Reddy, S. & Srinivasan, R., Effect of organic versus inorganic fluoride on enamel microhardness: An in vitro study, *J Conserv Dent* (2013), 16: 203–7.

8 Santos, A.P., Oliveira, B.H. & Nadanovsky, P., Effects of low and standard fluoride toothpastes on caries and fluorosis: Systematic review and meta-analysis, *Caries Res* (2013), 47(5): 382–90.

9 Thrash, W.J., Dodds, M.W. & Jones, D.L., The effect of stannous fluoride on dentinal hypersensitivity, *Int Dent J* (1994), 44(1, Suppl 1): 107–18.

10 Gerlach, R.W. & Amini, P., Randomized controlled trial of 0.454% stannous fluoride dentifrice to treat gingival bleeding, *Compend Contin Educ Dent* (2012), 33(2): 134–6, 138.

11 Feng, X., Chen, X., Cheng, R. et al., Breath malodor reduction with use of a stannous-containing sodium fluoride dentifrice: a meta-analysis of four randomized and controlled clinical trials, *Am J Dent* (2010), 23 Spec No B: 27B–31B.

12 Haguenauer, D., Welch, V., Shea B. et al., Fluoride for treating postmenopausal osteoporosis, *Cochrane Database Syst Rev* (2000),4: CD002825.

13 Schrauwen, I. & Van Camp, G., The etiology of otosclerosis: A combination of genes and environment, *Laryngoscope* (2010), 120(6): 1195–202.

14 Cruise, A.S., Singh, A. & Quiney, R.E., Sodium fluoride in otosclerosis treatment: Review, *J Laryngol Otol* (2010), 124(6): 583–6.

Therapeutic dose

Suggested doses of fluoride are as follows:

- *Caries protection:* fluoride supplementation is not required in areas supplied with fluoridated water. As fluoride is more protective when applied locally and many water supplies worldwide are fluoridated or contain natural fluoride, supplementation with fluoride tablets has largely been discontinued. All forms of fluoride should be used with caution, as they can lead to toxicity. Daily use of fluoridated toothpaste is recommended for general prevention of caries.
- *Osteoporosis:* 15–43 mg elemental fluoride per day. However, the use of fluoride is of limited benefit because it has not been shown to reduce bone fractures.
- *Otosclerosis:* sodium fluoride 60 mg/day initially, reducing to 20–25 mg on improvement.

Effects of excess

At high levels, fluoride acts as a cellular poison by binding calcium, interfering with the activity of proteolytic and glycolytic enzymes, and inhibiting Na/K-ATPase. It inhibits protein metabolism, alters signalling pathways involved in cell proliferation and apoptosis, induces the formation of ROS and reduces cellular antioxidant defences. Acute fluoride poisoning can occur at doses of 140–210 mg/70 kg body weight, and the lethal dose is 32–64 mg fluoride/kg weight. Acute toxicity symptoms include vomiting, diarrhoea, abdominal pain, cyanosis (blueness of the skin), severe weakness, breathlessness, seizures, muscle spasms, paralysis, kidney damage, ventricular fibrillation, convulsions, coma and possibly death. HF is highly corrosive, and inhalation can cause chemical burns in the respiratory tract, coughing, choking and pulmonary oedema. Skin contact with HF causes severe burns, and inhalation or skin exposure can be fatal. Chronic industrial exposure to inhaled aluminium fluoride may cause asthma. Chronic, prolonged ingestion of excessive doses of fluoride is a more common condition, and is an acknowledged risk related to water fluoridation. It causes impaired tooth enamel formation (dental fluorosis) in children, and impaired bone metabolism (skeletal fluorosis) in adults.

Dental fluorosis

Chronic exposure to excessive fluoride during tooth development can lead to fluorosis, affecting tooth enamel in children in the first eight years of life. It causes reduced mineralisation in the enamel, leading to increased porosity, loss of enamel translucency and increased opacity. Mild fluorosis causes white flecks or patches on teeth, frosty edges or fine, lacy chalk-like lines. More severe fluorosis is less common, and causes weak, crumbling teeth with brown discolouration and pitting. A higher level of fluoride in the water supply is associated with a higher prevalence of dental fluorosis. A US survey found that 8 per cent of twelve- to fifteen-year-olds have mild fluorosis and 5 per cent have moderate fluorosis. A review of 214 studies of water fluoridation found a dose-dependent increase in dental fluorosis and that, at a fluoride level of 1 ppm, an estimated 12.5 per cent of people would have fluorosis that would be aesthetically concerning.

To minimise dental fluorosis, the Australian and New Zealand upper level of intake (UL) for fluoride is 1.3 mg/day for children aged one to three years, and 2.2 mg/day for children aged four to eight years. There is some evidence that the use of fluoride toothpaste in children under twelve months of age may be associated with increased risk of fluorosis.

Skeletal fluorosis

Excess fluoride deposits in bones, and accumulates over many years, leading to bone abnormalities, disturbed calcium metabolism and hyperparathyroidism. Initially, skeletal fluorosis may appear as an increase in bone mineral density (osteosclerosis) of the vertebrae and the pelvis, which is detectable by x-ray. As it progresses, bone density increases further, and bones become thicker, bony outgrowths appear and calcium deposits form in ligaments, tendons and muscle insertions. Bones become brittle and fracture more easily. The joints of the hands, feet, knees and spine become stiff and painful. In severe cases—usually linked to industrial exposure—movement of the spine and lower limbs is impaired. Calcification of the ligaments may cause a fused, immobile spine ('poker back'), and outgrowths of bony spurs in the joints may cause contractures of the hips and knees. Although fluorosis commonly causes increased bone mineral density, it is also associated with reduced bone mineral density, osteoporosis and osteomalacia. Nerve symptoms may include a tingling sensation in the fingers and toes, nervous tension and depression.

Skeletal fluorosis occurs through industrial exposure to fluoride, and in regions around the world where the fluoride content of water is naturally high (more than 8 mg/L), such as parts of the Middle East,

Africa, Afghanistan, India, northern Thailand and China. The World Health Organization (WHO) has concluded that there is a clear higher risk of adverse bone effects with a total fluoride intake of 14 mg/day or more, and there is suggestive evidence of an increased risk with a total intake of more than 6 mg/day. The Australian and New Zealand UL for fluoride intake for adults is 10 mg/day.

Neurological effects in children

Animals exposed to 1 ppm of fluoride in water have been found to have changes in brain structure, increased levels of aluminium in the brain and impaired learning and memory. It has been proposed that fluoride may be a developmental neurotoxin that has adverse effects on brain development in children at exposures well below those that can cause toxicity in adults. Children living in regions with high fluoride exposure have been shown to have lower IQ scores than those living in low-fluoride regions.

Thyroid dysfunction

Even relatively low levels of fluoride intake are associated with decreased levels of serum thyroid hormones T3 and T4, and impaired thyroid function in animals. People exposed to high-fluoride drinking water have been found to have impaired activity of thyroperoxidase, lower levels of T3 and T4 and elevated thyroid-stimulating hormone (TSH) in serum.

Cancer

There is some evidence that fluoride exposure is associated with cancer, in particular osteosarcoma (bone cancer). However, some studies have found no association, and there is insufficient evidence at present to reach a conclusion.

Case reports—fluoride toxicity

- *A woman, 48 years of age,* developed increasingly severe throbbing bone and joint pain affecting her elbows, wrists, hips, knees and ankles over ten years, which limited her mobility.[1] She was found to have curvature of the spine, osteosclerosis, low vitamin D levels and increased levels of parathyroid hormone and TSH. Radiological investigations revealed signs of skeletal fluorosis, and she was found to have elevated serum and urinary fluoride. Investigation of her diet found that she had been in the habit of drinking 4–7.5 litres of brewed orange-pekoe and pekoe-cut black tea daily since twelve years of age. She brewed the tea with fluoridated tap water that had been boiled in a Teflon-coated pot. It was calculated that her fluoride intake from tea ranged from 14.6–29.3 mg/day and totalled 18.5–36.9 mg/day when including the amount in her tap water. She was asked to stop drinking tea and to minimise exposure to fluoride, and was given vitamin D supplementation. After six months, she reported that her pain had almost completely disappeared, but she did not return for any follow-up investigations.
- *A woman, 28 years of age* and living in a region of endemic fluorosis, developed insidious, progressive pain in the right hip and difficulty walking.[2] Investigations revealed a fracture of the neck of the right femur, with features suggestive of a giant-cell tumour. An operation was performed to replace part of her hip. Four years later, she developed pain in her left hip, and weakness and pain in her ribs and back, and she was found to have a pseudo-fracture of the neck of the left femur and low bone density in the vertebrae and ribs. She was diagnosed with osteomalacia and treated with calcium and vitamin D, but her symptoms did not improve and, over the next year, she developed severe bone pains and had great difficulty in standing. Eventually a fluoride assay was carried out, and she was found to have dramatically elevated serum and urinary fluoride. Her drinking water was found to have 8.4 times the normal fluoride level. The revised diagnosis was fluorosis leading to secondary hyperparathyroidism and osteomalacia. Her response to treatment was not reported.

REFERENCES

1 Izuora, K., Twombly, J.G. & Whitford, G.M. et al., Skeletal fluorosis from brewed tea, *J Clin Endocrinol Metab* (2011), 96(8): 2318–24.

2 Chadha, M. & Kumar, S., Fluorosis-induced hyperparathyroidism mimicking a giant-cell tumour of the femur, *J Bone Joint Surg Br* (2004), 86(4): 594–6.

Supplements

Because fluoride is added to many water supplies and excess intake has adverse effects, it is not used in nutritional supplements. Fluoride in fluoride toothpaste is available as sodium fluoride, sodium monofluorophosphate or stannous fluoride. Sodium fluoride contains 45 per cent elemental fluoride, stannous fluoride contains 23 per cent and sodium monofluorophosphate contains 12.5 per cent. Chewable fluoride tablets contain 0.25 mg of sodium fluoride per tablet and, if taken with milk or food, bioavailability is reduced by about 30–40 per cent. Mouthwashes may contain about 200–1000 mg/kg of sodium fluoride. Adult toothpastes contain about 1000 mg/kg of fluoride and children's toothpastes contain 400–500 mg/kg. Fluoride compounds used for water fluoridation in Australia are sodium fluoride, sodium fluorosilicate and fluorosilicic acid.

- *Fluorosilicic acid* is derived from production of phosphate fertilisers. Fluoride-containing ore is heated with sulfuric acid to form a phosphoric acid-gypsum slurry, and HF and silicon tetrafluoride is recovered from the slurry and condensed to form fluorosilicic acid.
- *Sodium fluorosilicate* and *sodium fluoride* are produced by neutralising fluorosilicic acid with either sodium chloride or caustic soda.

Cautions

Fluoride supplements and dental products should be used with caution because of the risk of fluorosis. Fluoride toothpaste may cause dental fluorosis if used by infants less than twelve months of age. Young children should use low-fluoride toothpaste, and parents should ensure that only a pea-sized amount of toothpaste is used and that the paste is not swallowed. A high intake of tea made with fluoridated water is not recommended in the long term. Excess fluoride should be avoided in people with impaired thyroid function.

ULTRATRACE ELEMENTS

Boron

BORON STATUS CHECK

1 **Do you have osteoporosis or a family history of osteoporosis?**
2 **Do you have a chronic inflammatory disorder?**
3 **Do you have low levels of vitamin D?**
4 **Do you have low levels of sex hormones?**

'Yes' answers may indicate a benefit from improved boron status. Note that a number of nutritional deficiencies or health disorders can cause similar effects and further investigation is recommended.

FAST FACTS . . . BORON

- **Good sources of boron include fruit, vegetables, legumes, nuts, wine, cider and beer.**
- **Boron plays a role in cartilage and bone growth and maintenance, energy production, metabolism of ROS, immunity, cell membrane function and the response to steroid hormones and insulin.**
- **It may have potential for the prevention of osteoporosis and the treatment of arthritis and cancer.**
- **Boron deficiency has not been identified in humans.**
- **Excess boron is unlikely, but may be associated with irritability, seizures, nausea, vomiting, diarrhoea with blue-green faeces, inflammation, congestion, oedema, scaly dermatitis, exfoliation of mucous membranes and kidney and liver damage.**

Boron is a metalloid element that is found in rocks, soil and seawater bound to oxygen as boric acid or its salts (borates). Natural forms include borax (hydrated sodium borate, also known as sodium metaborate decahydrate), boric acid, borates, kernite, colemite, tourmeline and ulexite. Boric acid and borax were commonly used food preservatives prior to the early twentieth century.

Boron has the chemical symbol B, and was discovered in 1808 by the French chemists Joseph-Louis Gay-Lussac and Louis-Jaques Thénard, and, at the same time, by the English chemist Sir Humphry Davy. Its name is believed to come from the Arabic word *buraq*, or the Persian word *burah*, meaning 'borax'. Boron is an essential trace element for many plants, but initially was not thought to be essential in animals. In 1996, the WHO Expert Committee on Trace Elements in Human Nutrition concluded that boron is probably essential for humans and the United Kingdom Expert Group on Vitamins and Minerals (2003) concluded that boron is presumably essential because a deficiency causes changes in biological functions that are reversible by boron repletion. Boron has been found to enhance cell membrane function and stability, and regulate cell metabolism by inhibiting enzyme activity, competing with various compounds in the body and controlling a number of metabolic pathways.

Digestion, absorption and transport

Boron in food is found as borax, boric acid or organic borate compounds. As boric acid, it is absorbed rapidly and almost completely in the digestive tract. It was thought that absorption was by passive diffusion, but an electrogenic sodium-coupled borate transporter, NaBC1, has been identified in mammals that appears to be essential for cell growth and proliferation. Absorption of boron does not appear to reduce with increased intake. Boron is transported in the bloodstream as boric acid, orthoboric acid and the borate anion, and is distributed evenly to soft tissues, except for adipose tissue, and concentrates in bones, teeth, hair and nails.

Metabolism, storage and excretion

Boron is not metabolised in the body because a large amount of energy is required to break boron–oxygen bonds. Boron does not accumulate in soft tissue, and most of the body content is in bones, which may act as a storage site. Boron is excreted mainly in urine as boric acid, and 84–90 per cent of intake is excreted routinely. Urinary excretion appears to regulate body levels, but there is some evidence that boron intake affects boron status by altering the expression of NaBC1.

Functions

Boric acid has the ability to form diester bridges between cis-hydroxyl-containing molecules, and acts as a linking agent. It forms complexes with the hydroxyl groups of organic compounds such as S-adenosylmethionine, pyridoxine, riboflavin, dehydroascorbic acid and pyridine nucleotides. Boron appears to play a role in cartilage and bone growth and maintenance, energy production, metabolism of ROS, immunity, cell membrane function and the response to steroid hormones and insulin. It may be a negative regulator that influences a number of metabolic pathways by competitively inhibiting some key enzyme reactions. Compounds of boron have been shown to have anti-osteoporotic, anti-inflammatory, blood lipid-lowering, anticoagulant and anticancer activity in animals. The functions of boron are not well understood, but may include the following:

- *Enzyme inhibition.* Boron inhibits oxidoreductase (XOR) enzymes, such as aldehyde dehydrogenase, xanthine oxidase and cytochrome b5 reductase, by competitively binding to the NAD or flavin cofactor. The XOR system plays a role in detoxification and generation of protective ROS during immune reactions. Boron inhibits serine proteases, such as the clotting factors Xa, IXa, XIa, XIIa, activated Hageman factor and thrombin, which are important regulators of blood clotting. It also inhibits the enzymes glyceraldehyde-3-phosphate dehydrogenase and lactate dehydrogenase in the glycolytic pathway of energy production by competitive binding to the NAD cofactor.
- *Anti-inflammatory and immune activity.* Boron suppresses enzyme activities that promote inflammation. It reduces ROS generation by leukocytes by down-regulating leukocyte 6-phosphogluconate dehydrogenase, and enhances the scavenging of ROS by antioxidant enzymes.
- *Hormone activity.* Boron affects cell membrane function and influences transmembrane signalling, transmembrane movement of regulatory ions and the cell's response to hormones. Boron is required for the hydroxylation step in the formation of testosterone and oestradiol, and it appears to have oestrogen-like effects.
- *Vitamin D function.* Boron can moderate the effects of vitamin D deficiency, possibly by enhancing the utilisation of calcitriol or having a calcitriol-sparing action. It appears to affect the metabolism and utilisation of calcium, magnesium and copper.

Dietary sources

Good sources of boron include fruit, vegetables, legumes, nuts, wine, cider and beer. Peanut butter, avocado, wine, raisins, dried fruit and nuts are particularly high in boron, but dairy products, fish, meat and most grains are poor sources. Red and white Australian wines contain about 2.5 mg/L of boron. Absorption from food averages 83–94 per cent.

Boron is not included in the Food Standards Australia New Zealand nutrient database (NUTTAB).

Factors influencing body status

Boron is readily absorbed, and it is not known whether absorption is impaired by food or other factors. A vegetarian diet that is based on fruit, vegetables, nuts and legumes is likely to provide higher amounts of boron, and diets based around animal products provide less boron.

Daily requirement

The Australian and New Zealand governments' *Nutrient Reference Values for Australia and New Zealand Including Recommended Dietary Intakes* does not provide information on boron requirements. The basal requirement for boron is likely to be more than 0.25 mg/day, and there is some evidence that standard diets provide 0.5–3.1 mg/day. Beneficial effects of boron appear to be associated with intakes of 0.5–1.0 mg/day or more.

Deficiency effects

In animals, a low boron intake affects calcium and magnesium concentrations, plasma alkaline phosphatase activity and bone calcification. Deficiency effects vary according to body levels of aluminium, calcium, vitamin D, magnesium, methionine and potassium, and include depressed growth and a reduction in steroid hormone concentrations. Boron deficiency has not been identified in humans, but depletion and repletion studies have found effects on many aspects of metabolism. In a human trial, a low boron intake resulted in poorer performance during tasks involving hand–eye coordination, attention and memory when compared with a higher boron intake. Boron deficiency could be a contributing factor to Kashin-Beck disease, a joint disorder affecting children in China that is associated with selenium deficiency. A survey in China found that boron in scalp hair was lower in children with Kashin-Beck disease compared with healthy children.

Assessment of body status

Testing for boron deficiency is rarely performed because of the absence of evidence for deficiencies in humans. The reference range given by the Mayo Medical Laboratories in the United States for serum/plasma boron is less than 100 mcg/L. However, serum/plasma levels do not correlate well with clinical manifestations, and are difficult to interpret.

THERAPEUTIC USES OF BORON

In human studies, boron supplementation after a period of depletion has resulted in increased serum vitamin D levels, decreased serum glucose and creatinine, increased serum triglycerides, increased urinary hydroxyproline excretion, increased superoxide dismutase in red blood cells, increased serum ceruloplasmin and increased haemoglobin and mean corpuscular haemoglobin content.[1] In postmenopausal women, boron supplementation reduced urinary losses of calcium and magnesium, especially if magnesium was low, and increased serum 17-beta oestradiol and testosterone.[2] It is suggested that boron supplementation may be useful for chronic inflammation, vitamin D deficiency disorders, menopausal disorders, osteoporosis, elevated blood glucose and low haemoglobin concentrations.

Osteoporosis

Boron improves bone strength and mineral composition in animals fed a high-energy diet,[3] and may be of use for the prevention of osteoporosis. Boron supplementation has been shown to slightly increase bone mineral density in female athletes, but not in sedentary women.[4]

Arthritis

Boron has been proposed as a treatment for arthritis, based on the finding of lower boron concentrations in bones and synovial fluid in people with arthritis, a higher incidence of arthritis in regions where boron intake is low and relief of arthritis in animals given supplementary boron. A small study of arthritis patients found that 6 mg of boron daily resulted in symptom relief in half of the subjects compared with 10 per cent of those on a placebo.[5] Rheumatoid arthritis patients have been found to have lower serum boron levels than controls.[6] Calcium fructoborate (CF), a complex of calcium, fructose and boron found naturally in plants such as celery, broccoli, grapes and plums, has antioxidant and anti-inflammatory activity. CF has been found to improve bone mineral density in animals and increase vitamin D levels in humans.[7] A small, unpublished study reported that CF, 6–12 mg/day, relieved joint stiffness and pain in people with arthritis.[7]

Cancer

An epidemiological study suggested an inverse relationship between boron intake and the risk of developing prostate cancer,[8] but a subsequent study failed to find an association.[9] Boron and boron derivatives may have anticancer activity by inhibiting enzymes such as serine proteases and NAD-dehydrogenases, and helping to regulate cell division and apoptosis. Boric acid inhibits cancer growth and induces apoptosis in a variety of cancer cells. In animals with androgen-sensitive prostate cancer, boric acid treatment resulted in a 25–38 per cent decrease in tumour growth and an approximate 88 per cent reduction in prostate-specific antigen (PSA) levels.[10] Boronic acids are potent and selective inhibitors of cancer cell growth, and the drug bortezomib, a boronic acid derivative, disrupts the cell cycle and induces apoptosis in a range of cancer cells. Boromycin, a natural antibiotic produced by *Streptomyces antibioticus*, disrupts the cell cycle in cancer cells, and increases their susceptibility to anticancer agents. CF acts as an antioxidant, and induces apoptosis in cancer cells, and boranes, compounds of boron and hydrogen, inhibit cancer cell metabolism and have selective effects against cancer cells. Boron neutron capture therapy (BNCT) is used in the treatment of some cancers. It is a method of selectively irradiating cancer cells with irradiated boron compounds, such as sodium borocaptate and boronophenylalanine.

REFERENCES

1. Nielsen, F.H., Biochemical and physiologic consequences of boron deprivation in humans, *Environ Health Perspect* (1994), 102 (Suppl 7): 59–63.
2. Nielsen, F.H., Hunt, C.D., Mullen, L.M. & Hunt, J.R., Effect of dietary boron on mineral, estrogen, and testosterone metabolism in postmenopausal women, *FASEB J* (1987), 1(5): 394–7.
3. Hakki, S.S., Dundar, N., Kayis, S.A. et al., Boron enhances strength and alters mineral composition of bone in rabbits fed a high energy diet, *J Trace Elem Med Biol* (2013), 27(2): 148–53.
4. Meacham, S.L., Taper, L.J. & Volpe, S.L., Effects of boron supplementation on bone mineral density and dietary, blood, and urinary calcium, phosphorus, magnesium, and boron in female athletes, *Environ Health Perspect* (1994), 102 (Suppl 7): 79–82.
5. Newnham, R.E., Essentiality of boron for healthy bones and joints, *Environ Health Perspect* (1994), 102 (Suppl 7): 83–5.
6. Al-Rawi, Z.S., Gorial, F.I., Al-Shammary, W.A. at al., Serum boron concentration in rheumatoid arthritis: correlation with disease activity, functional class, and rheumatoid factor, *J Exp Integr Med* (2013), 3(1): 9–15.
7. Miljkovic, D., Scorei, R.I., Cimpoiaşu, V.M. & Scorei, I.D., Calcium fructoborate: Plant-based dietary boron for human nutrition, *J Diet Suppl* (2009), 6(3): 211–26.
8. Cui, Y., Winton, M.I., Zhang, Z.F. et al., Dietary boron intake and prostate cancer risk, *Oncol Rep* (2004), 11(4): 887–92.
9. Gonzalez, A., Peters, U., Lampe, J.W. & White, E., Boron intake and prostate cancer risk, *Cancer Causes Control* (2007), 18(10): 1131–40.
10. Scorei, R.I. & Popa, R. Jr, Boron-containing compounds as preventive and chemotherapeutic agents for cancer, *Anticancer Agents Med Chem* (2010), 10(4): 346–51.

Therapeutic dose

There is limited information on the optimal therapeutic dose of boron; doses of 3–10 mg daily have been used in clinical trials.

Effects of excess

Inorganic borates, including boric acid and sodium, ammonium, potassium and zinc borates, have low acute toxicity. It is estimated that an intake of 0.2 mg/kg/day of boron for life is unlikely to be associated with adverse effects, and the US Institute of Medicine has set the tolerable upper intake level (UL) at 20 mg/day for adults. Turkish populations living in boron rich environments may have a daily intake of more than 6–8 mg of boron, and some regions of Turkey have water supplies providing 29 mg/L of boron. No adverse effects have been reported from such high intakes.

The acute, lethal dose of boric acid is 3–6 g for infants and 15–20 g for adults. Boron toxicity can occur at doses of 100 mg to 55.5 g daily, depending on age and body weight. Toxicity effects may include irritability, seizures, nausea, vomiting, diarrhoea with blue-green faeces, inflammation, congestion, oedema, scaly dermatitis, exfoliation of mucous membranes, and kidney and liver damage. Boron toxicity can cause an intense red skin rash on the face, palms, soles, buttocks or scrotum within 24 hours of exposure, followed by skin loss in the affected area one to two days later. Developmental effects in animals include high prenatal mortality, reduced foetal weight and bone, eye, central nervous system and cardiovascular system abnormalities. Long-term exposure to boron in animal studies has been reported to cause reduced fertility, decreased sperm motility and testicular toxicity, but adverse effects on fertility have not been found in humans. N-acetylcysteine is a boron chelator that increases urinary excretion of boron, and may be useful to treat toxicity.

Case reports—boron toxicity

- *Seven infants, six to sixteen weeks of age*, were given dummies coated with a borax and honey mixture for four to ten weeks, providing an estimated daily ingestion of 143–429 mg of boron.[1] This estimation was later found to be false, and was recalculated to be 429–1287 mg/day.[2] The infants developed generalised or alternating focal seizure disorders, irritability, gastrointestinal disturbances, inflammation, congestion, oedema, scaly dermatitis, exfoliation of mucous membranes and damage to kidney tubules. The seizures stopped when the borax and honey mixture was discontinued, and there appeared to be no adverse long-term effects.
- *A woman, 32 years of age*, developed pancreatitis, loss of almost all her body and scalp hair, redness of the palms of her hands, severe fatigue, loss of appetite and mental confusion.[3] It was discovered that she had swallowed several bottles of boric acid-containing mouthwash daily for at least one year. She was found to have a serum boron level of 5600 mcg/L. After stopping ingestion of the mouthwash, her hair regrew.

REFERENCES

1 O'Sullivan, K. & Taylor, M., Chronic boric acid poisoning in infants, *Arch Dis Child* (1983), 58(9): 737–9.

2 US Environmental Protection Agency, *Toxicological review of boron and compounds* (CAS No. 7440–42–8), EPA, Washington, DC, 2004.

3 Stein, K.M., Odom, R.B., Justice, G.R. & Martin, G.C., Toxic alopecia from ingestion of boric acid, *Arch Dermatol* (1973), 108: 95–7.

Supplements

Boron salts can be extracted from boron-containing ores or seawater. Boron is available as tablets and capsules, and is found mainly in multivitamin and mineral formulations, and products that support bone health. The forms of boron permitted in oral supplements in Australia are borax, borax pentahydrate and sodium perborate. Bioavailability of boron from supplements is generally high.

The amount of elemental boron in a specific boron source is listed on the product container, and may vary between individual products. The approximate elemental boron content of some common forms is shown in Table 12.8.

Table 12.8 Elemental boron content of common forms

Form	Boron content (%)
Boric acid	17
Borax pentahydrate	15
Borax	11
Sodium perborate	11

- *Borax* is produced from sodium borate ores by crushing, heating, mechanical separation and selective crystallisation, followed by flotation of borax decahydrate or pentahydrate from the concentrate.

- *Sodium perborate* is produced by the reaction of disodium tetraborate pentahydrate, hydrogen peroxide and sodium hydroxide. It is an ingredient in some mouthwashes because it breaks down to release hydrogen peroxide when mixed with warm water, and helps to remove tooth stains and kill oral bacteria.
- *Boric acid* is produced by reacting borax or other borates with hydrochloric or sulfuric acid.

Cautions

Boron may increase oestrogen levels in the body. The effect of taking boron supplements with oestrogen drugs is not known.

Silicon

SILICON STATUS CHECK

1 Do you have osteoporosis or a family history of osteoporosis?
2 Do you have weak hair and nails?
3 Do you have sun-damaged skin?
4 Do you have an increased risk of Alzheimer's disease?

'Yes' answers may indicate a benefit from improved silicon status. Note that a number of nutritional deficiencies or health disorders can cause similar effects and further investigation is recommended.

FAST FACTS . . . SILICON

- Good sources of silicon include beer, wine and mineral water, especially mineral water from Malaysia and Fiji.
- Silicon plays a role in connective tissue structure and bone growth, and may reduce aluminium levels in the body.
- It may improve hair, skin and nail texture, and has potential for the prevention of osteoporosis and Alzheimer's disease.
- Silicon deficiency has not been identified in humans.
- Excess silicon is relatively non-toxic, but long-term use of magnesium trisilicate antacids has been associated with silica kidney stones.

Silicon is a highly reactive element, and readily forms compounds with other elements. It is found in the environment as silicon dioxide (silica) and silicates, and is present in water and sand, and in crystalline form in quartz rock. As rocks break down, silica reacts with water to form soluble silicic acid, a collective term for orthosilicic acid (monosilicic acid), disilicic acid, trisilicic acid and metasilicic acid. Orthosilicic acid is an uncharged molecule, also known as monomeric silica. Orthosilicic acid forms larger, charged silica species (polysilicic acid), also known as oligomeric or polymeric silica—especially at higher silicon concentrations. Polymerisation of silica reduces its solubility and hence its bioavailability.

Silicon has the chemical symbol Si, and was discovered in 1823 by the Swedish scientist Jöns Jacob Berzelius. Its name comes from the Latin word *silex* or *silicis*, meaning 'flint'. Silicon is present in pharmaceutical products such as anti-diarrhoea medication, antacids and analgesics such as aspirin and in cosmetics and toiletries as viscosity control agents and excipients. In human nutrition, silicon appears to be required for the structural integrity of connective tissue, and normal bone growth and development.

Digestion, absorption and transport

Silicon in food is mainly found as oligomeric silica in plants, and as monomeric silica in fluids. Absorption is dependent on the production of soluble and absorbable species of silica in the digestive tract. Insoluble oligomeric silica needs to be broken down to soluble monomeric silica that may be absorbed by the paracellular pathway or small-pore transcellular pathway. Oligomeric silica is charged, which causes it to interact more strongly with the mucus layer in the gut, and it is a large size that may reduce its ability to pass through the mucus layer to enable absorption to take place. Silicon is transported in the bloodstream as silicates and free orthosilicic acid, which readily diffuses into cells.

Metabolism, storage and excretion

Silica is concentrated in connective tissues such as bones, tendons and the skin, which may act as a storage site. It is readily excreted in urine, and does not appear to accumulate in the body. Silicon intake correlates with urinary concentrations, and urinary excretion appears to regulate body levels. There is evidence from animal studies that urinary excretion is reduced in silicon deficiency.

Functions

Silicon plays a role in the formation of connective tissue structures and bone, but it is not known whether it has other roles in the body. It may be protective against aluminium toxicity. Functions of silicon may include:

- *Connective tissue integrity.* Silicon may have a role in transcription of the type I collagen gene or as a cofactor for the enzyme prolyl hydroxylase that, together with iron and vitamin C, acts to incorporate the amino acid proline into procollagen to form mature collagen, the major structural protein in connective tissue. Silicon also has a structural role in glycosaminoglycans (GAGs), which make up the water-holding matrix (ground substance) in connective tissue. It is believed to be present as silanolate, a derivative of silicic acid, in GAGs, and may have a cross-linking effect, linking different polysaccharides together or linking GAGs to anchoring proteins. Silicon may improve the integrity of connective tissue in joint cartilage, ligaments, tendons, gums, blood vessel walls and skin, hair and nails.
- *Bone formation.* Silicon supports connective tissue formation in bone, and may enhance the deposition of calcium and phosphorus in bone tissue. It appears to support calcification of bone matrix; silicon levels in unmineralised bone matrix are 25 times greater than in surrounding areas, and the silicon content gradually declines as calcification occurs. It may be that silicon plays a role in the electrochemical process of mineralisation, but the precise function of silicon in bone development is not known.
- *Protection against aluminium toxicity.* Aluminium can cause damage to the nervous system, and is associated with Alzheimer's disease. The oligomeric forms of silicon found in food can bind aluminium and reduce its uptake in the digestive tract. Silicon also appears to help reduce transport of aluminium into the brain. Monomeric silica from beverages has less ability to bind aluminium, but there is evidence that drinking water containing monomeric silica also inhibits the absorption of dietary aluminium.

Dietary sources

Monomeric silica is water soluble, and is found in drinking water and beverages such as beer and wine. It is readily absorbed in the gastrointestinal tract. In food, silica is in an oligomeric form that has reduced solubility and lower bioavailability.

Good sources of well-absorbed monomeric silica are beer, wine and mineral water, especially mineral water from Malaysia and Fiji. The silicon concentration of European mineral waters ranges from 4–16 mg/L and the content in Malaysian and Fijian mineral waters ranges from 30–40 mg/L. On average, drinking water levels range from 1–100 mg/L. Absorption of silica from beverages averages 50 per cent.

Plants take up silicon from soils, and produce phytolithic silica, an oligomeric form, which provides structural strength. Some plants are silicon accumulators; these include cereals, grasses such as rice, and the herbs horsetail, borage, comfrey and nettle, which accumulate about 10–20 times more silicon than most other plants. Good sources of less well-absorbed oligomeric silica are oat bran, grains, lettuce, cabbage, onions, dark-green leafy vegetables, root vegetables, alfalfa, shellfish, kelp, pectin, dried fruit, apples and bananas. In absorption studies, silica in green beans, raisins and horsetail was well absorbed, in contrast to the silica in bananas, which was poorly absorbed. Absorption averages 41 per cent from solid foods.

The silicon compounds silica (551), calcium silicate (552), magnesium hydrogen metasilicate (talc) (553), sodium aluminosilicate (554), potassium aluminosilicate (555), calcium aluminium silicate (556), bentonite (558), aluminium silicate (kaolin) (559) and potassium silicate (560) are used in food processing as anti-caking agents, thickeners and stabilisers, clarifying agents in beer and wine, glazing, polishing and release agents in confectionery, dusting powder in chewing gum and coating agents in rice. Silicon additives are thought to be inert and not readily absorbed from the gastrointestinal tract; however, there is evidence that a portion may be converted to monomeric forms in the gut and absorbed.

The Food Standards Australia New Zealand nutrient database (NUTTAB) does not provide the amount of silicon in specific foods.

Factors influencing body status

A high fibre intake reduces absorption of silicon, and calcium and magnesium may bind with silicon and form insoluble silicates or compete for absorption pathways. There is some indication that body levels of silicon decrease with age, but the effect of ageing is not well understood.

Daily requirement

The Australian and New Zealand governments' *Nutrient Reference Values for Australia and New Zealand Including Recommended Dietary Intakes* does not provide information on silicon requirements. Daily intake of silicon averages 20–50 mg from standard diets, and the basal requirement is unknown. Vegetarian diets may provide higher silicon intakes.

Deficiency effects

Early studies of silicon deficiency in animals reported bone and joint abnormalities, including abnormal development of the skull and long bones, abnormal bone growth in joints, a reduced amount of joint cartilage, reduced bone mineral density, reduced collagen synthesis and increased collagen breakdown. However, more recent studies have found only mild alterations in bone metabolism, such as reduction in bone growth plate thickness, an increase in cartilage cell density, inhibition of growth plate closure and increased longitudinal growth. There are no recognised deficiency effects in humans.

Assessment of body status

Testing for silicon deficiency is rarely performed because of the absence of evidence for deficiencies in humans. The reference range given by the Mayo Medical Laboratories in the United States for serum/plasma silicon is less than 0.05 mg/dL. Levels of silicon in random urine samples from healthy men are reported to be 1.31–1.46 mg/dL.

THERAPEUTIC USES OF SILICON

Because it is involved in connective tissue and bone formation, silica has been recommended for arthritis, joint deformities, joint pain, spinal disc degeneration, bone weakness, osteoporosis, atherosclerosis, heart valve weakness, varicose veins, athletic injuries and poor texture of skin, hair and nails. However, there is limited evidence about its efficacy. Therapeutic uses of silicon may include:

Bone mineral density

Animal studies have found that silicon supplementation stimulates bone formation, increases bone mineral density (BMD) and bone strength, reduces bone injuries and decreases calcium excretion in urine.[1] A higher dietary silicon intake has been found to be associated with higher BMD at the hip in men and premenopausal women,[2] and also in postmenopausal women, but only in those on hormone replacement therapy (HRT).[3] A study from the 1970s reported that silicon supplementation (27.5 mg/week for three months) in women with osteoporosis resulted in increases in trabecular bone volume compared with control subjects.[4] In people with osteoporosis, silicon supplementation, as monomethylsilanetriol (MMST), resulted in increased bone volume and improved BMD in the thighbone and lumbar spine.[5] Choline-stabilised orthosilicic acid (Ch-OSA), providing 6 mg of silicon daily, was used in a study of osteoporosis patients, together with calcium and vitamin D, and resulted in a slightly greater increase in thigh bone BMD compared to subjects on calcium and vitamin D only.[6]

Bone implants

Silicon enhances bone formation when incorporated into calcium phosphate bioceramics used in bone implants, such as silicon-substituted hydroxyapatites and Bioglass™. It has been found to form an amorphous silicon layer on bone that supports gene expression, osteoblast proliferation and differentiation, formation of type I collagen and apatite formation.[7]

Alzheimer's disease

Aluminium is present in senile plaques and neurofibrillary tangles (NFTs) that are features of Alzheimer's disease (AD) and intake of aluminium increases expression in animals of amyloid-beta, an abnormal protein present in senile plaques in the brain in AD. Aluminium levels greater than 0.1 mg/L in drinking water have been found to double the risk of AD.[8] However, there is controversy about whether aluminium has a causative role in AD.

In AD models, silicates can cause NFTs and precipitated beta-pleated sheets of amyloid-beta to convert to soluble forms.[9] Oligomeric silica binds aluminium in the digestive tract, and reduces its absorption. A study of healthy volunteers found that oligomeric silica reduced the uptake of aluminium by 67 per cent compared with controls given aluminium without silica, but monomeric silica had no effect.[10]

A low silica concentration was associated with low cognitive performance in elderly women,[11] and an increase of 10 mg/day of dietary silica has been associated with an 11 per cent reduction in risk of dementia.[12] AD patients with an intake of up to 1 L of a silicon-rich mineral water each day for twelve weeks had increased urinary excretion of aluminium, and cognitive performance improved in three of fifteen subjects.[13]

Skin, hair and nail texture

A study of women with photo-damaged facial skin given 10 mg of silicon daily as Ch-OSA for 20 weeks found that skin roughness and elasticity improved, and nails and hair became less brittle.[14] Another study using the same supplement for nine months reported that it improved hair strength and thickness in women with fine hair.[15]

REFERENCES

1 Jugdaohsingh, R., Silicon and bone health, *J Nutr Health Aging* (2007), 11(2): 99.

2 Jugdaohsingh, R., Tucker, K.L., Qiao, N. et al., Dietary silicon intake is positively associated with bone mineral density in men and premenopausal women of the Framingham Offspring cohort, *J Bone Miner Res* (2004), 19(2): 297–307.

3 Macdonald, H.M., Hardcastle, A.E., Jugdaohsingh, R. et al., Dietary silicon intake is associated with bone mineral density in premenopasual women and postmenopausal women taking HRT, *J Bone Min Res* (2005), 20: S393.

4 Schiano, A., Eisinger, F., Detolle, P. et al., Silicium, bone tissue and immunity, *Revue du Rhumatisme et des Maladies Osteo-Articulaires* (1979), 46(7–9): 483–6.

5 Eisinger, J. & Clairet, D., Effects of silicon, fluoride, etidronate and magnesium on bone mineral density: A retrospective study, *Magnes Res* (1993), 6(3): 247–9.

6 Spector, T.D., Calomme, M.R., Anderson, S. et al., Effect of bone turnover and BMD of low dose oral silicon as an adjunct to calcium/vitamin D3 in a randomized placebo-controlled trial, *J Bone Min Res* (2005), 20: S172.

7 Arcos, D., Izquierdo-Barba, I. & Vallet-Regí, M., Promising trends of bioceramics in the biomaterials field, *J Mater Sci Mater Med* (2009), 20(2): 447–55.

8 Rondeau, V, Commenges, D., Jacqmin-Gadda, H. & Dartigues, J.F., Relation between aluminum concentrations in drinking water and Alzheimer's disease: An 8-year follow-up study, *Am J Epidemiol* (2000), 152(1): 59–66.

9 Fasman, G.D. & Moore, C.D., The solubilization of model Alzheimer tangles: Reversing the beta-sheet conformation induced by aluminum with silicates, *Proc Natl Acad Sci USA* (1994), 91(23): 11232–5.

10 Jugdaohsingh, R., Reffitt, D.M., Oldham, C. et al., Oligomeric but not monomeric silica prevents aluminum absorption in humans, *Am J Clin Nutr* (2000), 71(4): 944–9.

11 Gillette-Guyonnet, S., Andrieu, S., Nourhashemi, F. et al., Cognitive impairment and composition of drinking water in women: Findings of the EPIDOS Study, *Am J Clin Nutr* (2005), 81(4): 897–902.

12 Rondeau, V., Jacqmin-Gadda, H., Commenges, D. et al., Aluminum and silica in drinking water and the risk of Alzheimer's disease or cognitive decline: Findings from 15-year follow-up of the PAQUID cohort, *Am J Epidemiol* (2009), 169(4): 489–96.

13 Davenward, S., Bentham, P., Wright, J. et al., Silicon-rich mineral water as a non–invasive test of the 'aluminum hypothesis' in Alzheimer's disease, *J Alzheimers Dis* (2013), 33(2): 423–30.

14 Barel, A., Calomme, M., Timchenko, A. et al., Effect of oral intake of choline-stabilized orthosilicic acid on skin, nails and hair in women with photodamaged skin, *Arch Dermatol Res* (2005), 297(4): 147–53.

15 Wickett, R.R., Kossmann, E., Barel, A. et al., Effect of oral intake of choline-stabilized orthosilicic acid on hair tensile strength and morphology in women with fine hair, *Arch Dermatol Res* (2007), 299(10): 499–505.

Therapeutic dose

There is limited information on the optimal therapeutic dose of silicon; doses of up to 40 mg daily have been used in clinical trials.

Effects of excess

High doses of silicon have very few adverse effects. Two animal studies have reported small reductions in bone strength on a very high, prolonged intake of silicon. Ruminant animals consuming plants with a high content of silicon may develop silicate kidney stones, and a small number of people taking magnesium trisilicate as an antacid for several decades have also developed silicate kidney stones. A no observed adverse effects level (NOAEL) of 50 000 mg/L has been estimated for silica in drinking water, based on animal studies. The tolerable upper intake level (UL) for silicon is estimated to be 700–1750 mg/day. The European Expert Group on Vitamins and Minerals has estimated that a safe upper level for supplementation is 700 mg silicon/day for adults over a lifetime.

Industrial exposure to crystalline silica dust causes respiratory irritation and inflammation in the lungs, and eventually leads to small airway obstruction (silicosis). Acute exposure to high concentrations causes cough, shortness of breath and pulmonary alveolar lipoproteinosis, which is the accumulation of protein and fat in the air sacs of the lungs. Silica dust exposure is associated with tuberculosis, chronic bronchitis, small airway disease, emphysema, autoimmune diseases such as rheumatoid arthritis, scleroderma and systemic lupus erythematosus, and kidney disease, characterised by glomerular and tubular changes.

Case reports—silicon toxicity

- *A male infant, ten months of age*, developed acute pyelonephritis caused by silica kidney stones.[1] It was discovered that his formula had been made with silicon-rich spring water providing 172 mg silicon/L. The silicon concentration in the water was seven to 34 times higher than the average amount in tap water, and it was estimated that his silicon intake was 172–206 mg/day. The water used to make up his formula was changed, and he recovered after treatment to break down the stones.
- *A woman, 38 years of age*, developed episodic left-flank pain associated with the passage of gravel-like sediment in her urine.[2] She was found to have kidney stones composed of 100 per cent silicate. She had a history of Lyme disease, osteoarthritis, gallstones and irritable bowel syndrome, and she reported that her sister had a history of kidney stones of unknown cause. Her medications included cefuroxime (an antibiotic), oxycodone (an analgesic), vitamin B12 injections, methocarbamol (a muscle relaxant) and ibuprofen (an anti-inflammatory). No obvious source of silica could be found, and she had not used colloidal silica or magnesium trisilicate antacids. It was discovered that she was taking a range of health supplements, including a glucosamine and rice bran product, a digestive aid and a herbal product containing *Uncaria tomentosa* (cat's claw), each of which listed silica dioxide as an ingredient. She had been taking four capsules of the glucosamine product daily, one capsule of the digestive aid daily and two capsules of *Uncaria tomentosa* three times daily for two years. She was advised to discontinue these supplements and her symptoms resolved. When she resumed the supplements, her symptoms returned. Testing revealed that each product contained less than 2 per cent silicon in the form of silicon dioxide, but no other source of silicon was identified and it was concluded that the supplements had caused her silica stones.

REFERENCES

1 Nishizono, T., Eta, S., Enokida, H. et al., Renal silica calculi in an infant, *Int J Urol* (2004), 11(2): 119–21.

2 Flythe, J.E., Rueda, J.F., Riscoe, M.K. & Watnick, S., Silicate nephrolithiasis after ingestion of supplements containing silica dioxide, *Am J Kidney Dis* (2009), 54(1): 127–30.

Supplements

Silicon is extracted from quartz rock or sand. It is available as tablets, capsules and colloids, and is found mainly in products that support skin, hair, nail, bone and joint health. All forms of silica that require hydrolysis in the gut, such as silica in food, magnesium trisilicate, colloidal silica and Ch-OSA, are less well absorbed than the monomeric silica found in beverages. The forms of silicon permitted in oral supplements in Australia are colloidal anhydrous silica and silicon dioxide. The herb horsetail is also used as a silica supplement, and this form of silica appears to be well-absorbed. The amount of elemental silicon in a specific silicon source is listed on the product container and may vary between individual products; the approximate elemental silicon content of some common forms is shown in Table 12.9.

Table 12.9 Elemental silicon content of common forms

Form	Silicon content (%)
Silicon dioxide	47
Colloidal anhydrous silica	47

- *Silicon dioxide* is extracted from quartz or sand, and appears to be a well-absorbed form of silicon.
- *Colloidal silica* can be prepared by various methods, including ion exchange of aqueous silicates, hydrolysis and condensation of silicon compounds, direct oxidation of silicon and silica powder peptisation (shaking the powder with a dispersion medium in the presence of small amount of electrolyte). It is a precipitated and completely polymerised form of silica that has been shown to have a very low absorption of less than 2 per cent because it is very slowly broken down to monomeric silica in the digestive tract. However, it may be more effective than monomeric silica for binding aluminium.

Silicon supplements not available in Australia include MMST, in which a methyl group replaces one hydroxyl group of orthosilicic acid, which maintains silica in a small, monomeric and well-absorbed form, and Ch-OSA, in which choline protects the silica from extensive polymerisation and precipitation by maintaining it in aqueous suspension. Ch-OSA still needs to break down to monomeric silica in the digestive tract, and is not as well absorbed as MMST. A study of silicon absorption in humans found that absorption was 64 per cent for MMST and alcohol-free beer, 44 per cent for green beans, 43 per cent for an orthosilicic acid solution, 17 per cent for Ch-OSA; 4 per cent for bananas and magnesium trisilicate antacids; and 1 per cent for colloidal silica.

Cautions

Large amounts of magnesium trisilicate antacids used in the long term may increase the risk of kidney stones in susceptible people.

HOW MUCH DO I KNOW?

Choose whether the following statements are true or false. Then review this chapter for the correct answers.

	True (T)	False (F)
1 Brazil nuts are a good source of silicon.	T	F
2 Selenoproteins take part in antioxidant and redox reactions.	T	F
3 Kashin-Beck disease is caused by chromium deficiency.	T	F
4 Chromium may be useful for insulin resistance and diabetes.	T	F
5 Molybdenum may reduce sensitivity to sulfites and alcohol.	T	F
6 Fluoridated water contains about 10 mg/L fluoride.	T	F
7 Borax is a supplementary form of boron.	T	F
8 Selenium reduces absorption of aluminium.	T	F
9 Oligomeric silica is not well absorbed.	T	F
10 An adequate intake of molybdenum is 45 mcg/day for adults.	T	F

FURTHER READING

Braun, L. & Cohen, M., *Herbs & natural supplements: An evidence-based guide*, 3rd ed., Churchill Livingstone Elsevier, New York, 2010.

Gropper, S.S., Smith, J.L. & Groff, J.L., *Advanced nutrition and human metabolism*, 5th ed., Thomson Wadsworth, Belmont, CA, 2009.

Higdon, J., *An evidence-based approach to vitamins and minerals*, Thieme, New York, 2003.

Linus Pauling Institute, Micronutrient Research Center, website, available at <lpi.oregonstate.edu/infocenter>.

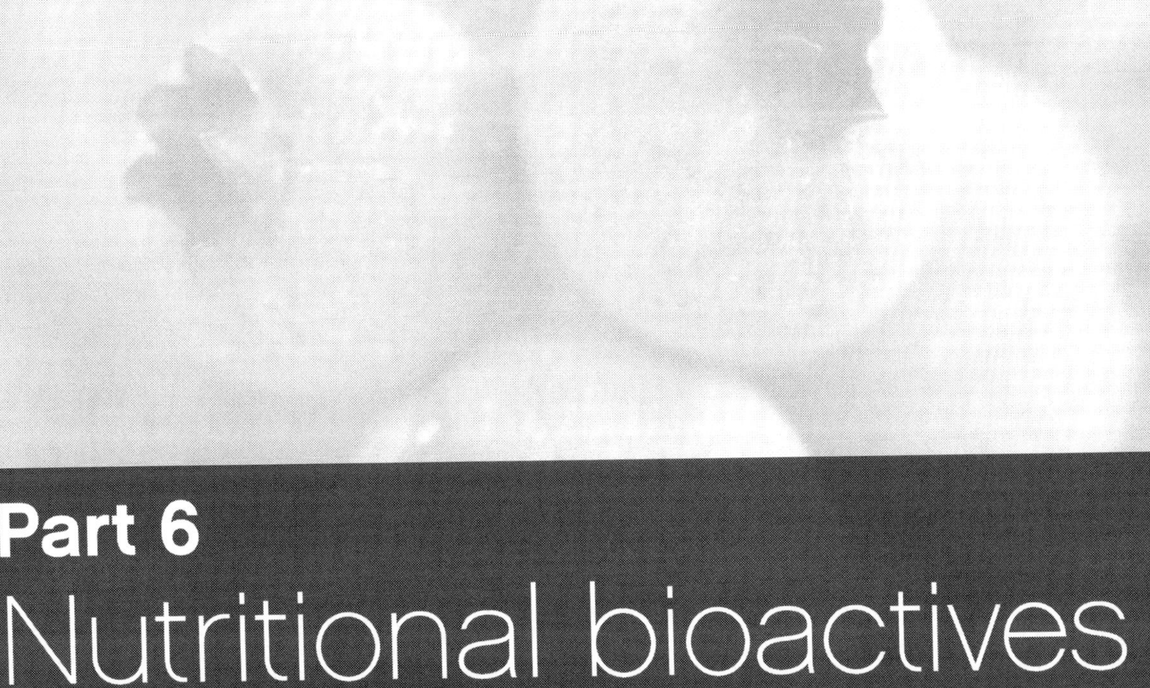

Part 6
Nutritional bioactives

13

Nutritional bioactives: coenzyme Q10, alpha-lipoic acid, phytochemicals and chlorophyll

Nutritional bioactives include naturally occurring components of food or diet-related substances that affect body function. They have health effects, and are used to support health and wellbeing, and prevent or treat health disorders; however, they are not regarded as essential nutrients because they do not appear to be essential for growth, development and life itself, or to have a defined deficiency syndrome that occurs with inadequate intake.

COENZYME Q10

FAST FACTS . . . COENZYME Q10

- **Coenzyme Q10 is a fat-soluble compound made in the body, which is also found in smaller amounts in food.**
- **It is required for energy production in mitochondria and antioxidant activity.**
- **It is particularly important for protecting mitochondria from oxidative damage.**
- **Supplementation may be helpful for muscle function and cardiovascular disorders.**

Coenzyme Q (also called ubiquinone) is a fat-soluble compound that is made up of a quinone ring and an isoprenoid side-chain containing a number of units. It was isolated from the mitochondria in beef heart by Dr Frederick Crane, a US researcher, in 1957. The predominant form of coenzyme Q in humans and many animals is coenzyme Q10 (CoQ10), also known as ubiquinone-10, containing ten units in the side-chain. The name ubiquinone is derived from the word 'ubiquitous', meaning 'present everywhere', as it is found in all cells. Q10 refers to its chemical structure: Q comes from the quinone ring and 10 from its ten side-chain units.

CoQ10 is not an essential dietary nutrient because it can be made in the body. It is found in all classes of lipoproteins, and in all cell membranes and membranes surrounding the organelles within cells, including the mitochondria. The body contains about 2 g of CoQ10, and about 500 mg is produced daily to maintain normal body levels. The average Western diet provides less than 5 mg a day, and production in the body is much more important than dietary intake. CoQ10 from the diet is taken up by chylomicrons, transported to the liver and incorporated into very low-density lipoproteins, where it acts as an antioxidant.

Synthesis

CoQ10 synthesis occurs in most body tissues, including the liver (see Figure 13.1). The first steps in making the side chains of CoQ10 require the enzyme HMG-CoA reductase and involve the conversion of acetyl coenzyme A to HMG-CoA, then to mevalonate and then to farnesyl pyrophosphate. These steps are also the first steps in the production of cholesterol. The amino acids phenylalanine or tyrosine, with the assistance of methyl groups from S-adenosylmethionine, produced during methionine metabolism, make the quinone ring to which the side chains attach. Vitamin C and vitamins B2, B3, B6 and folic acid are cofactors for enzymes required for CoQ10 production.

Functions

Functions of CoQ10 include:

- *Energy production*. CoQ10 is essential for the oxidative phosphorylation pathway that produces energy in mitochondria. It accepts and transfers electrons in Complex I and Complex II of the electron transport chain, a series of protein complexes embedded in the inner mitochondrial membrane. Electrons are transferred through these complexes, and protons are pumped across the membrane, generating a gradient that is used by the ATP synthase complex (Complex V) to synthesise ATP. CoQ10 transfers electrons and also transfers protons to create the proton gradient essential for ATP production.
- *Antioxidant activity*. CoQ10 can be converted to ubiquinol-10, the reduced form of ubiquinone, which is a potent fat-soluble antioxidant. Ubiquinol-10 is an efficient scavenger of free radicals within cell membranes, protecting membrane phospholipids, proteins and fats from oxidative damage, and also protecting lipoproteins and DNA. It appears to help protect the skin against UV-induced damage and wrinkling.

  Ubiquinol-10 has about the same effectiveness as vitamin E in reacting with free radicals and protecting membranes from oxidative stress. There is about ten

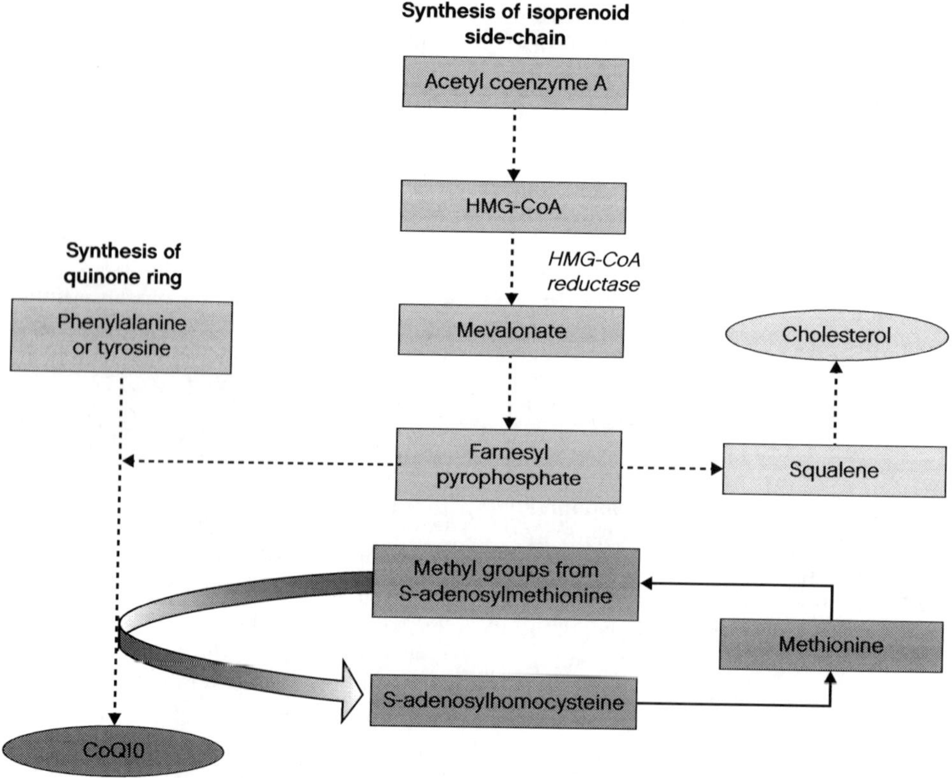

Figure 13.1 Synthesis of coenzyme Q10

times more ubiquinol-10 than vitamin E in the inner mitochondrial membranes, about equal amounts in other cell membranes and about twenty times less in lipoproteins. Ubiquinol-10 is used up before vitamin E, indicating that it is highly reactive with free radicals, and may act as a first line of defence for body lipids and cholesterol. It is much more efficient in inhibiting low-density lipoprotein (LDL) oxidation than lycopene, beta-carotene or vitamin E.

Ubiquinol-10 assists the antioxidant defence system by regenerating vitamin E from its radical form. CoQ10-facilitated electron transport across the cell membrane may help regenerate vitamin C in extracellular fluid from its radical form, whereas intracellular vitamin C is mainly regenerated by glutathione activity. Ubiquinol-10 is regenerated by dihydrolipoic acid, the thioredoxin system and enzymes in the mitochondrial electron transport chain.

- *Protection of DNA*. In animals, a lifelong intake of low-dose CoQ10 enhances plasma levels of CoQ10, vitamin A and vitamin E, and helps reduce DNA damage in blood cells and the age-related drop in the total antioxidant capacity of plasma. In cell studies, supplementary CoQ10 enhanced DNA resistance to hydrogen peroxide-induced damage in human lymphocytes. Oral CoQ10 has also been found to inhibit DNA damage in lymphocytes of healthy people, although several weeks of supplementation may be needed before protective effects are observed. The effects also lasted for several weeks after supplementation was discontinued.

  Mitochondrial DNA (mDNA) is more susceptible to damage than DNA in the cell nucleus and, if CoQ10 is inadequate, oxidative damage to mDNA accumulates. Decreased mitochondrial function reduces energy production and impairs cell function, which particularly affects the liver, heart and skeletal muscles, and is a feature of ageing. Mitochondrial malfunctions can cause muscle weakness and cramps, fatigue and exercise intolerance, and may be linked to many chronic degenerative diseases.
- *Sperm function*. In sperm cells, most of the CoQ10 is concentrated in the mitochondria of the mid-piece, where it is vital for producing the energy for movement and viability. Ubiquinol-10 prevents lipid peroxidation in sperm membranes and maintains sperm integrity.
- *Muscle function*. CoQ10 is important for energy production in muscles, including skeletal muscles, the heart and the smooth muscles in blood vessel walls.
- *Removal of waste material in cells.* Lysosomes, the waste-removal units in the cytoplasm of cells, use a CoQ10-dependent system to acidify the interior of the lysosome and activate enzymes to digest cellular debris.
- *Iron release in cells*. Iron bound to the transport protein transferrin in the bloodstream is engulfed by endosomes at the cell membrane, in which an acidic interior is generated that allows iron to split off and be released into the cytoplasm. It is believed that CoQ10 may act to acidify the interior of endosomes in a similar manner to its action in lysosomes.

Dietary sources

Very little CoQ10 is obtained from the diet, and it is poorly absorbed. The richest dietary sources are organ meats, such as heart, liver and kidneys, as well as beef, soy oil, canola oil, sardines, herrings, mackerel, nuts and seeds. The Food Standards Australia New Zealand nutrient database (NUTTAB) does not provide the amount of CoQ10 in specific foods.

Factors influencing body status

The ability to make CoQ10 appears to decrease progressively in various tissues with age, and levels in body organs may decrease by 30–60 per cent. Statin drugs used for cholesterol-lowering block the activity of HMG-CoA reductase, and may lead to lower body levels. Drugs for lowering blood glucose may decrease plasma levels of CoQ10 and reduce the effects of supplementation. Beta-blockers for lowering heart rate and blood pressure, some tranquillisers and some anti-depressants can inhibit CoQ10-dependent enzyme reactions.

Inadequate intake of B vitamins and vitamin C may impair CoQ10 synthesis. Selenium deficiency impairs function of thioredoxin reductase, an enzyme that regenerates ubiquinol-10. A selenium deficiency can cause levels of CoQ10 in the liver to decline by 50 per cent, and also decreases levels in the kidneys and heart but does not appear to lower muscle levels.

Daily requirement

CoQ10 is made in the body and is not an essential dietary nutrient. Therefore, no recommended daily intake has been established.

Assessment of body status

Plasma CoQ10 levels are an accepted measure in research settings, and reflect levels in platelets and white blood cells. CoQ10 testing is not widely available to the general public. Plasma levels are variable, with reported values ranging from 0.30–3.84 mcg/mL, and normal values have not yet been firmly established. A supplementary dose of 30 mg a day slightly elevates the plasma level and 100–150 mg daily can double it.

Deficiency effects

If CoQ10 status is inadequate, oxidative damage to the DNA of mitochondria accumulates and permanently and progressively impairs mitochondrial function. A lower level of CoQ10 may have adverse effects on the brain, heart, skeletal muscles and all organs and tissues. CoQ10 deficiency may contribute to poor memory, lack of concentration, fatigue, muscle pain and weakness, and poor stamina and endurance. Primary (genetic) and secondary (acquired) deficiencies have been identified. A primary deficiency is believed to be rare, and may be due to molecular defects in one or more of the nine genes that regulate CoQ10 biosynthesis.

Indicators of primary CoQ10 deficiency may include:

- encephalomyopathy, central nervous system (CNS) dysfunction, developmental delay, ataxia (inco-ordination) and seizures
- ragged red fibres in skeletal muscles, progressive muscle weakness (myopathy) and fatigue, exercise intolerance, myoglobin in the urine
- mitochondrial encephalomyopathy, lactic acidosis and stroke-like syndrome (MELAS)
- Kearns-Sayre syndrome (KSS), featuring progressive weakness of eye movements, eyelid droop, mild skeletal muscle weakness, heart block, short stature, hearing loss, ataxia, impaired cognitive function and diabetes.
- myoclonus epilepsy with ragged red fibres (MERRF), featuring sudden, brief, jerking spasms that can affect the arms and legs or the entire body, muscle weakness, ataxia, seizures, slow deterioration of intellectual function, short stature, degeneration of the optic nerve, hearing loss, cardiomyopathy and peripheral nerve damage
- severe infantile multisystemic disease, featuring growth retardation, ataxia and deafness
- cerebellar ataxia
- Leigh syndrome, usually occurring in infants, featuring poor feeding ability, ataxia, slow growth rate, deafness, loss of appetite, vomiting, irritability, crying, seizures, generalised weakness, lack of muscle tone and lactic acidosis, which can lead to impairment of respiratory and kidney function
- isolated myopathy.

Although CoQ10 can be made in the body, decreased levels have been detected, particularly in older people and in chronic disease states, such as heart disease, muscular dystrophies, Parkinson's disease, cancer, diabetes and HIV/AIDS. Children with food intolerances and allergies have been found to have decreased levels. The causes of these secondary deficiencies are not well understood, but may be due to impaired synthesis, increased requirements or increased utilisation.

Indicators of secondary CoQ10 deficiency may include:

- disorders associated with oxidative (free radical) damage
- muscle weakness, cramps, pain, fatigue, exercise intolerance
- cardiovascular disease (CVD), including congestive heart failure, chest pain, breathlessness, palpitations, high blood pressure
- diseases of ageing
- neurodegenerative diseases
- male infertility.

THERAPEUTIC USES OF COENZYME Q10

Exercise performance

CoQ10 supplementation may improve exercise endurance and reduce measures of oxidative damage after exercise training.[1]

Neuromuscular disorders

In children with Duchenne muscular dystrophy, CoQ10 used with prednisone therapy may increase muscle strength.[2] Supplementary CoQ10 may help relieve early symptoms of a primary deficiency, such as early-onset mitochondrial encephalomyopathies, and may have potential for slowing the progress of degenerative diseases, such as Huntington's disease, Parkinson's disease and Friedrich's ataxia.[3,4,5]

Alzheimer's disease

Supplementary CoQ10 has protective antioxidant effects, and has been shown to protect animals against amyloid-beta damage in the brain, which is associated with Alzheimer's disease.[6]

Cardiovascular disease

Supplementation with CoQ10 increases levels of ubiquinol-10 in lipoproteins and increases resistance of LDLs to lipid peroxidation. In animals on high-fat diets, CoQ10 decreases lipid hydroperoxide levels in atherosclerotic lesions and decreases lesion size.[7] CoQ10 supplementation may lower elevated blood pressure, improve heart function in cardiomyopathy and heart failure and relieve irregular heartbeat in diabetics.[8] It may also help prevent myocardial degeneration, assist repair of mitral valve prolapse, relieve angina and improve ischaemic heart disease (heart disease due to circulatory blockage). It has been used before heart surgery to reduce free radical damage and improve recovery.

Plasma CoQ10 levels have been found to be an independent predictor of mortality in cardiac patients.[9] In patients with coronary heart disease, CoQ10 (300 mg/day for one month) improved extracellular SOD activity and improved endothelial-derived vasodilation.[10] CoQ10 taken with conventional therapy has improved heart function and dramatically increased survival of cardiomyopathy patients compared with those on conventional treatment only.[11] CoQ10 supplementation in heart failure patients awaiting heart transplant has improved functional status, clinical symptoms and quality of life, but cardiac status was unchanged.[12] It has also reduced hospitalisations and the incidence of serious complications in heart failure.[13] However, not all trials have found that CoQ10 has benefits in heart failure, and a meta-analysis of seven trials concluded that there was insufficient evidence for its effectiveness.[14]

The key enzyme, HMG-CoA reductase, required for the initial steps in CoQ10 synthesis, is blocked by cholesterol-lowering statin drugs, with consequent adverse effects on mitochondrial and heart function. Statin therapy has been shown to lower serum CoQ10 levels, which can be prevented by supplementation.[15] Muscle pain is a side-effect of statin therapy, and CoQ10 supplementation (100 mg/day) has decreased pain severity in patients taking statins.[16] However, other studies have not shown beneficial effects.[17] It has been suggested that patients with familial elevated serum cholesterol levels, heart failure, high blood pressure and those at risk of heart disease or over 65 years of age on statin therapy may benefit from supplementary CoQ10.[18]

Diabetes

CoQ10 supplementation has been found to improve blood sugar control, blood pressure and blood glucose levels in diabetics.[19]

Male infertility

CoQ10 has improved fertility rates in men with low fertility and improved sperm motility in men with poor sperm motility.[20]

Migraine

CoQ10 has been found to reduce migraine frequency, duration and symptoms, and relieve headache-induced disability.[21,22]

Skin ageing

CoQ10 applied to the skin may help reduce the depth of wrinkles caused by excessive sun exposure and protect against damaging ultraviolet (UV) radiation.[23]

Visual disorders

CoQ10, when used with acetyl-L-carnitine, a form of the amino acid carnitine, plus omega-3 fats, was found to reduce visual deterioration in people with macular degeneration, a condition affecting older people that causes loss of central vision and leads to blindness.[24]

Gum disease

Applying CoQ10 to the gums has been found to strengthen gum tissue and speed healing in gum infections.[25]

REFERENCES

1 Vanfraecchem, J.H.P. & Folkers, K., Coenzyme Q10 and physical performance, in K. Folkers & Y. Yamamura (eds), *Biomedical and Clinical Aspects of Coenzyme Q, vol. 3*, Elsevier/North-Holland Biomedical Press, Amsterdam, 1981, pp. 235–41.

2 Spurney, C.F., Rocha, C.T., Henricson, E. et al., Cooperative International Neuromuscular Research Group Investigators, CINRG pilot trial of coenzyme Q10 in steroid-treated Duchenne muscular dystrophy, *Muscle Nerve* (2011), 44(2): 174–8.

3 Huntington Study Group, A randomized, placebo-controlled trial of coenzyme Q10 and remacemide in Huntington's disease, *Neurology* (2001), 57(3): 397–404.

4 Shults, C.W. et al., Effects of coenzyme Q10 in early Parkinson disease: Evidence of slowing of the functional decline, *Arch Neurol* (2002), 59(10): 1541–50.

5 Lodi, R. et al., Anti-oxidant treatment improves in vivo cardiac and skeletal muscle bioenergetics in patients with Friedreich's ataxia, *Ann Neurol* (2001), 49(5): 590–6.

6 Yang, X., Yang, Y., Li, G. et al., Coenzyme Q10 attenuates beta-amyloid pathology in the aged transgenic mice with Alzheimer presenilin 1 mutation, *J Mol Neurosci* (2008), 34(2): 165–71.

7 Witting, P.K., Pettersson, K., Letters, J. & Stocker, R., Anti-atherogenic effect of coenzyme Q10 in apolipoprotein E gene knockout mice, *Free Radic Biol Med* (2000), 29(3–4): 295–305.

8 Kumar, A., Kaur, H., Devi, P. & Mohan, V., Role of coenzyme Q10 (CoQ10) in cardiac disease, hypertension and Meniere-like syndrome, *Pharmacol Ther* (2009), 124(3): 259–68.

9 Molyneux, S.L., Florkowski, C.M., George, P.M. et al., Coenzyme Q10: an independent predictor of mortality in chronic heart failure, *J Am Coll Cardiol* (2008), 52(18): 1435–41.

10 Tiano, L., Belardinelli, R., Carnevali, P. et al., Effect of coenzyme Q10 administration on endothelial function and extracellular superoxide dismutase in patients with ischaemic heart disease: A double-blind, randomized controlled study, *Eur Heart J* (2007), 28(18): 2249–55.

11 Langsjoen, P.H., Folkers, K., Lyson, K. et al., Pronounced increase of survival of patients with cardiomyopathy when treated with coenzyme Q10 and conventional therapy, *Int J Tissue React* (1990), 12(3): 163–8.

12 Berman, M., Erman, A., Ben-Gal, T. et al., Coenzyme Q10 in patients with end-stage heart failure awaiting cardiac transplantation: A randomized, placebo-controlled study, *Clin Cardiol* (2004), 27(5): 295–9.

13 Morisco, C., Trimarco, B. & Condorelli, M., Effect of coenzyme Q10 therapy in patients with congestive heart failure: A long-term multicenter randomized study, *Clin Investig* (1993), 71 (8 Suppl): S134–6.

14 Madmani, M.E., Yusuf Solaiman, A., Tamr Agha, K. et al., Coenzyme Q10 for heart failure, *Cochrane Database Syst Rev* (2014), 6: CD008684.

15 Mortensen, S.A., Leth, A., Agner, E. & Rohde, M., Dose-related decrease of serum coenzyme Q10 during treatment with HMG-CoA reductase inhibitors, *Mol Aspects Med* (1997), 18 (Suppl): S137–44.

16 Caso, G., Kelly, P., McNurlan, M.A. & Lawson, W.E., Effect of coenzyme Q10 on myopathic symptoms in patients treated with statins, *Am J Cardiol* (2007), 99(10): 1409–12.

17 Schaars, C.F. & Stalenhoef, A.F., Effects of ubiquinone (coenzyme Q10) on myopathy in statin users, *Curr Opin Lipidol* (2008), 19(6): 553–7.

18 Levy, H.B. & Kohlhaas, H.K., Considerations for supplementing with coenzyme Q10 during statin therapy, *Ann Pharmacother* (2006), 40(2): 290–4.

19 Hodgson, J.M., Watts, G.F., Playford, D.A. et al., Coenzyme Q10 improves blood pressure and glycaemic control: A controlled trial in subjects with type 2 diabetes, *Eur J Clin Nutr* (2002), 56(11): 1137–42.

20 Balercia, G., Mancini, A. & Paggi, F. et al., Coenzyme Q10 and male infertility, *J Endocrinol Invest* (2009), 32(7): 626–32.

21 Hershey, A.D. et al., Coenzyme Q10 deficiency and response to supplementation in pediatric and adolescent migraine, *Headache* (2007), 47(1): 73–80.

22 Sandor, P.S. et al., Efficacy of coenzyme Q10 in migraine prophylaxis: A randomized controlled trial, *Neurology* (2005), 64(4): 713–15.

23 Hoppe, U., Bergemann, J., Diembeck, W. et al., Coenzyme Q10, a cutaneous anti-oxidant and energizer, *Biofactors* (1999), 9(2–4): 371–8.

24 Feher, J., Kovacs, B., Kovacs, I. et al., Improvement of visual functions and fundus alterations in early age-related macular degeneration treated with a combination of acetyl-L-carnitine, n-3 fatty acids, and coenzyme Q10, *Ophthalmologica* (2005), 219: 154–66.

25 Wilkinson, E.G. et al., Bioenergetics in clinical medicine. VI: Adjunctive treatment of periodontal disease with coenzyme Q10, *Res Commun Chem Pathol Pharmacol* (1976), 14: 715–19.

Therapeutic dose

As a general supplement for ageing, muscle weakness, cramps and fatigue, and for people on statin therapy, the dose range is 50–150 mg a day.

The following doses have been used for adults in clinical trials:

- *Diabetes:* 100–200 mg daily.
- *Heart disease:* 50–200 mg daily.
- *Cancer:* 90–390 mg daily.
- *Neuromuscular and neurodegenerative diseases:* 300–1200 mg daily; up to 3600 mg daily has been used for Parkinson's disease.

Supplements

CoQ10 (ubiquinone) is available as ubidecarenone (an alternative name for ubiquinone). It is fat soluble and is best absorbed when taken with a source of fat. Standard supplements contain CoQ10 powder in an oil suspension and are available as tablets or capsules. Pure CoQ10 has limited solubility in oils and fats and may have relatively poor bioavailability. Newer products are being developed that have enhanced solubility and are more bioavailable. Ubiquinol-10 is more bioavailable than ubiquinone. Idebenone is a synthetic form of CoQ10 that has similar functions in the body and may have similar beneficial effects, but more research is needed to establish its effectiveness. Most CoQ10 is made commercially in Japan by a microbial or yeast fermentation process. Some CoQ10 is made from solanesol obtained from plants of the *Solanaceae* family by a chemical process.

Cautions

Supplementary CoQ10 has few reported side-effects, with only mild gastrointestinal effects reported in less than 1 per cent of patients in clinical trials. However, these adverse effects may not be due to CoQ10 because there is no dose–response relationship—that is, there is no difference in incidence of reported effects between high doses or low doses. The observed safe level of CoQ10 supplementation is 1200 mg a day, and up to 3600 mg a day has been used without evidence of toxicity. However, blood levels do not increase at doses above 2400 mg. The safety of CoQ10 supplementation for pregnant or breastfeeding women, infants and children has not been established.

There is a suspected interaction between CoQ10 and blood-thinning drugs, such as warfarin, which may increase the risk of bleeding. However, a small trial of patients taking warfarin with 100 mg CoQ10 for four weeks found that it had no effect on clotting measures. Because there is a potential risk, the Therapeutic Goods Administration (TGA) in Australia requires the following warning on all retail products containing CoQ10:

'Not to be taken if on warfarin therapy without medical advice.'

People on warfarin who wish to take CoQ10 supplements should seek advice from their medical practitioner.

CoQ10 AND CANCER . . . A POTENTIAL NEW THERAPY?

Patients with breast, lung and pancreatic cancer have been found to have low plasma CoQ10, and CoQ10 levels have been found to be a powerful and independent predictor of risk of melanoma metastases.[1] Some studies have shown that CoQ10 provides some protection against cardiotoxicity or liver toxicity during cancer treatment, but better quality research is needed in this area.[2] Epidemiological studies have found that low plasma levels of CoQ10 have been linked to increased risk of breast cancer,[3] but another study found that higher CoQ10 levels may be associated with increased breast cancer risk in postmenopausal women.[4] Higher CoQ10 levels in plasma have been linked to a better prognosis in breast cancer patients.[5] As CoQ10 is made and utilised within cells, the significance of plasma levels is not well understood.

Breast cancer tissue has been found to have much lower levels of CoQ10 than normal tissue,[6] and case study reports on the use of CoQ10 in breast cancer have shown promising results. Thirty-two breast cancer patients who had received standard treatment were given 2850 mg vitamin C, 2500 IU vitamin E, 32.5 IU beta-carotene, 387 mcg selenium plus other vitamins and minerals, 1.2 g gamma-linolenic acid, 3.5 g omega-3 fatty acids and 90 mg CoQ10 per day for eighteen months.[7] On this therapy, no patients died, none showed metastases, quality of life improved with reduced use of pain killers and no weight loss, and six patients showed partial remission. In one of these six cases, CoQ10 was increased to 390 mg and mammography confirmed the absence of a tumour at two months. Another case was then treated with 300 mg CoQ10 and no residual tumour tissue was found at three months. In a further three case studies using 390 mg CoQ10 daily, numerous liver metastases disappeared in one patient, a tumour in the pleural cavity disappeared in another patient, and an older patient given a lumpectomy showed no residual cancer cells or metastases at follow-up.[8]

In another breast cancer study, 100 mg CoQ10, 10 mg riboflavin (vitamin B2) and 50 mg niacin (vitamin B3) were given with tamoxifen, which resulted in reduction of circulating tumour markers.[9] Tamoxifen therapy causes elevated serum triglyceride levels, and another study found that CoQ10 given with tamoxifen to breast cancer patients reduced lipid levels as well as reducing markers of angiogenesis, the process by which tumours create new blood vessels to allow them to grow and spread.[10]

Larger and better-designed trials are needed to properly evaluate the efficacy of CoQ10 in cancer. However, in view of its safety and potential benefits, it can be recommended as part of a nutritional support program for cancer patients.

REFERENCES

1 Rusciani, L., Proietti, I., Rusciani, A. et al., Low plasma coenzyme Q10 levels as an independent prognostic factor for melanoma progression, *J Am Acad Dermatol* (2006), 54(2): 234–41.

2 Roffe, L., Schmidt, K. & Ernst, E., Efficacy of coenzyme Q10 for improved tolerability of cancer treatments: A systematic review, *J Clin Oncol* (2004), 22(21): 4418–24.

3 Cooney, R.V., Dai, Q., Gao, Y.T. et al., Low plasma coenzyme Q(10) levels and breast cancer risk in Chinese women, *Cancer Epidemiol Biomarkers Prev* (2011), 20(6): 1124–30.

4 Chai, W., Cooney, R.V., Franke, A.A. et al., Plasma coenzyme Q10 levels and postmenopausal breast cancer risk: The multiethnic cohort study, *Cancer Epidemiol Biomarkers Prev* (2010), 19(9): 2351–6.

5 Jolliet, P., Simon, N., Barre, J. et al., Plasma coenzyme Q10 concentrations in breast cancer: Prognosis and therapeutic consequences, *Int J Clin Pharmacol Ther* (1998), 36: 506–9.

6 Portakal, O., Ozkaya, O., Erden Inal, M. et al., Coenzyme Q10 concentrations and anti-oxidant status in tissues of breast cancer patients, *Clin Biochem* (2000), 33: 279–84.

7 Lockwood, K., Moesgaard, S., Hanioka, T. & Folkers, K., Apparent partial remission of breast cancer in 'high risk' patients supplemented with nutritional anti-oxidants, essential fatty acids and coenzyme Q10, *Mol Aspects Med* (1994), 15 (Suppl): s231–40.

8 Lockwood, K., Moesgaard, S., Yamamoto, T. & Folkers, K., Progress on therapy of breast cancer with vitamin Q10 and the regression of metastases, *Biochem Biophys Res Commun* (1995), 212(1): 172–7.

9 Premkumar, V.G., Yuvaraj, S., Vijayasarathy, K. et al., Effect of coenzyme Q10, riboflavin and niacin on serum CEA and CA 15-3 levels in breast cancer patients undergoing tamoxifen therapy, *Biol Pharm Bull* (2007), 30(2): 367–70.

10 Sachdanandam, P., Antiangiogenic and hypolipidemic activity of coenzyme Q10 supplementation to breast cancer patients undergoing Tamoxifen therapy, *Biofactors* (2008), 32(1–4): 151–9.

ALPHA-LIPOIC ACID

FAST FACTS . . . ALPHA-LIPOIC ACID

- Alpha-lipoic acid is a naturally occurring sulfur-containing fatty acid that is made in the body and is also found in food.
- It has a special role as a 'super' or 'universal' antioxidant because, unlike other antioxidants, it acts in both the watery and the fatty compartments of the body.
- It is required for energy production in mitochondria and antioxidant activity.
- It helps protect the body against toxins.
- Supplementation may be helpful for diseases of ageing, nerve damage associated with diabetes and death-cap mushroom poisoning.

Alpha-lipoic acid (alpha-LA), also known as lipoic acid or thioctic acid, is a naturally occurring sulfur-containing fatty acid that is made in the body and is also found in food. It is an 8-carbon medium-chain fatty acid with sulfur atoms at C6 and C8 that was isolated by US researchers in 1951 from liver. Alpha-LA can exist in two forms, R-alpha-LA and S-alpha-LA, which are mirror images of each other; the 'R' form is made and utilised in the body and occurs naturally in food. Ingested alpha-LA is absorbed from the small intestine and distributed to the liver and various body tissues. It undergoes S-methylation and beta-oxidation during metabolism, and the main circulating metabolites are 4,6-bismethylthio-hexanoic acid and 2,4-bismethylthio-butanoic acid. It is fat-soluble and is easily transported across cell membranes, and can also cross the blood–brain barrier for delivery to brain cells. Once inside cells, it is converted to dihydrolipoic acid (DHLA). Both DHLA and alpha-LA are found within cells and mitochondria, and also in extracellular fluids. Alpha-LA acid is mainly excreted in bile, and some is excreted as conjugated forms in urine.

Synthesis

Alpha-LA is made in mitochondria from octanoic acid, an 8-carbon fatty acid, by the enzyme lipoic acid synthase. Sulfur atoms from the amino acid cysteine are added by the enzyme lipoyl synthase. Alpha-LA produced in the body is bound to proteins.

Functions

Key functions of alpha-LA include antioxidant protection and energy metabolism in mitochondria. Functions include:

- *Antioxidant activity.* Alpha-LA has a special role as a 'super' or 'universal' antioxidant because, unlike other antioxidants, it acts in both the watery and the fatty compartments of the body. It neutralises hydroxyl and peroxyl radicals, hypochlorous acid, singlet oxygen and peroxynitrite.

  DHLA has greater antioxidant activity than alpha-LA and is one of the most potent naturally occurring antioxidants. DHLA scavenges nitric oxide (NO), peroxynitrite, hypochlorous acid and superoxide, peroxyl and hydroxyl radicals without becoming a radical itself. It helps to regenerate glutathione, the body's primary water-soluble antioxidant, by promoting cellular uptake of cysteine, the rate-limiting amino acid for glutathione production. It also helps regenerate the antioxidants vitamin C, vitamin E and CoQ10 when they become inactive and helps repair oxidation damage. Alpha-LA and DHLA bind with metals that can enhance formation of free radicals; alpha-LA binds copper, zinc and lead but not iron, and DHLA binds copper, zinc, iron, lead, cadmium and mercury. Ingested alpha-LA can circulate unbound in plasma, and can chemically trap toxic metals and protect cells.

- *Energy production.* As alpha-lipoamide, alpha-LA is an essential cofactor for several mitochondrial enzyme complexes that act in the citric acid cycle and amino acid metabolism. It is a cofactor for the conversion of pyruvate to acetyl-CoA, and for the conversion of alpha-ketoglutarate to succinyl-CoA for use in the citric acid cycle. It also assists the breakdown of the branched-chain amino acids leucine, isoleucine and valine, which are used for energy in muscles. Alpha-LA is thought to support energy production during ageing by maintaining efficient mitochondrial function.
- *Glucose regulation.* Alpha-LA works with insulin to enable glucose to move from the bloodstream into cells, and may help maintain normal glucose metabolism. Alpha-LA and DHLA can bind to albumin and prevent glycation, a process by which glucose binds to proteins and prevents them from functioning—usually a consequence of elevated blood glucose levels.
- *Nervous system protection.* Alpha-LA can decrease lipid peroxidation and bind toxic metals in brain and nerve tissue, and may prevent glucose-related oxidative damage in diabetes. It has been found to suppress free radicals initiated by iron in the CNS. It helps protect the brain and nervous system from damage by reducing inflammation, scavenging free radicals and damaged fats in nervous tissue, protecting against alcohol damage and maintaining healthy nerve transmission.
- *Anti-inflammatory activity.* Alpha-LA suppresses inflammation by inhibiting the activity of pro-inflammatory chemicals, such as tumour necrosis factor-alpha (TNF-alpha) and nuclear factor kappaB (NF-kappaB).
- *Folic acid metabolism.* Alpha-LA is required for metabolism of 5,10-methylene tetrahydrofolate, a form of the B vitamin folic acid that is needed for producing nucleic acids for normal cell replication.

Dietary sources

There is limited information on food sources. Alpha-LA can be found bound to the amino acid lysine as lipoyl-lysine in food such as kidneys, heart, liver, spinach, broccoli, tomatoes, peas, Brussels sprouts, carrots, beets and rice bran. However, levels in food are much lower than the amount made in the body.

Daily requirement

Alpha-LA is made in the body, and is not an essential dietary nutrient. Therefore, no recommended daily intake has been established.

Assessment of body status

There is little information on optimal plasma levels of alpha-LA. In bioavailability studies, plasma levels of R-alpha-LA, the naturally occurring form, have been reported to be about 0.05 mcg/mL at baseline, increasing up to 45 mcg/mL after supplementation.

Deficiency effects

No specific deficiency syndrome has been identified for alpha-LA. However, a deficiency would be expected to increase oxidative stress and impair energy production.

THERAPEUTIC USES OF ALPHA-LA

Alpha-LA is used for disorders related to oxidative stress and mitochondrial dysfunction. Uses of alpha-LA include:

Protection against toxins

Toxic metals, such as lead, arsenic, mercury, cadmium and excess copper, can cause mitochondrial damage, inhibition of mitochondrial enzymes, suppression of protein synthesis and production of free radicals, and animal studies show that alpha-LA can bind toxic metals and reduce their damaging effects. Alpha-LA also maintains levels of the protective antioxidant glutathione and can mobilise heavy metals from body tissues, but has weaker activity than metal-chelating drugs.

Animal studies have shown that alpha-LA has protective activity against the toxic mould and food contaminant aflatoxin and the cancer drugs adriamycin, cisplatin and tamoxifen.[1,2,3] In animals, it protects the liver against damage by tamoxifen if used concurrently, but is less effective if used later to reverse tamoxifen-induced liver damage.[4] It helps protect the kidneys from cisplatin-induced damage by suppressing inflammation,[5] and cell studies indicate that it also may protect nerve cells.[6] In animals, alpha-LA protects mitochondria against damage to pigment cells in the retina of the eye caused by acrolein, a contaminant in over-heated cooking oils and cigarette smoke.[7]

Amanita phalloides (death cap) mushroom poisoning

This species of toxic fungi contains amanitin, which causes severe liver and kidney damage, leading to death in 50–90 per cent of cases. Alpha-LA is an effective therapy that has been shown to save lives. Reports from the United States claim that patients suffering from amanitin poisoning have all survived if given alpha-LA within two to three days after ingestion, and tissue damage has been reversed.[8] One patient who was given alpha-LA at a later stage did not survive. A further case report claims that a patient in a coma caused by amanitin poisoning survived after treatment with alpha-LA.[9]

Brain and nerve damage

Alpha-LA may be helpful for Alzheimer's disease and dementias, because it increases acetylcholine production, scavenges reactive oxygen species (ROS) and neurotoxic lipid peroxidation products and reduces inflammation. In animals, it has helped to prevent death of cells in the brain regions most affected in Parkinson's disease.[10] Long-term alpha-LA supplementation in a small number of patients with Alzheimer's disease appeared to stabilise cognitive function.[11] In patients with burning mouth syndrome (associated with nerve dysfunction), alpha-LA has relieved symptoms in some studies, and there are indications that it works best in patients who have not previously been treated with tranquillisers.[12]

Diabetes

Alpha-LA supplements have been shown to improve insulin sensitivity in patients with type 2 diabetes and reduce symptoms of diabetic neuropathy, such as pain, numbness and burning sensations.[13] In Germany, alpha-LA is an approved therapy for neuropathy caused by diabetes and alcohol, and for alcoholic liver disease. In obese patients with impaired glucose tolerance, iv alpha-LA improved insulin sensitivity and decreased plasma levels of free fatty acids, triglycerides, total cholesterol, LDL cholesterol, small dense LDL cholesterol, oxidised LDL cholesterol and VLDL cholesterol.[14] Markers of oxidation and inflammation decreased considerably.

Ageing

In animal studies, the increase in inflammation and oxidative stress in blood vessels that is associated with ageing is lessened by alpha-LA supplementation. It has improved mitochondrial structure and function, reduced oxidative damage, increased levels of antioxidants and slowed the progress of cognitive decline in older animals.[15] Alpha-LA given with acetyl-L-carnitine to aged rats decreased oxidant levels, lipid peroxidation, formation of protein carbonyls and DNA strand breaks.[16]

Polycystic ovarian syndrome

Women with polycystic ovarian syndrome (PCOS) taking a controlled release form of alpha-LA had improved insulin sensitivity, decreased serum triglyceride levels and improvements in LDL cholesterol, with some experiencing more regular menstrual cycles.[17]

REFERENCES

1 Karaman, M., Ozen, H., Tuzcu, M, et al., Pathological, biochemical and haematological investigations on the protective effect of alpha-lipoic acid in experimental aflatoxin toxicosis in chicks, *Br Poult Sci* (2010), 51(1): 132–41.

2 Balachandar, A.V., Malarkodi, K.P. & Varalakshmi, P., Protective role of DLalpha-lipoic acid against adriamycin-induced cardiac lipid peroxidation, *Hum Exp Toxicol* (2003), 22(5): 249–54.

3 Melli, G., Taiana, M., Camozzi, F. et al., Alpha-lipoic acid prevents mitochondrial damage and neurotoxicity in experimental chemotherapy neuropathy, *Exp Neurol* (2008), 214(2): 276–84.

4 Hesham, A., Lipoic acid attenuates DNA fragmentation, oxidative stress and liver injury induced by tamoxifen in rats, *Asian J Traditional Medicines* (2007), 2(5): 175–88.

5 Kang, K.P., Kim, D.H., Jung, Y.J. et al., Alpha-lipoic acid attenuates cisplatin-induced acute kidney injury in mice by suppressing renal inflammation, *Nephrol Dial Transplant* (2009), 24(10): 3012–20.

6 Gedlicka, C., Kornek, G.V., Schmid, K. & Scheithauer, W., Amelioration of docetaxel/cisplatin induced polyneuropathy by alpha-lipoic acid, *Ann Oncol* (2003), 14(2): 339–40.

7 Jia, L., Liu, Z., Sun, L. et al., Acrolein, a toxicant in cigarette smoke, causes oxidative damage and mitochondrial dysfunction in RPE cells: Protection by (R)-alpha-lipoic acid, *Invest Ophthalmol Vis Sci* (2007), 48(1): 339–48.

8 Becker, C.E., Tong, T.G., Boerner, U. et al., Diagnosis and treatment of Amanita phalloides-type mushroom poisoning: Use of thioctic acid, *West J Med* (1976), 125(2): 100–9.

9 Teutsch, C. & Brennan, R.W., Amanita mushroom poisoning with recovery from coma: A case report, *Ann Neurol* (1978), 3(2): 177–9.

10 Karunakaran, S., Diwakar, L., Saeed, U. et al., Activation of apoptosis signal regulating kinase 1 (ASK1) and translocation of death-associated protein, Daxx, in substantia nigra pars compacta in a mouse model of Parkinson's disease: Protection by alpha-lipoic acid, *FASEB J* (2007), 21(9): 2226–36.

11 Hager, K., Kenklies, M., McAfoose, J. et al., Alpha-lipoic acid as a new treatment option for Alzheimer's disease: A 48 months follow-up analysis, *J Neural Transm Suppl* (2007), 72: 189–93.

12 Femiano, F., Gombos, F. & Scully, C., Burning mouth syndrome: The efficacy of lipoic acid on subgroups, *J Eur Acad Dermatol Venereol* (2004), 18(6): 676–8.

13 Ziegler, D., Low, P.A., Litchy, W.J. et al., Efficacy and safety of anti-oxidant treatment with α-lipoic acid over 4 years in diabetic polyneuropathy: The NATHAN 1 trial, *Diabetes Care* (2011), 34(9): 2054–60.

14 Zhang, Y., Han, P., Wu, N. et al., Amelioration of lipid abnormalities by α-lipoic acid through antioxidative and anti-inflammatory effects, *Obesity (Silver Spring)* (2011), 19(8): 1647–53.

15 Liu, J., The effects and mechanisms of mitochondrial nutrient alpha-lipoic acid on improving age-associated mitochondrial and cognitive dysfunction: An overview, *Neurochem Res* (2008), 33(1): 194–203.

16 Sundaram, K. & Panneerselvam, K.S., Oxidative stress and DNA single strand breaks in skeletal muscle of aged rats: role of carnitine and lipoic acid, *Biogerontology* (2006), 7(2): 111–18.

17 Masharani, U., Gjerde, C., Evans, J.L. et al., Effects of controlled-release alpha lipoic acid in lean, nondiabetic patients with polycystic ovary syndrome, *J Diabetes Sci Technol* (2010), 4(2): 359–64.

Therapeutic dose

Oral doses used in research studies are 600–1800 mg daily, and it has been used iv in doses up to 1200 mg.

Supplements

Alpha-LA can be prepared by a chemical process that involves reacting 6,8 dichlorooctanoic acid with sodium disulphide. It is available as R-alpha-LA and R,S-alpha-LA. R,S-alpha-LA is a 50/50 mixture of R-alpha-LA and S-alpha-LA, and is commonly used in supplements. R-alpha-LA is the naturally occurring form, and it appears that it has better utilisation and retention in the body; plasma levels are 40–50 per cent higher after supplementation with the 'R' form compared with the 'S' form. There is some evidence that S-alpha-LA can impair the absorption and metabolism of R-alpha-LA. However, S-alpha-LA may stabilise R-alpha-LA in supplements. R-alpha-LA in a salt form (sodium R-alpha-lipoate) is more soluble and has been shown to be considerably more bioavailable than an equivalent dose of a 50/50 mixture of R-alpha-LA and S-alpha-LA. Alpha-LA supplements should be taken on an empty stomach 30 minutes before eating or two hours afterwards, because absorption is impaired if taken with food.

Cautions

Few effects of excess have been identified. Rarely, nausea and vomiting have been reported. In patients with amanitin poisoning, alpha-LA has been associated with hypoglycaemia, but this has not been reported in other studies. Use of alpha-LA may increase the need for the B vitamin biotin. Lipoic acid and biotin have a similar structure, and animal studies have found that lipoic acid competes with biotin and may reduce activity of biotin-dependent enzymes. There is a case report of loss of sense of taste after taking a combination herb and nutrient anti-ageing supplement containing alpha-LA that was reversed by high-dose biotin supplementation. The safety of alpha-LA supplementation for pregnant or breastfeeding women, infants and children has not been established.

PHYTOCHEMICALS

FAST FACTS . . . PHYTOCHEMICALS

- **Phytochemicals are plant compounds that have health effects in the body but are not essential nutrients.**
- **Many phytochemicals are poorly absorbed, and the portion that is absorbed is rapidly metabolised and excreted.**
- **Many phytochemicals have powerful antioxidant activity as well as anti-inflammatory and anticancer activity.**
- **Supplementation may be helpful for diseases related to oxidative stress, inflammation and ageing.**

Phytochemicals, also called phytonutrients, are chemicals produced by plants that affect body physiology but are not considered to be essential nutrients for human growth, development or survival. The term *phyto* comes from the Greek word for plant. Phenylpropanoids, derived from the amino acid phenylalanine, are the precursor molecules for production of phytochemicals. Phytochemicals provide plants with colour, flavour, smell and texture, and include compounds that have evolved to attract pollinators and to provide protection against exposure to UV radiation, toxins, pests and pathogens.

There are thousands of phytochemicals in plant foods, and only a limited number have been researched to date, although research in this area is expanding rapidly. It should be noted that phytochemicals do not exist in isolation in foods, and the health effects of phytochemical-rich foods may be due to their complex and diverse combinations of phytochemicals rather than to any individual phytochemical.

Bioactive dietary phytochemicals include:

- *carotenoids:*
  - *carotenes:* alpha-carotene, beta-carotene, gamma-carotene, lycopene
  - *xanthophylls:* lutein, zeaxanthin, beta-cryptoxanthin, canthaxanthin, astaxanthin, fucoxanthin, neoxanthin, violaxanthin, alloxanthin, crocoxanthin, monadoxanthin
- *polyphenolics:*
  - *phenolic acids:*
    - *hydroxycinnamic acids:* caffeic, ferulic and chlorogenic acids, curcumin
    - *hydroxybenzoic acids:* ellagic, gallic, vannilic and syringic acids
  - *flavonoids:*
    - *flavonols:* quercetin, quercitrin, rutin, kaempferol, myricetin, galangin, fisetin, isorhamnetin
    - flavones: apigenin, luteolin, chrysin, tangretin
    - *flavan-3-ols (flavanols):*
      - *monomers (catechins):* catechin, epicatechin, gallocatechin, epigallocatechin, epicatechin gallate, epigallocatechin-3-0-gallate (EGCG)
      - *dimers/polymers (oxidised catechins):* theaflavins, thearubigins
    - *flavanones:* hesperidin (hesperitin), citrin, naringenin, naringin
    - *anthocyanidins:* cyanidin, malvidin, pelargonidin, delphinidin, peonidin
    - *isoflavones (phytoestrogens):* genistein, daidzein, glycitein, formononetin, coumestans, lignans
    - *flavanolols:* silibinin, silymarin
  - *tannins:*
    - *condensed tannins (proanthocyanidins):* oligomeric proanthocyanidins (OPCs)
    - *hydrolysable tannins (polymers of gallic and ellagic acid):* tannic acid, ellagitannins
  - *stilbenes:* resveratrol, piceatannol, oxyresveratrol, pinosylvin, rhapontigenin, pterostilbene
  - *coumarins:* simple coumarins, furanocoumarins, pyranocoumarins, pyrone-substituted coumarins
- *organosulfur compounds:* indoles, indole-3-carbinol, allylic sulfur compounds, isothiocyanates, sulforaphane

- *alkaloids:*
  - *methylxanthines:* caffeine, theophylline, theobromine, nicotine
- *phytosterols:* betasitosterol, stigmasterol, campesterol, sitostanol, campestanol (see Chapter 4: Lipids).

About two-thirds of the total dietary intake of phytochemicals is made up of flavonoids, and phenolic acids make up most of the remaining third. The most abundant flavonoids in the diet are flavanols, anthocyanidins and their oxidation products. The main dietary sources are fruit, vegetables and beverages, such as fruit juice, wine, tea, coffee and beer. Total intake is about 1 g per day.

The actions of phytochemicals may include:

- antioxidant protection
- modulation of enzyme activity and biochemical reactions
- regulation of cell receptor activity
- hormonal effects
- enhancement of growth of beneficial bacteria in the colon, inhibition of growth of disease-causing bacteria and binding of toxins.

Absorption of phytochemicals

Absorption of phytochemicals is generally low, and appears to occur by passive diffusion and by various transporters, including solute carrier (SLC) transporters. The body protects itself against phytochemicals by the activity of phase I and phase II detoxification enzymes in enterocytes and the liver, which rapidly break them down to conjugated metabolites that are transferred to the bloodstream and delivered to the kidneys for excretion in urine. Some metabolites formed in the liver are secreted into the gut in bile and are either excreted in faeces or converted by microbial enzymes to simpler forms which may then be reabsorbed.

Overall, the body content of phytochemicals is very small. Phytochemicals such as isoflavones and most of the flavonoids can be absorbed in the small intestine, but larger compounds, such as condensed tannins and some phenolic acids, are poorly absorbed. Some phenolic acids pass into the colon, where they can be fermented by probiotics and then absorbed. Condensed tannins are not fermented and are excreted. Although more research is needed, it has been reported that gallic acid and isoflavones are the best absorbed polyphenols, followed by catechins, flavanones and quercetin glucosides. The least well absorbed appear to be proanthocyanidins (condensed tannins) and anthocyanidins. There is limited data on other phytochemicals. Even if absorbed, many phytochemicals are rapidly broken down in the body.

Some researchers believe that oral intake of many phytochemicals, especially those that are poorly water soluble or are larger and more complex, can have little impact on health. Although studies with cell cultures have shown that phytochemicals have potent health effects, many studies using oral supplementation have been unable to replicate these results. It is possible, however, that even low levels of phytochemicals may affect cell functions, such as cell signalling (the pathways that switch genes on or off to regulate the production of specific proteins in cells). Metabolites of phytochemicals may have health effects singly or synergistically that are not yet well understood. Also, poorly absorbed phytochemicals may have health benefits by protective activity within the digestive tract.

CAROTENOIDS

Carotenoids are fat-soluble orange, yellow and red pigments made by plants, algae and certain bacteria. In green plants, they are present in chloroplasts, and they act like natural sunscreens to help protect plant cells from the damaging effects of intense sunlight. There are several hundred different carotenoids in fruit and vegetables, but their colours may be masked by the presence of the green pigment chlorophyll. Carotenoids are 40-carbon structures that include carotenes and xanthophylls. Carotenes consist of hydrogen and carbon, and include alpha-carotene, beta-carotene, gamma-carotene and lycopene. Xanthophylls, which consist of carbon, hydrogen and oxygen, include lutein, zeaxanthin, beta-cryptoxanthin, canthaxanthin, astaxanthin, fucoxanthin, neoxanthin, violaxanthin alloxanthin, crocoxanthin and monadoxanthin. Metabolites of carotenoids contain fewer than 40 carbons, and are given the prefix 'apo'.

The term 'carotenoids' is derived from carrots (*Daucus carota*), and the term 'xanthophylls' is derived from the Greek words *xanthos* for yellow and *phyllon* for leaf. The main carotenoids that are nutritionally significant are the orange pigments beta-carotene and alpha-carotene, the red pigments lycopene and astaxanthin and the yellow pigments lutein and zeaxanthin. In general, the best carotenoid sources are green, orange and red vegetables and fruit, especially those that are brightly coloured, egg yolk, fish with red or pink flesh, crustaceans and seaweed.

Carotenoid absorption appears to occur via the transporter scavenger receptor class B type 1 (SR-B1), and requires the presence of fat in the intestine. Carotenoid supplements in an oil base appear to be more efficiently absorbed than carotenoids in foods. Dietary fat stimulates the secretion of pancreatic juices and bile, which are necessary for lipid digestion and the formation of mixed micelles, the fat and carotenoid-containing droplets that are absorbed by the intestine. Preserving vegetables in oil increases the bioavailability of carotenoids in food, and chopping, pureeing, juicing or cooking also improves bioavailability by breaking down some of the complex plant structures in which carotenoids are bound. Insufficient production of stomach acid or bile, plant sterols, drugs that reduce cholesterol or fat absorption, the fat substitute olestra and the epilepsy drug valproate may reduce absorption of carotenoids. Absorbed carotenoids are transported from the intestine to the liver in chylomicrons, and from the liver to cells in low-density lipoproteins (LDLs). Excess carotenoids are stored in the liver and adipose tissue, and deposited in the skin.

Beta-carotene, alpha-carotene and beta-cryptoxanthin can be converted to retinol (vitamin A) in the intestinal lining cells after absorption, with beta-carotene having the highest conversion rate, but the conversion is relatively inefficient and reduces if retinol status is high. The main carotenoids in plasma are beta-carotene, alpha-carotene, beta-cryptoxanthin, lutein, zeaxanthin and lycopene. Carotenoids have antioxidant activity in the body, and help detoxification, regulate cell proliferation, differentiation and communication, and protect the skin and eyes from UV light damage. Although carotenoids are antioxidants, they are relatively poorly absorbed, and are present in low concentrations in the body. Therefore, they are likely to play only a minor role in the antioxidant network compared with antioxidant enzymes and nutrients such as vitamins C and E.

Beta-carotene

Beta-carotene is an orange-coloured fat-soluble carotenoid found in fruit and vegetables that was originally isolated from carrots. Absorption from food ranges from 5–65 per cent. Beta-carotene exists in two forms, cis-beta-carotene and all-trans-beta-carotene. Cis forms found in the diet include 9-cis-, 13-cis- and 15-cis-beta-carotene. All-trans-beta-carotene is the main form that is converted into active vitamin A (all-trans-retinoic acid) in the body, and is the predominant form in many vegetables. Beta-carotene is stored in the liver, and also in adipose tissue, the kidneys, skin, lungs, adrenal glands, testes and mammary glands.

Functions

The functions of beta-carotene include:

- *Antioxidant activity.* Beta-carotene is incorporated into the interior of cell membranes, and works with vitamin E as a fat-soluble antioxidant. Carotenoids quench damaging singlet oxygen by absorbing its excess energy and releasing it as heat, thereby returning oxygen and the carotenoid back to their original states. In cell studies, beta-carotene reacts with peroxyl radicals, reducing lipid peroxidation. It scavenges ROS by hydrogen abstraction, electron transfer or by adding them to the unconjugated double bonds in its structure. It appears to work best in tissues where there is a low amount of oxygen, such as the smallest blood vessels in the peripheral areas of the body. Beta-carotene may protect against lipid peroxidation in blood lipids and cell membranes and, in the skin, acts as an antioxidant and blue light filter that helps protect against sun damage.
- *Vitamin A (retinol) formation.* Beta-carotene is the main carotenoid that is converted to retinol in the body, but absorption is inefficient and only a small amount of retinol is made in this way. After absorption, about 17–45 per cent of dietary beta-carotene is released into the blood stream intact, and the remainder is cleaved by enzyme activity in the intestinal lining. The enzyme beta,beta-carotene 15,15'-monooxygenase 1 (BCMO1) splits it in half to form two molecules of all-trans-retinal and the enzyme beta,beta-carotene 9',10'-dioxygenase (BCDO2) also splits it at a different point to form beta-apo-10'-carotenal and beta-ionone, which can ultimately be converted to one molecule of all-trans-retinal. Retinal can then be converted to retinoic acid, the active form of vitamin A. It is estimated that 12–21 mcg of dietary beta-carotene can produce 1 mcg of retinol, and 2 mcg of beta-carotene from an oil-based supplement can produce 1 mcg of retinol.

Retinoic acid binds to the nuclear retinoic acid receptor RAR, and is important for cell signalling and regulation of cell growth and development. The 9-cis form of beta-carotene is converted to 9-cis-retinoic acid in the intestine, which binds to the nuclear retinoid X receptor (RXR), and also controls cell signalling, and cell growth and development. Vitamin A helps maintain healthy eyes, skin, hair, nails and mucous membranes, and helps regulate cell replication, growth and immune responses.

- *Immunity.* Beta-carotene works with vitamin A to boost the immune response by supporting the growth of the thymus gland, increasing lymphocyte production, enhancing the activity of phagocytes, neutrophils and natural killer (NK) cells, and stimulating the production of immune-stimulating cytokines.
- *Cell communication.* Beta-carotene increases expression of the gene for connexin proteins that form pores in cell membranes (gap junctions), allowing cells to communicate through the exchange of small molecules. This type of intercellular communication is important for maintaining cells in a differentiated and functional state.

Dietary sources

Beta-carotene is found in dark-green, orange, yellow and red vegetables, including parsley, carrots, spinach, broccoli, pumpkin, alfalfa, sweet potato, turnip tops and watercress; seaweed and microalgae such as *Dunaliella* spp.; and yellow and orange fruit, including apricot, peach, mango, cantaloupe (rockmelon) and papaya (paw paw). Because it is fat-soluble, beta-carotene is best absorbed when food sources are eaten with about 3–5 g of fat.

The Food Standards Australia New Zealand nutrient database (NUTTAB) at <www.foodstandards.gov.au> provides the amounts found in specific foods.

HEALTH EFFECTS OF BETA-CAROTENE

Dietary beta-carotene is associated with a reduced risk of CVD, and higher serum beta-carotene concentrations are associated with decreased risk of CVD, total mortality and sudden cardiac death.[1,2] However, studies using beta-carotene supplementation have found positive and negative effects on CVD, and supplementation has been linked to an increase in risk of CVD mortality at doses of 20 and 30 mg/day.[3]

Although dietary beta-carotene is associated with protection against cancer, a meta-analysis found that beta-carotene supplements had no preventive effect on either cancer incidence or cancer mortality, and synthetic beta-carotene supplementation at a dose of 20 mg/day or more may increase the risk of lung and gastric cancer in smokers and people with a history of smoking or asbestos exposure.[4] Bowel polyps are associated with increased risk of bowel cancer. Beta-carotene (20 mg/day) was used in the Australian Polyp Prevention Project, and was shown to increase the risk of polyp recurrence in women.[5] However, another study found that beta-carotene had no effect on bowel polyp risk in male smokers.[6]

The reason for the possible cancer-promoting effect is unknown, but beta-carotene metabolism can lead to the formation of the beta-carotene radical that has the potential to act as a pro-oxidant, especially in the absence of other supporting antioxidants. Beta-carotene metabolism also generates carotenoid breakdown products such as highly reactive aldehydes and epoxides that are formed by its antioxidant activity. Vitamin C appears to be particularly important for converting the beta-carotene radical back to beta-carotene and vitamin C is low in people who smoke.

Supplementation with the algae *Dunaliella bardawil*, providing about 20 mg of beta-carotene daily, mainly as 9-cis-beta-carotene, has been found to increase the function of the retina in patients with retinitis pigmentosa, a genetic condition leading to blindness.[7] Beta-carotene (15 mg/day) may help to reduce the risk of age-related macular degeneration when used with vitamin C, vitamin E and zinc.[8]

Beta-carotene supplementation has been found to protect the skin against UV radiation, and to protect against immune suppression induced by UV exposure; however, it does not affect the risk of non-melanoma skin cancer. Supplementation protects against sunburn if used for a minimum of ten weeks.[9] Beta-carotene is used to reduce photosensitivity in patients with erythropoietic protoporphyria at doses up to 300 mg/day,[10] and *Dunaliella bardawil* supplementation in patients with mild, chronic, plaque-type psoriasis has led to improvements in skin lesions.[11] There is some evidence that beta-carotene may help to relieve symptoms of exercise-induced asthma[12] and cystic fibrosis.[13]

REFERENCES

1 Karppi, J., Laukkanen, J.A., Mäkikallio, T.H. et al., Low β-carotene concentrations increase the risk of cardiovascular disease mortality among Finnish men with risk factors, *Nutr Metab Cardiovasc Dis* (2012), 22(10): 921–8.

2 Karppi, J., Laukkanen, J.A., Mäkikallio, T.H. et al., Serum β-carotene and the risk of sudden cardiac death in men: A population-based follow-up study, *Atherosclerosis* (2013), 226(1): 172–7.

3 Mayne, S.T., Beta-carotene, carotenoids, and disease prevention in humans, *FASEB J* (1996), 10(7): 690–701.

4 Druesne-Pecollo, N., Latino-Martel, P., Norat, T. et al., Beta-carotene supplementation and cancer risk: A systematic review and metaanalysis of randomized controlled trials, *Int J Cancer* (2010), 127(1): 172–84.

5 Wahlqvist, M.L., Anti-oxidant relevance to human health, *Asia Pac J Clin Nutr* (2013), 22(2): 171–6.

6 Malila, N., Virtamo, J., Virtanen, M. et al., The effect of alpha-tocopherol and beta-carotene supplementation on colorectal adenomas in middle-aged male smokers, *Cancer Epidemiol Biomarkers Prev* (1999), 8(6): 489–93.

7 Rotenstreich, Y., Belkin, M., Sadetzki, S. et al., Treatment with 9-cis β-carotene-rich powder in patients with retinitis pigmentosa: A randomized crossover trial, *JAMA Ophthalmol* (2013), 131(8): 985–92.

8 Age-Related Eye Disease Study Research Group, A randomized, placebo-controlled, clinical trial of high-dose supplementation with vitamins C and E, beta carotene, and zinc for age-related macular degeneration and vision loss: AREDS report no. 8, *Arch Ophthalmol* (2001), 119(10): 1417–36.

9 Köpcke, W. & Krutmann, J., Protection from sunburn with beta-Carotene: A meta-analysis, *Photochem Photobiol* (2008), 84(2): 284–8.

10 Bayerl, C., Beta-carotene in dermatology: Does it help?, *Acta Dermatovenerol Alp Panonica Adriat* (2008), 17(4): 160–2, 164–6.

11 Greenberger, S., Harats, D., Salameh, F. et al., 9-cis-rich β-carotene powder of the alga Dunaliella reduces the severity of chronic plaque psoriasis: A randomized, double-blind, placebo-controlled clinical trial, *J Am Coll Nutr* (2012), 31(5): 320–6.

12 Neuman, I., Nahum, H. & Ben-Amotz, A., Prevention of exercise-induced asthma by a natural isomer mixture of beta-carotene, *Ann Allergy Asthma Immunol* (1999), 82(6): 549–53.

13 Renner, S., Rath, R., Rust, P. et al., Effects of beta-carotene supplementation for six months on clinical and laboratory parameters in patients with cystic fibrosis, *Thorax* (2001), 56(1): 48–52.

Supplements and dose

In Australia, the permitted forms of beta-carotene in supplements include beta-carotene and the marine microalga *Dunaliella salina,* a rich source of beta-carotene, as well as alpha-carotene, cryptoxanthin, zeaxanthin, lutein and lycopene. Beta-carotene may be derived from red palm oil, produced by the fungus *Blakeslea trispora*, or chemically synthesised by joining two or three smaller molecules to give the required 40-carbon structure. Natural beta-carotene in *Dunaliella salina* consists of about 50 per cent 9-cis-beta-carotene and 50 per cent all-trans-beta-carotene, and the natural beta-carotene in red palm oil contains more all-trans than 9-cis-beta-carotene. Synthetic beta-carotene supplements are 100 per cent all-trans-beta-carotene. Supplementary doses of beta-carotene range from 3-20 mg daily.

Cautions

Beta-carotene has limited conversion to retinol in the body, and does not cause vitamin A toxicity. It is used as a vitamin A supplement for pregnant women; up to 30 mg/day is not associated with adverse effects during pregnancy. However, high intakes (more than 30 mg/day) lead to a buildup of beta-carotene in the blood and skin, which causes a yellow-orange colouring, more noticeable in the palms of the hands, soles of the feet and around the nose and lips (beta-carotenaemia). The whites of the eyes do not turn yellow, which distinguishes beta-carotenaemia from jaundice caused by a liver disorder. The pigmentation is apparently harmless, and disappears two to three months after beta-carotene intake is reduced. Beta-carotenaemia may be associated with diabetes and hypothyroidism.

In general, food sources are preferred. High-dose synthetic beta-carotene supplements (20 mg or more) are not recommended for smokers and people with a history of smoking or asbestos exposure, because of a link to increased risk of cancer. Doses of 20 or 30 mg/day may increase risk of CVD mortality. No health issues have been linked to natural beta-carotene supplements at doses lower than 20 mg/day.

Lycopene

Lycopene is a red-coloured, fat-soluble carotenoid found in some varieties of red and pink fruits and vegetables, especially red tomatoes. Absorption from food ranges from 10 to 30 per cent. It exists in nature mainly as all-trans-lycopene, which is converted to cis-lycopene during cooking and processing. Cis forms are better absorbed, and include 5-cis-, 9-cis-, 13-cis- and 15-cis-lycopene. Dietary lycopene has no vitamin A activity, and is broken down by the enzyme BCO2 in the intestinal wall to apo-10'-lycopenoids or transferred intact to the bloodstream. About 50 per cent of the lycopene content of plasma is all-trans-lycopene and about 50 per cent is cis-lycopene. Lycopene is stored in the liver and also in adipose tissue, the adrenal glands, kidneys, lungs, ovaries, prostate gland and mammary glands. It has similar functions to beta-carotene in the body, but appears to have more potent antioxidant and anticancer activity.

Functions

The functions of lycopene include:

- *Antioxidant activity.* Cis-lycopene is the major antioxidant form of lycopene, and has double the antioxidant activity of beta-carotene because it contains more unconjugated double bonds that can interact with radicals. However, lycopene is more susceptible to oxidation than beta-carotene and may be used up more quickly. Lycopene quenches singlet oxygen and scavenges ROS and peroxyl radicals and, like beta-carotene, appears to work best in tissues where there is a low amount of oxygen. However, there are low concentrations in body tissues relative to other antioxidants like vitamin E, and some researchers believe that lycopene acts by altering gene expression rather than by direct antioxidant action. Oral and topical lycopene protect the skin against inflammation and damage after exposure to UV light.
- *Anti-inflammatory activity.* Lycopene has an inhibiting effect on key pro-inflammatory mediators, such as ROS, pro-inflammatory cytokines, signal transduction pathways and the enzymes cyclooxygenase (COX) and lipoxygenase (LOX), which produce inflammatory eicosanoids. It has been found to induce apoptosis in activated immune cells.
- *Detoxification.* Lycopene induces expression of phase II detoxification pathways that remove potentially harmful metabolites and xenobiotics (foreign and unwanted substances).
- *Anticancer activity.* Lycopene protects DNA from damage, and has been found to reduce cell proliferation, enhance differentiation, halt cell cycle progression and induce apoptosis in abnormal cells. It enhances gap junction inter-cell communication, and reduces production of insulin-like growth factor 1 (IGF-1), a promoter of tumour growth. Lycopene metabolites have been found to activate retinoid-mediated signalling and nuclear receptors, which may help promote normal cell growth and development. Lycopene reduces expression of the enzyme 5-alpha reductase that converts testosterone to the more active androgen dihydrotestosterone (DHT), which promotes cell growth in prostate tumour tissue. Lycopene also impairs oestrogen signalling and oestrogen-induced cell proliferation in the breast and endometrium but does not impair the beneficial effects of oestrogen on bone.
- *Cholesterol metabolism.* Lycopene has been found to inhibit activity of the enzyme HMG-CoA reductase that takes part in cholesterol synthesis in the body and reduces oxidation of LDL cholesterol.

Dietary sources

Lycopene is found in tomatoes, tomato-based products, pink grapefruit, papaya, watermelon and guava. Tomatoes cooked or processed in oil, such as tomato-based pasta sauces and sun-dried tomatoes in oil, are a particularly rich and well-absorbed source. The edible red berries of autumn olive (*Elaeagnus umbellata*) are an extremely rich source of lycopene, containing 15–54 mg per 100 g fresh fruit compared with about 3 mg/100 g in raw tomatoes. As lycopene is fat-soluble, it is best absorbed when taken with food containing some fat.

The Food Standards Australia New Zealand nutrient database (NUTTAB) at <www.foodstandards.gov.au> provides the amounts found in specific foods.

HEALTH EFFECTS OF LYCOPENE

A higher lycopene intake and plasma levels are associated with lower risk of prostate, breast, gastrointestinal, cervical, ovarian, pancreatic and liver cancer.[1] More than two servings of tomato products per week have been associated with a 23 per cent lower risk of prostate cancer compared with people eating less than one serve a month.[2] Prostate cancer patients eating tomato sauce providing 30 mg of lycopene/day for three weeks had a 20 per cent reduction in prostate-specific antigen (PSA) levels and reduced markers of oxidative stress.[3] Another study found that tomato products led to a 34 per cent decrease in PSA in prostate cancer patients.[4] A higher lycopene intake has also been associated with a lower risk of benign prostatic hyperplasia.[5] However, not all studies have shown benefits for cancer risk.

A higher intake of lycopene and higher plasma levels have been associated with a reduced risk of CVD, myocardial infarction (MI, heart attack) and markers of atherosclerosis.[6,7] Intake of tomato products or extract has led to reduced oxidation of serum lipids and LDL cholesterol, reduced serum LDL cholesterol and triglycerides, increased serum HDL cholesterol and reduced markers of inflammation in artery walls.[8] A meta-analysis of four clinical trials found that lycopene supplementation reduces systolic blood pressure in people with hypertension.[9] Lycopene has been reported to improve sperm count, quality and motility in infertile men.[10] Other disorders in which lycopene may be protective include sunburn protection, gingivitis (gum inflammation), asthma, emphysema and bone fractures in the elderly.[1]

REFERENCES

1 Story, E.N., Kopec, R.E., Schwartz, S.J. & Harris, G.K., An update on the health effects of tomato lycopene, *Annu Rev Food Sci Technol* (2010), 1: 189–210.

2 Giovannucci, E., Rimm, E.B., Liu, Y. et al., A prospective study of tomato products, lycopene, and prostate cancer risk, *J Natl Cancer Inst* (2002), 94(5): 391–8.

3 Bowen, P., Chen, L., Stacewicz-Sapuntzakis, M. et al., Tomato sauce supplementation and prostate cancer: Lycopene accumulation and modulation of biomarkers of carcinogenesis, *Exp Biol Med (Maywood)* (2002), 227(10): 886–93.

4 Kucuk, O., Sarkar, F.H., Sakr, W. et al., Phase II randomized clinical trial of lycopene supplementation before radical prostatectomy, *Cancer Epidemiol Biomarkers Prev* (2001), 10(8): 861–8.

5 Schwarz, S., Obermüller-Jevic, U.C., Hellmis, E. et al., Lycopene inhibits disease progression in patients with benign prostate hyperplasia, *J Nutr* (2008), 138(1): 49–53.

6 Jacques, P.F., Lyass, A., Massaro, J.M. et al., Relationship of lycopene intake and consumption of tomato products to incident CVD, *Br J Nutr* (2013), 110(3): 545–51.

7 Kohlmeier, L., Kark, J.D., Gomez-Garcia, E. et al., Lycopene and myocardial infarction risk in the EURAMIC Study, *Am J Epidemiol* (1997), 146(8): 618–26.

8 Riccioni, G., Mancini, B., Di Ilio, E. et al., Protective effect of lycopene in cardiovascular disease, *Eur Rev Med Pharmacol Sci* (2008), 12(3): 183–90.

9 Ried, K. & Fakler, P., Protective effect of lycopene on serum cholesterol and blood pressure: Meta-analyses of intervention trials, *Maturitas* (2011), 68(4): 299–310.

10 Gupta, N.P. & Kumar, R., Lycopene therapy in idiopathic male infertility: A preliminary report, *Int Urol Nephrol* (2002), 34(3): 369–72.

Supplements and dose

In Australia, the permitted form in supplements is lycopene. Natural lycopene may be derived from oleoresin from waste tomato products, such as skins, seeds and pulp, by solvent extraction or by high-pressure processing. Synthetic lycopene consists of about 70 per cent all-trans-lycopene, up to 23 per cent 5-cis-lycopene and small amounts of other cis isomers, and is produced from intermediates that are also used in the production of other carotenoids. Supplementary doses of lycopene range from 6–60 mg daily.

Cautions

No adverse effects have been observed for dietary or synthetic lycopene at intakes up to 3 g/kg body weight/day. Rarely, a long-term high intake of lycopene foods may lead to lycopenaemia, which is characterised by a harmless orange discolouration of the skin that disappears when lycopene intake is reduced. In general, food sources are preferred because most studies using food sources have shown positive health effects.

Lutein and zeaxanthin

Lutein and zeaxanthin are fat-soluble, yellow-orange carotenoids that are powerful antioxidants and blue light filters concentrated in the retina and lens of the eyes. They make up the macular pigments situated in the macula lutea (yellow spot), located in the central posterior portion of the retina. The macula has the highest concentration of photoreceptors in the eyes, and is responsible for central vision and visual acuity (sharpness). Lutein and zeaxanthin are the dominant carotenoids found in the brain, making up about 70 per cent of the total carotenoid concentration. They may help to protect against age-related macular degeneration, cataracts, abnormal cell replication and CVD. They do not convert to retinol in the body.

Lutein is found in food as all-trans-lutein in the free form and also esterified to fatty acids. The fatty acids are removed during digestion, and the free form is absorbed via SR-B1 and transported in the bloodstream in HDLs and LDLs. Beta-carotene and lutein use the same transport mechanisms, and may compete with each other for absorption. Lutein accumulates mainly in the eyes, and is also found in adipose tissue, mammary glands and the cervix. Uptake into the retina appears to be mediated by SR-B1.

Functions

Functions of lutein include:

- *Vision.* The macular pigments of the retina are lutein, zeaxanthin and meso-zeaxanthin, a metabolite of lutein. The highest concentration of macular pigment is near the fovea, the central-most part of the retina, that enables sharp central vision. Zeaxanthin is most concentrated in the central part of the fovea and lutein is found at the periphery of the macula. Lutein and zeaxanthin act as blue light filters to protect underlying retinal structures, such as photoreceptors, from light-induced damage.
- *Antioxidant activity.* Lutein and zeaxanthin quench singlet oxygen and scavenge ROS and peroxyl radicals. They protect DNA and the polyunsaturated fatty acid docosahexaenoic acid (DHA), which is found in high levels in the retina and brain, from oxidative damage. By scavenging ROS, lutein and zeaxanthin help suppress production of inflammatory chemicals and reduce cell apoptosis induced by oxidative stress.
- *Immunity.* Lutein and zeaxanthin appear to play a role in cellular and humoral immunity, possibly by regulating ROS levels. Lutein inhibits production of the inflammatory mediator NF-kappaB, and inhibits activity of the enzymes phospholipase A_2 and COX-2, which promote production of inflammatory eicosanoids.
- *Brain function.* Lutein and zeaxanthin affect brain function by improving cell-to-cell communication through gap junctions, modulating microtubule function in neurons and preventing breakdown of the proteins in synaptic vesicles that assist transmission of nerve impulses between nerve cells.

Dietary sources

Lutein and zeaxanthin are found in green vegetables such as broccoli, Brussels sprouts, kale, green beans and spinach; yellow-orange fruits such as apricot, peach, cantaloupe, honeydew melon, mango, tangerine, mandarin, orange and persimmon; yellow-orange vegetables such as squash, and red and yellow capsicum; and yellow corn, paprika and egg yolk. Lutein is present in the better-absorbed free form in egg yolks and green leafy vegetables, and as fatty acid esters in fruit and yellow corn. Free-range hens provide eggs with a higher amount of lutein. As lutein and zeaxanthin are fat soluble, they are best absorbed when taken with food containing some fat.

The Food Standards Australia New Zealand nutrient database (NUTTAB) at <www.foodstandards.gov.au> provides the amounts of lutein found in specific foods.

HEALTH EFFECTS OF LUTEIN AND ZEAXANTHIN

Lutein and zeaxanthin may be protective against eye disorders, such as sensitivity to glare, diabetic retinopathy, cataracts and age-related macular degeneration (ARMD), a major cause of central vision loss and blindness in the elderly. A dietary intake of 6–20 mg/day of lutein has been associated with a reduced risk of cataracts and ARMD.[1] Higher serum lutein and dietary lutein are correlated with improved macular pigment density (MPD). In ARMD patients, lutein supplementation was found to increase MPD, but had no effect on macular function or visual acuity.[1] Lutein (20 mg/day), and also lutein (10 mg/day) together with zeaxanthin (10 mg/day), has increased MPD and improved indicators of visual function in ARMD patients.[1] In the Australian Blue Mountains Eye Study, a higher intake of dietary lutein and zeaxanthin was found to reduce the risk of long-term incident ARMD.[2] However, in the Age-Related Eye Disease Study 2 (AREDS2), supplementation with 10 mg of lutein and 2 mg of zeaxanthin daily in addition to the standard AREDS formula of antioxidants and zinc did not provide further protection against ARMD than that provided by the original AREDS formula.[3] A meta-analysis of six studies found that dietary lutein and zeaxanthin was not associated with a reduced risk of early ARMD, but may be protective against late ARMD.[4] Neither the original AREDS formula nor the AREDS2 formula were shown to protect against cataracts, but a meta-analysis of six prospective studies found that dietary lutein and zeaxanthin were associated with a reduced risk of age-related nuclear cataract.[5] People with higher dietary or serum levels of lutein and zeaxanthin were found to have a 25 per cent lower risk of developing nuclear cataracts compared with people with the lowest levels, but no relationship was detected with other types of cataracts.

Topical and oral lutein (10 mg/day) and zeaxanthin (0.6 mg/day) has been found to improve skin hydration, elasticity and surface lipids, and protect against lipid peroxidation.[6] In patients with early atherosclerosis, lutein supplementation (20 mg/day) for three months decreased serum levels of LDL cholesterol, triglycerides and inflammatory markers.[7] Lutein may improve brain function in older adults. A study of centenarians found that zeaxanthin concentrations in the brain post-mortem were associated with measures of global cognitive function, memory retention, verbal fluency and dementia severity, and brain lutein levels have been found to be lower in people with mild cognitive impairment.[8] A study of older women found that lutein supplementation (12 mg/day), alone or together with DHA, improved verbal fluency scores, memory scores and learning ability.[8]

REFERENCES

1 Koushan, K., Rusovici, R., Li, W. et al., The role of lutein in eye-related disease, *Nutrients* (2013), 5(5): 1823–39.

2 Tan, J.S., Wang, J.J., Flood, V. et al., Dietary anti-oxidants and the long-term incidence of age-related macular degeneration: The Blue Mountains Eye Study, *Ophthalmology* (2008), 115(2): 334–41.

3 Age-Related Eye Disease Study 2 (AREDS2) Research Group, Lutein/zeaxanthin for the treatment of age-related cataract: AREDS2 randomized trial report no. 4, *JAMA Ophthalmol* (2013), 131(7): 843–50.

4 Ma, L., Dou, H.L., Wu, Y.Q. et al., Lutein and zeaxanthin intake and the risk of age-related macular degeneration: A systematic review and meta-analysis, *Br J Nutr* (2012), 107(3): 350–9.

5 Ma, L., Hao, Z.X., Liu, R.R. et al., A dose-response meta-analysis of dietary lutein and zeaxanthin intake in relation to risk of age-related cataract, *Graefes Arch Clin Exp Ophthalmol* (2013), 252(1): 6–70.

6 Palombo, P., Fabrizi, G., Ruocco, V. et al., Beneficial long-term effects of combined oral/topical anti-oxidant treatment with the carotenoids lutein and zeaxanthin on human skin: A double-blind, placebo-controlled study, *Skin Pharmacol Physiol* (2007), 20(4): 199–210.

7 Xu, X.R., Zou, Z.Y., Xiao, X. et al., Effects of lutein supplement on serum inflammatory cytokines, ApoE and lipid profiles in early atherosclerosis population, *J Atheroscler Thromb* (2013), 20(2): 170–7.

8 Johnson, E.J., A possible role for lutein and zeaxanthin in cognitive function in the elderly, *Am J Clin Nutr* (2012), 96(5): 1161S–5S.

Supplements and dose

In Australia, the permitted forms in supplements are lutein and zeaxanthin. Lutein and zeaxanthin can be produced synthetically or by extraction from marigold (*Tagetes erecta*) flower oleoresin. Vitamin C appears to enhance lutein absorption from supplements. The supplementary dose of lutein is 6–20 mg daily, and the zeaxanthin dose is 2–5 mg daily.

Cautions

Lutein has been used in doses up to 40 mg/day for two months and 25 mg/day for longer periods with no adverse effects. Carotenaemia from lutein and zeaxanthin is rare. It has been reported in some healthy subjects taking lutein in the form of mixed esters extracted from marigold flowers at a dose of 15 mg/day for four months, but has not been reported in patients with eye diseases taking about 25 mg/day of lutein for more than one year.

Astaxanthin

Astaxanthin is a red carotenoid made by bacteria, algae and fungi. It contains a hydroxyl group and a keto group on each end that gives it polar and non-polar properties. It is incorporated into cell membranes, where it aligns with structural phospholipids. Free astaxanthin is susceptible to oxidation, and it is found in foods bound to proteins or fatty acids as trans-astaxanthin. The proteins and fatty acids are removed during digestion and the free form is absorbed, possibly via SR-B1. It is transported in the bloodstream as free astaxanthin in LDLs and HDLs. Astaxanthin is better absorbed if taken with meals, and is about 40 per cent less bioavailable in smokers.

Functions

Functions of astaxanthin include:

- *Antioxidant activity*. Astaxanthin has two more oxygenated groups on each ring structure than the other carotenoids, which makes it a powerful antioxidant. It stabilises cell membranes and acts as an antioxidant on the surface and in the interior of the membrane, in contrast to other carotenoids that work mainly in the membrane interior. Astaxanthin quenches singlet oxygen and scavenges ROS and peroxyl and hydroxyl radicals, and is a more effective antioxidant than beta-carotene and alpha-tocopherol (vitamin E). As a quencher of singlet oxygen, it is eleven times more potent than beta-carotene and 550 times more potent than alpha-tocopherol. It protects against lipid peroxidation, protects the skin from photo-oxidation and increases activity of nuclear factor erythroid 2-related factor 2 (Nrf2), a gene transcription factor that regulates expression of antioxidant enzymes and proteins that control cell cycle and cell death.
- *Anti-inflammatory activity*. Astaxanthin inhibits the NF-kappaB pathway that stimulates production of inflammatory chemicals and enzymes.
- *Immunity*. Astaxanthin boosts lymphocyte proliferation and T and B cell numbers and increases NK cell activity.

Dietary sources

Astaxanthin is found in microalgae, especially the chlorophyte alga *Haematococcus pluvialis*, yeast, salmon, ocean trout, fish roe and crustaceans, including krill, shrimp, crayfish, lobster, crab and prawns.

HEALTH EFFECTS OF ASTAXANTHIN

Astaxanthin has shown anticancer activity in cell and animal studies,[1] and has improved markers of CVD, such as lipid peroxidation, inflammation, blood lipids, clotting and blood pressure, in animal studies.[2] In animals with atherosclerosis and elevated blood lipids, it has decreased infiltration of the atherosclerotic plaque by macrophages and improved plaque stability. Small human studies have found that astaxanthin decreases oxidation of fatty acids and LDL cholesterol, reduces serum triglycerides and increases serum HDL cholesterol.[2] It also increases levels of adiponectin, a protein that improves insulin function.[2] In animals fed a high-fat and high-fructose diet, astaxanthin has reduced insulin levels and improved insulin resistance.[3]

A preliminary study has suggested that astaxanthin may improve brain functions, such as cognition, attention, memory and information processing, in older people.[4] In patients with functional dyspepsia, 40 mg/day of astaxanthin reduced gastro-oesophageal reflux symptoms, but did not improve dyspepsia symptoms,[5] and cyclists receiving 4 mg/day of astaxanthin are reported to have improved performance on a time trial.[6] Astaxanthin has improved blood flow in the retina of the eyes in healthy people,[7] and has improved eye fatigue in a study of people working at visual display units.[8]

Astaxanthin is reported to have improved sperm velocity in infertile men and the pregnancy rate of their partners.[9] In men and women, astaxanthin supplementation has improved skin quality by reducing the appearance of wrinkles and age spots, and improving skin elasticity, texture and hydration.[10] A cell study found that astaxanthin inhibited the enzyme 5-alpha reductase that enhances prostate gland growth, reduced growth of prostate cancer cells and had an additive effect when used with the herb saw palmetto (*Serenoa repens*).[11]

REFERENCES

1 Guerin, M., Huntley, M.E. & Olaizola M., Haematococcus astaxanthin: applications for human health and nutrition, *TRENDS in Biotech* (2003), 21(5): 210–16.

2 Fassett, R.G. & Coombes, J.S., Astaxanthin in cardiovascular health and disease, *Molecules* (2012), 17(2): 2030–48.

3 Arunkumar, E., Bhuvaneswari, S. & Anuradha, C.V., An intervention study in obese mice with astaxanthin, a marine carotenoid—effects on insulin signaling and pro-inflammatory cytokines, *Food Funct* (2012), 3(2): 120–6.

4 Katagiri, M., Satoh, A., Tsuji, S. & Shirasawa, T., Effects of astaxanthin-rich Haematococcus pluvialis extract on cognitive function: A randomised, double-blind, placebo-controlled study, *J Clin Biochem Nutr* (2012), 51(2): 102–7.

5 Kupcinskas, L., Lafolie, P., Lignell, A. et al., Efficacy of the natural anti-oxidant astaxanthin in the treatment of functional dyspepsia in patients with or without *Helicobacter pylori* infection: A prospective, randomized, double blind, and placebo-controlled study, *Phytomedicine* (2008), 15(6–7): 391–9.

6 Earnest, C.P., Lupo, M., White, K.M. & Church, T.S., Effect of astaxanthin on cycling time trial performance, *Int J Sports Med* (2011), 32(11): 882–8.

7 Saito, M., Yoshida, K., Saito, W. et al., Astaxanthin increases choroidal blood flow velocity, *Graefes Arch Clin Exp Ophthalmol* (2012), 250(2): 239–45.

8 Takahashi, N. & Kajita, M., Effects of astaxanthin on accommodative recovery, *J Clin Ther & Med* (2005), 21(4): 431–6.

9 Schill, W.B., Schuppe, H.C., Weid, W. & Manning, M., Proceedings of the 7th Andrology Symposium: Treatment of male infertility—viewpoints, controversies, perspectives, *Andrologia* (2002), 34(5): 325–47.

10 Tominaga, K., Hongo, N., Karato, M. & Yamashita, E., Cosmetic benefits of astaxanthin on human subjects, *Acta Biochim Pol* (2012), 59(1): 43–7.

11 Anderson, M.L., A preliminary investigation of the enzymatic inhibition of 5alpha-reduction and growth of prostatic carcinoma cell line LNCap-FGC by natural astaxanthin and Saw Palmetto lipid extract in vitro, *J Herb Pharmacother* (2005), 5(1): 17–26.

Supplements and dose

Astaxanthin can be made by chemical synthesis from intermediates or other xanthophylls, or can be derived from natural sources, which include the green algae *Haematococcus pluvialis*, the red yeast *Xanthophyllomyces dendrorhous* (*Phaffia rhodozyma*) and crustacean by-products. *H. pluvialis* has the highest capacity to accumulate astaxanthin, and is the only form permitted in Australian supplements. The supplementary dose of astaxanthin is 6–12 mg daily.

Cautions

Animal studies using the human equivalent of 120 mg/day of astaxanthin have not shown adverse effects, and supplementation of 6 mg/day for eight weeks in a human trial was reported to have no adverse effects.

POLYPHENOLICS

Phenolic acids: Curcumin

Curcumin is a bright-yellow pigment found in the spice turmeric, which is derived from the rhizome of *Curcuma longa*, a plant related to ginger and commonly used in curry powder. The main bioactive in turmeric is curcumin, with smaller amounts of demethoxycurcumin (DMC), bisdemethoxycurcumin (BDMC) and cyclocurcumin, collectively known as curcuminoids. Curcuminoids are insoluble and not well absorbed, and the portion that is absorbed is rapidly broken down and eliminated in faeces via bile. Very little is excreted in urine. Absorption in humans is increased by 2000 per cent when curcumin is given with piperine, an alkaloid found in black pepper (*Piper nigrum*). Piperine reduces the breakdown of xenobiotics, including curcuminoids, by inhibiting the enzyme cytochrome P450 3A4 (CYP3A4), and also increases absorption of xenobiotics by inhibiting multi-drug resistance protein 1 (MDR1). More bioavailable forms of curcumin include curcumin combined with phospholipids or fatty acids, and metal-chelated, nanoparticle and bioconjugated formulations. Taking curcumin in the form of turmeric appears to improve the bioavailability of curcumin, possibly by the presence of curdione in essential oils in *Curcuma* spp. that acts to inhibit CYP3A4.

Metabolites of curcumin include tetrahydrocurcumin (THC), hexahydrocurcumin (HHC), octahydrocurcumin (OHC), curcumin glucuronide and curcumin sulfate. Some animal studies have shown that THC has greater anti-diabetic and antioxidant activity than curcumin, and others have shown that THC has much lower anti-inflammatory and anti-proliferative activity than curcumin. However, animal and human studies have found that oral doses of curcumin have beneficial effects on multiple pathways implicated in disease and cancer.

Functions

The functions of curcumin include:

- *Antioxidant activity.* Curcumin is a potent antioxidant that inhibits generation of ROS, and scavenges superoxide and hydroxyl radicals. THC has greater antioxidant potential than curcumin. Curcumin can also act as a pro-oxidant and generate ROS under certain conditions, which may contribute to its anticancer activity.
- *Anti-inflammatory activity.* Curcumin inhibits expression of the inflammatory transcription factor NF-kappaB. It inhibits numerous inflammatory pathways, including those involving TNF-alpha, interleukins, adhesion molecules and the enzymes COX-1 and COX-2, which produce inflammatory eicosanoids.
- *Anticancer activity.* Curcumin has been shown to have potent anticancer activity in animals, and can inhibit almost every stage of cancer development, including transformation, initiation, promotion, invasion, angiogenesis and metastasis. It interacts with genes to influence cell metabolism, growth and survival. It regulates cell-signalling pathways, inhibits inflammation, oxidation and expression of oncogenes (cancer-promoting genes), growth factors and cancer-promoting enzymes, regulates the cell cycle and enhances apoptosis of abnormal cells.
- *Immunity.* Curcumin can activate macrophages and NK cells, and modulate lymphocyte-mediated immune functions. It inhibits cell proliferation and induces apoptosis in viruses, bacteria and fungi.
- *Detoxification.* Curcumin has been found to inhibit the enzyme cytochrome P450 that produces potentially harmful chemicals in the liver during phase I detoxification and also increases the activity of phase II enzymes, such as glutathione S-transferases (GSTs), which help to convert xenobiotics into water-soluble forms for excretion in urine. Curcumin has also been found to inhibit GSTs in tumour tissue, in which over-expression of GSTs is associated with multi-drug resistance.

Dietary sources

Curcumin is found in turmeric rhizome and powder, curry powder and ginger. Turmeric contains about 2–9 per cent curcumin. It is present in some processed foods as the food colouring turmeric yellow (number 100).

Supplements, uses and dose

In Australian supplements, curcumin is available as turmeric extract (*Curcuma longa*), extracts of *Curcuma aromatica*, *Curcuma xanthorrhiza* or *Curcuma zedoaria*, or as curcumin. Curcumin is obtained by solvent extraction from the ground rhizomes of *Curcuma longa*. It is potentially useful for cancer prevention and treatment, chronic inflammatory diseases, inflammatory bowel disease, irritable bowel syndrome, arthritis, uveitis (inflammation of the middle layer of the eye), gastrointestinal ulcers, gastritis, idiopathic orbital inflammatory pseudotumour (eye inflammation), psoriasis, Alzheimer's disease, CVD, diabetes, diabetic complications, lupus nephritis (an auto-immune kidney disease), preventing rejection of kidney transplants, gall bladder disorders, liver damage and chronic bacterial prostatitis.[1] The supplementary dose is 1–3 g of curcumin daily, or up to 15 g of turmeric powder.

REFERENCE

1 Gupta, S.C., Patchva, S. & Aggarwal, B.B., Therapeutic roles of curcumin: Lessons learned from clinical trials, *AAPS J* (2013), 15(1): 195–218.

Cautions

Curcumin is generally well tolerated. In patients with an increased risk of cancer, 8 g/day of curcumin for three months was not associated with adverse effects. Curcumin was associated with diarrhoea, rash and yellow faeces in a small number of healthy people given 500–12 000 mg/day, but the effects were not dose-related.

FLAVONOIDS

Flavonoids, also called bioflavonoids, are a sub-class of polyphenol phytochemicals with a similar chemical structure, which features two or more aromatic rings containing at least one aromatic hydroxyl and connected by a carbon bridge. They are found as pigments in fruit, vegetables, nuts, seeds, herbs, spices, cocoa, tea and red wine. The flavonols quercetin, kaempferol, myricetin and isorhamnetin are white or yellow pigments that are the most common flavonoids in plant food. The first flavonoid was discovered in the 1930s in oranges, and was thought to be a new class of vitamin, called vitamin P. However, it was subsequently found to be the flavonoid rutin, which is not a vitamin. Over 4000 flavonoids have now been discovered.

Flavonoids have antioxidant activity, but there are only low concentrations in the body, and it seems that they play a minor role in the antioxidant network. The health benefits of flavonoids are now believed to be mainly related to their ability to affect cell-signalling pathways, and they appear to have biological activity even at low concentrations.

Functions

Functions of flavonoids include:

- *Antioxidant activity*. Flavonoids scavenge superoxide, hydroxyl, peroxyl and peroxynitrite radicals, in the process becoming relatively stable flavonoid radicals. They appear to act as chain-breaking antioxidants in a similar manner to vitamin E, and have vitamin E-sparing activity. Flavonoids also reduce the activity of enzymes that produce free radicals, and bind metals that help to generate them. They protect lipids and LDLs from oxidation damage. Quercetin is one of the most potent flavonoid antioxidants, and is able to chelate and stabilise iron to prevent iron-induced oxidation.
- *Regulation of cell function and anticancer activity*. Flavonoids and metabolites of flavonoids selectively inhibit kinase enzymes, which are cell-signalling proteins involved in regulating gene transcription and stimulating cell growth. Flavonoids help to regulate the cycle of cell division, and may induce apoptosis in cells with irreparably damaged DNA. They inhibit angiogenesis, reduce activity of mutated forms of p53 protein that are over-active in cancer tissue, reduce expression of heat shock proteins that work with mutated p53 to stimulate tumour growth, and reduce expression of Ras

proteins that act as oncogenes (cancer-promoting genes). Some flavonoids can bind oestrogen receptors, reducing the growth of some hormone-dependent cancers.

- *Anti-inflammatory activity.* Flavonoids inhibit the enzymes phospholipase A_2, COX and LOX that produce inflammatory eicosanoids from fatty acids in cell membranes. Some flavonoids—especially flavones—prevent activation of the genes that make inflammatory enzymes. In cell cultures, flavonoids inhibit production of inflammatory chemicals such as eicosanoids, cytokines, chemokines, adhesion molecules and C-reactive protein, and inhibit inflammatory transcription factors such as NF-kappaB.
- *Detoxification.* Flavonoids help activate phase II enzymes in the detoxification pathways that break down xenobiotics and cancer-causing agents.
- *Circulation.* Flavonoids, especially hesperidin, rutin and quercetin, strengthen the walls of blood vessels and reduce permeability (leakiness), which helps to prevent fluid buildup in tissues (oedema). Flavonoids help reduce oxidation damage to LDL cholesterol, inhibit abnormal blood clotting and dilate blood vessels to improve blood flow. They may help lower LDL cholesterol, increase HDL cholesterol and regulate blood pressure.
- *Immunity.* Flavonoids have antiviral, antibacterial and antifungal activity, and can help to boost immune defence. They may also be able to inactivate some bacterial toxins.
- *Modulation of oestrogen metabolism.* Isoflavones are flavonoids with a similar structure to female hormones. The main dietary isoflavones are daidzein and genistein. They can have oestrogenic activity at low levels and anti-oestrogenic activity at higher levels, and it is believed that they reduce oestrogen activity in premenopausal women and act as a substitute for oestrogen after menopause. Benefits appear to be greater in the 30–50 per cent of women who have gut bacteria that can metabolise daidzein to equol, which is more oestrogenic.

Dietary sources

In general, flavonoids are found in fruit and vegetables, including berries, spices, beans, onions, broccoli, spinach, parsley, celery, cherries, apples, grapes, pears and citrus fruit, as well as coffee, cocoa, chocolate, red wine and all types of tea, including green (unfermented), white (unfermented), oolong (partially unfermented) and black (fermented) tea.

Specific sources of some types of flavonoids are:

- *flavonols:* fruit, vegetables, onions, tea, and red wine
- *flavan-3-ol catechins:* green, white (unfermented) and oolong tea, berries, grapes, apples and chocolate
- *flavan-3-ol oxidised catechins:* black tea
- *flavanones*: citrus fruit
- *anthocyanidins:* red and purple fruit and vegetables, including bilberries, blueberries, blackberries, black and red currants, purple grapes, cherries, figs, olives and eggplant
- *isoflavones:* soybeans, chick peas and the herb red clover. The isoflavone content of soy products, such as soy milk and tofu, is reduced if alcohol-based processing methods are used.
- *flavanolols:* the herb milk thistle (*Silybum marianum*).

Supplements, uses and dose

- *Quercetin* is the form permitted in Australian supplements. It can be extracted from the bark of the oak tree *Quercus velutina* or the leaves of *Rhododendron cinnabarinum* Hook, *Ericaceae* or can be produced by chemical synthesis. It is potentially useful for inflammatory diseases, infections, allergies, asthma, anxiety, depression, diabetes, gastrointestinal ulcers, gastro-oesophageal reflux, high blood pressure, metabolic syndrome and the prevention of cancer, cataracts and CVD.[1,2] The supplementary dose is 150–1000 mg daily.
- *Citrus flavonoids* are available as hesperidin and rutin in Australian supplements. Hesperidin can be extracted from citrus fruit rind, and rutin can be extracted from the leaves of *Eucalyptus macrorhyncha*, buckwheat, rue, tobacco plants or forsythia. They are potentially useful for CVD and circulatory disorders, including varicose veins, haemorrhoids, poor circulation, bleeding, bruising, wound healing and fluid retention, and as a mild blood thinner.[3] The supplementary dose is 500–1000 mg daily.
- *Green tea catechins and epigallocatechin-3-0-gallate* (EGCG) are available in Australian supplements as extracts of green tea (*Camellia sinensis*) or the herb gambir (*Uncaria gambir*). They are potentially useful for diseases of ageing, prevention of CVD, diabetes, weight control, maintenance of healthy bones, cognitive function, circulation, immune defence and cancer prevention.[4] The supplementary dose is 200–800 mg daily.

- *Isoflavones* are available in Australian supplements as soy extracts or extracts of the herbs kudzu root (*Pueraria lobata*) or red clover (*Trifolium pratense*). They are potentially useful for menopausal symptoms, hot flushes, low bone mineral density, cognitive function, diabetic complications and prevention of CVD and cancer.[5] The supplementary dose is about 60 mg daily.

REFERENCES

1 Kelly, G.S., Quercetin monograph, *Altern Med Rev* (2011), 16(2): 172–94.
2 Lamson, D.W. & Brignall, M.S., Anti-oxidants and cancer III: Quercetin, *Altern Med Rev* (2000), 5(3): 196–208.
3 Benavente-García, O. & Castillo, J., Update on uses and properties of citrus flavonoids: New findings in anticancer, cardiovascular, and anti-inflammatory activity, *J Agric Food Chem* (2008), 56(15): 6185–205.
4 Zaveri, N.T., Green tea and its polyphenolic catechins: Medicinal uses in cancer and noncancer applications, *Life Sci* (2006), 78(18): 2073–80.
5 Wang, Q., Ge, X., Tian, X. et al., Soy isoflavone: The multipurpose phytochemical (review), *Biomedical Reports* (2013), 1: 697–701.

Cautions

Dietary flavonoids are generally well tolerated. However, they can affect transport pathways for prescription medication and the activity of enzymes that break down drugs. In particular, furanocoumarins and flavonoids in grapefruit juice inhibit expression of the detoxifying enzyme CYP3A4 in the intestinal wall, which increases the dose delivered to the body and potentially increases the risk of toxicity. People on prescription medication should seek medical advice before drinking grapefruit juice.

Green tea extracts have been associated with acute hepatitis in a small number of people. Quercetin has mutagenic potential, but most animal studies have not found an association with increased cancer risk. A single dose of 4 g of quercitin in humans and 500 mg taken twice daily for one month have not been associated with adverse effects. Isoflavone supplements are not recommended for pregnant women or women with oestrogen-sensitive breast cancer. The effects of soy-based formulas on infants are not well understood, but there is the possibility of endocrine effects.

TANNINS: OLIGOMERIC PROANTHOCYANIDINS

Proanthocyanidins are oligomers and polymers of flavan-3-ol monomer units. Oligomeric proanthocyanidins (OPCs) are a related group of red and blue plant pigments, also known as procyanidins, procyanidolic oligomers (PCOs), leucoanthocyanins and condensed tannins, that are found in the skin, bark and seeds of many plants, and have similar health effects to flavonoids. They bind to proteins and have an astringent effect, which causes a 'puckering' sensation when in contact with salivary proteins in the mouth. The absorption of OPCs is thought to be low. The OPC metabolite ethylcatechol is excreted in faeces via bile, and the metabolites hippuric acid, ethylcatechol and 3-hydroxyphenylproprionic acid are excreted in urine.

Functions

Functions of tannins include:

- *Antioxidant activity*. OPCs have potent antioxidant activity, estimated to be 20 times stronger than vitamin E and 50 times stronger than vitamin C, and appear to have a vitamin E-sparing effect. However, their relatively low absorption means that vitamin antioxidants are likely to be of more importance in the body. OPCs quench singlet oxygen and scavenge the hydroxyl radical and other radicals, inhibit lipid peroxidation and oxidation of LDL cholesterol, protect against DNA damage in the brain and liver in animals, and protect the skin from sun damage. OPCs also bind copper and iron, and reduce their potential to initiate oxidation and inhibit activity of the free radical generating enzymes cytochrome P450 2E1 (CYP2E1) and xanthine oxidase.
- *Anti-inflammatory activity*. OPCs inhibit the enzymes phospholipase A_2, COX and LOX, which produce

inflammatory eicosanoids, and inhibit production of inflammatory cytokines, interleukins and TNF-alpha.

- *Connective tissue strength.* OPCs have a particular affinity for proline-rich connective tissues, where they act to reinforce collagen cross-linking and inhibit the enzymes elastase, collagenase, hyaluronidase and beta-glucuronidase that break down connective tissue proteins and glycosaminoglycans (GAGs). They strengthen connective tissue in blood vessel walls, joint cartilage, spinal discs, ligaments, tendons, gums, bones and the skin, decrease blood vessel permeability and enhance capillary strength, vascular function and peripheral circulation.
- *Cardiovascular health.* OPCs can adhere to the surface of arteries and prevent oxidation damage, dilate blood vessels by increasing nitric oxide (NO) production and stimulate production of vascular endothelial growth factor, which helps repair damaged areas. OPCs help to regulate levels of serum lipids and cholesterol, reduce oxidation damage to serum lipids and cholesterol, and have anti-atherosclerosis effects. They appear to protect small blood vessels in the retina of the eye.
- *Anticancer activity.* Cell studies show that OPCs are toxic to cancer cells, but support the growth of normal cells. They can inhibit expression of the oncogene c-myc and modulate gene expression that regulates apoptosis. OPCs induce apoptosis of cancer cells, inhibit cancer metastasis in animals and inhibit aromatase, a key enzyme in oestrogen synthesis that plays a role in hormone-dependent breast cancer.
- *Antibacterial activity.* OPCs have protective activity against a range of bacteria. Cranberry proanthocyanidins are particularly effective for reducing the incidence of urinary tract infections. They act by inhibiting bacterial adhesion to the mucous membranes of the urinary tract, and by inhibiting bacterial growth by binding iron, making it unavailable for bacterial metabolism.

Dietary sources

OPCs are found in grape seeds, crab apples, apples, blackcurrants, cranberries, blueberries, bilberries, hawthorn berries, cola nuts, peanut skins, tea, red wine, hops, chocolate, rhubarb, rose hips, onions, parsley, barley and legumes.

Supplements, uses and dose

OPCs are available in Australian supplements as extracts of cranberry (*Vaccinium macrocarpon*), grape seed (*Vitis vinifera*), bilberry (*Vaccinium myrtillus*), sea bilberry (*Vaccinium bracteatum*), velvetleaf blueberry (*Vaccinium myrtilloides*), small cranberry (*Vaccinium oxycoccos*) and lingonberry (*Vaccinium vitis-idaea*), as well as the herb hawthorn (*Crataegus* spp.). OPCs are also available as the pine bark extracts Pycnogenol®, which uses an extraction method patented by French Professor Jacques Masquelier, and Enzogenol®, which is made by a patented process in New Zealand. OPCs can be extracted from the skins of peanuts, or from grape skins, pulp, seeds and stems that are the waste products of wine-making.

OPCs are potentially useful for chronic venous insufficiency (poor blood flow in veins), varicose veins, capillary fragility, bleeding, bruising, wound healing, fluid retention, prevention of cancer and CVD, atherosclerosis, high blood pressure, elevated serum cholesterol and lipids, abnormal blood clotting, diabetic retinopathy, pancreatitis, systemic lupus erythematosus, bacterial infections, disorders of the retina, asthma and skin protection against UV light.[1] The supplementary dose is 50–300 mg daily.

Cautions

Animal studies show that OPCs are well tolerated.

REFERENCE

1 [No authors listed], Oligomeric proanthocyanidins (OPCs) monograph, *Altern Med Rev* (2003), 8(4): 442–50.

STILBENES: RESVERATROL

Resveratrol is a fat-soluble phytochemical produced in some plants as a defence chemical (phytoalexin) against fungal attack, stress, injury and UV light. It occurs in nature as the cis and trans forms, but the cis form is very unstable. It is believed to be responsible for the protective effects of red wine on the cardiovascular system. Scientific interest in resveratrol was sparked when it was found to have anticancer activity, and to maintain healthy body function during ageing, rejuvenate older animals, counteract the health effects of a poor diet and dramatically extend the lifespan of cells and animals.

Resveratrol is mainly present as trans-resveratrol in food, and is well absorbed (about 70 per cent absorption), but it is rapidly broken down in the intestine and liver to the metabolites resveratrol sulfates, resveratrol glucuronides, resveratrol glucuronide-sulfates and piceatannol, some of which are in the cis form. Free trans-resveratrol and its metabolites are transported in the bloodstream bound to lipoproteins such as LDLs and albumin and excreted mainly in urine. There is some evidence that long-term intake is associated with an accumulation of resveratrol in the body, and it is speculated that resveratrol sulfate may serve as an inactive pool of resveratrol that is converted to the active form in target tissues.

Resveratrol metabolites and the resveratrol precursor piceid (also known as polydatin) and piceatannol, a naturally occurring hydroxylated analogue of resveratrol, may have similar health effects to resveratrol. Piceid is the more abundant form in foods, and it may be converted by enzymes in the colon or enterocytes to trans-resveratrol. Efforts are being made to produce forms of resveratrol supplements that have greater bioavailability and retention in the body.

Functions

Resveratrol may have life-extending, anti-ageing, anticancer, anti-inflammatory, anti-diabetic, anti-oxidant and anti-atherogenic properties. Functions of resveratrol include the following:

- *Antioxidant activity.* In cell studies, resveratrol is a potent antioxidant that scavenges hydroxyl radicals, superoxide radicals, superoxide anions, singlet oxygen, NO and hydrogen peroxide, protecting cell membranes, DNA and serum lipoproteins from oxidation damage. It appears to act as an antioxidant in normal cells and as a pro-oxidant in cancer cells. Resveratrol also binds iron and copper, and reduces their ability to enhance oxidation. Piceid appears to be more effective than resveratrol for scavenging hydroxyl radicals. Piceatannol is equal to vitamin C in antioxidant potency, and appears to be more potent than resveratrol in inhibiting copper-induced lipid peroxidation in LDLs and scavenging NO and hydrogen peroxide.
- *Anti-inflammatory activity.* Resveratrol helps regulate immunity and inflammation by reducing the production of inflammatory chemicals, and by regulating the immune system to suppress over-activity that contributes to inflammation. Resveratrol and piceatannol decrease NF-kappaB activation, which inhibits expression of the genes for numerous inflammatory chemicals and enzymes, including cell adhesion molecules (CAMs), TNF-alpha, interleukin-1 (IL-1), IL-8, inducible nitric oxide synthase (iNOS), and COX-1 and COX-2. Resveratrol enhances vasodilation, and inhibits platelet aggregation and COX-1 activity, in a similar manner to aspirin. Piceatannol inhibits COX-2 as well as tyrosine kinases, enzymes that activate mitogen-activated protein kinase (MAPK) and lead to the production of inflammatory chemicals and transcription factors. Piceatannol is a potent inhibitor of spleen tyrosine kinase (Syk), an enzyme implicated in asthma that promotes mast cell degranulation, bronchial constriction, bronchial oedema and anaphylaxis.
- *Anti-ageing and life extension activity.* Resveratrol appears to be able to switch on 'anti-ageing' genes that extend the lifespan of cells. These genes boost production of sirtuin (SIRT) proteins that regulate gene silencing, DNA repair, ageing, apoptosis and cell death, as well as reducing and repairing cell damage and extending lifespan. Resveratrol competitively inhibits phosphodiesterase enzymes that break down the cellular second messenger cyclic adenosine monophosphate (cAMP), thereby increasing cAMP levels and activating SIRT1.

  Resveratrol has been shown to extend the lifespan of various animal species in a similar manner to a long-term, very low-calorie diet. In a short-lived fish species, resveratrol increased average lifespan by 56 per cent, and old fish became more physically active and remained fertile, acting like much younger fish. In mice, a high-fat diet induced obesity and premature death, but mice given resveratrol together with a high-fat diet, although becoming obese, avoided the adverse health effects and had a longer lifespan and a 31 per cent reduction in death rate. The resveratrol-treated mice steadily improved their motor skills as they aged, had improved insulin sensitivity and glucose tolerance, more mitochondria in organ tissue and reduced heart, liver and pancreatic damage.
- *Anticancer activity.* Cell studies show that resveratrol can interfere with the development of cancers by blocking the activation of cancer-causing agents,

inhibiting the development and growth of tumours and causing abnormal cells to revert to normal. In cell studies, resveratrol has been found to protect normal cells and inhibit the growth of a variety of human cancer cell lines, including lymphoid and myeloid cancers, multiple myeloma, melanoma, head and neck squamous cell carcinoma, ovarian carcinoma, cervical carcinoma and cancers of the breast, prostate, stomach, colon, pancreas and thyroid. Resveratrol interacts with oestrogen receptors on breast cancer cells, and suppresses the growth-promoting effects of oestrogen. Resveratrol also inhibits inflammatory and oxidative processes that contribute to cancer, arrests cell cycle progression, increases expression of the antioxidant enzymes superoxide dismutase, catalase and glutathione peroxidase in cancer cells, and promotes cancer cell apoptosis. In animals, resveratrol blocks the cancer process at various stages by suppressing tumour initiation, promotion, progression and angiogenesis. Resveratrol also potentiates the apoptotic effects of cytokines, chemotherapeutic drugs and gamma-radiation. Piceid and piceatannol appear to have similar anticancer activity. Piceatannol inhibits the proliferation of a wide variety of cancer cells by cell cycle arrest and promotion of apoptosis.

- *Cardiovascular protection.* Resveratrol enhances the activity of endothelial nitric oxide synthase (eNOS), the enzyme that produces NO. NO dilates blood vessels and inhibits platelet aggregation and smooth muscle proliferation, which are features of atherosclerosis. Resveratrol reduces inflammation that is associated with atherosclerosis, improves blood flow and reduces oxidative damage to LDL and HDL cholesterol. It has been shown to enhance removal of cholesterol from macrophages in the artery wall. It enhances the repair process after a heart attack, and reduces the risk of heart disease.
- *Nerve and brain protection.* In humans, SIRT1 helps to protect neurons in Alzheimer's and Huntington's diseases. Resveratrol reduces inflammatory and oxidative damage to brain cells and markedly lowers levels of the peptide amyloid-beta that builds up in the brain in Alzheimer's disease. It has been shown to promote cleavage of the amyloid precursor protein to non-amyloid-beta peptides and to enhance the clearance of amyloid-beta.

Dietary sources

Resveratrol is found in grape skins and seeds, especially purple grapes, and in red wine, purple grape juice, cranberries, blueberries, bilberries, mulberries, peanuts, pine bark (Scots pine, Eastern white pine), Itadori tea (an Asian herbal tea used for heart disease and stroke), and the roots and stalks of giant knotweed (*Polygonum cuspidatum*), a herb used in Asian herbal medicine and also known as Japanese knotweed and tiger cane (Hu Zhang). Grape varieties that are particularly susceptible to fungal diseases, such as pinot noir, have higher resveratrol levels. Levels in Australian red wine range from 2–10 mg/L and Australian white wines contain about 1–2 mg/L. Piceid and piceatannol are found in foods and beverages that contain resveratrol, including grapes and giant knotweed. Piceatannol is also found in passionfruit seeds and sugar cane plants.

Supplements, uses and dose

Resveratrol is available in Australian supplements as extracts of the herb giant knotweed (*Polygonum cuspidatum*) and grape seed (*Vitis vinifera*). It is potentially useful for cancer prevention and treatment, diseases of ageing, life extension, chronic inflammatory diseases, neurodegenerative diseases, diabetes, heart disease, cerebral insufficiency, metabolic syndrome, type 2 diabetes, asthma and non-alcoholic and alcohol-induced fatty liver.[1] The supplementary dose has not been established, but doses of 5–5000 mg daily have been used in clinical trials. A giant knotweed extract providing 40 mg/day of resveratrol has been shown to suppress oxidative stress and inflammation in male athletes in a six-week human trial.[2]

REFERENCES

1 [No authors listed], Resveratrol monograph, *Altern Med Rev* (2010), 15(2): 152–8.

2 Zahedi, H.S., Jazayeri, S., Ghiasvand, R. et al., Effects of polygonum cuspidatum containing resveratrol on inflammation in male professional basketball players, *Int J Prev Med* (2013), 4(Suppl 1): S1–4.

Cautions

Animal studies show that resveratrol is well tolerated. In humans, no adverse effects have been reported in doses up to 5 g/day. A small number of people have reported frontal headaches at doses of 5 g daily.

COUMARINS

Coumarins are fragrant plant compounds that were first isolated from the tonka bean, a native of Central and South America. They include simple coumarins, furanocoumarins, pyranocoumarins and pyrone-substituted coumarins. The coumarin derivative dicoumarol, found in sweet clover that has become mouldy or damaged, inhibits production of vitamin K-dependent clotting factors in the liver, and dicoumarol derivatives are used as blood-thinning drugs. Coumarins are rapidly absorbed from the gastrointestinal tract and are rapidly and almost completely metabolised in the liver by cytochrome P450 enzymes, the main metabolite being 7-hydroxycoumarin which is excreted in urine. Coumarins have been regarded as toxic because they cause acute liver toxicity in rodents. However, research has shown that they are not hepatotoxic in humans, possibly because of efficient detoxification in the liver and excretion in urine.

Functions

Functions of coumarins include:

- *Antioxidant activity.* The coumarins scopoletin, aesculetin, fraxetin, umbelliferone and daphnetin have been found to have potent antioxidant activity by scavenging ROS and reactive nitrogen species (RNS) and inhibiting lipid peroxidation. Coumarins also inhibit production of the damaging superoxide anion.
- *Immune-boosting and anti-inflammatory activity.* Coumarins stimulate lymphocyte proliferation and activation, and increase secretion of interferon-gamma, a protein involved in immune and inflammatory responses, including the activation, growth and differentiation of T cells, B cells, macrophages and NK cells. Coumarins inhibit the LOX and COX pathways that produce inflammatory eicosanoids.
- *Anti-oedema activity*. Coumarins have been shown to reduce swelling in patients with high-protein oedema, in which there is an accumulation of protein in tissue following trauma or inflammation that leads to fluid leakage from capillaries into tissue spaces. Coumarins have been found to relieve lymphoedema caused by breast cancer surgery and radiotherapy.
- *Anticancer activity.* Coumarins have antioxidant, anti-inflammatory and immune-enhancing properties, and inhibit cell cycle progression and induce apoptosis in cancer cells. They have been shown to inhibit growth of leukaemia, kidney, breast, prostate and lung cancer cells, and to inhibit the growth of drug-sensitive and multi-drug-resistant cancer cell lines. 7-hydroxycoumarin inhibits the release of cyclin D1, a regulator of cell proliferation that is over-expressed in many types of cancer.

Dietary sources

Coumarins are found in bilberries, green tea and chicory. The richest plant sources are the Rutaceae (rue or citrus family), including oranges, lemons, mandarins, grapefruit and the herbs rue and prickly ash, and Umbelliferae (carrot or parsley family), including carrots, celery, coriander, fennel and parsley.

Supplements, uses and dose

Coumarins are not used as supplements, but coumarin derivatives are used as prescription medications. Dicoumarol has anticoagulant activity, but other coumarins in food or herbs do not. Warfarin (coumadin) is a synthetic coumarin used as a potent blood-thinning drug. Coumarins are found in medicinal herbs such as *Aesculus hippocastanum* (horse chestnut seed), *Angelica sinensis* (dong quai), *Ruta graveolens* (rue) and *Trifolium pratense* (red clover). Coumarins have antioxidant, immune-boosting, anti-inflammatory, anti-oedema and anticancer activity.[1]

REFERENCE

1 Jain, P.K., & Joshi, H., Coumarin: Chemical and pharmacological profile, *J Appl Pharm Sci* (2012), 2(06): 236–40.

Cautions

Many furanocoumarins cause phototoxicity by sensitising the skin to UV light. Furanocoumarins and flavonoids in grapefruit juice affect the metabolism of some drugs by inhibiting expression of the detoxifying enzyme CYP3A4 in the intestinal wall, which increases the dose delivered to the body and potentially increases the risk of toxicity. People on prescription medication should seek medical advice before using grapefruit juice.

ORGANOSULFUR COMPOUNDS

Organosulfur compounds (OCs) give a pungent taste and smell to foods, and include glucosinolates, cysteine sulfoxides and diallylsulfides. Glucosinolates such as glucoraphanin are found in cabbage-family vegetables (cruciferous or brassica plants), and are broken down by the enzyme myrosinase to the active metabolites indole-3-carbinol (I3C) and isothiocyanates, which include sulforaphane (SFN). Myrosinase is present in OC-containing plants, and is released when the plant is chopped or chewed; myrosinase is also present in gut bacteria. I3C is absorbed in the small intestine as diindolylmethane (DIM) and the main metabolite in serum is 2-(indol-3-ylmethyl)-3,3'-diindolylmethane (LTr-1).

Raw onion and garlic (allium) vegetables are rich in OCs such as gamma-glutamyl-S-allylcysteine (GSAC) and S-allyl-L-cysteine sulfoxides (alliin), which are broken down to other bioactive compounds when garlic is processed. The enzyme alliinase breaks down alliin during chewing, crushing or chopping to form allicin, which rapidly breaks down to other sulfur-containing compounds.

Allicin was originally thought to be the active principle in garlic but it is now believed that its metabolites are responsible for the beneficial effects. These include the water-soluble compounds S-allylmercaptocysteine (SAMC), S-allylcysteine (SAC), S-ethylcysteine (SEC), S-propylcysteine (SPC), gamma-glutamyl-S-methylcysteine (GSMC) and gamma-glutamyl-S-propylcysteine (GSPC), as well as the fat-soluble compounds ajoene, vinyl dithiin, diallylsulfide (DAS), diallyldisulfide (DADS) and diallyltrisulfide (DATS).

Functions

The functions of OCs include:

- *Antioxidant activity.* OCs, including SAC and other garlic compounds, are potent antioxidants that can protect cell DNA from damage by scavenging ROS, stimulating activity of the cellular antioxidant enzymes superoxide dismutase, catalase and glutathione peroxidase, and increasing production of glutathione. OCs inhibit lipid peroxidation and oxidative damage to LDL cholesterol, protect DNA against free radical-mediated damage and mutations, inhibit carcinogenesis and protect against ionising radiation and UV-induced tissue damage. SFN can reverse the age-associated decline in immune function in old animals by switching on genes that have antioxidant effects in immune cells. It has been shown to protect the pigmented epithelial cells of the retina in the eyes from photo-oxidation, and to protect nerve cells from oxidative and inflammatory damage.
- *Anti-inflammatory activity.* OCs can inhibit the activity of inflammatory enzymes and immune cells. DATS from garlic oil appears to have the most potent effect of all the OCs in garlic on inhibiting the inflammatory enzymes COX and iNOS. DATS inhibits the MAPK and NF-kappaB inflammatory pathways and also activates Nrf2, a transcription factor that reduces levels of ROS that promote inflammation. SFN has similar inhibiting effects to DATS on COX and NF-kappaB inflammatory pathways. I3C also inhibits the NF-kappaB pathway.
- *Detoxification.* OCs boost glutathione production that is needed for phase II detoxification activity in the liver. I3C can boost the activity of phase I and phase II detoxification enzymes, and SFN is a potent inducer of numerous enzymes involved in detoxification. The garlic oil constituent DAS is converted to diallyl sulfoxide and then to diallyl sulfone by the enzyme CYP2E1 in the liver. These compounds inhibit activation of cancer-causing agents during phase I detoxification, and have anticancer activity.
- *Anticancer activity.* OCs inhibit the growth of tumour cells and induce apoptosis of abnormal cells. I3C and ajoene have been found to cause cell cycle arrest and enhance apoptosis in tumour cells. SAMC and SFN inhibit the enzyme histone deacetylase; inhibition of this enzyme reactivates genes that are switched off in cancer cells, triggering cell cycle arrest and apoptosis. SFN has shown a remarkable ability to

prevent cancer growth in cell studies. Human colon cancer cells stop growing in the presence of SFN and, in bladder cancer cells, 80 per cent of cells stop growing and die within three hours. Similar results have been found in breast cancer cells. In mice with prostate cancer, SFN inhibits tumour growth by 50–70 per cent. DIM, a metabolite of I3C, has been shown to bind to oestrogen receptors, and has the potential to act as an oestrogen antagonist in hormone-dependent breast cancer.

- *Regulation of cholesterol synthesis.* Garlic OCs, especially SAC, inhibit the enzyme HMG-CoA reductase that produces cholesterol in the body. SAC, SEC and SPC have been found to inhibit cholesterol synthesis by 40–60 per cent compared with 20–35 per cent by GSAC, GSMC and GSPC. The effect of multiple garlic compounds was found to be greater than that of any individual compound.
- *Cardiovascular activity.* Garlic extracts have been found to inhibit platelet aggregation and reduce blood clotting, and allicin and thiosulfinates appear to be the most active components. This anti-platelet activity is strongest in raw garlic extracts and lowest in whole, cooked garlic cloves. Crushing garlic before moderate cooking helps retain this activity. Garlic OCs have a mild blood pressure-lowering effect.
- *Antimicrobial activity.* Cell studies show that garlic OCs can act against a variety of bacteria, fungi, viruses and parasites. Ajoene has antifungal and anti-parasitic effects and SFN has been shown to reduce the growth in the stomach of *Helicobacter pylori*, the bacteria responsible for stomach ulcers.

Dietary sources

Good sources of glucosinolates include broccoli, Brussels sprouts, cabbage, cauliflower, collard greens, kale, kohlrabi, mustard, rutabaga, turnips, bok choy, Chinese cabbage, rocket, horseradish, radishes, wasabi and watercress. Broccoli sprouts are extremely rich in SFN, having between ten and 100 times more than a mature broccoli plant. Good sources of alliin include garlic as well as onions, leeks, chives and shallots. OCs are water-soluble, and can be depleted by water processing and cooking methods.

Supplements, uses and dose

OCs are available as brassica extracts or dried or fresh garlic extracts, garlic powder, garlic oil or aged garlic extract (AGE). To produce garlic extracts, whole or sliced garlic cloves are soaked in an extracting solution, such as purified water and diluted alcohol, for varying amounts of time. OCs in garlic supplements vary according to the manufacturing process. Dehydrated garlic powder is made by drying and pulverising crushed garlic cloves, and contains oil-soluble sulfur compounds derived from allicin. AGE has been extracted and aged for about twenty months, reducing its strong taste and odour and increasing the content of water-soluble OCs such as SAC and SAMC. Deodorised garlic also contains SAC. Garlic oil is made by grinding whole garlic cloves in water and using heat distillation or solvent extraction to remove the oil. It contains ajoene, vinyl dithiin, DAS, DADS and DATS.

All types of garlic products appear to have potent antioxidant and antimicrobial activity, but most of the research has been carried out on AGE. Enteric-coated garlic tablets deliver the active constituents directly to the intestine to avoid breakdown in stomach acid and to minimise 'garlic breath'. An Australian study using an enteric-coated garlic powder supplement found that it was effective in lowering total and LDL cholesterol, but the garlic odour was detectable on subjects' breath.[1]

OCs are potentially useful for chronic inflammatory diseases, cervical dysplasia, cancer prevention, gastric ulcers, age-related macular degeneration, neuro-degenerative diseases, elevated blood cholesterol, CVD, detoxification and infections.[2,3,4]

The supplementary dose of SFN is 50–100 mg daily, and the dose of I3C is 200–400 mg daily. The supplementary dose of alliin is 4–12 mg daily. Garlic products that are standardised for alliin content may be preferable. The dose of raw garlic is 2–5 g daily (crushed or chewed first), 0.4–1.2 g daily of dried powder and 2–5 mg daily of garlic oil. The dose for aged garlic is 1–7.2 g daily.

REFERENCES

1 Kannar, D., Wattanapenpaiboon, N., Savige, G.S. & Wahlqvist, M.L., Hypocholesterolemic effect of an enteric-coated garlic supplement, *J Am Coll Nutr* (2001), 20(3): 225–31.

2 Tsai, C.W., Chen, H.W., Sheen, L.Y. & Lii, C.K., Garlic: Health benefits and actions, *BioMed* (2012), 2(1): 17–29.
3 [No authors listed], Sulforophane glucosinolate monograph, *Altern Med Rev* (2010), 15(4): 352–60.
4 [No authors listed], Indole-3-carbinol monograph, *Altern Med Rev* (2005), 10(4): 337–42.

Cautions

Animal studies show that OCs are generally well tolerated. However, raw garlic can irritate the gut, and the irritating constituents can be eliminated or reduced by soaking the garlic in alcohol, wine, milk or vinegar before use. AGE is generally lower in irritating constituents. Enteric-coated garlic supplements may cause digestive upsets in some people. High doses of garlic may have a blood-thinning effect; people on blood thinning medication should seek advice from a healthcare practitioner before taking high-dose garlic supplements, and high-dose garlic supplements should be discontinued ten days before surgery. People who are allergic to garlic should avoid garlic products.

ALKALOIDS: METHYLXANTHINES

Dietary methylxanthines (MXs) include caffeine (1,3,7-trimethylxanthine), theophylline (1,3-dimethyl-xanthine) and theobromine (3,7-dimethylxanthine), which have very similar bioactive properties. Caffeine is rapidly absorbed and distributed throughout body tissues, and is extensively metabolised to paraxanthine (1,7-dimethylxanthine) in the liver by the enzyme CYP1A2, a member of the cytochrome P450 family of detoxifying enzymes. Other metabolites include theobromine, theophylline and 1,3,7-trimethyluric acid. Theophylline is broken down mainly to 1,3-dimethyluric acid and smaller amounts of caffeine, 1-methylxanthine and 3-methylxanthine. Theobromine is broken down mainly to 6-amino-5-(N-methylformylamino)-1-methyluracil, with smaller amounts of 3-methylxanthine, 7-methylxanthine and 3,7-dimethyluric acid. Infants up to the age of eight or nine months have a greatly reduced ability to metabolise MXs. Metabolism is also reduced in pregnancy, and in users of the oral contraceptive pill, and is increased in smokers. The major excretory pathway of MXs and their metabolites is via urine.

Dietary sources

Caffeine is found in coffee, cola drinks, sports and energy drinks, with smaller amounts in tea, cocoa and chocolate. It is a constituent of the herbs guaraná (*Paullinia cupana*), yerba maté (*Ilex paraguariensis*) and kola (*Cola acuminata*). Theophylline is the major MX in tea and theobromine is the major MX in cocoa and chocolate. The amount of caffeine in a 250 mL cup of instant coffee is about 93 mg, and there is about 160 mg per 250 mL cup of cappuccino and 57 mg per 250 mL cup of black tea.

The Food Standards Australia New Zealand nutrient database (NUTTAB) at <www.foodstandards.gov.au> provides the amounts found in specific foods and beverages.

Actions

MXs and their metabolites are antagonists of adenosine receptors (ARs) but theobromine has much weaker activity than caffeine and theophylline. Adenosine is a purine that binds to ARs and acts to modulate cell function by altering the levels of signalling molecules such as cAMP and cyclic guanosine monophosphate (cGMP) within cells. In the CNS, adenosine binding to ARs modifies nerve cell responses to neurotransmitters. The effect of inhibitory neurotransmitters is increased, resulting in a slowing down of metabolic activity and drowsiness, fatigue and sleep. MXs bind to ARs and prevent adenosine from binding, increasing the effects of excitatory neurotransmitters and catecholamines (dopamine, noradrenaline and adrenaline), which speed up metabolic activity and promote a continued state of alertness. MXs increase heart and breathing rate and modulate intracellular calcium handling, and at high doses, inhibit cyclic nucleotide phosphodiesterases (PDEs), enzymes that break down signalling molecules in cells.

In general, caffeine is the most potent MX and theobromine is the weakest. Theophylline is a potent diuretic and bronchodilator, and theobromine has similar but weaker effects and very little effect on the CNS. MXs enhance thinking ability and mood, reduce sleepiness and potentiate the effects of analgesics. Even at low doses (100 mg/day or less), caffeine can stimulate cognitive performance, mood and thirst. MXs constrict peripheral blood vessels, stimulate cardiac muscle, temporarily increase heart rate and blood pressure, and dilate coronary arteries. In the respiratory system, MXs increase breathing rate and have a bronchodilator action. MXs act as diuretics by increasing the rate of blood flow through the kidneys, and also have anti-histamine effects, increase gastric acid secretions and increase fat oxidation. Maximal effects of MXs occur about an hour after ingestion, and effects may last four to six hours.

Effects of excess[1]

Excess theophylline increases serum calcium, creatine kinase, myoglobin and leukocyte count, and decreases serum phosphate and magnesium. Chronic or acute overdose of theophylline medication can cause agitation, hyperventilation, headache, convulsions, abnormal heart rhythm, thirst, nausea, persistent vomiting and diarrhoea, and may be lethal.

The acute lethal dose of caffeine in adults is about 10 g, and mild effects have been observed at doses of 200–300 mg/day. Effects of caffeine may include tremors, anxiety, nervousness, irritability, insomnia, sensory disturbances, abnormal heart rhythm, heart palpitations, faster breathing rate, restlessness, restless legs, frequent urination, excess acid in the stomach, stomach inflammation, nausea, indigestion, abdominal colic, diarrhoea and irritable bowel syndrome. Excessive consumption of energy drinks high in caffeine has caused seizures. Caffeine has been found to increase intraocular pressure in patients with glaucoma or ocular hypertension. In children, caffeine intake is associated with fidgety, jittery and restless behaviour, anxiety, nervousness, hyperactivity and difficulty sleeping, and high doses can lead to frequent urination, severe vomiting, fast heartbeat and agitation. Chronic exposure to caffeine induces tolerance to some of the stimulant effects. A high daily intake (more than 500–600 mg of caffeine) may lead to 'caffeinism', which features restlessness, anxiety, irritability, agitation, muscle tremor, insomnia, headache, frequent urination, tinnitus (noises in the ears), abnormal heart rhythm, nausea, vomiting and diarrhoea.

In women, more than 400 mg/day of caffeine may increase the risk of developing an overactive ('irritable') bladder and lower doses may aggravate symptoms in women with this disorder. Consumption of 500 mg of caffeine/day or more has been associated with an increased risk of CVD in some studies. Caffeine has adverse effects on bone metabolism if calcium intake is low, but intakes of less than 400 mg/day of caffeine do not appear to affect bone status or calcium balance in people taking at least 800 mg of calcium/day. A caffeine intake of 300 mg/day or more may reduce fertility in women, and may have adverse effects on foetal development in pregnant women. A limited amount of evidence suggests that intake of more than 400 mg/day may decrease sperm motility in men. Very high doses of caffeine cause birth defects in animals, but there is little evidence for such an effect in humans. Although studies have found inconsistent results, caffeine does not appear to increase the risk of cancer at doses of less than 500 mg of caffeine/day. In general, MXs have few adverse effects on health at doses of less than 300 mg/day.

Supplements, uses and dose

Caffeine is available in prescription and non-prescription medication, and in the herbs guaraná, yerba maté and kola. Caffeine is used for the management of fatigue and orthostatic hypotension (a drop in blood pressure when changing posture),[2] and for the short-term treatment of apnoea (breathing difficulties) in premature infants.[3] It may be neuroprotective in spinal cord injury, stroke and neurodegenerative diseases such as Parkinson's and Alzheimer's diseases.[4] It has been used as a weight loss aid because of its stimulant effects on body metabolism and fat oxidation,[5] and low doses enhance athletic performance, possibly by increasing the utilisation of fat and reducing the use of glycogen or by direct effects on muscles and the nervous system that enhance endurance.[6] Benefits do not increase with increasing doses, and the effect varies between individuals. Theophylline is available as prescription medication and is used as a diuretic and for chronic lung diseases, such as asthma, emphysema and chronic bronchitis.[7] Theobromine has been used as a vasodilator, diuretic and heart stimulant.[8] Low doses of caffeine are 80–250 mg/day and moderate doses are 300–400 mg/day. Caffeine is used in doses of 100–200 mg every three to four hours for adult fatigue.

REFERENCES

1 Nawrot, P., Jordan, S., Eastwood, J. et al., Effects of caffeine on human health, *Food Addit Contam* (2003), 20: 1–30.

2 Ahmad, R.A. & Watson, R.D., Treatment of postural hypotension: A review, *Drugs* (1990), 39(1): 74–85.
3 Aranda, J.V., Beharry, K., Valencia, G.B., Natarajan, G. & Davis, J., Caffeine impact on neonatal morbidities, *J Matern Fetal Neonatal Med* (2010), 23(Suppl 3): 20–3.
4 Rivera-Oliver, M. & Díaz-Ríos, M., Using caffeine and other adenosine receptor antagonists and agonists as therapeutic tools against neurodegenerative diseases: A review, *Life Sci* (2014), 101(1–2): 1–9.
5 Heckman, M.A., Weil, J. & Gonzalez de Mejia, E., Caffeine (1, 3, 7-trimethylxanthine) in foods: A comprehensive review on consumption, functionality, safety, and regulatory matters, *J Food Sci* (2010), 75(3): R77–87.
6 Burke, L.M., Caffeine and sports performance, *Appl Physiol Nutr Metab* (2008), 33(6): 1319–34.
7 Barnes, P.J., Theophylline, *Am J Respir Crit Care Med* (2013), 188(8): 901–6.
8 Smit, H.J., Theobromine and the pharmacology of cocoa, *Handb Exp Pharmacol* (2011), 200: 201–34.

Cautions

An abrupt reduction or cessation of caffeine intake is associated with headaches, fatigue, anxiety, irritability, depressed mood and difficulty concentrating. Caffeine intake should be restricted to less than 300 mg/day in pregnant women, and in women trying to conceive and their partners. Caffeine intake should be avoided in children, people with glaucoma or ocular hypertension, and women with an overactive bladder. People with epilepsy, anxiety, nervous tension, insomnia, abnormal heart rhythm, elevated blood pressure, heart disease or excess stomach acid should limit their caffeine intake.

CHLOROPHYLL

FAST FACTS . . . CHLOROPHYLL

- **Chlorophyll is a green plant pigment required by plants for light absorption and photosynthesis.**
- **It is poorly absorbed, but cell studies show that it has antioxidant, anti-inflammatory, immune-enhancing and anticancer activity.**
- **Supplementation may be helpful for wound healing, reduction of body odour and cancer prevention.**

Chlorophyll is a green pigment that is a magnesium-containing porphyrin synthesised by plants. It has a similar structure to haem in red blood cells, but, in haem, iron takes the place of magnesium. The function of chlorophyll in plants is to absorb light, the energy of which, together with water and carbon dioxide, is used to produce oxygen and carbohydrates—a process known as photosynthesis. Chlorophyll selectively absorbs light in the red and blue regions, and therefore emits a green colour. At least six different chlorophyll molecules have been identified: chlorophyll a and b in higher plants; chlorophyll c, d and e in algae; and bacteriochlorophylls in photosynthetic bacteria.

Chlorophyll in plants is in chloroplasts, where it is complexed with phospholipids, polypeptides and tocopherols, and protected by a hydrophobic membrane. Derivatives of chlorophyll found in plants include chlorophyllide a and b, pheophytin a and b and pheophorbide a and b. When chlorophyll is extracted for commercial use, its magnesium ion becomes unstable, and may be displaced easily, and often copper is substituted for magnesium in order to create a more stable form, which is known as chlorophyllin. Most research studies have used sodium copper chlorophyllin (SCC), which consists of copper-chlorin e4 (derived from chlorophyll a) and copper-chlorin e6 (derived from chlorophyll b).

Chlorophyll is poorly absorbed, but the magnesium contained in chlorophyll is released during digestion and is bioavailable. Exposure of chlorophyll to hydrochloric acid in the stomach causes removal of magnesium and its replacement with hydrogen ions, forming pheophytins a and b, about 5–10 per cent of which are absorbed. Chlorophyll and its derivatives are lipophilic, and absorption may be enhanced if taken with a source of dietary fat. Copper-chlorophyllin is water-soluble, but its bioavailability appears to be low and an animal study found that only copper-chlorin e_4 was absorbed. The main serum metabolite in people taking copper-chlorophyllin was found to be copper-chlorin e_4 ethyl ester.

The breast cancer resistance protein (BCRP), a member of the ABC transporter family, transports the chlorophyll derivative pheophorbide, and is a highly efficient inhibitor of its absorption in the gut. Pheophorbide is potentially harmful because it forms oxygen in tissues such as the skin when exposed to light, causing oxidative damage to cell membranes (phototoxicity). The majority of chlorophyll derivatives are exported back into the digestive tract after uptake by epithelial cells, possibly as a protective mechanism against phototoxicity.

Functions

Although early studies suggested that chlorophyll and its derivatives may play a role in the formation of blood cells in the body, subsequent research has found that this is not the case. Functions of chlorophyll include the following:

- *Anticancer activity.* Chlorophyll binds to and reduces the absorption and activity of several mutagenic substances, including polyaromatic hydrocarbons, heterocyclic amines, 2-amino-3-methylimidazo[4,5-*f*] quinoline and the mycotoxin aflatoxin B1. When compared with retinol, beta-carotene and vitamins C and E, chlorophyllin was the most effective anti-mutagen when all substances were used in the same concentration. Chlorophyllin may also have anti-mutagenic effects by inhibiting cytochrome P450 enzymes that can produce mutagens during detoxification processes, inducing protective phase II detoxification enzymes and protecting DNA from damage. The metal-free chlorophyll derivatives pheophytins and pheophorbides also have anti-mutagenic activity. SCC has been found to induce apoptosis in human cancer cells.
- *Antioxidant activity.* Chlorophyllin protects against lipid peroxidation, and protects DNA from damaging gamma radiation, possibly by scavenging ROS and reducing production of the superoxide anion and peroxyl and hydroxyl radicals. It is suggested that the copper component may be important for the antioxidant effects.
- *Immune and anti-inflammatory activity.* In cell studies, chlorophyllin stimulated humoral and cell-mediated immune responses, and inhibited the activation of inflammatory transcription factors and NF-kappaB.

Dietary sources

Good sources of chlorophyll include green leafy vegetables, wheatgrass, alfalfa, green tea, parsley, micro-algae such as chlorella and spirulina, and many herbs. During heat processing and cooking, the bright-green colour changes to an olive-green, which is a result of the conversion to magnesium-free chlorophyll derivatives such as pheophytins and pyropheophytins.

Supplements, uses and dose

The forms permitted in Australia for use in supplements are chlorophyll, chlorophyll-copper complexes and chlorophyllin-copper complex. Supplements are available as liquid, powder, capsule or tablet formulations. Commercial chlorophyll is extracted from dried alfalfa by breaking down cell structures by grinding, homogenisation, ultrasound or sonication (agitation by sound), followed by organic solvent extraction or supercritical fluid extraction using carbon dioxide. It can also be extracted from microalgae such as chlorella. Chlorophyllin is manufactured by reacting a chlorophyll extract with a strong alkali, resulting in water soluble magnesium chlorophyllin. The magnesium is then replaced by copper for stability.

Chlorophyll and copper complexes of chlorophyll are used as natural food colourings (numbers 140 and 141). Topical application of ointment containing chlorophyllin, papain and urea has been found to promote wound healing.[1] In the 1950s, chlorophyll was promoted for reducing bad breath, vaginal and menstrual odours, and odours from skin ulcers, faecal incontinence and colostomy bags, based on a limited number of cases.[2] Chlorophyllin (180 mg/day for three weeks) is effective for reducing body odour in people with the genetic disorder trimethylaminuria, which is an inability to metabolise trimethylamine to trimethylamine N-oxide, causing a strong body odour similar to that of rotting fish.[3] It appears to act by binding trimethylamine in the gut and reducing absorption. In people exposed to aflatoxin-containing foods, 100 mg of SCC three times daily for four months led to a 50–55 per cent reduction in a urinary marker of aflatoxin-damaged DNA.[4] Chlorophyll can act as a photosensitiser, and can be useful for the photodynamic therapy of cancer.[5] In animal models of skin cancer, SCC and pheophytins a and b have suppressed tumour promotion and progression.[6,7] In humans, increased chlorophyll consumption is associated with a decreased risk of colorectal cancer.[8] In an animal model of calcium oxalate kidney stones, iv SCC was found to inhibit the deposition and growth of calcium oxalate crystals.[9] The supplementary dose of chlorophyll is 100–300 mg/day.

REFERENCES

1 Smith, R.G., Enzymatic debriding agents: An evaluation of the medical literature, *Ostomy Wound Manage* (2008), 54(8): 16–34.

2 Weingarten, M. & Payson, B., Deodorization of colostomies with chlorophyll, *Rev Gastroenterol* (1951), 18(8): 602–4.

3 Yamazaki, H., Fujieda, M., Togashi, M. et al., Effects of the dietary supplements, activated charcoal and copper chlorophyllin, on urinary excretion of trimethylamine in Japanese trimethylaminuria patients, *Life Sci* (2004), 74(22): 2739.

4 Egner, P.A., Muñoz, A. & Kensler, T.W., Chemoprevention with chlorophyllin in individuals exposed to dietary aflatoxin, *Mutat Res* (2003), 523–24: 209–16.

5 Kessel, D. & Smith, K., Photosensitization with derivatives of chlorophyll, *Photochem Photobiol* (1989), 49(2): 157–60.

6 Park, K.K. & Surh, Y.J., Chemopreventive activity of chlorophyllin against mouse skin carcinogenesis by benzo[a]pyrene and benzo[a]pyrene-7,8-dihydrodiol-9,10-epoxide, *Cancer Lett* (1996), 102: 143–9.

7 Nakamura, Y., Murakami, A., Koshimizu, K. & Ohigashi, H., Inhibitory effect of pheophorbide a, a chlorophyll-related compound, on skin tumor promotion in ICR mice, *Cancer Lett* (1996), 108: 247–55.

8 Balder, H.F., Vogel, J., Jansen, M.C. et al., Heme and chlorophyll intake and risk of colorectal cancer in the Netherlands cohort study, *Cancer Epidemiol Biomarkers Prev* (2006), 15(4): 717–25.

9 Tawashi, R., Cousineau, M. & Sharkawi, M., Effect of sodium copper chlorophyllin on the formation of calcium oxalate crystals in rat kidney, *Invest Urol* (1980), 18(2): 90–2.

Cautions

Chlorophyll appears to be generally well tolerated. Diarrhoea and green discolouration of faeces or urine have been reported. Topical applications may cause skin irritation. In Japan, use of chlorella has been associated with phototoxicity in a small number of cases, featuring swelling and reddish-purple lesions on sun-exposed skin. The chlorella supplement responsible was found to contain 8.2 mg/g of pheophorbide. Subsequently, the Japanese government limited the amount of total pheophorbide permitted in algal supplements to 1.2 mg/g. People with low or absent BCRP activity may be at increased risk of developing phototoxicity from dietary or supplementary chlorophyll.

HOW MUCH DO I KNOW?

Choose whether the following statements are true or false. Then review this chapter for the correct answers.

	Statement	True (T)	False (F)
1	Coenzyme Q10 protects mitochondrial function.	T	F
2	The natural form of alpha-lipoic acid is S-alpha-lipoic acid.	T	F
3	Phytochemicals are essential dietary nutrients.	T	F
4	Carotenoids are fat-soluble antioxidants.	T	F
5	Yellow corn is a good source of lycopene.	T	F
6	Astaxanthin is found in microalgae and crustaceans.	T	F
7	Isoflavonoids have oestrogenic activity.	T	F
8	Resveratrol is found in turmeric root.	T	F
9	Garlic contains alliin that breaks down to other sulfur-containing compounds.	T	F
10	Xanthines are central nervous system depressants.	T	F

FURTHER READING

Braun, L. & Cohen, M., *Herbs & natural supplements: An evidence-based guide*, 3rd ed., Churchill Livingstone Elsevier, New York, 2010.

Gropper, S.S., Smith, J.L. & Groff, J.L., *Advanced nutrition and human metabolism*, 5th ed., Thomson Wadsworth, Belmont, CA, 2009.

Higdon, J., *An evidence-based approach to dietary phytochemicals*, Thieme, New York, 2007.

14

Nutritional bioactives: digestive enzymes, probiotics, arthritis bioactives, fungi, algae and bee products

DIGESTIVE ENZYMES

FAST FACTS . . . DIGESTIVE ENZYMES

- **Digestive enzymes are proteins that break down complex food molecules into small, absorbable molecules.**
- **They include proteases, amylase, lipase, bromelain, papain, lactase and cellulase.**
- **Supplementation may be helpful for heartburn, reflux, stomach pain, abdominal pain, nausea, bloating, burping, flatulence, constipation and diarrhoea.**

Digestive enzymes are proteins produced in the body that are released into the gastrointestinal tract in response to eating. They break down complex food molecules into small molecules that are able to be absorbed across the gut wall (see Chapter 1: Digestion). Poor digestion impairs the ability to absorb essential nutrients, and causes sub-optimal nutrition and associated health disorders. Digestive impairment occurs in ageing, chronic alcohol abuse, pancreatic disorders, stomach inflammation, inflammatory bowel disease, liver or bile disorders, cystic fibrosis, food intolerances and after gastrointestinal surgery to treat obesity. Digestive enzyme supplements are used to support digestive function and improve absorption of essential nutrients.

Supplements and dose

- *Hydrochloric acid and pepsin* support stomach function. Inadequate stomach acid can impair pepsin function and protein digestion, and cause bloating, abdominal discomfort, heartburn and reflux after meals, especially after a high-protein food such as meat. It can also lead to impaired absorption of nutrients—particularly vitamin B12, folic acid, iron and calcium—and increased risk of infections from ingested pathogens. A lack of stomach acid is more common in older people, and is associated with bacterial overgrowth in the small intestine. Hydrochloric acid is available in buffered form as betaine hydrochloride together with pepsin. Betaine hydrochloride is made synthetically by reacting chloroacetic acid with sodium carbonate and then adding liquid trimethylamine, followed by hydrochloric acid. Pepsin is a protein-digesting enzyme derived from animals—usually pigs or cattle. The supplementary dose of betaine hydrochloride is 300–600 mg per meal, combined with about 100 mg pepsin.

- *Pancreatic enzymes* include amylase, which digests starch, protein-splitting enzymes (proteases) and lipase, which digests fats and oils. Proteases and amylase may be derived from animal pancreatic secretions—usually pigs or cattle—and lipase is produced by micro-organisms such as *Aspergillus oryzae* and *Rhizopus arrhizus*. Inadequate pancreatic enzyme secretion can cause weight loss, loss of appetite, abdominal bloating and pain, flatulence and changes in the appearance and frequency of stools. Diarrhoea and steatorrhoea (fat in the faeces) are common, and faeces may be pale, bulky, foul-smelling and float in the toilet bowl.

  Pancreatic enzymes are usually enteric-coated, to enable them to pass through the stomach intact and be viable in the duodenum. However, if stomach pH temporarily rises above 6.0, the enteric coating disintegrates and releases the enzymes. Pancreatic lipase becomes irreversibly inactivated at a pH of less than 4.0, and can be destroyed if it is released prematurely and stomach pH subsequently falls. Patients with abdominal pain caused by chronic pancreatitis have reported greater pain relief on non-enteric coated preparations, which are usually given with stomach acid-inhibiting medication. The dose of pancreatic enzymes, measured by lipase content, is 25 000–80 000 lipase units (LipU) per meal for adults with pancreatic insufficiency. For infants and children, the dose is 500–10 000 LipU, and the maximum daily dose is 10 000 LipU/kg/bodyweight.
- *Bromelain* is a naturally occurring protein-digesting enzyme derived from the stems of pineapple plants, which appears to be absorbed intact and also may produce systemic effects. Bromelain remains active in a pH of 4.5–9.8 and the supplementary dose is 1000–1600 mg daily.
- *Papain* is a naturally occurring protease derived from paw paw (papaya) fruit latex. It is also available as a powder for tenderising meat before cooking because it helps to break down tough meat fibres. The supplementary dose is not well established.
- *Lactase* is useful for people with lactose intolerance who cannot produce the enzyme lactase. It is available as tilactase, which is commercially derived from the fungus *Aspergillus oryzae* by fermentation. It can be added to milk and milk products, or taken as a supplement with meals to reduce flatulence, bloating, abdominal pain and diarrhoea caused by undigested lactose in the digestive tract. The supplementary dose varies with individual needs.
- *Cellulase* refers to a class of enzymes that break down the plant fibre cellulose to beta-glucose. Humans cannot produce cellulases; they are produced chiefly by fungi, protozoa and bacteria. Fungi such as *Aspergillus oryzae* and bacteria are used for the commercial production of cellulase. The supplementary dose is not well established.

ACTIVITY MEASUREMENT

The Food Chemical Codex (FCC) has developed standardised units of measurement for digestive enzyme activity. In supplements, the activity of a specific enzyme is more important than the amount by weight.

- ***Amylase*** **activity is measured by dextrinising units (DU). One DU of amylase activity is defined as the amount of enzyme that will break down (dextrinise) soluble starch at the rate of 1 g per hour at 30°C.**
- ***Bromelain and papain*** **activity is measured by papain units (PU). One PU is the amount of enzyme that liberates the equivalent of 1 mcg of the amino acid tyrosine per hour from a casein (milk protein) substrate at pH 6.0 and 40°C.**
- ***Cellulase*** **activity is measured by cellulase units (CU). One CU is the amount of enzyme that will produce a relative fluidity change of one in five minutes in a fibre substrate at pH 4.5 and 40°C.**
- ***Lactase/tilactase*** **activity is measured by acid lactase units (ALU). One ALU is defined as the amount of enzyme that will liberate one micromole (μmol) of ortho-nitrophenol per minute from ortho-nitrophenyl-beta-D-galactopyranoside at pH 4.5 and 37°C.**
- ***Lipase*** **activity is measured by lipase units (LipU). One LipU is defined as the amount of enzyme that will liberate the equivalent of one μmol of acid per minute from an olive oil substrate at pH 6.5 and 30°C.**
- ***Protease*** **activity is measured by haemoglobin units on a tyrosine basis (HUT). One HUT is defined as the amount of enzyme that produces a hydrolysate from denatured haemoglobin in one minute at pH 4.7 and 40°C, which is similar to a hydrolysate produced by a specific solution of tyrosine and hydrochloric acid.**

Digestive function testing

Bowel bacteria produce hydrogen and methane when exposed to unabsorbed sugars and other carbohydrates, and these are absorbed and exhaled. The hydrogen/methane breath test is used to measure the amount of these gases breathed out, which rises when digestion is compromised. During the test, a base level of breath gases is measured and then gases are measured again after ingestion of a sugar. High breath gases can indicate an intolerance to dietary sugars such as lactose, lactulose, sucrose, fructose and sorbitol, an over-growth of bacteria in the small intestine, or an excessively rapid passage of food through the intestine.

Uses

Betaine hydrochloride and digestive enzymes are used to support digestion and relieve digestive disorders, including heartburn, reflux, stomach pain, abdominal pain, nausea, bloating, burping, flatulence, constipation and diarrhoea, and may relieve digestive symptoms of food intolerances and mild food allergies.[1] Digestive enzymes are used for cystic fibrosis, gastritis, pancreatitis, bile insufficiency, small bowel bacterial overgrowth, irritable bowel syndrome (IBS)—especially if diarrhoea is a prominent feature—inflammatory bowel diseases, diabetes, human immunodeficiency virus (HIV) and nutritional anaemias, and also after bowel or stomach surgery. Older people may benefit from digestive support because stomach acid and pancreatic enzyme production often decline with age. In coeliac patients, digestive enzymes may be useful together with a gluten-free diet to improve absorption of nutrients during the period when the small intestine is recovering from gluten toxicity.

In people with non-anaphylactic food allergies, pancreatic enzymes have markedly reduced the severity of food-induced symptoms, especially digestive symptoms.[2] Proteases reduce inflammation and pain, possibly by improving the breakdown of allergenic proteins in the diet. In patients with rheumatic diseases, proteases have been found to have pain-relieving and anti-inflammatory effects, and pancreatic enzymes, papain and bromelain are potentially useful for the relief of chronic inflammatory disorders such as arthritis.[3] Bromelain has anti-inflammatory activity, and helps to maintain a healthy cardiovascular system and immune response.[4] It can also help recovery after surgery, remove damaged tissue in wounds, enhance wound healing, relieve fluid retention and sinusitis, and dissolve clots, and has anticancer activity in cell and animal studies.[5] Papain appears to have similar activity to bromelain.[6] The betaine component of betaine hydrochloride acts as a methyl donor, and betaine is used to lower homocysteine levels by enhancing its conversion to methionine.[7]

REFERENCES

1. Roxas, M.,The role of enzyme supplementation in digestive disorders, *Altern Med Rev* (2008), 13(4): 307–14.
2. Raithel, M. et al., Pancreatic enzymes: A new group of antiallergic drugs?, *Inflamm Res* (2002), 51(Suppl 1): S13–14.
3. Leipner, J., Iten, F., & Saller, R., Therapy with proteolytic enzymes in rheumatic disorders, *BioDrugs* (2001), 15(12): 779–89.
4. Kelly, G., Bromelain: A literature review and discussion of its therapeutic applications, *Altern Med Rev* (1996), 1(4): 243–57.
5. Maurer, H.R., Bromelain: Biochemistry, pharmacology and medical use, *Cell Mol Life Sci* (2001), 58(9): 1234–45.
6. Mamboya, E.A.F., Papain, a plant enzyme of biological importance: A review, *Am J Biochem Biotech* (2012), 8(2): 99–104.
7. McRae, M.P., Betaine supplementation decreases plasma homocysteine in healthy adult participants: A meta-analysis, *J Chiropr Med* (2013), 12(1): 20–5.

Cautions

Betaine hydrochloride and digestive enzymes should be taken during a meal so that they mix well with the food ingested. Digestive enzymes are generally well tolerated if taken as directed, and should be stored in cool conditions to ensure viability. Betaine hydrochloride and digestive enzymes have no effect on food allergies that trigger anaphylactic reactions, and people with these types of food allergies must avoid the allergenic food completely. Betaine hydrochloride and pepsin supplements are best taken with a regular-sized meal because they can cause heartburn if taken on an empty stomach or with only a small amount of food. They are not recommended for people on proton pump-inhibiting drugs (drugs designed to suppress stomach acid production) or people with a gastric ulcer because they increase stomach acid. If a burning sensation occurs after taking betaine hydrochloride, it can be relieved by drinking one or two glasses of water or soda water to dilute the acid. Bromelain has a blood-thinning effect, and should be used with caution before surgery and in people on blood-thinning medication.

PROBIOTICS

FAST FACTS . . . PROBIOTICS

- **Probiotics are live micro-organisms that live in the digestive tract and provide health benefits.**
- **They include coliforms, bacteroides, lacto-bacilli and enterococci.**
- **Supplementation may be helpful for maintaining bowel health, and for relieving diarrhoea, *Helicobacter pylori* stomach infections, irritable bowel syndrome and colitis.**

Probiotics are live micro-organisms that inhabit the digestive tract and provide health benefits. They survive digestion and pass into the colon, where they grow, fermenting indigestible carbohydrates, such as fibre, for energy. Probiotics are named according to the genus, the species and the strain, which usually consists of letters and/or numbers—for example, *Lactobacillus* (genus name) *rhamnosus* (species name) GG (strain name).

To act as a probiotic, a micro-organism must be able to:

- resist destruction by stomach acid and bile
- adhere to the gastrointestinal tract
- remain metabolically active in the gastrointestinal tract
- inhibit the growth of disease-causing (pathogenic) bacteria, and
- make the colon more acidic (reduce colon pH).

Common microbes that meet these criteria are the bacteria lactobacilli, bifidobacteria and *Streptococcus thermophilus*, and the yeast *Saccharomyces cerevisiae*.

Bacteria found in the healthy digestive system

The healthy upper gastrointestinal tract contains a much lower count of bacteria than the colon because gastric acid, bile salts and digestive enzymes suppress growth, and the more vigorous digestive tract movements reduce the ability of bacteria to adhere to the lining. Upper intestinal tract bacteria consist mainly of small amounts of lactobacilli and enterococci. The lower part of the small intestine contains greater numbers of bacteria, such as coliforms, bacteroides, lactobacilli and enterococci. The colon has the most bacteria, the predominant species being anaerobic bacteroides, anaerobic methanogenic bacteria and anaerobic lactic acid bacteria of the genus bifidobacterium (*Bifidobacterium bifidum*), with smaller numbers of enterococci, clostridia and lactobacilli.

Colonisation of the digestive tract

At birth, the entire intestinal tract is sterile and bacterial colonisation begins with the first feed. In breastfed infants, more than 90 per cent of bowel bacteria are bifidobacteria, with small amounts of enterobacteriaceae and enterococci, and only traces of bacteroides, staphylococci, lactobacilli and clostridia. Breast milk contains a growth factor that enhances growth of bifidobacteria, which then competitively inhibits growth of pathogens. In contrast, bifidobacteria are not the main species present in formula-fed infants. As solid foods and cow's milk are introduced, enterics, bacteroides, enterococci, lactobacilli and clostridia levels increase.

Actions

Probiotics have the following actions in the body:

- *Colon health*. Probiotic fermentation produces short-chain fatty acids (SCFAs), and also lactic acid, methane, hydrogen and carbon dioxide. SCFAs support the health of the colon lining cells (colonocytes) by providing a fuel source and helping to regulate their growth. Butyric acid produced by probiotic fermentation in the gut helps maintain normal cell development and induces apoptosis of abnormal cells.

- *Immunity enhancement, suppression of pathogens.* Probiotics boost immune defence by increasing production of protective mucin that reduces the ability of pathogens to adhere to the gut wall and invade tissues, and by binding to the bowel lining and triggering activity of immune defence cells and production of antibodies. Probiotics produce pathogen-inhibitory substances, such as defensins, bacteriocins, microcins, hydrogen peroxide and nitric oxide (NO), which stimulate immune defence and inhibit bacterial signalling, pathogen growth and attachment to the bowel lining, and the action of microbial toxins. They compete with pathogens for nutrients and for adherence to the bowel lining, and maintain the integrity of the bowel, helping to protect against 'leaky gut', a condition in which the gut is more permeable to microbes, toxins and allergens. Probiotics can inhibit growth of pathogens such as *Clostridium perfringens* and *Escherichia coli*, common causes of bowel infections, *Helicobacter pylori*, responsible for stomach inflammation and ulcers, and *Candida albicans*, responsible for thrush infections.
- *Anti-inflammatory and anti-allergy activity.* Probiotics have anti-inflammatory activity in the bowel by inhibiting the expression of genes for inflammatory cytokines and chemokines, and inhibiting the nuclear factor kappaB (NF-kappaB) pathway that promotes inflammation. Probiotics such as lactobacilli or bifidobacteria may relieve hypersensitivity reactions by breaking down or altering the structure of allergy-triggering substances (antigens), suppressing production of inflammatory chemicals and assisting the normal development of the immune system in infants after birth.
- *Protection against urinary tract and vaginal infections.* Oral lactobacilli and bifidobacteria species have been shown to have protective effects in the urinary tract and vagina. They can help restore normal vaginal bacteria and suppress the growth of pathogens in the urinary and reproductive tracts.
- *Nutrient production and preservation.* Probiotics can help preserve antioxidants and vitamins ingested in food, and some species can synthesise vitamins B1, B2, B6, B12 and K in the gut. However, these vitamins may not be well absorbed from the colon and may be lost in faeces.

Dietary sources

Probiotics are found in cultured dairy products, such as yoghurt, sour milk, buttermilk, leben, fromage frais, quark and kefir, and other fermented foods, such as tempeh and sauerkraut. Probiotics ferment indigestible components of plant foods in order to obtain energy. Food components that are fermented by probiotics are called prebiotics, and include soluble dietary fibre, sugar alcohols, resistant starch and oligosaccharides, such as fructans, fructo-oligosaccharides and inulin. Prebiotics have beneficial effects by selectively stimulating the growth and/or activity of probiotics. Whole grains, legumes, nuts, seeds, fruit and vegetables are good sources of prebiotics.

Supplements, uses and dose

Probiotic supplements are mainly available as lactobacillus and bifidobacterium species and *Saccharomyces cerevisiae* in powder and capsule formulations. Most products containing live organisms should be kept refrigerated to ensure viability. Some products contain probiotics that are micro-encapsulated with natural plant material, and can remain viable when stored at room temperature. The supplementary daily dose is not well established, but is likely to be one billion (10^9) to one trillion (10^{12}) or more live organisms, referred to as colony-forming units (CFU). Doses used in clinical trials are one billion (10^9) to 100 billion (10^{11}) CFU two or three times daily.

The results of clinical trials relate to the specific strain of probiotics used, and may not be applicable to all organisms of the same species. Lactobacilli are associated with vaginal health in women, and probiotics have been found to have anti-tumour activity in animals. Probiotics may be useful for the prevention of diarrhoea, including childhood, traveller's and antibiotic-induced diarrhoea.[1,2] The most effective strains appear to be *Lactobacillus* GG and *Saccharomyces boulardii*, and *S. boulardii*, and a mixture of *Lactobacillus acidophilus* and *Bifidobacterium bifidum* has been shown to prevent traveller's diarrhoea. Probiotics may relieve some symptoms of *Helicobacter pylori* stomach infections, and *S. boulardii* appears to help eradicate the infection.[3] *Bifidobacterium infantis* 35624 has been found to relieve IBS symptoms.[3] Patients with ulcerative colitis (UC) have been found to have reductions in bifidobacteria and lactobacilli in the colon, and *Lactobacillus paracasei* has anti-inflammatory activity in UC.[3] A probiotic mixture containing lactobacilli, bifidobacteria and *S.*

thermophilus (VSL#3) used with orthodox treatment has induced remission in UC patients.[3] A combination of bifidobacteria and *Lactobacillus acidophilus* has reduced the incidence and mortality rate of severe intestinal inflammation (necrotising enterocolitis) in premature infants.[3] *Lactobacillus* GG used in pregnant and lactating women has been shown to reduce the risk of eczema in infants, but there is insufficient evidence about the effects of probiotics on other allergic diseases.[3] *Streptococcus thermophilus*, *Lactobacillus bulgaricus* and other lactobacilli used in fermented milk products can provide sufficient lactase to enable lactose digestion in people with lactose intolerance.[4] *Lactobacillus sporogenes* has been associated with a reduction in total and LDL cholesterol in a human study.[4]

Cautions

Probiotics are generally well tolerated.

REFERENCES

1 Guandalini, S., Probiotics for prevention and treatment of diarrhea, *J Clin Gastroenterol* (2011), 45 (Suppl): S149–53.

2 McFarland, L.V., Meta-analysis of probiotics for the prevention of traveler's diarrhea, *Travel Med Infect Dis* (2007), 5(2): 97–105.

3 Gogineni, V.K., Morrow, L.E. & Malesker, M.A., Probiotics: Mechanisms of action and clinical applications, *J Prob Health* (2013), 1(1): 1–11.

4 Parvez, S., Malik, K.A., Ah Kang, S. & Kim, H.Y., Probiotics and their fermented food products are beneficial for health, *J Appl Microbiol* (2006), 100(6): 1171–85.

ARTHRITIS BIOACTIVES

FAST FACTS . . . ARTHRITIS BIOACTIVES

- **Arthritis bioactives include glucosamine, chondroitin sulfate, methylsulfonylmethane and green-lipped mussel.**
- **Glucosamine and chondroitin sulfate are part of connective tissue structures in joint cartilage.**
- **Methylsulfonylmethane is a sulfur-containing substance that has anti-inflammatory activity.**
- **Green-lipped mussel has anti-inflammatory and antioxidant activity.**
- **Arthritis bioactives may be useful for relieving the symptoms of osteoarthritis, such as joint pain, swelling and stiffness.**

Arthritis bioactives include glucosamine, chondroitin sulfate (CS), methylsulfonylmethane (MSM) and green-lipped mussel. They help to maintain the integrity of connective tissue structures in joint cartilage and reduce inflammation. Joint cartilage is a tough, smooth substance that covers the ends of bones in joints, and allows smooth and flexible joint movements (see Figure 14.1). It is made up of cells (chondrocytes) that produce a surrounding matrix of strengthening collagen and carbohydrate–protein complexes (proteoglycans) that attract and trap water. Chondrocytes also secrete enzymes that stimulate the breakdown of old tissue and replacement with new.

Proteoglycans in cartilage consist of glycosaminoglycans (GAGs, previously called mucopolysaccharides) attached to proteins (see Figure 14.2). GAGs include CS, keratan sulfate and hyaluronic acid, and are made up of chains of glucosamine, galactose and glucuronic acid units (see Figure 14.3). GAGs are made by chondrocytes and are secreted into the extracellular matrix, in which CS and keratan sulfate attach to protein chains to form proteoglycans. Proteoglycans have a structure similar to a bottlebrush, with chondroitin sulphate and keratan sulphate making up the bristles, and they function to attract and trap water. Proteoglycans are anchored to long chains of hyaluronic acid and interwoven with rope-like collagen fibres. Cartilage does not have a blood supply, and receives nutrients through a process of diffusion, in which nutrients diffuse out from blood vessels in the synovial membranes (membranes lining the joint cavity).

In early osteoarthritis (OA), chondrocytes begin dividing excessively, and become very active, producing increased amounts of proteoglycans and cartilage that fails to mature normally. As the disease progresses,

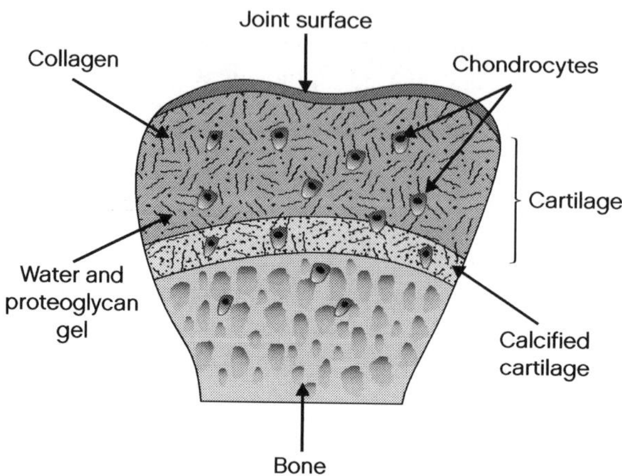

Figure 14.1 Joint cartilage

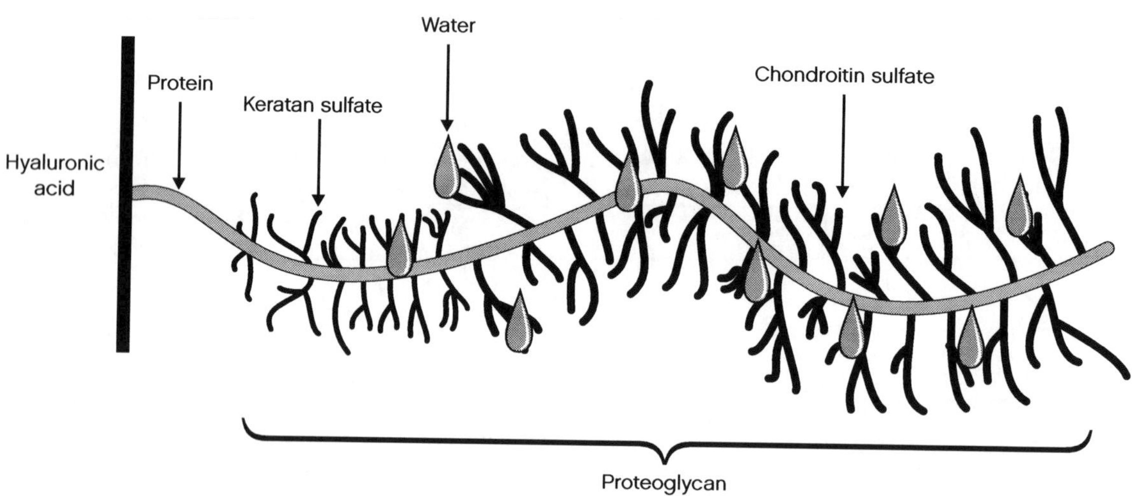

Figure 14.2 Structure of a proteoglycan

inflammatory cytokines and eicosanoids are produced and enzymes that break down cartilage become overactive. Eventually, more cartilage is broken down than can be repaired, bone surfaces become exposed, bone spurs develop and the inflammatory process continues, causing ongoing tissue destruction, swelling, pain, stiffness and loss of movement.

Glucosamine

Glucosamine is a naturally occurring substance made from glucose and the amino acid glutamine by connective tissue cells in the body. It is required for the synthesis of GAGs in the connective tissue that is part of tendons, ligaments, cartilage, synovial fluid, mucous membranes, the eyes, blood vessels and heart valves.

Actions

Glucosamine is responsible for joint cartilage maintenance and repair in the body. In cell studies, glucosamine has been shown to stimulate proteoglycan and GAG production in joint tissue, normalise cartilage metabolism, rebuild experimentally damaged cartilage,

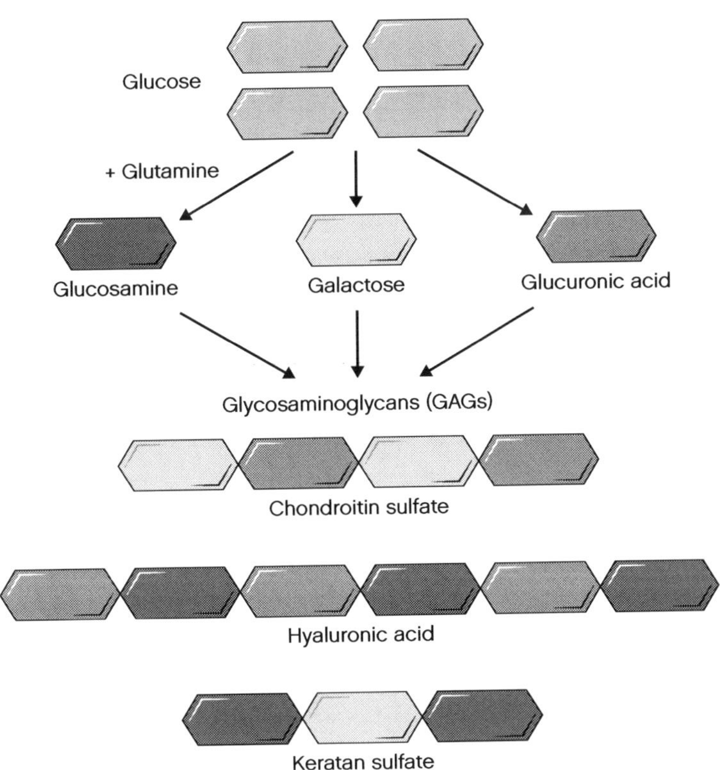

Figure 14.3 Synthesis of glycosaminoglycans

and to have antioxidant and anti-inflammatory properties. It inhibits inflammatory mediators such as NF-kappaB, NO, cyclooxygenase-2 (COX-2) and matrix metalloproteinases in OA tissue, and prevents expression of genes for osteoclasts that break down the bone surrounding joints.

Dietary sources

There is very little in the diet because the main source of glucosamine is the inedible shells of shellfish.

Supplements, uses and dose

Glucosamine is available as glucosamine sulfate or glucosamine hydrochloride, and is extracted from chitin found in the shells of crustaceans, such as crabs, prawns and lobsters. Glucosamine is also a constituent of shark cartilage. The manufacturing process involves extraction of the protein component of the shells by alkalis or enzymes, and removal of minerals and lipids. Glucosamine is extracted from the resulting chitosan by hydrochloric acid, and filtered to remove pigments, forming glucosamine hydrochloride crystals. Glucosamine sulfate is made from glucosamine hydrochloride by adding either potassium or sodium sulfate. Glucosamine can also be produced by fermentation using genetically engineered micro-organisms. Vegetarian glucosamine is usually manufactured from glucose extracted from maize starch or by microbial fermentation.

Glucosamine sulfate is unstable, and requires the incorporation of potassium chloride or sodium chloride to reduce oxidation and water absorption during storage. Glucosamine hydrochloride does not need an added stabiliser, and therefore provides a more concentrated dose of glucosamine—about 24 per cent more than in the glucosamine sulfate potassium chloride form. Glucosamine sulfate, glucosamine sulfate–potassium chloride complex, glucosamine sulfate–sodium chloride complex and glucosamine hydrochloride are oral supplements permitted for use in Australia, and acetylglucosamine is permitted for topical use only.

Glucosamine itself appears to be the active component, not the salt carrier. The sulfate or hydrochloride salt is split off in the stomach, leaving the glucosamine base that is absorbed into enterocytes. Most clinical trials to date have used glucosamine sulfate, while most veterinary studies have used the hydrochloride form. A study of glucosamine sulfate and glucosamine hydrochloride found that both forms of glucosamine were equally effective in osteoarthritis of the knee, and both forms have equal absorption rates.[1] However, the bioavailability of glucosamine is believed to be low (about 26 per cent). The metabolism of glucosamine in the body is not well understood.

Glucosamine has been used in a large number of clinical trials for OA, some of which have shown that it relieves pain and stiffness, and reduces progressive loss of cartilage. Studies sponsored by a European producer of glucosamine sulfate (Rottapharm, Italy) have reported positive results, but a meta-analysis that excluded these studies found that glucosamine had no effect on symptoms of OA.[2] However, this meta-analysis did report some positive results. In four trials that compared glucosamine with non-steroidal anti-inflammatories, a glucosamine preparation was found to be superior in two and equivalent in two, and the same preparation was able to slow radiological progression of OA of the knee over a three-year period. A comparison trial of glucosamine and the non-steroidal anti-inflammatories ibuprofen and piroxicam for OA found that glucosamine was effective and better tolerated.[3] A review of clinical trials that measured changes in joint structure has found evidence that glucosamine can reduce the risk of progression of OA by 54 per cent.[4] Researchers have recommended that glucosamine and chondroitin should be used as viable first-line treatment options for knee OA, especially for patients who are sensitive to anti-inflammatory medication.[5]

In the Glucosamine/Chondroitin Arthritis Intervention Trial (GAIT) of patients with knee OA, overall results showed that glucosamine hydrochloride and CS were not significantly better than placebo in reducing knee pain by 20 per cent.[6] However, there was a significant improvement in a sub-group of patients with moderate to severe knee pain who took glucosamine with chondroitin, and a trend towards a greater rate of response to glucosamine (3.9 per cent greater), chondroitin (5.3 per cent greater) and combined glucosamine with chondroitin (6.5 per cent greater) than for placebo. Limitations of this study include the use of subjective measures of effectiveness, the selection of an arbitrary 20 per cent improvement in symptom scores and the subjects' relatively mild degree of OA pain. The authors subsequently admitted that the outcome measures did not behave as rigorously as expected, and may not have been sensitive enough to measure mild pain.[7]

Overall, the use of glucosamine for OA is controversial. Anecdotal reports are that it is very effective in some, but not all, individuals with OA. The supplementary dose is 1500 mg daily, and it may be more effective when taken in combination with CS. It is slow acting and should be trialled for up to three months before an assessment of its effectiveness is made.

REFERENCES

1. Owens, S., Wagner, P. & Vangsness, C.T. Jr, Recent advances in glucosamine and chondroitin supplementation, *J Knee Surg* (2004), 17(4): 185–93.
2. Towheed, T.E., Maxwell, L., Anastassiades, T.P. et al., Glucosamine therapy for treating osteoarthritis, *Cochrane Database Syst Rev* (2005), 2: CD002946.
3. Matheson, A.J. & Perry, C.M., Glucosamine: A review of its use in the management of osteoarthritis, *Drugs Aging* (2003), 20: 1041–60.
4. Poolsup, N., Suthisisang, C., Channark, P. & Kittikulsuth, W., Glucosamine long-term treatment and the progression of knee osteoarthritis: Systematic review of randomized controlled trials, *Ann Pharmacother* (2005), 39(6): 1080–7.
5. Richy, F., Bruyere, O., Cucherat, M. et al., Structural and symptomatic efficacy of glucosamine and chondroitin in knee osteoarthritis, *Arch Intern Med* (2003), 163: 1514–22.
6. Clegg, D.O., Reda, D.J., Harris, C.L. et al., Glucosamine, chondroitin sulphate, and the two in combination for painful knee osteoarthritis, *N Engl J Med* (2006), 354(8): 795–808.
7. Clegg, D.O. & Reda, D.J., Glucosamine and chondroitin sulfate for knee osteoarthritis: correspondence—authors' reply, *N Engl J Med* (2006), 354(20): 2184–5.

Cautions

Glucosamine generally appears to be well tolerated. Side-effects are mild, and include nausea, heartburn, diarrhoea and constipation, and—rarely—drowsiness, skin reactions and headache. People on low-potassium or low-sodium diets should use glucosamine hydrochloride, which does not contain potassium or sodium chloride. People with shellfish allergy should use vegetarian glucosamine. Almost all studies to date have been on OA of the knee, and it is not known whether glucosamine is of benefit for other types of OA.

In cell studies and studies of rats using infused (but not oral) glucosamine, it has increased activity of the hexosamine biosynthesis pathway that modulates insulin sensitivity and glucose uptake in peripheral tissues. This has led to concerns that glucosamine may adversely affect glucose metabolism in people with impaired glucose tolerance or diabetes. A review of eleven human studies found that four studies reported decreased insulin sensitivity or increased fasting glucose in subjects taking glucosamine, but there were limitations in the design of the studies and, overall, the reviewers were not able to come to a conclusion. Other reviews have concluded that, on the available evidence, glucosamine does not affect glucose or insulin metabolism.

Chondroitin sulfate

Chondroitin sulfate (CS) is a naturally occurring substance consisting of galactosamine and glucuronic acid, which is made in the body by connective tissue cells. It is a GAG that is part of the water-holding proteoglycans in the extracellular matrix of joint cartilage. CS is commonly used with glucosamine for OA.

Actions

CS has the following actions in the body:

- *Maintenance and repair of joint cartilage.* CS works with the other GAGs, keratan sulfate and hyaluronic acid, to hold water in the cartilage of joints and maintain cartilage integrity. It has beneficial effects on the metabolism of chondrocytes, synoviocytes (cells in the synovial lining in joints) and bone cells surrounding joints. It promotes chondrocyte survival, increases synthesis of type II collagen and proteoglycans by chondrocytes, and reduces activity of enzymes that break down cartilage.
- *Anti-inflammatory activity.* CS inhibits the activation of NF-kappaB and its translocation to the nucleus, thereby reducing the expression of inflammatory genes.
- *Nerve function support.* CS proteoglycans, as part of the extracellular matrix, play a role in nervous tissue structure, cell signalling, the development and survival of nerve cells and central nervous system (CNS) function.

Dietary sources

CS is found in the gristle of meat and the bones of sharks, and is not present in significant quantities in food.

Supplements, uses and dose

Most CS supplements are extracted from shark cartilage or bovine (cow) trachea by chemical hydrolysis, breakdown of the proteoglycan core, elimination of proteins, and recovery and purification of CS. CS can also be sourced from birds, sheep and pigs. About 70 per cent of oral CS is absorbed after first being broken down to saccharides during digestion. Absorption of intact CS is low, ranging from zero to 12 per cent, depending on the molecular weight of the type of chondroitin used. Bovine tracheal CS has a lower molecular weight, whereas shark cartilage CS has a higher molecular weight. It is estimated that 5 per cent of a 4 g dose of bovine CS and 2.5 per cent of a 4 g dose of shark CS is absorbed. CS and calcium, sodium and potassium salts of CS derived from bovine or shark sources are permitted in Australian supplements. Special approval is required for the use of bovine CS if sourced from countries where bovine spongiform encephalopathy ('mad cow' disease) has occurred.

In animal models of OA, CS inhibits oedema, synovitis and destruction of joint cartilage in a dose-dependent manner and slows arthritis progression.[1] Human trials have reported that CS relieves symptoms of OA, such as pain and loss of function, and causes a small reduction in the rate of deterioration of joint cartilage.[2] CS intake is associated with an average 50 per cent improvement in symptoms, such as pain, walking time, pain medication use and joint mobility.[3] Avian CS (1000 mg/day) and bovine CS (1200 mg/day) have been shown to be equally effective for pain relief and functional improvement in patients with knee OA.[4] Improvements were noted at week six and persisted over the six-month study period.

The anti-inflammatory activity of CS may be useful for inflammatory bowel and skin diseases, atherosclerosis, Parkinson's disease, Alzheimer's disease, multiple sclerosis, amyotrophic lateral sclerosis (motor neurone disease), rheumatoid arthritis and systemic lupus erythematosus.[5]

In eleven patients with OA and psoriasis, CS (800 mg daily for two months) led to dramatic skin improvements, including reduced swelling, redness, flaking and itching, and increased skin hydration and softness, with psoriasis completely clearing in one patient.[6] A larger study of patients with OA and psoriasis found that CS (800 mg daily for three months) relieved both OA and skin symptoms.[7] Animal studies have found that CS may benefit inflammatory bowel disease and prevent post-surgical adhesions.[8] The supplementary dose is 800–1200 mg daily, and a single daily dose appears to have the same efficacy as divided doses. It is a slow-acting supplement, and should be used for at least three months before assessing its efficacy.

REFERENCES

1 Volpi, N., Anti-inflammatory activity of chondroitin sulphate: New functions from an old natural macromolecule, *Inflammopharmacology* (2011), 19(6): 299–306.

2 Hochberg, M., Chevalier, X., Henrotin, Y. et al., Symptom and structure modification in osteoarthritis with pharmaceutical-grade chondroitin sulfate: What's the evidence? *Curr Med Res Opin* (2013), 29(3): 259–67.

3 Leeb, B.F., Schweitzer, H., Montag, K. & Smolen, J.S., A metaanalysis of chondroitin sulfate in the treatment of osteoarthritis, *J Rheumatol* (2000), 27(1): 205–11.

4 Fardellone, P., Zaim, M., Saurel, A.S. & Maheu, E., Comparative efficacy and safety study of two chondroitin sulfate preparations from different origin (avian and bovine) in symptomatic osteoarthritis of the knee, *Open Rheumatol J* (2013), 7: 1–12.

5 Vallières, M. & du Souich, P., Modulation of inflammation by chondroitin sulfate, *Osteoarthritis Cartilage* (2010), 18(Suppl 1): S1–6.

6 Vergés, J., Montell, E., Herrero, M. et al., Clinical and histopathological improvement of psoriasis with oral chondroitin sulfate: A serendipitous finding, *Dermatol Online J* (2005), 11(1): 31.

7 Möller, I., Pérez, M., Monfort, J. et al., Effectiveness of chondroitin sulphate in patients with concomitant knee osteoarthritis and psoriasis: A randomized, double-blind, placebo-controlled study, *Osteoarthritis Cartilage* (2010), 18(Suppl 1): S32–40.

8 [No authors listed], Chondroitin sulfates monograph, *Altern Med Rev* (2006), 11(4): 338–43.

Cautions

CS is well tolerated, and adverse effects, which include mild dyspepsia or nausea, are rare. People with seafood allergy should not use CS derived from shark cartilage.

Methylsulfonylmethane

Methylsulfonylmethane (MSM), also known as dimethyl sulfone and methyl sulfone, is the oxidised form of dimethyl sulfoxide (DMSO). DMSO and MSM occur naturally in the environment, and are taken up by plants from soil. MSM is about 34 per cent sulfur, which may be useful for the formation of sulfur-containing structures in joint cartilage. The main use of MSM is for the relief of OA symptoms.

Actions

MSM has shown anti-inflammatory, pain-relieving and antioxidant activity in the body. In cell studies, MSM significantly inhibited activity of the key inflammatory mediator NF-kappaB, which led to reduced expression of the inflammatory enzymes inducible nitric oxide synthase (iNOS) and COX-2 and reduced production of prostaglandin E_2 (PGE_2), interleukin-6 (IL-6) and tumour necrosis factor-alpha (TNF-alpha).

Dietary sources

MSM is found in cow's milk, coffee, beer, tomatoes, tea, silverbeet, corn, alfalfa and the herb horsetail (*Equisetum arvense*).

Supplements, uses and dose

MSM is the supplement form, which is commercially produced from DMSO derived from wood pulp. MSM is produced from a reaction between DMSO and hydrogen peroxide. In an animal model of OA, MSM intake for thirteen weeks has been shown to decrease degeneration of the cartilage in knee joints in a dose-dependent manner.[1] Several human studies have found that MSM relieves symptoms of mild to moderate OA of the knee. However, a trial of patients with knee OA who took MSM for twelve weeks found that it improved pain and physical function only slightly, which may not have been clinically relevant.[2] A meta-analysis of three clinical trials that used DMSO or MSM found that there was a slight improvement in pain in two trials and no effect in the other.[3] Overall, no effect was found on pain relief, but the studies had limitations, including inadequate trial length. A clinical trial found that individual and combination therapy with glucosamine and MSM produced relief of symptoms in osteoarthritis.[4] MSM and glucosamine used together were more effective in reducing pain and swelling, and improving joint mobility, and relief was more rapid than individual use.

A preliminary study found that MSM supplementation (2600 mg daily for 30 days) reduced symptoms associated with hayfever,[5] and MSM has reduced damage to the colon in an animal model of colitis.[6] Other animal studies show that MSM has potential for protecting the liver against toxins[7] and protecting against the development of autoimmune disease.[8] The supplementary dose is 4–6 g daily and, because it is a slow-acting supplement, three months' intake is recommended before assessing efficacy.

REFERENCES

1 Ezaki, J., Hashimoto, M., Hosokawa, Y. & Ishimi, Y., Assessment of safety and efficacy of methylsulfonylmethane on bone and knee joints in osteoarthritis animal model, *J Bone Miner Metab* (2013), 31(1): 16–25.

2 Debbi, E.M., Agar, G., Fichman, G. et al., Efficacy of methylsulfonylmethane supplementation on osteoarthritis of the knee: A randomized controlled study, *BMC Complement Altern Med* (2011), 11: 50.

3 Brien, S., Prescott, P. & Lewith, G., Meta-analysis of the related nutritional supplements dimethyl sulfoxide and methylsulfonylmethane in the treatment of osteoarthritis of the knee, *Evid Based Complement Alternat Med* (2011): 528403.

4 Usha, P.R. & Naidu, M.U.R., Randomised, double-blind, parallel, placebo-controlled study of oral glucosamine, methylsulfonylmethane and their combination in osteoarthritis, *Clin Drug Invest* (2004), 24: 353–63.

5 Barrager, E., Veltmann, J.R. Jr, Schauss, A.G. & Schiller, R.N., A multicentered, open-label trial on the safety and efficacy of methylsulfonylmethane in the treatment of seasonal allergic rhinitis, *J Altern Complement Med* (2002), 8(2): 167–73.

6 Amirshahrokhi, K., Bohlooli, S. & Chinifroush, M.M., The effect of methylsulfonylmethane on the experimental colitis in the rat, *Toxicol Appl Pharmacol* (2011), 253(3): 197–202.

7 Kamel, R. & El Morsy, E.M., Hepatoprotective effect of methylsulfonylmethane against carbon tetrachloride-induced acute liver injury in rats, *Arch Pharm Res* (2013), 36(9): 1140–8.

8 Morton, J.I. & Siegel, B.V., Effects of oral dimethyl sulfoxide and dimethyl sulfone on murine autoimmune lymphoproliferative disease, *Proc Soc Exp Biol Med* (1986), 183: 227–30.

Cautions

MSM is generally well tolerated. Adverse effects are uncommon, but may include mild digestive upsets and skin rashes. Animal toxicity studies have shown only minor adverse effects at levels of intake that are five to seven times more than the human dose range. One case report has associated intake of multiple supplements, including MSM, with bilateral acute angle closure, a type of glaucoma. It was suggested that MSM may act like sulfonamides (sulfa drugs) that are known to precipitate this condition.

Green-lipped mussel

Green-lipped mussel (GLM) is a type of shellfish (*Perna canaliculus*) grown in New Zealand waters. Extracts of GLM may contain protein, peptides, lipids, minerals, betaine and connective tissue GAGs, including chondroitin sulfate, which are important for joint health. Lipids in GLM include sterols, sterol esters, triglycerides, phospholipids and free fatty acids, including the omega-3 fatty acids eicosapentaenoic acid (EPA) and docosahexaenoic acid (DHA). A family of polyunsaturated fatty acids (PUFAs) structurally related to omega-3 PUFAs has been identified in GLM lipids, including stearidonic acid (C18:4 n-3) and its derivative eicosatetraenoic acid (ETA) (C20:4 n-3), also found in echium (*Echium plantagineum*) oil and blackcurrant seed oil. ETA is a structural isomer of the omega-6 PUFA arachidonic acid (AA) (C20:4 n-6) and may competitively inhibit omega-6 metabolism. Furan fatty acids (F-acids), found in algae and salmon, have been discovered in GLM.

Actions

GLM is mainly used for the relief of symptoms of OA. It has the following actions in the body:

- *Anti-inflammatory activity.* In cell and animal studies, lipid extracts of GLM have been shown to reduce levels of inflammatory chemicals by competitively inhibiting AA metabolism, and have more potent anti-inflammatory activity than flaxseed, evening primrose or fish oils. The free fatty acid fraction and purified PUFA extracts of GLM are potent inhibitors of the enzymes COX-1 and COX-2, which produce inflammatory eicosanoids, such as PGE_2, from AA in cell membranes. GLM lipids also inhibit the enzyme 5-lipoxygenase (5-LOX), and thereby inhibit production of inflammatory leukotrienes. F-acids have potent free radical-scavenging activity, and may be more effective anti-inflammatories than EPA.
- *Antioxidant and anti-ageing activity.* Mussel oligopeptides may protect against cellular ageing induced by hydrogen peroxide by increasing production of the antioxidant enzyme glutathione peroxidase, improving mitochondrial function and stimulating expression of the antioxidant peroxiredoxin 1 (Prx1) and the expression of sirtuin 1 (SIRT1). SIRT1 is a protein that stimulates mitochondrial metabolism and antioxidant protection, and has life extension effects on cells.

Supplements, uses and dose

Perna canaliculus mussels are grown in licensed marine farms in New Zealand. Supplements include freeze-dried concentrated powder and lipid extracts, which can be produced by steaming the shells to open the mussels and then freeze-drying and grinding the meat; grinding the entire mussel and shell, separating out the shell by centrifuging and freeze-drying the meat; or mechanical removal of the meat and cold extraction, which preserves the activity of the lipids. Stabilisation, which may utilise oxalic acid or tartaric acid, is an important step for preserving beneficial lipids because the lipid fraction oxidises quickly after harvesting.

GLM has antimicrobial, blood pressure-lowering, blood-thinning, immune-modulating and anti-inflammatory activity. GLM has been found to help reduce pain, swelling and stiffness, and improve joint function in people with rheumatoid arthritis (RhA) and OA. A study of OA and RhA patients compared stabilised GLM powder (1150 mg/day) and stabilised GLM lipid extract (210 mg/day) for three months.[1] Both interventions led to improvements in morning stiffness and measures of joint tenderness and joint function in OA and RhA patients. In a pilot study of OA patients, GLM extract (3000 mg/day for eight weeks) improved knee joint pain, stiffness and mobility, as well as improving gastrointestinal function.[2] A review of clinical trials found that only two trials met the reviewers' criteria, and these indicated that GLM was effective for relieving symptoms of mild to moderate OA.[3]

In an animal model of colitis, stabilised GLM lipid extract reduced inflammatory damage to the bowel, and may have potential for relieving symptoms of inflammatory bowel disease.[4] Freeze-dried GLM powder has reduced damage to the gastric mucosa in animals caused by several non-steroidal anti-inflammatory drugs.[5] Stabilised GLM lipid extract taken by asthmatics has been found to relieve daytime wheeze, reduce the concentration of exhaled hydrogen peroxide and increase morning peak expiratory flow, a measure of breathing capacity.[6]

Lyprinol® is a patented stabilised lipid extract that contains 50 mg of GLM lipids and 100 mg olive oil per capsule, and the dose is 100–200 mg/day. The dose of GLM freeze-dried powder is about 1000 mg/day. In general, beneficial effects are noted after two to four weeks of treatment.

REFERENCES

1 Gibson, S.L.M. & Gibson, R.G., The treatment of arthritis with a lipid extract of Perna canaliculus: A randomized trial, *Complem Ther Med* (1998), 6(3): 122–6.

2 Coulson, S., Vecchio, P., Gramotnev, H. & Vitetta, L., Green-lipped mussel (Perna canaliculus) extract efficacy in knee osteoarthritis and improvement in gastrointestinal dysfunction: A pilot study, *Inflammopharmacology* (2012), 20(2): 71–6.

3 Brien, S., Prescott, P., Coghlan, B. et al., Systematic review of the nutritional supplement Perna canaliculus (green-lipped mussel) in the treatment of osteoarthritis, *QJM* (2008), 101(3): 167–79.
4 Tenikoff, D., Murphy, K.J., Le, M. et al., Lyprinol (stabilised lipid extract of New Zealand green-lipped mussel): A potential preventative treatment modality for inflammatory bowel disease, *J Gastroenterol* (2005), 40(4): 361–5.
5 Rainsford, K.D. & Whitehouse, M.W., Gastroprotective and anti-inflammatory properties of green lipped mussel (Perna canaliculus) preparation, *Arzneimittelforschung* (1980), 30(12): 2128–32.
6 Emelyanov, A., Fedoseev, G., Krasnoschekova, O. et al., Treatment of asthma with lipid extract of New Zealand green-lipped mussel: A randomised clinical trial, *Eur Respir J* (2002), 20(3): 596–600.

Cautions

GLM is generally well tolerated. Adverse effects are rare, and include mild gastrointestinal upsets. People with shellfish allergy should avoid GLM products.

FUNGI

FAST FACTS . . . FUNGI

- **Fungi used as health supplements include cordyceps, the mushrooms coriolus, maitake, reishi and shiitake, and brewer's yeast.**
- **Fungi contain potent immune-stimulating polysaccharides such as beta-glucans.**
- **Fungi may be useful for their immune-boosting, antimicrobial and anticancer activity.**

Fungi used as health supplements include the fungus cordyceps (*Ophiocordyceps sinensis*, also called *Cordyceps sinensis*), the mushrooms coriolus (*Coriolus versicolor*), maitake (*Grifola frondosa*), reishi (*Ganoderma lucidum*) and shiitake (*Lentinula edodes*), and brewer's yeast (*Saccharomyces cerevisiae*). In biology, yeasts belong to the fungi kingdom. Fungi are mainly used as general tonics, immune stimulants, for boosting mental and physical performance, for infections, immune disorders, diabetes, abnormal blood lipids and diseases of ageing, and to support cancer therapy.

Cordyceps (*Ophiocordyceps sinensis*)

Cordyceps, also called caterpillar fungus, is a fungus parasite that grows within a caterpillar, and is found mainly in North America, Europe and Asia. The caterpillar carcase and fungus is dried and used for medicinal purposes in Asia, where it is revered as a tonic to strengthen mind and body and aid recuperation, and for its anti-ageing activity. Bioactive ingredients in cordyceps include:

- extracellular and intracellular polysaccharides, including beta-glucans, that have immune, anti-oxidant and anti-tumour effects
- the immune-modulating nucleosides cordycepin, guanosine and adenosine
- the antioxidant and anti-inflammatory peptide cordymin
- the immune inhibitor myriocin
- the fatty acids pentadecanoic acid and palmitic acid, which may have a role in insulin release and immunity
- anti-inflammatory cordysinins
- the sterols sitosterol and ergosterol (provitamin D2) and a range of sterol esters that have cytotoxic and anti-tumour effects.

Actions

Cordyceps has a wide range of effects in the body, including heart, nerve, liver and kidney protection; improved function of the endocrine, cardiovascular and immune systems; and blood glucose and blood lipid regulation. It also has antioxidant, anti-ageing, anti-inflammatory, anti-thrombosis, anti-arrhythmia, anti-hypertension, performance-enhancing and anti-cancer properties.

Actions include:

- *Anticancer activity.* The anticancer activity of cordyceps includes direct cytotoxicity, immune stimulation, stimulation of anti-tumour natural killer (NK) cells, promotion of apoptosis, selective inhibition of RNA and protein synthesis, and antioxidant and antiviral activity. Cordyceps inhibits angiogenesis (the development of new blood vessels to supply a tumour) and tumour metastasis (spread of a tumour to other tissues of the body). In cell studies, cordycepin has inhibited cancer cell division by 55 per cent, with little effect on normal cells.

- *Immune modulation.* Cordyceps has both potentiating and suppressive effects on the immune system by regulating innate and adaptive immunity and modulating the gastrointestinal immune system.
- *Antioxidant activity.* Cordyceps has potent antioxidant activity, inhibiting lipid peroxidation and scavenging damaging superoxide anions and hydroxyl radicals in cell studies.
- *Blood glucose-lowering activity.* Cordyceps increases insulin sensitivity, lowers fasting serum glucose levels and diminishes insulin secretion after a carbohydrate challenge in animal studies.
- *Reproductive function.* Cordyceps is reported to have enhanced testosterone release in plasma, stimulated libido and sexual activity, and restored reproductive function in both sexes in human studies.
- *Anti-stress activity.* In animals, cordyceps has improved resistance to stress, increased efficiency of oxygen utilisation and decreased fatigue.

Supplements, uses and dose

Naturally occurring cordyceps is very rare, and natural substitutes such as *C. militaris*, *C. liangshanensis*, *C. gunnii* and *C. cicadicola*, as well as cultured *O. sinensis* and *C. militaris*, are used in supplements. It is cultured by surface and submerged fermentation processes. Cordyceps sinensis is approved for use in Australian supplements. Cordyceps has wide-ranging uses, particularly in Asian countries, where it is traditionally used to strengthen the lungs, kidneys and bone marrow, and for excess mucus, cough, anaemia, lower back pain, low libido, impotence, infertility, irregular menstruation, night sweats and weakness in the elderly. It is also used for elevated blood glucose, and respiratory, kidney, cardiovascular and liver disorders.

Most reports on the use of cordyceps are from studies conducted in China and Japan, and the results are summarised below.[1] It is reported that cordyceps, given with standard cancer treatment, has reduced tumour size in cancer patients and maintained white blood cell count, and has also increased the number of NK cells in leukaemia patients by 400 per cent. Older patients with fatigue are reported to show improvements in fatigue, cold intolerance, dizziness, frequent night urination, tinnitus, libido and memory, and increases in energy output and oxygen capacity during exercise. Cordyceps has reduced blood pressure and protein in the urine in patients with kidney disease, and assisted recovery of kidney function in patients with gentamicin-induced kidney damage. Diabetic patients have shown improved glucose tolerance on cordyceps treatment, and patients with liver disease have had improvements in liver function. Cordyceps has lowered total cholesterol by up to 21 per cent and triglycerides by up to 26 per cent, and increased HDL cholesterol by up to 30 per cent. The supplementary dose of cordyceps is 3–4.5 g/day, except in cases of severe liver disease, in which the dose is 6–9 g/day. It is generally used in conjunction with orthodox medical treatment.

REFERENCE

1 Holliday, J., Cleaver, M., Tajnik, M. et al., Cordyceps, *Encyclopedia of Dietary Supplements,* 2nd ed., CRC Press, Boca Raton, FL, 2010.

Cautions

Cordyceps is generally well tolerated. Rarely, dry mouth, nausea and diarrhoea have been reported. No toxicity has been reported in humans or animals. Cordyceps is priced by weight, and collectors of wild cordyceps have been known to insert lead or other metals to boost its weight; there are reported cases of lead poisoning from wild cordyceps products, but not from cultivated products.

Mushrooms

Mushrooms contain a range of bioactives that are antioxidants, vascular support agents, immune-system enhancers, and anticancer and anti-inflammatory agents. The fibre component of mushrooms is made up of potent immune-boosting polysaccharides—in particular, beta-glucans such as lentinan, schizophyllan, active hexose-correlated compound (AHCC), polysaccharide-peptide (PSP) and polysaccharide-K (PSK). Various types of beta-glucans are found in fungi, algae and the bran of oats and barley. Beta-glucans increase immune defence by interacting with cell surface receptors, activating the complement system and enhancing macrophage and NK cell activity. Beta-glucans have anticancer activity by protecting against carcinogens and mutagenesis, stimulating immune activity and reducing angiogenesis, tumour proliferation and metastasis. Lentinan and schizophyllan are poorly absorbed orally, and are used iv or by injection, but PSP and PSK can be used orally. AHCC appears to be similar in effect to PSP and PSK, although there is less research on its effectiveness. Mushrooms also contain ergosterol that is converted to vitamin D2 if exposed to UV radiation.

Mushroom supplements include whole mushroom powders, mushroom spore powders and extracts in tablet or capsule form. Mushroom spores are not bioavailable unless the indigestible outer shell has been broken down by grinding. Most mushroom supplements are derived from traditional hot water extraction, microwave-assisted extraction, ultrasonic extraction or enzyme-assisted extraction of the dried fruit body (the cap of the mushroom), followed by centrifugation, precipitation and spray drying. Most whole mushroom powder supplements contain 20–30 per cent polysaccharides, whereas mushroom extracts have polysaccharides that are about six to fifteen times more concentrated. Extracts are more commonly used in clinical trials.

Coriolus mushroom (*Coriolus versicolor*)

The coriolus mushroom, also known as *Trametes versicolor* or 'turkey tail', grows on tree trunks and dead wood in China, Japan and North America, and is popular in Asian traditional medicine. It has antioxidant activity, and is a good source of PSP and PSK which boost immune cell production and have powerful antimicrobial, anti-viral and anti-tumour properties. Both coriolus PSK and PSP have demonstrated inhibitory effects against HIV-1 in cell studies, and PSK has been shown to dramatically increase NK cell numbers.

Supplements, uses and dose

Supplements are produced by fermentation of the mushroom to the mycelium stage. *Trametes versicolor* and *Trametes versicolor* proteoglycan are approved for use as supplements in Australia. The Japanese government has approved the use of coriolus-derived PSP and PSK for treating several types of cancer, for which it is used as a prescription medication in conjunction with orthodox treatment at a dose of 3 g/day. PSK has been shown to increase survival rates in gastric, oesophageal, colorectal, nasopharyngeal and lung cancer.[1,2,3,4,5]

REFERENCES

1 Sukamoto, J., Morita, S., Oba, K. et al., Efficacy of adjuvant immunochemotherpay with polysaccharide K for patients with curatively resected colorectal cancer: A meta-analysis of centrally randomised controlled clinical trials, *Cancer Immunol Immunother* (2006), 55: 404–11.

2 Hayakawa, H., Mitsuibashi, N., Saito, Y. et al., Effect of Krestin (PSK) as adjuvant treatment on the prognosis after radical radiotherapy in patients with non-small lung cancer, *Anticancer Res* (1993), 13: 1815–20.

3 Nakazato, H., Koike, A., Saji, S. et al., Efficacy of immunotherapy as adjuvant treatment after curative resection of gastric cancer, *Lancet* (1994), 343: 1122–6.

4 Ogoshi, K., Satou, H., Isono, K. et al., Possible predictive markers of immunotherapy of oesophageal cancer retrospective analysis of a randomised study. The Co-operative Study Group for Oesophageal Cancer in Japan, *Cancer Invest* (1995), 13: 363–9.

5 Go, P. & Chung, C.H., Adjuvant PSK immunotherapy in patients with carcinoma of the nasopharynx, *J Int Med Res* (1989), 17: 141–9.

Cautions

Coriolus is generally well tolerated. Rarely, coughing, nail pigmentation, nausea, constipation and diarrhoea have been reported, mainly from use of whole mushroom powder.

Maitake mushroom (*Grifola frondosa*)

Maitake is a large mushroom that grows in mountainous areas of Asia. It is traditionally used as a general tonic and adaptogen that enhances the body's ability to adapt to physical and mental stress. Maitake reduces buildup of fats in the liver, and lowers blood glucose—possibly by activating glucose receptors. Maitake beta-glucans have immune stimulating activity by enhancing the activity of NK cells and cytotoxic T cells. The D-fraction (beta-D-glucan), a standardised form of isolated beta-glucan polysaccharides, has a unique and complex structure, and is particularly potent as an immune-boosting supplement. Subsequent research on the D-fraction has identified an MD-fraction, which appears to be more bioactive.

Supplements, uses and dose

Maitake is not approved for use in Australian supplements. A number of animal studies have found that maitake has anticancer activity, and can improve lipid metabolism, protect the liver, reduce blood pressure and lower blood glucose.[1] In a human study, maitake powder together with the MD-fraction was found to be of benefit in breast, liver and lung cancer.[2] Maitake is best used with chemotherapy, and appears to be particularly effective in reducing pain and the side-effects of chemotherapy. Patients with HIV have reported an improved sense of wellbeing.[1] The supplementary dose is not well established, but may be 0.5–1.0 mg/kg/body weight/day of the D-fraction and 200–2500 mg of the whole powder.

Cautions

Maitake is generally well tolerated. No toxicity has been observed in animals fed large quantities of maitake or the D-fraction.

REFERENCES

1 Mayell, M., Maitake extracts and their therapeutic potential, *Altern Med Rev* (2001), 6(1): 48–60.

2 Kodama, N., Komuta, K. & Nanba, H., Can maitake MD-fraction aid cancer patients? *Altern Med Rev* (2002), 7(3): 236–9.

Reishi mushroom (*Ganoderma lucidum*)

Reishi mushroom, also called Lingzhi, grows on decaying logs and tree stumps in Asia and North America. Black and red varieties appear to have the most important health-enhancing effects. Reishi is a revered traditional Chinese medicine, known as the 'elixir of immortality' and claimed to promote calmness, harmony, inner awareness and strength. It is believed to affect the *qi* (energy flow) of the heart, increase mental function and improve memory.

Bioactives include terpene and polysaccharide fractions that have antioxidant activity, the alkaloid cyclo-octasulfur that has heart tonic effects, the triterpene ganodermadiol that lowers blood pressure, ganoderic acids that lower blood pressure and inhibit cholesterol synthesis, beta-D-glucan that supports macrophage function and Ling Zhi-8, a triterpene that appears to be an immune regulator and anti-allergy agent.

Supplements, uses and dose

Ganoderma lucidum is approved for use in Australian supplements. It appears to have cardiovascular and liver-protecting, immune-boosting, anti-ageing, anti-diabetic, antiviral, antibacterial and anticancer effects, and is used for many disorders, including arthritis, cardiovascular disease (CVD), menopausal symptoms, diseases of ageing, immune deficiency, cancer and fatigue disorders. Reishi is reported to have reduced pain and accelerated healing after shingles, and to have accelerated healing in genital and oral herpes in a small number of patients.[1,2] In cancer patients, reishi (1800 mg/day for twelve weeks) has improved markers of cellular immunity, including NK cell numbers.[3] Diabetic patients given reishi (1800 mg three times daily for twelve weeks) had lower blood glucose concentrations and reduced levels of glycated haemoglobin (HbA_{1C}), a marker of glucose-induced red blood cell damage.[4] The supplementary dose appears to be 1800 mg/day or more.

REFERENCES

1 Hijikata, Y. & Yamada, S., Effect of Ganoderma lucidum on postherpetic neuralgia, *Am J Chin Med* (1998), 26: 375–81.
2 Hijikata, Y., Yamada, S. & Yasuhara, A., Herbal mixtures containing the mushroom Ganoderma lucidum improve recovery time in patients with herpes genitalis and labialis, *J Altern Complement Med* (2007), 13: 985–7.
3 Gao, Y.H., Zhou, S.F., Jiang, W.Q. et al., Effects of Ganopoly (a Ganoderma lucidum polysaccharide extract) on immune functions in advanced-stage cancer patients, *Immunol Invest* (2003), 32: 201–15.
4 Gao, Y., Lan, J., Dai, X. et al., A phase I/II study of Lingzhi mushroom Ganoderma lucidum (W. Curt.: Fr.) Lloyd (Aphyllophoromycetideae) extract in patients with type II diabetes mellitus, *Int J Med Mushrooms* (2004), 6: 33–40.

Cautions

Reishi is generally well tolerated.

Shiitake mushroom (*Lentinula edodes*)

Shiitake mushrooms grow on dead wood in the warm, humid climate of Southeast Asia, and are used as food and medicine. Like other mushrooms, they are a source of bioactive polysaccharides, including beta-glucans such as lentinan. Lentinan has anticancer activity by activating macrophages, T helper cells and NK cells, and stimulating production of interleukins and TNF-alpha. Shiitake mushroom contains eritadenine, also called lentinacin or lentysine, which lowers serum cholesterol and lipids, reduces buildup of fats in the liver and lowers blood pressure in animals. Lentinan and its derivatives also have antimicrobial and anti-parasitic activity. Dried and heated mushrooms contain compounds that block the formation of carcinogenic N-nitroso compounds produced from dietary nitrates and nitrites, such as sodium nitrite preservatives in cured meats.

Supplements, uses and dose

Shiitake is not approved for use in supplements in Australia. Supplements are usually derived from a dried water extract of the mycelia or fruiting body. Shiitake has been used for cancer, heart disease, elevated serum lipids and cholesterol, high blood pressure, infections, allergies, liver disease and urinary incontinence. Usually, iv or im injections of lentinan are used in cancer. In animals with cancer, intraperitoneal injections of lentinan are reported to have led to an 80 per cent reduction in tumour size or complete regression of the tumour.[1] Oral lentinan given to animals before introduction of human cancer cells was found to reduce tumour size, and lymphocytes from animals given lentinan retarded the development of tumours when they were transferred to other animals before cancer introduction.[2] Lentinan injections have prolonged survival time, improved immunity and caused tumour regression in some cancer patients on chemotherapy, and lentinan is reported to have greater activity if used before chemotherapy is commenced.[3] Response to lentinan may vary with the ability of an individual to mount an immune response. Small studies of oral lentinan in post-operative breast cancer patients on chemotherapy, breast cancer patients on hormone therapy and gastric cancer patients on chemotherapy have reported improved quality of life and markers of immunity.[4,5]

The standard dose of the dried mushroom in tea or in mushroom dishes is 6–16 g/day, which is equivalent to about 90 g of fresh mushroom. The supplementary dose of shiitake extract is 4–8 g/day, and the dose of *Lentinula edodes* mycelium extract (LEM) is 1–3 g three times daily.

REFERENCES

1 Wasser, S.P., *Encyclopedia of dietary supplement*, CRC Press, Boca Raton, FL, 2005.
2 Ng, M.L. & Yap, A.T., Inhibition of human colon carcinoma development by lentinan from shiitake mushrooms (Lentinus edodes), *J Altern Complement Med* (2002), 8(5): 581–9.
3 Shah, S.K., Walker, P.A., Moore-Olufemi, S.D. et al., An evidence-based review of a Lentinula edodes mushroom extract as complementary therapy in the surgical oncology patient, *J Parenter Enteral Nutr* (2011), 35(4): 449–58.

4 Yamaguchi, Y., Miyahara, E. & Hihara, J., Efficacy and safety of orally administered Lentinula edodes mycelia extract for patients undergoing cancer chemotherapy: A pilot study, *Am J Chin Med* (2011), 39(3): 451–9.

5 Suzuki, N., Takimoto, Y., Suzuki, R. et al., Efficacy of oral administration of Lentinula edodes mycelia extract for breast cancer patients undergoing postoperative hormone therapy, *Asian Pac J Cancer Prev* (2013), 14(6): 3469–72.

Cautions

Shiitake is generally well tolerated. Adverse effects include mild diarrhoea and a skin rash, which usually disappears with continued use. The skin rash (shiitake dermatitis) features whip-like, linear, red weals on the skin, which appear one to two days after consuming raw or cooked shiitake mushrooms. Shiitake has blood-thinning activity, and should be used with caution in people on anticoagulant medication. Excessive amounts may depress immune responses.

Brewer's yeast (*Saccharomyces cerevisiae*)

Brewer's and baker's yeast (*Saccharomyces cerevisiae*) is a single-celled yeast. Different strains are used commercially for making beer and bread because they have the ability to ferment starch to ethanol and carbon dioxide. Brewer's yeast is a deactivated form of *S. cerevisiae* derived from the brewing industry that is used as a health supplement. Although it has a strong, bitter taste, it was popularly used as a rich source of nutrients before high-strength vitamin and mineral supplements became available. Popular forms of brewer's yeast extracts include Vegemite, Marmite and Promite®.

Other yeast supplements include torula yeast and nutritional yeast. Torula yeast is a deactivated form of the yeast *Candida utilis*, and has a long history of use commercially as a nutritional supplement in animal feeds. Nutritional yeast is usually a deactivated form of *S. cerevisiae*, but can be other species of yeast, and is available as savoury yeast flakes. These forms of yeast have a milder flavour than brewer's yeast.

Brewer's yeast is a rich source of protein, lysine, minerals and trace elements, including phosphorus, potassium, magnesium, copper, chromium, zinc, iron, manganese and selenium, as well as most B vitamins, but is lacking in vitamin B12 unless the yeast has been fortified with B12 during manufacture. Brewer's yeast can be grown in an environment enriched with chromium, molybdenum or selenium, which become incorporated into the yeast cell. The resulting enriched yeast is used as an organic, bioavailable source of these essential trace elements. A low-molecular weight chromium-binding substance has recently been identified in brewer's yeast that consists of glutamic acid, glycine, cysteine, nicotinic acid and chromium, and a high-molecular weight binding substance has also been identified. Torula yeast is a poor source of chromium.

Brewer's yeast contains 4.4 per cent lipids, which consist of squalene, triglycerides, phosphatidylcholine, sterols, steryl esters and free fatty acids. Squalene makes up 33 per cent of total lipids. Squalene is a polyprenyl compound found in the diet and made in the body as an intermediate in cholesterol synthesis. It has antioxidant and immune-boosting activity, and helps to eliminate xenobiotics. The yeast cell wall consists of beta-glucans, proteins and mannan, with small amounts of chitin. Beta-glucans maintain the rigidity and shape of the yeast cell, and are important bioactives.

Actions

Brewer's yeast has the following physiological actions:

- *Immune-stimulating and anticancer activity.* Beta-glucans in yeast have similar immune-stimulating properties to those in other fungi, which include interacting with cell surface receptors, activating the complement system and enhancing macrophage and NK cell activity. They have antimicrobial and anticancer activity. In cell studies, brewer's yeast has induced apoptosis in breast cancer cells, and ergosterol from yeast has inhibited breast cancer cell growth.
- *Blood glucose regulation.* Brewer's yeast is a good source of bioavailable chromium that supports insulin function. Chromium from brewer's yeast has been shown to have better retention in the body than inorganic chromium chloride.
- *Cardiovascular support.* Brewer's yeast may reduce the risk of CVD by normalising blood lipids and cholesterol, and helping to control blood glucose levels.

Supplements, uses and dose

The forms of brewer's yeast permitted in Australian supplements are high-selenium (high-Se) yeast, high-chromium (high-Cr) yeast, high-molybdenum (high-Mo) yeast and dried brewer's yeast. The amount of molybdenum in high-Mo yeast is restricted to 62.5 mcg per daily dose. Brewer's yeast is a by-product of the brewing process, and is grown on malted barley. After use, it is debittered and dried to form a powder for use as a supplement in powder, capsule or tablet formulations. Other forms of nutritional yeasts and torula yeast are cultivated using molasses, wood cellulose or brewing by-products. When harvested, the yeast is killed by pasteurisation and dried to form a powder. Because supplementary forms of yeast do not contain live organisms, they do not have any capacity for fermentation or probiotic effects in the digestive tract.

Brewer's yeast can assimilate selenium from enriched media, and convert it to selenomethionine, which is incorporated into yeast proteins or cell wall constituents. In the body, selenium from high-Se yeast increases selenoenzyme activity, and can be stored as selenomethionine in tissues. It has greater retention in the body, and causes higher tissue selenium concentrations than inorganic selenium. Supplementation with high-Se yeast in patients with a history of non-melanoma skin cancer did not affect skin cancer, but was found to reduce total cancer incidence by 25 per cent and prostate cancer incidence by 52 per cent.[1] A small study of young and middle-aged men found that high-Se yeast for nine months led to a 32 per cent increase in blood glutathione levels, and a significant decrease in prostate specific antigen (PSA), a marker of prostate disease.[2]

High-Se yeast has decreased markers of inflammation in an animal model of rheumatoid arthritis (RhA).[3] In a small pilot study of patients with recent-onset RhA, high-Se yeast providing 200 mcg selenium/day taken for three months was associated with reduced pain and joint inflammation.[4] However, a study using 256 mcg of selenium from high-Se yeast in patients with more advanced RhA showed no benefit.[5] High-Se yeast has decreased growth of brain metastatic tumours and improved survival in animal models of cancer,[6] and has inhibited the deposition of amyloid-beta plaques in animal models of Alzheimer's disease.[7]

Brewer's yeast (9 g/day providing 15 mcg of chromium) has resulted in improvements in serum total cholesterol, triglyceride and HDL cholesterol levels.[8] Brewer's yeast, 1.8 g/day, was found to reduce blood pressure in patients with type 2 diabetes.[9] In another study of type 2 diabetics, both brewer's yeast, providing 23.3 mcg of chromium/day, and chromium chloride, providing 200 mcg of chromium/day, given separately, led to decreased fasting blood glucose and triglyceride levels and increased HDL cholesterol levels, and patients on insulin were able to reduce or discontinue insulin use.[10] Compared with inorganic chromium chloride, brewer's yeast chromium was better retained in the body, and improvements in triglycerides and HDL cholesterol were maintained for longer after stopping supplementation. Some patients who had discontinued insulin had to resume use when brewer's yeast supplementation was stopped. In elderly people, 9 g/day of high-Cr brewer's yeast improved glucose tolerance, insulin sensitivity and serum lipids, but chromium-poor torula yeast had no effect.[11] Brewer's yeast has been shown to boost activity in an animal model of chronic fatigue syndrome.[12]

REFERENCES

1 Duffield-Lillico, A.J., Reid, M.E., Turnbull, B.W. et al., Baseline characteristics and the effect of selenium supplementation on cancer incidence in a randomized clinical trial: A summary report of the Nutritional Prevention of Cancer Trial, *Cancer Epidemiol Biomarkers Prev* (2002), 11: 630–9.

2 El-Bayoumy, K., Richie, J.P. Jr, Boyiri, T. et al., Influence of selenium-enriched yeast supplementation on biomarkers of oxidative damage and hormone status in healthy adult males: A clinical pilot study, *Can Epidemiol Biomarkers Prev* (2002), 11: 1459–65.

3 Vieira, A.T., Silveira, K.D., Arruda, M.C. et al., Treatment with Selemax®, a selenium-enriched yeast, ameliorates experimental arthritis in rats and mice, *Br J Nutr* (2012), 108(10): 1829–38.

4 Peretz, A., Néve, J., Duchateau, J.P. & Famaey, J.P., Adjuvant treatment of recent onset rheumatoid arthritis by selenium supplementation: Preliminary observations, *Br J Rheumatol* (1992), 31: 281–6.

5 Tarp, U., Overvad, K., Thorling, E.B. et al., Selenium treatment in rheumatoid arthritis, *Scand J Rheumatol* (1985), 14(4): 364–8.
6 Wrobel, J.K., Seelbach, M.J., Chen, L. et al., Supplementation with selenium-enriched yeast attenuates brain metastatic growth, *Nutr Cancer* (2013), 65(4): 563–70.
7 Lovell, M.A., Xiong, S., Lyubartseva, G. & Markesbery, W.R., Organoselenium (Sel-Plex diet) decreases amyloid burden and RNA and DNA oxidative damage in APP/PS1 mice, *Free Radic Biol Med* (2009), 46(11): 1527–33.
8 Wang, M.M., Fox, E.A., Stoecker, B.J. et al., Serum cholesterol of adults supplemented with brewer's yeast or chromium chloride, *Nutr Res* (1989), 9(9): 989–98.
9 Hosseinzadeh, P., Djazayery, A., Mostafavi, S.A. et al., Brewer's yeast improves blood pressure in type 2 diabetes mellitus, *Iran J Public Health* (2013), 42(6): 602–9.
10 Bahijiri, S.M., Mira, S.A., Mufti, A.M. & Ajabnoor, M.A., The effects of inorganic chromium and brewer's yeast supplementation on glucose tolerance, serum lipids and drug dosage in individuals with type 2 diabetes, *Saudi Med J* (2000), 21(9): 831–7.
11 Offenbacher, E.G. & Pi-Sunyer, F.X., Beneficial effect of chromium-rich yeast on glucose tolerance and blood lipids in elderly subjects, *Diabetes* (1980), 29(11): 919–25.
12 Takahashi, T., Yu, F. & Zhu, S.J. et al., Beneficial effect of brewers' yeast extract on daily activity in a murine model of chronic fatigue syndrome, *Evid Based Complement Alternat Med* (2006), 3(1): 109–15.

Cautions

Brewer's yeast can cause nausea, vomiting, intestinal bloating, flatulence and diarrhoea, and should be introduced into the diet gradually. It contains salicylates, histamine and tyramine, which can cause adverse reactions in susceptible individuals, including migraine-like headaches and hypersensitivity reactions such as skin rash, itching, swelling and angio-oedema. Monoamine oxidase inhibitor drugs (MAOIs) inhibit the breakdown of dietary amines. People on MAOIs should not take brewer's yeast supplements because the high tyramine content may cause high blood pressure, nausea, vomiting, heart palpitations and severe headaches, and may possibly lead to brain haemorrhage and severe hypertensive crisis. Brewer's yeast may lower blood glucose levels in diabetics, and people on diabetic medication may need to lower the dose if blood glucose drops. High-Se yeast has not been associated with selenium toxicity at intakes of up to 800 mcg/day of selenium long-term. However, the TGA in Australia recommends that the maximum daily dose of selenium from dietary supplements should not exceed 150 mcg.

ALGAE

Algae used as health supplements include brown, red and green marine macroalgae (seaweeds) and green and blue-green varieties of freshwater microalgae.

FAST FACTS . . . ALGAE

- **Algae used as health supplements include marine macroalgae and freshwater micro-algae.**
- **Marine macroalgae (seaweeds) contain carotenoids, flavonoids, peptides, brominated phenols, alkaloids, sterols and sulfated polysaccharides that have health-promoting effects.**
- **Green and blue-green microalgae are used as a nutrient source, and for their antioxidant, anti-inflammatory and immune-stimulating activity.**

Marine macroalgae

Marine macroalgae are marine plants that include brown (*Phaeophyceae*), red (*Rhodophyceae*) and green (*Chlorophyceae*) varieties. Red algae used as food include dulse (*Palmaria palmata*), nori, also called laver (*Porphyra* spp.), ogonori (*Gracilaria* spp.), Irish moss (*Chondrus crispus*) and coralline algae (*Corallina officinalis*), which secrete calcium carbonate on to the surface of their cells and can be used as a calcium source. Brown algae used as food and a source of iodine include kelp and kombu (*Laminaria* spp.), bull kelp (*Durvillaea antarctica*), Norwegian kelp (*Ascophyllum nodosum*), winged kelp (*Alaria esculenta*), bladderwrack (*Fucus vesiculosus*), hijiki (hiziki, *Sargassum fusiforme*), sea bamboo (*Ecklonia maxima*), wakame (*Undaria pinnatifida*), mozuku (*Cladosiphon okamuranus*) and sea palm (*Postelsia palmaeformis*). Green algae used as food include anori (green laver) (*Monostroma* and *Enteromorpha* spp.), sea lettuce (*Ulva* spp.) and sea grapes (*Caulerpa* spp.).

Algae are sources of fermentable polysaccharides (dietary fibre), protein, lipids, including omega-3 and omega-6 PUFAs, minerals, including iron and iodine, and vitamins A, B, C, D, E and K. Dried wakame is a particularly rich source of vitamin K. Dried green and purple lavers (nori and anori) contain substantial amounts of bioavailable vitamin B12, equivalent to the amount in liver, although other edible algae contain none or only traces of vitamin B12. The protein content varies: brown algae is less than 15 per cent protein, green algae is up to 20 per cent protein and red algae is 35–47 per cent protein in some species. However, the protein content is unlikely to contribute greatly to protein intake in the amount commonly eaten in Western countries. Beneficial phytochemicals in macroalgae include carotenoids, flavonoids, peptides, brominated phenols, alkaloids, sterols and sulfated polysaccharides.

Actions

Marine macroalgae contain the following bioactives:

- *Carotenoids and flavonoids.* Carotenoids in algae include beta-carotene, alpha-carotene, lutein and xanthophylls, including zeaxanthin, neoxanthin, fucoxanthin, violaxanthin, alloxanthin, crocoxanthin and monadoxanthin. Carotenoids have antioxidant activity in the body and help detoxification, regulate cell proliferation, differentiation and communication, and protect the skin and eyes from UV light damage. The main flavonoid found in algae is hesperidin, with rutin, catechol, morin, myricetin, caffeic acid and quercitrin present in varying amounts. Flavonoids have antioxidant activity and affect cell-signalling pathways.
- *Peptides.* Algal peptides have antioxidant, blood-thinning, immune-stimulating and anticancer activity. They can protect against UV-induced skin damage and inhibit angiotensin-I-converting enzyme (ACE-I) that converts angiotensin I to angiotensin II, the active peptide that stimulates vasoconstriction and raises blood pressure.
- *Brominated phenols.* Algal brominated phenols (BPs) have antioxidant, anti-inflammatory, blood-thinning, antibacterial, antiviral and antifungal activity, stimulate immune responses and have cytotoxic activity in cancer cells. BPs suppress hydrogen peroxide-induced cellular apoptosis and activate cellular antioxidant enzymes. They have anti-diabetic activity by inhibiting tyrosine-protein phosphatase non-receptor type 1 (PTPN1) and the enzyme alpha-glucosidase. PTPN1 suppresses the insulin-signalling pathway, and enhances storage of triglycerides in fat tissue, and alpha-glucosidase takes part in digestion of carbohydrates. Some BPs also inhibit aldose reductase, the enzyme that converts glucose to fructose. Fructose plays an important role in the development of diabetic complications. BPs can inhibit HMG-CoA reductase, the key enzyme in cholesterol synthesis in the body.
- *Alkaloids.* Phenylethylamine (PEA) is an alkaloid found in some varieties of brown and red macroalgae that acts as a neuromodulator and a neurotransmitter in the brain, and has potent anti-depressant activity. Hordenine is an algal alkaloid that is a diuretic, modulates CNS activity and stimulates heart function in high doses. Caulerpin is an alkaloid in green and red macroalgae that has antimicrobial activity, but also has potential for neurotoxicity, causing numbness of the lips and tongue. Halogenated indole alkaloids in red macroalgae appear to have antimicrobial properties.
- *Sterols.* Red macroalgae primarily contain cholesterol as well as desmosterol and 22-dehydrocholesterol. Brown macroalgae primarily contain fucosterol, and green macroalgae contain chondrillasterol, poriferasterol, 28-isofucosterol, ergosterol and cholesterol. In general, sterols in macroalgae reduce serum cholesterol and inhibit a buildup of fats in the liver.
- *Sulfated polysaccharides.* Algal sulfated polysaccharides (SPs) are types of dietary fibre used commercially as food thickeners, stabilisers and texturisers. Red macroalgae contains carrageenan, agar, agarose and furcellaran, and brown macroalgae contains fucoidans and laminarins. SPs have antiviral, blood-thinning and anti-ulcer activity. Carrageenan reacts with the mucous lining of the stomach to provide a protective layer that prevents damage from pepsin and hydrochloric acid. Fucoidans have potent antioxidant and blood-thinning effects, and immune-boosting, antiviral, anti-inflammatory and anticancer properties. In animals with abnormal blood lipids, fucoidan from *Laminaria japonica* dramatically reduced serum total cholesterol,

triglycerides and LDL cholesterol, and increased serum HDL cholesterol. Laminarin is a beta-glucan that is a fermentable form of dietary fibre with prebiotic effects in the gut, and antioxidant, anti-inflammatory, immune-stimulating, anticancer, antibacterial, antiviral, blood-thinning, blood glucose-lowering and liver-protecting activity.

Dietary sources

Seaweed products are used in Japanese cuisine in foods such as dashi (miso soup base), salads, sauces, soups, fried dishes, rice dishes, sushi, sashimi dishes, pickles, beverages and Japanese kombucha tea, made from kombu (the name kombucha tea is also used for a tea made from a fungus that does not contain seaweed). Some Chinese dishes may contain sea palm. Alginates derived from macroalgae are food additives used as emulsifiers, stabilisers and thickeners in sauces, syrups, pie fillings, ice cream, cake mixes, instant milk desserts, jellies and canned meat and vegetables.

Supplements, uses and dose

Macroalgae supplements are available in tablets, capsules and powders. The macroalgae approved for use by the TGA in Australian supplements include *Laminaria cloustoni*, *L. digitata*, *L. japonica*, *Chondrus crispus*, *Corallina officinalis*, *Fucus vesiculosus* (kelp), *Undaria pinnatifida* and *Ulva lactuca*. Most supplements contain imported seaweeds that may be from wild seaweed or farmed crops. Alginates are used as laxatives, appetite suppressants, vegetarian gelatin substitutes, food additives and clarifying agents in brewing. SPs have potential as immune-enhancing, anti-tumour, anti-clotting, anti-mutagenic, anti-inflammatory, antimicrobial and antiviral agents, but there is limited research in this area.[1] Algal peptides have potential for lowering elevated blood pressure,[2] and *Laminaria* spp. have been found to reduce fat absorption in animals, possibly acting in a similar way to other types of dietary fibre, and may have potential in diabetes, CVD and obesity.[3] Fucoidans have a number of potential benefits, including treating infections, abnormal blood lipids, blood clots, cancer, ischaemia (impaired blood supply), transplant arteriosclerosis following heart transplant, oxalate kidney stones and nephritis, but research is very limited.[4] Topical use of seaweed oligosaccharides derived from the polysaccharide membrane of *Laminaria digitata*, and a novel seaweed oligosaccharide-zinc complex (SOZC) may relieve symptoms of acne by reducing sebum production and skin bacteria.[5] The supplementary dose of macroalgae depends on the amount of iodine contained in the product, and should not exceed the RDI amount (see Chapter 11: Iodine, Table 11.5) unless supervised by a health professional.

REFERENCES

1 Mišurcová, L., Škrovánková, S., Samek, D. et al., Health benefits of algal polysaccharides in human nutrition, *Adv Food Nutr Res* (2012), 66: 75–145.

2 Jiménez-Escrig, A., Gómez-Ordóñez, E. & Rupérez, P., Seaweed as a source of novel nutraceuticals: Sulfated polysaccharides and peptides, *Adv Food Nutr Res* (2011), 64: 325–37.

3 Shirosaki, M. & Koyama, T., Laminaria japonica as a food for the prevention of obesity and diabetes, *Adv Food Nutr Res* (2011), 64: 199–212.

4 Li, B., Lu, F., Wei, X. & Zhao, R., Fucoidan: Structure and bioactivity, *Molecules* (2008), 13(8): 1671–95.

5 Ruxton, C.H. & Jenkins, G., A novel topical ingredient derived from seaweed significantly reduces symptoms of acne vulgaris: A general literature review, *J Cosmet Sci* (2013), 64(3): 219–26.

Cautions

Macroalgae, particularly brown algae, are known to accumulate toxic metals such as cadmium, lead, mercury, arsenic and aluminium, and are used as indicators of environmental pollution. In Australia, supplements are tested for toxic metals and other contaminants, and must comply with permitted levels for food.

Macroalgae, especially brown varieties, are rich in iodine, and over-consumption may reduce binding of iodine by the thyroid gland and result in hypothyroidism and goitre. Iodine sensitivity varies between individuals. The average seaweed intake in Japan is 4–7 g/day, and it is suggested that habitual use throughout life may lead to immunity from the adverse effects of excessive iodine. Following 2009 reports of iodine toxicity from a brand of soy milk that contained kombu, an Australian survey was undertaken and found that iodine concentrations in dried brown seaweeds were high, but the amount in wakame and nori in Australia was generally low, as was the amount in other commercial seaweed-containing beverages such as rice and soy milk. Products containing more than 1000 mg iodine/kg dried weight are banned from importation to Australia by the Australian Quarantine and Inspection Service (AQIS).

Red macroalgae are rich in arachidonic acid (AA) and eicosapentaenoic acid (EPA), which can be metabolised to form eicosanoids. The red macroalgae *Gracilaria* and *Gracilariopsis* spp. synthesise the same eicosanoids that are produced in humans, including the inflammatory eicosanoids PGE_2 and leukotriene B_4, and consumption of raw *Gracilaria verrucosa* has been associated with toxicity, referred to as ogonori poisoning. Symptoms include nausea, vomiting and diarrhoea, which appear 30–60 minutes after ingestion and may progress to very low blood pressure, shock and death. *Gracilaria foliifera*, *Gracilaria coronopifolia* and *Gracilaria edulis* may also have toxic effects. Cooking the macroalgae denatures the eicosanoids and prevents toxicity.

Gracilaria corticata has been reported to act as a post-coital contraceptive by enhancing pre-implantation loss of the embryo, and *Gracilaria edulis* contains spermicidal compounds that disrupt the plasma membrane of sperm and inhibit sperm motility. Kainic acid, found in low levels in some red macroalgae, is a potent CNS stimulant, structurally similar to the neurotransmitter glutamate. It has potent activity against intestinal parasitic worms, but in high levels can induce seizures in experimental animals.

Microalgae

Microalgae, which include diatoms (Bacillariophyta), dinoflagellates (Dinophyceae), green algae (Chlorophyta) and blue-green algae (also known as blue-green bacteria or Cyanobacteria), grow in freshwater lakes. Green microalgae include *Dunaliella salina*, which accumulates up to 14 per cent of its dry weight as beta-carotene and is used as a beta-carotene supplement, and chlorella (*Chlorella vulgaris*), which has the highest concentration of the green pigment chlorophyll of any plant. Chlorella has strong cell walls, and is indigestible unless it has been processed to break down the cell walls prior to ingestion. Blue-green microalgae used as food include *Nostoc* spp., spirulina (*Arthrospira maxima*, *A. platensis*) and *Aphanizomenon flos-aquae* (AFA). They have digestible cell walls and characteristics of both bacteria and algae, but are more closely related to bacteria.

Microalgae have been used as food in the traditional cultures of the Philippines, China, Chad and Mexico. Blue-green microalgae contain about 60–70 per cent protein by weight, and this is of higher quality than most plant protein sources but not as high as meat or dairy proteins. The limiting amino acids in spirulina are methionine, cysteine and lysine. The total lipid content is about 6 per cent, of which about 40 per cent is polyunsaturated, mainly consisting of the omega-6 fatty acids linoleic acid (LA) and gamma-linolenic acid (GLA), together with omega-3 PUFAs, including small amounts of EPA and DHA. Blue-green microalgae are rich in pigments, including chlorophyll, carotenoids and phycobiliproteins, which include C-phycocyanin (C-PC), R-phycocyanin and allophycocyanin. Spirulina contains beta-carotene, beta-sitosterol, phenol compounds, vitamin E and B vitamins, and is a rich source of potassium, sodium, calcium, phosphorus and magnesium, as well as bioavailable forms of trace elements. It is claimed that spirulina is a rich source of vitamin B12 because early research identified corrinoid compounds that are B12 analogues (look-alikes). However, subsequent research has concluded that only about 17 per cent of the corrinoids in spirulina is active vitamin B12 in humans. AFA appears to contain only inactive B12 analogues.

Chlorella is 48 per cent protein and 13 per cent lipids. It has only trace amounts of GLA, but contains higher amounts of PUFAs and much higher DHA (21 per cent of total lipids) compared with blue-green algae. Chlorella is rich in calcium, magnesium, phosphorus, sodium, potassium and especially iron (259.1 mg/100 g compared with 95.4 mg/100 g of iron in spirulina). It also contains polysaccharides, the carotenoids canthaxanthin and astaxanthin, and a range of trace elements and vitamins. Chlorella contains a water-soluble growth-promoting substance known as chlorella growth factor (CGF) that is made up of amino acids, peptides, proteins, vitamins, sugars and nucleic acids. Although microalgae are nutrient dense, they provide low levels of nutrients in the amounts commonly consumed compared with food sources.

Actions

Microalgae have the following physiological actions:

- *Antioxidant, anti-inflammatory and anticancer activity.* C-PC has been found to be a potent inhibitor of NADPH oxidase activity, an enzyme that contributes to oxidation damage and inflammation. C-PC has antioxidant, radical-scavenging, anticancer, gene-regulating and liver-protecting properties. It inhibits the key inflammatory enzyme COX-2 that produces inflammatory eicosanoids and inhibits NF-kappaB activity, leading to reduced expression of inflammatory cytokines. C-PC is a potent inhibitor of platelet aggregation in cell studies, and inhibits cell proliferation and induces apoptosis in cancer cells. Sulfated polysaccharides (SPs) in microalgae have antioxidant, anti-inflammatory, anticancer and immune-enhancing activity. Calcium spirulan, an intracellular polysaccharide produced by spirulina, inhibits tumour spread in cell studies by inhibiting adhesion and invasion in basement membranes and the breakdown of heparan sulfate in connective tissue.
- *Blood lipid and glucose regulation.* Microalgal SPs inhibit intestinal cholesterol absorption, reduce expression of liver genes that enhance lipid synthesis and can lower plasma total cholesterol and triglycerides. They also reduce insulin and glucose levels in diabetic animals.
- *Immunity.* Chlorella and blue-green microalgae have immune-stimulating and antimicrobial effects. Blue-green microalgae have been shown to boost the phagocytic activity of macrophages, stimulate the production of antibodies and immune chemicals, and increase the activity of white blood cells, such as T cells, B cells and NK cells. Cyanovirin-N (CV-N) is a protein in microalgae that inhibits immunodeficiency viruses. SPs in microalgae have antiviral activity and inhibit the ability of pathogens to adhere to cell surfaces. In cell studies, calcium spirulan has been found to inhibit replication of viruses by preventing penetration of the virus into the host cell, and is effective against herpes simplex type I, human cytomegalovirus, measles, mumps, influenza A and HIV-1 viruses in cell studies. Lipopeptides from microalgae have antimicrobial effects, as well as cytotoxic, anticancer and enzyme-inhibiting properties.

Supplements, uses and dose

Forms of microalgae permitted in Australian supplements are *Arthrospira platensis* (*Spirulina platensis*), *Arthrospira maxima* (*Spirulina maxima*) and *Chlorella vulgaris*, which are available in powder, tablet or capsule forms. Microalgae grow naturally in lakes in Africa and Mexico, and are commercially grown in closed photobioreactors or in open ponds in tropical or sub-tropical regions around the world. They are grown using food-grade fertilisers and are harvested, washed and spray-dried to form a powder. Most commercial microalgae are grown in open ponds, and are at risk of contamination. They can accumulate heavy metals, such as mercury, cadmium and lead, if grown in contaminated waters, and may become contaminated with liver toxins produced by other blue-green microalgae, such as *Microcystis aeruginosa* that produces microcystin toxin and *Nodularia spumigena* that produces nodularin toxins. AFA appears to be susceptible to microcystin toxin because Lake Klamath, Oregon, USA, where AFA is grown, has a history of overgrowth of *Microcystis aeruginosa*. Cultivation in closed photo-bioreactors helps to prevent contamination. Microalgae are tested for toxins and contaminants during the production process.

Microalgae have been found to have immune-boosting, antimicrobial, anticancer, antioxidant, anti-inflammatory, anti-allergic, anti-diabetic, lipid-lowering and blood-thinning properties. Spirulina has been used as an effective nutritional supplement for under-nourished children,[1] and as a source of beta-carotene in regions of vitamin A deficiency.[2] It has improved markers of oxidation and inflammation in human studies.[3] A small study found that athletes supplemented with spirulina had an increase in exercise performance, fat oxidation and glutathione levels, and less exercise-induced oxidative damage to lipids in body tissues.[4]

In patients with abnormal blood lipids, 1 g/day of spirulina for twelve weeks resulted in a lowering of serum triglycerides by 16.3 per cent, LDL cholesterol by 10.1 per cent, total cholesterol by 8.9 per cent, and the ratio of total cholesterol to HDL cholesterol by 11.5 per cent, despite no change in weight and body mass index.[5] Elevated levels of blood fats after a meal (postprandial lipaemia) are associated with atherosclerosis, insulin resistance and obesity. A study of runners given 5 g/day of spirulina for fifteen days found that postprandial blood lipids were lower after a fatty meal.[6] Spirulina supplementation for twelve weeks has improved markers of iron status and immune function in elderly people.[7] Spirulina supplementation has relieved nasal discharge, sneezing, nasal congestion and itching in patients with allergic rhinitis.[8]

There is limited research on *Chlorella vulgaris*. Supplementation with chlorella (3.6 g/day for six weeks) has improved antioxidant status and reduced lipid peroxidation in cigarette smokers.[9] Chlorella supplementation in addition to standard treatment in patients with non-alcoholic fatty liver disease has improved markers of liver function.[10] *C. pyrenoidosa* has been found to maintain immunity in cancer patients, relieve symptoms of fibromyalgia and ulcerative colitis, reduce blood pressure and lower serum cholesterol.[11] The supplementary dose of microalgae used in clinical trial is 1–10 g daily.

REFERENCES

1 Simpore, J., Kabore, F., Zongo, F. et al., Nutrition rehabilitation of undernourished children utilizing Spiruline and Misola, *Nutr J* (2006), 5: 3–7.

2 Seshadri, C.V., *Large scale nutritional supplementation with Spirulina alga. All India Coordinated Project on Spirulina*, Shri Amm Murugappa Chettiar Research Center (MCRC), Madras, 1993.

3 Deng, R. & Chow, T.J., Hypolipidemic, antioxidant, and antiinflammatory activities of microalgae Spirulina, *Cardiovasc Ther* (2010), 28(4): e33–45.

4 Kalafati, M., Jamurtas, A.Z., Nikolaidis, M.G. et al., Ergogenic and antioxidant effects of spirulina supplementation in humans, *Med Sci Sports Exerc* (2010), 42(1): 142–51.

5 Mazokopakis, E.E., Starakis, I.K., Papadomanolaki, M.G. et al., The hypolipidaemic effects of Spirulina (Arthrospira platensis) supplementation in a Cretan population: A prospective study, *J Sci Food Agric* (2014), 94(3): 432–7.

6 Torres-Durán, P.V., Ferreira-Hermosillo, A., Ramos-Jiménez, A. et al., Effect of Spirulina maxima on postprandial lipemia in young runners: A preliminary report, *J Med Food* (2012), 15(8): 753–7.

7 Selmi, C., Leung, P.S., Fischer, L. et al., The effects of Spirulina on anemia and immune function in senior citizens, *Cell Mol Immunol* (2011), 8(3): 248–54.

8 Cingi, C., Conk-Dalay, M., Cakli, H. & Bal, C., The effects of spirulina on allergic rhinitis, *Eur Arch Otorhinolaryngol* (2008), 265(10): 1219–23.

9 Panahi, Y., Mostafazadeh, B., Abrishami, A. et al., Investigation of the effects of Chlorella vulgaris supplementation on the modulation of oxidative stress in apparently healthy smokers, *Clin Lab* (2013), 59(5–6): 579–87.

10 Panahi, Y., Ghamarchehreh, M.E., Beiraghdar, F. et al., Investigation of the effects of Chlorella vulgaris supplementation in patients with non-alcoholic fatty liver disease: A randomized clinical trial, *Hepatogastroenterology* (2012), 59(119): 2099–103.

11 Merchant, R.E. & Andre, C.A., A review of recent clinical trials of the nutritional supplement Chlorella pyrenoidosa in the treatment of fibromyalgia, hypertension, and ulcerative colitis, *Altern Ther Health Med* (2001), 7(3): 79–91.

Cautions

Spirulina and chlorella are generally well tolerated. Mild nausea, flatulence and abdominal cramps have been reported, but these disappear with continued use. Animals fed dried spirulina at a dose of 10 g/kg body weight showed no toxic effects. There is one case report of dermatomyositis (skin and muscle inflammation and muscle necrosis) and another case report of rhabdomyolysis (muscle necrosis), both apparently associated with spirulina supplementation.

Chlorella supplementation has been associated with phototoxicity in a small number of cases, featuring swelling and reddish-purple lesions on sun-exposed skin. This was reported to be caused by pheophorbide a, a product of chlorophyll breakdown.

BEE PRODUCTS

Bee products that are used as health supplements include honey, bee pollen, propolis and royal jelly. Honey is produced by honey bees from nectar collected from flowers and other plant parts that is brought to the hive, where it is thickened and stored in the cells of honeycomb for ripening. Bees also collect honeydew, which comes from droplets that form on flowers in the

FAST FACTS . . . BEE PRODUCTS

- **Bee products that are used as health supplements include honey, bee pollen, propolis and royal jelly.**
- **They have immune-stimulating, anti-microbial, antioxidant and anti-inflammatory activity.**
- **They are used primarily for infections and wound healing, and as a nutrient source.**

morning, and this can be made into honey. Bee pollen is pollen from the stamens of flowers that sticks to the bees' legs. It is mixed with bee saliva and transported to the hive, where it is processed and put into honeycomb cells to ripen into bee bread. Royal jelly is produced from secretions from young bees that are added to bee bread to make bee milk and royal jelly. Royal jelly is the most nutrient-rich bee milk, which is fed to the queen bee to increase her growth and longevity. Propolis is made by bees from collected tree gums, glues, waxes and resins mixed with beeswax and saliva. It is used by bees to seal, repair and sterilise the hive, and embalm any invaders. Bee products should be used with caution in people with allergies—especially asthmatics.

Honey

Honey is composed mainly of the sugars fructose and glucose, together with oligosaccharides and traces of phytochemicals, enzymes (lysozyme, amylase, sucrase, glucose oxidase, catalase), vitamin C, vitamin E, carotenoids, minerals, hydrogen peroxide, organic acids, amino acids, proteins and pollen. It is not a good source of essential nutrients in the amounts commonly eaten compared with food sources. Phytochemicals in honey include phenolic acids and the flavonoids flavones, flavonols and flavanones, including quercetin, kaempferol, galangin, apigenin, chrysin and luteolin. Hydrogen peroxide is produced from oxidation of glucose by glucose oxidase during ripening in the hive. Biological activity appears to be highest in fresh and raw honey.

Actions

Honey has the following physiological actions:

- *Antimicrobial activity.* Honey has a low pH, high sugar concentration and low available moisture content that inhibits the growth of bacteria, and hydrogen peroxide, lysozyme, phenolic acids and flavonoids have antimicrobial activity. Honey has been found to inhibit viruses, bacteria and the Leishmania parasite. Manuka honey from the New Zealand tea tree (*Leptospermum scoparium*) has very high antibacterial activity, which appears to be due to the non-hydrogen peroxide constituents methyl syringate and syringic acid, as well as methylglyoxal produced from the dihydroxyacetone present in manuka nectar. Honey from the Australian plants jelly bush (*Leptospermum polygalifolium*), marri (*Corymbia calophylla*) and jarrah (*Eucalyptus marginata*) have also been found to have high antibacterial activity. In these honeys, the hydrogen peroxide antimicrobial activity decreased during storage but the non-hydrogen peroxide antimicrobial activity increased. Microbial resistance to honey has not been reported.
- *Antioxidant activity.* Antioxidants in honey include flavonoids, phenolic acids, glucose oxidase, catalase, vitamin C, vitamin E, organic acids, Maillard reaction products (products of glucose and protein interactions during heating), amino acids and proteins. The antioxidant activity varies according to the flower source. In cell studies, honey has inhibited ROS production and cell membrane oxidation. Honey has increased the antioxidant capacity of serum and increased vitamin C, beta-carotene, uric acid and glutathione reductase levels in humans. Prolonged storage appears to reduce the antioxidant effect.
- *Anti-inflammatory and anticancer activity.* Honey reduces oxidant-induced inflammation, inhibits COX-2 activity, and reduces $PGF_{2\alpha}$ and PGE_2 production. Honey has been found to have anti-mutagenic properties in cell studies, induces cell cycle arrest and apoptosis of tumour cells, and appears to potentiate the activity of some chemotherapies.
- *Immune-stimulating and wound-healing activity.* Honey stimulates B and T lymphocytes, neutrophils, monocytes, eosinophils and NK cells, and enhances antibody production. Topically, honey maintains a protective barrier against infection, and its osmotic properties keep moisture in wounds, which assists healing. It is reported to assist debridement (removal of dead or infected tissue), reduce inflammation and tissue damage during wound healing, decrease swelling in damaged skin and promote tissue regeneration. Honey may reduce the pain of burns and prevent superficial burns from converting to full-thickness burns.

- *Digestive system support*. Honey reduces gastric acidity, inhibits the growth of *Helicobacter pylori* and has prevented gastric ulcer development and enhanced healing of gastric ulcers in an animal model of gastric ulcers. Honey is protective against bacterial diarrhoea, and honey oligosaccharides have prebiotic effects in the gut.

Supplements, uses and dose

Commercial honey is extracted from the honeycomb, excess moisture is removed, and it is heat-treated to prevent fermentation and crystallisation before filtering to remove impurities. Honey can also be creamed by moderate heating and stirring. Manuka honey is available as honey and honey dressings for wounds and burns, and has an activity rating based on non-peroxide antibacterial activity. Most studies have used manuka honey with a rating of 12 or higher.

Honey has been used in oral rehydration products and as a dressing for wounds, burns and skin grafts. Soft alginate dressings are recommended for keeping honey in contact with the wound and about 25 mL of honey is used for a 10 cm^2 dressing. However, a rigorous review of 25 clinical trials found that honey dressings are not effective for venous leg ulcers when used with compression therapy, and honey may delay healing in burns in comparison to early excision and grafting, and also delay healing in skin Leishmaniasis when used with standard drug treatment.[1] The reviewers found that honey might be superior to some conventional dressings, but there is insufficient evidence to form a conclusion.

A topical mixture of honey, beeswax and olive oil has been used for nappy rash, eczema and tinea with promising results.[2,3,4] Diluted honey applied to affected skin every second day was found to dramatically enhance healing of seborrhoeic dermatitis and dandruff.[5] Topical application of honey for oral and genital herpes has reduced pain and the mean duration of the outbreak, and enhanced crusting and healing more effectively than the antiviral medication aciclovir.[6] A review of three trials of honey for protection from the effects of radiation-induced oral mucositis, a complication of radiation therapy for cancer, found that honey reduced the risk of mucositis by 80 per cent, although the trials were not considered to be of sufficient quality to enable firm conclusions to be reached.[7]

Honey, given as 250 mL of water containing 75 g of natural honey, decreased triglycerides, LDL cholesterol, homocysteine and C-reactive protein, and increased HDL cholesterol in a small study of normal and hyperlipidaemic people.[8] Honey also had less effect on blood glucose levels than glucose and sucrose in diabetics.[8] Honey may be more effective for nocturnal coughs in children with upper respiratory infections compared with diphenhydramine.[9] The optimal dose is not known, but may be several teaspoons daily.

REFERENCES

1. Jull, A.B., Walker, N. & Deshpande, S., Honey as a topical treatment for wounds, *Cochrane Database Syst Rev* (2013), 2: CD005083.
2. Al-Waili, N.S., Clinical and mycological benefits of topical application of honey, olive oil and beeswax in diaper dermatitis, *Clin Microbiol Infect* (2005), 11(2): 160–3.
3. Al-Waili, N.S., Topical application of natural honey, beeswax and olive oil mixture for atopic dermatitis or psoriasis: Partially controlled, single-blinded study, *Complement Ther Med* (2003), 11(4): 226–34.
4. Al-Waili, N.S., An alternative treatment for pityriasis versicolor, tinea cruris, tinea corporis and tinea faciei with topical application of honey, olive oil and beeswax mixture: An open pilot study, *Complement Ther Med* (2004), 12(1): 45–7.
5. Al-Waili, N.S., Therapeutic and prophylactic effects of crude honey on chronic seborrheic dermatitis and dandruff, *Eur J Med Res* (2001), 6(7): 306–8.
6. Al-Waili, N.S., Topical honey application vs. acyclovir for the treatment of recurrent herpes simplex lesions, *Med Sci Monit* (2004), 10(8): MT94–8.
7. Song, J.J., Twumasi-Ankrah, P. & Salcido, R., Systematic review and meta-analysis on the use of honey to protect from the effects of radiation-induced oral mucositis, *Adv Skin Wound Care* (2012), 25(1): 23–8.

8 Al-Waili, N.S., Natural honey lowers plasma glucose, C-reactive protein, homocysteine, and blood lipids in healthy, diabetic, and hyperlipidemic subjects: Comparison with dextrose and sucrose, *J Med Food* (2004), 7(1): 100–7.

9 Oduwole, O., Meremikwu, M.M., Oyo-Ita, A. & Udoh, E.E., Honey for acute cough in children, *Cochrane Database Syst Rev* (2012), 3: CD007094.

Cautions

Honey is usually well tolerated, and allergies to honey are relatively uncommon. However, honey allergy, caused by allergy to traces of plant or bee proteins, can result in coughs, itching in the throat and face, swelling of the throat or lips, rhinitis, headache, redness of the skin or life-threatening anaphylaxis, especially in patients with a history of allergies. Large amounts of honey have a mild laxative effect, caused by the fructose content. People with fructose intolerance should avoid honey. Oral intake of honey should be used in moderation because it is a concentrated source of sugar that may cause tooth decay or affect blood glucose levels. Honey is less cariogenic than sucrose or fruit juice.

Honey may contain pyrrolizidine alkaloids, toxic compounds from plants such as Paterson's Curse (Salvation Jane) (*Echium plantagineum*) and rhododendron and laurel spp., and this is generally controlled by banning honey production in areas where these plants are found, and by blending different batches of honey to reduce the amount of toxins present. Symptoms of honey poisoning include dizziness, nausea, vomiting, convulsions, headache, palpitations and, rarely, death. Toxins in honey identified include tutin (from tutu) and hyenanchin (from passion-vine hopper), both more common in New Zealand honey, and euphorbic acid (from *Euphorbia* spp.), acetylandromedol (from rhododendron and laurel) and ericolin (from bearberry).

Honey should not be given to infants under one year of age because it may contain spores of the bacterium *Clostridium botulinum*, which may activate in the infant's gut to produce botulinum toxin, a potent neurotoxin that can cause muscle weakness, poor muscle tone, floppiness, constipation, listlessness, lethargy, difficulty suckling and swallowing, weak crying and loss of head control. An infant is much more susceptible to *C. botulinum* toxin than older children and adults. Infant botulism is very rare, and most affected infants recover completely. The TGA in Australia requires the following advisory statement on medicinal products containing honey: '*Not suitable for infants under 12 months.*'

Bee pollen

Bee pollen contains the male reproductive cells of seed plants, and is collected by a screen over the hive opening that squeezes pollen from the bees' pollen sacs during entry. The major constituents of bee pollen are proteins, amino acids, polysaccharides, sugars and lipids, including waxes, sterols, saturated fats and unsaturated fats, such as alpha-linolenic acid. Pollen also contains glucose oxidase, vitamins (mainly water-soluble vitamins; it is low in fat soluble vitamins), minerals and trace elements, phenylpropanoids (precursors of polyphenolic compounds) and phytochemicals such as carotenoids, phenolic acids and flavonoids, including flavonols, flavones and anthocyanins. The constituents of bee pollen vary widely according to the plants on which the bees forage. Floral pollen is rich in flavonoids and phenolic acids. Most pollens contain all the essential amino acids, but some types may be low in phenylalanine and/or tryptophan. In a simulated human digestion study, only 48–59 per cent of pollen protein was digestible. The nutrient content deteriorates with prolonged storage. Pollen can boost nutritional intake, but is not a rich source of essential nutrients in the amounts commonly ingested when compared with food sources.

Actions

Bee pollen has the following physiological actions:

- *Antioxidant activity.* Phenylpropanoids, flavonoids, hydroxycinnamic acids and caffeic acid in bee pollen appear to have potent antioxidant activity, and are protective against lipid peroxidation. Animal studies have found that bee pollen increases levels of glutathione, and enhances the activity of the antioxidant enzymes glutathione peroxidase and glutathione reductase.
- *Anti-inflammatory activity.* Ethanolic extracts of bee pollen containing isorhamnetin, kaempferol and quercetin and their metabolites have been found to be potent inhibitors of NO and COX-2 that promote inflammation.

- *Anticancer activity.* A steroid fraction of bee pollen has been found to induce apoptosis in prostate cancer cells.
- *Immune and antimicrobial activity.* Bee pollen has been found to stimulate humoral immunity and inhibit the activation of mast cells in allergic reactions. It can inhibit the growth of a variety of bacteria, including *Staphylococcus aureus* and fungi, including *Candida* spp., but activity varies between types of pollen.
- *Bone support.* Bee pollen has been found to increase the calcium and DNA content of bone and increase activity of alkaline phosphatase, an enzyme involved in bone growth, in an animal study.

Supplements, uses and dose

Bee pollen is available as granules, powders and capsules. Commercial bee pollen is processed after collection by drying and purifying. Freeze drying appears to preserve the bioactives better than oven drying. Freezing followed by storage in liquid nitrogen at −20°C has been recommended for preserving pollen bioactives long-term (up to 6 months). Because pollen contains moisture and is an ideal medium for growth of bacteria, yeasts and moulds, it should be collected while fresh and dried shortly after collection to reduce the moisture content and protect against contamination by mycotoxins (toxins made by moulds).

In general, bee pollen is used as a source of essential nutrients, and to assist weight loss, increase energy and endurance, reduce hay fever symptoms, relieve digestive disorders, inflammation, infections and anaemia, and improve immunity, but there is limited supporting research. Two studies have found that bee pollen does not improve athletic performance.[1,2] Bee pollen extract from rye-grass pollen (*Secale cereale*) improved self-rated urinary symptoms in men with benign prostatic hyperplasia (BPH),[3] and was reported to improve urine flow and markers of inflammation in men with chronic prostatitis.[4] The pollen polysaccharide LBPP has been found to reduce tumour formation, increase the activity of NK cells and phagocytes, increase lymphocyte proliferation and improve anaemia in an animal model of cancer.[5] In female animals, bee pollen has decreased release of insulin-like growth factor and increased secretion of progesterone and oestradiol.[6] The optimal dose of bee pollen is not known, but may be 5–10 g/day or more.

REFERENCES

1 Maughan, R.J. & Evans, S.P., Effects of pollen extract upon adolescent swimmers, *Br J Sports Med* (1982), 16: 142–5.
2 Woodhouse, M.L., Williams, M. & Jackson, C., The effects of varying doses of orally ingested bee pollen extract upon selected performance variables, *Athletic Training* (1987), 22(1): 26–8.
3 MacDonald, R., Ishani, A., Rutks, I. & Wilt, T.J., A systematic review of cernilton for the treatment of benign prostatic hyperplasia, *BJU Int* (2000), 85(7): 836–41.
4 Rugendorff, E.W., Weidner, W., Ebeling, L. et al., Results of treatment with pollen extract (cernilton N) in chronic prostatitis and prostatodynia, *Br J Urol* (1993), 71: 433–8.
5 Yang, X., Guo, D., Zhang, J. & Wu, M., Characterization and anti-tumor activity of pollen polysaccharide, *Int Immunopharmacol* (2007), 7(3): 401–8.
6 Kolesarova, A., Bakova, Z., Capcarova, M. et al., Consumption of bee pollen affects rat ovarian functions, *J Anim Physiol Anim Nutr (Berl)* (2013), 97(6): 1059–65.

Cautions

Bee pollen should be used cautiously, especially in people with known allergies. It may cause asthma, hives, itching, swelling and life-threatening anaphylaxis. Bee pollen may contain liver-damaging pyrrolizidine alkaloids if bees forage on plants that contain these alkaloids. Bee pollen is susceptible to contamination by *Aspergillus* spp., types of moulds that produce the potent mycotoxins aflatoxin and ochratoxin that cause liver damage and liver cancer. Bee pollen may potentiate the blood-thinning drug warfarin, requiring a reduction in warfarin dose. There are case reports of acute kidney failure, eosinophilia and liver dysfunction associated with bee pollen supplementation.

Propolis

Propolis consists mainly of resins, waxes, essential oils and pollen, together with phytochemicals, sterols, vitamins, minerals, sugars, enzymes, aldehydes, ketones and alcohols. The main phytochemicals in propolis are flavones, flavonols and flavanones, which include pinocembrin, acacetin, chrysin, rutin, catechin, naringenin, galangin, luteolin, kaempferol, apigenin, myricetin, quercetin, cinnamic acid, caffeic acid and resveratrol. An important constituent is caffeic acid phenethyl ester (CAPE), a phytochemical that has potent antioxidant, anti-inflammatory and anticancer properties.

Actions

Propolis has antioxidant, anti-inflammatory, immunomodulatory, antimicrobial, anticancer, cardioprotective and neuroprotective properties. The actions of propolis include the following:

- *Antioxidant activity.* CAPE in propolis inhibits production of ROS by suppressing NF-kappa B and iNOS activation, and protects against cell membrane lipid peroxidation, DNA strand breakages and protein damage. The phytochemical propolin C in propolis is a potent free radical scavenger and tectochrysin from propolis increases the activity of the antioxidant enzymes cytosolic superoxide dismutase (SOD), catalase and glutathione peroxidase in animals exposed to liver toxins.
- *Anti-inflammatory activity.* Ethanolic extract of propolis has potent anti-inflammatory effects. Chrysin can suppress COX-2 expression, and CAPE can inhibit NF-kappaB and the 5-LOX pathway that produces inflammatory leukotrienes. CAPE and propolin C are inhibitors of xanthine oxidase activity, which may reduce uric acid levels and protect against gout.
- *Immune activity.* Propolis activates macrophages, enhances NK cell activity and stimulates antibody production. It has an inhibiting effect on the proliferation of lymphocytes that may be associated with anti-inflammatory effects.
- *Antimicrobial activity.* Propolis has antiviral, antifungal and antibacterial properties, and extracts with a high content of polyphenols (at least 59 per cent) have been associated with more potent effects. Propolis has multiple antibacterial effects that include inhibiting bacterial protein synthesis and cell division, and disrupting bacterial cytoplasm, cytoplasmic membranes and cell walls. Ethanolic extract of propolis has been found to inhibit the growth of 60 strains of yeasts and 38 strains of fungi. Propolis extracts were active against *Trypanosoma cruzi* (the parasite that causes Chagas disease, which is endemic in Latin America) and lethal to *Trichomonas vaginalis*, a sexually transmitted disease that infects the genital tract.
- *Anticancer activity.* In cell studies, CAPE inhibits growth of precancerous lesions, inhibits enzyme activities associated with colon cancer and induces apoptosis in cancer cells. A semi-synthetic derivative of CAPE, phenethyl caffeate benzoxanthene lignan (PCBL), induces DNA damage and apoptosis in tumour cells, and appears to inhibit processes that contribute to cancer spread, such as angiogenesis and activity of matrix metalloproteinases and vascular endothelial growth factor. Artepillin C, a hydroxycinnamic acid derivative in propolis, has potent immune-stimulating and cancer-inhibiting properties, and the propolis phytochemicals PM-3 and propolin C also have anticancer activity.
- *Liver support.* Propolis inhibits phase I enzymes and induces phase II enzymes in liver detoxification pathways; it also has liver-protecting effects.
- *Nerve protection.* CAPE and pinocembrin, a propolis flavonoid, protect brain tissue from reperfusion injury (damage caused by restoration of blood supply) after circulatory blockage. CAPE also protects nerve cells from inflammation and glutamate-induced excitotoxicity (excessive stimulation that kills nerves). Chrysin protects nerves from inflammatory damage by inhibiting expression of iNOS, COX-2 and NF-kappaB signalling, and suppressing the release of NO.

Supplements, uses and dose

The permitted forms of propolis in Australian supplements are propolis and propolis balsam, dry extract, liquid extract, resin and tincture. Supplements include capsules, tablets, liquids and sprays. Propolis is also found in mouthwashes, toothpaste, lozenges, ointments and cosmetics. After collection, bioactives from raw propolis are extracted by solvents such as ethanol, glycol, water or oil, and the solvent is then removed by freeze-drying, vacuum distillation or evaporation.

Propolis is used for infections, oral health, burns and wound healing, cancer prevention, immune and cardiovascular support, digestive tract disorders, and liver and nerve protection. Propolis is used topically for ulcers, wounds and burns, and has been found to accelerate skin repair and reduce healing time.[1] CAPE has shown anticancer activity in melanoma, as well as colon, lung and prostate cancer, in cell studies.[2] In an animal model of diabetes, bee propolis extracts decreased fasting blood glucose and serum total cholesterol, triglycerides and LDL cholesterol, and increased serum HDL cholesterol and SOD.[3] A Russian report of twelve patients with chronic sinusitis caused by *Candida albicans* claims that an alcohol–oil emulsion of propolis applied to the sinuses after saline irrigation led to improvement in symptoms and recovery in 75 per cent of subjects.[4] Propolis may be of benefit in dentistry as an antiseptic, and for the management of caries, tooth sensitivity, plaque formation, tooth, mouth and gum infections, mouth ulcers, vital pulp therapy (an alternative to root canal treatment that keeps dental pulp alive), denture stomatitis (mouth inflammation associated with denture use) and the repair of surgical wounds.[5]

REFERENCES

1 Ramos, A.F. & Miranda, J.L., Propolis: A review of its anti-inflammatory and healing actions, *J Venom Anim Toxins incl Trop Dis* (2007), 13(4): 697–710.

2 Ozturk, G., Ginis, Z., Akyol, S. et al., The anticancer mechanism of caffeic acid phenethyl ester (CAPE): Review of melanomas, lung and prostate cancers, *Eur Rev Med Pharmacol Sci* (2012), 16(15): 2064–8.

3 Fuliang, H.U., Hepburn, H.R., Xuan, H. et al., Effects of propolis on blood glucose, blood lipid and free radicals in rats with diabetes mellitus, *Pharmacol Res* (2005), 51(2): 147–52.

4 Kovalik, P.V., Use of propolis for treatment of chronic sinusitis of fungal etiology, *Vestn Otorinolaringol* (1979), 6: 60–2.

5 Parolia, A., Thomas, M.S., Kundabala, M. & Mohan, M., Propolis and its potential uses in oral health, *Int J Med Sci* (2010), 2(7): 210–15.

Cautions

Propolis can cause allergies such as skin irritation, itching and rash, swelling and itching of the mouth or throat, oral lesions and anaphylaxis, and may trigger asthma attacks in sensitive people. Contact dermatitis is observed in bee keepers. A fixed drug eruption, a type of allergy in which skin lesions recur in the same location after each ingestion of the allergen, has reportedly been associated with propolis use. The main allergens in propolis are believed to be caffeate esters. There is one case report of liquid propolis causing lung tumours after being applied to the nasal mucosa for a period of six months. The tumours were apparently comprised of propolis particles that had been breathed into the lungs.

Common contaminants in propolis are lead and synthetic acaricides used as pesticides against varroa mites (bee parasites). Varroa is not present in Australia, but is predicted to cross from New Zealand and Papua New Guinea in the future. Australian supplements are routinely tested for contaminants.

The TGA in Australia requires the following advisory statements to be included on propolis product labels:

For external use, *'WARNING: Propolis may cause skin irritation. Test before use'*; and for internal use, *'WARNING: Propolis may cause allergic reactions. If irritation or swelling of the mouth or throat occurs—discontinue use.'*

Royal jelly

Royal jelly consists of water, proteins, peptides, amino acids, carbohydrates, fructose, glucose, lipids, sterols, minerals, water-soluble vitamins, enzymes, and hormones, including testosterone, progesterone, prolactin and oestradiol, together with a range of bioactive phytochemicals that have immune-stimulating and antibacterial properties. Royal jelly is not a good source of essential nutrients in the amounts commonly eaten when compared with food. Royalactin is a royal jelly protein that stimulates expression of epidermal growth factor receptors, and has been identified as the growth-promoting factor in the queen bee. Royal jelly is a rich source of vitamin B5, and contains unusual hydroxy acids with 10 carbon atoms, such as 10-hydroxydecenoic acid and 10-hydroxy-2-decenoic acid (10H2DA), that are identifying markers. 10H2DA has anticancer, antibiotic, immune-modulating, oestrogenic and neurogenic properties, and royal jelly proteins and peptides have antioxidant, immune-modulating, antibacterial and anti-inflammatory effects.

Actions

Royal jelly is reported to have antioxidant, anticancer, antimicrobial, anti-inflammatory, oestrogenic, tonic and anti-ageing effects, and to support the function of the nervous system, cardiovascular system and liver. Actions of royal jelly include:

- *Antioxidant activity.* Royal jelly has been found to scavenge free radicals such as the superoxide anion and hydroxyl radical, inhibit lipid peroxidation and protect DNA against oxidative damage. Polyphenolic compounds and protein fractions in royal jelly are believed to be the main antioxidants.
- *Antimicrobial activity.* Antibacterial peptides (jelleines) and 10H2DA in royal jelly are active against a range of bacteria and yeasts, such as *Candida* and *Trichosporon* spp. Major royal jelly proteins (MRJPs) have immune modulating activity. The royal jelly protein royalisin possesses antibiotic properties against Gram-positive bacteria. It appears that the antibacterial activity of royal jelly is less effective than the ether-soluble extract.
- *Anti-inflammatory activity.* 10H2DA inhibits NF-kappaB activation and suppresses NO production. MRJP3 is a protein that suppresses the production of interleukins and interferon-gamma, and may have anti-allergy effects.
- *Nervous system support.* Adenosine monophosphate N1 oxide (AMP N1-oxide) and 10H2DA in royal jelly enhance growth of nerve cells, astroglia and oligodendrocytes, and stimulate nerve cell differentiation.
- *Oestrogenic activity.* Royal jelly interacts with oestrogen receptors and stimulates gene expression, causing oestrogenic effects. It competes with 17beta-oestradiol for binding to human oestrogen receptors, but has weaker affinity than diethylstilboestrol and phyto-oestrogens.

Supplements, uses and dose

The permitted forms of royal jelly in Australian supplements are royal jelly, fresh or lyophilised (freeze-dried), and it is available in its natural form or as capsules. Fresh royal jelly is a milky-white or pale yellowish, paste-like substance. After harvesting, it is filtered to remove traces of wax or larvae, and chilled or frozen to protect the bioactives and to prevent it from hardening and browning.

Royal jelly may be used for allergies, inflammatory disorders, infections, fatigue, menopausal disorders, nerve and liver protection, diseases of ageing, elevated blood glucose and lipids, and sports performance. It is also used as a general health tonic, immune stimulant and anti-ageing supplement. Topically, royal jelly is used as a skin treatment and hair-growth stimulant. However, human research is limited.

In animal models of dermatitis, royal jelly decreased itching, skin inflammation and the development of lesions.[1,2] Royal jelly has reduced markers of oxidative damage to DNA and extended lifespan in an animal study.[3] In an animal model of systemic lupus erythematosus, royal jelly decreased production of auto-antibodies, delayed onset of the disease and extended lifespan.[4] Royal jelly has also improved endurance in an animal study,[5] and 100 mg/kg/body weight in animals has counteracted the adverse effects of anabolic steroid treatment on plasma testosterone levels and sperm count, maturation and motility.[6] Royal jelly protein isolate has been found to inhibit ACE-1, and to have a prolonged blood pressure-lowering effect in animals.[7] In animals, loss of muscle mass and strength that occurs with ageing was reduced by royal jelly, the regenerating capacity of injured muscles was improved, and serum insulin-like growth factor-1 levels increased.[8] Royal jelly maintained spatial learning and memory in an animal model of Alzheimer's disease.[9] In an animal model of menopause, royal jelly maintained bone calcium and phosphate levels, and reduced bone loss in the lumbar spine and proximal femur.[10] Royal jelly has enhanced collagen production in the skin in female animals with oestrogen deficiency.[11]

A meta-analysis of Russian studies using royal jelly in people with abnormal blood lipids found that it reduced total serum lipids and cholesterol levels, and normalised HDL and LDL cholesterol.[12] The meta-analysis concluded that Royal jelly (about 50–100 mg/day) decreased total serum cholesterol levels by about 14 per cent and total serum lipids by about 10 per cent. A small study of healthy people found that a one-off dose of royal jelly (20 g) reduced blood glucose levels during a glucose-tolerance test.[13] Healthy people given 3 g of royal jelly/day for six months were found to have increased serum testosterone, red blood cell count and haematocrit, and improved glucose tolerance and mental health score.[14] The optimal dose is unknown, but doses of 50–100 mg have been used for abnormal blood lipids, and up to 20 g/day has been used in research studies.

REFERENCES

1 Taniguchi, Y., Kohno, K., Inoue, S. et al., Oral administration of royal jelly inhibits the development of atopic dermatitis-like skin lesions in NC/Nga mice, *Int Immunopharmacol* (2003), 3(9): 1313–24.

2 Yamaura, K., Tomono, A., Suwa, E. & Ueno, K., Topical royal jelly alleviates symptoms of pruritus in a murine model of allergic contact dermatitis, *Pharmacogn Mag* (2013), 9(33): 9–13.

3 Inoue, S., Koya-Miyata, S., Ushio, S. et al., Royal jelly prolongs the life span of C3H/HeJ mice: Correlation with reduced DNA damage, *Exp Gerontol* (2003), 38(9): 965–9.

4 Mannoor, M.K., Shimabukuro, I., Tsukamotoa, M. et al., Honeybee royal jelly inhibits autoimmunity in SLE-prone NZB × NZW F1 mice, *Lupus* (2009), 18(1): 44–52.

5 Kamakura, M., Mitani, N., Fukuda, T. & Fukushima, M., Antifatigue effect of fresh royal jelly in mice, *J Nutr Sci Vitaminol (Tokyo)* (2001), 47(6): 394–401.

6 Zahmatkesh, E., Najafi, G., Nejati, V. & Heidari, R., Protective effect of royal jelly on the sperm parameters and testosterone level and lipid peroxidation in adult mice treated with oxymetholone, *Avicenna J Phytomed* (2014), 4(1): 43–52.

7 Takaki-Doi, S., Hashimoto, K., Yamamura, M. & Kamei, C., Antihypertensive activities of royal jelly protein hydrolysate and its fractions in spontaneously hypertensive rats, *Acta Med Okayama* (2009), 63(1): 57–64.

8 Niu, K., Guo, H., Guo, Y. et al., Royal jelly prevents the progression of sarcopenia in aged mice in vivo and in vitro, *J Gerontol A Biol Sci Med Sci* (2013), 68(12): 1482–92.

9 Zamani, Z., Reisi, P., Alaei, H. & Pilehvarian, A.A., Effect of Royal jelly on spatial learning and memory in rat model of streptozotocin-induced sporadic Alzheimer's disease, *Adv Biomed Res* (2012), 1: 26.

10 Kafadar, I.H., Güney, A., Türk, C.Y. et al., Royal jelly and bee pollen decrease bone loss due to osteoporosis in an oophorectomized rat model, *Eklem Hastalik Cerrahisi* (2012), 23(2): 100–5.

11 Park, H.M., Cho, M.H., Cho, Y. & Kim, S.Y., Royal jelly increases collagen production in rat skin after ovariectomy, *J Med Food* (2012), 15(6): 568–75.

12 Vittek, J., Effect of royal jelly on serum lipids in experimental animals and humans with atherosclerosis, *Experientia* (1995), 51(9–10): 927–35.

13 Münstedt, K., Bargello, M. & Hauenschild, A., Royal jelly reduces the serum glucose levels in healthy subjects, *J Med Food* (2009), 12(5): 1170–2.

14 Morita, H., Ikeda, T., Kajita, K. et al., Effect of royal jelly ingestion for six months on healthy volunteers, *Nutr J* (2012), 11: 77.

Cautions

Royal jelly should be used with caution. It is an allergenic substance, and can cause itching, skin rashes, eczema, eyelid and facial swelling, conjunctivitis, runny nose and breathing difficulties, and trigger asthma. Rarely, it may lead to acute severe asthma, anaphylaxis and death in susceptible people. Topical applications can cause contact dermatitis. Pregnant women, women with a history of hormone-sensitive breast cancer and people with a history of asthma or allergy—especially to bee pollen or bee venom—should not use royal jelly. There is one case report of haemorrhagic colitis associated with use of royal jelly. Royal jelly may increase the effects of warfarin and a lower dose may be required. The TGA in Australia requires that the following advisory statement is included on product labels:

'This product contains royal jelly which has been reported to cause severe allergic reactions and in rare cases fatalities—especially in asthma and allergy sufferers.'

HOW MUCH DO I KNOW?

Choose whether the following statements are true or false. Then review this chapter for the correct answers.

	True (T)	False (F)
1 Amylase is a protease enzyme.	T	F
2 Probiotics enhance immunity and have anti-inflammatory effects.	T	F
3 Glucosamine is part of glycosaminoglycans in connective tissue.	T	F
4 Methylsulfonylmethane is used to relieve the symptoms of osteoarthritis.	T	F
5 The adverse effects of cordyceps include a whip-like, linear skin rash.	T	F
6 High-selenium brewer's yeast may improve glucose tolerance.	T	F
7 Alginates from seaweed are used as food additives.	T	F
8 Spirulina may be useful for reducing elevated blood lipids and cholesterol.	T	F
9 Honey is used as a wound dressing.	T	F
10 Propolis has antioxidant, anti-inflammatory and antimicrobial activity.	T	F

FURTHER READING

Braun, L. & Cohen, M., *Herbs & natural supplements: An evidence-based guide*, 3rd ed., Churchill Livingstone Elsevier, New York, 2010.

Appendix
Nutrient tables

AUSTRALIAN AND NEW ZEALAND NUTRIENT REFERENCE VALUES AND ESTIMATED ENERGY REQUIREMENTS

Table A.1 ANZ Nutrient Reference Values (NRVs) for proteins, fats, carbohydrates, fibre, water

Age range	Protein (g/day)			Dietary fats[a]: Linoleic (n-6) (g/day)		Dietary fats[a]: α-linolenic (n-3) (g/day)		Dietary fats[a]: LC n-3 (DHA/EPA/DPA) (mg/day)		Carbohydrate (g/day)		Dietary fibre (g/day)		Total water[b] (figure in brackets is fluid component only) (L/day)	
	AI		UL	AI	UL	AI	UL	AI	UL	AI	UL	AI	UL	AI	UL
Infants[c]															
0–6 months	10		BM	4.4	BM	0.5[a]	BM	–	NP	60	BM	NP	NP	0.7 (0.7)	NP
7–12 months	14		B/F	4.6	B/F	0.5[a]	B/F	–	NP	95	B/F	NP	NP	0.8 (0.6)	NP
	EAR	RDI	UL	AI	UL	AI	UL	AI	UL	AI	UL	AI	UL	AI	UL
Children															
1–3 years	12	14	NP	5	NP	0.5	NP	40	3000			14	NP	1.4 (1.0)	NP
4–8 years	16	20	NP	8	NP	0.8	NP	55	3000			18	NP	1.6 (1.2)	NP
Boys															
9–13 years	31	40	NP	10	NP	1.0	NP	70	3000			24	NP	2.2 (1.6)	NP
14–18 years	49	65	NP	12	NP	1.2	NP	125	3000			28	NP	2.7 (1.9)	NP
Girls															
9–13 years	24	35	NP	8	NP	0.8	NP	70	3000			20	NP	1.9 (1.4)	NP
14–18 years	35	45	NP	8	NP	0.8	NP	85	3000			22	NP	2.2 (1.6)	NP
Men															
19–30 years	52	64	NP	13	NP	1.3	NP	160	3000			30	NP	3.4 (2.6)	NP
31–50 years	52	64	NP	13	NP	1.3	NP	160	3000			30	NP	3.4 (2.6)	NP
51–70 years	52	64	NP	13	NP	1.3	NP	160	3000			30	NP	3.4 (2.6)	NP
71+ years	65	81	NP	13	NP	1.3	NP	160	3000			30	NP	3.4 (2.6)	NP
Women															
19–30 years	37	46	NP	8	NP	0.8	NP	90	3000			25	NP	2.8 (2.1)	NP
31–50 years	37	46	NP	8	NP	0.8	NP	90	3000			25	NP	2.8 (2.1)	NP
51–70 years	37	46	NP	8	NP	0.8	NP	90	3000			25	NP	2.8 (2.1)	NP
71+ years	46	57	NP	8	NP	0.8	NP	90	3000			25	NP	2.8 (2.1)	NP
Pregnancy															
14–18 years	47[d]	58[d]	NP	10	NP	1.0	NP	110	3000			25	NP	2.4 (1.8)	NP
19–30 years	49[d]	60[d]	NP	10	NP	1.0	NP	115	3000			28	NP	3.1 (2.3)	NP
31–50 years	49[d]	60[d]	NP	10	NP	1.0	NP	115	3000			28	NP	3.1 (2.3)	NP
Lactation															
14–18 years	51	63	NP	12	NP	1.2	NP	140	3000			27	NP	2.9 (2.3)	NP
19–30 years	54	67	NP	12	NP	1.2	NP	145	3000			30	NP	3.5 (2.6)	NP
31–50 years	54	67	NP	12	NP	1.2	NP	145	3000			30	NP	3.5 (2.6)	NP

Abbreviations: AI, adequate intake; BM, amount normally received from breast milk; B/F, amount in breast milk and food; EAR, estimated average requirement; RDI, recommended dietary intake; NP, not possible to set—may be insufficient evidence or no clear level for adverse effects; UL, upper level of intake.

[a] Recommendation for total n-6 and total n-3; total fat AI also set at 30–31 g/day for infants.

[b] Total water includes water from foods as well as fluids.

[c] AI recommendations for infants are based on amounts in breast milk.

[d] In second and third trimesters only.

Table A.2 ANZ Nutrient Reference Values (NRVs) for vitamins

Age range	Thiamin (mg/day)			Riboflavin (mg/day)			Niacin[a] (mg/day niacin equivalents)			Vitamin B6 (mg/day)			Vitamin B12 (µg/day)			Folate[b] (as dietary folate equivs) (µg/day)		
	AI		UL	AI		UL	AI		UL	AI		UL[c]	AI		UL	AI		UL
Infants[d]																		
0–6 months	0.2		NP	0.3		BM	2		BM	0.1		BM	0.4		BM	65		BM
7–12 months	0.3		NP	0.4		B/F	4		B/F	0.3		B/F	0.5		B/F	80		B/F
	EAR	RDI	UL	EAR	RDI	UL	EAR	RDI	UL	EAR	RDI	UL	EAR	RDI	UL	EAR[e]	RDI[e]	UL
Children																		
1–3 years	0.4	0.5	NP	0.4	0.5	NP	5	6	10	0.4	0.5	15	0.7	0.9	NP	120	150	300
4–8 years	0.5	0.6	NP	0.5	0.6	NP	6	8	15	0.5	0.6	20	1.0	1.2	NP	160	200	400
Boys																		
9–13 years	0.7	0.9	NP	0.8	0.9	NP	9	12	20	0.8	1.0	30	1.5	1.8	NP	250	300	600
14–18 years	1.0	1.2	NP	1.1	1.3	NP	12	16	30	1.1	1.3	40	2.0	2.4	NP	330	400	800
Girls																		
9–13 years	0.7	0.9	NP	0.8	0.9	NP	9	12	20	0.8	1.0	30	1.5	1.8	NP	250	300	600
14–18 years	0.9	1.1	NP	0.9	1.1	NP	11	14	30	1.0	1.2	40	2.0	2.4	NP	330	400	800
Men																		
19–30 years	1.0	1.2	NP	1.1	1.3	NP	12	16	35	1.1	1.3	50	2.0	2.4	NP	320	400	1000
31–50 years	1.0	1.2	NP	1.1	1.3	NP	12	16	35	1.1	1.3	50	2.0	2.4	NP	320	400	1000
51–70 years	1.0	1.2	NP	1.1	1.3	NP	12	16	35	1.4	1.7	50	2.0	2.4	NP	320	400	1000
71+ years	1.0	1.2	NP	1.3	1.6	NP	12	16	35	1.4	1.7	50	2.0	2.4	NP	320	400	1000
Women																		
19–30 years	0.9	1.1	NP	0.9	1.1	NP	11	14	35	1.1	1.3	50	2.0	2.4	NP	320	400	1000
31–50 years	0.9	1.1	NP	0.9	1.1	NP	11	14	35	1.1	1.3	50	2.0	2.4	NP	320	400	1000
51–70 years	0.9	1.1	NP	0.9	1.1	NP	11	14	35	1.3	1.5	50	2.0	2.4	NP	320	400	1000
71+ years	0.9	1.1	NP	1.1	1.3	NP	11	14	35	1.3	1.5	50	2.0	2.4	NP	320	400	1000
Pregnancy																		
14–18 years	1.2	1.4	NP	1.2	1.4	NP	14	18	30	1.6	1.9	40	2.2	2.6	NP	520	600	800
19–30 years	1.2	1.4	NP	1.2	1.4	NP	14	18	35	1.6	1.9	50	2.2	2.6	NP	520	600	1000
31–50 years	1.2	1.4	NP	1.2	1.4	NP	14	18	35	1.6	1.9	50	2.2	2.6	NP	520	600	1000
Lactation																		
14–18 years	1.2	1.4	NP	1.3	1.6	NP	13	17	30	1.7	2.0	40	2.4	2.8	NP	450	500	800
19–30 years	1.2	1.4	NP	1.3	1.6	NP	13	17	35	1.7	2.0	50	2.4	2.8	NP	450	500	1000
31–50 years	1.2	1.4	NP	1.3	1.6	NP	13	17	35	1.7	2.0	50	2.4	2.8	NP	450	500	1000

Abbreviations: AI adequate intake; BM, amount normally received from breast milk; B/F, amount in breast milk and food; EAR, estimated average requirement; RDI, recommended dietary intake; NP, not possible to set—may be insufficient evidence or no clear level for adverse effects; UL, upper level of intake.

[a] The UL for niacin refers to nicotinic acid. For supplemental nicotinamide, the UL is 900 mg/day for men and non-pregnant women, 150 mg/day for 1–3-year-olds, 250 mg/day for 4–8-year-olds; 500 mg/day for 9–13-year-olds and 750 mg/day for 14–18-year-olds. It is not possible to set a UL for nicotinamide for infancy (intake should be only breast milk, formula or foods) or pregnancy and lactation (source should be food only).

[b] For folate, the UL is for intake from fortified foods and supplements as folic acid.

[c] For vitamin B6, the UL is set for pyridoxine.

[d] All infant AIs are based on milk concentrations in healthy women and average volumes.

[e] This is for dietary intake. For pregnant women, it does not include the additional supplemental folic acid required to prevent neural tube defects.

Pantothenic acid (mg/day)		Biotin (µg/day)		Vitamin A (retinol equivalents) (µg/day)			Vitamin C (mg/day)			Vitamin D (µg/day)		Vitamin E (α-tocopherol equivalents[f]) (mg/day)		Vitamin K (µg/day)		Choline (mg/day)	
AI	UL	AI	UL	AI		UL[g]	AI		UL[h]	AI	UL	AI	UL	AI	UL	AI	UL
1.7	BM	5	BM	250 (as retinol)		600	25		BM	5	25	4	BM	2	BM	125	BM
2.2	B/F	6	B/F	430		600	30		B/F	5	25	5	B/F	2.5	B/F	150	B/F
AI	UL	AI	UL	EAR	RDI	UL	EAR	RDI	UL	AI	UL	AI	UL	AI	UL	AI	UL
3.5	NP	8	NP	210	300	600	25	35	NP	5	80	5	70	25	NP	200	1000
4.0	NP	12	NP	275	400	900	25	35	NP	5	80	6	100	35	NP	250	1000
5.0	NP	20	NP	445	600	1700	28	40	NP	5	80	9	180	45	NP	375	1000
6.0	NP	30	NP	630	900	2800	28	40	NP	5	80	10	250	55	NP	550	3000
4.0	NP	20	NP	420	600	1700	28	40	NP	5	80	8	180	45	NP	375	1000
4.0	NP	25	NP	485	700	2800	28	40	NP	5	80	8	250	55	NP	400	3000
6.0	NP	30	NP	625	900	3000	30	45	NP	5	80	10	300	70	NP	550	3500
6.0	NP	30	NP	625	900	3000	30	45	NP	5	80	10	300	70	NP	550	3500
6.0	NP	30	NP	625	900	3000	30	45	NP	10	80	10	300	70	NP	550	3500
6.0	NP	30	NP	625	900	3000	30	45	NP	15	80	10	300	70	NP	550	3500
4.0	NP	25	NP	500	700	3000	30	45	NP	5	80	7	300	60	NP	425	3500
4.0	NP	25	NP	500	700	3000	30	45	NP	5	80	7	300	60	NP	425	3500
4.0	NP	25	NP	500	700	3000	30	45	NP	10	80	7	300	60	NP	425	3500
4.0	NP	25	NP	500	700	3000	30	45	NP	15	80	7	300	60	NP	425	3500
5.0	NP	30	NP	530	700	2800	38	55	NP	5	80	8	300	60	NP	415	3000
5.0	NP	30	NP	550	800	3000	40	60	NP	5	80	7	300	60	NP	440	3500
5.0	NP	30	NP	550	800	3000	40	60	NP	5	80	7	300	60	NP	440	3500
6.0	NP	35	NP	780	1100	2800	58	80	NP	5	80	12	300	60	NP	525	3000
6.0	NP	35	NP	800	1100	3000	60	85	NP	5	80	11	300	60	NP	550	3500
6.0	NP	35	NP	800	1100	3000	60	85	NP	5	80	11	300	60	NP	550	3500

[f] One α-tocopherol equivalent is equal to 1 mg RRR α- (or d-α-) tocopherol, 2 mg β-tocopherol, 10 mg γ-tocopherol or 3 mg α-tocotrienol. The relevant figure for synthetic all-rac-α-tocopherols (dl-α-tocopherol) is 14 mg.

[g] A UL cannot be established for supplemental β-carotene use and is not required for food use.

[h] Not possible to establish a UL for vitamin C from available data, but 1000 mg/day would be a prudent limit.

Table A.3 ANZ Nutrient Reference Values (NRVs) for minerals

Age range	Calcium[a] (mg/day)			Phosphorus (mg/day)			Zinc (mg/day)			Iron (mg/day)			Magnesium (mg/day)		
	AI		UL	AI		UL	AI		UL	AI		UL	AI		UL[b]
Infants															
0–6 months	210		BM	100		BM	2		4	0.2		20	30		BM
							EAR	RDI	UL	EAR	RDI	UL			
7–12 months	270		B/F	275		B/F	2.5	3	5	7.0	11	20	75		B/F
	EAR	RDI	UL	EAR	RDI	UL	EAR	RDI	UL	EAR	RDI	UL	EAR	RDI	UL
Children															
1–3 years	360	500	2500	380	460	3000	2.5	3	7	4.0	9	20	65	80	65
4–8 years	520	700	2500	405	500	3000	3.0	4	12	4.0	10	40	110	130	110
Boys															
9–13 years	800–1050	1000–1300	2500	1055	1250	4000	5.0	6	25	6.0	8	40	200	240	350
14–18 years	1050	1300	2500	1055	1250	4000	11.0	13	35	8.0	11	45	340	410	350
Girls															
9–13 years	800–1050	1000–1300	2500	1055	1250	4000	5.0	6	25	6.0	8	40	200	240	350
14–18 years	1050	1300	2500	1055	1250	4000	6.0	7	35	8.0	15	45	300	360	350
Men															
19–30 years	840	1000	2500	580	1000	4000	12.0	14	40	6.0	8	45	330	400	350
31–50 years	840	1000	2500	580	1000	4000	12.0	14	40	6.0	8	45	350	420	350
51–70 years	840	1000	2500	580	1000	4000	12.0	14	40	6.0	8	45	350	420	350
71+ years	1100	1300	2500	580	1000	3000	12.0	14	40	6.0	8	45	350	420	350
Women															
19–30 years	840	1000	2500	580	1000	4000	6.5	8	40	8.0	18	45	255	310	350
31–50 years	840	1000	2500	580	1000	4000	6.5	8	40	8.0	18	45	265	320	350
51–70 years	1100	1300	2500	580	1000	4000	6.5	8	40	5.0	8	45	265	320	350
71+ years	1100	1300	2500	580	1000	3000	6.5	8	40	5.0	8	45	265	320	350
Pregnancy															
14–18 years	1050	1300	2500	1055	1250	3500	8.5	10	35	23.0	27	45	335	400	350
19–30 years	840	1000	2500	580	1000	3500	9.0	11	40	22.0	27	45	290	350	350
31–50 years	840	1000	2500	580	1000	3500	9.0	11	40	22.0	27	45	300	360	350
Lactation															
14–18 years	1050	1300	2500	1055	1250	4000	9.0	11	35	7.0	10	45	300	360	350
19–30 years	840	1000	2500	580	1000	4000	10.0	12	40	6.5	9	45	255	310	350
31–50 years	840	1000	2500	580	1000	4000	10.0	12	40	6.5	9	45	265	320	350

Abbreviations: AI, adequate intake; BM, amount normally received from breast milk; B/F, amount in breast milk and food; EAR, estimated average requirement; RDI, recommended dietary intake; NP, not possible to set—may be insufficient evidence or no clear level for adverse effects; UL, upper level of intake.

[a] For calcium, there are separate recommendations for children aged 9–11 years and 12–13 years because of growth needs. 9–11-year-olds who are growing and maturing at much greater rates than average may need the intakes recommended for 12–13-year-olds.

[b] Note that all of the ULs listed for magnesium refer to supplements.

[c] 920 mg sodium/day is equivalent to 40 mmol/day; 2300 mg sodium/day is equivalent to 100 mmol/day.

[d] Intake of manganese beyond that normally found in food and beverages could represent a health risk, but there are insufficient data to set a UL.

[e] A level of no more than 1600 mg sodium/day (70 mmol) is recommended for older, overweight hypertensives and for those wishing to maintain low blood pressure over the lifespan.

f For potassium, supplements should be taken only under medical supervision.

Iodine (μg/day)			Selenium (μg/day)			Molybdenum (μg/day)			Copper (mg/day)		Chromium (μg/day)		Manganese (mg/day)		Fluoride (mg/day)		Sodium (mg/day)[c]		Potassium (mg/day)	
AI	UL		AI	UL		AI	UL		AI	UL	AI	UL	AI	UL[d]	AI	UL	AI	UL[e]	AI	UL[f]
90	BM		12	45		2	BM		0.2	BM	0.2	NP	0.003	BM	0.01	0.7	120	NP	400	NP
110	B/F		15	60		3	B/F		0.22	B/F	5.5	NP	0.6	B/F	0.5	0.9	170	NP	700	NP
EAR	RDI	UL	EAR	RDI	UL	EAR	RDI	UL	AI	UL	AI	UL	AI	UL	AI	UL	AI	UL	AI	UL
65	90	200	20	25	90	13	17	300	0.7	1	11	NP	2.0	NP	0.7	1.3	200–400	1000	2000	NP
65	90	300	25	30	150	17	22	600	1.0	3	15	NP	2.5	NP	1.0	2.2	300–600	1400	2300	NP
75	120	600	40	50	280	26	34	1100	1.3	5	25	NP	3.0	NP	2.0	10.0	400–800	2000	3000	NP
95	150	900	60	70	400	33	43	1700	1.5	8	35	NP	3.5	NP	3.0	10.0	460–920	2300	3600	NP
75	120	600	40	50	280	26	34	1100	1.1	5	21	NP	2.5	NP	2.0	10.0	400–800	2000	2500	NP
95	150	900	50	60	400	33	43	1700	1.1	8	24	NP	3.0	NP	3.0	10.0	460–920	2300	2600	NP
100	150	1100	60	70	400	34	45	2000	1.7	10	35	NP	5.5	NP	4.0	10.0	460–920	2300	3800	NP
100	150	1100	60	70	400	34	45	2000	1.7	10	35	NP	5.5	NP	4.0	10.0	460–920	2300	3800	NP
100	150	1100	60	70	400	34	45	2000	1.7	10	35	NP	5.5	NP	4.0	10.0	460–920	2300	3800	NP
100	150	1100	60	70	400	34	45	2000	1.7	10	35	NP	5.5	NP	4.0	10.0	460–920	2300	3800	NP
100	150	1100	50	60	400	34	45	2000	1.2	10	25	NP	5.0	NP	3.0	10.0	460–920	2300	2800	NP
100	150	1100	50	60	400	34	45	2000	1.2	10	25	NP	5.0	NP	3.0	10.0	460–920	2300	2800	NP
100	150	1100	50	60	400	34	45	2000	1.2	10	25	NP	5.0	NP	3.0	10.0	460–920	2300	2800	NP
100	150	1100	50	60	400	34	45	2000	1.2	10	25	NP	5.0	NP	3.0	10.0	460–920	2300	2800	NP
160	220	900	55	65	400	40	50	1700	1.2	8	30	NP	5.0	NP	3.0	10.0	460–920	2300	2800	NP
160	220	1100	55	65	400	40	50	2000	1.3	10	30	NP	5.0	NP	3.0	10.0	460–920	2300	2800	NP
160	220	1100	55	65	400	40	50	2000	1.3	10	30	NP	5.0	NP	3.0	10.0	460–920	2300	2800	NP
190	270	900	65	75	400	35	50	1700	1.4	8	45	NP	5.0	NP	3.0	10.0	460–920	2300	3200	NP
190	270	1100	65	75	400	36	50	2000	1.5	10	45	NP	5.0	NP	3.0	10.0	460–920	2300	3200	NP
190	270	1100	65	75	400	36	50	2000	1.5	10	45	NP	5.0	NP	3.0	10.0	460–920	2300	3200	NP

Table A.4 ANZ Estimated Energy Requirements (EERs) of infants and young children

Age (months)	Reference weight (kg)		EER (kJ/day)	
	Boys	Girls	Boys	Girls
1	4.4	4.2	2000	1800
2	5.3	4.9	2400	2100
3	6.0	5.5	2400	2200
4	6.7	6.1	2400	2200
5	7.3	6.7	2500	2300
6	7.9	7.2	2700	2500
7	8.4	7.7	2800	2500
8	8.9	8.1	3000	2700
9	9.3	8.5	3100	2800
10	9.7	8.9	3300	3000
11	10.0	9.2	3400	3100
12	10.3	9.5	3500	3200
15	11.1	10.3	3800	3500
18	11.7	11.0	4000	3800
21	12.2	11.6	4200	4000
24	12.7	12.1	4400	4200

Source: National Health and Medical Research Council.

Table A.5 ANZ Estimated Energy Requirements (EERs) of children and adolescents using BMR, predicted from weight, height and age

Age guide[a] (years)	Reference weight[b] (kg)	Reference height (m)	BMR[c] (MJ/day)	Physical activity level (PAL)					
				1.2[d]	1.4[d]	1.6[d]	1.8[d]	2[d]	2.2[d]
				Bed rest	Very sedentary	Light	Moderate	Heavy	Vigorous
Boys									
3	14.3	0.95	3.4	4.2	4.9	5.6	6.3	6.9	7.6
4	16.2	1.02	3.6	4.4	5.2	5.9	6.6	7.3	8.1
5	18.4	1.09	3.8	4.7	5.5	6.2	7.0	7.8	8.5
6	20.7	1.15	4.1	5.0	5.8	6.6	7.4	8.2	9.0
7	23.1	1.22	4.3	5.2	6.1	7.0	7.8	8.7	9.5
8	25.6	1.28	4.5	5.5	6.4	7.3	8.2	9.2	10.1
9	28.6	1.34	4.8	5.9	6.8	7.8	8.8	9.7	10.7
10	31.9	1.39	5.1	6.3	7.3	8.3	9.3	10.4	11.4
11	35.9	1.44	5.4	6.6	7.7	8.8	9.9	11.0	12.0
12	40.5	1.49	5.8	7.0	8.2	9.3	10.5	11.6	12.8
13	45.6	1.56	6.2	7.5	8.7	10.0	11.2	12.4	13.6
14	51.0	1.64	6.6	8.0	9.3	10.6	11.9	13.2	14.6
15	56.3	1.70	7.0	8.5	9.9	11.2	12.6	14.0	15.4
16	60.9	1.74	7.3	8.9	10.3	11.8	13.2	14.7	16.2
17	64.6	1.75	7.6	9.2	10.7	12.2	13.7	15.2	16.7
18	67.2	1.76	7.7	9.4	10.9	12.5	14.0	15.6	17.1
Girls									
3	13.9	0.94	3.2	3.9	4.5	5.3	5.8	6.4	7.1
4	15.8	1.01	3.4	4.1	4.8	5.5	6.1	6.8	7.5
5	17.9	1.08	3.6	4.4	5.1	5.7	6.5	7.2	7.9
6	20.2	1.15	3.8	4.6	5.4	6.1	6.9	7.6	8.4
7	22.8	1.21	4.0	4.9	5.7	6.5	7.3	8.1	8.9
8	25.6	1.28	4.2	5.2	6.0	6.9	7.7	8.6	9.4
9	29.0	1.33	4.5	5.5	6.4	7.3	8.2	9.1	10.0
10	32.9	1.38	4.7	5.7	6.7	7.6	8.5	9.5	10.4
11	37.2	1.44	4.9	6.0	7.0	8.0	9.0	10.0	11.0
12	41.6	1.51	5.2	6.4	7.4	8.5	9.5	10.6	11.6
13	45.8	1.57	5.5	6.7	7.8	8.9	10.0	11.1	12.2
14	49.4	1.60	5.7	6.9	8.1	9.2	10.3	11.5	12.6
15	52.0	1.62	5.8	7.1	8.2	9.4	10.6	11.7	12.9
16	53.9	1.63	5.9	7.2	8.4	9.5	10.7	11.9	13.1
17	55.1	1.63	5.9	7.2	8.4	9.6	10.8	12.0	13.2
18	56.2	1.63	6.0	7.3	8.5	9.7	10.9	12.1	13.3

[a] The height and/or weight to age ratio may differ markedly in some ethnic groups. In this case, if BMI is in the acceptable range, it would be more relevant to use body weight as the main guide to current energy needs.

[b] Reference weights from Kuczmarski et al (2000), available at <www.cdc.gov/growthcharts>. See also FNB:IOM (2002), available at <www.nal.usda.gov/fnic/DRI/DRI_Energy/energy_full_report.pdf>.

[c] Estimated using Schofield (1985) equations for weight, height and age group 3–10, 10–18, available at <www.ncbi.nlm.nih.gov/pubmed/4044297>.

[d] PALs (Physical Activity Levels) incorporate relevant growth factor for age.

Source: National Health and Medical Research Council.

Table A.6 ANZ Estimated Energy Requirements (EERs) of adults, predicted BMR x PAL

Age (years)	BMI = 22.0[a]		BMR (MJ/day)	Physical activity level (PAL)[b] Males (MJ/day)						BMR (MJ/day)	Physical activity level (PAL)[b] Females (MJ/day)					
	Height (m)	Weight (kg)	Male	1.2	1.4	1.6	1.8	2.0	2.2	Female	1.2	1.4	1.6	1.8	2.0	2.2
19–30	1.5	49.5	–	–	–	–	–	–	–	5.2	6.1	7.1	8.2	9.2	10.2	11.2
	1.6	56.3	6.4	7.7	9.0	10.3	11.6	12.9	14.2	5.6	6.6	7.7	8.8	9.9	11.1	12.2
	1.7	63.6	6.9	8.3	9.7	11.0	12.4	13.8	15.2	6.0	7.2	8.4	9.6	10.8	12.0	13.2
	1.8	71.3	7.4	8.9	10.3	11.8	13.3	14.8	16.3	6.5	7.7	9.0	10.3	11.6	12.9	14.2
	1.9	79.4	7.9	9.5	11.1	12.6	14.2	15.8	17.4	7.0	8.4	9.7	11.1	12.5	13.9	15.3
	2.0	88.0	8.4	10.1	11.8	13.5	15.2	16.9	18.6	–	–	–	–	–	–	–
31–50	1.5	49.5	–	–	–	–	–	–	–	5.2	6.3	7.3	8.4	9.4	10.4	11.5
	1.6	56.3	6.4	7.6	8.9	10.2	11.4	12.7	14.0	5.5	6.5	7.6	8.7	9.8	10.9	12.0
	1.7	63.6	6.7	8.0	9.4	10.7	12.1	13.4	14.8	5.7	6.8	8.0	9.1	10.3	11.4	12.5
	1.8	71.3	7.1	8.5	9.9	11.3	12.7	14.2	15.6	6.0	7.2	8.3	9.5	10.7	11.9	13.1
	1.9	79.4	7.5	9.0	10.4	11.9	13.4	14.9	16.4	6.2	7.5	8.7	10.0	11.2	12.5	13.7
	2.0	88.0	7.9	9.5	11.0	12.6	14.2	15.8	17.3	–	–	–	–	–	–	–
51–70	1.5	49.5	–	–	–	–	–	–	–	4.9	6.0	6.9	7.9	8.9	9.8	10.9
	1.6	56.3	5.8	7.0	8.2	9.3	10.4	11.5	12.7	5.2	6.2	7.3	8.3	9.3	10.4	11.4
	1.7	63.6	6.1	7.3	8.6	9.8	11.1	12.3	13.6	5.4	6.5	7.6	8.7	9.8	10.7	12.0
	1.8	71.3	6.5	7.8	9.1	10.4	11.7	13.1	14.4	5.7	6.9	8.0	9.1	10.3	11.4	12.6
	1.9	79.4	6.9	8.3	9.6	11.1	12.4	13.8	15.2	6.0	7.2	8.4	9.6	10.8	12.0	13.2
	2.0	88.0	7.3	8.8	10.2	11.7	13.2	14.7	16.1	–	–	–	–	–	–	–
> 70	1.5	49.5	–	–	–	–	–	–	–	4.6	5.6	6.5	7.4	8.3	9.3	10.2
	1.6	56.3	5.2	6.3	7.3	8.3	9.4	10.4	11.5	4.9	5.9	6.9	7.8	8.8	9.8	10.8
	1.7	63.6	5.6	6.7	7.8	8.9	10.0	11.2	12.3	5.2	6.2	7.2	8.3	9.3	10.3	11.4
	1.8	71.3	6.0	7.1	8.3	9.5	10.7	11.9	13.1	5.5	6.6	7.7	8.7	9.8	10.9	12.0
	1.9	79.4	6.4	7.6	8.9	10.2	11.4	12.7	14.0	5.8	6.9	8.1	9.2	10.4	11.5	12.7
	2.0	88.0	6.8	8.1	9.5	10.8	12.2	13.5	14.9	–	–	–	–	–	–	–

[a] A BMI of 22.0 is approximately the mid-point of the WHO (1998) healthy weight range (BMI 18.5–24.9).

[b] Physical activity level (PAL) of 1.2 (bed rest) to 2.2 (very active or heavy occupational work). PALs of 1.75 and above are consistent with good health. PALs below 1.4 are not compatible with moving around freely or earning a living. PALs above 2.5 are difficult to maintain for long periods.

Note: The original Schofield equations from which these tables were derived (Schofield 1985), available at <www.nal.usda.gov/fnic/DRI/DRI_Energy/energy_full_report.pdf>, used 60+ years as the upper age category. For people aged 51–70 years, the estimates were derived by averaging those for the younger (19–30 years) and older (>70 years) adults.

Source: National Health and Medical Research Council.

US DIETARY REFERENCE INTAKES

Table A.7 US Dietary Reference Intakes (DRIs): Recommended dietary allowances and adequate intakes—vitamins
Food and Nutrition Board, Institute of Medicine, National Academies

Life stage group	Vitamin A (µg/d)[a]	Vitamin C (mg/d)	Vitamin D (µg/d)[b,c]	Vitamin E (mg/d)[d]	Vitamin K (µg/d)	Thiamin (mg/d)	Riboflavin (mg/d)	Niacin (mg/d)[e]	Vitamin B6 (mg/d)	Folate (µg/d)[f]	Vitamin B12 (µg/d)	Pantothenic acid (mg/d)	Biotin (µg/d)	Choline (mg/d)[g]
Infants														
0–6 months	400*	40*	10	4*	2.0*	0.2*	0.3*	2*	0.1*	65*	0.4*	1.7*	5*	125*
6–12 months	500*	50*	10	5*	2.5*	0.3*	0.4*	4*	0.3*	80*	0.5*	1.8*	6*	150*
Children														
1–3 years	300	15	15	6	30*	0.5	0.5	6	0.5	150	0.9	2*	8*	200*
4–8 years	400	25	15	7	55*	0.6	0.6	8	0.6	200	1.2	3*	12*	250*
Males														
9–13 years	600	45	15	11	60*	0.9	0.9	12	1.0	300	1.8	4*	20*	375*
14–18 years	900	75	15	15	75*	1.2	1.3	16	1.3	400	2.4	5*	25*	550*
19–30 years	900	90	15	15	120*	1.2	1.3	16	1.3	400	2.4	5*	30*	550*
31–50 years	900	90	15	15	120*	1.2	1.3	16	1.3	400	2.4	5*	30*	550*
51–70 years	900	90	15	15	120*	1.2	1.3	16	1.7	400	2.4[h]	5*	30*	550*
> 70 years	900	90	20	15	120*	1.2	1.3	16	1.7	400	2.4[h]	5*	30*	550*
Females														
9–13 years	600	45	15	11	60*	0.9	0.9	12	1.0	300	1.8	4*	20*	375*
14–18 years	700	65	15	15	75*	1.0	1.0	14	1.2	400[i]	2.4	5*	25*	400*
19–30 years	700	75	15	15	90*	1.1	1.1	14	1.3	400[i]	2.4	5*	30*	425*
31–50 years	700	75	15	15	90*	1.1	1.1	14	1.3	400[i]	2.4	5*	30*	425*
51–70 years	700	75	15	15	90*	1.1	1.1	14	1.5	400	2.4[h]	5*	30*	425*
> 70 years	700	75	20	15	90*	1.1	1.1	14	1.5	400	2.4[h]	5*	30*	425*
Pregnancy														
14–18 years	750	80	15	15	75*	1.4	1.4	18	1.9	600[j]	2.6	6*	30*	450*
19–30 years	770	85	15	15	90*	1.4	1.4	18	1.9	600[j]	2.6	6*	30*	450*
31–50 years	770	85	15	15	90*	1.4	1.4	18	1.9	600[j]	2.6	6*	30*	450*
Lactation														
14–18 years	1200	115	15	19	75*	1.4	1.6	17	2.0	500	2.8	7*	35*	550*
19–30 years	1300	120	15	19	90*	1.4	1.6	17	2.0	500	2.8	7*	35*	550*
31–50 years	1300	120	15	19	90*	1.4	1.6	17	2.0	500	2.8	7*	35*	550*

continues

Table A.7 US Dietary Reference Intakes (DRIs): Recommended dietary allowances and adequate intakes—vitamins *continued*

Notes: This table (taken from the DRI reports, see <www.nap.edu>) presents Recommended Dietary Allowances (RDAs) in **bold type** and Adequate Intakes (AIs) in ordinary type followed by an asterisk (*). An RDA is the average daily dietary intake level, sufficient to meet the nutrient requirements of nearly all healthy individuals in a group (97–98%). It is calculated from an estimated average requirement (EAR). If sufficient scientific evidence is not available to establish an EAR, and thus to calculate an RDA, an AI is usually developed. For healthy breastfed infants, an AI is the mean intake. The AI for other life stage and gender groups is believed to cover the needs of all healthy individuals in the groups, but lack of data or uncertainty in the data prevent being able to specify with confidence the percentage of individuals covered by this intake.

[a] As retinol activity equivalents (RAEs). 1 RAE = 1 μg retinol, 12 μg β-carotene, 24 μg α-carotene, or 24 μg β-cryptoxanthin. The RAE for dietary provitamin A carotenoids is two-fold greater than retinol equivalents (RE), whereas the RAE for preformed vitamin A is the same as RE.

[b] As cholecalciferol. 1 μg cholecalciferol = 40 IU vitamin D.

[c] Under the assumption of minimal sunlight.

[d] As α-tocopherol. α-tocopherol includes *RRR*-α-tocopherol, the only form of α-tocopherol that occurs naturally in foods, and the *2R*-stereoisomeric forms of α-tocopherol (*RRR-*, *RSR-*, *RRS-* and *RSS*-α-tocopherol) that occur in fortified foods and supplements. It does not include the *2S*-stereoisomeric forms of α-tocopherol (*SRR-*, *SSR-*, *SRS-* and *SSS*-α-tocopherol), also found in fortified foods and supplements.

[e] As niacin equivalents (NE). 1 mg of niacin = 60 mg of tryptophan; 0–6 months = preformed niacin (not NE).

[f] As dietary folate equivalents (DFE). 1 DFE = 1 μg food folate = 0.6 μg of folic acid from fortified food or as a supplement consumed with food = 0.5 μg of a supplement taken on an empty stomach.

[g] Although AIs have been set for choline, there are few data to assess whether a dietary supply of choline is needed at all stages of the life cycle, and it may be that the choline requirement can be met by endogenous synthesis at some of these stages.

[h] Because 10–30 % of older people may malabsorb food-bound B12, it is advisable for those older than 50 years to meet their RDA mainly by consuming foods fortified with B12 or a supplement containing B12.

[i] In view of evidence linking folate intake with neural tube defects in the foetus, it is recommended that all women capable of becoming pregnant consume 400 μg from supplements or fortified foods in addition to intake of food folate from a varied diet.

[j] It is assumed that women will continue consuming 400 μg from supplements or fortified food until their pregnancy is confirmed and they enter prenatal care, which ordinarily occurs after the end of the periconceptional period—the critical time for formation of the neural tube.

Sources: Dietary Reference Intakes for Calcium, Phosphorous, Magnesium, Vitamin D, and Fluoride (1997); *Dietary Reference Intakes for Thiamin, Riboflavin, Niacin, Vitamin B6, Folate, Vitamin B12, Pantothenic Acid, Biotin, and Choline* (1998); *Dietary Reference Intakes for Vitamin C, Vitamin E, Selenium, and Carotenoids* (2000); *Dietary Reference Intakes for Vitamin A, Vitamin K, Arsenic, Boron, Chromium, Copper, Iodine, Iron, Manganese, Molybdenum, Nickel, Silicon, Vanadium, and Zinc* (2001); *Dietary Reference Intakes for Water, Potassium, Sodium, Chloride, and Sulfate* (2005); and *Dietary Reference Intakes for Calcium and Vitamin D* (2011). These reports may be accessed via <www.nap.edu>.

Table A.8 US Dietary Reference Intakes (DRIs): Recommended dietary allowances and adequate intakes—elements
Food and Nutrition Board, Institute of Medicine, National Academies

Life stage group	Calcium (mg/d)	Chromium (µg/d)	Copper (µg/d)	Fluoride (mg/d)	Iodine (µg/d)	Iron (mg/d)	Magnesium (mg/d)	Manganese (mg/d)	Molybdenum (µg/d)	Phosphorus (mg/d)	Selenium (µg/d)	Zinc (mg/d)	Potassium (g/d)	Sodium (g/d)	Chloride (g/d)
Infants															
0–6 months	200*	0.2*	200*	0.01*	110*	0.27*	30*	0.003*	2*	100*	15*	2*	0.4*	0.12*	0.18*
6–12 months	260*	5.5*	220*	0.5*	130*	11	75*	0.600*	3*	275*	20*	3	0.7*	0.37*	0.57*
Children															
1–3 years	700	11*	340	0.7*	90	7	80	1.2*	17	460	20	3	3.0*	1.0*	1.5*
4–8 years	1000	15*	440	1*	90	10	130	1.5*	22	500	30	5	3.8*	1.2*	1.9*
Males															
9–13 years	1300	25*	700	2*	120	8	240	1.9*	34	1250	40	8	4.5*	1.5*	2.3*
14–18 years	1300	35*	890	3*	150	11.0	410	2.2*	43	1250	55	11	4.7*	1.5*	2.3*
19–30 years	1000	35*	900	4*	150	8	400	2.3*	45	700	55	11	4.7*	1.5*	2.3*
31–50 years	1000	35*	900	4*	150	8	420	2.3*	45	700	55	11	4.7*	1.5*	2.3*
51–70 years	1000	30*	900	4*	150	8	420	2.3*	45	700	55	11	4.7*	1.3*	2.0*
> 70 years	1200	30*	900	4*	150	8	420	2.3*	45	700	55	11	4.7*	1.2*	1.8*
Females															
9–13 years	1300	21*	700	2*	120	8	240	1.6*	34	1250	40	8	4.5*	1.5*	2.3*
14–18 years	1300	24*	890	3*	150	15	360	1.6*	43	1250	55	9	4.7*	1.5*	2.3*
19–30 years	1000	25*	900	3*	150	18	310	1.8*	45	700	55	8	4.7*	1.5*	2.3*
31–50 years	1000	25*	900	3*	150	18	320	1.8*	45	700	55	8	4.7*	1.5*	2.3*
51–70 years	1200	20*	900	3*	150	8	320	1.8*	45	700	55	8	4.7*	1.3*	2.0*
> 70 years	1200	20*	900	3*	150	8	320	1.8*	45	700	55	8	4.7*	1.2*	1.8*
Pregnancy															
14–18 years	1300	29*	1000	3*	220	27	400	2.0*	50	1250	60	12	4.7*	1.5*	2.3*
19–30 years	1000	30*	1000	3*	220	27	350	2.0*	50	700	60	11	4.7*	1.5*	2.3*
31–50 years	1000	30*	1000	3*	220	27	360	2.0*	50	700	60	11	4.7*	1.5*	2.3*
Lactation															
14–18 years	1300	44*	1300	3*	290	10	360	2.6*	50	1250	70	13	5.1*	1.5*	2.3*
19–30 years	1000	45*	1300	3*	290	9	310	2.6*	50	700	70	12	5.1*	1.5*	2.3*
31–50 years	1000	45*	1300	3*	290	9	320	2.6*	50	700	70	12	5.1*	1.5*	2.3*

Note: This table (taken from the DRI reports, see <www.nap.edu>) presents recommended dietary allowances (RDAs) in **bold type** and adequate intakes (AIs) in ordinary type followed by an asterisk (*). An RDA is the average daily dietary intake level, sufficient to meet the nutrient requirements of nearly all healthy individuals in a group (97–98%). It is calculated from an estimated average requirement (EAR). If sufficient scientific evidence is not available to establish an EAR, and thus to calculate an RDA, an AI is usually developed. For healthy breastfed infants, an AI is the mean intake. The AI for other life-stage and gender groups is believed to cover the needs of all healthy individuals in the groups, but lack of data or uncertainty in the data prevent being able to specify with confidence the percentage of individuals covered by this intake.

Sources: Dietary Reference Intakes for Calcium, Phosphorous, Magnesium, Vitamin D, and Fluoride (1997); *Dietary Reference Intakes for Thiamin, Riboflavin, Niacin, Vitamin B6, Folate, Vitamin B12, Pantothenic Acid, Biotin, and Choline* (1998); *Dietary Reference Intakes for Vitamin C, Vitamin E, Selenium, and Carotenoids* (2000); and *Dietary Reference Intakes for Vitamin A, Vitamin K, Arsenic, Boron, Chromium, Copper, Iodine, Iron, Manganese, Molybdenum, Nickel, Silicon, Vanadium, and Zinc* (2001); *Dietary Reference Intakes for Water, Potassium, Sodium, Chloride, and Sulfate* (2005); and *Dietary Reference Intakes for Calcium and Vitamin D* (2011). These reports may be accessed via <www.nap.edu>.

Table A.9 US Dietary Reference Intakes (DRIs): Recommended dietary allowances and adequate intakes—total water and macronutrients

Food and Nutrition Board, Institute of Medicine, National Academies

Life stage group	Total water[a] (L/d)	Carbohydrate (g/d)	Total fiber (g/d)	Fat (g/d)	Linoleic acid (g/d)	α-linolenic acid (g/d)	Protein[b] (g/d)
Infants							
0–6 months	0.7*	60*	ND[c]	31*	4.4*	0.5*	9.1*
6–12 months	0.8*	95*	ND	30*	4.6*	0.5*	**11.0**
Children							
1–3 years	1.3*	**130**	19*	ND[c]	7.0*	0.7*	**13.0**
4–8 years	1.7*	**130**	25*	ND	10.0*	0.9*	**19.0**
Males							
9–13 years	2.4*	**130**	31*	ND	12.0*	1.2*	**34.0**
14–18 years	3.3*	**130**	38*	ND	16.0*	1.6*	**52.0**
19–30 years	3.7*	**130**	38*	ND	17.0*	1.6*	**56.0**
31–50 years	3.7*	**130**	38*	ND	17.0*	1.6*	**56.0**
51–70 years	3.7*	**130**	30*	ND	14.0*	1.6*	**56.0**
> 70 years	3.7*	**130**	30*	ND	14.0*	1.6*	**56.0**
Females							
9–13 years	2.1*	**130**	26*	ND	10.0*	1.0*	**34.0**
14–18 years	2.3*	**130**	26*	ND	11.0*	1.1*	**46.0**
19–30 years	2.7*	**130**	25*	ND	12.0*	1.1*	**46.0**
31–50 years	2.7*	**130**	25*	ND	12.0*	1.1*	**46.0**
51–70 years	2.7*	**130**	21*	ND	11.0*	1.1*	**46.0**
> 70 years	2.7*	**130**	21*	ND	11.0*	1.1*	**46.0**
Pregnancy							
14–18 years	3.0*	**175**	28*	ND	13.0*	1.4*	**71.0**
19–30 years	3.0*	**175**	28*	ND	13.0*	1.4*	**71.0**
31–50 years	3.0*	**175**	28*	ND	13.0*	1.4*	**71.0**
Lactation							
14–18 years	3.8*	**210**	29*	ND	13.0*	1.3*	**71.0**
19–30 years	3.8*	**210**	29*	ND	13.0*	1.3*	**71.0**
31–50 years	3.8*	**210**	29*	ND	13.0*	1.3*	**71.0**

Notes: This table (taken from the DRI reports, see <www.nap.edu>) presents recommended dietary allowances (RDA) in **bold type** and adequate intakes (AI) in ordinary type followed by an asterisk (*). An RDA is the average daily dietary intake level, sufficient to meet the nutrient requirements of nearly all healthy individuals in a group (97–98%). It is calculated from an estimated average requirement (EAR). If sufficient scientific evidence is not available to establish an EAR, and thus to calculate an RDA, an AI is usually developed. For healthy breastfed infants, an AI is the mean intake. The AI for other life stage and gender groups is believed to cover the needs of all healthy individuals in the groups, but lack of data or uncertainty in the data prevent it being possible to specify with confidence the percentage of individuals covered by this intake.

[a] Total water includes all water contained in food, beverages and drinking water.

[b] Based on g protein per kg of body weight for the reference body weight, e.g., for adults 0.8 g/kg body weight for the reference body weight.

[c] Not determined.

Sources: Dietary Reference Intakes for Energy, Carbohydrate, Fiber, Fat, Fatty Acids, Cholesterol, Protein, and Amino Acids (2002/2005) and *Dietary Reference Intakes for Water, Potassium, Sodium, Chloride, and Sulfate* (2005). The report may be accessed via <www.nap.edu>.

Table A.10 US Dietary Reference Intakes (DRIs): Acceptable macronutrient distribution ranges—fat, carbohydrate and protein
Food and Nutrition Board, Institute of Medicine, National Academies

	Range (% energy)		
Macronutrient	Children (1–3 years)	Children (4–18 years)	Adults
Fat	30–40	25–35	20–35
n-6 polyunsaturated fatty acids[a] (linoleic acid)	5–10	5–10	5–10
n-3 polyunsaturated fatty acids[a] (α-linolenic acid)	0.6–1.2	0.6–1.2	0.6–1.2
Carbohydrate	45–65	45–65	45–65
Protein	5–20	10–30	10–35

[a] Approximately 10% of the total can come from longer-chain n-3 or n-6 fatty acids.

Source: Dietary Reference Intakes for Energy, Carbohydrate, Fiber, Fat, Fatty Acids, Cholesterol, Protein, and Amino Acids (2002/2005). The report may be accessed via <www.nap.edu>.

Table A.11 US Dietary Reference Intakes (DRIs): Acceptable macronutrient distribution ranges—dietary cholesterol, trans fatty acids, saturated fatty acids and added sugars
Food and Nutrition Board, Institute of Medicine, National Academies

Macronutrient	Recommendation
Dietary cholesterol	As low as possible while consuming a nutritionally adequate diet
Trans fatty acids	As low as possible while consuming a nutritionally adequate diet
Saturated fatty acids	As low as possible while consuming a nutritionally adequate diet
Added sugars[a]	Limit to no more than 25% of total energy

[a] Not a recommended intake. A daily intake of added sugars that individuals should aim for to achieve a healthful diet was not set.

Source: Dietary Reference Intakes for Energy, Carbohydrate, Fiber, Fat, Fatty Acids, Cholesterol, Protein, and Amino Acids (2002/2005). The report may be accessed via <www.nap.edu>.

Table A.12 US Dietary Reference Intakes (DRIs): Tolerable upper intake levels—vitamins
Food and Nutrition Board, Institute of Medicine, National Academies

Life stage group	Vitamin A (µg/d)[a]	Vitamin C (mg/d)	Vitamin D (µg/d)	Vitamin E (mg/d)[b,c]	Vitamin K	Thiamin	Riboflavin	Niacin (mg/d)[c]	Vitamin B6 (mg/d)	Folate (µg/d)[c]	Vitamin B12	Pantothenic acid	Biotin	Choline (g/d)	Carotenoids[d]
Infants															
0–6 months	600	ND[e]	25	ND	ND	ND	ND	ND	ND	ND	ND	ND	ND	ND	ND
6–12 months	600	ND	38	ND	ND	ND	ND	ND	ND	ND	ND	ND	ND	ND	ND
Children															
1–3 years	600	400	63	200	ND	ND	ND	10	30	300	ND	ND	ND	1.0	ND
4–8 years	900	650	75	300	ND	ND	ND	15	40	400	ND	ND	ND	1.0	ND
Males															
9–13 years	1700	1200	100	600	ND	ND	ND	20	60	600	ND	ND	ND	2.0	ND
14–18 years	2800	1800	100	800	ND	ND	ND	30	80	800	ND	ND	ND	3.0	ND
19–30 years	3000	2000	100	1000	ND	ND	ND	35	100	1000	ND	ND	ND	3.5	ND
31–50 years	3000	2000	100	1000	ND	ND	ND	35	100	1000	ND	ND	ND	3.5	ND
51–70 years	3000	2000	100	1000	ND	ND	ND	35	100	1000	ND	ND	ND	3.5	ND
> 70 years	3000	2000	100	1000	ND	ND	ND	35	100	1000	ND	ND	ND	3.5	ND
Females															
9–13 years	1700	1200	100	600	ND	ND	ND	20	60	600	ND	ND	ND	2.0	ND
14–18 years	2800	1800	100	800	ND	ND	ND	30	80	800	ND	ND	ND	3.0	ND
19–30 years	3000	2000	100	1000	ND	ND	ND	35	100	1000	ND	ND	ND	3.5	ND
31–50 years	3000	2000	100	1000	ND	ND	ND	35	100	1000	ND	ND	ND	3.5	ND
51–70 years	3000	2000	100	1000	ND	ND	ND	35	100	1000	ND	ND	ND	3.5	ND
> 70 years	3000	2000	100	1000	ND	ND	ND	35	100	1000	ND	ND	ND	3.5	ND
Pregnancy															
14–18 years	2800	1800	100	800	ND	ND	ND	30	80	800	ND	ND	ND	3.0	ND
19–30 years	3000	2000	100	1000	ND	ND	ND	35	100	1000	ND	ND	ND	3.5	ND
31–50 years	3000	2000	100	1000	ND	ND	ND	35	100	1000	ND	ND	ND	3.5	ND
Lactation															
14–18 years	2800	1800	100	800	ND	ND	ND	30	80	800	ND	ND	ND	3.0	ND
19–30 years	3000	2000	100	1000	ND	ND	ND	35	100	1000	ND	ND	ND	3.5	ND
31–50 years	3000	2000	100	1000	ND	ND	ND	35	100	1000	ND	ND	ND	3.5	ND

Note: A tolerable upper intake level (UL) is the highest level of daily nutrient intake that is likely to pose no risk of adverse health effects to almost all individuals in the general population. Unless otherwise specified, the UL represents total intake from food, water and supplements. Due to a lack of suitable data, ULs could not be established for vitamin K, thiamin, riboflavin, vitamin B12, pantothenic acid, biotin and carotenoids. In the absence of a UL, extra caution may be warranted in consuming levels above recommended intakes. Members of the general population should be advised not to routinely exceed the UL. The UL is not meant to apply to individuals who are treated with the nutrient under medical supervision or to individuals with predisposing conditions that modify their sensitivity to the nutrient.

[a] As pre-formed vitamin A only.

[b] As α-tocopherol; applies to any form of supplemental α-tocopherol.

[c] The ULs for vitamin E, niacin and folate apply to synthetic forms obtained from supplements, fortified foods or a combination of the two.

[d] β-carotene supplements are advised only to serve as a provitamin A source for individuals at risk of vitamin A deficiency.

[e] ND = Not determinable due to lack of data of adverse effects in this age group and concern with regard to lack of ability to handle excess amounts. Source of intake should be from food only to prevent high levels of intake.

Sources: Dietary Reference Intakes for Calcium, Phosphorous, Magnesium, Vitamin D, and Fluoride (1997); *Dietary Reference Intakes for Thiamin, Riboflavin, Niacin, Vitamin B6, Folate, Vitamin B12, Pantothenic Acid, Biotin, and Choline* (1998); *Dietary Reference Intakes for Vitamin C, Vitamin E, Selenium, and Carotenoids* (2000); *Dietary Reference Intakes for Vitamin A, Vitamin K, Arsenic, Boron, Chromium, Copper, Iodine, Iron, Manganese, Molybdenum, Nickel, Silicon, Vanadium, and Zinc* (2001); and *Dietary Reference Intakes for Calcium and Vitamin D* (2011). These reports may be accessed via <www.nap.edu>.

Table A.13 US Dietary Reference Intakes (DRIs): Tolerable upper intake levels—elements
Food and Nutrition Board, Institute of Medicine, National Academies

Life stage group	Arsenic[a]	Boron (mg/d)	Calcium (mg/d)	Chromium	Copper (μg/d)	Fluoride (mg/d)	Iodine (μg/d)	Iron (mg/d)	Magnesium (mg/d)[b]
Infants									
0–6 months	ND[e]	ND	1000	ND	ND	0.7	ND	40	ND
6–12 months	ND	ND	1500	ND	ND	0.9	ND	40	ND
Children									
1–3 years	ND	3	2500	ND	1000	1.3	200	40	65
4–8 years	ND	6	2500	ND	3000	2.2	300	40	110
Males									
9–13 years	ND	11	3000	ND	5000	10	600	40	350
14–18 years	ND	17	3000	ND	8000	10	900	45	350
19–30 years	ND	20	2500	ND	10000	10	1100	45	350
31–50 years	ND	20	2500	ND	10000	10	1100	45	350
51–70 years	ND	20	2000	ND	10000	10	1100	45	350
> 70 years	ND	20	2000	ND	10000	10	1100	45	350
Females									
9–13 years	ND	11	3000	ND	5000	10	600	40	350
14–18 years	ND	17	3000	ND	8000	10	900	45	350
19–30 years	ND	20	2500	ND	10000	10	1100	45	350
31–50 years	ND	20	2500	ND	10000	10	1100	45	350
51–70 years	ND	20	2000	ND	10000	10	1100	45	350
> 70 years	ND	20	2000	ND	10000	10	1100	45	350
Pregnancy									
14–18 years	ND	17	3000	ND	8000	10	900	45	350
19–30 years	ND	20	2500	ND	10000	10	1100	45	350
31–50 years	ND	20	2500	ND	10000	10	1100	45	350
Lactation									
14–18 years	ND	17	3000	ND	8000	10	900	45	350
19–30 years	ND	20	2500	ND	10000	10	1100	45	350
31–50 years	ND	20	2500	ND	10000	10	1100	45	350

Notes: A Tolerable Upper Intake Level (UL) is the highest level of daily nutrient intake that is likely to pose no risk of adverse health effects to almost all individuals in the general population. Unless otherwise specified, the UL represents total intake from food, water and supplements. Due to a lack of suitable data, ULs could not be established for vitamin K, thiamin, riboflavin, vitamin B12, pantothenic acid, biotin and carotenoids. In the absence of a UL, extra caution may be warranted in consuming levels above recommended intakes. Members of the general population should be advised not to routinely exceed the UL. The UL is not meant to apply to individuals who are treated with the nutrient under medical supervision or to individuals with predisposing conditions that modify their sensitivity to the nutrient.

[a] Although the UL was not determined for arsenic, there is no justification for adding arsenic to food or supplements.

[b] The ULs for magnesium represent intake from a pharmacological agent only and do not include intake from food and water.

[c] Although silicon has not been shown to cause adverse effects in humans, there is no justification for adding silicon to supplements.

[d] Although vanadium in food has not been shown to cause adverse effects in humans, there is no justification for adding vanadium to food and vanadium supplements should be used with caution. The UL is based on adverse effects in laboratory animals and this data could be used to set a UL for adults but not children and adolescents.

[e] ND = Not determinable due to lack of data of adverse effects in this age group and concern with regard to lack of ability to handle excess amounts. Source of intake should be from food only to prevent high levels of intake.

Sources: Dietary Reference Intakes for Calcium, Phosphorous, Magnesium, Vitamin D, and Fluoride (1997); *Dietary Reference Intakes for Thiamin, Riboflavin, Niacin, Vitamin B6, Folate, Vitamin B12, Pantothenic Acid, Biotin, and Choline* (1998); *Dietary Reference Intakes for Vitamin C, Vitamin E, Selenium, and Carotenoids* (2000); *Dietary Reference Intakes for Vitamin A, Vitamin K, Arsenic, Boron, Chromium, Copper, Iodine, Iron, Manganese, Molybdenum, Nickel, Silicon, Vanadium, and Zinc* (2001); *Dietary Reference Intakes for Water, Potassium, Sodium, Chloride, and Sulfate* (2005); and *Dietary Reference Intakes for Calcium and Vitamin D* (2011). These reports may be accessed via <www.nap.edu>.

Manganese (mg/d)	Molybdenum (μg/d)	Nickel (mg/d)	Phosphorus (g/d)	Selenium (μg/d)	Silicon[c]	Vanadium (mg/d)[d]	Zinc (mg/d)	Sodium (g/d)	Chloride (g/d)
ND	ND	ND	ND	45	ND	ND	4	ND	ND
ND	ND	ND	ND	60	ND	ND	5	ND	ND
2	300	0.2	3.0	90	ND	ND	7	1.5	2.3
3	600	0.3	3.0	150	ND	ND	12	1.9	2.9
6	1100	0.6	4.0	280	ND	ND	23	2.2	3.4
9	1700	1.0	4.0	400	ND	ND	34	2.3	3.6
11	2000	1.0	4.0	400	ND	1.8	40	2.3	3.6
11	2000	1.0	4.0	400	ND	1.8	40	2.3	3.6
11	2000	1.0	4.0	400	ND	1.8	40	2.3	3.6
11	2000	1.0	3.0	400	ND	1.8	40	2.3	3.6
6	1100	0.6	4.0	280	ND	ND	23	2.2	3.4
9	1700	1.0	4.0	400	ND	ND	34	2.3	3.6
11	2000	1.0	4.0	400	ND	1.8	40	2.3	3.6
11	2000	1.0	4.0	400	ND	1.8	40	2.3	3.6
11	2000	1.0	4.0	400	ND	1.8	40	2.3	3.6
11	2000	1.0	3.0	400	ND	1.8	40	2.3	3.6
9	1700	1.0	3.5	400	ND	ND	34	2.3	3.6
11	2000	1.0	3.5	400	ND	ND	40	2.3	3.6
11	2000	1.0	3.5	400	ND	ND	40	2.3	3.6
9	1700	1.0	4.0	400	ND	ND	34	2.3	3.6
11	2000	1.0	4.0	400	ND	ND	40	2.3	3.6
11	2000	1.0	4.0	400	ND	ND	40	2.3	3.6

UK DIETARY REFERENCE VALUES

Table A.14 UK reference nutrient intakes for vitamins

Age	Thiamin (mg/day)	Riboflavin (mg/day)	Niacin (nicotinic acid equivalent) (mg/day)	Vitamin B6# (mg/day)	Vitamin B 12 (µg/day)	Folate (µg/day)	Vitamin C (mg/day)	Vitamin A (µg/day)	Vitamin D (µg/day)
0–3 months	0.2	0.4	3	0.2	0.3	50	25	350	8.5
4–6 months	0.2	0.4	3	0.2	0.3	50	25	350	8.5
7–9 months	0.2	0.4	4	0.3	0.4	50	25	350	7.0
10–12 months	0.3	0.4	5	0.4	0.4	50	25	350	7.0
1–3 years	0.5	0.6	8	0.7	0.5	70	30	400	7.0
4–6 years	0.7	0.8	11	0.9	0.8	100	30	500	–
7–10 years	0.7	1.0	12	1.0	1.0	150	30	500	–
Males									
11–14 years	0.9	1.2	15	1.2	1.2	200	35	600	–
15–18 years	1.1	1.3	18	1.5	1.5	200	40	700	–
19–50 years	1.0	1.3	17	1.4	1.5	200	40	700	–
50+ years	0.9	1.3	16	1.4	1.5	200	40	700	**
Females									
11–14 years	0.7	1.1	12	1.0	1.2	200	35	600	–
15–18 years	0.8	1.1	14	1.2	1.5	200	40	600	–
19–50 years	0.8	1.1	13	1.2	1.5	200	40	600	–
50+ years	0.8	1.1	12	1.2	1.5	200	40	600	–
Pregnancy	+0.1***	+0.3	*	*	*	+100	+10	+100	10.0
Lactation									
0–4 months	+0.2	+0.5	+2	*	+0.5	+60	+30	+350	10.0
4+ months	+0.2	+0.5	+2	*	+0.5	+60	+30	+350	10.0

* No increment, ** after age 65 years the RNI is 10 µg/day for men and women, *** for last trimester only, # based on protein providing 14.7% of EAR for energy.

Data from Department of Health, Crown copyright reproduced with the permission of the Controller of Her Majesty's Stationery Office.

Source: Department of Health, *Dietary Reference Values for Food Energy and Nutrients*, Report of the Panel on Dietary Reference Values of the Committee on Medical Aspects of Food Policy. Report on Health and Social Subjects 41. London: HMSO, 1991.

Table A.15 UK reference nutrient intakes for minerals

Age	Calcium (mg/day)	Phosphorus[a] (mg/day)	Magnesium (mg/day)	Sodium[b] (mg/day)	Potassium[c] (mg/day)	Chloride[d] (mg/day)	Iron (mg/day)	Zinc (mg/day)	Copper (mg/day)	Selenium (µg/d)	Iodine (µg/d)
0–3 months	525	400	55	210	800	320	1.7	4.0	0.2	10	50
4–6 months	525	400	60	280	850	400	4.3	4.0	0.3	13	60
7–9 months	525	400	75	320	700	500	7.8	5.0	0.3	10	60
10–12 months	525	400	80	350	700	500	7.8	5.0	0.3	10	60
1–3 years	350	270	85	500	800	800	6.9	5.0	0.4	15	70
4–6 years	450	350	120	700	1100	1100	6.1	6.5	0.6	20	100
7–10 years	550	450	200	1200	2000	1800	8.7	7.0	0.7	30	110
Males											
11–14 years	1000	775	280	1600	3100	2500	11.3	9.0	0.8	45	130
15–18 years	1000	775	300	1600	3500	2500	11.3	9.5	1.0	70	140
19–50 years	700	550	300	1600	3500	2500	8.7	9.5	1.2	75	140
50+ years	700	550	300	1600	3500	2500	8.7	9.5	1.2	75	140
Females											
11–14 years	800	625	280	1600	3100	2500	14.8[e]	9.0	0.8	45	130
15–18 years	800	625	300	1600	3500	2500	14.8[e]	7.0	1.0	60	140
19–50 years	700	550	270	1600	3500	2500	14.8[e]	7.0	1.2	60	140
50+ years	700	550	270	1600	3500	2500	8.7	7.0	1.2	60	140
Pregnancy	*	*	*	*	*	*	*	*	*	*	*
Lactation											
0–4 months	+550	+440	+50	*	*	*	*	+6.0	+0.3	+15	*
4+ months	+550	+440	+50	*	*	*	*	+2.5	+0.3	+15	*

* No increment, [a] phosphorus RNI is set equal to calcium in molar terms, [b] 1 mmol sodium = 23 mg, [c] 1 mmol potassium = 39 mg, [d] corresponds to sodium 1 mmol = 35 5 mg, [e] insufficient for women with high menstrual losses where the most practical way of meeting iron requirements is to take iron supplements.

Data from Department of Health, Crown copyright reproduced with the permission of the Controller of Her Majesty's Stationery Office.

Source: Department of Health, *Dietary Reference Values for Food Energy and Nutrients*, Report of the Panel on Dietary Reference Values of the Committee on Medical Aspects of Food Policy. Report on Health and Social Subjects 41. London: HMSO, 1991.

Table A.16 UK dietary reference values for fat and carbohydrate for adults as a percentage of daily total energy intake (percentage of food energy)

	Individual minimum	Population average	Individual maximum
Saturated fatty acids		10 (11)	
Cis-polyunsaturated fatty acids	n-3: 0.2 n-6: 1.0	6 (6.5)	10
Cis-mono-unsaturated fatty acids		12 (13)	
Trans fatty acids		2 (2)	
Total fatty acids		30 (32.5)	
TOTAL FAT		33 (35)	
Non-milk extrinsic sugars	0	10 (11)	
Intrinsic and milk sugars and starch		37 (39)	
TOTAL CARBOHYDRATE		47 (50)	
NON-STARCH POLYSACCHARIDE (g/day)	12	18	24

The average percentage contribution to total energy does not total 100% because figures for protein and alcohol are excluded. Protein intakes average 15% of total energy which is above the RNI. It is recognised that many individuals will derive some energy from alcohol, and this has been assumed to average 5% approximating to current intakes. However, the Panel allowed that some groups might not drink alcohol and that, for some purposes, nutrient intakes as a proportion of food energy (without alcohol) might be useful. Therefore, average figures are given as percentages both of total energy and, in brackets, of food energy.

Data from Department of Health, Crown copyright reproduced with the permission of the Controller of Her Majesty's Stationery Office.

Source: Department of Health, *Dietary Reference Values for Food Energy and Nutrients*, Report of the Panel on Dietary Reference Values of the Committee on Medical Aspects of Food Policy. Report on Health and Social Subjects 41. London: HMSO, 1991.

Table A.17 UK safe intakes for nutrients for which insufficient information exists to set DRVs

Nutrient	Safe intake
Vitamins	
Pantothenic acid	
Adults	3–7 mg/day
Infants	1.7 mg/day
Biotin	10–200 μg/day
Vitamin E	
Men	Above 4 mg/day
Women	Above 3 mg/day
Infants	0.4 mg/g polyunsaturated fatty acids
Vitamin K	
Adults	1 μg/kg/day
Infants	10 μg/day
Minerals	
Manganese	
Adults	1.4 mg (26 μmol)/day
Infants and children	16 μg (0.3 μmol)/day
Molybdenum	
Adults	50–400 μg/day
Infants, children and adolescents	0.5–1.5 μg/kg/day
Chromium	
Adults	25 μg (0.5 μmol)/day
Children and adolescents	0.1–1.0 μg (2–20 μmol)/kg/day
Fluoride (for infants only)	0.05 mg (3 μmol)/kg/day

Data from Department of Health, Crown copyright reproduced with the permission of the Controller of Her Majesty's Stationery Office.

Source: Department of Health, *Dietary Reference Values for Food Energy and Nutrients*, Report of the Panel on Dietary Reference Values of the Committee on Medical Aspects of Food Policy. Report on Health and Social Subjects 41. London HMSO, 1991.

Table A.18 UK revised Estimated Average Requirements (EAR) for infants 1–12 months

Age (months)	EAR[a]					
	Breast-fed		Breast milk substitute-fed		Mixed feeding or unknown[b]	
	MJ/kg per day (kcal/ kg per day)	MJ/day (kcal/day)	MJ/kg per day (kcal/ kg per day)	MJ/day (kcal/day)	MJ/kg per day (kcal/ kg per day)	MJ/day (kcal/day)
Boys						
1–2	0.4 (96)	2.2 (526)	0.5 (120)	2.5 (598)	0.5 (120)	2.4 (574)
3–4	0.4 (96)	2.4 (574)	0.4 (96)	2.6 (622)	0.4 (96)	2.5 (598)
5–6	0.3 (72)	2.5 (598)	0.4 (96)	2.7 (646)	0.3 (72)	2.6 (622)
7–12	0.3 (72)	2.9 (694)	0.3 (72)	3.1 (742)	0.3 (72)	3.0 (718)
Girls						
1–2	0.4 (96)	2.0 (478)	0.5 (120)	2.3 (550)	0.5 (120)	2.1 (502)
3–4	0.4 (96)	2.2 (526)	0.4 (96)	2.5 (598)	0.4 (96)	2.3 (550)
5–6	0.3 (72)	2.3 (550)	0.4 (96)	2.6 (622)	0.3 (72)	2.4 (574)
7–12	0.3 (72)	2.7 (646)	0.3 (72)	2.8 (670)	0.3 (72)	2.7 (646)

[a] Calculated as TEE + energy deposition (kJ/day).

[b] These figures should be applied for infants when there is mixed feeding and the proportions of breast milk and breast milk substitute are not known.

Source: Department of Health, *Dietary Reference Values for Food Energy and Nutrients*, Report of the Panel on Dietary Reference Values of the Committee on Medical Aspects of Food Policy. Report on Health and Social Subjects 41. London: HMSO, 1991.

Table A.19 UK revised population Estimated Average Requirements (EAR) for children aged 1–18 years[a]

Age (years)	PAL[b]	EAR MJ/d (kcal/d) Boys	Girls
1	1.40	3.2 (765)	3.0 (717)
2	1.40	4.2 (1004)	3.9 (932)
3	1.40	4.9 (1171)	4.5 (1076)
4	1.58	5.8 (1386)	5.4 (1291)
5	1.58	6.2 (1482)	5.7 (1362)
6	1.58	6.6 (1577)	6.2 (1482)
7	1.58	6.9 (1649)	6.4 (1530)
8	1.58	7.3 (1745)	6.8 (1625)
9	1.58	7.7 (1840)	7.2 (1721)
10	1.75	8.5 (2032)	8.1 (1936)
11	1.75	8.9 (2127)	8.5 (2032)
12	1.75	9.4 (2247)	8.8 (2103)
13	1.75	10.1 (2414)	9.3 (2223)
14	1.75	11.0 (2629)	9.8 (2342)
15	1.75	11.8 (2820)	10.0 (2390)
16	1.75	12.4 (2964)	10.1 (2414)
17	1.75	12.9 (3083)	10.3 (2462)
18	1.75	13.2 (3155)	10.3 (2462)

[a] Calculated from BMR x PAL. BMR values are calculated from the Henry equations, using weights and heights indicated by the 50th centiles of the UK-WHO Growth Standards (ages 1–4 years) and the UK 1990 reference for children and adolescents.

[b] Physical activity level.

Source: Department of Health, *Dietary Reference Values for Food Energy and Nutrients*, Report of the Panel on Dietary Reference Values of the Committee on Medical Aspects of Food Policy. Report on Health and Social Subjects 41. London: HMSO, 1991.

Table A.20 UK revised population Estimated Average Requirements (EAR) values for adults

Age range (years)	Men		Women	
	Height cm[a]	EAR MJ/d (kcal/d)[b]	Height cm[a]	EAR MJ/d (kcal/d)[b]
19–24	178	11.6 (2772)	163	9.1 (2175)
25–34	178	11.5 (2749)	163	9.1 (2175)
35–44	176	11.0 (2629)	163	8.8 (2103)
45–54	175	10.8 (2581)	162	8.8 (2103)
55–64	174	10.8 (2581)	161	8.7 (2079)
65–74	173	9.8 (2342)	159	8.0 (1912)
75+	170	9.6 (2294)	155	7.7 (1840)
All adults	175	10.9 (2605)	162	8.7 (2079)

[a] Values for illustration derived from mean heights in 2009 for England (Health Survey for England 2009) (NHS IC, 2010).

[b] Median PAL = 1.63.

Source: Department of Health, *Dietary Reference Values for Food Energy and Nutrients*, Report of the Panel on Dietary Reference Values of the Committee on Medical Aspects of Food Policy. Report on Health and Social Subjects 41. London: HMSO, 1991.

Index

Page numbers in **bold** refer to tables
Page numbers in *italic* refer to figures